KELLY VANA'S NURSING LEADERSHIP AND MANAGEMENT

KELLY VANA'S NURSING LEADERSHIP AND MANAGEMENT

FOURTH EDITION

Edited by

Patricia Kelly Vana, RN, MSN

Professor Emerita
Purdue University Northwest
College of Nursing
Hammond, Indiana
Faculty
Health Education Systems, Inc. (HESI)
Houston, Texas

Janice Tazbir, RN, MS, CS, CCRN, CNE, RYT

Consultant,
Anderson Continuing Education
Sacramento, California
Staff Nurse,
University of Chicago Medicine
Chicago, Illinois
Faculty
Health Education Systems, Inc. (HESI)
Houston, Texas
Professor (retired)
Purdue University Northwest
College of Nursing
Hammond, Indiana

WILEY Blackwell

Registered Office(s)
John Wiley & Sons, Inc., 111 River Street, Hoboken, NJ 07030, USA
John Wiley & Sons Ltd, The Atrium, Southern Gate, Chichester, West Sussex, PO19 8SQ, UK

Editorial Office
9600 Garsington Road, Oxford, OX4 2DQ, UK

For details of our global editorial offices, customer services, and more information about Wiley products visit us at www.wiley.com

Wiley also publishes its books in a variety of electronic formats and by print-on-demand. Some content that appears in standard print versions of this book may not be available in other formats.

Library of Congress Cataloging-in-Publication Data

Names: Vana, Patricia Kelly, 1941- editor. | Tazbir, Janice, editor.
Title: Kelly Vana's Nursing Leadership and Management
  / edited by Patricia Kelly Vana, Janice Tazbir.
Other titles: Nursing leadership & management | Nursing leadership and
  management
Description: Fourth edition. | Hoboken, NJ : Wiley-Blackwell, 2021. |
  Preceded by Nursing leadership & management / [edited] by Patricia
  Kelly. 3rd ed. 2012. | Includes bibliographical references and index.
Identifiers: LCCN 2020021964 (print) | LCCN 2020021965 (ebook) | ISBN
  9781119596615 (paperback) | ISBN 9781119596622 (adobe pdf) | ISBN
  9781119596639 (epub)
Subjects: MESH: Nursing Services—organization & administration | Nursing
  Care—organization & administration | Nurse Administrators | Leadership
  | United States
Classification: LCC RT89 (print) | LCC RT89 (ebook) | NLM WY 105 | DDC
  362.17/3—dc23
LC record available at https://lccn.loc.gov/2020021964
LC ebook record available at https://lccn.loc.gov/2020021965

Cover Design: Wiley
Cover Images: © Marje/Getty Images

Set in 10/12pt and TimesLTStd by SPi Global, Chennai

SKYD472366C-B384-476B-9635-F7BBBDD22AF0_022621

Patricia would like to dedicate this book to the memory of Dr. Joyce Ellis. Joyce was a born leader and manager. She was Pat's Faculty as a student, and her "boss," Department Head, mentor and friend as a Faculty member. Janice would like to dedicate this book to the memory of Dr. Gloria Smokvina. Gloria was Janice's Professor and Dean as a student and her "boss," Dean, mentor and friend as a faculty member. Joyce and Gloria taught that leadership begins with personal integrity, honesty, and the desire to do the right thing. Their lives were an example of the kind of leader and manager nursing (and we all) really need. We ask you, the next generation of nursing, to be more like Dr. Ellis and Dr. Smokvina. Have courage and maintain your integrity in all circumstances, be honest and trustworthy, and always try to do the right thing.

CONTENTS

CONTRIBUTORS

Forward

Mary A. Dolansky, PhD, RN, FAAN
Sarah C. Hirsh Professorship in Nursing,
Associate Professor
Frances Payne Bolton School of Nursing
Case Western Reserve University
Cleveland, Ohio
Nurse Adviser,
National VA Quality Scholars Program (VAQS)
Senior Nurse Fellow VAQS,
Louis Stokes Cleveland VA
Director, QSEN Institute

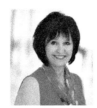

Unit 1
Nursing Leadership
and Management

01
Nursing Leadership,
Management, and
Motivation

Linda Searle-Leach, RN, PhD, NEA-BC
Director of Nursing Research and Innovation
Azusa Pacific University, Azusa, CA, USA,
Huntington Hospital
Pasadena, California

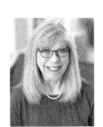

02
The Health Care
Environment

Ronda Hughes, PhD, MHS, RN, CLNC, FAAN
Director, Center for Nursing Leadership
Director, Executive Doctorate of Nursing Practice
Associate Professor
University of South Carolina
Columbia, South Carolina

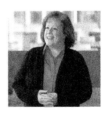

Janice Tazbir, RN, MS, CS, CCRN, CNE, RYT
Consultant
Anderson Continuing Education
Sacramento, California
Staff Nurse
University of Chicago Medicine
Chicago, Illinois
Faculty
Health Education Systems, Inc. (HESI)
Houston, Texas
Professor (retired)
Purdue University Northwest
College of Nursing
Hammond, Indiana

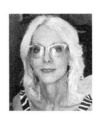

03
Nursing Leadership
and Management
in a Historical
Context

Brigid Lusk, PhD, RN, FAAN
Adjunct Clinical Professor and Director
Midwest Nursing History Research Center
University of Illinois at Chicago College of
Nursing
Chicago, Illinois

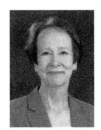

04
Organization of
Patient care in High
Reliability Health
Care Organizations

Patti Ludwig-Beymer, PhD, RN, CTN-A, NEA-BC,
CPPS, FAAN
Associate Professor
Purdue University Northwest
College of Nursing
Hammond, Indiana

05
Organization and
Staffing of Patient
Care at the Unit
Level

Diane Spoljoric. PhD, RNC, FNP
Associate Professor of Nursing
Purdue University Northwest
College of Nursing
Westville Campus
LaPorte, Indiana
Nurse Practitioner
Walker Medical Clinic
LaPorte, Indiana

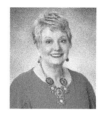

Marsha M. King, DNP, MBA, RN, NEA-BC, CNE
Dean of the University of Saint Francis
Crown Point Site, Indiana
Associate Professor

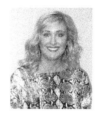

06
Health Care
Economics

Lanette Stuckey, PhD, MSN, RN, CNE, CMSRN,
CNEcl, NEA-BC
Dean of Nursing
Associate Professor
Lakeview College of Nursing
Danville Campus
Danville, Illinois

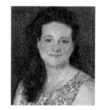

Debra A Cherubini, PhD, RN
Chair, Department of Nursing
Assistant Professor
Salve Regina University
Newport, Rhode Island

Samuel A. Sacco, Jr., BA, MCRP
Lecturer
Salve Regina University
Newport, Rhode Island

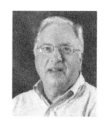

07
Hospital,
Department, and
Unit
Budgets

Isabelle Clarke Garibaldi, DNP, RN, NEA-BC,
CENP, CPPS
Vice President, Patient Care Services and Chief
Nursing Officer
LifePoint-Sumner Regional Medical Center
Gallatin, Tennessee

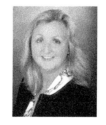

Unit 2
Leadership and
Management of
Patient-Centered
Care

08
Patient-Centered
Care

Tom Blodgett, PhD, RN, AGACNP-BC
Assistant Professor
Duke University
Durham, North Carolina

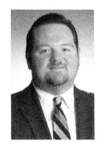

Nicole Petsas Blodgett, PhD, RN
Assistant Professor
Duke University
Durham, North Carolina

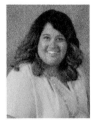

09
Patient and Health
Care Education

Rochelle R. Flayter, MSN, RN, CCRN-K, TCRN
Senior Director, Trauma Services UC Health
Southern Colorado
Memorial Hospital
Colorado Springs, Colorado

Lisa Kidin, MHA, MSN, RN, CPHQ, NEA-BC
Director of Professional Development
UCHealth
Colorado Springs, Colorado

Monika S. Schuler, PhD, RN, CNE
Assistant Professor
NFLP Program Director
College of Nursing
University of Massachusetts, Dartmouth
North Dartmouth, Massachusetts

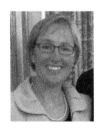

10
Patient Outcomes
and Evidence-
Based Health Care

Parul Patel, MS, MBA, BSN, RN
Director of Healthcare Services-Utilization
Management
Molina Healthcare
Oakbrook, Illinois

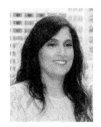

11
Searching for the
Evidence

Charlotte Beyer, MSIS, AHIP
Library Director
Boxer Library
Lecturer
Interprofessional Healthcare Studies
Rosalind Franklin University of Medicine and
Science
North Chicago

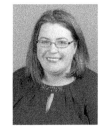

12
Quality
Improvement of
Patient Care

Christine Rovinski-Wagner, MSN, ARNP
National Transformational Coach Captain
Office of Veterans Access to Care
Veterans' Health Administration
Washington, DC

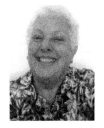

Catherine C. Alexander DNP, MPH, RN
Performance Improvement Specialist
San Francisco VA Medical Center
San Francisco, CA

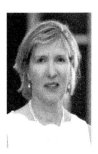

13
Improving Quality
at the Bedside

Christine Rovinski-Wagner, MSN, ARNP
National Transformational Coach Captain
Office of Veterans Access to Care
Veterans Health Administration
Washington, DC

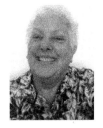

Catherine C. Alexander DNP, MPH, RN
Performance Improvement Specialist
San Francisco VA Medical Center
San Francisco, CA

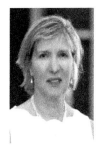

14
Safety, Patient and
Health Care Team

Christine Rovinski-Wagner, MSN, ARNP
National Transformational Coach Captain
Office of Veterans Access to Care
Veterans' Health Administration
Washington, DC

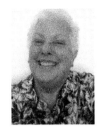

Peter D. Mills, PhD, MS
Director
VA National Center for Patient Safety Field Office
Veterans Affairs Medical Center
White River Junction, Vermont
Adjunct Associate Professor of Psychiatry
The Geisel School of Medicine at Dartmouth
Hanover, New Hampshire

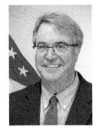

15
Nursing
Informatics

Rebecca Rankin, MS, RN, CPHQ, PMP
Director, Nursing Informatics
UW Health
Madison, Wisconsin

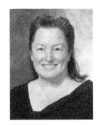

Unit 3
Nursing and the
Interprofessional
Team

16
Interprofessional
Teamwork and
Collaboration

Dianne J. Hoekstra, MS, RN, ACNS-BC, ACUE
Clinical Assistant Professor
College of Nursing
Purdue University Northwest
Hammond, Indiana

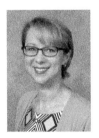

Janet Chaney, DNP(c)
Assistant Clinical Professor
College of Nursing
Purdue University Northwest
Hammond, Indiana

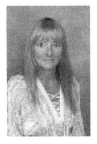

17
Members of the
Interprofessional
Team

Patrick D. Reed, RN, DNP, MSN, MSHCM, MBA,
CPHQ
Adjunct Faculty
College of Nursing
Purdue University Northwest
Hammond, Indiana

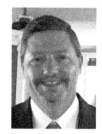

Bryan J. Camus, RN, MSN, CCRN
Instructor
Charity/Delgado School of Nursing
New Orleans, LA

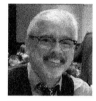

18
Delegation,
Assignment, and
Supervision of
Patient Care

Ruth Hansten, RN BSN MBA PhD FACHE
Hansten Healthcare
Santa Rosa, California

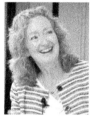

Patricia Kelly Vana, RN, MSN
Professor Emerita
Purdue University Northwest
College of Nursing
Hammond, Indiana
Faculty
Health Education Systems, Inc. (HESI)
Houston, Texas

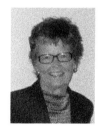

19
Time Management
and Setting Patient
Care Priorites

Patrick Joswick, DNP, RN
Director of Nursing
Kalamazoo Valley Community College
Kalamazoo, Michigan

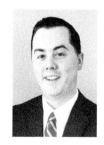

20
Change, Clinical
Decision Making
and Innovation

Patricia Keresztes, PhD, RN, CCRN
Associate Professor
Saint Mary's College
Department of Nursing Science
Notre Dame, Indiana

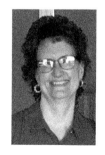

21
Power and Politics

Richard J. Maloney, EdD, MA, MAHRM, BS
Lecturer
School of Nursing and Healthcare Leadership
University of Washington Tacoma
Tacoma, Washington
Partner
Policy Governance Associates
Tacoma, Washington

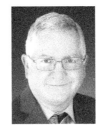

Patsy Maloney, EdD, RN, MSN, MA, NPD-BC,
NEA-BC, CEN
Teaching Professor
School of Nursing and Healthcare Leadership
University of Washington Tacoma
Tacoma, Washington
Professor Emeritus
Pacific Lutheran University

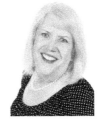

22
Legal Aspects of
Nursing

Carol L. Wallinger, BSN, JD
Clinical Professor
Rutgers Law School &
Rutgers School of Nursing
Camden, New Jersey
Adjunct Professor
Cooper Medical School
Camden, New Jersey

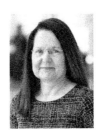

23
Ethical Aspects of
Nursing

Joan Dorman, RN, MSN, CEN
Clinical Associate Professor
Purdue University Northwest
College of Nursing
Hammond, Indiana

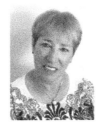

24
Culture,
Generational
Differences, and
Spirituality

Amanda Kratovil, PhD, RN
Assistant Professor
Purdue University Northwest
College of Nursing
Hammond, Indiana

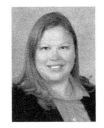

Unit 4
Leadership and
Management of the
Self and the Future

25
NCLEX Preparation

Janice Tazbir, RN, MS, CS, CCRN, CNE, RYT
Consultant
Anderson Continuing Education
Sacramento, California
Staff Nurse
University of Chicago Medicine
Chicago, Illinois
Faculty
Health Education Systems, Inc. (HESI)
Houston, Texas
Professor (retired)
Purdue University Northwest
College of Nursing
Hammond, Indiana

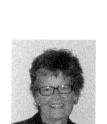

Patricia Kelly Vana, RN, MSN
Professor Emerita
Purdue University Northwest
College of Nursing
Hammond, Indiana
Faculty
Health Education Systems, Inc. (HESI)
Houston, Texas

26
Entry into the
Profession—
Your First Job

Dianne J. Hoekstra, MS, RN, ACNS-BC, ACUE
Clinical Assistant Professor
College of Nursing
Purdue University Northwest
Hammond, Indiana

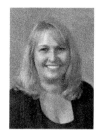

27
Career Planning
and Professional
Development

Angela Schooley, PhD, RN, CNE
Associate Professor of Nursing
Purdue University Northwest
College of Nursing
Hammond, Indiana

28
Healthy Living:
Balancing a Healthy
Personal and
Professional Life

Cheryl Moredich, DNP, RN
Director, Online Programs
Purdue University Northwest
College of Nursing
Hammond, Indiana

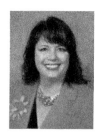

29
Nursing Career
Opportunities

Jade Tazbir, RN BSN
Staff Nurse
University of Chicago Medicine
Chicago, Illinois

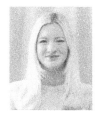

Janice Tazbir, RN, MS, CS, CCRN, CNE, RYT
Consultant
Anderson Continuing Education
Sacramento, California
Staff Nurse
University of Chicago Medicine
Chicago, Illinois
Faculty
Health Education Systems, Inc. (HESI)
Houston, Texas
Professor (retired)
Purdue University Northwest
College of Nursing
Hammond, Indiana

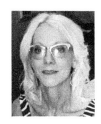

Appendix

Preparation to
Assume New
Position
as Bedside Staff
Nurse Leader
and Manager of
Patients on Labor
and Delivery Unit

and

Daily RN Shift
Timeline for
Nursing Care of
Patients on Labor
and Delivery (L&D)
Unit

Beth L. A. Richard, RN MSN C-EFM
Clinical Shift Coordinator
Northwestern Medicine Delnor Hospital
Geneva, Illinois
Waubonsee Community College
Adjunct Professor School of Nursing
Aurora, Illinois

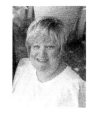

Preparation to
Assume New
Position as Bedside
Staff Nurse Leader
and Manager of
Various Types of
Patients

and

Daily RN Shift
Timeline for
Nursing Care
of Patients on
Medical, Surgical,
Intensive/Critical
Care and Stepdown
Units, Labor and
Delivery, Mother/
Baby, Pediatric, and
Psychiatric Units

Carolyn Ruud, DNP, RN, CNE®cl, CCRN, CVRN
-BC, SCRN
Rapid Response Nurse
Northwestern Medicine Delnor Hospital
Geneva, Illinois
Visiting Professor
Chamberlain College of Nursing
Addison, Illinois
Adjunct Faculty
Aurora University
Aurora Illinois

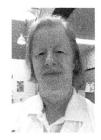

Former Contributors to the Third Edition

Rinda Alexander, PhD, RN, CS
Professor Emeritus, Nursing
College of Nursing
Purdue University Northwest
Hammond, Indiana

Kim Siarkowski Amer, PhD, RN
Associate Professor
Department of Nursing
DePaul University
Chicago, Illinois

Margaret M. Anderson, EdD, RNa
Professor of Nursing and Past Chair
College of Health Professions, Department of Advanced Nursing
  Studies
Northern Kentucky University
Highland Heights, Kentucky

Ida M. Androwich, PhD, RN, BC, FAAN
Professor and Director, Health Systems Management
Niehoff School of Nursing
Loyola University Chicago
Chicago, Illinois

Crisamar J. Anunciado, RN, MSN, FNP-BC
Inpatient Nurse Practitioner
Sharp Chula Vista Medical Center Chula Vista, California
and
Adjunct Faculty
Southwestern Community College
Associate Degree Nursing Program
Chula Vista, California

Anne Bernat, RN, MSN, CNAA
Vice President of Patient Care Services (Retired)
Arlington, Virginia

Nancy Braaten, RN, MS
Adult Health Clinical Nurse Specialist
Clinical Analyst, Nursing Information Systems
Northeast Health Acute Care Division
Troy, New York

Sister Kathleen Cain, OSF, JD
Attorney
Franciscan Legal Services
Baton Rouge, Louisiana

Carolyn Christie-McAuliffe, PhD, FNP
Director of Research
Hematology Oncology Associates of CNY
East Syracuse, New York
and
Assistant Professor, SUNY Institute of Technology
Utica, New York

**Martha Desmond, RN, MS, Post Masters Certificate
  in Nursing Education**
Clinical Nurse Specialist in Critical Care
Northeast Health Acute Care Division
Troy, New York
and
Adjunct Faculty
Excelsior College
Albany, New York

Joan Dorman, RN, MS, CEN
Clinical Assistant Professor
Purdue University Northwest
Hammond, Indiana

Deborah Erickson, PhD, RN
Assistant Professor
Bradley University
Peoria, Illinois

Barbara K. Fane, MS, RN, APRN-BC
Clinical Nurse Specialist, Critical Care
Northeast Health Acute Care Division
Troy, New York
and
Adjunct Clinical Faculty
Southern Vermont College
Bennington, Vermont

Mary L. Fisher, PhD, RN, CNAA, BC
Professor and Department Chair
Environments for Health
Indiana University School of Nursing
Indianapolis, Indiana

Charlene C. Gyurko, PhD, RN, CNE
Assistant Professor
Purdue University Northwest
College of Nursing
Hammond, Indiana

Corinne Haviley, MS, RN
Associate Chief Nursing Officer
Central DuPage Hospital
Winfield, Illinois

Paul Heidenthal, MS
Senior Curriculum Developer
Texas Department of Health and Human Services
Austin, Texas

Sara Anne Hook, JD, MLS, MBA
Professor of Informatics, Indiana University School of Informatics
Indianapolis, Indiana
and
Adjunct Professor of Law, Indiana University School of Law
Indianapolis, Indiana

Karen Houston, RN, MS
Director of Quality and Continuum of Care
Albany Medical Center
Albany, New York

Ronda G. Hughes, PhD, MHS, RN
Senior Health Scientist Administrator
Senior Advisor on End-of-Life Care
Center for Primary Care, Prevention, and Clinical Partnerships
Agency for Healthcare Research and Quality
Rockville, Maryland

Mary Anne Jadlos, MS, ACNP-BC, CWOCN
Coordinator—Wound, Skin and Ostomy Nursing Service
Northeast Health Acute Care Division
Samaritan Hospital
Troy, New York
and
Albany Memorial Hospital
Albany, New York

Josette Jones, PhD, RN
Assistant Professor
Indiana University School of Informatics
School of Nursing
Indianapolis, Indiana

Stephen Jones, MS, RN, CPNP ET
Pediatric Clinical Nurse Specialist/Nurse Practitioner
The Children's Hospital at Albany Medical Center
Albany, New York
and
Founder, Pediatric Concepts
Averill Park, New York

Patricia Kelly Vana, RN, MSN
Professor Emerita
Purdue University Northwest
College of Nursing
Hammond, Indiana
Faculty
Health Education Systems, Inc. (HESI)
Houston, Texas

Glenda B. Kelman, PhD, ACNP-BC
Associate Professor and Chair
Nursing Department
The Sage Colleges
Troy, New York
and
Acute Care Nurse Practitioner
Wound, Skin, and Ostomy Nursing Service
Northeast Health Acute Care Division
Samaritan Hospital
Troy, New York
and
Albany Memorial Hospital
Albany, New York

Mary Elaine Koren, RN, PhD
Associate Professor of Nursing
Area Coordinator
Northern Illinois University
School of Nursing and Health Studies
DeKalb, Illinois

Lyn LaBarre, MS, RN
Patient Care Service Director
Critical Care, Specialty and Emergency Services
Albany Medical Center
Albany, New York

Linda Searle Leach, PhD, RN, NEA-BC
Assistant Professor
UCLA School of Nursing
Los Angeles, California

Camille B. Little, MS, RN, BSN
Instructional Assistant Professor (Retired)
Mennonite College of Nursing
Illinois State University
Normal, Illinois

Sharon Little-Stoetzel, RN, MS, CNE
Associate Professor of Nursing
MidAmerica Nazarene University
Independence, Missouri

Miki Magnino-Rabig, PhD, RN
Assistant Professor
University of St. Francis
Joliet, Illinois

Patsy L. Maloney, EdD, MSN, MA, RN-BC, NEA-BC
Professor and Director, Continuing Nursing Education
School of Nursing
Pacific Lutheran University
Tacoma, Washington

Richard J. Maloney, EdD, MA, MAHRM, BS
Partner
Policy Governance Associates
Tacoma, Washington

Maureen T. Marthaler, RN, MS
Associate Professor
College of Nursing
Purdue University Northwest
Hammond, Indiana

Judith W. Martin, RN, JD
Attorney
Franciscan Legal Services
Baton Rouge, Louisiana

Edna Harder Mattson, RN, BN, BA(CRS), MDE
Doctoral Student in Education
University of Phoenix
and
President
International Nursing Consultation and Tutorial Services
Winnipeg, Manitoba, Canada

Mary McLaughlin, RN, MBA
Assistant Director for Case Management and Social Work
Albany Medical Center
Albany New York

Terry W. Miller, PhD, RN
Dean and Professor
Pacific Lutheran University
School of Nursing
Tacoma, Washington

Leslie H. Nicoll, PhD, MBA, RN, BC
President and Owner
Maine Desk, LLC
Portland, Maine

Laura J. Nosek, PhD, RN
Doctor of Nursing Practice Faculty
The Bolton School of Nursing
Case Western Reserve University
Cleveland, Ohio
and
Adjunct Associate Professor of Nursing
Marcella Niehoff School of Nursing
Loyola University Chicago
Chicago, Illinois
and
Course Facilitator
Excelsior College
Albany, New York

Amy Androwich O'Malley, MSN, RN
Education and Program Manager
Medela, Inc.
McHenry, Illinois

Kristine E. Pfendt, RN, MSN
Associate Professor
College of Health Professions
Department of Advanced Nursing Studies
Northern Kentucky University
Highland Heights, Kentucky

Karin Polifko-Harris, PhD, RN, CNAA
Vice President
Organization Development and Research
Naples Community Healthcare System
Naples, Florida

Chad Priest, RN, MSN, JD
Chief Executive Officer
MESH, Inc.
Indianapolis, Indiana

Jacklyn Ludwig Ruthman, PhD, RN
Associate Professor, Retired
Bradley University
Peoria, Illinois

Patricia M. Lentsch Schoon, MPH, RN
Adjunct Associate Professor
School of Graduate and Professional Programs
St. Mary's University, Minneapolis, Minnesota
and
Clinical Instructor
School of Nursing
University of Wisconsin Oshkosh, Oshkosh, Wisconsin

Kathleen F. Sellers, PhD, RN
Associate Professor
School of Nursing and Health Systems
SUNY Institute of Technology
Utica, New York

Susan Abaffy Shah, MS, ACNP-BC
Division of Cardiology
Albany Medical Center
Albany, New York

Maria R. Shirey, PhD, MBA, RN, NEA-BC, FACHE, FAAN
Associate Professor
University of Southern Indiana
College of Nursing and Health Professions
Evansville, Indiana

Tanya L. Sleeper, GNP-BC, MSN, MSB
Assistant Professor
Division of Nursing
University of Maine at Fort Kent
Fort Kent, Maine

Nancy S. Sisson, MS, RN
Adult Health Clinical Nurse Specialist
Clinical Nurse Specialist—Telemetry
Northeast Health Acute Care Division
Albany, New York

Erin C. Soucy, MSN, RN
Director, Division of Nursing
Assistant Professor of Nursing
University of Maine at Fort Kent
Fort Kent, Maine

Sara Swett, RN, BSN, MSN
Clinical Instructor
Pacific Lutheran University
School of Nursing
Tacoma, Washington

Janice Tazbir, RN, MS, CCRN, CS, CNE
Professor of Nursing
Purdue University Northwest
College of Nursing
Hammond, Indiana

Beth A. Vottero, PhD, RN, CNE
Assistant Professor of Nursing
Purdue University Northwest
College of Nursing
Hammond, Indiana

Karen Luther Wikoff, RN, PhD
Assistant Professor
California State University, Stanislaus
Turlock, California

PREFACE

Nurses are committed to safe, high-quality, patient-centered care. Nurses demonstrate leadership and management skills in the provision of patient care, both interdependently with physicians and other members of the interprofessional team, and independently as nursing professionals. Various theories about Leadership and Management have been developed, as discussed in Chapter 1 of this book. These Leadership and Management theories are utilized by nurses in their personal life and from Day 1 of their clinical nursing practice. Millions of Americans turn to nurses for delivery of primary health care services, health care education. and health advice and counseling. The Gallup Poll (Brenan, 2018) has consistently found the nursing profession to be ranked as the Number One trusted profession in its annual polls of Americans. Suzanne Gordon is a journalist who has been writing about nursing issues since 1986. She writes,

"Nurses are regarded as honest and ethical but their breadth of skill is not known. When I was at the Beth Israel hospital, I was on the oncology clinic and followed these nurses for two years. Doctor comes in one day. Had a patient with breast cancer and the patient died. The husband gives him a trip around the world. What does he give the two nurses who cared for her? A scarf. The woman died, so it didn't work. The people who cared for her were the nurses. I happen to know the doctor, he was a, you're dying, I'm disappearing, kind of guy. The people who took care of her were her nurses. He gets the trip around the world, they get scarves. I think that says it all" (Maggi, 2001, p. 2).

Typically, professions are distinguished by certain specific characteristics. These include, but are not limited to:

- Formal educational requirements,

- Autonomy of practice,

- Adherence to an established code of ethics,

- Expansion of the level of knowledge, and

- A common culture and values present among members (Joel & Kelly, 2002).

Professions progress through an expected evolutionary process. This consists of:

- Expanding the scientific base,

- Creating technical workers to share in the essential mission of the field,

- Standardizing and up-grading education for entry into practice, and

- Moving forward with specialization.

Nursing's progression has been spotty and incomplete, largely because of the influence of external communities of interest, and the fact that nurses have resisted and personalized decisions that are necessary for future generations (Joel & Kelly, 2002). A profession must have a clear educational pathway into the practice and a constantly growing body of knowledge within institutions of higher learning (Blais & Hayes, 2011). Currently, there are many pathways for nursing education, ranging from 2-year degree programs to Bachelor to direct-entry Masters and Doctorate programs. For around 100 years, nurses have debated entry into practice. The result has been a myriad of programs with graduates used interchangeably in the real world. This absence of consensus within the discipline of nursing causes consumer confusion and seriously compromises our ability to serve the public (Joel & Kelly, 2002). Despite the variety of nursing programs and the range of advanced degrees they offer, all students have their basic professional nursing skills assessed by The National Council of State Boards of Nursing Licensure Exam (NCLEX).

Successful completion of the NCLEX exam permits any RN to practice under the nursing practice act of an individual state, regardless of the level of education attained, though more and more health care institutions are choosing to give RNs with a Bachelor degree priority in the hiring process.

In 1999, a National Academy of Sciences, Institute of Medicine (IOM) Report, *To Err Is Human: Building a Safer Health Care System* (Kohn, Corrigan, & Donaldson, 1999), shocked the nation and called attention to the adverse events that occur in many acute care hospitalizations. The IOM Report stated that the annual estimated cost of medical errors was between $17 billion and $29 billion at hospitals across the country, with between 44,000 and 98,000 deaths yearly, more than die from motor vehicle accidents, breast cancer, or AIDS.

In 2004, another IOM Report, *Keeping Patients Safe: Transforming the Work Environment of Nurses* (Institute of Medicine, 2004), found that, "how we are cared for by nurses affects our health, and sometimes can be a matter of life and death . . . nurses are indispensable to our safety." Nurses play a crucial role in protecting patient safety and providing quality health care. This finding has since been confirmed by several research studies (Aiken et al., 2017; Aiken et al., 2014; Cho, et al., 2016; Cho, Kim, Yeon, You, & Lee, 2015; Harrison et al., 2019; Kim & Bae, 2018; McHugh et al., 2016; You et al., 2013). The 2004 IOM Report concluded that education for the health professions was in need of a major overhaul.

In 2005, the Robert Wood Johnson Foundation funded a national project to educate nurses about patient safety and quality. The project developed Quality and Safety Education for Nurses (QSEN) Competencies, which identify the knowledge, skills, and attitudes needed for safety, quality, patient-centered care, informatics, teamwork and collaboration, and evidence-based practice to provide safe and effective quality nursing care. Today, QSEN Competencies are being integrated into nursing curricula, research, accreditation, and licensing to address the gap between nursing education and nursing practice.

In 2010, the Report, *Unmet Needs: Teaching Physicians to Provide Safe Patient Care* by the Lucian Leape Institute (2010) at the National Patient Safety Foundation highlighted the need for medical schools to integrate systems analysis, quality improvement, and patient-centered care into their curricula. The Report emphasized the importance of a culture of safety in teaching hospitals, stressing that unprofessional behavior and authority gradients prevent physician trainees from reporting and learning from errors (Ranji, 2014).

In 2016, Henry reported that improving quality and safety has been a focal point in medical education for more than a decade, but improvements have not been dramatic. Some medical schools are changing their curriculum—and cultures—to make greater strides through their work with the American Medical Association's *Accelerating Change in Medical Education Consortium* (Henry, 2016).

Makary & Daniels (2016) found that more than 250,000 people in the United States die every year because of medical mistakes, making medical mistakes the third leading cause of death after heart disease and cancer. Makary & Daniels (2016), define a death due to medical error as a death that is caused by inadequately skilled staff, an error in judgment or care, a system defect, or a preventable adverse effect. These deaths include deaths from mix-ups with the dose or type of medications administered to patients, surgical complications that go undiagnosed, and computer breakdowns. Makary & Daniels (2016), also noted that death certificates in the U.S., used to compile national statistics, have no way to identify medical error and that the reporting system should be revised to facilitate better understanding of deaths due to medical error. In 2019, the Institute for Healthcare Improvement (IHI) noted that health care delivery continues to be unsafe and that substantive improvements in patient safety will be difficult to achieve without major medical education reform at the medical school and residency training program levels (Gandhi et al., 2018).

The Robert Wood Johnson Foundation (RWJF) partnered with the Institute of Medicine (IOM) in 2010 and released a Report on The Future of Nursing: Leading Change, Advancing Health (National Academy of Science, 2011). This Report offered a series of recommendations to advance nursing's contributions to the health care environment, as follows:

- Nurses should achieve higher levels of education and training through an improved education system that promotes seamless academic progression.

- Nurses should be full partners, with physicians and other health care professionals, in redesigning health care in the United States.

- Nurses should practice to the full extent of their education and training.

- Effective workforce planning and policy making require better data collection and information infrastructure.

Following this Report, the American Association of Retired Persons (AARP) and RWJF launched the Future of Nursing: Campaign for Action to shepherd the implementation of the Report's recommendations. The Future of Nursing: Campaign for Action coordinated through the Center to Champion Nursing in America (CCNA), works nationally and through state Action Coalitions to advance its goals. The Future of Nursing: Campaign for Action Dashboard 2017 yearly progress report on the 2010 IOM Recommendations on The Future of Nursing: Leading Change, Advancing Health Report notes the following progress on the goals:

- Goal: Increase the proportion of nurses with a Baccalaureate Degree to 80% by 2020. 2017 Dashboard reports 56% of employed nurses hold a Baccalaureate (or higher) degree in nursing.

- Goal: Double the number of nurses with a Doctorate by 2020. 2017 Dashboard reports 28,004 employed nurses have a Doctoral degree.

- Goal: Advanced Practice Registered Nurses should be able to practice to the full extent of their education and training.

2017 Dashboard reports Advanced Practice Registered Nurses are able to practice to the full extent of their education and training in approximately one-third of U.S. states.

- Goal: Expand opportunities for nurses to lead and disseminate collaborative improvement effort. Unfortunately, the 2017 Dashboard reports that the number of health professions courses that include both RN students and graduate students of other health professions has decreased.

- Goal: Health care decision makers should ensure leadership positions are available to and filled by nurses. 2017 Dashboard reports 6,532 nurses have reported serving on non-Nursing Boards.

(Future of Nursing: Action Dashboard, available at, https://campaignforaction.org/wp-content/uploads/2019/07/Dashboard-Indicator-Updates_7.9.19.pdf, accessed July 22, 2017.) and The Nurses on Boards Coalition, available at, (https://www.nursesonboardscoalition.org/, accessed August 31, 2019).

Following passage of the Affordable Care Act of 2010, the Center for Medicare and Medicaid Services (CMS) invested in patient safety by tying hospital reimbursement to patient and family satisfaction, patient outcomes, and quality and safety.

As mentioned earlier, Leadership and Management theories are utilized by nurses from Day 1 of their clinical practice. This text, *Nursing Leadership & Management*, Fourth Edition, is edited by Patricia Kelly Vana and Janice Tazbir. It explores the Leadership and Management theories and skills that beginning nurses need in order to collaborate with the interprofessional team and structure the patient care environment to meet patient needs. Nurses use informatics and apply evidence-based, safe, high-quality standards and develop and monitor work processes and staffing, etc., to achieve high quality, safe, patient-centered care outcomes.

The Editors, Patricia and Janice, believe that all nurses, regardless of their role, are leaders and managers. Nursing Leadership and Management begins at a personal level when the new nurse reviews their career and life goals, such as goals for education and certification, type and quality of hospital for employment, desired type of patient care unit to work on, work benefits, financial goals, home purchase goals, etc. Nursing Leadership and Management continues with the staff nurse at the bedside. This bedside staff nurse is responsible for assuring that the evidence-based health care structures and processes needed to achieve safe, high quality patient-centered outcomes are available to patients. The staff nurse at the bedside demonstrates this commitment to patient care quality and safety with the utilization of evidence-based care, development of a high quality, safe, patient care environment, safe staffing, review of quality patient care guidelines and medications, and the development of professional communication, speech, and dress that strengthens the nurse's ability to manage and collaborate with the interprofessional team and lead patients to safe, high quality, patient-centered outcomes. In addition, the bedside staff nurse recognizes that many factors in the environment and

health care system influence the development of evidence-based, safe, high-quality, patient-centered outcomes. Accordingly, this bedside staff nurse recognizes the importance of developing personal, professional, and political power and joining nursing, hospital, and community committees, associations, Boards of Directors, etc., to assure the development of evidence-based, safe, high-quality, patient-centered outcomes.

Nursing Leadership & Management, Fourth Edition reviews information from the Agency for Healthcare Quality and Research, The Joint Commission, the Leapfrog Group, the National Quality Forum, and the Institute for Healthcare Improvement (IHI), among others, all focused on improvement of the quality and safety of patient care.

The chapter contributors to this Fourth Edition include many different types of nurses and members of the interprofessional team including: staff, educators, administrators, faculty informaticists, historians, quality scholars, clinical nurse specialists, nurse lawyers, nurse practitioners, entrepreneurs, physicians, librarians, psychologists, and others. These contributors are from all sections of the United States, illustrating a broad view of nursing leadership and management. There are chapter contributors and interviews from California, Colorado, Florida, Illinois, Indiana, Kentucky, Maine, Maryland, Massachusetts, Michigan, Minnesota, Missouri, New Hampshire, New Orleans, New York, New Jersey, Ohio, Rhode Island, South Carolina, Texas, Vermont, Washington, and Wisconsin.

1 Organization

Nursing Leadership & Management, Fourth Edition, consists of 29 chapters organized in a Conceptual Framework. This Conceptual Framework highlights nursing leadership and management responsibilities to the patient, to the community, to the interprofessional health care team, to the institution, and to self. The Four Units of the Conceptual Framework provide beginning nurse leaders and managers with the knowledge needed in today's health care environment.

Unit 1 introduces Kelly Vana's Nursing Leadership and Management. This unit discusses Nursing Leadership and Management in the Health Care Environment and reviews Nursing Leadership and Management in a Historical Context, and Nursing in a High Reliability Health Care Organization. It discusses Organization and Staffing of Patient Care at the Unit Level, as well as Health Care Economics and the Hospital, Department, and Unit Budget. Unit 2 discusses Leadership and Management of Patient-Centered Care. This Unit reviews Patient and Health Care Education, Evidence-Based Practice, Searching for the Evidence, Quality Improvement, and Improving Quality at the Unit Level, along with Safety for the Patient and Health Care Team. Lastly, Informatics is also discussed. Unit 3 discusses Nursing Leadership and the Interprofessional Team. This Unit reviews Interprofessional Teamwork and Collaboration and Members of the Interprofessional Team. It discusses Delegation, Assignment, and

Supervision of Patient Care, Time Management and Setting Priorities, Change, Critical Thinking and Clinical Reasoning. Power and Politics, Legal Aspects of Nursing, Ethical Aspects of Nursing, and Culture, Generational Differences, and Spirituality are also discussed. Unit 4 discusses Leadership and Management of Self and the Future. This Unit discusses NCLEX-RN Preparation, Entry into the Profession—Your First Job, Career Planning and Achieving Balance, Balancing A Healthy Personal and Professional Life, and Nursing Career Opportunities. Numerous additions and supplemental offerings have been made to the text to increase understanding and broaden your learning experience. Some of these are outlined below.

All chapters have been revised to reflect current practice.

- A strong foundation for evidence-based health care with attention to high-quality, safe care is emphasized throughout the text.

- The role of the entry level staff nurse in nursing leadership and management at the bedside is emphasized and provides a framework for understanding how the new nurse is a leader and manager and can make a difference within the health care system.

- Quality and Safety in Education (QSEN) competencies have been emphasized, with chapters on each of the 6 QSEN competencies, i.e., Quality Improvement, Patient-Centered Care, Evidence-Based Care, Informatics, Teamwork and Collaboration, and Safety, as well as an additional chapter on Searching for the Evidence in the Literature.

Chapters on Nursing Leadership and Management in a Historical Context and Organization of Patient Care in High Reliability Health Care Organizations have been added.

- All chapters have been updated to include new information from national and state health care and nursing organizations, e.g., the Institute for Healthcare Improvement (IHI) and The Joint Commission (TJC) on patient quality and safety.

- Content on delegation, setting patient care priorities, budgeting, and health care economics, has been significantly reworked and expanded.

- The chapter on NCLEX-RN licensure preparation helps students ensure that they are prepared for licensure by including a mini-nutrition chart, mini-medication chart, tips on preparing for the Next Generation NCLEX-RN licensure examination, and information on clinical reasoning, available at http://www.ncsbn.org/14172.htm, accessed June 16, 2020.

- Review questions are included in all chapters to help students test their knowledge and prepare for course exams. Review question formats include single choice and multiple option style questions.

- The Appendix include a Glossary of Key Terms and Answers to Chapter Review Questions for student and Faculty use.

- Several Appendix documents illustrating Preparation for new nurses and hour-by-hour schedules for a Labor and Delivery (L & D) patient care unit and various other patient care units are provided. There are also photos illustrating various elements of patient care.

A new website, accessed at www.wiley.com/go/kelly-Nursing-Leadership, is provided including:

- Faculty resources

- Additional online review questions with answers for each chapter

- Student resources Online

- PowerPoint for each chapter

- Tables and Figures for all chapters

- Chapter Review question answers

- Glossary of Key Terms

1.1 Chapter Features

Several standard chapter features are utilized throughout the text, which provide the reader with a consistent format for learning and an assortment of resources for understanding and applying the knowledge presented. Chapter features include the following:

- Health care or nursing quote related to chapter content

- Objectives that state the chapter's learning goals

- Opening scenario, a mini entry-level nursing case study that relates to the chapter, with critical thinking questions, which are discussed at the end of each chapter

- Photos, Figures, and Tables to clarify chapter content

- Key Concepts, a listing of the primary understandings the reader is to take from the chapter

- Key Terms, a listing of important new terms defined in the chapter

- NCLEX-RN style Review Questions at the end of each chapter. Answers available to students at the end of each chapter

- Review Activities, a reflection of chapter content applied to entry-level real-world nursing situations

- Discussion Points, critical thinking elements for discussion in student groups and/or the classroom

- Exploring the Web, websites related to chapter content

- Informatics, website exercise to develop informatics skill of student, including one website exercise that takes the student to the Quality and Safety in Nursing (**QSEN**) website, www.qsen.org

- Lean Back, questions related to chapter that encourage reflective thinking

- References for chapter

- Suggested Reading for further development of thinking related to chapter

Special elements are sprinkled throughout the chapters to enhance student learning and encourage critical thinking. These include:

- Evidence from the Literature with synopsis of key findings from nursing and health care literature

- Real World Interviews with health care leaders and managers, including nursing staff, clinicians, administrators, quality improvement staff, faculty, nursing and medical practitioners, patients, nursing assistive personnel (**NAP**), librarians, and lawyers

- Critical Thinking exercises regarding an ethical, legal, cultural, spiritual, delegation, or quality improvement nursing or health care topic

- Case Studies to provide the entry-level nurse with a clinical nursing leadership/management situation calling for critical thinking to solve a health care problem

1.2 How To Use This Book

QUOTE

- A nursing or health care theorist quote gives a professional's perspective regarding the topic at hand; read this as you begin each new chapter and see whether your opinion matches or differs, or whether you are in need of further information.

OBJECTIVES

- These statements indicate the performance-based, measurable objectives that are targeted for mastery upon completion of the chapter.

OPENING SCENARIO

- This mini case study with related critical thinking questions should be read prior to delving into the chapter; it sets the tone for the material to come and helps you identify your knowledge base and perspective. Discussion answers of the questions are included near the end of each chapter.

CASE STUDIES

- These short case studies with related questions present a beginning clinical nursing leadership or management situation calling for judgment, decision making, or analysis in solving an open-ended problem. Familiarize yourself with the types of situations and settings you will later encounter in nursing practice and challenge yourself to devise solutions that will result in the best outcomes for all parties, within the boundaries of legal and ethical nursing practice.

EVIDENCE FROM THE LITERATURE

- Study these key evidence findings from nursing and health care research, theory, and the literature. Ask yourself how they will influence your nursing practice. Do you see ways in which your nursing could be affected by these evidence findings? Do you agree with the implications identified by the author?

CRITICAL THINKING EXERCISES

- Ethical, cultural, spiritual, legal, delegation, and performance improvement considerations are highlighted in these exercises. Before beginning a new chapter, page through and read the Critical Thinking Exercises. Jot down your comments or reactions, then see whether your perspective changes after you complete the chapter.

REAL WORLD INTERVIEWS

- Interviews with nursing and many other interprofessional health care leaders and managers are included as well as interviews with hospital administration leaders, patients, family members, and others. As you read these interviews, ask yourself whether you had ever considered that individual's point of view on the given topic. How will knowing another person's point of view affect the care you deliver?

DISCUSSION POINTS

- These are critical thinking questions related to chapter content for discussion in student groups or the classroom.

INFORMATICS

- These include website exercises to develop the informatics skill of student, including one exercise that takes the student to the Quality and Safety in Nursing (QSEN) website.

LEAN BACK

- These are questions that encourage reflective thinking on chapter content.

EXPLORING THE WEB

- These are websites related to chapter content.

KEY CONCEPTS

- This bulleted list of key chapter concepts serves as a review and study tool for you as you complete each chapter.

KEY TERMS

- Study this list prior to reading the chapter, and then once again as you complete a chapter to test your understanding of the key terms covered in the chapter. Refer to the chapter's key terms in the Glossary in the Appendix to thoroughly appreciate the material of the chapter.

REVIEW QUESTIONS

- These questions will challenge your comprehension of objectives presented in the chapter and will allow you to demonstrate content mastery, build critical thinking skills, and prepare for the NCLEX-RN. Answers are found in the textbook Appendix.

REVIEW ACTIVITIES

- These thought-provoking activities at the close of a chapter invite you to approach a problem or scenario critically and apply the knowledge you have gained.

EXPLORING THE WEB

- Internet activities encourage you to use your computer and reasoning skills to search the Web for additional information on quality, safety, and nursing leadership and management.

REFERENCES

- Evidence-based research, theory, and literature, as well as nursing, medical, and health care sources, are included in these reference lists. Refer to them as you read the chapter to verify the content and findings.

- These entries invite you to pursue additional topics, articles, and information in related resources.

PHOTOS, TABLES, AND FIGURES

- These items illustrate key concepts and offer visual reinforcement of the concepts.

2 Instructor Resources (IR)

Chapter PowerPoints are available to Faculty and students online. They are designed to assist the faculty in presenting to nursing students the essential skills and information that are needed to help them secure a position as a beginning nursing manager and leader. The IR will assist faculty in planning and developing their programs and classes for the most efficient use of time and resources. The IR includes several must-have components:

1. Lecture Slides in PowerPoint™ serve as guides for presentation in the classroom.

2. An Online Test Bank for Faculty offers question sets by chapters, reviewing the 29 chapters, in multiple-choice and multiple response NCLEX-RN style formats. Complete answers including detailed rationales are also provided for Faculty.

3. An Image Library includes photos, diagrams, figures, and tables from the text, which can be imported into classroom presentations.

REFERENCES

Aiken, L. H., Sloane, D. M., Bruyeel, L., Van den Heede, K., Griffiths, P., et al. (2017). Hospitals; Mortality in nine European countries: A retrospective observational study. *The Lancet, 6736*(13), 62631–62638. doi:10.1016/S0140-6736(13)62631-8

Aiken, L. H., Sloane, D., Griffiths, P., Rafferty, A. M., Bruyeel, L., et al. (2014). Nursing skill mix in European hospitals: Cross-sectional study of the association with mortality, patient ratings, and quality of care. *The Lancet, 383*(9931), 1824–1830.

Brenan, M. (2018). *Nurses again outpace other professions for honesty, ethics.* https://news.gallup.com/poll/245597/nurses-again-outpace-professions-honesty-ethics.aspx.

Cho, E., Lee, N. J., Kim, E. Y., Kim, S., Lee, K., et al. (2016). Nurse staffing level and overtiome associated with patient safety, quality of care and care left undone in hospitals: A cross-sectional study. *International Journal of Nursing Studies, 60*, 263–271. doi:10.1016/j.ijnurstu.2016.05.009

Cho, S. H., Kim, Y. S., Yeon, K. N., You, S. J., &. Lee, I. D. (2015). Effects if increasing nurse staffing on missing nursing care. *International Nursing Review, 62*(2), 267-274. 10.1111/inr.12173

Gandi, T., Kaplan, G., Leape, L., Berwick, D., Edgman-Levitan, S., Edmondson, A., Meyer, G. S., Michaels, D., Morath, J. M., Vincent, C., & Wachter, R. (July 17, 2018). Transforming concepts in patient safety: A progress report. *BMJ Quality & Safety, 27*(12), 1019–1026. doi:10.1136/bmjqs-2017-007756

Harrison, J. M., Aiken, L. H., Sloane, D. M., Brooks Carthon, J. M., Merchant, R. M., et al. (2019). In hospitals with more nurses who have Baccalaureate degrees, better outcomes for patients after cardiac arrest. *Health Aff (Millwood), 38*(7), 1087–1094. doi:10.1377/h1thaff.2018.05064

Henry, T. A. (2016). *Accelerating change in medical education: Med schools focus on quality improvement, patient safety.* American Medical Association. Available at www.ama-assn.org/education/accelerating-change-medical-education/med-schools-focus-quality-improvement-patient

Institute of Medicine. (2004). *Keeping patients safe: Transforming the work environment of nurses.* Washington, DC: National Academies Press. doi: 10.17226/11151

Institute of Medicine. (2011). *The future of nursing: Leading change, advancing health.* Washington, DC: The National Academies Press. doi: 10.17226/12956

Joel, L. A., & Kelly, L. (2002). *The nursing experience: Trends, challenges, and transitions.* New York: McGraw-Hill.

Kim, C. G., & Bae, K. S. (2019). Relationship between nurse staffing level and adult nursing-sensitive outcomes in tertiary hospitals in Korea: Retrospective observational study. *International Journal of Nursing Studies, 80*, 155–164. doi:10.1016/j.ijnurstu.2018.01.001

Kohn, L. T., Corrigan, J. M., & Donaldson, M. S. (1999). *To err is human: building a safer health system.* Washington, DC: National Academy Press, Institute of Medicine.

Lucian Leape Institute. (2010). *Unmet needs: Teaching physicians to provide safe patient care.* Boston, MA: National Patient Safety Foundation.

Maggi, L. (2001). *A conversation with Suzanne Gordon.* Available at https://prospect.org/article/conversation-suzanne-gordon/, accessed June 16, 2020.

Makary, M. A., & Daniel, M. (2016). Medical error: The third leading cause of death in the U.S. *British Medical Journal, 353*, i2139. doi:10.1136/bmj.i2139

McHugh, M. D., Rochman, M. F., Sloane, D. M., Berg, R. A., Mancini, M. E., et al. (2016). Better nurse staffing environments associated with increase survival of in-hospital cardiac arrest patients. *Medical Care, 54*(1), 74–80. doi:10.1097/MLR.0000000000000456

Ranji, S. R. (2014). A piece of my mind. What gets measured gets (micro) managed. *Journal of the American Medical Association, 312*(16), 1637–1638. doi:10.1001/jama.2014.11268.PMID: 25335143

You, L. M., Aiken, L. H., Sloane, D. M., Liu, K., He, G. P., et al. (2013). Hospital nursing, care quality, and patient satisfaction: Cross-sectional surveys of nurses and patients in hospitals in China and Europe. *International Journal of Nursing Studies, 50*(2), 154–161. doi:10.1097/MLR.0000000000000456

FOREWORD

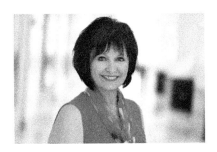

Kudos to Professors Kelly Vana and Tazbir for publishing the 4th edition of the book *Kelly Vana's Nursing leadership and management!* This book is a valuable educational resource not only for undergraduate nursing students but also for bedside nurses, managers, educators, and clinical specialists. Nursing students <u>and</u> nurses will benefit from the content of the book that includes perspectives from bedside nurses, faculty, educators, directors of nursing, nursing historians, lawyers, psychologists, and others. The book provides the content needed to lead at every level of nursing, emphasizing leadership from the bedside to the boardroom. The "call to action" is for every nurse, as a leader, to value that "everyone in healthcare really has two jobs when they come to work every day: to do their work and to improve it" (Batalden & Davidoff, 2007). Leadership is required to meet this "call to action" and transform health care to ensure that every patient receives high-quality, safe care every time.

The book includes chapters on the Quality and Safety for Nurses (**QSEN**) competencies: patient-centered care, teamwork and collaboration, evidence-based practice, quality improvement, safety and informatics (Cronenwett et al., 2007). These competencies provide the guide for the knowledge, skills, and attitudes that are needed to ensure the delivery of high-quality and safe care. The essential ingredient in integrating and implementing the QSEN competencies is leadership. Leadership to stand up and deliver nursing care that aligns with high-quality standards. This takes courage and strength as often the status quo is to "get through the shift," missing the opportunity to be an authentic leader. Being an authentic leader requires time to pause and be reflective in order to understand the values and strengths of yourself and others and the context of our work environments (Cooper, Scandura, & Schriesheim, 2005).

We can look to our country's great leaders to inspire us. Abraham Lincoln rises to the top of my list. I have always been impressed with President Lincoln and his ability to overcome failure and persist. Among the many leadership principles that President Lincoln lived by, the one that resonates the most with me is to "preach a vision and continually reaffirm it" (Phillips, 1992). It is our call in nursing to preach the vision of high-quality and safe care and continually reaffirm it. Thanks to Professors Kelly Vana and Tazbir for providing this book that helps us on the leadership journey to get us there.

MARY A. DOLANSKY, PHD, RN, FAAN
SARAH C. HIRSH PROFESSORSHIP IN NURSING
ASSOCIATE PROFESSOR
FRANCES PAYNE BOLTON SCHOOL OF NURSING
ASSOCIATE PROFESSOR, SCHOOL OF MEDICINE
CASE WESTERN RESERVE UNIVERSITY
CLEVELAND, OH

ASSOCIATE DIRECTOR
NURSE ADVISOR, NATIONAL VA QUALITY SCHOLARS PROGRAM (VAQS)
SENIOR NURSE FELLOW VAQS
LOUIS STOKES CLEVELAND VA
DIRECTOR, QSEN INSTITUTE

REFERENCES

Batalden, P. B., & Davidoff, F. (2007). What is "quality improvement" and how can it transform healthcare? *BMJ Quality Safe Health Care*, *16*(1), 2–3. doi:10.1136/gshc.2006.022046

Cooper, C. D., Scandura, T. A., & Schriesheim, C. A. (2005). Looking forward but learning from our past: Potential challenges to developing authentic leadership theory and authentic leaders. *The Leadership Quarterly*, *16*(3), 475–493. doi:10.1016/j.leaqua.2005.03.008

Cronenwett, L., Sherwood, G., Barnsteiner, J., et al. (2007). Quality and safety education for nurses. *Nursing Outlook*, *55*(3), 122–131.

Phillips, D. T. (1992). *Lincoln on leadership: Executive strategies for tough times*. Illinois: DTP/Companion Book.

CHAPTER FEATURES

Several standard chapter features are utilized throughout the text, which provide the reader with a consistent format for learning and an assortment of resources for understanding and applying the knowledge presented. Chapter features include the following:

- Health care or nursing quotes related to chapter content.
- Objectives that state the chapter's learning goals.
- Opening scenario: a mini entry-level nursing case study that relates to the chapter, with critical thinking questions, which are discussed at the end of each chapter.
- Photos, Figures, and Tables to clarify chapter content.
- Key Concepts: a listing of the primary understandings the reader is to take from the chapter.
- Key Terms: a listing of important new terms defined in the chapter.
- NCLEX-RN style Review Questions at the end of each chapter. Answers are available to students at the end of the chapter-no more flipping back and forth for answers!
- Review Activities: a reflection of chapter content applied to entry-level real-world nursing situations.
- Discussion Points: critical thinking elements for discussion in student groups and/or the classroom.
- Exploring the Web: websites related to the chapter content.
- Informatics: website exercises to develop the informatics skill of student, including one website exercise that takes the student to the Quality and Safety in Nursing (QSEN) website, www.qsen.org
- Lean Back: questions related to the chapter that encourage reflective thinking.
- References for the chapter.
- Suggested Readings for further development of thinking related to the chapter.

Special elements are sprinkled throughout the chapters to enhance student learning and encourage critical thinking. These include:

- Evidence from the Literature: with synopsis of key findings from nursing and health care literature.
- Real World Interviews: with health care leaders and managers, including nursing staff, clinicians, administrators, quality improvement staff, faculty, nursing and medical practitioners, patients, nursing assistive personnel (NAP), librarians, and lawyers.
- Critical Thinking: exercises regarding an ethical, legal, cultural, spiritual, delegation, or quality improvement nursing or health care topic.
- Case Studies: to provide the entry-level nurse with a clinical nursing leadership/management situation calling for critical thinking to solve a health care problem.

ABOUT THE EDITORS

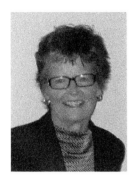

Patricia Kelly Vana earned a Diploma in Nursing from St. Margaret Hospital School of Nursing, Hammond, Indiana; a Baccalaureate in Nursing from DePaul University in Chicago, Illinois; and a Master's Degree in Nursing from Loyola University in Chicago, Illinois. Pat is Professor Emerita, Purdue University Northwest, Hammond Indiana. She has worked as a staff registered nurse, charge nurse, school nurse, nurse educator, travel nurse, industrial nurse, per diem nurse, and nurse volunteer in six states, i.e., Indiana, Illinois, Wisconsin, Oklahoma, Texas, and Pennsylvania. Pat loves to travel and has traveled extensively in the United States, Canada, Europe, Mexico, South America, Asia, and Puerto Rico. She has taught conferences for The Joint Commission, Resource Applications, Pediatric Concepts, and Kaplan, Inc. She has served as a Disaster Volunteer for the American Red Cross; as a volunteer nurse with a health care team of nurses, doctors, pharmacists, and lay people on a health care trip to Nicaragua; as a nursing volunteer at a free clinic in Chicago; and as a volunteer at church food pantries in Austin, Texas, and in Chicago, Illinois. Pat currently teaches national three-day NCLEX-RN reviews for Evolve Testing & Remediation/Health Education Systems, Inc. (HESI), Houston, Texas, and volunteers part time in the Emergency Department at Advocate Christ Medical Center, Oak Lawn, Illinois, and at Lee Memorial Hospital, Fort Meyers, Florida.

Pat was Director of Quality Improvement at the University of Chicago Hospitals and Clinics. She has taught at Wesley-Passavant School of Nursing in Chicago, Chicago State University, and was Associate Degree Program Coordinator at Purdue University Northwest in Hammond Indiana. She has taught Fundamentals of Nursing, Adult Nursing, Nursing Leadership and Management, Nursing Issues, Nursing Trends, Quality Improvement, and Legal Aspects of Nursing. Pat has been a member of Sigma Theta Tau, the American Nurses Association, and the Emergency Nurses Association. She has been listed in *Who's Who in American Nursing*, 2000 *Notable American Women*, and the *International Who's Who of Professional and Business Women*.

Pat has served on the Board of Directors of Tri City Mental Health Center, St. Anthony's Home, and the Quality Connection Journal.

Pat is the Editor with Dr. Beth Vottero and Dr. Carolyn Christie-McAuliffe of *Introduction to Quality and Safety Education for Nurses*, First and Second Editions, by Kelly, Vottero and Christie-McAuliffe, Springer Publications (2018 and 2014). She is also the Editor with Dr. Beth Vottero and Dr. Geralyn Altmiller, of *Quality and Safety Education for Nurses*, Third Edition, Springer Publications (2021) Pat is the Editor of *Nursing Leadership & Management*, First, Second, and Third Editions, Delmar Cengage Learning Publications (2012, 2008, and 2003), which has been adapted for use in Canada, i.e., *Nursing Leadership and Management* by Patricia Kelly and Heather Crawford, First and Second Editions (2013 and 2008) Nelson Publications; and *Nursing Leadership and Management*, by Patricia Kelly and Heather Quesnelle, Third Edition (2016). The text is also used in India.

Pat is the Editor of *Essentials of Nursing Leadership & Management*, First Edition, by Kelly-Heidenthal, 2003, Elsevier Publications. She is also the Editor with Professor Tazbir of *Essentials of Nursing Leadership & Management* with Janice Tazbir, Fourth Edition, 2021, by Kelly and Tazbir, Wiley Publications (2021). She co-edited *Nursing Delegation, Priority Setting, and Making Patient Care Assignments*, with Maureen Marthaler, First and Second Editions, Delmar Cengage Learning Publications (2011 and 2005). In this Fourth Edition of *Nursing Leadership and Management*, Pat is the chapter co-author with Dr. Ruth Hansten of "Nursing Delegation," and the chapter co-author with Janice Tazbir of "NCLEX-RN Preparation." Pat also contributed many chapters on various topics to most of the above textbooks.

Pat also contributed a chapter on "Obstructive Lung Disease: to Daniels, R. *Medical Surgical Nursing*, Delmar Cengage Learning (2010), and a chapter on "Preparing the Undergraduate Student and Faculty to Use Quality Improvement" in *Practice to Improving Quality*, Second Edition, by Meisenheimer. She has written several articles, including "Chest X-Ray Interpretation" and many articles on quality improvement. Throughout most of her career, she has taught nursing at the university level. Pat has traveled extensively in the United States, Canada, China, Europe, and Mexico, and has been licensed and worked part-time throughout her career in Emergency Departments or other patient care units in Indiana, Illinois, Wisconsin, Texas, Oklahoma, and Philadelphia. She currently lives with her husband, Ron, part of the year in Oak Lawn, IL and part of the year in Meyers, FL. Pat may be contacted at patkelly777@aol.com.

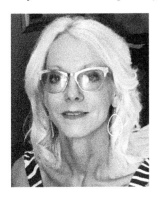

JANICE TAZBIR

Janice Tazbir earned an Associate Degree in Science in Nursing at Purdue University Calumet beginning her career as an RN at the age of 19. She furthered her education, earning a Bachelor's Degree and then a Master's Degree as a Clinical Nurse Specialist in Critical Care. Her clinical nursing background is in critical care nursing and she has worked the entirety of her career, currently in critical care at the University of Chicago Medicine in the Level 1 Trauma ICU. Her husband, Johnny, and daughter, Jade, are RNs as well, working at the University of Chicago Medicine. Jade is a newly graduated RN and is the primary chapter author for Chapter 29 in this text. Another daughter, Joule, is a 2020 graduate of the University of Alabama (with a 4.0 GPA) in Accounting. Janice has maintained a clinical practice as staff nurse her entire nursing career. Her teaching career has been at Purdue University Northwest, Hammond, Indiana from 1997 to 2019, where she has taught advanced medical surgical nursing, pathophysiology, critical care, capstone in nursing, care of the older adult, physical assessment, and NCLEX-RN preparation. Janice attained the status of Professor of Nursing in 2011 at Purdue University Northwest. She was awarded the Teaching Excellence Award at Purdue University Northwest in 2006. She has been a Certified Nurse Educator (**CNE**) since 2012. Janice is a member of many professional organizations including Sigma Theta Tau, the American Association of Critical Care Nurses, and the American Association of Neuroscience Nurses. She has published numerous refereed articles and book chapters over her career. She has presented locally and nationally, authored/edited four previous books including: *Clinical Companion to Accompany Contemporary Medical Surgical Nursing*. Tazbir, J. (2007), *Medical Surgical Atlas* (First Edition). Tazbir, J., & Keresztes, P. (2008), *Clinical Companion to Accompany Contemporary Medical Surgical Nursing* (Second Edition). Tazbir, J. (2010) and *Essentials of Nursing Leadership and Management* (Third Edition). Kelly, P., & Tazbir, J. (2014).

Janice publishes on current topics in critical care* (see selected publications).

She teaches NCLEX reviews for Evolve Testing & Remediation/Health Education Systems, Inc. (HESI), Houston, Texas as a Live Review Instructor and has been a Peer Advisor and Consultant, is an expert on NCLEX and HESI exams, including test writing, test analysis, teaching faculty regarding NCLEX, and presenting on NCLEX* (see selected presentation). She currently is a Consultant for Anderson Continuing Education in Sacramento, California as well as a staff nurse at University of Chicago Medicine.

Janice's administrative and committee involvement includes serving as past Undergraduate Program Coordinator at Purdue University Northwest, Hammond Campus. In her over 20 years of progressive teaching and administrative contributions to the PNW, she has made many key contributions that include (but are not limited to): appointed to Faculty Senate for multiple terms, Chairperson for multiple committees, including Faculty Affairs and Curriculum and Educational Policy and the Ad Hoc Promotion and Tenure Committee. She represented faculty in key University strategic initiatives such as mentoring, evaluations, promotion and tenure, strategic planning, experiential learning, first year experience, and unification. She was a key leader for Purdue University Northwest College of Nursing initiatives including NCLEX success and preparation, mentoring faculty and students, HESI coordination, testing center collaboration, testing, strategic planning and Purdue University Northwest College of Nursing unification efforts, where Purdue University Calumet and Purdue Westville combined universities as well as colleges of nursing.

Her passions include her family, traveling, and yoga. She has traveled the world from Egypt to Iceland and continues to travel and grow. She is a Registered Yoga Teacher (**RYT**) and practices yoga on and off the mat. Contact her at jtazbir1@gmail.com

Selected publications:

*Tazbir, J., & Wickheim, M. (2014). Hands when you want them, staffing when you need it. *Critical Care Nurse*. doi: http://dx.dio.org/10.4037/ccn2014902.

*Tazbir, J. (2012).Sepsis Early Recognition and Treatment in the Medical-Surgical Setting. July/August 2012, *MEDSURG Nursing*.

*Keresztes, P., & *Tazbir, J. (2005). CSF drainage after thoracic aneurysm repair. *Program and Proceedings, National Teaching Institute & Critical Care Exposition*.

*Keresztes, P., & Tazbir, J. (2005). The PFA-100: Analysis and interpretation of a platelet function measurement. *Journal of Cardiovascular Nursing, 20*, 405–407.

*Tazbir, J., Marthaler, M., Moredich, C., & Keresztes, P. (2005). Decompressive hemicraniectomy with duraplasty: A treatment for large-volume ischemic stroke. *Journal of Neuroscience Nursing, 37*, 194–197.

*Tazbir, J. (2004). Sepsis overview and the role of protein c. *Critical Care Nurse, 24*, 40–45.

Selected presentations:

*Tazbir, J., Landrum, J., & Cooke, C. (2016). Acing the Test: Creating a Testing Committee Nursing Education Conference in the Rockies Breckenridge, CO.

*Davis, J., Blodgett, N., Garwood, B., Ott, V., & Tazbir, J. (2016). Passing the NCLEX—What's the Evidence. Queen's Joanna Briggs Collaboration Conference, Kingston, Ontario, Canada.

*Davis, J., Tazbir, J., & Garwood, B. (2016). NCLEX—looking beyond passing. The Joanna Briggs Institute 20th Anniversary Conference Adelaide, Australia.

Tazbir, J., & *Zweighart, E. (2016). HESI Over Time: What the Research Demonstrates and Applications to Improving Student Outcomes. Evolve Elsevier. Las Vegas, NV.

Tazbir, J. (2014, March). *HESI implementation throughout the curriculum: Using Teamwork & Collaboration to Improve Outcomes*. Elevate the Outcomes with Evolve, Evolve Elsevier. Las Vegas, NV.

*Tazbir, J. (2011). Our Evolve experience at PUC. Hesi User Conference. Oakbrook, IL

ACKNOWLEDGMENTS

A book such as this requires great effort and the coordination of many people with various areas of expertise. We would like to thank all of the contributors for their time and effort in sharing their knowledge gained through years of experience in both the clinical and academic setting. All of the contributing authors worked within tight time frames to accomplish their work. Special thanks go to Corinne Haviley, RN, MS, PhD, Beth L. A. Richard RN MSN C-EFM, and Carolyn Ruud, DNP, RN, CNE®cl, CCRN, CVRN -BC, SCRN, Northwestern Medicine Delnor Hospital, Geneva, Illinois, for their help in developing some of the nursing information for the Appendix. Jane Woodruff McDaniel, Hobart, Indiana, supported the process with her computer expertise.

We thank the reviewers for their time spent critically reviewing the manuscript and providing the valuable comments that have enhanced this text.

Pat would like to give special thanks to Ron Vana, her husband, for his ongoing support and for the happiness he brings to her life. Thanks also go to her Dad and Mom, Ed and Jean Kelly; her sisters, Tessie Kelly Dybel and Kathy Kelly Milch; her Aunt Pat (who convinced her to start writing), and Uncle Bill Kelly; her Aunt Verna and Uncle Archie Payne; her nieces, Natalie Dybel Bevil, Melissa Milch Arredondo, and Stacey Milch Monks; her nephew, John Milch; her grandnephew, Brock Bevil; her grandniece, Reese Bevil; her nephews-in-law, Tracy Bevil, Peter Arredondo, and Derek Monks; and her dear friends, Patricia Wojcik, Florence Lebryk, Lee McGuan, Dolores Wynen, and Joan Fox, who have supported her throughout her development of this book. Special thanks to Pat's wonderful nursing friends, Zenaida Corpuz, Dr. Mary Elaine Koren, Dr. Barbara Mudloff, Dr. Patricia Padjen, Jane McKeon, Nancy Weber, Kerrie Ellingsen, and Dorothy Daniel Smith. Special thanks also to Pat's dear friends and nursing classmates of 58 years, Sylvia Komyatte, Gerri Kane, Julie Martini, Ivy Schmude, Anna Fizer, Judy Ilijanich, Janice Klepitch, Trudy Keilman, Mary Kay Moredich, Judy Rau, Lillian Rau, and Jenny Hawk, who have supported her during their years together as nurses. Special thanks also go to Pat's Co-Editor on this and other texts, Janice Tazbir, a great nurse, friend, and Co-Editor., and to Pat's Faculty mentors, Dr. Imogene King and Dr. Joyce Ellis.

Janice would like to gratefully acknowledge her family: Jade and Joule, her beautiful daughters-inside and out, and her husband of 25 years, Johnny, who is her best friend. Her family is a continual source of joy. Her gratitude extends to the students at Purdue University Northwest (PNW) for the years of inspiration, joy and driving her passion. She would also like to acknowledge her University of Chicago Medicine (UCM) colleagues that remind her of the incredible work and passion it takes to face critical care situations day in and out and provide excellent care and to Peggy Zemansky for being a living example of a great manager. Special thanks to Pat Kelly-Vana, a mentor and friend through the years (she was one of Janice's first professors) and to Catherine Ashton, fellow-yogi, friend and mentor; may your light shine forever-Namaste.

We would like to acknowledge and sincerely thank the team at Wiley who have worked to make this book a reality. Jennifer Seward, (Senior Project Editor), Tom Marriott (Editorial Assistant), P. Sathishwaran, our Content Refinement Specialist, Reference and Trade, and our Publisher, Magenta Styles.

ABOUT THE COMPANION WEBSITE

This book is accompanied by a companion website:

www.wiley.com/go/kelly-Nursing-Leadership

The website includes:
Instructor Resources Online

- Additional online review questions with answers for each chapter
- Lecture PowerPoint for each chapter
- Tables and figures for all chapters

Student Resources Online

- Lecture PowerPoint for each chapter
- Tables and figures for all chapters
- Chapter Review question answers
- Glossary of Key Terms

Scan this QRcode to visit the companion website:

Nursing Leadership, Management, and Motivation

1

Linda Searle-Leach

Azusa Pacific University, Azusa, CA, USA, and Huntington Hospital, Pasadena, CA, USA

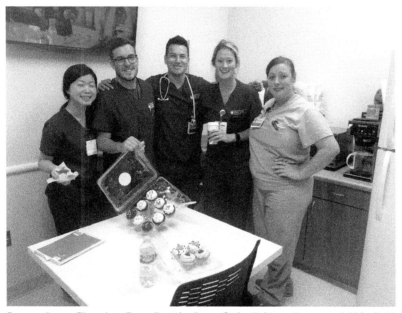

Source: Jenny Chenying, Ryan Beattie, Jason Ortiz, Brittany Bryne, and Abigail Alund.

Leadership is not about titles, positions or flowcharts. It is about one life influencing another.

(*John Maxwell,* 1997)

OBJECTIVES

Upon completion of this chapter, the reader should be able to:

1. Define and differentiate between leadership and management.

2. Distinguish characteristics of effective leaders.

3. Identify leadership theories.

4. Explain emotional intelligence.

5. Identify direct care nurses as Knowledge Workers and first-line leaders of patient care delivery.

6. Apply knowledge of leadership theory in carrying out the nurse's role as a leader.

7. Describe the management process.

8. Explain frontline, middle and executive level management roles that nurses fulfill in an organization.

9. Relate management theories.

10. Summarize motivation theories.

Kelly Vana's Nursing Leadership and Management, Fourth Edition. Edited by Patricia Kelly Vana and Janice Tazbir
© 2021 John Wiley & Sons Ltd. Published 2021 by John Wiley & Sons Ltd.
Companion Website: www.wiley.com/go/kelly-Nursing-Leadership

OPENING SCENARIO

Ed Harley was admitted to the cardiac observation unit earlier in the day. He had been diagnosed previously with heart disease and had experienced episodes of ventricular arrhythmias. His cardiologist had determined the need to change his antiarrhythmic medication to reduce the side effects Mr. Harley was experiencing. That evening, while Mr. Harley was talking to his wife on the phone and as his nurse, Maria, was walking to his bedside, he suddenly stopped talking and went into ventricular fibrillation and cardiac arrest. Maria reacted instinctively and started Advanced Cardiac Life Support (ACLS) defibrillating him immediately. Normal sinus rhythm appeared on the monitor before anyone else could respond to the code. Mr. Harley was then transferred to the Coronary Care Unit (CCU).

*Maria had been a Registered Nurse (RN) for less than one year at the time, and although she had participated in Code arrests a few times, she had never witnessed one occur right before her eyes. Her knowledgeable action saved this patient's life. In nursing, **Cardiopulmonary Resuscitation (CPR) and ACLS are mandatory** skills and considered part of a nurse's ordinary work. Yet it is quite extraordinary work.*

Everything had happened so quickly that evening that Maria did not have a chance to talk to the patient before he was transferred. She entered his room the next morning in CCU, as the sun was just rising. As he awoke, Maria spent that quiet time with him. While he embraced the start of a new day, his thoughts were intense. What he chose to share was this acknowledgment: "You saved my life. Thank you." This precious moment was a celebration of both of their lives.

What leadership characteristics did Maria demonstrate in preventing a nurse-sensitive outcome of cardiac arrest?

Why is Maria considered a leader, even though she is not in a formal leadership or management position?

For all nurses, their knowledge of nursing and ability to apply that knowledge, is the basis of their leadership. Many people think that leaders are only top corporate executives and administrators, political representatives, military generals, or those who head an organization. This is because these leaders are highly visible and hold high-profile positions. However, leaders are needed at all levels of an organization. With the advent of the information age, many professionals, including nurses, became known as knowledge workers. Nurses' education and specialized clinical preparation develops their expertise and leadership ability. Nursing knowledge workers are leaders. This idea of nursing knowledge workers contrasts with the manufacturing age, where the manager was the most knowledgeable person and closely supervised employees to carry out routine work. Leadership however is a basic competency for all nursing professionals. Leadership development is a necessary part of the preparation of nurses.

Nurses make a critical difference every day in the lives of their patients and patients' families, yet nurses believe those accomplishments are part of their ordinary work. Nurses are leaders, and by using their expert knowledge, they coordinate patient care and lead patients and families through health care journeys. Nurses lead themselves as they develop in their career and nurses lead change to improve patient outcomes and the quality of care. Nurses are leaders and lead without being in a management position.

Leadership and management are different. Leadership influences or inspires the actions and goals of others. One does not have to be in a position of authority to demonstrate leadership. Not all leaders are managers. Leaders have been characterized as people who do the right thing whereas managers are viewed as people who do things right (Drucker, 1993). Both leadership and management are crucial but different.

This chapter lays the groundwork for the development of knowledge about nursing leadership and management. Many concepts touched on in this chapter will be developed in depth in the chapters that follow. This chapter discusses leadership and provides a framework to differentiate leadership and management and explain emotional intelligence. Leadership characteristics, styles of leadership, and leadership theories are described emphasizing transformational leadership and complexity leadership. The chapter introduces the process of management and explains management and motivation theories. The content is developed for the beginning nurse preparing to graduate from a pre-licensure program and enter the profession in the role of registered nurse. Benner's work describing skill acquisition of nurses uses a framework called, "From Novice to Expert" and labels this new graduate nurse as an advanced beginner (Benner, Tanner, & Chesla, 2009).

Definition of Leadership

Leadership is commonly defined as a process of influence in which the leader influences others toward goal achievement (Yukl, 2006). Nurses function as leaders when they lead themselves and influence others toward goal achievement.

Influence is an instrumental part of leading others and leaders influence others, often by inspiring, enlivening, and engaging others to participate. Leadership can occur personally. It can occur between the leader and another individual; between the leader and a group; or between a leader and an organization, a community, or a society. Defining leadership as a process helps us understand more about leadership than the traditional view of a leader being in a position of authority, exerting command, control, and power over subordinates. There are many more leaders in organizations than those who are in positions of authority. Each person has the potential to set goals and enact leadership. What this means for nurses as professionals is that nurses set goals and are leaders.

Leadership can be **formal leadership**, as when a person is in a position of authority or in a sanctioned, assigned role within an organization that connotes influence, such as a nurse manager (Northouse, 2018). The traditional formal leadership roles in nursing include clinical supervisor, unit/department manager, director of nursing and the top-level nurse executive, usually called the chief nurse executive or chief nursing officer. Other formal leader roles in nursing include the charge nurse of a patient care unit, the Chief Operating Officer, of a hospital the nurse who leads interprofessional team rounds and the nurse who represents her unit/department at an event or meeting.

An **informal leader** is a person who demonstrates leadership outside the scope of a formal leadership role or as a member of a group rather than as the head or leader of the group. The informal leader is considered to have emerged as a leader when she is accepted by others, is an opinion leader, and is perceived to have influence. Informal leader roles in nursing include examples such as the staff nurse who regularly sets personal, proffessional, and patient care goals, assuring the delivery of safe, evidence-based, patient-centered, high quality care, including responding quickly to a code.

Leaders and Followers

Leaders and followers are both necessary roles. Nurses are alternately leaders and followers when they work with other health care team members to achieve patient care goals, participate in meetings, and so forth. The most valuable followers are skilled, self-directed employees who participate actively in setting the group's direction and who invest time and energy in the work of the team or group, thinking critically and advocating for new ideas (Grossman & Valiga, 2013). Good followers communicate and work well with others, being supportive, yet thoughtful, in their approach to new ideas.

Leaders Versus Managers

Kotter (1990a) describes the differences between leadership and management in the following way: Leadership is about creating change. He says that leaders establish direction, align people through empowerment, and motivate and inspire others toward achieving a vision and creating meaningful change; whereas managers focus on managing, defined as planning and budgeting, organizing and staffing, problem solving, and controlling complexity. Complexity has to do with interdependence; being dependent on others to carry out our work. Interdependence requires coordination and cooperation. Managers engage in controlling complexity to produce predictability, stability, and order (Kotter, 1990b).

Nurses function as leaders when they demonstrate leadership characteristics in their personal and professional roles and work with other nurses and health care staff to lead patients, families, and communities to their best health. See Table 1.1 for examples of selected nursing leadership characteristics and personal and professional role activities.

Leadership Characteristics

One popular way of characterizing leadership is by describing it as **authentic leadership**. The American Association of Critical Care Nurses in their landmark work, AACN *Standards for Establishing Healthy Work Environments: A Journey to Excellence,* cite authentic leadership as one of the key standards necessary for establishing a healthy work environment. AACN's belief is that to establish and sustain healthy work environments for nurses, leadership that is authentic is a critical element. Authentic leadership requires skill in the core competencies of self-knowledge, strategic vision, risk taking and creativity, interpersonal and communication effectiveness, and inspiration (American Association of Critical Care Nurses (AACN), 2004; Raso, 2019).

Leaders are also described by fundamental qualities that effective leaders have been found to share (Bennis & Nanus, 1985). The first quality is a guiding vision. Leaders focus on a professional and purposeful vision that provides direction toward a preferred future. The second quality is passion. Passion expressed by the leader involves the ability to inspire and align people toward the promises of life. Passion is an inherent quality of the nurse leader. The third quality is integrity that is based on knowledge of self, honesty, and maturity developed through experience and growth. Other leadership qualities include self-awareness—knowing our strengths and weaknesses—that can allow us to use feedback and learn from our mistakes (McCall, 1998). Daring and curiosity are also basic ingredients of leadership that leaders draw on to take risks, learning from what works as much as from what does not work (Bennis & Nanus, 1985).

Certain characteristic traits are commonly attributed to leaders. These traits are considered desirable and seem to contribute to the perception of being a leader; intelligence, self-confidence, determination, integrity, and sociability (Stodgill, 1948, 1974). Research among 46 hospitals designated as Magnet® Hospitals by the **American Nurses Center for Certification** (ANCC) for their success in attracting and retaining registered nurses reported that nurse leaders who are visionary and enthusiastic, are supportive and knowledgeable,

Table 1.1   Nursing Leadership Characteristics and Role Activities

Nursing leadership characteristics.	Examples of personal and professional nursing role activities,
Leadership establishes direction.	Nurses set personal, professional, and patient care goals.
Leadership aligns people through empowerment.	Nurses demonstrate leadership when they model high quality practices as they work to empower and mentor other nurses.
Leadership motivates and inspires others toward achieving a vision and creating meaningful change.	Nurses motivate members of the interprofessional health care team toward the delivery of safe, evidence-based, patient-centered, high quality care
Leadership is about service.	Service is helping others or doing work for others. The profession of nursing is founded on serving others in need of health care. Leadership is serving others through leading. This concept has been popularized as servant leadership (Greenleaf, 1970/2008; Keith, 2016). The premise is that servant leaders want to serve first, whereas other leaders lead first.
Leadership is about people and relationships.	Nurses demonstrate leadership and play roles in patient outcomes when they build relationships with patients and their significant others (Wong & Cummings, 2007).
Leadership is contextual.	Nurses demonstrate leadership when they adjust their leadership styles, to achieve nursing goals. A major context evolves around the interrelationships that nurses have with others (Spence Laschinger, Finegan, & Wilk, 2009).
Leadership is about using communication that inspires others.	Nurses demonstrate leadership when they monitor the meaning of what is being communicated, both verbally and nonverbally, and manage the situation to achieve goals for all involved, using communication that is clear and inspiring
Leadership is about balancing.	Nurses demonstrate leadership when they multitask and balance all that they do to achieve nursing goals. Leadership is also about pursuing a work and life balance in order to sustain one's personal and professional self and be available for others.
Leadership is about continuous learning and improvement.	Nurses demonstrate leadership by developing personal and professional goals and continuing to grow their knowledge and expertise.
Leadership is about effective decision making.	Nurses demonstrate leadership when they make effective, evidence-based decisions. Nurses must be autonomous in their decision making yet also work with other health care team members to assure the best care for their patients (Wong & Cummings, 2009).
Leadership is a political process.	Nurses demonstrate leadership when they participate in the hospital and in the community, join hospital and community Boards of Directors, and participate in various political processes locally and globally.
Leadership is about integrity.	Nurses demonstrate leadership when they consistently model integrity, honesty, fairness, and morality.

Note: Adapted from Moore, J. (2004). *Leadership: Lessons learned.* Terre Haute, Indiana, and the author's personal observations.

have high standards and expectations, value education and professional development, demonstrate power and status in the organization, are visible and responsive, communicate openly, and are active in professional associations are valued (Kramer, 1990; Kramer & Schmalenberg, 2005; McClure & Hinshaw, 2002; McClure, Poulin, Sovie, & Wandelt, 1983). Research findings from other studies on nurses revealed

that caring, respectability, trustworthiness, and flexibility were the leadership characteristics most valued. In one study, nurse leaders identified managing the dream, mastering change, designing organization structure, learning, and taking initiative as leadership characteristics (Murphy & DeBack, 1991). Research by Kirkpatrick and Locke (1991) concluded that leaders are different from non-leaders across six traits: drive, the desire to lead, honesty and integrity, self-confidence, cognitive ability, and knowledge of the business. Although no set of traits is definitive and reliable in determining who is a leader or who is effective as a leader, many people still rely on many of these traits to describe and define leadership characteristics.

Leadership Theories

Many believe that the critical factor needed to maximize people's involvement is leadership (Bennis & Nanus, 1985). A more in-depth understanding of leadership can be gleaned from a review of leadership theories. Leadership theories can be classified various ways. These are summarized in Table 1.2.

Behavioral Approach

Leadership studies from the 1930s by Kurt Lewin and colleagues at Iowa State University conveyed information about three leadership styles based on the leader's behavior that are still widely recognized today: autocratic, democratic, and laissez-faire leadership (Lewin, 1939; Lewin & Lippitt, 1938; Lewin, Lippitt, & White, 1939). **Autocratic leadership** involves centralized decision making, with the leader making decisions and using power to command and control others. **Democratic leadership** is participatory leadership, with authority delegated to others. To be influential, the democratic leader uses expert power and the power base afforded by having close, personal relationships. The third leadership style, **laissez-faire leadership**, is passive and permissive, and the leader defers decision making. Lewin (1939) contrasted these styles and concluded that autocratic leaders were associated with high-performing groups, but that close supervision was necessary and feelings of hostility were often

Table 1.2 Leadership Theories

Behavioral Leadership Theories (Three Approaches)	**Autocratic** Centralized decision making: Leaders make decisions and use power to command and control others.
	Democratic Participative: Leaders use expert power and the power that emanates from close, personal relationships to involve others and make decisions.
	Laissez-faire Passive and permissive: Leaders defer making decisions
Two Basic Leader Behaviors	**Job-centered behaviors** Leaders focus on schedules, costs, and efficiency; minimal attention given to develop work groups and high-performance goals.
	Employee-centered behaviors Leaders focus on human needs of employees.
Two Dimensions of Leader Behavior	**Initiating structure** Emphasis is on the work to be structured; focus on task and production. Concern is how the work is organized and achieving goals. Leaders plan, direct others, establish deadlines, and give details of how work is to be done.
	Consideration Focus is on consideration of the employee and relating and getting along with people. Leaders attend to the well-being of others; show empathy and interest in others; work on creating relationships to promote communication and trust.

(Continued)

Table 1.2 (Continued)

Contingency Leadership Theories (Four types)	**Contingency Theory of Leader Effectiveness** Leader behavior is dependent or contingent on the interaction of the leader and the needs of the situation. By developing good or poor leader-member relations, high or low task structure, and high or low position power, the leader matches the most favorable leadership style to the situation.
	Situational Leadership Theory Focus is on the situation in determining leadership style: Telling style is high task, low relationship; Selling style is high task, high relationship; Participating style is low task, high relationship; Delegating style is low task and low relationship style.
	Path-Goal Theory Leaders make the path toward the goal easier for followers by selecting an appropriate style of leadership: Directive style focuses on the task; Supportive style is relationship focused and encouraging; Participative style involves followers in decision making; Achievement-oriented style focuses on high structure and direction with high support and consideration.
	Substitutes for Leadership Substitutes for leadership are variables that may take the place of leadership behaviors and have influence on followers to the same degree as the leader's behavior. Examples included routine work, intrinsic satisfaction in the work, cohesiveness of the group, low position power, and rigid adherence to the rules.
Contemporary Leadership Theories (Five types)	**Charismatic Theory** Leaders convey an inspirational quality that promotes an emotional connection with followers. Leader qualities include self-confidence, strength of convictions, communicating a vision, and high expectations.
	Transformational Leadership Theory Transformational leaders empower others to become involved in a collective purpose, inspired by a vision of a preferred future; they motivate others to contribute and take action.
	Knowledge Workers Knowledge workers bring specialized expertise to an organization. Valued for what they know, they are at the frontlines with expertise and information to take action; they are the organization's leaders.
	Complexity Leadership Complexity leadership is relationship-based. Leaders facilitate information flow, context, circumstances, and interaction to create the structure for change using systems thinking and complex adaptive systems as a foundation for leading.
	Servant Leadership Servant Leadership is a leadership philosophy that emphasizes service to others, a holistic approach to work, and promotes a sense of community and sharing of power in decision making (Spears & Lawrence, 2004).

present in these groups. Democratic leaders engendered positive feelings in their groups and performance was strong, whether the leader was present or not. Low productivity and feelings of frustration were associated with laissez-faire leaders.

Behavioral leadership studies from the University of Michigan and from Ohio State University led to the identification of two basic leader behaviors: job-centered behaviors and employee-centered behaviors. Effective leadership was described as having a focus on the human needs of subordinates and was called

employee-centered leadership (Griffin & Moorhead, 2014). **Job-centered leaders** were viewed as less effective because of their focus on schedules, costs, and efficiency, resulting in a lack of attention to developing work groups and high-performance goals (Griffin & Moorhead, 2014).

The researchers at Ohio State focused their efforts on two dimensions of leader behavior: initiating structure and consideration. **Initiating structure** involves an emphasis on the work to be done, a focus on the task, and production. Leaders who focus on initiating structure are concerned with how work is organized and on the achievement of goals. Leader behavior includes planning, directing others, and establishing deadlines and details of how work is to be done. For example, a nurse demonstrating the leader behavior of initiating structure could be a charge nurse who, at the beginning of a shift, makes out a patient assignment.

The dimension of **consideration** involves activities that focus on the employee and emphasize relating and getting along with people. Leader behavior focuses on the well-being of others. The leader is involved in creating a relationship that fosters communication and trust as a basis for respecting other people and their potential contributions. A nurse demonstrating consideration behavior will take the time to talk with coworkers, be empathetic, and show an interest in them as people.

The leader behaviors of initiating structure and consideration define four leadership styles:

* Low initiating structure, low consideration

* High initiating structure, low consideration

* High initiating structure, high consideration

* Low initiating structure, high consideration

The Ohio State University studies associate the high initiating structure–high consideration leader behaviors with better performance and satisfaction outcomes than the other styles. This leadership style is considered effective, although it is not appropriate in every situation.

Real World Interview

It is important that beginning nurses see themselves as leaders. Leadership doesn't mean you have to have an administrative title. The central task of leadership is catalyzing others to achieve shared values in a complex world that is constantly changing and requiring us to design new ways of achieving our goals. This is a description of what is required of nurses each day, every day.

Angela Barron McBride, PhD, RN, FAAN
Distinguished Professor-Dean Emerita
Indiana University School of Nursing
Indianapolis, Indiana

Evidence from the Literature

Citation: Buresh, B. and Gordon, S. (2013). From silence to voice: What nurses know and must communicate to the public (The culture and politics of health care work). 3rd ed. Ithaca, NY: ILR Press.

Discussion: In this book by Suzanne Gordon and Bernice Buresh, the authors convey their journalistic perspectives and experience in writing about health care work. They provide an informative insight that nurses need to do a better job of accurately describing what nurses do and how nurses use expert knowledge acquired through scientific and technical mastery. They caution that nurses fail to articulate the value of the contribution nurses make to successful patient outcomes. Their message to nurses is that there is a reason that the public has such little understanding of nursing and the importance of our work. The reason is twofold: traditional stereotypes about nursing cloud the reality of nursing as it is currently practiced, and nurses have been patterned to describe their contribution to health care in self-sacrificing and anonymous ways.

Implications for Practice: Nurses need to be clear about why it is important for the public to know what nurses do and how nurses use specialized knowledge based on science to deliver health care. This book is an important vehicle from which nurses can begin to examine their own words and ways of discussing what nurses do and reflect upon the historical religious and societal practices that interfere with a clear, accurate, and realistic image of modern nursing. It is important for nurses to be clear about the value of nursing—their assessments, decisions, knowledgeable actions, ability to educate, emergency responses, and therapeutic compassion. What nurses often think of as their ordinary work is really quite extraordinary. Nurses use scientific knowledge, expert judgment, and complex skills to make critical decisions that affect patient outcomes. Nurses need to be able to articulate how they do their work and the difference it makes in the lives of patients and families, their communities and to the health of the nation.

Real World Interview

I have been a nurse for almost 60 years. I have come to realize that leadership and a happy life begins with me. As new nurses beginning your career, I suggest you assume leadership and identify your professional and personal goals. Select and add to the professional and personal goals and leadership strategies below. Identify your completion timeframe also.

Professional Goals	Leadership Strategy	Completion Timeframe
Pass NCLEX-RN	• Take NCLEX-RN review course • Check out, https://ncsbn-external.myabsorb.com/#/public-dashboard, accessed January 31, 2020 • Practice 60 questions daily and review weak content areas identified on exit exam • Relieve anxiety with music, exercise, laughter	Take NCLEX-RN within 2 months of graduation
Get first nursing job	• Apply to 3 favorite, high quality hospitals • Practice interviewing with friend	Within 3 months of graduation
Orient to assigned nursing unit	• Review evidence-based patient care guidelines and 10 most common medications for type of patients you will care for • Identify a mentor to guide your clinical development	
Obtain nursing certification in your clinical practice	• Review partial list of certifications at, https://nurse.org/articles/nursing-certifications-credentials-list, accessed January 31, 2020	
Identify nursing goals	• Obtain higher nursing degree, e.g., BSN, MSN, APN, Ph.D. • Become an advanced practice nurse, e.g., www.allnursingschools.com/specialties/advanced-practice-nurse, accessed January 31, 2020 • Become a travel nurse, e.g., https://blog.bluepipes.com/best-travel-nursing-companies-2019, accessed January 31, 2020 • Start independent Nursing business, e.g., Jon Haws RN, at, https://nursing.com/contact, accessed January 31, 2020 • Join hospital or community Board of Directors • Join a professional nursing association and contribute to the strength of the nursing profession.	
Personal Goals	• Dream Big! Choose your goals and lead yourself to the life of your dreams. Your life is waiting! • Buy home in safe area. Check there are good schools in area to add to home value • Grow your Net Worth. Calculate it yearly at, www.kiplinger.com/tool/saving/T063-S001-net-worth-calculator-how-to-calculate-net-worth/index.php, accessed January 31, 2020 • Enroll in 401K, Roth IRA, or other investment program, earning at a good percentage rate with low fees. Deposit and let your money grow. Don't touch it until you are 65+. Do this and many become a millionaire! • Read investment article in Kiplinger's, Consumer Report, Barron's, other, once monthly to build financial investing knowledge. • Get at least 150 minutes of moderate aerobic activity or 75 minutes of vigorous aerobic activity a week. Do strength training exercises for all major muscle groups at least two times a week www.mayoclinic.org/healthy-lifestyle/fitness/expert-answers/exercise/faq-20057916, accessed January 31, 2020 • Run for Public Office and improve health care, www.dummies.com/education/politics-government/the-requirements-to-run-for-public-office, accessed January 31, 2020 • Help others, e.g., volunteer at a food pantry monthly • Volunteer as a short-term Medical Mission Nurse, e.g., www.volunteerhq.org/blog/medical-mission-trips, accessed January 31, 2020 • Travel the world, enjoy new hobbies, take educational and fun courses, laugh often, enjoy friends and family, etc.	Enroll in 10% automatic payroll deposit immediately in your first job.

Remember, leadership and a happy life begins with you. Set your goals and lead yourself to a wonderful life!

Patricia Kelly Vana
Professor Emerita
Purdue University Northwest
Hammond, Indiana

Contingency Approach

Another approach to leadership is **contingency theory**. Contingency theory acknowledges that factors in the environment influence outcomes as much as leadership style and that leader effectiveness is contingent upon or depends upon something other than the leader's behavior. The premise is that different leader behavior patterns will be effective in different situations.

Fielder's Contingency Theory

Fielder (1967) is credited with the development of the contingency model of leadership effectiveness. Fielder's theory of leadership effectiveness views the pattern of leader behavior as dependent upon the interaction of the personality of the leader and the needs of the situation. The needs of the situation or how favorable the situation is toward the leader involves leader-member relationships, the degree of task structure, and the leader's position of power (Fielder, 1967). **Leader-member relations** are the feelings and attitudes of followers regarding acceptance, trust, and credibility of the leader. Good leader-member relations exist when followers respect, trust, and have confidence in the leader. Poor leader-member relations reflect distrust, a lack of confidence and respect, and dissatisfaction with the leader by the followers

Task structure refers to the degree to which work is defined, with specific procedures, explicit directions, and goals. High task structure involves routine, predictable, clearly defined work tasks. Low task structure involves work that is not routine, predictable, or clearly defined, such as creative, artistic, or qualitative research activities.

Position power is the degree of formal authority and influence associated with the leader. High position power is favorable for the leader, and low position power is unfavorable. When all dimensions—leader-member relations, task structure, and position power—are high, the situation is favorable to the leader. When these dimensions are low, the situation is not favorable to the leader. In both circumstances, Fielder showed that a task-directed leader, concerned with task accomplishment, was effective. When the range of favorableness is intermediate or moderate, a human relations leader, concerned about people, was most effective. These situations need a leader with interpersonal and relationship skills to foster group achievement. Fielder's contingency theory is an approach that matches the organizational situation to the most favorable leadership style for that situation.

Situational Approach

Situational leadership theory addresses the follower characteristics in relation to effective leader behavior.

Hersey and Blanchard's Situational Theory

Whereas Fielder examines the situation, Hersey and Blanchard consider follower readiness as a factor in determining leadership style. Rather than using the words, *initiating structure* and *contingency,* they use the words, *task behavior* and *relationship behavior. Task behavior* is used to identify behaviors focused on tasks. The words, *relationship behavior,* are used to identify behaviors focused on relationships

High task behavior and low relationship behavior is called a *telling leadership* style. A high task, high relationship style is called a *selling leadership* style. A low task and high relationship style is a *participating leadership* style. A low task and low relationship style is a *delegating leadership* style.

Follower readiness, called maturity, is assessed to select one of the four leadership styles for a situation. For example, according to Hersey and Blanchard's situational leadership theory (2000), groups with low maturity, whose members are unable or unwilling to participate or are unsure, need a leader to use a telling leadership style to provide direction and close supervision. The selling leadership style is a match for groups with low to moderate maturity who are initially unable to do the task but willing and confident and need clear direction and supportive feedback to get the task done. Participating leadership style is recommended for groups with moderate to high maturity who are able but unwilling to do a task or are unsure and who need support and encouragement. The leader should use a delegating leadership style with groups of followers with high maturity who are able to do a task and ready to participate and can engage in the task without direction or support.

An additional aspect of situational leadership theory is the idea that the leader not only changes leadership style according to followers' needs but also develops followers over time to increase their level of maturity (Schindler, 2015). Use of these four leadership styles helps a nurse manager lead effectively and assign work to others.

Path-Goal Theory

In this leadership approach, the leader works to motivate followers and influence goal accomplishment. The seminal author on path-goal theory is Robert House (1971). By using the appropriate style of leadership for the situation (i.e., directive, supportive, participative, or achievement oriented), the leader makes the path toward the goal easier for the follower. The *directive* style of leadership provides structure through direction and authority, with the leader focusing on the task and getting the job done. The *supportive* style of leadership is relationship oriented, with the leader providing encouragement, interest, and attention. *Participative* leadership means that the leader focuses on involving followers in the decision-making process. The *achievement-oriented* style provides high structure and direction as well as high support through consideration behavior. The leadership style is matched to the situational characteristics of the followers, such as the desire for authority, the extent to which the control of goal achievement is internal or external, and the ability of the follower to be involved. The leadership style is also matched to the situational factors in the environment, including the routine nature or complexity of the task, the power associated with the leader's position, and the work group relationship. This alignment of leadership style with the needs of followers is motivat-

ing and believed to enhance performance and satisfaction. The path-goal theory is based on expectancy theory, which holds that people are motivated when they, (a) believe they are able to carry out the work, (b) think their contribution will lead to the expected outcome, and (c) believe that the rewards for their efforts are valued and meaningful (Northouse, 2018).

Substitutes for Leadership

Substitutes for leadership are variables that may influence followers to the same extent as the leader's behavior. Kerr and Jermier (1978) investigated situational variables and identified substitutes that eliminate the need for leader behavior and other aspects that act as neutralizers and nullify the effects of the leader's behavior. Some of these variables include follower characteristics, such as the presence of structured routine tasks, the amount of feedback provided by the task, and the presence of intrinsic satisfaction in the work; and organizational characteristics, such as the presence of a cohesive group, a formal organization, a rigid adherence to rules, and low position power. For example, an individual's experience substitutes for task-direction leader behavior (Kerr & Jermier, 1978). Nurses and other professionals with a great deal of experience already have knowledge and judgment and do not need direction and supervision to perform their work. Thus, their experience serves as a leadership substitute. Another substitute for leader behavior is intrinsic satisfac-

---

Real World Interview

Beginning nurses show leadership by bringing their understanding of **evidence-based practices** (EBP) and by implementing them at the bedside. They are part of committees and have a voice about unit and hospital policies. Every nurse, no matter if brand new or seasoned, brings leadership qualities to the bedside. In the Intensive Care Unit where I work, assessing changes in the patient's condition, communicating with physicians, and making

sure something gets done to help the patient in a matter of minutes requires leadership. This is what we do to make sure patients get the best care.

Johnny Tazbir, RN, BSN
Crown Point, Indiana

Critical Thinking 1.1

Several characteristics attributed to leaders include:

- Intelligence
- Self-confidence
- Determination
- Integrity
- Sociability

- Caring
- Respectability
- Trustworthiness
- Flexibility

Review each of these characteristics attributed to leaders. Are these the characteristics you think are important for nurse leaders? To what extent do you portray each of these leadership characteristics?

Critical Thinking 1.2

Can professional nursing standards, such as the Code of Ethics for nurses, https://www.nursingworld.org/coe-view-only, accessed January 31, 2020, serve as a substitute for leadership?

tion that emerges from just doing the work. Intrinsic satisfaction occurs frequently among nurses when they provide care to patients and families. Intrinsic satisfaction substitutes for the support and encouragement of relationship-oriented leader behavior.

Contemporary Approach

Contemporary approaches to leadership address the leadership functions necessary to develop learning organizations. Contemporary leadership approaches include charismatic theory, transformational leadership theory, knowledge workers, complexity leadership, and servant leadership.

Charismatic Leadership Theory

A charismatic leader has an inspirational quality that promotes an emotional connection from followers. House (1971) developed a theory of charismatic leadership that described how charismatic leaders behave as well as distinguishing characteristics and situations in which such leaders would be effective. Charismatic leaders display self-confidence, have strength in their convictions, and communicate high expectations and their confidence in others. They have been described as emerging during a crisis, communicating vision, and using personal power and unconventional strategies (Conger & Kanungo, 1987). One consequence of this type of leadership is a belief in the charismatic leader that is so strong that it becomes almost an obsession that takes over, and the leader is worshipped as if superhuman. Charismatic leaders can have a positive and powerful effect on people and organizations. Martin Luther King, Lee Iacocca, former **chief executive officer** (CEO) of Chrysler Corporation, and Herb Kelleher, former CEO of Southwest Airlines, are all described as charismatic leaders. This type of leader can contribute significantly to an organization, even though all the leaders in an organization are not charismatic leaders. There are also effective leaders who do not exhibit all the qualities associated with charismatic leadership. Charisma seems to be a special and valuable quality that some people have while others do not.

Transformational Leadership Theory

Transformational leadership is one of the most prominent contemporary leadership theories. Transformational leadership is defined as a process in which "leaders and followers raise one another to higher levels of motivation and morality" (Burns, 1978, p. 21). Transformational leadership theory is based on the idea of empowering others to engage in pursuing a collective purpose by working together to achieve a vision of a preferred future. This kind of leadership can influence0 both the leader and the follower to a higher level of conduct and achievement that transforms them both (Burns, 1978). Burns maintained that there are two types of leaders: the traditional manager concerned with day-to-day operations, called the **transactional leader**, and the leader who is committed to a vision that empowers others, called the **transformational leader**.

Transformational leaders motivate others by behaving in accordance with values, providing a vision that reflects mutual values, and empowering others to contribute. Bennis and Nanus (1985) describe this leader as a person who "commits people to action, who converts followers into leaders, and who converts leaders into agents of change" (p. 3). According to research by Tichy and Devanna (1986), effective transformational leaders identify themselves as change agents; are courageous; believe in people; are value driven; are lifelong learners; are able to negotiate complexity, ambiguity, and uncertainty; and are visionaries. Yet transformational leadership may be demonstrated by anyone in an organization regardless of his position (Burns, 1978). The interaction that occurs between individuals can be transformational and motivate both to a higher level of performance (Bass, 1985).

Transformational leadership at the organizational level is about innovation and change. The transformational leader uses vision based on shared values to align people and inspire

Case Study 1.1

A nurse is making rounds on her new postoperative laryngectomy patient. As the nurse enters the room, the patient begins to bleed from his neck incision. The nurse applies direct pressure to the patient's carotid artery with one hand and calls for assistance. Help arrives, and the patient is taken to surgery, with the nurse still maintaining pressure on the bleeding site. The patient's condition is stabilized and the patient is discharged to home a few days later.

How does nursing leadership and management on a patient care unit ensure good patient care in an emergency?

How can you develop your leadership and management skills to improve your ability to care for a group of patients?

growth and advancement. It is both the inspiration and the empowerment aspects of transformational leadership that lead to commitment beyond self-interest, commitment to a vision, and commitment to action that creates change. Transformational leadership theory suggests that the relationship between the leader and the follower inspires and empowers an individual toward commitment to the organization.

Nurse researchers have described nurse executives according to transformational leadership theory and have used this theory to measure leadership behavior among nurse executives and nurse managers (Dunham-Taylor, 2000; Leach, 2005; McDaniel & Wolf, 1992; Wolf, Boland, & Aukerman, 1994; Young, 1992). Additionally, transformational leadership theory has been the basis for the nursing administration curriculum and for investigation of relationships such as relationships between a nurse's commitment to an organization (Leach, 2005) and productivity in a hospital setting (McNeese-Smith, 1997) and the ethical aspects of transformational leadership (Cassidy & Koroll, 1998). Barker (1990) also comprehensively discussed nursing in terms of transformational leadership theory. Of the contemporary theories of leadership, transformational leadership has been a popular approach in nursing and is well suited to the rapidly changing health care environment.

Most recently, the **National Academy of Medicine** (NAM) identified transformational leadership theory as a precursor to any change initiative and stated that transformational leadership can be a crucial approach toward achieving work environments that optimize patient safety (NAM, 2003).

Knowledge Workers

Nurses are **knowledge workers**. Knowledge workers are those who bring specialized, expert knowledge to an organization (Drucker, 2006, 1993, 1959). They are valued for what they know. Knowledge organizations, in which the knowledge worker is at the front lines with the expertise and the information to act, have become the dominant organizational type in the information age (Drucker, 2006, 1993; Helgesen, 1995). The knowledge organization shares, provides, and grows the information necessary to work efficiently and effectively. In organizations such as these, the ideas of leadership at the top and leadership equated with the power of a position are obsolete notions. Knowledge workers with the expertise and information to act are the organization's leaders. They provide the service, interact with the customer, represent the organization, and accomplish its goals.

Knowledge workers work in the information age, where the rapid, instant access to information makes information the medium of exchange. Knowledge workers are valued for what they know. The development of new knowledge and innovation and meaningful interpretation and application becomes the source for transactions with patients and staff. Nursing's transition to the information age has occurred in the context of rapidly advancing technology and nanotechnology and been influenced by three key trends: mobility, virtuality, and user-driven practices (Porter O'Grady, 2001).

Mobility refers to the ability to do work in convenient places using telehealth rather than working at fixed places, which may or may not be convenient. Technology has enabled mobility with the development of the small computer chip. Nurses work in a variety of settings today and use portable computers in wireless phones and computers at the bedside.

Virtuality means working through virtual means using digital networks, where the worker may be far from the patient but present in a digital reality. Telemetry monitoring and telehealth care by nurses are examples of virtuality.

User-driven practices mean that, at a time when digital mediums have given us more access to information and therefore more choices, the individual acts more independently and is increasingly accountable for those choices and actions. Nurses use electronic devices for self and patient education and teach patients to use digital monitors for self-care.

Nursing leadership practices are evolving to match nurses' work within this mobile, changing environment, with nurses as knowledge workers who can make decisions and take action. This is facilitated by the growth and sophistication of nursing research, the application of nursing science, and the translation of available evidence into evidence-based nursing practice. Nurses are able to display the rich and valuable contribution that their knowledge and expertise make to the quality of patient care and to quality health care outcomes.

Using Knowledge

Good nursing leadership and management of patients includes getting to know the patients; spending time assessing normal behavior, physiological and psychological responses to illness and hospitalization; and using knowledge to recognize even subtle changes in the patients' conditions and further evaluate them. Another key aspect of using knowledge is developing the ability to anticipate patient care problems. When a nurse intervenes with a postoperative patient who is bleeding from his incision by applying pressure at the site, the nurse minimizes the amount of bleeding. Using knowledge and anticipating such complications assists a nurse to intervene correctly. Thinking in advance about what should be done if a particular complication should occur, and then monitoring the patient to assess and identify complications early or, when possible, to prevent them, is one way that nurses apply their knowledge. Another aspect of using knowledge for good leadership and management on the patient care unit is to have the right type of personnel and the right amount of personnel; in other words, having patient care unit staffing with enough registered nurses, licensed practical nurses, or nursing assistants on the unit, so that they all can fulfill their roles appropriately with enough people to adequately care for the patients.

Nurses develop their leadership and management skills with continuing education and by increasing their knowledge and expertise in caring for a group of patients by taking care of those patients regularly. The more experience a nurse gains in caring for a population of patients, the more opportunity the nurse has to learn to recognize patterns that occur with these patients. These patterns can include the type of symptoms that are common, possible complications or emergencies, and actions that can help prevent complications or negative outcomes. Planning in advance, prioritizing time and attention, determining actions needed and what can be delegated to others are ways that nurses manage a group of patients.

Knowledgeable nursing leadership and management on a nursing unit fosters good patient care by providing a supportive environment for nurses to deliver care. A supportive leadership and management environment is characterized by a clear chain of command, clear job descriptions, evidence-based patient care standards, appropriate staffing, accessible Internet and library resources, and continuing education support. This allows the nurse to set goals, seek a mentor, and continue employment in a setting that is supportive of high quality, safe, patient-centered care.

Complexity Leadership

Margaret Wheatley, in *Leadership and the New Science* (1999), says, "There is a simpler way to lead organizations, one that requires less effort and produces less stress than the current practices." She presents a new view of leadership, one encompassing connectedness and self-organizing systems that follow a natural order of both chaos and uncertainty, which is different from a linear order in a hierarchy. The leader's function is to guide an organization using vision, to make choices based on mutual values, and to engage in the culture to provide meaning and coherence. This type of leadership fosters growth within each of us as individuals and as members of a group. A new model of leadership and understanding health care organizations and patient care units as **Complex Adaptive Systems** (CAS) has emerged from these ideas. CAS are complex, nonlinear, interactive and self-organizing systems with the capacity for self-renewal. The environment in a CAS is unpredictable and control is distributed with simple rules as the basis of operation. CAS are able to learn and adapt as a network of interacting, interdependent agents who cooperate in common goals and create new patterns of operating (Plowman & Duchon, 2008).

Complexity leadership is the new model where leadership is described as transformational, collaborative, self-reflective, and relationship based. Complexity leaders see people in organizations as self-organizing and self-renewing and envision work occurring through relationships. This optimizes autonomy at all levels because the relationships among the individual and the whole are strong. For nursing, such relationships might provide the infrastructure that will foster inter-professional decision making and strengthen the connection with other health co-workers.

In Wheatley's subsequent book, *Finding Our Way: Leadership for an Uncertain Time* (2005), she discusses how humans learn best when they are engaged in relationships with others and can exchange knowledge and expertise through informal, self-organized communities. Wheatley refers to these as communities of practice and encourages us to develop new leaders using communities of practice. Her notion of a community of practice represents several elements nurses are familiar with, that is, forming informal groups, using a group process of organizing, using principles of learning, and sharing information. What is unique in her description of these communities of practice is that they form via self-organization. They come together naturally. What makes these communities of practice different from informal groups is Wheatley's characterization of a community of practice built from relationships and participation in a way that connects nurses and allows the creation of meaning from information or the exchange of knowledge. One example of the concept of a community of practice is a group of nurses and physicians who work together to identify the best evidence to establish efficient patient flow through the emergency department to admission to the hospital. In work done for the Center of Creative Leadership, communities of practice are described as being different from the ideas or experiences we have had with groups, teams, and collective forming, because communities of practice emerge from shared activity, shared knowledge, and ways of knowing that create meaning and thus a culture of engagement, participation, and relationships (Drath & Palus, 1994). Wheatley directs nurses to name these communities of practice that bring people together, support these connections, nourish the community, and illuminate their work. These exciting notions hold great promise for health professionals as we learn how to collaborate within and across disciplines and countries to advance health care practices.

Servant Leadership

Servant Leadership is a leadership philosophy that emphasizes service to others, a holistic approach to work, and promotes a sense of community and sharing of power in decision-making (Spears & Lawrence, 2004). Some common features of servant leadership are that the servant leader considers the needs of employees first, commits to helping employees develop expertise and improve performance, and insists that the organization make a positive contribution to society. While not losing their focus on a healthy bottom line, servant leaders make sure an organization improves its community, region, and nation.

Emotional Intelligence

Emotional intelligence is a component of leadership and refers to the capacity to accurately perceive and express emotion, to use feelings to inform and guide thinking, to understand the meanings of emotions and to manage emotions for personal and social growth (Goleman, 1998). Emotional intelligence consists of social and emotional skills enabling the capacity to interact with understanding and respect, resolve conflicts, withstand stress and adversity to persevere. Better performance and job success have been attributed to emotional intelligence, whereas problems with interpersonal relationships and difficulty adapting occur when emotional intelligence is low or absent. Emotional intelligence is necessary for nurses to maintain a calm and professional demeanor in emergency situations, to participate effectively in teams and groups and to navigate interpersonal issues and adversity.

Emotional intelligence includes five basic emotional and social competencies: i.e., Self-awareness, Self-regulation, Motivation, Empathy, and Social skills (Table 1.3).

Nursing Leadership during the Pandemic

The COVID-19 Pandemic began as an active crisis in 2020, causing thousands of deaths. Now more than ever, nurses, as leaders and managers, were responding to protect patients, family, friends, the public, and members of the interprofessional health care team, including nurses. Situations not

thought plausible had become reality. The American Nurses Association Response to the COVID-19 Pandemic document highlights Nursing's response and illustrates one of the ways that nurses have always answered the call to serve their patients, their country, and communities during times of crisis.

Doctors and nurses were dying because of lack of **personal protective equipment** (PPE) supplies; not just in one country, but in many. Nurses were being fired for voicing truths, such as hospital PPE shortages; how could we protect transparency and patient safety? Nurses had to demonstrate leadership in safeguarding their patients and themselves.

This situation has put a magnifying glass on the errors in many world health care systems and shows that some health care systems and governments prepared and responded better than others. The Pandemic has brought a plethora of opportunities and critical needs for nursing and also underscores our need for data-driven decisions. Nurses' voices need to be heard and this is a call for you to use yours. An incomplete list of opportunities and critical needs for nursing leaders includes: (see COVID-19 and disaster planning p. 15)

Table 1.3 Emotional Intelligence (EI)

Emotional and social competencies		Examples for a beginning nurse leader
Self-awareness	Knowing what you are feeling in the moment and using your preferences to guide your decision making; having a realistic assessment of your own abilities and a well-grounded sense of self-confidence	Recognizing fatigue and feeling a bit drained after admitting a new patient and getting another patient off to surgery; rather than skipping a break, thinking that the break time will help with catching up, the EI nurse uses self-awareness to decide it would be best to take the break. She checks in with the charge nurse and then hands-off assigned patients and uses the time to rest and refresh.
Self-regulation	Handling your emotions so that they facilitate rather than interfere with the task at hand; being conscientious and delaying gratification to pursue goals; and recovering well from emotional distress	Discovering that a medication error has occurred can create emotional distress ranging from fear of what peers will think, fears that you did something that might have caused patient harm, to feeling less than adequate as a nurse. The EI nurse will manage those emotions in the moment to focus on reporting the error, examining how it happened, and being open to learning and taking action to prevent a future occurrence.
Motivation	Using your deepest preferences to move and guide you toward your goals, to help you take initiative and strive to improve, and to persevere in the face of setbacks and frustrations	A goal for a new nurse is to pursue becoming board certified in a selected area of nursing. For example, the certification for critical care nurses is the Critical Care Registered Nurse (CCRN); for oncology nurses, the certification is **Oncology Certified Nurse** (OCN). After completing a review course and taking the certification exam, a nurse receives results that show she didn't pass the exam. At first, she is embarrassed and feels that she isn't smart enough. As an EI nurse, she realizes that this setback isn't going to prevent her from reaching her goals. She also takes initiative and asks for help to guide her preparation to retake the exam in the future.
Empathy	Sensing what people are feeling; being able to take their perspective; cultivating rapport and being in tune with a broad diversity of people	As the nurse walks into the patient's room planning to change the patient's dressing, the patient begins to cry. The EI nurse realizes that the patient's emotional distress is a priority and she takes time to comfort the patient and acknowledge the patient's need to express her feelings.
Social Skills	Handling emotions in relationships well and accurately reading social situations and networks; interacting smoothly; using these social skills to persuade, lead, negotiate, and settle disputes, and for cooperation and teamwork	Interacting smoothly at change of shift can require the EI nurse to recognize when the situation with a peer is not going well. It's important to not take it personally but rather to acknowledge if another's expectations were not met. Then say what you can/will do and explore what you need to do for continued teamwork.

Real World Interview

Transformational leadership encourages the retention of nurses through job satisfaction. Initially, it is important for a beginning nurse to have structure and supportive supervision. The nurse leader should be visible and approachable. The younger generation generally wants meaningful work, feedback, continuous learning, and flexibility for balancing activities. Transformational leadership fosters healthy staff-focused workplaces through such techniques as shared organizational goals, learning opportunities for career development, rewards and recognition, empowerment, autonomy, employee health programs, and shared governance. That facilitates quality of care, and consequently, job satisfaction and nurse retention.

Anne Marriner-Tomey, PhD,RN
Author, Guide to Nursing Management
and Leadership Professor Emerita
Indiana State University-College of Nursing
Terre Haute, Indiana

COVID-19 and Disaster Planning

- Nursing Membership on Boards of Directors and other Decision-Making Groups
- Ensuring protection and safety for all health care workers
- Disaster Preparedness and Preparedness Training
- Telemedicine
- Organization of patient care for large groups of patients
- Global disease management
- Supply chain issues
- Information and communication
- Community health nursing
- Nursing education
- Advanced practice
- Racism and blaming
- Economic impacts on healthcare
- Population Health
- Mental Health Care Management, e.g., Post Traumatic Stress Disorder, Depression, Anxiety, Addiction, Abuse, etc.
- Ethical issues
- Political, social, and community activism
- Review of National health care systems versus private health care
- Patients with health disparities
- Employment protection for health care workers
- Entrepreneurial ventures
- Ensuring the basics- food, water, air, shelter, and safety
- Eldercare, nursing homes, and long-term healthcare
- Women, reproductive rights, childbearing and children
- Healthcare disparities

Note. American Nurses Association. ANA Response to COVID-19 Pandemic, available at, www.nursingworld.org/practice-policy/work-environment/health-safety/disaster-preparedness/coronavirus/ana-covid-19-statement, Accessed April 2, 2020.

Definition of Management

Management is defined as a process of coordinating actions and allocating resources to achieve organizational goals. It is a process of planning, organizing and staffing, leading, and controlling actions to achieve goals. Planning involves setting goals and identifying ways to meet them. Organizing and staffing is the process of ensuring that the necessary human and physical resources are available to achieve the planning goals. It also involves assigning work to the right person or group and specifying who has the authority to accomplish certain tasks. Finally, controlling is comparing actual performance to a standard and revising the original plan as needed to achieve the goals. The daily activities of managers are diverse and fast paced, with regular interruptions. Priority activities are integrated among inconsequential ones. In the scope of one morning, a nurse manager may make serious decisions about a critically ill patient, a staff or patient complaint, a shortage of nurse staffing, and so forth. A nurse manager's work is driven by problems that emerge in random order and that have a range of importance and urgency. These circumstances create an image of the nurse manager as a *firefighter* involved in immediate and operational concerns. A significant proportion of a manager's time is spent in interaction with others, and more of the work is concerned with handling information than in making decisions (McCall, Morrison, & Hannan, 1978). Nurse managers constantly interact with other members of a health care administrative team. This administrative team can include nurses, various clinical practitioners, unit staff, and staff from other departments who share information and assure that quality patient outcomes are achieved.

Managerial Roles

One of the most frequently referenced taxonomies of managerial roles is from an in-depth, month-long study of five chief executives by Henry Mintzberg. A **taxonomy** is a system that orders principles into a grouping or classification. Mintzberg's observations led to the identification of three categories of managerial roles: (a) information-processing role, (b) interpersonal role, and (c) decision-making role (Mintzberg, 1973).

A role includes behaviors, expectations, and recurrent activities within a pattern that is part of the organization's structure (Katz & Kahn, 1978). Specific or distinct roles are part of each of the three categories of managerial roles. The *information-processing roles* are monitor, disseminator, and spokesperson, each of which is used to manage the information needs that people have. The *interpersonal roles* are §head, leader, and liaison, and each of these roles is used to manage relationships with people. The *decision-making roles* are the entrepreneur, disturbance handler, allocator of

Real World Interview

Newly graduated nurses are concerned about their abilities to perform as nurses. They are worried about their skills and abilities and about advancing to independently manage a full patient load. New graduate nurses also deal with the emotional and physical realities of full-time work and the transition from the role of student into professional nurse. To help support this transition, all new nurses are included in our year-long Nurse Residency Program. This program provides them with a monthly opportunity to learn new skills and affirm their current skills and abilities through a variety of learning activities, including simulation. The new nurses also discuss their challenges and experiences when discussing tales

from the bedside. They learn how to take the theory of EBP and apply it to a unit-based issue. They create change within the Medical Center through their EBP projects! This often is the highlight of the first year of transition.

Katherine Pakieser-Reed, PhD, RN
Director, Center for Nursing Professional
Practice and Research
University of Chicago Medical Center
Chicago, Illinois

resources, and negotiator roles that managers use to act when making decisions.

The Management Process

In the early 1900s, an emphasis on management as a discipline emerged with a focus on the science of management and a view that management is the art of accomplishing things through people (Follet, 1924). Henri Fayol, a manager, wrote a book in 1917 called *General and Industrial Management*. He described the functions of planning, organizing, coordinating, and controlling as the **management process** (Fayol, 1917/1949). His work has become a classic in the way that we define the process of managing. Two other individuals, Gulick and Urwick, in some part resulting from their esteemed status as informal advisers to President Franklin D. Roosevelt, defined the management process further according to seven principles (Fayol, 1917/1949). Their principles form the acronym POSDCORB, which stands for Planning, Organizing, Staffing, Directing, Coordinating, Reporting, and Budgeting (Fayol, 1917/1949;

Gulick & Urwick, 1937). Their work is also considered to be a classic description of management and is still a relevant description of how the management process is carried out today.

More recently, Yukl (2013) and colleagues (Kim & Yukl, 1995; Yukl, Wall, & Lepsinger, 1990) followed this classic work by describing 13 management functions that address two broad aspects of the management process: managing the work and managing relationships. The management functions for *managing the work* are planning and organizing, problem solving, clarifying roles and objectives, informing, monitoring, consulting, and delegating. The management functions for *managing relationships* are networking, supporting, developing and mentoring, managing conflict and team building, motivating and inspiring, and recognizing and rewarding.

The amount of time managers spend on particular roles or functions varies by the level of their positions in organizations, ranging from the first-level management positions, to the middle-level management positions, to the executive-level management positions. A first-level managerial role or function in health care organizations is the nurse manager at the

Critical Thinking 1.3

Select three opportunities to observe interactions by the nurse manager of the unit where you are doing your clinical rotation or where you are a new graduate nurse. These opportunities could be during a unit staff meeting, when the nurse manager makes rounds, and during conversation with others at the nurses' station. Which of the following nurse management functions do you see your unit nurse manager performing?

– **Managing the work**

  – **Planning and organizing**
  – **Problem solving**
  – **Clarifying roles and objectives**

– **Informing**
– **Monitoring**
– **Consulting**
– **Delegating**

– **Managing relationships**

  – **Networking**
  – **Supporting**
  – **Developing and mentoring**
  – **Managing conflict and team building**
  – **Motivating and inspiring**
  – **Recognizing and rewarding**

clinical bedside. First-level nurse managers spend the majority of time directly managing patient care and supervising others as they deliver care. The next highest percentage of their time is spent in planning. The rest of first-level nurse managers' functions typically take fewer than 10% or less of their time: planning and organizing, problem solving, clarifying roles and objectives, informing, monitoring, consulting, and delegating.

In contrast, middle-level managers, usually called nursing directors, spend less time in direct supervision and more time in the other managerial roles or functions, particularly, planning and coordinating. At the highest level of the organization, usually described as the executive level, planning and being a generalist are greatly expanded role functions. Direct supervision is not a major aspect of the executive role as it is in the other two levels. Nurses in executive-level roles in health care organizations usually have the title Chief Nurse Executive or Chief Nursing Officer or, in acute care hospitals, the title may be Vice President of Patient Care Services.

Management Theories

The current management practices have evolved from earlier theories. Management practices were part of the governance in ancient Samaria and Egypt as far back as 3,000 B.C. (Daft & Marcic, 2015). Most of our current understanding of management, however, is based on theories of management that were introduced during the industrial age as factories developed and manufacturing flourished. Some of these theories are discussed in Table 1.4.

Scientific Management

While practicing managers, such as Fayol, who was mentioned earlier, were describing the functions of managers, a man named Frederick Taylor was focusing his attention on the operations within an organization by exploring production at the worker level. Taylor is acknowledged as the Father of Scientific Management for his use of the scientific method and as the author of *Principles of Scientific Management* (1911). Productivity was the area of focus in Scientific Management. Taylor, an engineer, introduced precise procedures based on systematic investigation of specific situations. The underlying point of view of Scientific Management is that the organization is a machine to be run efficiently to increase production. Scientific Management pioneered studies of time and motion that emphasized efficiency and culminated in "one best way" of carrying out work.

Bureaucratic Management

Max Weber is the German theorist recognized for the management theory of Bureaucracy. Weber's beliefs were in stark contrast to the typical European organization that was based on a family-type structure in which employees were loyal to an individual, not to the organization. Weber, however, believed efficiency is achieved through impersonal relations within a formal structure, competence should be the basis for hiring and promoting an employee, and decisions should be made in an orderly and rational way based on rules and regulations. Organizations were bureaucracies based on a hierarchy

Table 1.4   Management Theories

Management theory	Key aspects
Scientific Management Gulick & Urwick (1937), Mooney & Reiley (1939), Taylor (1947)	Focuses on goals and productivity; organization is a machine to be run efficiently to increase production. Selects the right person to do the job; provides the proper tools, training, and equipment to work efficiently. Uses time and motion studies to make the work efficient.
Bureaucratic Management Weber (1864)	Focuses on hierarchical superior-subordinate communication transmitted from top to bottom via a clear chain of command. Uses rational, impersonal management; distributes activities among personnel. Uses merit and skill as basis for promotion and/or reward. Uses rules and regulations; focuses on exacting work processes and technical competence. Limits personal freedom. Emphasizes career service, salaried managers.
Human Relations Argyris (1964), Barnard (1938), Likert (1967), McGregor (1960) Roethlisberger & Dickson (1939)	Focuses on empowerment of the individual worker as the source of control, motivation, and productivity in meeting the organization's goals. Emphasizes that participatory decision making increases worker autonomy and provides training to improve work. Studies at the Hawthorne Western Electric plant in Cicero, Illinois, led to the belief that human relations between workers and managers and among workers are the main determinants of efficiency. The Hawthorne effect refers to the phenomena of how being observed or studied results in a change in behavior.

Note. Compiled with information from Burns, L. R., Bradley, E. H., & Weiner, B. J. (2020). *Shortell & Kaluzny's health care management: Organization design and behavior.* 6th ed. Chapter 4: Motivating People). Boston, MA: Cengage Learning.

with clear superior-subordinate communication and relations, based on positional authority, in which orders from the top were transmitted down through the organization via a clear chain of command.

Human Relations Management

Management that focused on human relations began by examining employee responses to conditions through a series of studies called the Hawthorne experiments. In contrast to the science of exact procedures, rules and regulations, and formal authority that characterized Scientific Management, theories from the Human Relations Management school of thought espoused the individual worker as the source of control, motivation, and productivity in organizations. During the 1930s, labor unions became stronger and were instrumental in advocating for the human needs of employees. During this time, experiments were conducted at the Hawthorne plant of the Western Electric Company in Chicago that led to a greater understanding of the influence of human relations in organizations.

Electricity had become the preferred power source over gas; the Hawthorne plant experiments were run to show people that more light was necessary for greater productivity. This approach was designed to increase the use of electricity. Researchers Mayo (1933) and Roethlisberger and Dickson (1939) measured the effects on production of altering the intensity of lighting. They found that, with more and brighter light, production increased as expected. However, production also increased each time they reduced the light, even when the light was extremely dim. Their research findings led to the conclusion that something else besides the light was motivating these workers.

The notion of social facilitation, or the idea that people increase their work output in the presence of others, was a result of the Hawthorne experiments. The researchers also concluded that the effect of being watched and receiving special attention could alter a person's behavior. The phenomena of being observed or studied, resulting in changes in behavior, is now called the **Hawthorne Effect**. Also emerging from this study was the concept that people benefit and are more productive and satisfied when they participate in decisions about their work environments.

Motivation Theories

The human relations perspective in management theory grew from the conclusion that worker output was greater when the worker was treated humanely. This spawned a human relations point of view and a focus on the individual as a source of motivation. Motivation is not explicitly demonstrated by people but rather is interpreted from their behavior. **Motivation** is a source of influence for personal choices. Motivation is a process that occurs internally to influence and direct our behavior in order to satisfy needs (Lussier & Achua, 2015). Motivation theories are not management theories per se; however, they are frequently considered along with management theories.

There are many theories of motivation, e.g., Maslow's Hierarchy of Needs; Aldefer's **Expectancy-Relatedness-Growth (ERG) Theory** and Model of Growth Needs, Relatedness Needs, and Existence Needs; Herzberg's Two-Factor Theory; and McClelland's Theory and Model of Achievement, Power, and Affiliation. Table 1.5 discusses several of these Motivation Theories, including Maslow's Hierarchy of Needs, Herzberg's Two-Factor Theory, McGregor's Theory X and Theory Y, Ouchi's Theory Z, and Vroom's Expectancy Theory.

Maslow's Hierarchy of Needs

One of the most well-known theories of motivation is Maslow's Hierarchy of Needs. Maslow (1970) developed a Hierarchy of Needs that shows how an individual is motivated. Motivation, according to Maslow, begins when a need is not met. For example, when a person has a basic physiological need, such as thirst, this unmet need has to be satisfied before a person is motivated to pursue the next higher-level needs. Certain needs have to be satisfied first, beginning with basic physiological needs, then safety needs, then social belonging needs, then self-esteem needs, and finally self-actualization needs. After each level of these needs is met, an individual is motivated by needs at the next level. The need for self-actualization drives people to the pinnacle of performance and achievement.

Herzberg's Two-Factor Theory

Frederick Herzberg (1968) contributed to research on motivation and developed the Two-Factor Theory of Motivation. He analyzed the responses of accountants and engineers and concluded that there are two sets of factors associated with motivation. One set of motivation factors must be maintained to avoid job dissatisfaction. These factors include such items as salary, working conditions, status, quality of supervision, relationships with others, and so on. These factors have been labeled **Hygiene Maintenance Factors**.

Other **Motivation Factors**, such as achievement, recognition, responsibility, advancement, and so on, also contribute to job satisfaction. These factors are intrinsic and serve to satisfy or motivate people. Herzberg proposed that, when these Motivation Factors are present, people are very motivated and satisfied with their jobs. When these Motivation Factors are absent from a work setting, people have a neutral attitude about their organizations. In contrast, when the Hygiene Maintenance Factors are absent, people are dissatisfied. Herzberg believed that, by providing the Hygiene Maintenance Factors, job dissatisfaction could be avoided, but that Hygiene Maintenance Factors alone will not motivate people.

Table 1.5 Selected Motivation Theories

Motivation theories	Key aspects	Application to beginning nurse leader/manager
Hierarchy of needs Maslow	Motivation occurs when needs are not met. Certain needs have to be satisfied first. The hierarchy of needs starts with Physiological needs, then Safety and security needs, then Social needs, followed by Self-esteem needs. Then Self-actualization needs can be met. Needs at one level must be satisfied before one is motivated by needs at the next higher level.	A new graduate nurse understands that needs change, but if needs are unmet, then an individual may not be able to attend to the next higher level need until the lower level needs are met. A co-worker who does not feel safe from violence at work would not be able to fully engage in socializing until her safety and security needs were met.
Two-Factor Theory: Hygiene Maintenance Factors and Motivator Factors Herzberg	**Hygiene Maintenance Factors** can prevent *job dissatisfaction* or be a source of job dissatisfaction if absent. These include adequate salary, job security, quality of supervision, safe and tolerable working conditions, and relationships with others. These factors by themselves do not lead to job *satisfaction*. **Motivator Factors** do contribute to *job satisfaction* and include meaningful work, opportunities for development and advancement, responsibility and recognition.	New graduate nurses can consider salary, working conditions, and quality of supervision when applying and interviewing for a job, as these Hygiene Maintenance Factors are needed to avoid job dissatisfaction. Motivator Factors should also be evaluated when considering a job opportunity to ensure that there are adequate opportunities for responsibility, recognition, advancement, and support for achievement.
Theory X and Y McGregor	**The Theory X** view is that motivation results from leaders who direct and control their employees; the underlying notion is that people prefer security, direction, and minimal responsibility so that coercion and threats are necessary for people to do their work. In contrast, the **Theory Y** view is that people have self-control and discipline and enjoy/are motivated by involvement in work and creative opportunities. Leaders must remove work obstacles to enable involvement so that people can carry out their work.	Individuals working in a group or a team of diverse individuals might have different motivators. A nurse leader can adjust their leadership style to work both with **Theory Y** people who display self-control and discipline as well as to work with other **Theory X** people who prefer more direction, less responsibility, and more supervision.
Theory Z Ouchi	**The Theory Z** view is that collective decision making, long-term employment, being mentored, and working in quality circles to manage service and quality is a humanistic style of motivating workers; studied in Japanese organizations.	New graduate nurses can pursue opportunities to be involved in the organization if the aspects of Theory Z are desirable. A nurse can seek out a mentor and would want to have a leader who fosters employee involvement and quality circles.
Expectancy Theory Vroom	The equation of *Force = Valence (x) Expectancy* can help to predict an individual's motivation as negative, neutral, or positive. Force equals the amount of effort that will be exerted to reach a goal. Valence is the level of attractiveness or unattractiveness of the goal. Expectancy is the perception that the goal will be achieved.	One way to apply this theory when deciding what groups to become involved in is to identify if a group's motivation is negative, neutral, or positive that the goal will be achieved.

New graduate nurses can use Herzberg's Two-Factor Theory by evaluating the Hygiene Maintenance Factors present in health care organizations when they apply for jobs. The pay, working conditions, and the beginning relationship that has been established with a supervisor are aspects of a job that the nurse should consider. If these Hygiene Maintenance Factors are not adequate to begin with, then the nurse may become easily dissatisfied with the job. The higher-level needs that Herzberg describes as Motivation Factors should also be evaluated by the nurse before joining an organization. Are there opportunities for the nurse to achieve professional growth, to take on new responsibilities, to advance and be recognized for the contribution he has made?

It is important to recognize that not all employees respond to the same motivation factors. For example, a manager might be surprised to learn that some personnel will not respond to opportunities for autonomy and personal growth on the job. Rather, they may view their jobs as a means of providing income and seek various forms of personal fulfillment off-the-job through their families and leisure activities (Burns, Bradley & Weiner, 2020).

McGregor's THEORY X AND THEORY Y

Continuing the emphasis on factors that stimulate job satisfaction and what motivates people to be involved and contribute productively at work, McGregor capitalized on his experience as a psychologist and university president to develop Theory X and Theory Y (McGregor, 1960). Theory X and Theory Y identify two different views of how to motivate or influence others based on underlying attitudes about human nature. Each view reflects different attitudes about the nature of humans. **Theory X** identifies how, in bureaucratic organizations, employees prefer security, direction, and minimal responsibility. Coercion, threats, or punishment are necessary because people do not like the work to be done. These employees are not able to offer creative solutions to help the organizations advance.

The assumptions of **Theory Y** are that, in the context of the right conditions, people enjoy their work; can show self-control and discipline; are able to contribute creatively; and are motivated by ties to the group, the organization, and the work itself. In essence, this view espouses the belief that people are intrinsically motivated by their work. Theory Y was a guide for managers to take advantage of the potential of each person, which McGregor thought was being only partially utilized, and to provide support and encouragement to employees to do good work (McGregor, 1960).

OUCHI'S THEORY Z

Theory Z was developed by William Ouchi (1981) based on his years of study of organizations in Japan. He identified that Japanese organizations had better productivity than organizations in the United States and that they were managed differently with their use of quality circles to pursue better productivity and quality. Theory Z focuses on a better way of motivating people through their involvement. The organization invests in its employees and considers both home and work issues when creating a path for career development. Democratic leaders, who are skilled in interpersonal relations, foster employee involvement (Ouchi, 1981).

Vroom's Expectancy Theory

Vroom's Expectancy Theory of Motivation centers around what people want and their prospect of getting it (Vroom, 1964). There are three variables in Vroom's motivation theory. They are force, valence, and expectancy. Force describes the amount

Table 1.6   Common Employee Motivation Problems and Potential Solutions

Motivation problems	Potential solutions
1. Inadequate performance definition (i.e., lack of goals, inadequate job descriptions, inadequate performance standards, inadequate performance assessment)	1. Well-defined job descriptions ○ Goal setting ○ Well-defined performance standards ○ Clear feedback on performance ○ Improved employee selection ○ Job redesign or enrichment
2. Impediments to performance (i.e., bureaucratic or environmental obstacles, inadequate support or resources, poor employee-job matching, inadequate job information)	2. Enhanced Hygiene Maintenance Factors (i.e., safe and clean environment, good salary, future education reimbursement, fringe benefits, job security, good staffing, time off job, good equipment, pay for performance, clear job descriptions, good hiring practices,
3. Inadequate performance-reward linkages (i.e., inappropriate or inadequate job rewards, poor timing of rewards, low probability of receiving rewards, inequity in distribution of rewards)	3. Enhanced job achievement or growth rewards (i.e., increased employee involvement and participation, job redesign or enrichment, career planning, professional development opportunities) ○ Enhanced job esteem or power factors (i.e., job autonomy or personal control, self-management, modified work schedule, recognition, praise or awards, opportunity to display skills or talents, opportunity to mentor or train others, promotions in rank or position, clear information concerning organization or department, preferred work activities or projects, letters of recommendation, preferred work space) ○ Enhanced affiliation or relatedness factors (i.e., recognized work teams and task groups; opportunities to attend conferences, social activities, and professional nursing, hospital, and community committees and join a Board of Directors)

Source: Compiled with information from Burns, L. R., Bradley, E. H., & Weiner, B. J. (2020). *Shortell & Kaluzny's health care management: Organization design and behavior.* 6th ed. Chapter 4: Motivating People). Boston, MA: Cengage Learning. Bradley, E. H., & Weiner, B. J. (2020).

of effort one will exert to reach one's goal. Valence speaks to the level of attractiveness or unattractiveness of the goal. Valence is graded between +*1*, an outcome that is highly attractive to the individual, and −*1*, a highly unattractive goal. A valence of 0 indicates the goal does not interest the individual. Expectancy is the perceived possibility that the goal will be achieved. Expectancy is evaluated between *1 and 0*. A score of *1* indicates assurance that the goal will be achieved, and a score of *0* indicates that the individual sees the goal as impossible to achieve. Vroom's theory appears in the form of an equation as *Force = Valence × Expectancy*. Vroom proposes that this equation can help to predict the motivation of an individual to achieve a goal as negative, neutral, or positive based on the underlying notion that our expectations affect our motivation.

Motivation theories are useful because they help explain why people act the way they do and how a manager can relate to individuals as human beings and workers. When you are interested in creating change, influencing others, and managing patient care outcomes, it is helpful to understand the motivation that is reflected in a person's behavior. Motivation is a critical part of leadership because we need to understand each other to lead effectively. See Table 1.6 for common motivation problems and potential solutions.

KEY CONCEPTS

- Nurses are leaders and make a difference through their contributions of expert knowledge and leadership to patients and to health care organizations.

- Leadership development is a necessary component of preparation as a health care provider.

- All nurses are leaders because they have expert knowledge that they contribute to coordinate and provide patient care.

- Leadership is a process of influence that involves the leader, the follower, and their interaction. Followers can be individuals, groups of people, communities, and members of society in general.

- Leadership can be formal or informal. It can occur by being in a position of leadership and authority in an organization, such as a manager. Leadership can also occur outside the scope of a formal leadership role, such as when an individual or member of a group moves to assume leadership.

- Nurses are leaders. They lead nursing practice. Nurses lead other nurses, and they lead patients and communities toward improved health.

- Leadership styles are described as autocratic, democratic, and laissez-faire. They have been studied by examining job-centered or task-oriented leadership approaches versus employee-centered or relationship-oriented leadership approaches.

- Contingency theories of leadership acknowledge that other factors in the environment, in addition to the leader's behavior, affect the effectiveness of the leader. Variables that substitute for leadership eliminate the need for leadership or nullify the effect of the leader's behavior. Charismatic Leadership Theory describes leader behavior that displays self-confidence, passion, and communication of high expectations and confidence in others. These types of leaders often emerge in a crisis with a vision, have an appeal based on their personal power, and often use unconventional strategies and their emotional connections to succeed.

- Transformational leadership theory involves two styles of leadership: the transactional leader and the transformational leader. Transactional leaders focus on organizational operations and short-term goals. Transformational leaders inspire and motivate others to excel and participate in a vision that goes beyond self-interests. Transformational leadership is believed to empower followers and contribute to their commitment to action and change.

- Management is a process used to achieve organizational goals. Management roles are classified as the information-processing role, the interpersonal role, and the decision-making role. Managers use these roles to manage the work and to manage relationships with people to accomplish the work.

- The management process involves planning, coordinating, organizing, and controlling. The RN uses this process to manage patient care.

- Scientific Management, based on the work of Taylor and others, viewed industrial organizations as machines where work was to be carried out in the most scientifically exact and efficient way to increase production.

- Bureaucratic Theory discusses the idea of organizations as bureaucracies with a formal organizational structure, impersonal relations, a hierarchy based on positional authority, and a clear chain of command.

- Motivation is an internal process that contributes to behavior in an effort to satisfy needs. Maslow's Hierarchy of Needs reflects the belief that the needs that motivate individuals have a priority order. Lower-level needs have to be satisfied first or individuals will not be motivated to address higher-level needs.

- Herzberg's Two-Factor Theory of Motivation identifies hygiene maintenance factors, such as security and salary, that are needed to prevent job dissatisfaction, and motivator factors, such as job development and opportunities to advance, that contribute to job satisfaction.

- Vroom's Expectancy Theory focuses very simply yet specifically on the assessment of the desires of what people desire/expect and their prospect of getting it.

- Organizations need to be viewed as living, self-organizing systems where what initially looks like chaos and uncertainty is indeed part of a larger coherence and a natural order.

- Future directions for nurses in organizations will continue to be influenced by technology and by the notions of mobility, virtuality, and user-driven practices.

- Knowledge Workers, with specialized knowledge and expertise, are more self-directed. Future leadership practices need to adapt to knowledge workers and to changing work environments and circumstances.

- Nursing has transitioned to the knowledge age where nursing research advances nursing science, and nursing science is translated into evidence-based nursing practice.

KEY TERMS

Authentic leadership	Hygiene factors	Motivation factors
Autocratic leadership behavior	Informal leader	Position power
Complex adaptive systems	Initiating structure	Situational leadership
Complexity leadership	Job-centered leaders	Substitutes for leadership
Consideration	Knowledge workers	Task structure
Contingency theory	Laissez-faire leadership behavior	Theory X
Democratic leadership behavior	Leader-member relations	Theory Y
Emotional intelligence	Leadership	Theory Z
Employee-centered leadership	Hygiene maintenance factors management	Transformational leadership
Formal leadership	Management process	Transactional leader
Hawthorne effect	Motivation	Transformational leader

REVIEW QUESTIONS

1. Management is a process that is used today by nurses and nurse managers in health care organizations and is best described as which of the following?
   a. Scientific management.
   b. Decision making.
   c. Commanding and controlling others using hierarchical authority.
   d. Planning, organizing, coordinating, and controlling.

2. A participative leadership style is appropriate for employees who do which of the following?
   a. Are not able to get the task done and are less mature.
   b. Are able to contribute to decisions about getting the work done.
   c. Are unable and unwilling to participate.
   d. Need direction, structure, and authority.

3. When the concepts of Theory Y are used to describe nurses, which of the following statements are the best description?
   a. Nurses prefer to be directed and want job security more than other things.
   b. Nurses use self-direction and self-control to achieve work objectives in which they believe.
   c. Nurses have a hard time accepting responsibility, but they learn to do this over time.
   d. Nurses don't really want to work and would quit if they could.

4. Nurse retention is an important focus for health care organizations as we face a growing shortage of health care professionals in the future. According to Herzberg's motivation factors, which of the following would most likely contribute to increased job satisfaction?
   a. The organization recognizes and rewards those nurses who advance their education and achieve certification, such as the Critical Care Registered Nurse (CCRN) certification for critical care RNs.
   b. Hiring bonuses of up to $5,000 are given to nurses to reduce the vacant positions and prevent short-staffing.

   c. Nurse managers place an emphasis on establishing effective relationships with the nurses who work for them.
   d. Salary is increased.

5. The factors that are present which may serve as a substitute for leadership from your nurse manager include which of the following? Select all that apply
   a. Your desire for a promotion and an increase in pay.
   b. Professional nursing standards, code of ethics, and the intrinsic reward you get from this important work.
   c. Your manager spends time telling you exactly what to do and how to do it.
   d. Your nurse manager is inspiring and highly motivating to work for.

6. Leadership is defined as which of the following?
   a. Being in a leadership position with authority to exert control and power over subordinates.
   b. A process of interaction in which the leader influences others toward goal achievement.
   c. Being able to manage collaboration.
   d. Being self-confident and democratic.

7. The reason that leadership development is important for nurses, even if they are not in a management position, is which of the following?
   a. Nurses don't get education on leadership in nursing school.
   b. Nurses are knowledge workers with expert knowledge of patient care.
   c. Nurse leaders leave their jobs sooner for other positions.
   d. Nurses who lead are less satisfied in their jobs.

8. The motivation theory that allows the student to determine the probability of achieving one's goal is which of the following?
   a. Maslow's Hierarchy of Needs Theory
   b. Herzberg's Two-Factor Theory
   c. Vroom's Expectancy Theory
   d. Theory Y

9. Leadership characteristics are important for the nurse to master to assure effective management of patients? Which of the following are leadership characteristics? Select all that apply.
   a. Develop a professional and purposeful vision that provides direction toward the preferred future.
   b. Portray a passion that involves the ability to inspire and align people toward the goal.
   c. Display integrity that is based on knowledge of self, honesty, and maturity.
   d. Know your strengths and weaknesses.

10. Emotional intelligence is the capacity to interact with understanding and respect. Which of the following are basic social and emotional competencies? Select all that apply.
    a. Self-awareness
    b. Self-regulation
    c. Management
    d. Compassion
    e. Social skills

REVIEW QUESTION ANSWERS

1. Answer: D is correct.
   Rationale: The management process is defined as encompassing planning, organizing, coordinating, and controlling. While nurses and managers do use decision making (B) as a component of their work, decision making is not the best answer to describe the management process. Commanding and controlling others using hierarchical authority (C) is not a description of the management process. It is one way that managers have carried out their role in organizations (typically bureaucracies) where commanding is the style used to manage subordinates. While controlling is one aspect of the management process, it is not a complete answer.

2. Answer: B is correct
   Rationale: A participative leadership style engages people. To be effective using this style, employees need to be willing and have the ability to contribute. It is not the best style when employees are less mature (A) and/or unwilling (C). Nor is a participative style useful when employees need direction to understand the task and how to proceed, and when structure is needed (D).

3. Answer: B is correct
   Rationale: Theory Y is a description of people who can direct themselves, are motivated to achieve work objectives and have self-discipline. Theory X is a view of people who need direction and want job security (A). Neither Theory X or Theory Y focuses on accepting responsibility, thus answer (C) is not correct and (D) is too general a statement about nurses to accept that it is factual. Nor would this be an accurate description of Theory Y behaviors.

4. Answer: D is correct
   Rationale: Herzberg's theory explains motivation through two factors: hygiene maintenance factors and motivator factors. Motivator factors contribute to job satisfaction. These factors are achievement, recognition, responsibility, advancement, and they contribute to job satisfaction

5. Answer: B is correct.
   Rationale: Substitutes for leadership include standards and procedures that provide guidance, direction, and convey expectations.

6. Answer: B is correct.
   Rationale: Leadership is defined as influencing others toward goals and goal achievement. It also is fundamentally about relational aspects of interacting with other individuals and/or groups.

7. Answer: C is correct
   Rationale: Vroom's expectancy theory explains how to identify the likelihood or probability that a group will exert the effort to reach goals, that the goals are attractive or unattractive, and individuals see the goals as being possible to reach. Other theories do not use goals to explain motivation.

8. Answer: All answers are leadership characteristics. Selecting all is correct: A, B, C, and D.
   Rationale: Vision of a preferred future is a defining element of transformation leadership along with inspiring others and aligning them toward a goal. Additional characteristics that are necessary to be credible as a leader include honesty and maturity. Emotionally intelligent leaders acquire a knowledge of themselves that contributes to self-awareness and self-regulation and the ability to identify/assess strengths and weaknesses. Nurses as leaders need all of these characteristics to make decisions, act in emergencies, collaborate and advocate for patients, and influence care delivery.

9. Answer: A, B, and D are the correct answers. Motivation and empathy are not part of the definition of emotional intelligence.
   Rationale: The capacity to interact with understanding and respect involves the basic social and emotional competencies of self-awareness, self-regulation, and social skills. Motivation and empathy are not part of the definition of emotional intelligence.

10. Answer: A, B, and E are the correct answers. Management and compassion are not part of the definition of emotional intelligence.

REVIEW ACTIVITIES

1. Take the opportunity to learn about yourself by reflecting on five predominant factors identified as being influential in a nurse's leadership development: self-confidence, innate leader qualities or tendencies, progression of experiences and success, influence of significant others, and personal life factors. Consider which of these five factors reinforces your confidence in yourself. What innate qualities or tendencies do you have that contribute to your development as a leader? Consider what professional experiences, mentors, and personal experiences or events can help you influence and change nursing practice, when needed.

2. Describe the type of leader you want to be as a nurse in a health care organization. Identify specific behaviors you plan to use as

a leader. In what way does transformational leadership theory and complexity leadership theory inform your development as a leader?

3. Rate each of these 12 motivating or hygiene maintenance factors job factors that contribute to job satisfaction by placing a number from 1 to 5 on the line before each factor, with 5 being Very important, and 1 being Not important.

Very Important	Somewhat Important	Not Important		
5	4	3	2	1

_____ 1. An interesting job I enjoy doing

_____ 2. A good manager who treats people fairly

_____ 3. Getting praise and other recognition and appreciation for the work I do

_____ 4. A satisfying personal life

_____ 5. The opportunity for advancement

_____ 6. A prestigious or status job

_____ 7. Job responsibility that gives me freedom to do things my way

_____ 8. Good working conditions (safe environment, nice office, cafeteria)

_____ 9. The opportunity to learn new things

_____ 10. Sensible company rules, regulations, procedures, and policies

_____ 11. A job I can do well and succeed at

_____ 12. Job security and benefits

Write the number from 1 to 5 that you selected for each factor. Total each column for a score between 12 and 60 points. The closer to 60 your score is, the more important these factors (Motivating or Hygiene Maintenance Factors) are to you.

Motivating Factors	Hygiene Maintenance Factors
1._____	2._____
3._____	4._____
5._____	6._____
7._____	8._____
9._____	10._____
11._____	12._____
Totals _____	_____

Source: From. Lussier, R.N, and Achua, C.F. (2015) Leadership: Theory, Application, Skill Development Cincinnati, OH: South-Western College Publishing.)

1. What would a health care organization be like if it more closely resembled a self-organizing system and more holistic environment? How different would it be from a bureaucratic and more structured organization?

2. As nurses have become more self-directed, what kind of leadership practices are most effective?

3. What quality improvement projects are nurses in your work setting involved in? How is evidence being used to improve nursing practice? What sources of evidence from nursing science are you exploring through journals, attending educational conferences, the Internet, and participating in professional nursing associations?

DISCUSSION POINTS

• How can you use the characteristics, models, and theories presented in this chapter to recognize the leadership behaviors and styles of leading displayed by the nurses you work with such as your nurse manager, your charge nurse, and the most experienced nurses in your setting?

DISCUSSION OF OPENING SCENARIO

1. _What leadership characteristics did Maria demonstrate in preventing a nurse-sensitive outcome of cardiac arrest?'_

2. _Why is Maria considered a leader, even though she is not in a leadership or management position?_

• Consider the differences between management and leadership and begin to note when you observe managing functions and when you observe leadership.

• Why do you think it is important to learn about leadership as a nurse?

Maria is not in a formal leadership or management position, yet she is considered a leader because she is a Knowledge Worker and is educated with specialized knowledge and expertise. This positions Maria to lead not only herself as a professional but also to assume leadership in guiding patients and families toward the goal of health.

EXPLORING THE WEB

Search the Web, checking the following sites:

• American Association of Critical Care Nurse's Standards for Establishing and Sustaining Healthy Work Environments: www.aacn.org.

Under Priority Issues, click Healthy Work Environments. Accessed April 25, 2019. How does your unit or clinical site measure up to the standards?

- www.mindtools.com. Essential skills in leadership, management, and personal effectiveness to assist in building an excellent career. Accessed February 19, 2019. Take a leadership test and see how you measure up.

- American Organization of Nurse Executives Competencies: www.aone.org Click Resource Center and then click AONE Nurse Exec Competencies. Accessed December 3, 2019. What competencies surprised you?

- American Nurses Association Magnet Status Hospitals: www.nursecredentialing.org. Accessed March 4, 2019. Is your hospital

Magnet? If not, what improvements could be made to move in that direction?

- This site on classic management functions can keep you busy all week: http://www.1000ventures.com Review your character and personality and click on other areas of interest. Accessed April 5, 2019.

- Joanna Briggs Institute for Evidence Based Nursing: www.joannabriggs.edu.au Accessed February 18, 2019. Search for evidence in your area of interest.

INFORMATICS

1. Find the American Nurses Association Magnet Status Hospitals: www.nursecredentialing.org. Accessed February 19, 2019. Go to ANCC and then scroll down to Certification. Find and read the information on Certification in Informatics and Certification for Nurse Executives.

2. Find the **Institute for Healthcare Improvement (IHI)** web site at www.ihi.org. Accessed February 25, 2019. Go to online

learning and find the Leadership 101 course Introduction to Health Care Leadership. Register for a free account at IHI to explore the leadership lessons and consider all the relevant resources on this site.

3. Go to http://qsen.org Accessed April 1, 2019. Click on QSTUDENT and read, Leadership in Health Care.

LEAN BACK

- To what extent will using nursing leadership, management, and motivation concepts provide you with the knowledge to learn how to work with people and understand situations at work?

- How can the knowledge gained about nursing leadership enable you to advocate for patients and families?

- Leadership is about influencing others and leading change. Improving the way care is delivered is an ongoing challenge. How do effective leaders gain acceptance for needed changes?

REFERENCES

American Association of Critical Care Nurses. (2004). *AACN standards for establishing and sustaining healthy work environments: A journey to excellence*. Retrieved from www.aacn.org/WD/HWE/Docs/HWEStandards.pdf

American Nurses Association. (2020). ANA response to COVID-19 Pandemic. www.nursingworlld.org/ractice-policy/work environment/healthsafety/disasterpreparedness/coronavirus/ana-covid-19statement. Accessed April, 2, 2020.

Argyris, C. (1964). *Integrating the individual and the organization*. Hoboken, NJ: Wiley.

Barker, A. (1990). *Transformational nursing leadership: A vision for the future*. Baltimore: Williams & Wilkins.

Barnard, C. (1938). *The functions of the executive*. Boston, MA: Harvard University Press.

Bass, B. (1985). *Leadership and performance beyond expectations*. New York: Free Press.

Benner, P., Tanner, C., & Chesla, C. (2009). *Expertise in nursing practice: Caring, clinical judgment, and ethics* (2nd ed.). New York: Springer Publishing.

Bennis, W., & Nanus, B. (1985). *Leaders: The strategies for taking charge*. New York: Harper & Row.

Burns, L. R., Bradley, E. H., & Weiner, B. J. (2020). Chapter 4: Motivating People. In *Shortell & Kaluzny's health care management: Organization design and behavior* (7th ed.). Boston, MA: Cengage Learning.

Burns, J. M. (1978). *Leadership*. New York: Harper & Row.

Cassidy, V., & Koroll, C. (1998). Ethical aspects of transformational leadership. In E. Hein (Ed.), *Contemporary leadership behavior: Selected readings* (5th ed., pp. 79–82). Philadelphia, NJ: Lippincott.

Conger, J., & Kanungo, R. (1987). Toward a behavioral theory of charismatic leadership in organizational settings. *Academy of Management Review*, *12*, 637–647.

Daft, R. L., & Marcic, D. (2015). *Understanding management* (8th ed.). Cincinnati, OH: South-Western College Publications.

Drath, W. H., & Palus, C. J. (1994). *Making common sense: Leadership as meaning-making in a community of practice*. Retrieved from www.ccl.org/leadership/pdf/publications/readers/reader156ccl.pdf

Drucker, P. F. (1959). *The landmarks of tomorrow*. New York: Harper & Row.

Drucker, P. F. (1993). *Management tasks, responsibilities, practices*. New York: Harper Business.

Drucker, P. F. (2006). *The practice of management*. New York: Harper Business.

Dunham-Taylor, J. (2000). Nurse executive transformational leadership found in participative organizations. *Journal of Nursing Administration*, *30*(5), 241–250.

Fayol, H. (1917). *Administration industrielle et générale*. Paris: Dunod.

Fayol, H. (1916/1949). (C. Storrs, Trans.). *General and industrial management*. London: Pitman.

Fielder, F. (1967). *A theory of leadership effectiveness*. New York: McGraw-Hill.

Follet, M. (1924). *Creative experience*. London: Longmans, Green.

Goleman, D. (1998). *Working with emotional intelligence*. New York: Bantam Books.

Greenleaf, R. K. (1970/2008). *The servant as leader*. Westfield, IN: Greenleaf Center for Servant Leadership.

Griffin, R. W., & Moorhead, G. W. (2014). Organizational behavior: managing people and organizations. In *Leadership Models and Concepts*. Mason, OH: South-Western Cengage Learning.

Grossman, S. C., & Valiga, T. M. (2013). *The new leadership challenge: creating the future of nursing*. F.A Davis Company.

Gulick, L., & Urwick, L.. (Eds.). (1937). *Papers on the science of administration*. New York: Institute of Public Administration.

Helgesen, S. (1995). *The female advantage: womens ways of leadership*. New York: Doubleday Currency.

Herzberg, F. (1968). One more time: How do you motivate employees? *Harvard Business Review*, *46*(1), 53–62.

House, R. H. (1971). A path-goal theory of leader effectiveness. *Administrative Science Quarterly*, *16*, 321–338.

Katz, D., & Kahn, R. L. (1978). *The social psychology of organizations* (2nd ed.). New York: John Wiley.

Keith, K. M. (2016). *The contemporary servant as leader*. Atlanta, GA: The Greenleaf Center.

Kerr, S., & Jermier, J. (1978). Substitutes for leadership: Their meaning and measurement. *Organizational Behavior and Human Performance*, *22*, 374–403.

Kim, H., & Yukl, G. (1995). Relationships of self-reported and subordinate-reported leadership behaviors to managerial effectiveness and advancement. *Leadership Quarterly*, *6*, 361–377.

Kirkpatrick, S. A., & Locke, E. A. (1991). Leadership: Do traits matter? *The Executive*, *5*, 48–60.

Kotter, J. (1990a). *A force for change: How leadership differs from management*. Glencoe, IL: Free Press.

Kotter, J. (1990b). What leaders really do. *Harvard Business Review*, *68*, 104.

Kramer, M. (1990). The magnet hospitals: Excellence revisited. *Journal of Nursing Administration*, *20*(9), 35–44.

Kramer, M., & Schmalenberg, C. E. (2005). Best quality patient care: A historical perspective on magnet hospitals. *Nursing Administration Quarterly*, *29*(3), 275–287.

Leach, L. S. (2005). Nurse executive leadership and organizational commitment among nurses. *Journal of Nursing Administration*, *35*(5), 228–237.

Lewin, K. (1939). Field theory and experiment in social psychology: Concepts and methods. *Journal of Sociology*, *44*, 868–896.

Lewin, K., & Lippitt, R. (1938). An experimental approach to the study of autocracy and democracy: A preliminary note. *Sociometry*, *1*, 292–300.

Lewin, K., Lippitt, R., & White, R. (1939). Patterns of aggressive behavior in experimentally created social climates. *Journal of Social Psychology*, *10*, 271–299.

Likert, R. (1967). *The human organization: Its management and value*. New York: McGraw-Hill.

Lussier, R. N., & Achua, C. F. (2015). *Leadership: Theory, application, skill development*. Cincinnati, OH: South-Western College Publications.

Maslow, A. (1970). *Motivation and personality* (2nd ed.). New York: Harper & Row.

Maxwell, J. (1997). *Becoming a person of influence: How to positively impact the lives of others*. Nashville, TN: Thomas Nelson, Inc.

Mayo, E. (1933). *The human problems of an industrial civilization*. New York: Macmillan.

McCall, M. W., Jr. (1998). *High flyers: Developing the next generation of leaders*. Boston, MA: Harvard Business School Press.

McCall, M. W., Morrison, A. M., & Hannan, R. L. (1978). *Studies of managerial work: results and methods*. Greensboro, NC: Center for Creative Leadership.

McClure, M., & Hinshaw, A.. (Eds.). (2002). *Magnet hospitals revisited*. Washington, DC: American Nurses Publishing.

McClure, M., Poulin, M., Sovie, M., & Wandelt, M. (1983). *Magnet hospitals: Attraction and retention of professional nurses*. Kansas City, MO: American Nurses Association.

McDaniel, C., & Wolf, G. (1992). Transformational leadership in nursing service. *Journal of Nursing Administration*, *12*(4), 204–207.

McGregor, D. (1960). *The human side of enterprise*. New York: McGraw-Hill.

McNeese-Smith, D. (1997). The influences of manager behavior on nurses' job satisfaction, productivity, and commitment. *Journal of Nursing Administration*, *27*(9), 47–55.

Mintzberg, H. (1973). *The nature of managerial work*. New York: Harper & Row.

Mooney, J. D., & Reiley, A. C. (1939). *Principles of organization*. New York, NY: Harper & Row.

Murphy, M., & DeBack, V. (1991). Today's nursing leaders: Creating the vision. *Nursing Administration Quarterly*, *16*(1), 71–80.

National Academy of Medicine. (Ed.). (2003). *The Future of the Public Health in the 21st Century*. doi:10.17226/10548

Ouchi, W. (1981). *Theory Z: How American business can meet the Japanese challenge*. Reading, MA: Addison-Wesley.

Plowman, D. A., & Duchon, D. (2008). Dispelling the myths about leadership: From cybernetics to emergence. *Complexity Leadership*, 129–153.

Porter-O'Grady, T. (2001). Profound change: 21st century nursing. *Nursing Outlook*, *49*(4), 182–186. doi:10.1067/mno.2001.112789

Raso, R. (2019). Be you! Authentic leadership. *Nursing Management (Springhouse)*, *50*(5), 18–25. doi:10.1097/01.numa.0000557619.96942.50

Roethlisberger, J. F., & Dickson, W. J. (1939). *Management and the worker*. Cambridge, MA: Harvard University Press.

Schindler, A. (2015). *Ambidextrous Leadership - the role of opening and closing leadership behaviors for team innovative outcome in the case of management consultancies*. doi:10.13140/RG.2.1.1447.0560

Spears, L., & Lawrence, M.. (Eds.). (2004). *Practicing servant leadership: Succeeding through trust, bravery, and forgiveness*. Jossey-Bass.

Spence Laschinger, H., Finegan, J., & Wilk, P. (2009). Context matters: The impact of unit leadership and empowerment on nurses' organizational commitment. *The Journal of Nursing Administration*, *39*(5), 228–235.

Stodgill, R. M. (1948). Personal factors associated with leadership: A survey of the literature. *Journal of Psychology*, *25*, 35–71.

Stodgill, R. M. (1974). *Handbook of leadership: A survey of theory and research*. New York: Free Press.

Taylor, F. W. (1911). *The principles of scientific management*. New York: Harper & Brothers.

Taylor, F. W. (1947). *Scientific management*. New York: Harper and Brothers.

Tichy, N., & Devanna, D. (1986). *Transformational leadership*. New York: Wiley.

Vroom, V. (1964). *Work and motivation*. New York: Wiley.

Wheatley, M. J. (1999). *Leadership and the new science: Learning about organization from an orderly universe*. San Francisco: Berrett-Koehler Publishers.

Wolf, G., Boland, S., & Aukerman, M. (1994). A transformational model for the practice of professional nursing. Part 1. *Journal of Nursing Administration, 24*(4), 51–57.

Wong, C., & Cummings, G. (2007). The relationship between nursing leadership and patient outcomes: A systematic review. *Journal of Nursing Management, 15*, 508–521.

Wong, C., & Cummings, G. (2009). Authentic leadership: A new theory for nursing or back to basics. *Journal of Health Organization and Management, 23*(5), 522–538.

Young, S. (1992). Educational experiences of transformational nurse leaders. *Nursing Administration Quarterly, 17*(1), 25–33.

Yukl, G. (2006). *Leadership in organizations* (6th ed.). Upper Saddle River, NJ: Pearson-Prentice Hall.

Yukl, G. (2013). *Leadership in organizations* (8th ed.). New York: Pearson.

Yukl, G., Wall, S., & Lepsinger, R. (1990). Preliminary report on validation of the managerial practices survey. In K. E. Clarke & M. B. Clark (Eds.), *Measures of leadership* (pp. 223–238). West Orange, NJ: Leadership Library of America.

SUGGESTED READINGS

Aiken, L. H., Clarke, S. P., Sloane, D. M., Sochalski, J., & Silber, J. H. (2002). Hospital nurse staffing, patient mortality, nurse burnout, and job dissatisfaction. *Journal of American Medical Association, 288*(16), 1987–1993.

Akerjordet, K., & Severinsson, E. (2010). The state of the science of emotional intelligence related to nursing leadership: An integrative review. *Journal of Nursing Management, 18*(4), 363–382.

Alloubani, A., Akhu-Zaheya, L., Abdelhafiz, I. M., & Almatari, M. (2019). Leadership styles' influence on the quality of nursing care. *International Journal of Health Care Quality Assurance, 32*(6), 1022–1033.

American Association of Critical Care Nurses. (2003). *Written testimony to the IOM Committee on work environment of nurses and patient safety*. Retrieved from www.aacn.org

Amerson, R. (2010). The impact of service-learning on cultural competence. *Nursing Education Perspectives, 31*(1), 18–22.

Barkhordari-Sharifabad, M., & Mirjalili, N. S. (2019). Ethical leadership, nursing error and error reporting from the nurses' perspective. *Nursing Ethics, 27*(2), 609–620. 969733019858706

Bennis, W., Spreitzer, G. M., & Cummings, T. G. (2001). *The future of leadership*. San Francisco: Jossey-Bass.

Bergstedt, K., & Wei, H. (2020). Leadership strategies to promote frontline nursing staff engagement. *Nursing Management February, 51*(2), 48–53.

Bishop, V. (2010). Coalition in leadership. Politics the big picture and the big game. *Journal of Research in Nursing, 15*(4), 291–293.

Bittner, A. (2019). Mentoring millennials for nursing leadership. *Nursing, 49*(10), 53–56.

Blake, R. R., & Mouton, J. S. (1985). *The managerial grid III*. Houston, TX: Gulf.

Bodine, J. L. (2019). Preparing nurse leaders in nursing professional development: Association for Nursing Professional Development Leadership Academy. *Journal of Nurses Professional Development, 35*(6), 351–353.

Bolman, L., & Deal, T. (2003). *Reframing organizations: Artistry, choice, and leadership* (3rd ed.). San Francisco, CA: Jossey-Bass.

Brady, G., & Cummings, G. (2010). The influence of nursing leadership on nurse performance: A systematic literature review. *Journal of Nursing Management, 18*(4), 425–439.

Buresh, B., & Gordon, S. (2013). *From silence to voice: What nurses know and must communicate to the public (the culture and politics of health care work)* (3rd ed.). Ithaca, NY: ILR Press.

Burns, L., Bradley, E., & Weiner, B. (2019). *Shortell & Kaluzny's health care management: Organization design and behavior* (7th ed.). Clifton Park, NY: Cengage Learning.

Collins, E., Owen, P., Digan, J., & Dunn, F. (2019). Applying transformational leadership in nursing practice. *Nursing Standards*.

Covey, S. R. (2013). *The seven habits of highly effective people*. New York: Simon & Schuster.

Disch, J. (2019). Nursing leadership in policy formation. *Nursing Forum, 55*(1), 4–10. doi:10.1111/nuf.12375

Donley, R. (2005). *Reflecting on 30 years of nursing leadership: 1975–2005*. Indianapolis, IN: Sigma Theta Tau International.

Gallup P. (2019). Retrieved from https://news.gallup.com/poll/274673/nurses-continue-rate-highest-honesty-ethics.aspx

George, B. (2015). *True north: Discover your authentic leadership*. San Francisco, CA: Jossey-Bass.

Gilbreth, F. (1912). *Primer of scientific management*. New York: Van Nostrand.

Haddad, L. M., & Geiger, R. A. (2019). Nursing ethical considerations. In *StatPearls* [Internet]. Retrieved from www.ncbi.nlm.nih.gov/books/NBK526054

Hales, C. P. (1986). What managers do: A critical review of the evidence. *Journal of Management Studies, 23*, 88–115.

Hallock, A. B. (2019). A Case for leadership development in nursing practice. *Nephrology Nursing Journal, 46*(3), 325–328.

Hersey, P., & Blanchard, K. (2000). *Management of organizational behavior* (8th ed.). Englewood Cliffs, NJ: Prentice Hall.

Institute of Medicine. (2003). *Health professions education: A bridge to quality*. Washington, DC: The National Academies Press.

Joel, L. (2002). Education for entry into nursing practice: Revisited for the 21st century. *Online Journal of Issues in Nursing, 7*(2), Manuscript 4. Available at www.nursingworld.org/MainMenuCategories/ANAMarketplace/ANAPeriodicals/OJIN/TableofContents/Volume72002/No2May2002/EntryintoNursingPractice.aspx

Kelly, P., Vottero, B. A., & Christie-McCauliffe, C. (2018). *Introduction to quality and safety education for nurses* (2nd ed.: Core Competencies for Nursing Leadership and Management). New York: Springer Publishing.

Laschinger, H. K. S., Almost, J., & Tuer-Hodes, D. (2003). Workplace empowerment and magnet hospital characteristics: Making the link. *Journal of Nursing Administration, 33*(7/8), 410–422.

Leach, L. S. (2012). Leadership and management. In P. Kelly (Ed.), *Nursing Leadership & Management* (33rd ed.). Clifton Park, NY: Cengage Learning.

Machon, M., Cundy, D., & Case, H. (2019). Innovation in nursing leadership: A skill that can be learned. *Nursing Administration Quarterly, 43*(3), 267–273.

Miles, J. M., & Scott, E. S. (2018). A new leadership development model for nursing education. *Journal of Professional Nursing, 35*(1), 5–11.

Moore, J. (2004). Leadership: Lessons learned. In *Power point presentation to Indiana State University PhD educational leadership and foundation students*. Indianapolis: Indiana. Non published PowerPoint presentation

National League for Nursing. (2010). *Core values*. Retrieved from www.nln.org/about/core-values

Northouse, P. (2015). *Leadership: Theory and practice* (8th ed.). Thousand Oaks, CA: Sage Publishing.

Northouse, P. G. (2018). *Leadership: Theory and practice.* (8th ed.). Thousand Oaks, CA: Sage Publishing.

Plowman, D., & Lichtenstein, B. B. (2009). The leadership of emergence: A complex systems leadership theory of emergence at successive organizational levels. *Leadership Quarterly, 20*(4), 617–630.

Porter O'Grady, T. (2015). *Leadership in nursing practice: Changing the landscape of health care* (2nd ed.). Burlington, MA: Jones & Bartlett Learning.

Richardson, A., & Storr, J. (2010). Patient safety: A literature review on the impact of nursing empowerment, leadership and collaboration. *International Nursing Review, 57*(1), 12–21.

Salvage, J., & White, J. (2019). Nursing leadership and health policy: everybody's business. *International Nursing Review, 66*(2), 147–150.

Scott, J. G., Sochalski, J., & Aiken, L. (1999). Review of magnet hospital research: Findings and implications for professional nursing practice. *Journal of Nursing Administration, 29*(1), 9–19.

Taylor, F. (1911). *Principles of scientific management*. New York: Harper & Row.

Thusini, S., & Mingay, J. (2019). Models of leadership and their implications for nursing practice. *British Journal of Nursing, 28*(6), 356–360.

Tortorice, J. (2014). *Ten of the most influential nurses in history*. Available from https://ceufast.com/blog/ten-of-the-most-influential-nurses-in-history

Warshawsky, N. E. (2019). Nursing leadership: State of the science. *Journal of Nursing Administration, 49*(5), 229–230.

Weber, M. (1864), as reported in Mommsen, W. J. (1992)). *The political and social theory of Max Weber: Collected essays*. Chicago: University of Chicago Press.

Wheatley, M. J. (2005). *Finding our way: Leadership for an uncertain time*. San Francisco, CA: Berrett-Koehler Publishers.

The Health Care Environment

Ronda G. Hughes[1], Janice Tazbir[2, 3, 4, 5]

[1] Center for Nursing Leadership, Executive Doctorate of Nursing Practice, University of South Carolina, Columbia, SC, USA
[2] University of Chicago Medicine, Chicago, IL, USA
[3] Anderson Continuing Education, Sacramento, CA, USA
[4] Retired, Purdue University Northwest, College of Nursing, Hammond, IN, USA
[5] Health Education Systems, Inc. (HESI), Houston, TX, USA

2

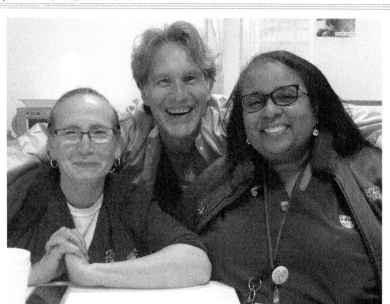

Nurses work together to provide high-quality care and to seek opportunities for improvement.
Source: Tish Watts, Johnny Tazbir & Venita Chew.

Health care in the twenty-first century will require a new kind of health professional: someone who is equipped to transcend the traditional doctor–patient relationship to reach a new level of partnership with patients; someone who can lead, manage, and work effectively in a team and organizational environment; someone who can practice safe, high-quality care but also constantly see and create the opportunities for improvement.

(Donaldson, 2001)

OBJECTIVES

Upon completion of this chapter, the reader should be able to:

1. Discuss how health care is organized and financed in the United States.

2. Compare U.S. health care with that of other industrialized countries.

3. Identify major issues facing health care.

4. Relate efforts for improving the quality, safety, and access to health care.

OPENING SCENARIO

Your neighbor calls, asking you to come over and advise her as to what to do with her grandchild who is sick. Finding the 3-year-old child with a runny nose, a slight fever, and a congested cough, you recommend that she take the child to her primary care clinician for an office visit, especially if the fever continues or rises, and if her symptoms seem worse. Your neighbor feels that there is no urgency because of the high cost of the office visit co-pay, her difficulty in getting the child to the clinician during the limited hours that don't coincide with her work schedule, and she can't get an appointment until 2 weeks later because her grandchild is covered by Medicaid. She opts to wait until

a couple of days later when she gets home from work and finds that her grandchild seems more fussy, and then takes the child to the emergency department (ED) where she will have no co-pay and can get seen right away. By the time they arrive at the hospital, the child has a temperature of 104°F (40°C) and is subsequently hospitalized for a week in the pediatric intensive care unit.

1. *Do you think this type of scenario is uncommon in the United States?*

2. *What are the advantages of everyone having access to health care regardless of type of insurance?*

The U.S. health care system consists of a mix of different types of health care providers from either nonprofit or for-profit organizations in both the public government and private sectors. These providers and organizations provide more than 300 million American citizens with access to cost-effective, quality health care. Reimbursement for health care services is paid in one or a combination of these four ways:

- Private insurers
- Public government-funded payers
- Charitable entities
- Out-of-pocket payment by patients and their families

Public government health care programs such as Medicare and Medicaid, **State Children's Health Insurance Program** (SCHIP), Department of Veterans Affairs, and other programs (e.g., for the military, **American Indians** (AI), and federal prisoners) provide health care services primarily funded through a percentage of dollars collected through Federal taxes. **National health care expenditures** (NHE) grew 3.9% to 3.5 trillion in 2017 and accounted for 17.9% of the **gross domestic product** (GDP) (NHE, 2019). Many Americans are surprised that the Federal Government already funds almost half of health care services, yet verbalize reluctance to move toward a government run health care program for all citizens.

This chapter discusses a selected history of American health care. It discusses health care in various settings, disease management, and the influence of external forces on health care. The chapter reviews how health care is organized, funded, and accredited. It explores health care disparities and clinical variation, and reviews reports of the **Institute of Medicine** (IOM) Committee on Health Care. Finally, the chapter discusses issues regarding quality health care and the education of health care professionals. **Patient Protection and Affordable Care Act** (PPACA) of 2010 and the **Health Care and Education Reconciliation Act** (HCERA) of 2010. We will explore how

health care is organized and financed in the United State, compare U.S. health care with that of other industrialized countries, identify major issues facing health care, and relate efforts for improving the quality, safety, and access to health care.

Most Americans are in good health, but many children, elderly, sick, and disabled are in need of better access to quality health care services at a reasonable cost. The need for accessible, high-quality, safe, and reasonable priced care has driven various initiatives to improve health care in the past and present. Some of the key initiatives include the 1935 passage of the Social Security Act; the 1946 passage of the Hill-Burton Act; and the 1965 passage of Medicare and Medicaid. The 2010 passage of both the PPACA and the HCERA was a recent attempt to improve health care access for the millions of Americans without health care coverage.

The U.S. spends 17.9% (an average of $10,224 per person) of its GDP on health care, more than any other wealthy country, all of whom provide health care insurance for all their citizens (Papanicolas, Woskie, & Jha, 2018). Many wealthy countries in the world spend less on health care, for example, Canada ($4.902), Germany ($5,728), Sweden ($5,511), and the United Kingdom ($4,246), yet provide **Universal Health Care** (UHC) to their citizens (Sawyer & Cox, 2018). In these countries, per capita spending on health care is considerably less than in the U.S., yet health care outcomes for such things as infant mortality, immunization rates, and life expectancy in the U.S. are poorer by comparison (Nolte & McKee, 2008). Perhaps Americans need to study what other countries have done in health care and modify it to fit. Throughout the history of the U.S., efforts to implement a UHC program have been resisted, with costly social and economic consequences.

To avoid the financial burden of health care costs, many Americans delay obtaining care. Their contact with the health care system is episodic and usually in acute care settings. Even after their symptoms have progressed and are well-advanced, many Americans are likely to obtain only irregular, sporadic care. This means that they lack consistent care from a health care provider whom they see regularly, whether for health promotion, illness prevention, early detection, or health restoration.

Inability to pay for recommended treatments and medications also compromises adherence to health care recommendations, which in turn affects recovery. Medical debt is now the number one reason for personal bankruptcy in the U.S. The majority of people declaring bankruptcy because of medical debt are employed and have health insurance (Himmelstein, Warren, Thorne, & Woolhandler, 2005). A cascading effect occurs for patients with soaring costs, high incidence of medical bankruptcy, progressively worsening health outcomes, and a high incidence of medical malpractice claims.

Spending on health care services is concentrated in disproportionate ways, which also adds to health care costs. For example, 90% of health care costs are on chronic conditions (Centers for Disease Control and Prevention (CDC), 2019). In 2016, half of all health spending was on 5% of the population. The 5% of people who spend the most on health care spend an average of around $50,000 annually; people in the top 1% have average spending of over $109,750. The 50% of the population with the lowest spending accounted for only 3% of all total health spending; the average spending was $276 (Sawyer, Claxton, & Kaiser, 2016).

The fight to achieve quality health care for all continues. Schulte (2011) recommends the development of evidence-based guidelines by the nursing and medical professional associations as one way to tackle the health care problem. Adherence to these guidelines then could be regularly monitored on electronic health records to note the outcomes, improve both patient care and evidence-based guidelines, and decrease the incidence of medical malpractice.

In 2010, 47 million uninsured people in the United States did not have health care insurance. This led to many discussions of rights to health care, access, fairness, sustainability, safety, quality, and discussions of the amount of money spent by the government on health care. The PPACA (Public Law 111–148) (Kaiser Family Foundation, 2010) was signed into law by President Barack Obama on March 23, 2010. Along with the HCERA of 2010 (Public Law 111–152), signed March 30, the Acts are a product of the health care reform efforts of the 111th Congress and the Obama administration (Office of the Legislative Counsel. 111th Congress, 2d Session. May, 2010). PPACA and HCERA required most U.S. citizens and legal residents to have health insurance and introduced many insurance market reforms over the next few years. They prohibited insurers from establishing annual insurance coverage caps and provide funds for medical research. They created a new insurance marketplace with state-based American Health Benefit Insurance Exchanges through which individuals can purchase insurance coverage, with premium- and cost-sharing credits available to individuals and families with income between 133% and 400% of the **federal poverty level** (FPL) (the poverty level was $18,310 for a family of three in 2009).

PPACA and HCERA created separate state Insurance Exchanges through which small businesses can purchase insurance coverage. They subsidized insurance premiums for people making up to 400% of the FPL ($88,000 for a family of four in 2010), so their maximum *out-of-pocket* payment for annual premiums will be from 2% to 9.8% of income, providing incentives for businesses to provide health care benefits, prohibiting denial of coverage and denial of claims based on pre-existing conditions, prohibiting insurers from establishing annual coverage caps, and giving support for medical research. The costs of these provisions are offset by a variety of taxes, fees, and cost-saving measures, such as new Medicare taxes for those in high-income brackets, taxes on indoor tanning, cuts to the Medicare Advantage program in favor of traditional Medicare, and fees on medical devices and pharmaceutical companies. There is also a tax penalty for those who do not obtain health insurance, unless they are exempt due to low income or other reasons. The Congressional Budget Office estimated that the net effect of both Acts will be a reduction in the federal deficit by $143 billion over the first decade.

PPACA included fundamental changes to Medicare, expansion of the Medicaid program, and reforms to Part D, closing the Medicare donut hole by 2020. It includes initiatives to prevent fraud and abuse; includes more health **information technology** (IT); and promotes disease prevention programs across the health care system. HCERA makes a number of health-related financing and revenue changes to the PPACA of 2010. HCERA is divided into two titles, one addressing health care reform and the other addressing student loan reform. It was anticipated that PPACA and HCERA would impact health care significantly, and it was estimated that the net effect of both PPACA and HCERA would be a reduction in the federal deficit by $143 billion over the first decade. A fast-forward of changes since the ACA was enacted (Collins, Bhupal, & Doty, 2019). Today, 45% of U.S. adults aged 19–64 are inadequately insured (almost the same as in 2010)

- Compared to 2010, many fewer adults are uninsured today.

- Despite actions by the Trump administration and Congress to weaken the ACA, the adult uninsured rate was 12.4% in 2018.

- More people who have coverage are underinsured now than in 2010.

History of Health Care

Florence Nightingale observed that noise, food, rest, light, fresh air, and cleanliness were instrumental in health and illness patterns. Thus, she maintained, the aim of nursing was to put the patient in the best condition for nature to act upon her or him (Nightingale, 1865/1970). Nightingale also discovered the link between adverse patient outcomes and a lack of cleanliness and hand washing. Yet generations after the insights of Nightingale were first set forth, sporadic adherence by health care providers to hand washing continues. Although significant progress has been made in preventing some health care-associated infection types, there is much more work to be done. On any given day, about one in 31 hospital patients has at least one health care-associated infection. Three percent of hospitalized patients in the 2015 survey had one or more HAIs. There were an estimated 687,000 HAIs in U.S. hospitals in 2015. About 72,000 hospital patients with HAIs died during their hospitalizations (CDC, 2018b).

One hundred years ago, illnesses such as tuberculosis or pneumonia required lengthy hospitalizations and were often catastrophic for individuals and families. Today, such illnesses are preventable and are often easily treated. Vaccination programs have been used extensively to prevent the spread of communicable diseases. Additionally, surgical interventions in hospitals (e.g., tonsillectomies, appendectomies, and reproductive procedures) have improved to treat otherwise debilitating or mortal conditions. Health care is delivered by professional nursing and medical practitioners who are science based and who use evidence-based practice. Health care is primarily directed at preventing and treating chronic and behavioral diseases. Health care advances have extended life expectancy, with the consequence of more elderly people requiring more health care for chronic and complex health problems. The majority of clinical care is still provided in hospitals, but length of stay is much shorter, and a variety of innovative models of care are now used to provide cost-effective care for people with acute, community, and long-term clinical needs (Health Workforce Solutions LLC & Robert Wood Johnson Foundation, 2008).

Health care-associated infections currently result in increased length of stay, mortality, and health care costs. In addition, a Centers for Disease Control and Prevention (CDC, 2018) report estimates that the overall annual direct medical costs of health care-associated infections in U.S. hospitals ranges from $28.4 to $33.8 billion. These infections are most often attributed to invasive supportive measures such as endotracheal intubation and the placement of intravascular lines and urinary catheters. Several studies have noted that health care-associated infections can be prevented through a number of multidisciplinary, evidence-based interventions, reducing the incidence of infection by as much as 70% (Anderson et al., 2007; Harbarth, & Gastmeir, 2003; Muto et al., 2005).

Structuring Hospitals Around Nursing Care

Nightingale also described the importance of structuring hospitals around nursing care. The initial design of hospitals followed that advice by building large wards where nurses could easily monitor and observe their patients. Later, hospital design evolved to placing patient rooms surrounding centrally located nursing stations. Then, as today, the physical environment of hospitals can create stress for patients, their families, and clinical staff. Research is finding links between the physical environment and patient outcomes, patient safety, and patient and staff satisfaction (Hamilton, 2003). Studies show that such elements of hospital design as exposure to natural light, private rooms, and facilities that are staff friendly and have less noise contribute to improved patient outcomes (Ulrich, Quan, Zimring, Joseph, & Choudhary, 2004).

Although little is known about how to best design the hospital environment to facilitate clinical advances and care delivery, an estimated $200 billion will be expended for new hospital construction across the United States during the next 10 years (Institute of Medicine (IOM), 2004a). The **Robert Wood Johnson Foundation** (RWJF), the nation's largest philanthropy devoted exclusively to health and health care, has provided funding to the Center for Health Design, a nonprofit research organization, for the Designing the twenty-first Century Hospital Project, which is the most extensive review of the evidence-based approach to hospital design ever conducted. Launched in 2000, the Pebble Project is a joint research effort between the Center for Health Design and health care providers. The project engages health care providers that are building new health care facilities or renovating old ones using an evidence-based design. The project uses the latest available evidence to inform design innovations and then measure the outcomes of the innovations through carefully designed research projects. The results are shared with the larger health care community to promote change. The Pebbles Project is an example of facility design to improve quality of care (The Center for Health Design, 2011).

Collecting Data

Nightingale also astutely recognized the importance of collecting and using data to assess the quality of health care. She employed coxcomb diagrams to present visual images of the number of preventable deaths during the Crimean war (Figure 2.1) and then later in London hospitals.

Today, data is collected through patient records, surveys, and administrative systems. From these, reports are developed, such as *To Err is Human* (IOM, 1999); the CDC National Vital Statistics Reports (Martin, Hamilton, Sutton, & Ventura, 2006); and The **National Healthcare Disparities Report** (NHDR) (**Agency for Healthcare Research and Quality** (AHRQ), 2005). These reports provide invaluable information, and data is displayed with charts and pictures to emphasize the successes and failures of health care throughout our nation. Evidence of significant disparities and low quality continue to demonstrate the need for significant health care improvement.

Influence of External Forces on Health Care

Recognizing the influence of external forces on care delivery and scope of practice, Nightingale also kept informed of the activities of practitioners and government policy makers (Dossey, Selanders, & Beck, 2005). With health care being the

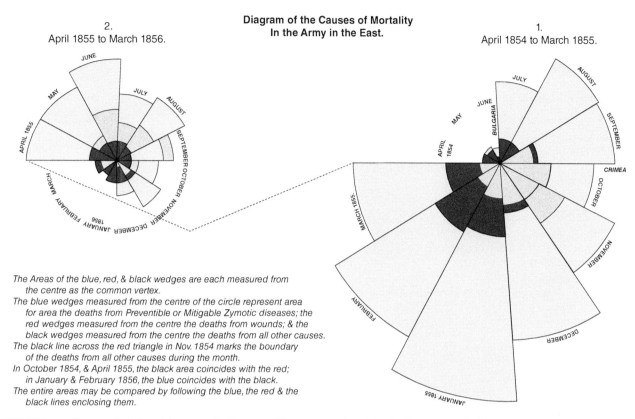

Diagram of the Causes of Mortality In the Army in the East.

2.
April 1855 to March 1856.

1.
April 1854 to March 1855.

The Areas of the blue, red, & black wedges are each measured from
   the centre as the common vertex.
The blue wedges measured from the centre of the circle represent area
   for area the deaths from Preventible or Mitigable Zymotic diseases; the
   red wedges measured from the centre the deaths from wounds; &the
   black wedges measured from the centre the deaths from all other causes.
The black line across the red triangle in Nov. 1854 marks the boundary
   of the deaths from all other causes during the month.
In October 1854, & April 1855, the black area coincides with the red;
   in January & February 1856, the blue coincides with the black.
The entire areas may be compared by following the blue, the red & the
   black lines enclosing them.

FIGURE 2.1   Florence Nightingale's coxcomb diagram of the causes of mortality in the army in the East.
Source: Florence Nightingale (1820–1910). [Public domain].

largest sector of our economy, employers, clinicians, managers, and patients all have vested interests in proposed changes to health care financing, organization, and the responsibilities and scope of practice for clinicians. Today, nursing leaders, managers, and staff need to be aware of and involved in the ongoing processes of making health policy.

Organization of Health Care

Health care systems have three main components: structure, process, and outcome. The **structure component of health** care includes resources or structures needed to deliver quality health care, for example, human and physical resources, such as nurses and nursing and medical practitioners, hospital buildings, medical records, and pharmaceuticals. The **process component of health** care includes the quality activities, procedures, tasks, and processes performed within the health care structures, such as hospital admissions, surgical operations, and nursing and medical care delivery following standards and guidelines to achieve quality outcomes. The **outcome component of health** care refers to the results of good care delivery achieved by using quality structures and quality processes and includes the achievement of outcomes such as patient satisfaction, good health and functional ability, and the absence of health care acquired infections and morbidity. See Table 2.1 for examples of structure, process, and outcome performance measures in clinical care, financial management, and human resources management. The

American Nurses Association's (ANA) Nursing Care Report Card for Acute Care (1995) also uses the structure, process, outcome framework for its indicators of quality.

It would be naïve to consider health care in the United States, as it is currently being delivered, as being an effective system of care. If that were true, it would imply that health care is based on shared values and goals; is organized around the patient; utilizes all pertinent information; ensures value-based and quality-based care; rewards quality care; is universally standardized and simplified; is available to everyone regardless of income, race, ethnicity, or education; is affordable; and reflects effective collaboration among clinicians and with patients. The **World Health Organization** (WHO) has put forth primary goals for what good health care should do: improve equity in health, reduce health risks, promote healthy lifestyles and settings, and respond to the underlying determinants of health (World Health Organization (WHO), 2019).

Consistent with these goals, Healthy People 2020 has also developed overarching goals to increase quality and years of healthy life and eliminate health disparities. These goals are:

- Attain high-quality, longer lives, free of preventable disease, disability, injury, and premature death.

- Achieve health equity, eliminate disparities, and improve the health of all groups.

Table 2.1 **Examples of Performance Measures by Category**

	Clinical care	Financial management	Human resources management
Structure	*Effectiveness* Percent of nurses and physicians who are certified JC (formerly JCAHO) accreditation Presence of council for quality improvement planning Presence of magnet recognition	*Effectiveness* Qualifications of administrators in finance department Use of preadmission criteria Presence of an integrated financial and clinical information system and clinical decision-making technology	*Effectiveness* Ability to attract desired nursing and medical practitioners and other health professionals Size or growth of nursing and medical staff Salary and benefits competitive with competitors Quality of in-house staff education
Process	*Effectiveness* Ratio of medication errors Ratio of nurse-sensitive complications Ratio of health care-acquired infection Ratio of postsurgical wound infection Ratio of normal tissue removed during surgery	*Effectiveness* Days in accounts receivable Use of generic drugs and drug formulary Market share Size (or growth) of shared service arrangements	*Effectiveness* Number and type of staff grievances Number of promotions Organizational climate
	Productivity Ratio of total patient days to total full-time equivalent (FTE) nurses Ratio of total admissions to total FTE staff Ratio of patient visits to total FTE nursing and medical practitioners	*Productivity* Ratio of collections to FTE financial staff Ratio of total admissions to FTE in finance department Ratio of new capital acquisitions to fund-raising staff	*Productivity* Ratio of front-line staff to managers
	Efficiency Average cost per admission Average cost per surgery	*Efficiency* Average cost per debt collection Debt/equity ratio	*Efficiency* Recruitment costs
Outcome	*Effectiveness* Case-severity-adjusted mortality Patient satisfaction Patient functional health status Number of deaths from medical errors	*Effectiveness* Return on assets Operating margins Size and growth of federal, state, and local grants for teaching and research Bond rating	*Effectiveness* Staff turnover rate Number of absenteeism days Staff satisfaction

Source: Compiled with information from Shortell, S. M., & Kaluzny, A. D. (2006). *Health care management* (5th ed.). Clifton Park, NY: Delmar Cengage Learning.

- Create social and physical environments that promote good health for all.

- Promote quality of life, healthy development, and healthy behaviors across all life stages (Healthy People 2020, 2010).

Health Care Rankings

Despite having the most expensive health care, the United States ranks last overall among the 11 countries on measures of health system equity, access, administrative efficiency, care delivery, and health care outcomes. While there is room for improvement in every country, the U.S. has the highest costs and lowest overall performance of the nations in the study, which included Australia, Canada, France, Germany, the Netherlands, New Zealand, Norway, Sweden, Switzerland, and the United Kingdom. The U.S. spent $9,364 per person on health care in 2016, compared to $4,094 in the U.K., which ranked first on performance overall (Commonwealth Fund, 2017). An overall score of 64% was recently given to the United States for its achievement across 42 core health indicators related to long, healthy, and productive lives; quality; access; efficiency; and equity of health care (Commonwealth Fund, 2012) (see Figure 2.2).

Real World Interview

What can be said about the United States health care system is that it is not really a system, but rather a hodge-podge of systems, some great, some not so great, with a "sometimes" desire for universal service, but with also the fierce energy of independent individuals seeking autonomy.

Ellyn Stecker, MD
Shipshewana, Indiana

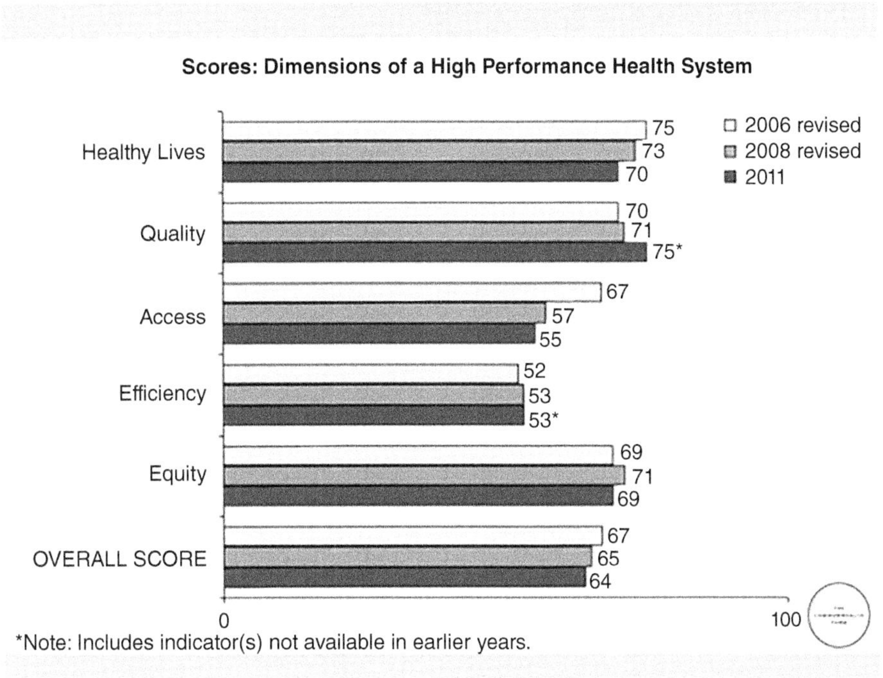

Scores: Dimensions of a High Performance Health System

*Note: Includes indicator(s) not available in earlier years.

FIGURE 2.2   U.S. scorecard on health system performance.
Source: The Commonwealth Fund. (2012, January 15). Scores Dimensions of a High Performance Health System. Retrieved from https://www.commonwealthfund.org/chart/scores-dimensions-high-performance-health-system.

Some major findings from the U.S. Scorecard include the following (Radley, Hayes, & Collins, 2019):

- Rising death rates, high levels of obesity, and gaps in care are pressing challenges for states

- The rise in deaths from suicide, alcohol, and drug overdose is a national crisis

- Regional differences in performance persist, as do within-state disparities

- Many states are not getting good value for their health care dollars

- States made progress in areas that were the target of efforts to improve

- Per capita spending growth in employer plans is outpacing that in Medicare

Access to Health Care for All

The United States is one of only a few large countries in the world without a universal system of health care. The U.S. has higher prices for most health care services and prescription drugs, according to available internationally comparable data. Meanwhile, utilization of several services, including physician consultations and hospital stays, is lower than in many comparable countries. Use of some services, such as C-sections and knee replacements, is higher in the U.S. than in similar countries (Sawyer, McDermott, & Kaiser, 2019). In the US we have

fewer office visits and shorter average hospital stays, yet the U.S. overall spends twice as much per person on health care than do comparable countries (Sawyer et al., 2019).

Health Care Payment in Other Countries

Note that some countries, such as Britain, New Zealand, and Cuba, provide health care in government hospitals, with the government paying the bills. Others (e.g., Canada and Taiwan) rely on private-sector providers, paid for by government-run insurance. Many other wealthy countries (e.g., Germany, the Netherlands, Japan, and Switzerland) provide universal coverage using private doctors, private hospitals, and private insurance plans. In some ways, health care is less *socialized* overseas than in the United States, where almost all Americans sign up for government Medicare insurance at age 65. In Germany, Switzerland, and the Netherlands, seniors stick with private insurance plans for life. Meanwhile, the U.S. Department of Veterans Affairs is one of the world's purest examples of government-run health care (Reid, 2009).

Hospital Care

The number of acute care hospital beds in the United States is 6,210 and in 2016, there were about 35.7 million hospital stays with a mean length of stay of 4.6 days and a mean cost of $11,700 per stay (AHA, 2019). From 1980 to 2015, the overall mortality rate in the United States fell by 29%, compared to

---

Critical Thinking 2.1

Think about how you could improve the delivery of health care delivery with limited funding and clinicians. Why are people in the United States not as healthy as they are in other countries? Health care that focuses on more delivery of prevention and primary care would increase health and decrease disease throughout the U.S. How can you work individually and with your community to begin to accomplish this?

Real World Interview

As a nurse practitioner, there are many things about the American health care system that I really value. There are minimal wait times and there are lots of specialties.

I like that a patient whom I refer with a serious diagnosis can be seen by a specialist within 2 weeks. We develop and make top-notch technology available and we have great health care standards. For all of these reasons, we keep the world on track and it follows our lead. I'm also aware every day of the shortcomings of the health care system. It's far too expensive, there are too many special interest groups, and it's all going to collapse under its own weight, a classic example of capitalism gone amuck. For example, health insurance companies have too much power, and I hate how all the insurance hoops prevent me and my colleagues from giving the best care to our patients. We need a national health policy, and if the American people make enough noise, politicians will get behind it, too. I'm in favor of a national health plan, one that will ensure that all Americans have access to care. It needs to be one that incorporates what we already do best with what's useful from other countries such as Japan and Canada. We have a lot to learn from what they do well that we don't do.

Nadine Lamoreau, RN, MSN, FNP, APRN-C
Fort Fairfield, Maine

---

a 54% decline in comparable countries. **Disability adjusted life years** (DALYs) are a measure of disease burden and the rate per 100,000 shows the total number of years lost to disability and premature death. Though DALYs have declined in the U.S. and comparable countries since 2000, the U.S. continues to have higher age-adjusted rates than those of comparable countries. In 2017, the DALYs rate was 31% higher in the U.S. than the comparable country average (Sawyer et al., 2019).

When you look at a group of 1,000 people, it is estimated that 800 of them will experience symptoms of some disease or condition. Of this group of 800, 265 people will be seen in a practitioner's office or hospital outpatient department or emergency department, or they will use home health care. Only eight will eventually be hospitalized. The majority of the people don't need hospitalization and would benefit from more resources available for primary health care delivery outside the hospital (Green, Gryer, Yawn, Lanier, & Dovery, 2000). This finding seems odd when considering where the research dollars are targeted and where the majority of health care dollars are devoted, that is, acute care settings in hospitals. Note that a consistent focus on illness and injury, often referred to as a downstream focus, means fewer dollars are invested in upstream efforts. A focus on upstream efforts would be directed at keeping the population well through health promotion and illness prevention strategies and would be less costly.

Need for Primary Health Care

The majority of patient care and health care occurs in communities outside acute care settings. Primary care "which provides integrated, accessible health care services by clinicians who are accountable for addressing a large majority of personal health care needs, developing a sustained partnership with patients, and practicing in the context of family and community" (IOM, 1996, p. 1), should be better understood and appreciated for the role it has in improving patient's health status and health outcomes. The key foundations of primary care (Starfield, 1998) can be applied across the health care continuum and across organizational settings, because **primary care** emphasizes seven important features: care that is continuous, comprehensive, coordinated, community oriented, family centered, culturally competent, and begun at first contact with the patient. According to Starfield (1998), patients and clinicians need to work together to appropriately utilize services, based on the following four foundations of primary care:

- *First Contact:* Conduct the initial evaluation and define the health dysfunction, treatment options, and health goals.

- *Longitudinality:* Sustain a patient–clinician relationship continuously over time, throughout the patient's illness, acute need, and disease management.

- *Comprehensiveness:* Manage the wide range of health care needs, across health care settings and among different health care professionals.

- *Coordination:* Build upon longitudinality. Care received through referrals and other providers is followed and integrated, averting unnecessary services and duplication of services.

Case Study 2.1

You work in an Emergency Department (ED) that sees 6,000 patients a month. Patients are charged at least $200.00 per visit plus charges for tests and medications. Thus, these 6,000 patients can generate $1,200,000 in gross revenue for the hospital. Consider that there are 15 RNs making $30.00 hr and 6 MDs, making $150.00 hr working each shift. Salaries for the RNs total $324,000. Salaries for the MDs total $648,000. The total salary for these two groups is $972,000. Of the 6,000 patients, 50% have Medicare/Medicaid, 45% are covered by managed care or insurance, and 5% have no insurance. Thus, just 95% of patients can pay their bills. The other 5% of patient's bills are written off by the hospital as bad debt.

Medicare/Medicaid/Managed Care/Insurance companies often pay only 55% of the bills for these patients. They may deny payment for 45% of the bills. Thus, for the $1,140,000 billed (95% of $1,200,000), the hospital will receive approximately $627,000 (55% of the $1,140,000 billed). Approximately $513,000 of the bill will not be paid by Medicare/Medicaid/Managed Care/Insurance. Consider the following:

What other expenses besides salary must the hospital pay out of the $627,000 that it receives? Consider hospital space, liability insurance, technology costs, and so on.

Notice the effect that increasing the volume of patients has on your budget figures. What happens to your budget if the patient volume goes to 8,000 patient ED visits per month and staffing stays the same?

Are patients receiving useful information about future illness prevention and healthy living practices in the ED?

Is this a cost-effective way to deliver health care?

How could we better serve the health care needs of Americans?

Primary care clinicians, which primarily include both medical and nursing practitioners, can be a patient's greatest asset in negotiating the health care system and improving patient outcomes. It is through understanding the patient's past and present that future health care needs can be anticipated. Primary care interventions, such as health promotion and timely preventive care and medication administration, can reduce the need for hospitalizations, improve the health of patients, and avert adverse morbidity and mortality outcomes. Patients and their families can communicate with clinicians to understand their health care needs, how to achieve the best possible health, and how to partner with clinicians to improve decision making. This is what patient-centered care is based on, both primary care and patient decision making. The World Health Report (2008b), *Primary Health Care: Now More than Ever*, underscores the need for primary health care. The report cites a disproportionate focus on specialist hospital care, fragmentation of health systems, and the proliferation of unregulated commercial care. The WHO (2010b) has also identified key elements in improving health status through primary care strategies aimed at reducing disparities through universal access, enhancing coordination and delivery of care, and increasing stakeholder participation at multiple levels.

The Federal Government

The federal government is a major driver of health care organization and delivery. Distinct, major divisions of the U.S. **Department of Health and Human Services** (DHHS) include the following:

- *Agency for Healthcare Research and Quality (AHRQ):* Funds health services research on the effectiveness of health care services and outcomes of care.

- *Centers for Disease Control and Prevention (CDC):* Promotes health and quality of life by preventing and controlling disease, injury, and disability.

- *Centers for Medicare and Medicaid Services (CMS):* Administers the Medicare program and regulates the Medicaid program.

- *Food and Drug Administration (FDA):* Monitors the safety of food, the safety of cosmetic products, the safety and efficacy of drugs, and the safety and efficacy of medical devices.

- *Health Resources and Services Administration (HRSA):* Administers training programs for health care clinicians, funding for pregnant women and children, programs for persons with HIV/AIDS, and programs serving low-income, underserved, and rural populations.

- *Indian Health Service (IHS):* Maintains health services provided to American Indians and Alaska Natives (ANs).

- *National Institutes of Health (NIH):* Funds biomedical research through 18 research institutes primarily organized according to specific diseases.

- *Substance Abuse and Mental Health Services Administration (SAMHSA):* Provides leadership in services, policy, and information dissemination for mental health and substance abuse treatment and prevention.

State and Local Levels

Public health services at the state and local levels include boards of health and state and local health departments. Even with the 1988 IOM Report on public health, the ability of public health departments to engage in improving the health of the public has become limited (Tilson & Berkowitz, 2006). In addition, efforts for bioterrorism and disaster preparedness have brought the nation's infrastructure desolation to light, causing increased funding for this nation's disaster preparedness efforts, with little money focused on public health care funding and infrastructure redevelopment.

Home Health Care

The location of care delivery is continually changing to adapt to technologies and patient needs. The use of home health care services continues to grow as more and more individuals access these services in the community setting, in lieu of institutional care. According to the Centers for Medicare and Medicaid Services (CMS) (2018), home health care expenditures were 3% of national health care expenditures in 2017, of the overall spending of having reached $3.5 trillion. This increase has been primarily driven by higher growth in Medicaid spending, partly due to Medicaid's continued shifting of long-term care from institutional to home settings. In light of an aging population, home health care services will continue to serve an integral role in health care delivery.

Health Care Disparities and Social Determinants of Health

Inequalities in such things as gender, age, ethnicity, etc. (Figure 2.3) have been recognized as great influences on health outcomes. Socioeconomic status is the number one predictor of poor health. The 2018 NHDR found from 2000 to 2017 (AHRQ, 2019):

- More than half of access measures showed improvement.
- One-third of access measures did not show improvement.
- Fourteen percent showed worsening.
- Blacks, American Indians and Alaska Natives (AI/ANs), and **Native Hawaiians/Pacific Islanders** (NHPIs) received worse care than Whites for about 40% of quality measures.

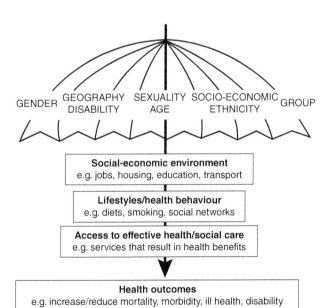

FIGURE 2.3   The spectrum of inequality.
Source: https://www.nationalarchives.gov.uk/doc/open-government-licence/version/3/ Contains Parliamentary information licensed under the Open Parliament Licence v3.0

- Hispanics received worse care than Whites for about 35% of quality measures.
- Asians received worse care than Whites for 27% of quality measures, but better care than Whites for 28% of quality measures

The report also noted, even when the overall quality of care improves, health care disparities often still persist across socioeconomic groups, racial and ethnic populations, and geographical areas (AHRQ, 2019). In addition, not enough health care delivery and attention is directed toward the top underlying causes of death in the United States (Table 2.2).

Quality of health care improved overall from 2000 through 2016–2017, but the pace of improvement varied by priority, which are (AHRQ, 2019):

Person-Centered Care: Almost 70% of measures were improving.

Patient Safety: More than 60% of measures were improving.

Healthy Living: Almost 60% of measures were improving.

Effective Treatment: Almost half of measures were improving.

Care Coordination: One-third of measures were improving.

Care Affordability: No care affordability measures changed.

Overalls, as one ages, more health care services are utilized; women use health care services more frequently than men; and whites have greater health care access, and therefore higher utilization rates, than do patients of color as reported by the National Healthcare Disparities Report (NHDR), 2018; (AHRQ, 2019). Both financial and nonfinancial barriers to care delivery result in lack of attention to health care disparities and factors contributing to the underlying causes of death, which affects health outcomes. In-depth information on national health care disparities is reported in the annual National Health Disparities Report (AHRQ, 2019).

For example, disparities in infant morbidity and mortality, cardiovascular and pulmonary disease, diabetes, communicable disease, cancer, and disease prevention (i.e., immunization and health screening) are more likely to be experienced by people disadvantaged by poverty, age, skin color, or ability to speak English. Such differences are further aggravated by miscommunication and misunderstanding, stereotyping, discrimination, and prejudice between patients and providers. Lifestyle behaviors that contribute to illness are higher among vulnerable groups. Because of their financial difficulties and other difficulties in accessing the health care system, vulnerable people often postpone health care. They are more likely to use the acute care system when their illness symptoms are advanced. Use of emergency departments and other acute care facilities for treatment is the most expensive way to obtain health care. In countries with a national health care system, health disparities also exist, but virtually everyone in those countries, regardless of socioeconomic background, is assured

Table 2.2 Top 10 Actual Causes of Death in the United States in 2000

1. Tobacco	4. Alcohol	7. Motor vehicle crashes	9. Sexual behaviors
2. Poor diet	5. Microbial agents	8. Firearms	10. Illicit drug use
3. Physical inactivity	6. Toxic agents		

Source: CDC. "FastStats - Deaths and Mortality." *Centers for Disease Control and Prevention,* Centers for Disease Control and Prevention, 21 June 2019, www.cdc. gov/nchs/fastats/deaths.htm.

of equal access to quality health care. Health care is associated with 10–20% of the modifiable contributors to healthy patient outcomes (Magnan, 2017). The other 80–90% are dependent on health behaviors (e.g., tobacco use, diet/exercise, and alcohol use), social/economic factors (e.g., education, income, and employment), and the individual's physical environment (e.g., air quality, housing, and transit) (Magnan, 2017). These "social determinants" are so important when it comes to health that they have been called the "causes of causes."

Social determinants of health (SDOH) include access to health care, culture, language, education/literacy, access to transportation, crime rates, and safe housing. Research studies indicate that SDOH do matter and can have a significant impact on a population's health (CDC, 2018).

Health Care Spending

In the United States, health insurance has been generally employment-based, so long as it is affordable for the employer to offer this health care coverage to employees. The higher one's income in this country, the greater the likelihood of having health insurance coverage. The opposite is true for those with low incomes, especially those with poverty-level incomes. Patients who are at poverty levels often cannot afford insurance premiums nor can they afford, in the majority of instances, out-of-pocket health care costs. Since the inception of private health insurance in the late 1920s following the development of hospitals as the *center* of health care and subsequent rising health care costs (Starr, 1983), private health insurance from third-party payers such as insurance companies has been generally voluntarily offered as a benefit to employees and sometimes their families. Patients may make payments to providers of health care and third-party payers. Providers of health care deliver service to patients and bill third-party payers. Third-party payers may make payments to providers as direct payment fees for individuals, capitated payment for services for a group of patients, or as prospective payments for future patients. Health insurance distributes health care funds from the healthy to the sick (Figure 2.4).

Medicare and Other Health Care Costs

One reason proposed for the steady incline in health care costs is that the elderly have virtually UHC coverage through Medicare. This UHC coverage indicates that the United States will likely experience very rapid growth in overall health

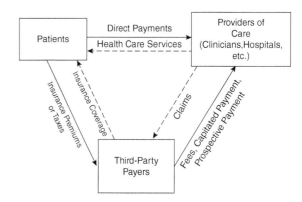

FIGURE 2.4 Economic relationships in the health care delivery system.
Source: Adapted from "What Can Americans Learn from Europeans?" by U. E. Reinhardt, 1989, Health Care Financing Review [Supplement], pp. 97–103.

expenditures in the coming years, as the population continues to age. Other sources of health care funding, and where it went, are shown in Figures 2.5 and 2.6.

Health Care Insurance

In the United States, health care insurance is one of the most significant factors in facilitating access to health care services. Recently, the number of people covered by insurance as well as the breadth and depth of health insurance coverage has decreased. According to data from the Kaiser Family Foundation-Health Research and Educational Trust Annual Employer Survey (2018), the average yearly costs for employer-sponsored health insurance in 2018 are $6,896 for single coverage and $19,616 for family coverage. The average single premium increased by 3% and the average family premium increased by 5% in the last year. Workers' wages increased by 2.6% and inflation increased by 2.5% over the past year. The average insurance premium for family coverage has increased by 20% since 2013 and by 55% since 2008.

In the past, American health insurance companies have routinely rejected applicants with a *preexisting condition.* The insurance companies often denied claims. If a customer was hit by a truck and faced big medical bills, the insurance company dug through the records looking for grounds to cancel the policy, often while the victim was still in the hospital (Reid, 2009). Foreign health insurance companies, in contrast, must accept all applicants, and they can't cancel insurance as long as premiums are paid. Everyone is mandated to buy

THE NATION'S HEALTH DOLLAR ($3.5 TRILLION), CALENDAR YEAR 2017:
WHERE IT CAME FROM

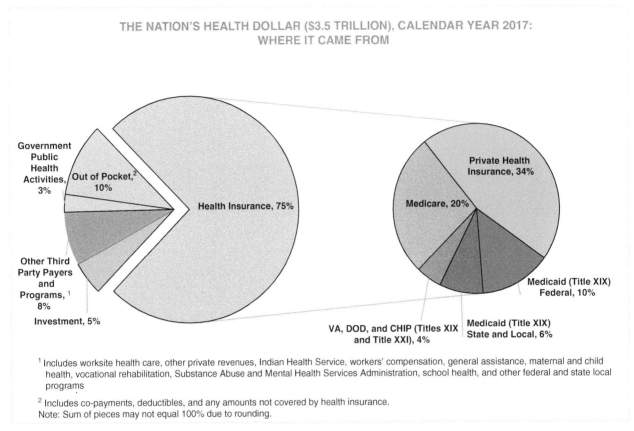

¹ Includes worksite health care, other private revenues, Indian Health Service, workers' compensation, general assistance, maternal and child health, vocational rehabilitation, Substance Abuse and Mental Health Services Administration, school health, and other federal and state local programs

² Includes co-payments, deductibles, and any amounts not covered by health insurance.
Note: Sum of pieces may not equal 100% due to rounding.

FIGURE 2.5 The nation's health dollar, calendar year 2017 where it came from. Centers for Medicaid and Medicare (CMS), Office of the Actuary, National Health Statistics
Source: Centres for Medicaid and Medicare (CMS), Office of the Actuary, National Health Statistics Group.

insurance to give the plans an adequate pool of rate payers. The key difference is that foreign health insurance plans exist only to pay people's medical bills, not to make a profit. ***The United States is the only developed country that lets insurance companies profit from basic health coverage***. In many ways, foreign health care models are not really *foreign* to America, because our health care system uses elements of

all of them. In Britain, the government provides health care, funding it through general taxes, and patients get no bills. In Germany, premiums are split between workers and employers, and private insurance plans pay private doctors and hospitals. In Canada; everyone pays premiums for an insurance plan run by the government, and the public plan pays private doctors and hospitals according to a set fee schedule. In the world's

Real World Interview

I was admitted to the hospital in December for what was later diagnosed as angina. After being stabilized in the emergency room, I was admitted to the cardiac care unit. A series of tests were ordered by my cardiologist to determine enzyme levels in my blood. This would show if I had suffered a heart attack. Blood was drawn every 8 hr for 24 hr. The news was good—no heart attack—until I received the bill. My insurance company said the enzyme tests for angina were frivolous and not necessary, and they would not pay. I had my cardiologist write a letter of explanation, saying the tests he ordered were routine for determining a diagnosis. After this second appeal, the insurance company rejected my payment claim again. After several more appeals, my

insurance company ultimately paid the laboratory bill for these tests but would not pay the pathologist for his interpretation of the blood tests. It has now been six months since I received my initial bill, and the hospital and pathologist's office have turned my case over to a collection agency. They did not take into consideration the fact that I was appealing the bill. They wanted me to pay upfront and then appeal. That was not going to happen.

Kathleen A. Milch
Patient
Whiting, Indiana

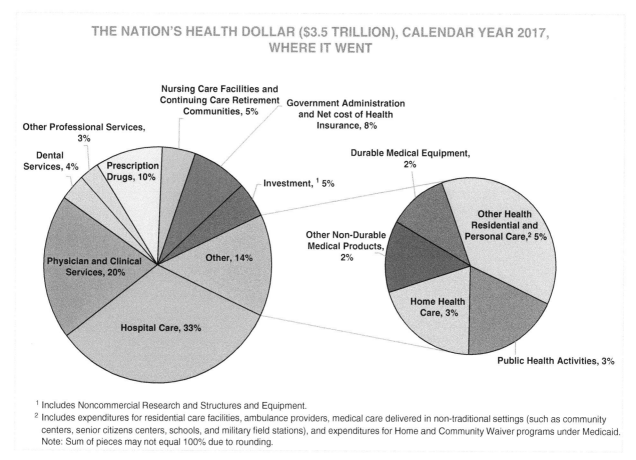

THE NATION'S HEALTH DOLLAR ($3.5 TRILLION), CALENDAR YEAR 2017, WHERE IT WENT

Nursing Care Facilities and Continuing Care Retirement Communities, 5%

Government Administration and Net cost of Health Insurance, 8%

Other Professional Services, 3%

Dental Services, 4%

Prescription Drugs, 10%

Durable Medical Equipment, 2%

Investment, [1] 5%

Other Health Residential and Personal Care,[2] 5%

Other Non-Durable Medical Products, 2%

Physician and Clinical Services, 20%

Other, 14%

Home Health Care, 3%

Hospital Care, 33%

Public Health Activities, 3%

[1] Includes Noncommercial Research and Structures and Equipment.

[2] Includes expenditures for residential care facilities, ambulance providers, medical care delivered in non-traditional settings (such as community centers, senior citizens centers, schools, and military field stations), and expenditures for Home and Community Waiver programs under Medicaid. Note: Sum of pieces may not equal 100% due to rounding.

FIGURE 2.6 The nation's health dollar, calendar year 2017, where it went to.
Source: Centers for Medicare and Medicaid Services, Office of the Actuary, National Health Statistics Group.

poor nation, sick people pay out of pocket for medical care; those who can't pay, stay sick or die. Seven hundred thousand Americans are forced into bankruptcy each year because of medical bills. In France, the number of medical bankruptcies is zero; Britain, zero; Japan, zero; and Germany, zero (Reid, 2009).

Canadians have their choice of health care providers. In Austria and Germany, if a doctor diagnoses a person as *stressed*, medical insurance pays for weekends at a health spa. Canada does make patients wait weeks or months for nonemergency care, as a way to keep costs down. But studies by the Commonwealth Fund and others report that many nations—Germany, Britain, Austria—outperform the United States on measures such as waiting times for appointments and for elective surgeries (Reid, 2009).

Many gaps have existed in insurance programs in the United States, including incomplete health care coverage, need for copayments and deductibles, lack of provider choice, need for preauthorization, and other difficulties in maneuvering through the insurance company requirements. **Copayments** are a fixed health care fee paid by the patient to the health care

provider at the time of service; this amount is paid in addition to the money the health care provider will receive from the insurance company. **Deductibles** are a predetermined out-of-pocket fee paid by a patient for health care services before reimbursement through health insurance begins to be paid. For example, if an insurance plan has a $50 copayment and a $1,000 deductible, the patient is responsible for paying the $50 at each health care visit plus paying the first $1,000 of health care costs, after which costs will be reimbursed as allowed by the patients' health insurance plan. Preauthorization requires that approval be obtained from the insurance company before care or treatment, such as hospitalization or diagnostic testing, is initiated if such services are to be reimbursed by the patients' health insurance plan.

Medicare and Medicaid

Because the United States does not have a national/UHC program, public health care programs are intended to help fill the gap. Beginning in 1965 under Titles XVIII (Medicare) and XIX (Medicaid) of the Social Security Act, eligibility for public insurance has been based on age (Medicare for those age 65 and older) or based on having a low income and/or having a disability (Medicaid). Medicare and Medicaid programs ensure access to many needed services for patients. Medicare is the largest federal program. Medicare Part A is an insurance plan for hospital, hospice, home health, and skilled nursing care that is paid through Social Security taxes. Nursing home care that is mainly custodial is not covered. Medicare Part B is an optional insurance that covers physician services, medical equipment, and diagnostic tests. Part B is funded through federal taxes and monthly premiums paid by the recipients. Part D is optional coverage for outpatient medications.

Medicaid, a state program financed by federal and state funds, pays for services provided to persons who are medically indigent, blind, or disabled and to children with disabilities. The federal government pays between 50% and 83% of total Medicaid costs based on the per capita income of the state. Services funded by Medicaid vary from state to state but must include services provided by hospitals, physicians, laboratories, radiology, prenatal and preventive care, and nursing home and home health care services.

Other Public Programs

Other large public insurance programs are associated with American Indian and Alaska Native heritage, and the Military Services, that is, veteran's health and insurance for active military personnel and their families. The IHS, under the U.S. DHSS, provides health services to American Indians and Alaska natives enrolled in more than 500 tribes, villages, and pueblos (U.S. Department of Health and Human Services, 2010). The Indian Self-Determination Act of 1975 gave many tribal organizations the responsibility for the provision of health care services. IHS maintains some hospitals and clinics, yet recent legislation has severely cut funding for these sites of care.

The **Department of Defense** (DOD) finances and manages TRICARE, the triple option benefit care plan available for military families, formerly called the **Civilian Health and Medical Program of the Uniformed Services** (CHAMPUS), for enlisted military personnel and their military dependents as well as for retirees and their dependents and survivors. The Department of Veterans Affairs, established in 1921,

finances and manages the Veterans Health Administration (VHA). This program is available for U.S. veterans if they need any medical, prescription, surgical, and rehabilitation care services.

State Regulation of Health Insurance

Three key pieces of federal legislation set forth national standards that the individual states use to regulate health insurance. First, the **Employee Retirement Income Security Act** (ERISA) of 1974 provides a framework for states to regulate health insurers. Second, the **Consolidated Omnibus Budget Reconciliation Act** (COBRA) of 1985 ensures that employees who resigned, were laid off, were terminated, or lost their jobs due to family-related reasons, can retain their health insurance coverage for up to 18 months and, in some cases, up to a maximum of 36 months if they are deemed qualified and pay the full premiums. A third piece of legislation, the **Health Insurance Portability and Accountability Act** (HIPAA) of 1996, imposed restrictions on limitations and exclusions of insurance coverage for those with preexisting conditions and restricted other attempts to exclude employees from insurance coverage. It also provides protection of insurance coverage as employees change employers, and it provides tax exclusions for medical savings accounts.

International Perspective

To the extent that the United States is similar economically and socio-politically to countries such as France, Canada, and Japan, an examination of the health systems in those countries is useful. The differences in health care spending in the United States as compared to other countries as a percent of GDP are graphically displayed in Figure 2.7 (Table 2.3).

The UK is rated as number one (and spends 9.6% of its GDP on health care), followed respectively by Australia (10.3%), the Netherlands (10.1%), New Zealand (9.0%), Norway (10.4%), Sweden (10.9%), Switzerland (12.3%), Germany (11.3%), Canada (10.4%), France (11.3%), and trailing at 11th with 17.2% of the GDP spent on health care, the United States Papanicolas (2018). The U.S. ranks last overall on health care outcomes. Compared to other countries, the U.S. comes in last on infant mortality, life expectancy at age 60, and deaths that

---

Critical Thinking 2.2

You work in a large health care system. One of your patients is not following his health care regime. You wonder what thought processes this patient is using to justify continuing an activity that presents risk to his health.

How can you best assist the patient in your health care system and community? What kinds of structures, processes, and

outcomes will your system want to develop to improve care to this patient and the population of patients that your system serves? How could you work in the community to enhance the population's choices for diet, exercise, or lifestyle?

SPENDING & COSTS

Health Care Spending per Capita by Source of Funding, 2017

Adjusted for Differences in Cost of Living
Dollars ($US)

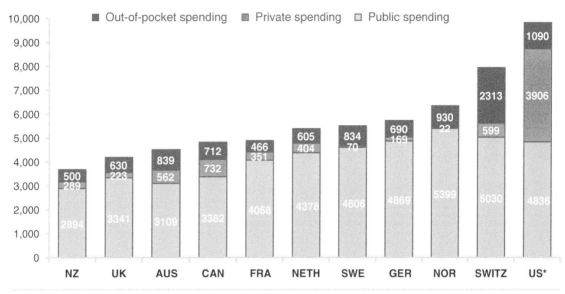

FIGURE 2.7   International health care spending per capita by source of funding. Tikkanen, 2018.
Source: Tikkanen, R. (2018). Multinational Comparisons of Health Systems Data, 2018. Retrieved October 6, 2019, from https://www.commonwealthfund.org/sites/default/files/2018-12/Multinational Comparisons of Health Systems Data 2018_RTikkanen_final.pdf.. (Commonwealth, 2017)

Table 2.3 HIPAA Privacy Regulations

- Allows patient to review and request amendments to their medical records
- Gives consumers control over how their personal health information is used and limits the release of information without a patient's consent
- Restricts the amount of patient information shared between physicians and other caregivers to the *minimum necessary*
- Requires privacy-conscious business practices, such as hiring a privacy officer and training employees about patient confidentiality
- Requires that paper records and oral communications be protected from privacy breaches.

Source: Compiled with information from U.S. Department of Health & Human Services. (1996). Summary of the Health Insurance Portability and Accountability Act (HIPAA) Privacy Rule, available at www.hhs.gov/ocr/privacy

were potentially preventable with timely access to effective health care Papanicolas (2018).

France

France, ranked as having the tenth best health care system in the world, spends 11.3% of its GDP on health care Papanicolas, (2018). This is almost one-half of what the United States spends on health care per person. Comprehensive health care is guaranteed for all citizens and legal residents in France. Similar to the United States, health care in France is provided

through private and government insurance. Unlike Canada and Britain, there are no lengthy wait times in France. Unlike the United States, everyone is insured in France, and there are no additional patient charges for health insurance plan deductibles (Shapiro, 2008). Employed residents are covered by a national health insurance plan, referred to as *Sécurité sociale*, which includes spouses and children. Another plan, *couverture maladie universelle* (CMU), provides coverage for those people who do not qualify for the *sécurité sociale* program, and is free to some people whose income is below a certain level. The national health insurance plan is funded through private and public means, with employees paying up to 21% of their incomes to the national health care system and employers making similar contributions. By comparison, Americans pay fewer taxes but pay more for health care (e.g., through paying health insurance premiums and other out-of-pocket expenses not covered by their insurance plans). In France, costs are dependent upon the type of provider seen; for example, a general practitioner is less expensive than a specialist. Likewise, it is more expensive to seek treatment at night, on the weekend, or on public holidays. Hospital care is reimbursed through the national health plan, and a percentage of the cost of prescription drugs is also reimbursed to the patient. Essentially, the sicker a person is, the more coverage is allowed, including for expensive drugs and experimental cancer treatments. Reducing cost and improving efficiency are the challenges for this system. Waste, such as *doctor shopping*, whereby a patient seeks treatment from more than one health care provider for the same ailment, and overuse of prescription drugs, are partly responsible for high health care costs in France (National Coalition on Health Care (NCHC), 2008; Shapiro, 2008).

Canada

Annually, the Canadian government spends 10% of its GDP on its national health care system Papanicolas, (2018). The Canadian health care system is administered by each Canadian provincial or territorial government. Seventy percent of health spending is publicly funded through federal and provincial taxation of individuals and corporations, and the remaining 30% is paid through private and out-of-pocket sources for additional services such as prescription medications or dental and vision care (Canadian Institute for Health Information (CIHI), 2006). All Canadians have equal access to the same quality and quantity of health care. Under the Canada Health Act of 1984, comprehensive health care is publicly administered, portable between provinces, and accessible to all. Primary care is provided by physicians and nurse practitioners, who may work in private clinics or public institutions. These health care providers are reimbursed on a fee-for-service basis, which allows them to be reimbursed by each provincial or territorial health plan for each health care service rendered to a patient.

Unlike the privatized health care system in the United States, extra billing, deductibles, and copayments are not allowed. The health care provider bills the provincial or territorial health plan and is reimbursed with an agreed-upon amount for each health service given. No additional charges or costs can be billed to or recovered from the patient. With only one insurance payer, referred to as a single-payer system, many of the problems embedded within the American health care system are eliminated. The problem currently facing the Canadian health care system is the lengthy wait times to access family practitioners, specialists, emergency room services, diagnostic tests, and surgical procedures (NCHC, 2008). To help remedy this issue, Canada has established benchmarks for treatment and waiting times. 2018 data for the Canadian

Institute for Health Information reveals that the Canadian benchmark for hip replacement is 182 days and they are currently at 75% compliance with the benchmark. In the U.S., patients cannot imagine a "standard" wait time of 6 months to have a hip replacement. With more life threatening issues such as a hip fracture, their benchmark for a hip fracture repair speeds up to 48 hr and they are at an impressive 88% compliance with the benchmark (Canadian Institute for Health Information, 2018). This illustrates that wait times in Canada are circumvented based on the gravity of a patient's condition, but this solution aggravates the waiting time for less urgent cases. In a geographically vast country with a small population compared to the United States, some Canadians in rural or isolated locales often travel long distances to obtain specialized services (Canadian Institute for Health Information, 2018).

As an example of the comprehensiveness and affordability of the Canadian health care service, a 51-year-old Canadian nurse working in the United States recently returned with her spouse and 15-year-old child to her home province of Alberta for 1 year. During that time, the family enrolled in the Alberta Health Care Insurance Plan for a cost of $88 per month (Alberta Health and Wellness, 2004). Health care for the nurse included an annual physical examination, lab tests, mammogram, bone density testing, and a routine colonoscopy. The colonoscopy required a 5-month wait. Her husband underwent elective day surgery, which was booked 7 months in advance. Her daughter was immunized at school, and she was once treated at a community health center for a persistent respiratory infection. Beyond payment of their monthly premium, the family was issued no bills for the health care they received.

Japan

To pay for its national health care system, Japan spends 10.2% of its GDP on health care Papanicolas, (2018). This is less than France, Canada, or the United States, and Japan enjoys the longest life expectancy of all 83.98 years as of 2016 (World Bank, 2018). The government regulates close to all aspects of health care in Japan. The Universal **Statutory Health Insurance System** (SHIS) requires by law that the national and local governments provide efficient, quality medical care Papanicolas, (2018). Citizens are mandated to enroll in one of the SHIS plans based on age, employment status, or place of residence. Non-citizens, immigrants, and visitors are not covered. The majority of the Japan has some form of private health insurance, only as a supplementary or complementary role.

All SHIS plans provide the same benefits package that is decided by the government. The package covers hospital, primary, specialty, and mental health care, approved prescription drugs, home care services by medical institutions, hospice care, physiotherapy, and most dental care Papanicolas, (2018). Plan participants have to pay a 30% coinsurance for services and goods received and there are zero deductibles. In 2013, out-of-pocket payments for cost-sharing accounted for 13% of current health expenditures Papanicolas, (2018).

The Japanese health care system provides comprehensive care and is one of the most advanced in the world. Physicians and hospitals are predominantly run as private businesses, and costs for care are reimbursed through the national health care system. Patients' health care costs are reimbursed at a fixed amount determined by the government. Refusal of coverage by insurers is impossible, and personal medical debt is nonexistent.

Factors contributing to lower health care costs in Japan include healthier diets and lifestyles, with a lower incidence of chronic diseases. Reimbursement rates for health care services are low, but reimbursement strategies for quantity rather than quality of services erodes the advantage a healthier lifestyle might have in terms of curbing costs. Despite cost containment efforts, health care expenses are increasing, especially with the earthquakes of 2011. A shortage of physicians also means the wait time to access the health system is an issue. With an aging population and shrinking workforce, concerns as to how access, affordability, and quality will continue in the future are being voiced (National Coalition Health Care, 2008; Reid, 2009).

The Rising Cost of Health Care

Health care costs are measured as part of the U.S. GDP. The **GDP** is an economic measure of a country's national income and output within a year and reflects the market value of goods and services produced within the country. The GDP is used as a barometer of the national economy. Health care costs in the U.S. were increased by 3.9% percentage points in 2017 (CMS, 2018). Employer-based health care premiums have doubled since 2000, yet those who are insured incur greater financial burdens as they pay for more out-of-pocket expenses.

U.S. national health care expenditures were $3.5 trillion in 2017 (CMS, 2018). Health spending totaled $74.6 billion in 1970. In 2000, health expenditures had increased to about $1.4 trillion, and in 2017 the amount spent on health had more than doubled to $3.5 trillion (CMS, 2018). Health care spending continues to increase faster than the overall U.S. economy and analysts project this number to keep rising.

Factors Contributing to Rising Health Care Costs

There are many factors contributing to the rising costs of health care. The five key factors include population growth, population aging, disease prevalence or incidence, service utilization, and service price and intensity (Dieleman, 2017). Between 1996 and 2013, inflation-adjusted spending on inpatient, ambulatory, retail pharmaceutical, nursing facility, emergency department, and dental care increased at 3.5% annually, from $1.2 trillion to $2.1 trillion (Dieleman, 2017). The areas with the highest increases were in emergency departments (6.4%) and on medications (5.6%). Diabetes as a whole had the greatest increase in cost at an annual rate of 6.1–7.0%, translating into $57.9–$70.6 billion (Dieleman, 2017). Back

and neck pain had the second-largest increase in spending, at an annual rate of 6.5% (or $57.2 billion) between 1996 and 2013. During the same time frame, the treatment of hypertension rose to $47.6 billion, the treatment of hyperlipidemia to $41.9 billion, and depressive disorders to $30.8 billion annually (Dieleman, 2017).

Aging Population

More and more baby boomers are turning 65, and the average life expectancy is increasing, with the elderly are becoming the largest group in the population. The U.S. Census Bureau (2019) reports:

* The number of Americans ages 65 and older is projected to nearly double from 52 million in 2018 to 95 million by 2060.

* The older population is becoming more racially and ethnically diverse.

* Older adults are working longer. By 2018, 24% of men and about 16% of women aged 65 and older were in the labor force.

* Obesity rates among adults aged 60 and older have been increasing, standing at about 41% in 2015–2016.

* Wide economic disparities are evident across different population subgroups. Among adults aged 65 and older, 17% of Latinos and 19% of African Americans lived in poverty in 2017—more than twice the rate among older non-Hispanic whites (7%).

* More older adults are divorced compared with previous generations. The share of divorced women aged 65 and older increased from 3% in 1980 to 14% in 2018, and for men from 4% to 11% during the same period.

* The aging of the baby boom generation could fuel more than a 50% increase in the number of Americans aged 65 and older requiring nursing home care, to about 1.9 million in 2030 from 1.2 million in 2017.

* The number of Americans living with Alzheimer's disease, could more than double by 2050 to 13.8 million, from 5.8 million today.

Increased Utilization of Pharmaceuticals

The CMS (2019) published a National Health Expenditures Report 2018–2027. Prescription drug spending was projected to have grown by 3.3% in 2018. This is due to an increase in new drug introductions. Prescription drug spending growth was projected to increase to 4.6% in 2019, because of faster utilization growth from both existing and new drugs, as well as a modest increase in drug price growth. For the reminder of the projection, 2020–2027, prescription drug spending is projected to grow by 6.1% per year on average, or by 1.5 percentage points more rapidly than in 2019, influenced by new drugs and efforts to encourage patients with chronic conditions to consistently treat their disease (CMS, 2019).

Technological Advances

Although technological advances have helped with earlier diagnoses and better treatment of disease, factors such as the greater availability of new technology drive per capita expenditures higher (Boddenheimer, 2005b). Treatment for the five most expensive health conditions include septicemia, osteoarthritis, complications of device, implant or graft, newborn care, and acute myocardial infarction (AHA, 2019). These require the use of expensive medications and technologies. While use of some technologies such as electronic record keeping may reduce costs, the presumed success of sophisticated drugs and technologies shapes consumer expectations of what the health care system can deliver (Woo, Ranji, Lundy, & Chen, 2007). Health care consumers, including both patients and providers, also contribute to the cost of health care. These consumers' demands for intense services, despite the lack of definite clinical need, strains health care spending. Mikulic (2019) reports that the number of **magnetic resonance imaging** (MRI) machines per million population is 37.56 in the U.S., 34.49 in Germany, 29.08 in Korea, and 28.4 in Italy. Yet the United States lags behind these same countries with respect to patient care outcomes (Commonwelth Fund, 2006).

The United States is home to groundbreaking medical research, but so are other countries with much lower cost structures. Any American who has had a hip or knee replacement is standing on French innovation. Deep-brain stimulation to treat depression is a Canadian breakthrough. Many of the wonder drugs promoted endlessly on American television, including Viagra, come from British, Swiss, or Japanese labs. Overseas, strict cost controls actually drive innovation. Under the pressure of cost controls, Japanese researchers found ways to perform the same diagnostic technique for one-fifteenth of the American price and still make a profit (Reid, 2009).

Rising Hospital Costs

A large proportion of health care dollars are devoted to hospital care. The Hill-Burton Act of 1946 funded the development of the nation's infrastructure of hospitals. Today, there are 6,210 hospitals nationwide (AHA, 2019). As technology and scientific knowledge grow and patients live longer, there has been a greater severity of illness in the hospitalized population. Hospital services contribute to the rise in health care costs due to the increased utilization of expensive technologies, high labor costs, the shortage of nurses, rising malpractice premiums, and increased costs of hospitalization. Given the aging hospital infrastructure and increases in hospital reimbursements, future building of new hospital beds will also increase health care costs (Bazzoli, Gerland, & May, 2006) (Table 2.4).

Practitioner Availability and Behavior

Defensive medicine and the high cost of medical malpractice insurance all add to increasing physician costs. Malpractice claims in the United States are filed 50% more often than in Great Britain and 350% more often than in Canada (Anderson, Hussey, Frogner, & Waters, 2005). Two-thirds of claims in the

Table 2.4   Cost of Selected Medications

Drug and doses cost	
Accutane	$1,182.04
Acyclovir-90	$53.33
Ampicillin	$39.30
Demser	$20,197.11
Epipen	$388.14
Lipitor-90	$127.16
Lasix-40	$11.55
Lorazepam-90	$24.03
Norco	$114.85
Simponi	$5,453.81

Source: GoodRx. (2019). Prescription Prices, Coupons & Pharmacy Information. Retrieved from www.goodrx.com. October 5, 2019.

United States are dropped, which results in a similar distribution of claim settlements among these countries. Regardless, the need for medical malpractice insurance to protect American physicians against such claims contributes to the cost of physician care. There are many calls for malpractice reform.

The U.S. has less fewer doctors, especially psychiatrists per capita in the U.S. than there are in most comparably wealthy countries and the U.S. has a similar number of nurses per capita (Sawyer, Sroczynski, & Kaiser, 2016). This shortage is most pronounced in certain practice specialties, for example, family practice physicians and geriatric physicians. Physician shortages are also apparent in rural areas. U.S. physicians earn more than physicians in most countries. A physician specialist who makes $300,000 in the U.S or a family physician whose income is $175,000 per year in the U.S. would, on average, earn approximately 25–50% less in Canada (Eisenberg, 2006) (Table 2.5).

Physicians can be extremely persuasive in health care and hospitals as they advise patients where to go for treatment. The physician represents the primary source of patients for most hospitals. A physician affiliated with two or three hospitals can steer patients toward any of those hospitals. This power over admissions is one of the most important forces in the hospital. Physician control over admissions also affects nursing home admissions, home care agency patient referrals, and referrals to other physician specialists.

Cost Shifting

The popular practice of **cost shifting**, whereby health care providers raise prices for the privately insured to offset the lower health care payments from both Medicare and Medicaid as well as the often nonpayment of health care premiums from the uninsured, continues to raise the cost of health care. Medicare and Medicaid payments are less than 50% of what private insurers pay. Health care providers shift charges for health care costs to the private insurance sector. Some estimates of

Table 2.5 Health Care Compensation

	Annual salary
Allergan CEO Brent Saunders	$6,624,473
GlaxoSmithKline CEO Emma Walmsley	$7,662,210
UnitedHealth Group CEO David Wichmann	$18,107,356
Cigna CEO David Cordani	$18,944,045
CVS Health CEO Larry Merlo	$21,953,040
Chief Executive Officer (CEO)–Non-MD	$158,193
Chief Executive Officer (CEO)–MD	$275,123
Director of Human Resources	$96,388
Medical Director	$222,229
Director of Nursing	$84,922
Nurse Practitioner	$93,281
Physical Therapist	$70,568
Cardiologist	$254,945
Anesthesiologist	$291,631
General Surgeon	$270,741
Family Medicine MD	$182,882
Emergency Care MD	$220,642

Source: Salary Comparison, Salary Survey, Search Wages. (2019). Retrieved October 5, 2019, from www.payscale.com and Ramsey, L. (2019, May 16). Health care CEOs make as much as $26 million a year. Here's what the industry's top executives earned in 2018. Retrieved from www.businessinsider.com/pharma-and-healthcare-ceo-compensation-2018-2019-4.

the cost shift are being valued at $6 billion annually. Cost shifting increases the cost of all health care. The health care facility or the health care professional shifts the cost of health care to other patients with health insurance or to those patients who can afford to pay. Costs to the public for these programs continue to increase. Almost two-thirds of all Medicaid spending for services goes to the elderly and those with disabilities. The elderly and those with disabilities made up less than one-quarter of all Medicaid enrollees as of 2014 (Rudowitz, Orgera, &

Hinton, 2019). Dual eligible beneficiaries alone account for almost 40% of all spending, mostly for long-term care. The 5% of Medicaid beneficiaries with the highest costs drive more than half of all Medicaid spending (Rudowitz et al., 2019). The high costs are due to their needs, acute care, long-term care, or often both. Higher costs for prescription drugs, long-term services and supports, and behavioral health services, as well as state policy decisions to implement targeted provider rate increases, have been recently cited as factors putting upward pressure on Medicaid spending (Rudowitz et al., 2019).

Administrative Costs

According to Boddenheimer (2005a), the cost of administration of U.S. health care in 1999 was 24% of the nation's health care expenditures. In an attempt to reduce these costs, providers such as practitioners' offices, clinics, hospitals, and so on, have invested in Information Technology (IT). IT has played a role in improving quality through availability of the electronic medical record, aiding with HIPAA compliance, and streamlining insurance coding and billing services. Because of the increased demand for such systems, the administrative cost of implementation has also gone up.

It may seem to Americans that U.S.-style free enterprise (i.e., private-sector, for-profit health insurance) is naturally the most cost-effective way to pay for health care. But, in fact, many other countries' payment systems are more efficient than ours. U.S. health insurance companies have the highest administrative costs in the world. The CMS (2019) estimates project that $496 billion will be spent on administrative costs in the U.S. alone. Himmelstein (2014) reports that administrative costs account for about one-fourth of the US hospital spending and this is more than spent in Canada (12%), England (16%), and the Netherlands (20%). Interestingly, Himmelstein found that there is no apparent link between higher administrative costs and better quality care (2014).

U.S. hospital administrative costs rose from 23.5% of total hospital costs ($97.8 billion) in 2000 to 25.3% ($215.4 billion) in 2011. During that period, the hospital administration share of national GDP rose from 0.98% to 1.43%. Canada spends

Real World Interview

Several years ago, I went to the hospital with excruciating pain. They admitted me to the hospital, and I had tests and X-rays for 9 days before they found the cause. I had cancer in my left kidney, and I needed immediate surgery. I had the surgery and was discharged on my 18th hospital day. Thank heaven, I was now cancer free.

The hospital bill for this stay was $18,689.20. The radiologist and surgeon submitted additional bills. I was glad that I had Medicare and Blue Cross insurance, which paid it all. The only charge I had to pay was $25.00 per day for a private room. When I looked

at the hospital bill, there were many charges for medications and treatments I never received. There were even charges for the day after I was discharged. I wonder how the hospital makes out the bill. I also wonder how people with no insurance pay these kinds of hospital bills.

Leona McGuan
Patient
Schererville, Indiana

0.41% of their GDP on health care administrative costs. The rising spending on administrative costs need to be addressed at every level and corporate greed addressed.

Other Factors Contributing to Rising Health Care Costs

Americans could narrow the life-expectancy gap between the United States and other countries by adopting a healthier lifestyle. It is estimated that sticking to five low-risk lifestyle-related factors could prolong life expectancy at age 50 years by 14.0 and 12.2 years for female and male US adults, respectively, compared with individuals who adopted zero low-risk lifestyle factor (Li et al., 2018). The five lifestyle related factors include diet, smoking, physical activity, alcohol consumption, and **body mass index** (BMI). Unhealthy lifestyles counterbalance the gain in life expectancy, particularly the increasing obesity epidemic and decreasing physical activity levels. Three-quarters of premature CVD deaths and half of premature cancer deaths in the U.S. could be attributed to lack of adherence to a low-risk lifestyle (Li et al., 2018). Prevention should be a top priority for national health policy, and preventive care should be an integral part of the US health care system. A healthy diet pattern, moderate alcohol consumption, nonsmoking, a normal weight, and regular physical activity are each associated with a low risk of premature mortality. Smoking is a strong independent risk factor of cancer, diabetes mellitus, CVDs, and mortality (Li et al., 2018). Physical activity and weight control significantly reduce risks of diabetes mellitus, cardiac disease, and breast cancer. Changing lifestyles is the most cost-effective way to prevent illness and increase quality of life, yet it seems to be the most difficult for Americans. Note other factors that can both increase and decrease utilization, as listed in Table 2.6.

Cost Containment Strategies

Research has suggested the hazards and ethical problems in the overuse of services in fee-for-service settings (where payment is made based on service rendered to individuals for individual services) rather than service underuse in capitated care (where payment is made based on service rendered to a group of patients) (Berwick 1994; Leape et al., 1990). Over the years, cost containment strategies have targeted the financing and reimbursement sides of health care. Financing strategies have used health services regulation and limitation by means of taxes or insurance premiums and encouraged competition such as managed competition. Reimbursement containment strategies have used regulatory and competitive price controls and utilization controls, such as capitation, patient cost sharing, and utilization management. Capitation and prospective payment have had some of the most significant impacts on cost containment.

Capitation

Even though legislation creating managed care was passed in 1973 (the Health Maintenance Organization Act), managed care did not become a major player or driving force in health care until the late 1980s. In an effort to reduce the number of hospitalizations and control profit incentives for health care providers, managed care plans offered hospitals and practitioners a capitated set fee for office visits and hospitalizations for a group of patients. Capitation is the payment of a fixed dollar amount, per person, for the provision of health services to a patient population for a specified period of time, for example, 1 year. Under capitation, health care organizations benefit from using their financial resources to keep people well. Otherwise, health care providers bear the financial loss. Then in the mid-1990s, the U.S. population had quality concerns with this system and *backlashed* against managed care organizations.

Prospective Payment

Reacting to rapidly increasing costs to Medicare, the **Tax Equity and Fiscal Responsibility Act** (TEFRA) passed in 1982 mandated the **Prospective Payment System** (PPS) to control health care costs. For Medicare Part A services, PPS uses Medicare's administrative data to develop and continually refine PPS payments based on **diagnosis-related groups** (DRGs), that is, patients with similar diagnoses. The PPS is a method of reimbursement in which Medicare payment is made based on a predetermined, fixed amount for reimbursement to acute inpatient hospitals, home health agencies, hospices, hospital outpatient and inpatient psychiatric facilities, inpatient rehabilitation facilities, long-term care hospitals, and skilled nursing facilities. For Medicare Part B services, the **Resource-Based Relative Value Scale** (RBRVS) is used to determine reimbursement amounts for practitioner services. The major problem that the CMS has encountered with funding prospective payment is DRG creep, in which health care providers *up code* or over bill a patient to indicate a need for financial reimbursement for more expensive health care services to recoup what the health care provider believes is a more equitable payment.

Health Care Quality

The health care report *To Err Is Human,* confronted health care clinicians and managers with concerns about the poor quality of health care attributable to misuse, overuse, and underuse of resources and procedures, which was responsible for thousands of deaths (IOM, 1999). The health care report, *Crossing the Quality Chasm* (IOM, 2001), and several large studies (McGlynn et al., 2003; Thomas et al., 2000), have shown that the quality of health care in the United States is at an unexpected low level and needs improvement in many dimensions, given the amount of money the United States spends on health care (Table 2.7). One implication is that if a measure is

Table 2.6   Forces that Affect Overall Health Care Utilization

Force	Factors that may decrease health services utilization	Factors that may increase health services utilization
Financial incentives that reward practitioners and hospitals for performance (e.g., pay for performance (P4P) programs that reward quality practice)	Changes in clinician practice patterns (e.g., encouraging patient self-care and healthy lifestyles; reduced length of hospital stay)	Changes in clinician practice patterns (e.g., more aggressive treatment of the elderly)
Increased accountability for performance	Consensus documents or guidelines that recommend decreases in utilization	Consensus documents or guidelines that recommend increases in utilization
Technological advances in the biological and clinical sciences	Better understanding of the risk factors of diseases and prevention initiatives (e.g., smoking-prevention programs, cholesterol-lowering drugs)	New procedures and technologies (e.g., hip replacement, stent insertion, magnetic resonance imaging (MRI)) New drugs, expanded use of existing drugs Increased supply of services (e.g., ambulatory surgery centers, assisted living residences)
Increase in chronic illness	Aging of the population Discovery and implementation of treatments that cure or eliminate diseases Public health and sanitation advances (e.g., quality standards for food and water distribution)	Growing elderly population: • more functional limitations associated with aging • more illness associated with aging • more deaths among the increased number of elderly (the elderly are correlated with high utilization of services)
Increased ethnic and cultural diversity of the population	Lack of insurance coverage Low income	Growth in national population Efforts to eliminate disparities in access and outcomes
Changes in the supply and education of health professionals	Decreased supply (e.g., hospital closures, large numbers of nursing and medical practitioners and nurses retiring) Shifts to other sites of care may cause declines in utilization of staff at the original sites: • as technology allows shifts (e.g., ambulatory surgery) • as alternative sites of care become available (e.g., assisted living)	Increase in chronic conditions Growth in national population
Social morbidity (e.g., increased AIDS, drugs, violence, disasters)	Disparities in access to health services and outcomes	New health problems (e.g., HIV/AIDS, bioterrorism, earthquakes)
Access to patient information	Changes in consumer preferences (e.g., home birthing, more self-care, alternative medicine)	Changes in consumer demand
Globalization and expansion of the world economy	Growth in uninsured population	Growth in national population
Cost control and competition for limited resources	Insurance payer pressures to reduce costs	Increased health insurance coverage Consumer and employee pressures for more comprehensive insurance coverage Changes in consumer preferences and demand (e.g., cosmetic surgery, hip and knee replacements, direct marketing of pharmaceuticals)

Source: Adapted from Bernstein, A. B., Hing, E., Moss, A. J., Allen, K. F., Siller, A. B., Tiggle, R. B. (2003). *Health care in America: Trends in utilization.* Hyattsville, MD: National Center for Health Statistics; and Shortell, S. M., & Kaluzny, A. D. (2006). *Health care management* (5th ed.). Clifton Park, NY: Delmar Cengage Learning. And CDC. (2018). *National Center for Health Statistics. Health, United States, 2017: With special feature on mortality.. National Center for Health Statistics. Health, United States, 2017: With special feature on mortality.* Retrieved from www.cdc.gov/nchs/data/hus/hus17.pdf

Table 2.7   Health Care Dimensions Needing Improvement

Health Care Should Be	Health Care Should
1. Safe: Avoid injuries from care intended to help patients.	1. Offer care based on continuous healing relationships: Make care available every day through face-to-face visits, telephone, Internet, and other means.
2. Effective: Provide services based on scientific knowledge to all who could benefit, and refrain from providing services to those not likely to benefit (avoid overuse and underuse).	2. Customize care based on patient needs and values: Provide care responsive to patient needs and preferences.
3. Patient centered: Provide respectful and responsive care to individuals; patient preferences, needs, and values must guide clinical decision making.	3. Have the patient as source of control: Foster patient empowerment and autonomy through information and shared decision making.
4. Timely: Reduce wait time and harmful delays for those who receive and give care.	4. Share knowledge and free flow of information: Facilitate patient access to his or her own medical information and to available clinical knowledge.
5. Efficient: Avoid waste, for example, of equipment, supplies, ideas, energy, and other costly resources.	5. Use evidence-based decision making: Provide consistent quality of care based on best available scientific knowledge.
6. Equitable: Provide care consistent in quality irrespective of gender, ethnicity, geographical, and socioeconomic factors.	6. Develop safety as a systems property: Develop systems of safety that mitigate error, promote patient safety, and reduce risk of injury.
	7. Be transparent: Make information available to patients and families about health plans, hospitals, clinical practice, and alternative treatment options, including performance related to their safety, evidence-based practice, and patient satisfaction.
	8. Anticipate needs: Anticipate patient needs rather than respond to events.
	9. Continuously decrease waste: Use limited resources wisely.
	10. Cooperate among clinicians: Collaborate and coordinate care between clinicians and institutions.

Source: Compiled with information from the Institute of Medicine. (2001). *Crossing the quality chasm: A new health system for the 21st century.* Washington, DC: National Academy Press; and Berwick, D. M. (2002). A user's manual for the IOM's 'Quality Chasm' report. *Health Affairs, 2* (3), 80–90.

described in a way that is clear and understandable, people are more likely to value the measure (AHRQ, 2011).

Health Care Variation

Groundbreaking research beginning in the 1970s and continuing into the 1990s demonstrated that there was significant variation in utilization of specific health care services associated with geographical location, provider preferences and training, type of health insurance, and patient-specific factors such as age and gender (Adams, Fraser, & Abrams, 1973; Greenfield et al., 1992; Leape, 1992; Safran, Rogers, Tarlov, McHorney, & Ware Jr., 1997; Wennberg & Gittelsohn, 1973). Associations between utilization rates of health care services have been found with availability of services and technologies, for example, MRIs, hospital beds, practitioners (Joines, Hertz-Picciotto, Carey, Gesler, & Suchindran, 2003), prevalence and severity of morbidities (Dunn, Lyman, & Marx, 2005; AHRQ, 2008b), race or ethnicity (AHRQ, 2008b), patient adherence, health-seeking behaviors of patients (Calvocoressi et al., 2004), and many other factors. Variation in the delivery and quality of health services is also associated with socio-demographics, hospital types (e.g., urban and rural, teaching and nonteaching), and clinical areas (e.g., heart disease, diabetes, pneumonia, and clinical preventive services). Regions of the country and health

care providers with more resources had higher rates of use and cost. Efforts to decrease the variation of health care practices through standardization of care with quality, evidence-based guidelines are important to improve clinical decision making, care delivery, health outcomes, and cost efficiency.

Achieving **health care transparency** or truth in reporting is the ability to discover information about health care costs, medical errors, or practice preferences, preferably before receiving the service. Transparency is being encouraged by the CMS, though transparency can be hampered by the fear of litigation or reprisal against the health care provider. The Patient Safety and Quality Improvement Act of 2005 addresses such concerns by encouraging health care providers to participate in developing and implementing evidence-based improvement initiatives. The Act also highlights the importance of recognizing and responding to the underlying hazards and risks to patient safety. Establishing national health benchmarks, such as those in Healthy People 2020 (USDHHS, 2010), is another strategy by which to achieve and measure quality improvement.

Highly Reliable Health Care: Improvements to Standardize Care

Using the example of the management of heart disease, recent research findings illustrate the need for significant improvements to standardize the process of health care delivery. Each year, heart disease contributes to thousands of deaths. When evidence-based standards are used to guide the care of the patient with heart disease. and aspirin and beta-blockers are given to patients who have had a myocardial infarction, it can lower health care dollars and save lives associated with heart disease (Schulte, 2011). This is true, even if it is because aspirin use is being measured to assess provider performance (Williams, Schmaltz, Morton, Koss, & Loeb, 2005). Standardization of patient care can change the list of the top ten health care conditions, both in cost and mortality, by making patient care delivery more reliable (Table 2.8).

Performance and Quality Measurement

Performance and quality measurement is an essential component of health care improvement efforts. Performance and quality are measured to determine resource allocation, organize care delivery, assess clinician competency, and improve health care delivery processes. Hospitals and practitioners have been given past and present financial incentives to score well on measures of quality from both public and private health care payers. When the quality of care is measured, it improves (Brook, Kamberg, & McGlynn, 1996; Chassin & Galvin, 1998). possibly largely due to the Hawthorne effect, which has illustrated that observed activity shows improvement. Ramirez (2019) reports that more people receive **evidence-based care** (EBC) for heart attack when they arrive at a hospital, hospital-acquired conditions decreased from 2014 to 2017, that medicare 30-day hospital readmission rates have declined, and that mortality rates within 30 days after hospital admission for heart attack, stroke, and pneumonia have decreased.

From 2003 to 2013, the mortality rate for deaths amenable to health care in the U.S. declined by about 17%. More recently, the rate has increased slightly.

Nursing leaders have also recognized the need to establish classifications that can be used to measure nursing care. Selected classifications are listed in Table 2.9.

Note that setting standards for appropriate care and guideline development should have a basis in validated measures of quality, using reliable performance data, and making appropriate adjustments in care delivery. Reliable methods and measures need to be developed and tested. Some practitioners have been resistant to their care delivery being measured because they have believed that it would interfere with their professionalism and autonomy. If this belief persists, the majority of health care delivery will not be measured.

Table 2.8   Top 10 Causes of Death—Cost and Death

Heart disease: 199 billion
Cancer: 174 billion
Accidents: 75 billion
Chronic lower respiratory conditions: 36 billion
Stroke: 34 billion
Alzheimer's disease: 215 billion
Diabetes: 237 billion
Influenza and pneumonia: 8.7 billion
Nephritis, nephrotic syndrome and nephrosis :124 billion
Intentional self-harm: 69 billion

Source: CDC. (2019). FastStats—Deaths and Mortality. Retrieved from www.cdc.gov/nchs/fastats/deaths.htm.

Table 2.9   Selected Classification Systems (List compiled by R. Hughes).

North American Nursing Diagnosis Association (NANDA): www.nanda.org

Home Health Care Classification (HHCC): www.sabacare.com

PeriOperative Nursing Data Set: www.aorn.org

National Quality Forum-Endorsed Nursing-Sensitive Consensus Standards: www.qualityforum.org

Omaha System: www.omahasystem.org

ABC Codes: www.alternativelink.com

Logical Observation Identifiers Names and Codes: www.loinc.org

Nursing Interventions Classification: www.nursing.uiowa.edu

Nursing Outcomes Classification: www.nursing.uiowa.edu

National Database of Nursing Quality Indicators (NDNQI): www.nursingworld.org. (Search for NDNQI.)

SNOMED CT: www.snomed.org

International Classification of Nursing Practice: www.icn.ch

Malcolm Baldridge National Quality Award

Health care organizations are eligible to consider another framework for health care quality and to apply for the Malcolm Baldridge National Quality Award. The Health Care Criteria of the Malcolm Baldridge National Quality Award explores a hospitals mission and key objectives in seven critical areas: Leadership, Strategy, Customers, Measurements, Workforce, Operations, and Results. The Baldrige framework is based on core values and concepts that represent beliefs and behaviors found in high-performing organizations. Baldrige works with public and private sector partners to address critical national needs related to long-term success and sustainability, including cybersecurity risk management and excellence in US communities (Eastman, 2019).

Outcome Measurement

Outcome measurements can be done indicating an individual's clinical state, such as the severity of illness, course of illness, and the effect of interventions on the individual's clinical state. Outcome measures involving a patient's functional status evaluate a patient's ability to perform activities of daily living (ADLs). These can include measures of physical health in terms of function, mental and social health, cost of care, health care access, and general health perceptions. The measures can distinguish the concepts of physical and mental health and identify the five indicator categories of clinical status, functioning, physical symptoms, emotional status, and patient/family evaluation, and in Canada perceptions about quality of life. Selected quality-of-life measures include **quality-adjusted life years** (QALYs), **quality-adjusted life expectancy** (QALE), and **quality-adjusted healthy life years** (QUALYs) (Drummond, Stoddart, & Torrance, 1994).

Other Health Assessment Tools

The assessment of **health-related quality of life** (HR-QOL) is an essential element of health care evaluation. Many generic and specific HR-QOL instruments have been developed and include the Medical Outcomes Study 36-Item Short Form (SF-36) health survey; the **Nottingham Health Profile** (NHP); the **Sickness Impact Profile** (SIP); the Dartmouth Primary Care **Cooperative Information Project** (COOP) Charts; the **Quality of Well-Being** (QWB) Scale; the **Health Utilities Index** (HUI); and the EuroQol Instrument (EQ-5D) (Coons, Rao, Keininger, & Hays, 2000). The U.S. News & World Report (2019) reports that the country with the best quality of life is Canada, followed by Sweden and Denmark. The U.S. lags in sixth place.

Public Reporting of Performance

Public reporting of organizational performance and quality information is being driven by several forces. As more data about quality become available electronically, individuals reporting the data and those wanting to make comparisons among organizations want the data analyzed and the findings reported. This information can be used to determine where there are health care inefficiencies and poor quality of care. Performance reporting is also used to influence clinician and patient utilization behavior. It also moves health care toward a population-based approach, as opposed to focusing on individual patient care.

Institute of Medicine Health Care Reports

The IOM, established in 1970 under the charter of the National Academy of Sciences, provides independent, objective, evidence-based advice to policymakers, health professionals, the private sector, and the public. In 1996, the IOM launched a concerted, ongoing effort focused on assessing and improving the nation's quality of care. The *Ensuring Quality Cancer Care Report* (1999) documented the wide gulf that exists between ideal cancer care and the reality many Americans with cancer experience.

Other reports released by the IOM on the quality of health care include:

To Err is Human; Building A Safer Health System (1999);

Crossing the Quality Chasm: A New Health System for the Twenty-first Century (2001);

Strategies for Addressing the Evolving Nursing Crisis (2002);

Patient Safety: Achieving a New Standard for Care (2003);

Keeping Patients Safe: Transforming the Work Environment of Nurses (2003);

Health Professions Education: A Bridge to Quality (2003);

Priority Areas for National Action: Transforming Health Care Quality (2003);

Performance Measurement: Accelerating Improvement (2005);

Preventing Medication Errors (2006); and

The Future of Nursing: Leading Change, Advancing Health (2010).

A complete listing of IOM Reports is available at www.iom.edu/Reports.aspx

Eight principles are integral to health care reform, as envisioned by the IOM (2008). These eight principles are:

* Accountability

* Efficiency

* Objectivity

* Scientific rigor

* Consistency

* Feasibility

* Responsiveness

* Transparency

These principles are consistent with a professional nursing agenda, which states that all persons are entitled to affordable, quality health care services (American Nurses Association (ANA), 2010). The *Quality Chasm* report described broader quality issues, defined six aims, and highlighted ten rules for care delivery redesign (Table 2.7) (IOM, 2001).

Other National Public Quality Reports

Several key national public quality sources of interest for health care and nursing leaders and managers for purposes of performance measurement and benchmarking or comparison are as follows:

- *AHRQ National Healthcare Quality Report 2009* Available at www.ahrq.gov/qual/nhqr09/nhqr09.htm

- *AHRQ National Healthcare Disparities Report 2009* Available at www.ahrq.gov/qual/qrdr09.htm

- *Healthy People 2010:* Available at www.healthypeople.gov

- *Health Grades for Hospitals and Physicians:* Available at healthgrades.com

- *Leapfrog:* Available at www.leapfroggroup.org

- *The National Quality Forum:* Available at www.qualityforum.org

- *Health Plan and Employer Data and Information Set (HEDIS) & Quality Measurement, National Committee for Quality Assurance (NCQA):* Available at www.ncqa.org

- *Consumer Assessment of Healthcare Providers and Systems (CAHPS), Agency for Healthcare Research and Quality (AHRQ):* Available at www.cahps.ahrq.gov/default.asp

- *Medicare Hospital Compare:* Available at www.hospital-compare.hhs.gov.

- *The Thomson Reuters 100 Top Hospitals®*: Available at www.100tophospitals.com/top-national-hospitals

- *U.S. News and World Report Best Hospitals, annual ranking:* Available at http://health.usnews.com/best-hospitals

Public reporting of quality performance has been shown to improve care. While providers and policymakers do seek out these public quality reports, the general public does not search them out, does not understand them, distrusts them, and fails to make use of them (Marshall, Hiscock, & Sibbald, 2002). In many respects, hospitals are providing quality care. Data to assess clinical performance from the **Joint Commission** (JC) core measures program, which uses standardized, evidence-based measures, and data from the Medicare program, show improvements in the quality of care in hospitals (Williams et al., 2005).

Disease Management

According to the The Care Continiuum Alliance (2010), **disease management** is a system of coordinated health care interventions and communications for populations with conditions in which patient self-care is significant. What makes caring for patients with chronic diseases problematic is that the patients usually have multiple chronic conditions (e.g., the patient with congestive heart failure who also has hypertension, diabetes, emphysema, urinary incontinence, and chronic pain). Heart disease, stroke, cancer, chronic respiratory diseases, and diabetes are the leading cause of mortality in the world (WHO, 2019). Common, modifiable risk factors underlie the major NCDs. They include tobacco, harmful use of alcohol, unhealthy diet, insufficient physical activity, overweight/obesity, raised blood pressure, raised blood sugar, and raised cholesterol (WHO, 2019).

Balanced Scorecards

Another type of results reporting that is used by organizations is the balanced scorecard. A **balanced scorecard** is a framework to implement and manage strategy. It links a vision to strategic objectives, measures, targets, and initiatives. It balances financial measures with performance measures and

Evidence From the Literature

Source: Adapted from Yong, P., Saunders, R., & Olsen, L. (2010). Healthcare Imperative: Lowering Costs and Improving Outcomes: Workshop Series Summary [National Institutes of Health]. doi: http://www.nap.edu/catalog/12750.html

Discussion: The IOM's Roundtable on Value & Science-Driven Health Care has been convened to help transform the way evidence on clinical effectiveness is generated and used to improve health and health care. Participants have set a goal that, by the year 2020, 90% of clinical decisions will be supported by accurate, timely, and up-to-date clinical information, and will reflect the best available evidence.

This summary highlights the presentations and discussions from these workshops, delving into the major causes of excess spending, waste, and inefficiency in health care. The ideas and observations presented are offered in the truism that health reform, now and in the future, will benefit from identifying actionable options to lower health care costs in ways that maximize value.

Implications for Practice: This series delves into the major causes of excess spending, waste, and inefficiency in health care. By understanding where waste exists, nurses can help reduce waste and improve patient and cost outcomes.

objectives related to all other parts of the organization. They are used to monitor customer perspective; financial perspective; internal processes and human resources; and learning and growth for strategic management and as a way to examine performance throughout the organization. This examination allows the organization to review multiple key areas of performance, selected on the basis of their importance to the organization's strategic plan for quality.

Evidence-Based Practice

The body of evidence supporting clinical practice is steadily growing. However, even when evidence-based quality care guidelines are available for numerous conditions, for example, diabetes, congestive heart failure, and asthma, they have not been fully implemented in actual patient care, and variation in clinical practice is abundant (IOM, 2001; McGlynn et al., 2003; Timmermans & Mauck, 2005). Health care knowledge continues to expand. This requires practice guidelines and the measures of quality on which they are based to be continually updated. It also requires attention to continuing to develop health care quality.

Accreditation and Patient Safety

Health care accreditation is a mechanism used to ensure that organizations meet certain national standards. Hospitals and other organizations seek accreditation to demonstrate their abilities to meet national quality standards. The Joint Com-

mission (JC), formerly known as the **Joint Commission on Accreditation of Healthcare Organizations (JCAHO)**, is the preeminent regulatory body overseeing health care quality. Its review processes are extensive, and payments to a hospital by government insurers of health care (CMS) are dependent on the organization's ability to meet JC standards with a high degree of compliance (Table 2.10). In addition, other federal, state, local, and voluntary regulatory agencies oversee the quality of specific organizational components such as pharmacy, laboratory, long-term care, rehabilitative care, dietary, behavioral health, and fire safety. Accreditation, which signifies that the organization meets the standards for practice of these oversight agencies, influences market perception about the quality of health care that the organization provides and engenders trust and confidence in the organization.

Improving Quality Through Health Professions Education

There is a need to focus on retooling the health care workforce with new knowledge and requisite skills to function in better, redesigned health care systems. To begin to realize the quality agenda set forth by the IOM (2001), a subsequent report, *Health Professions Education: A Bridge to Quality* (IOM, 2003c), delineates a needed *overhaul* of the curriculum of health professionals' education to transform current skills and knowledge (IOM, 2003c, p. 1). This curriculum includes training clinicians to develop:

Table 2.10 Hospital Accreditation Standards Overview

• Environment of care	• Life safety	• Performance improvement
• Emergency management	• Medication management	• Record of care, treatment, and services
• Human resources	• Medical staff	• Rights and responsibilities of the individual
• Infection prevention and control	• National patient safety goals	• Transplant safety
• Information management	• Nursing	• Waived testing
• Leadership	• Provision of care, treatment, and services	

Source: © Joint Commission: *CAMH: 2010 Comprehensive Accreditation Manual for Hospitals.* Oakbrook Terrace, IL: Joint Commission, 2011, available at www.jcrinc.com/Joint-Commission-Requirements/Hospitals

---

Critical Thinking 2.3

Review the case studies on reducing harm to patients at, www.commonwealthfund.org/Innovations/Case-Studies.aspx

What can each staff member do to improve the quality of care, especially the safety of patient care?

How can we work toward a culture of continual improvement for those issues and situations that cause errors and almost lead to errors?

How much control do nurses have in identifying errors and reporting them?

What can you do to improve the quality of care afforded in your organization?

1. *Ability to provide patient-centered care:* Patient-centered care emphasizes recognition of the patient or designee as the source of control and full partner in providing compassionate and coordinated care based on respect for the patient's preferences, values, and needs. It builds knowledge of effective communication approaches that allows patient access to information and achieves patient understanding. Patient-centered care respects patients' individuality, values, and needs, and uses related population-based strategies to improve appropriate utilization of health care services. Patient-centered care is important, because research continues to find that involving patients in decision making about their care results in higher functional status, better outcomes, and lower costs.

2. *Ability to effectively work in interprofessional teams:* This competency calls for functioning effectively within nursing and interprofessional teams and fostering open communication, mutual respect, and shared decision making to achieve quality patient care. Interprofessional teams have been shown to enhance quality and lower costs, even though this training is challenged by differences in communication norms across disciplines and power and turf controversies among disciplines.

3. *Understanding of evidence-based practices:* Evidence-based practice integrates the best current research evidence with clinical expertise and patient and family preferences and values for delivery of optimal health care. To actively provide EBC, clinicians need the following knowledge and skills: how to locate the best sources of evidence, how to formulate clear clinically-based questions, and how to determine when and how to translate new knowledge into practice.

4. *Ability to measure the quality of care:* Clinicians need to be able to use data to monitor the outcomes of care processes and use improvement methods to design and test changes to continuously improve the quality and safety of health care systems. Clinicians must use comparison benchmarks to identify opportunities for improvement; design, test, and assess quality improvement interventions; identify current and potential errors in care; and implement safety design principles such as recognizing human factors and the need for standardization.

5. *Ability to use health information technology:* Health care informatics applications use information and technology to communicate, manage knowledge, mitigate errors, and support decision making. They enhance patient safety by driving standardization, as well as by facilitating knowledge management and communication. As more technology becomes available, database systems are linked within and across health care settings. As our evidence-based measures and decision-making tools improve, clinicians will need to be able to fully utilize health information technology to improve the quality of health care delivery.

Quality and Safety Education for Nurses (QSEN)

The IOM's 2004 *Report on Patient Safety* was the first in a series of three reports published since the year 2000 to emphasize the connections among nursing, patient safety, and quality of care. *Keeping Patients Safe* sets forth the structures and processes that health care workers use in the delivery of care and emphasizes the need to design the nurses' environments to promote the practice of safe nursing care (IOM, 2004b). The importance of organizational management practices, strong nursing leadership, and adequate nurse staffing for providing a safe care environment is critical (Laschinger & Leiter, 2006). The IOM Report (2010) *The Future of Nursing Leading Change Advancing Health* suggest that nurses should practice to the full extent of their education and training, achieve higher levels of education and training through an improved education system that promotes seamless academic progression, and be full partners with physicians and other health care professionals.

In 2008, the **American Association of Colleges of Nursing (AACN)** and the **National League for Nursing (NLN)** embraced the inclusion of quality improvement systems thinking, change strategies, and patient safety, etc., into undergraduate and graduate nursing education curricula. In 2005, the RWJF funded the University of North Carolina at Chapel Hill School of Nursing on a long-term project aimed at increasing the inclusion of quality in nursing education and the development of well-prepared faculty to teach the quality and safety competencies recommended by the IOM to make health care safe, effective, patient centered, timely, efficient, and equitable (IOM, 2001). In 2009, the AACN lent its support to this **Quality and Safety Education for Nurses** (QSEN) project (www.qsen.org) (Kovner et al., 2010).

The QSEN website is now a comprehensive resource for teaching strategies, etc., for the development of quality and safety competency in nursing.

Never Conditions

In 2008, the CMS identified hospital-acquired conditions (never conditions) for which they will not reimburse hospitals for a higher DRG payment (i.e., pressure ulcers; fractures, dislocations, intercranial injury, crushing injury, and burns; catheter-associated urinary tract infections; vascular catheter-associated infections, object left in patient during surgery, air embolism, blood incompatibility, and mediastinitis after coronary artery bypass graft). Medicare no longer pays hospitals for these conditions (Waxman, 2008). Clearly the nurse of the future must be educated about never events. The term "Never Event" was first introduced in 2001 by Ken Kizer,

---

Critical Thinking 2.4

Think about the competencies needed to improve health care education:

1. Patient-centered care delivery
2. Interdisciplinary teamwork
3. Evidence-based practice
4. Measurement of the quality of care
5. Health information technology skill
6. Culture of safety

How can you improve your education and experience in each of the competencies now and throughout your career?

MD, former CEO of the **National Quality Forum** (NQF), in reference to gross medical errors like wrong-site surgery that should never occur. Over time, the term's use has expanded to signify adverse events that are clearly identifiable and measurable, resulting in death or significant disability, and usually preventable. Since the initial never event list was developed in 2002, it has been revised multiple times, and now consists of 29 "serious reportable events" grouped into seven categories (Abimanyi-Ochom, Jones, & Cheng, 2019). The latest list from 2016 includes:

1. Surgical or invasive procedure events

2. Product or device events

3. Patient protection events

4. Care management events

5. Environmental events

6. Radiological events

7. Potential criminal events

A complete listing, including the subcategories, is available at www.qualityforum.org

Nurse Shortages

Until recently, shortages of nurses have been cyclical. These nurse shortages are associated with increased demand for patient care services at a time of falling nursing school enrollment, salary compression, and nominal increases in wages. The U.S. is projected to experience a **shortage** of Registered **Nurses** (RNs) that is expected to intensify as Baby Boomers age. According to a 2018 survey conducted by the National Council of State Boards of Nursing and The Forum of State Nursing Workforce Centers, 50.9% of the RN workforce is age 50 or older. The HRSA projects that more than 1 million registered nurses will reach retirement age within the next 10–15 years. The **RN** workforce was expected to grow from 2.9 million in 2016 to 3.4 million in 2026, an increase of 438,100 or 15% (ANA, 2019). According to the Bureau of Labor Statistics' Employment Projections 2016–2026, it projects the need for an additional 203,700 new RNs each year through 2026 to fill newly created positions and to replace retiring nurses. The current nursing workforce has 56% of RNs prepared at the baccalaureate or graduate degree level. The AACN reported a 3.7% enrollment increase in baccalaureate programs in nursing in 2018. According to AACN's report on 2018–2019 Enrollment and Graduations in Baccalaureate and Graduate Programs in Nursing, U.S. nursing schools turned away more than 75,000 qualified applicants from baccalaureate and graduate and nursing programs in 2018. Changing demographics signal a need for more nurses to care for our aging population. Issued in May 2014, the U.S. Census Bureau report on An Aging Nation: The Older Population in the United States, found that by 2050 the number of U.S. residents aged 65 and over is projected to be 83.7 million, almost double its estimated population of 43.13 million in 2012. With larger numbers of older adults, there will be an increased need for geriatric care, including care for individuals with chronic diseases and comorbidities. With an aging nursing workforce (Norman et al., 2005), more nursing faculty is needed to train larger numbers of students.

American Nurses Association

The ANA is a full service, professional organization representing the nation's entire RN population. The ANA represents the 4 million RNs in the United States through its 54 constituent state and territorial associations. The ANA's mission is to work for the improvement of health standards and availability of

---

Case Study 2.2

Review the ratings of hospitals in your area of the country at www.healthgrades.com, www.hospitalcompare.hhs.gov, www.100tophospitals.com/top-national-hospitals, and the U.S. News & World Report Best Hospitals, annual ranking, available at http://health.usnews.com/best-hospitals

What kinds of ratings are given to hospitals in your area?

Review the criteria and evaluation system used to rate the hospitals. Is it valid and reliable?

Will you choose a hospital for your own family's care using a rating system like this?

health care services for all people, foster high standards for nursing, stimulate and promote the professional development of nurses, and advance their economic and general welfare (ANA, 2019).

The **National Labor Relations Board** (NLRB) recognizes the ANA as a collective bargaining agent. The fact that the ANA has a dual role of being a professional organization and a collective bargaining agent causes controversy. Some nurses believe that unionization is not professional and that the ANA cannot truly support nursing as a profession if it is also a collective bargaining agent. Nurse managers are excluded from union membership. The ANA lobbies Congress and regulatory agencies on health care issues affecting nurses and the general public. The ANA initiates many policies involving health care

reform. It also publishes its position on issues, ranging from whistle blowing to patients' rights. The **American Nurses Credentialing Center** (ANCC), a subsidiary of the ANA, created the Magnet Recognition Program to recognize health care organizations that provide the very best in nursing care. Since 1994, many institutions have received this award.

In this chapter, we have explored how health care is organized and financed in the United State, compared U.S. Health care with that of other industrialized countries, identified major issues facing health care, and related efforts for improving the quality, safety, and access to health care. Staying abreast of U.S. health care and health care in other countries is part of being a registered nurse and understanding the environment in which we work.

KEY CONCEPTS

- Health care reports provide invaluable information that emphasizes the successes and failures of health care throughout our nation.

- Evidence of significant disparities and low quality continue to demonstrate the need for significant health care improvement.

- Today, leaders, managers, and staff need to be aware of and involved in the ongoing processes of the making of health policy.

- Health care systems have three simple components: structure, process, and outcome.

- The United States is one of only a few advanced countries in the world without a universal system of health care.

- In the United States, the emphasis on acute care health care services has successfully driven health care costs higher, but has not necessarily improved the quality of care or patient outcomes.

- **Primary care** provides integrated, accessible health care services by clinicians who are accountable for addressing a large majority of personal health care needs, developing a sustained partnership with patients, and practicing in the context of family and community.

- Patients and clinicians need to work together to appropriately utilize services based on the following four foundations of primary care: First Contact, Longitudinality, Comprehensiveness, and Coordination.

- The federal government is a major driver of health care organization and delivery.

- Today, almost as many persons receive health care in the home as receive health care in acute-care settings.

- Enabling factors such as income, type of insurance coverage, gender, race or ethnicity, geographical proximity, and system characteristics affect a person's ability to have access to health care.

- The 2010 passage of The Patient Protection and Affordable Care Act and the HCERA has made changes in the U.S. health care system.

- The elderly have a form of UHC coverage through Medicare.

- Because the United States does not have national/UHC insurance, public health care programs are intended to fill the gap.

- Health care spending continues to increase faster than the overall U.S. economy.

- There are many contributing factors to the rising costs of health care. The key factors include the aging of the population with growth in the demand for health care, increased utilization of pharmaceuticals, expensive new technologies, rising hospital care costs, practitioner behavior, cost shifting, and administrative costs.

- Because rising health care costs are based on utilization, it is important to understand other factors that can both increase and decrease utilization.

- Capitation and prospective payment have had some of the most significant impacts on cost containment.

- The report *To Err Is Human,* confronted health care clinicians and managers with concerns about the poor quality of health care attributable to misuse, overuse, and underuse of resources and procedures, which was responsible for thousands of deaths (IOM, 1999).

- The report, *Crossing the Quality Chasm* (IOM, 2001) and several large studies (McGlynn et al., 2003; Thomas et al., 2000) have shown that the quality of health care in the United States is at an unexpected low level and needs improvement in many dimensions, given the amount of money the United States spends on health care.

- Groundbreaking research, beginning in the mid-1980s and continuing in the 1990s, demonstrated that there was significant variation in utilization of specific health care services associated with geographical location, provider preferences and training, type of health insurance, and patient-specific factors such as age and gender.

- Recent research findings illustrate the need for significant improvements in the process of health care delivery.

- Health care performance and quality are measured to determine resource allocation, organize care delivery, assess clinician competency, and improve health care delivery processes.

- Public reporting of organizational performance and quality information is being driven by several forces.

- Several key national public quality reports of interest for health care and nursing leaders and managers for purposes of performance measurement and benchmarking are available.

- A key challenge for health care is the numerous deficiencies in the delivery of care of patients with chronic conditions.

- Evidence-based practice involves supplementing clinical expertise with the judicious and conscientious implementation of the most current and best evidence along with patient values and preferences to guide health care decision making.

- Health care accreditation is a mechanism used to ensure that organizations meet certain national standards.

- There is a need to focus on retooling the health care workforce with new knowledge and requisite skills to function in better, redesigned health care systems.

- Health professionals' education to transform current skills and knowledge includes training clinicians to effectively work in inter-disciplinary teams; have an educational foundation in informatics; and deliver patient-centered care, fully exploiting evidence-based practice, quality improvement approaches, and informatics.

- The IOM's 2004 *Report on Patient Safety* was the first in a series of reports published since the year 2000 to emphasize the connections among nursing, patient safety, and quality of care.

KEY TERMS

Balanced scorecards	Disease management	Outcome measurements
Co-payments	Gross domestic product (GDP)	Primary care
Cost shifting	Health care transparency	Process component of health
Deductibles	Outcome component of health	Structure component of health

---

REVIEW QUESTIONS

1. The national organization that accredits health care organizations is known as which of the following?
   a. American Nurses Association
   b. Health Professions Commission
   c. Agency for Health Care Research and Quality
   d. Joint Commission

2. The largest purchaser of health care in America is which of the following?
   a. Private individuals
   b. Private insurance companies
   c. Health Maintenance Organizations
   d. Medicare, Medicaid, and other governmental programs

3. Who identified a structure, process, and outcome framework for quality?
   a. Nightingale
   b. Donabedian
   c. Starr
   d. Lohr

4. What is the top underlying cause of health care disparity in the United States?
   a. Socioeconomic status
   b. Age
   c. Geographical location
   d. Chronic illness

5. Payment for health care services as a fixed dollar amount per member over a period of time is referred to as which of the following?
   a. Traditional fee for services
   b. Prospective payment system
   c. Capitation
   d. Diagnosis-related groupings

6. The Patient Protection and Affordable Care Act provides comprehensive health care reform through a number of initiatives, including which of the following? Select all that apply.
   a. Restricting in-patient hospital stays
   b. Expanding health insurance coverage
   c. Targeting fraud, abuse, and waste in health care
   d. Increasing access to primary care services
   e. Promoting preventive health strategies

7. Key factors contributing to rising health care costs in the United States include which of the following? Select all that apply.
   a. An aging population
   b. Advancements in technology
   c. Increased utilization of pharmaceuticals
   d. Rising costs of primary care
   e. Administrative costs

8. The competencies for the education of health care professionals recommended by the Institute of Medicine to improve the quality of health care include all but which of the following?
   a. Primary care settings
   b. A patient-centered approach
   c. Use of health information technology
   d. Evidence-based practice

9. The link between adverse patient outcomes and cleanliness was discovered by:
   a. W. Edwards Deming
   b. Florence Nightingale
   c. Isabel Hampton Robb
   d. Dorothea Dix

10. Three components of health care systems are:
   a. strategy, outcome, and performance
   b. process, strategy, and opportunity
   c. structure, process, and outcome
   d. outcome, procedure, and structure

REVIEW QUESTION ANSWERS

1. Answer: D is correct.
   Rationale: The national organization that accredits health care organizations is known as (D) Joint Commission. (A) The ANA is the professional nurses association. (B) Health professions Commission, and (C) the Agency for Health Care Research and Quality do not accredit health care organizations.

2. Answer D: is correct.
   Rationale: The largest purchaser of health care in America is (D) Medicare, Medicaid, and other governmental programs. (A) Private individuals, (B) Private insurance companies, and (C) Health Maintenance Organizations are not the largest purchaser.

3. Answer: B is correct.
   Rationale: (B) Donabedian identified a structure, process, and outcome framework for quality. The others, (A) Nightingale, (C) Starr, and (D) Lohr did not.

4. Answer: A is correct.
   Rationale: (A) Socioeconomic status is the top underlying cause of health care disparity in the United States, so (B) age, (C) geographical location, or (D) chronic illness are all incorrect.

5. Answer: A is correct.
   Rationale: Payment for health care services as a fixed dollar amount per member over a period of time is referred to as (A) traditional fee for services, so not (B) prospective payment system, (C) capitation, or (D) diagnostic related groupings.

6. Answer: B, C, D, E, and F are correct answers.
   Rationale: The Patient Protection and Affordable Care Act provides comprehensive health care reform through a number of initiatives, including all except (A) restricting in-patient hospital stays. (B) Expanding health insurance coverage, (C) targeting fraud, abuse, and waste in health care, (D) increasing access to primary care services, and (E) promoting preventive health strategies, are all correct.

7. Answer: A, B, C, D, and E are correct answers.
   Rationale: Key factors contributing to rising health care costs in the United States include (A) an aging population, (B) advancements in technology, (C) increased utilization of pharmaceuticals, (D) rising costs of primary care, and (E) administrative costs.

8. Answer: A is correct.
   Rationale: The competencies for the education of health care professionals recommended by the Institute of Medicine to improve the quality of health care include all except (A) primary care settings. They do include (B) a patient-centered approach, (C) use of health information technology, or (D) evidence-based practice.

9. Answer: B is correct.
   Rationale: The link between adverse patient outcomes and cleanliness was discovered by (B) Florence Nightingale, not (A) W. Edwards Deming, (C) Isabel Hampton Robb, or (D) Dorthea Dix.

10. Answer: C is correct.
    Rational: The three components of health care systems are: (1) *structure* (resources or "structures" required to deliver health care), (2) *process* (quality activities, procedures, and tasks performed to deliver quality health care), and (3) *outcome* (the results of good health care delivery). Therefore (A), (B), and D are all incorrect.

REVIEW ACTIVITIES

1. Although it is difficult to modify the entire structure of health care in the U.S., what could you do to modify the process of health care delivery to improve health care quality in your organization?

2. What strategies can be used to ensure patient access to appropriate health care services in public and private health care agencies?

3. How can the five IOM health professions competencies and the need for safe, high-quality care be achieved in health care organizations?

DISCUSSION POINTS

1. Are all adverse events inevitable?

2. How is the FDA involved in improving patient safety?

3. Do sentinel events have to be reported to TJC?

4. What are the similarities in the measures of patient safety and the measures of quality of care?

5. Should only events that harm patients be reported to external quality and safety organizations?

6. Do patients have better outcomes when they stay in the hospital longer?

7. Name three of the QSEN competencies.

8. Does blaming a nurse for an error improve patient safety?

9. Name the six aims of the health care system from the IOM Crossing the Quality Chasm 2001 report.

10. Is improving quality and patient safety expensive?

DISCUSSION OF OPENING SCENARIO

With the ongoing debate about the cost and importance of everyone throughout the nation having access to health care, regardless of ability to pay, concern continues among the disadvantaged or low income groups about their future ability to access health care services. Unfortunately, this is a common scenario for all too many Americans. As the only industrialized nation in the world without UHC, the rising costs of health care, and the challenges of being able to access care at any time or any place, many in our nation will continue to be exposed to situations where the outcomes could have been better. As nurses, we may assume that patients will do the right thing when it comes to their health or the health of those that depend upon them. With experience and understanding of health care research, we know this is not always the case. We have tremendous opportunities to make needed changes in how health care can be accessed and payed for, as well as helping patients understand how they can best navigate the health care system.

EXPLORING THE WEB

FEDERAL GOVERNMENT:

- Agency for Healthcare Research and Quality (AHRQ): www.ahrq.gov

- Centers for Disease Control and Prevention (CDC): www.cdc.gov

- Centers for Medicare and Medicaid Services (CMS): www.cms.gov

- Department of Defense (DOD) TRICARE program: www.tricare.mil

- Food and Drug Administration (FDA): www.fda.gov

- Health Resources and Services Administration (HRSA): www.hrsa.gov

- Indian Health Service (IHS): www.ihs.gov

- National Center for Health Statistics: www.cdc.gov. Search for National Center for Health Statistics.

- National Guidelines Clearinghouse: www.guidelines.gov

- National Institutes of Health (NIH): www.nih.gov

- Substance Abuse and Mental Health Services Administration (SAMHSA): www.samhsa.gov

- Veterans' Health Administration (VHA): www.va.gov

PRIVATE FOUNDATIONS AND ORGANIZATIONS:

- Commonwealth Fund: www.cmwf.org

- Henry J. **Kaiser Family Foundation** (KFF): www.kff.org

- Joint Commission (JC): www.jointcommission.org

- National Committee for Quality Assurance (NCQA): www.ncqa.org

- National Quality Forum (NQF): www.qualityforum.org

- Robert Wood Johnson Foundation (RWJF): www.rwjf.org

- **Malcolm Baldridge Quality Award** (MBQA): www.quality.nist.gov

INFORMATICS

- **Visit the** Centers for Medicare and Medicaid Services Innovation Center: https://innovation.cms.gov and review the innovation models and see where the partners are located. You can share your ideas here as well.

LEAN BACK

- Although it is difficult to modify the structure of health care, what could you do to implement a system to continually modify the process of health care delivery to improve health care quality in your organization?

- What are strategies to ensure patient access to appropriate health care services in public and private health care agencies?

- How can the five IOM health professions competencies and the need for safe, high-quality care be achieved in the current workplace?

REFERENCES

Abimanyi-Ochom, A., Jones, M., & Cheng, H. (2019). *Never events*. Retrieved from https://psnet.ahrq.gov/primer/never-events

Adams, D. F., Fraser, D. B., & Abrams, H. L. (1973). The complications of coronary arteriography. *Circulation, 48*(3), 609–618.

Agency for Healthcare Research and Quality (AHRQ). (2008b). National healthcare quality report. Rockville, MD: Author. Retrieved August 4, 2008, from HYPERLINK "http://www.ahrq.gov/qual" http://www.ahrq.gov/qual/qrdr07.htm#toc

Agency for Healthcare Research and Quality. (2019, September). *National Healthcare Disparities Report, 2018* (Rep. No. AHRQ Pub. No. 19-0070-EF). Retrieved https://www.ahrq.gov/sites/default/files/wysiwyg/research/findings/nhqrdr/2018qdr-final.pdf

AHA. (2019). *Fast facts on U.S. Hospitals, 2019: AHA*. Retrieved from https://www.ahrq.gov/sites/default/files/wysiwyg/research/findings/nhqrdr/2018qdr-final.pdf

AHRQ. (2006). *National healthcare disparities report, 2005*. Retrieved from https://archive.ahrq.gov/qual/nhdr05/fullreport/Index.htm

AHRQ. (2011). *Types of health care quality measures*. Retrieved from www.ahrq.gov/talkingquality/measures/types.html

AHRQ. (2019). *2018 National healthcare quality and disparities report*. Retrieved from www.ahrq.gov/research/findings/nhqrdr/nhqdr18/index.html

Alberta Health and Wellness. (2004). *Health care insurance plan*. Edmonton, AL: Government of Alberta. Retrieved from www.health.alberta.ca

American Nurses Association (ANA). (1995). *Nursing care report card for acute care*. Washington, DC: American Nurses Association.

Anderson, D. J., Kirkland, K. B., Kayes, K. S., Thacker, P. A., Kanafani, Z. A., & Sexton, D. J. (2007). Under-resourced hospital infection control and prevention programs: Penny wise, pound foolish? *Infection Control and Hospital Epidemiology, 28*(7), 767–773. doi:10.1086/518518

Anderson, G. F., Hussey, P. S., Frogner, B. K., & Waters, H. R. (2005). Health spending in the United States and the rest of the industrialized world. *Health Affairs, 24*(4), 903–914.

Bazzoli, G. J., Gerland, A., & May, J. (2006). Construction activity in U.S. hospitals. *Health Affairs, 25*(3), 783–791.

Berwick, D. M. (1994). Eleven worthy aims for clinical leadership of health system reform. *Journal of the American Medical Association, 272*, 797–802.

Boddenheimer, T. (2005a). High and rising health care costs. Part 1: Seeking an explanation. *Annals of Internal Medicine, 142*(10), 847–854.

Boddenheimer, T. (2005b). High and rising health care costs. Part 2: Technologic innovation. *Annals of Internal Medicine, 142*(11), 932–937.

Brook, R. H., Kamberg, C., & McGlynn, E. (1996). Health System Reform and Quality. *JAMA: The Journal of the American Medical Association, 276*(6), 476. doi:10.1001/jama.1996.03540060052035

Calvocoressi, L., Kasl, S. V., Lee, C. H., Stolar, M., Claus, E. B., & Jones, B. A. (2004). A prospective study of perceived susceptibility to breast cancer and nonadherence to mammography screening guidelines in African American and white women ages 40 to 79 years. *Cancer Epidemiology Biomarkers Preview, 13*(12), 2096–2105.

Canadian Institute for Health Information (CIHI). (2006). *CIHI looks at how Canada measures up in health spending*. Ottawa, ON: Canadian Institute for Health Information. Retrieved from www.cihi.ca/cihiweb/en/downloads/Dir_Wint06_ENG.pdf

Canadian Institute for Health Information. (2018). *Wait Times for Priority Procedures in Canada, 2018: Technical Notes* (ISBN 978-1-77109-677-5 (PDF), pp. 1–10, Rep.). Ottawa, ON: Canadian Institute for Health Information. Retrieved June 19, 2020, from https://secure.cihi.ca/free_products/wt2018-tech-notes-2018-en-web.pdf

Centers for Disease Control and Prevention (CDC). (2018a). *Data portal | HAI | CDC*. Retrieved from www.cdc.gov/hai/data/portal/index.html

CDC. (2018b). *Data portal | HAI | CDC*. Retrieved from www.cdc.gov/hai/data/portal/index.html

CDC. (2019). *FastStats: deaths and mortality*. Retrieved from www.cdc.gov/nchs/fastats/deaths.htm

Chassin, M. R., & Galvin, R. W. (1998). The urgent need to improve health care quality: Institute of Medicine National Roundtable on Health Care Quality. *The Journal of the American Medical Association, 280*, 1000–1005.

CMS. (2018). *Population predictions*. Retrieved from www.cms.gov/Research-Statistics-Data-and-Systems/Statistics-Trends-and-Reports/NationalHealthExpendData

CMS. (2019). *CMS office of the actuary releases 2018-2027 projections of national health expenditures*. Retrieved from www.cms.gov/newsroom/press-releases/cms-office-actuary-releases-2018-2027-projections-national-health-expenditures

Collins, S. R., Bhupal, H., & Doty, M. (2019). *Health insurance coverage eight years after the ACA: commonwealth fund*. Retrieved from www.commonwealthfund.org/publications/issue-briefs/2019/feb/health-insurance-coverage-eight-years-after-aca

Commonwealth Fund. (2006). *International comparison: Access and timeliness*. New York: Commonwealth Fund. Retrieved from www.commonwealthfund.org/snapshotscharts/snapshotscharts_show.htm?doc_id=409110

Commonwealth Fund. (2012). *Scores dimensions of a high performance health system*. Retrieved from www.commonwealthfund.org/chart/scores-dimensions-high-performance-health-system

Commonwealth Fund. (2017). *New 11-country study: U.S. health care system has widest gap between people with higher and lower incomes*. Retrieved from www.commonwealthfund.org/press-release/2017/new-11-country-study-us-health-care-system-has-widest-gap-between-people-higher

Coons, S. J., Rao, S., Keininger, D. L., & Hays, R. D. (2000). *A comparative review of generic quality-of-life instruments*. Retrieved from www.ncbi.nlm.nih.gov/pubmed/10747763

Dieleman, J. L. (2017). *Factors associated with increases in US health care spending, 1996-2013*. Retrieved from https://jamanetwork.com/journals/jama/fullarticle/266157

Dossey, B., Selanders, L., & Beck, D. (2005). *Florence Nightingale today: Healing, leadership, global action*. Washington, DC: American Nurses Publishing.

Drummond, M. F., Stoddart, F. L., & Torrance, G. W. (1994). *Methods for the economic evaluation of health care programmes*. Oxford, UK: Oxford University Press.

Dunn, W. R., Lyman, S., & Marx, R. G. (2005). Small area variation in orthopedics. *Journal of Knee Surgery, 18*(1), 51–56.

Eastman, M. (2019). *Baldrige excellence framework (health care)*. Retrieved from www.nist.gov/baldrige/publications/baldrige-excellence-framework/health-care

Eisenberg, M. J. (2006). An American physican in the Canadian health care system. *Archives of Internal Medicine, 166*, 281–282.

GoodRx. (2019). Prescription prices, coupons & pharmacy information. Retrieved from www.goodrx.com

Green, L. A., Gryer, G. E., Yawn, B. P., Lanier, D., & Dovery, S. M. (2000). The ecology of medical care revisited. *New England Journal of Medicine, 344*, 2021–2025.

Greenfield, S., Nelson, E. C., Zubkoff, M., Manning, W., Rogers, W., Kravitz, R. L., Keller, A., Tarlov, J. E., & Ware, J. (1992). Variations in resource utilization among medical specialties and systems of care. Results from the medical outcomes study. *Journal of the American Medical Association, 267*(12), 1624–1630.

Hamilton, K. (2003). The four levels of evidence based practice. *Healthcare Design, 3*, 18–26.

Harbarth, S., & Gastmeier, P. (2003). The preventable portion of nosocomial infections: An overview of published reports. *Journal of Hospital Infection, 53*(4), 258–266.

Health Workforce Solutions LLC & Robert Wood Johnson Foundation. (2008). *Innovative care models.* Retrieved from www.innovativecaremodels.com/about/about

Healthy People 2020. (2010). *U.S. Department of Health and Human Services.* Retrieved from www.healthypeople.gov/2020/about/default.aspx

Himmelstein, D. U. (2014). *A comparison of hospital administrative costs in eight nations: U.S. costs exceed all others by far.* Retrieved from www.commonwealthfund.org/publications/journal-article/2014/sep/comparison-hospital-administrative-costs-eight-nations-us

Himmelstein, D. U., Warren, E., Thorne, D., & Woolhandler, S. (2005). Illness and injury as contributors to bankruptcy. *Health Affairs*, W5–63. Retrieved from http://content.healthaffairs.org/cgi/content/abstract/hlthaff.w5.63v1

Institute of Medicine (IOM). (1996). *Primary care: America's health in a new era.* Washington, DC: National Academy Press.

IOM. (1999). *To err is human.* Washington, DC: National Academy Press.

IOM. (2001). *Crossing the quality chasm: A new health system for the 21st century.* Washington, DC: National Academy Press.

IOM. (2003b). *Health professions education: A bridge to quality.* Available at www.iom.edu/?id=35961

IOM. (2004a). *Evidence-based hospital design improves healthcare outcomes for patients, families, and staff.* Washington, DC: National Academy Press.

IOM. (2004b). *Insuring America's health: Principles and recommendations.* Washington, DC: National Academy Press.

IOM. (2008). Committee on reviewing evidence to identify highly effective clinical services). *Knowing what works in health care: A roadmap for the nation* (pp. 1–276). Washington, DC: National Academies Press. 978-0-309-11356-4

IOM. (2010). *The healthcare imperative: Lowering costs and improving outcomes: Workshop series summary.* Washington, DC: The National Academies Press. doi:10.17226/12750

Joines, J. D., Hertz-Picciotto, I., Carey, T. S., Gesler, W., & Suchindran, C. (2003). A spatial analysis of count-level variation in hospitalization rates for low back problems in North Carolina. *Social Science and Medicine, 56*(12), 2541–2553.

Kaiser Family Foundation (KFF). (2010). *Focus on health reform.* Summary of New Health Reform law, Patient Protection and Affordable Care Act (P.L. 111-148). March 26, 2010. Retrieved from www.kff.org/healthreform/8061.cfm

Kaiser Family Foundation. (2018). Kaiser Family Foundation-Health Research and Educational Trust Annual Employer Survey (Rep.). Retrieved October 20, 2020, from Kaiser Family Foundation website: http://files.kff.org/attachment/Report-Employer-Health-Benefits-Annual-Survey-2018

Kovner, E. T., Brewer, C. S., Yingrengreung, S., Fairchild, S., et al. (2010). New nurses: views of quality improvement education. *Joint Commission Journal of Quality and Patient Safety.* January 26, 29–35.

Laschinger, H. K. S., & Leiter, M. P. (2006). The impact of nursing work environments on patient safety outcomes: The mediating role of burnout/engagement. *Journal of Nursing Administration, 36*(5), 259–267.

Leape, L. L. (1992). Unnecessary surgery. *Annual Review of Public Health, 13*, 363–383.

Leape, L. L., Park, R. E., Solomon, D. H., Chassin, M. R., Kisecoff, J., & Brook, R. H. (1990). Does inappropriate use explain small area variations in the use of health care services? *Journal of the American Medical Association, 263*, 669–672.

Li, Y., Hu, Y. L. F. B., Liu, X., Dhana, K., Franco, O. H., et al. (2018). *Impact of healthy lifestyle factors on life expectancies in the US population.* Retrieved from www.ahajournals.org/doi/full/10.1161/CIRCULATIONAHA.117.032047

Magnan, S. (2017). *Social determinants of health 101 for health care: Five plus five.* NAM Perspectives. Retrieved from https://nam.edu/social-determinants-of-health-101-for-health-care-five-plus-five

Marshall, M. N., Hiscock, J., & Sibbald, B. (2002). Attitudes to the public release of comparative information on the quality of general practice care: A qualitative study. *British Medical Journal, 325*(7375), 1278.

Martin, J. A., Hamilton, B. E., Sutton, P. D., & Ventura, S. J. (2006). *Births: Final data for 2004.* National vital statistics reports, 55(1). Hyattsville, MD: National Center for Health Statistics.

McGlynn, E. A., Asch, S. M., Adams, J., Keesey, J., Hicks, J., DeCristofaro, A., Kerr, E. A. (2003). The quality of health care delivered to adults in the United States. *New England Journal of Medicine, 348*, 2635–2645.

Mikulic, M. (2019). MRI units density by country 2017. Retrieved from www.statista.com/statistics/282401/density-of-magnetic-resonance-imaging-units-by-country

Muto, C., Harrison, E., Edward, J. R., Horan, T., Andus, M., Jernigan, J. A., & Kutty, P. K. (2005). Reduction in central line-associated bloodstream infections among intensive care units—Pennsylvania, April 2001–March 2005. *MMWR. Morbidity and Mortality Weekly Report, 54*(40), 1013–1016. Retrieved from /www.cdc.gov/mmwr/preview/mmwrhtml/mm5440a2.htm

National Coalition on Health Care (NCHC). (2008). *World health care data.* Retrieved from www.nchc.org/facts/world/shtml

NHE. (2019). *NHE-fact-sheet.* Retrieved from www.cms.gov/research-statistics-data-and-systems/statistics-trends-and-reports/nationalhealthexpenddata/nhe-fact-sheet.html

Nightingale, F. (1865/1970). *Notes on nursing.* Princeton: NJ: Vertex.

Nolte, E., & McKee, C. M. (2008). Measuring the health of nations: Updating an earlier analysis. *Health Affairs, 27*(1), 58–71.

Norman, L. D., Donelan, K., Buerhaus, P. I., Willis, G., Williams, M., Ulrich, B., et al. (2005). The older nurse in the workplace: Does age matter? *Nursing Economics, 23*(6), 282–289, 279

Office of the Legislative Counsel. 111th Congress, 2d Session. (2010). Compilation of the patient protection and affordable care act, as amended through May 1, 2010, including the patient protection and affordable care act and health related portions of the health care and education reconciliation act of 2010, Retrieved from http://docs.house.gov/energycommerce/ppacacon.pdf.

Organization of Economic Co-operation and Development (OECD). (2019). *Health at a glance 2019: OECD indicators.* Paris: OECD Publishing. doi:10.1787/4dd50c09-en

Papanicolas, I., Woskie, L.R., & Jha, A. (2018). *Health care spending in the United States and other high-income countries.* The Commonwealth Fund.

Retrieved from www.commonwealthfund.org/publications/journal-article/2018/mar/health-care-spending-united-states-and-other-high-income

Pruitt, S. D., & Epping-Jordan, J. E. (2005). Preparing the 21st century global healthcare workforce. *British Medical Journal, 330*(7492), 637–639. doi:10.1136/bmj.330.7492.637

Radley, D., Hayes, S. L., & Collins, S. R. (2019). 2019 Scorecard on state health system performance: Deaths from suicide, alcohol, drugs on the rise; Progress expanding health care coverage stalls. In *Health Costs Are a Growing Burden*. Retrieved from www.commonwealthfund.org/publications/fund-reports/2019/jun/2019-scorecard-state-health-system-performance-deaths-suicide

Ramirez, M. (2019). *How has the quality of the U.S. healthcare system changed over time?* Retrieved from www.healthsystemtracker.org/chart-collection/how-has-the-quality-of-the-u-s-healthcare-system-changed-over-time/#item-start

Ramsey, L. (2019). *Healthcare CEOs make as much as $26 million a year.* Here's what the industry's top executives earned in 2018. Retrieved from www.businessinsider.com/pharma-and-healthcare-ceo-compensation-2018-2019

Reid, T. R. (2009). *5 myths about health care around the world.* Sunday, August 23, 2009. The Washington Post Company. Retrieved from www.washingtonpost.com/wp-dyn/content/article/2009/08/21/AR2009082101778.html

Rudowitz, R., Orgera, K., & Hinton, E. (2019). Medicaid financing: The basics. Retrieved from https://www.kff.org/medicaid/issue-brief/medicaid-financing-the-basics/view/print

Safran, D. G., Rogers, W. H., Tarlov, A. R., McHorney, C. A., & Ware, J. E., Jr. (1997). Gender differences in medical treatment: The case of physician-prescribed activity restrictions. *Social Science & Medicine, 45*(5), 711–722.

Salary Comparison, Salary Survey, Search Wages. (2019). Retrieved from www.payscale.com

Sawyer, B., Claxton, G., & Kaiser, G. (2016). *How do health expenditures vary across the population?*. Retrieved from www.healthsystemtracker.org/chart-collection/health-expenditures-vary-across-population

Sawyer, B., & Cox, C. (2018). *How does health spending in the U.S. compare to other countries?* Peterson-Kaiser Health System Tracker. Accessible at www.healthsystemtracker.org/chart-collection/health-spending-u-s-compare-countries

Sawyer, B., McDermott, D. & Kaiser, G. (2019). *How does the quality of the U.S. healthcare system compare to other countries?* Retrieved from www.healthsystemtracker.org/chart-collection/quality-u-s-healthcare-system-compare-countries/#item-start

Sawyer, B., Sroczynski, N., & Kaiser, G. (2016). *How do U.S. health care resources compare to other countries?* Retrieved from www.healthsystemtracker.org/chart-collection/u-s-health-care-resources-compare-countries/#item-u-s-fewer-acute-care-hospital-beds-per-capita-many-comparable-countries

Schulte, M. F. (2011). *Healthcare Delivery in the U.S.A.: An Introduction.* Productivity Press.

Shapiro, J. (2008). *Health care lessons from France.* Washington,DC: National Public Radio. Retrieved from www.npr.org/templates/story/story.php?storyId=91972152

Starfield, B. (1998). *Primary care: Balancing health needs, services, and technology.* New York: Oxford University Press.

Starr, P. (1983). *The social transformation of American medicine.* Jackson, TN: Basic Books.

The Center for Health Design. 2011. *Pebble project.* Available at www.healthdesign.org/research/pebble/overview.php

The Joint Commission. (2008). *Improving America's Hospitals The Joint Commission's Annual Report on Quality and Safety 2008* (pp. 1–134, Rep.). OakbrookTerrace, IL: The Joint Commission. Retrieved from www.jointcommission.org/-/media/tjc/documents/accred-and-cert/pathway-to-accreditation/hospital/annual-report/2008_annual_reportpdf.pdf?db=web&hash=893DE75B9CC367CC6CAADBAAE35F67D3.

The WorldBank. (2018). *Life expectancy at birth, total (years) 2018 Data.* Retrieved from https://data.worldbank.org/indicator/SP.DYN.LE00.IN

Thomas, E. J., Studdert, D. M., Burstin, H. R., Orav, E. J., Zeena, T., et al. (2000). Incidence and types of adverse events and negligent care in Utah and Colorado. *Medical Care, 38*, 261–271.

Tikkanen, R. (2018). Multinational comparisons of health systems data, 2018. Retrieved from www.commonwealthfund.org/sites/default/files/2018-12/MultinationalComparisons of Health Systems Data 2018_RTikkanen_final.pdf

Tilson, H., & Berkowitz, B. (2006). The public health enterprise: Examining our twenty-first century policy challenges. *Health Affairs, 25*(4), 900–910.

Timmermans, S., & Mauck, A. (2005). The promises and pitfalls of evidence-based medicine. *Health Affairs, 24*(1), 18–28.

U.S. Department of Health and Human Services. (1996). *Summary of the health insurance portability and accountability act (HIPAA) privacy rule*, available at www.hhs.gov/ocr/privacy

U.S. Department of Health and Human Services. (2010). Healthy people 2020. ODPHP Publication No. B0132 [Brochure]. Retrieved from www.healthypeople.gov/sites/default/files/HP2020_brochure_with_LHI_508_FNL.pdf

Ulrich, R., Quan, X., Zimring, C., Joseph, A., & Choudhary, R. (2004). *The role of the physical environment in the hospital of the 21st century.* Concord, CA: Center for Health Design.

US Census Bureau. (2019). *Population projections.* Retrieved from www.census.gov/programs-surveys/popproj.html

US News & World Report. (2019). *The 80 countries with the highest quality of life.* Retrieved from www.usnews.com/news/best-countries/quality-of-life-rankings

Waxman, K. T. (2008). *A practical guide to finance and budgeting: Skills for nurse managers* (2nd ed.). Marblehead, MA: HCPro.

Wennberg, J. E., & Gittelsohn, A. M. (1973). Small area variations in health care delivery. *Science, 182*(117), 1102–1108.

WHO. (2010). *Chronic disease and health promotion.* Retrieved from www.who.int/chp/en

WHO. (2019). About us. Retrieved from www.who.int/healthpromotion/about/goals/en

Williams, S. C., Schmaltz, S. P., Morton, D. J., Koss, R. G., & Loeb, J. M. (2005). Quality of care in U.S. hospitals as reflected by standard measures, 2003–2004. *New England Journal of Medicine, 353*(3), 255–264.

Woo, A., Ranji, U., Lundy, J., & Chen, F. (2007). *Prescription drug costs.* Menlo Park: Kaiser Family Foundation. Retrieved from www.kaiseredu.org/topics_im.asp?id=352&parentID=68&imID=1

World Health Organization (WHO). (2008). *The world health report: 2008 primary health care—Now more than ever.* Retrieved from www.who.int/whr/2008/whr08_en.pdf

SUGGESTED READINGS

Administration of Aging. (2010). *Health System Reform: Nursing's Goal of High Quality, Affordable Care for All [Brochure].* Silver Spring, MD: Administration of Aging. Retrieved from www.nursingworld.org/~4afd55/globalassets/practiceandpolicy/health-policy/health-system-reform---final--haney---6-10-10.pdf

Administration of Aging American Nurses Association. (2019). *About ANA.* American Nurses Association. Accessible at www.nursingworld.org/ana/about-ana

Agency for Healthcare Research and Quality (AHRQ). (2008a). *National healthcare disparities report.* Rockville, MD: Agency for Healthcare Research and Quality. Retrieved from www.ahrq.gov/qual/qrdr07.htm

AHRQ. (2008b). *National healthcare quality report.* Rockville, MD: Agency for Healthcare Research and Quality. Retrieved from www.ahrq.gov/qual/qrdr07.htm#toc

American Association for Accreditation of Ambulatory Surgery Facilities (AAAASF). (2001). *About AAAASF.* Retrieved from, www.aaaasf.org/aboutAAAAst/about.cfm

American Nurses Association (ANA). (1995). *Nursing care report card for acute care.* Washington, DC: American Nurses Association.

Anderson, R. M., Rice, T. H., & Kominski, G. F. (2007). *Changing the U.S. health care system: Key issues in health services policy and management* (3rd ed.). San Francisco, CA: Jossey-Bass.

Brown, M. A., Draye, M. A., Zimmer, P. A., Magyary, D., Woods, S. L., et al. (2006). Developing a practice doctorate in nursing: University of Washington perspectives and experience. *Nursing Outlook, 54*(3), 130–138.

Baldridge National Quality Program. (2010). *Health care criteria for performance excellence.* Gaithersburg, MD: Baldridge National Quality Program.

Berwick, D. M. (2002). A user's manual for the IOM's "quality chasm" report. *Health Affairs, 21*(3), 80–90.

Buerhaus, P. I., & Staiger, D. O. (1999). Trouble in the nurse labor market? Recent trends and future outlook. *Health Affairs, 18*(1), 214–222.

CDC. (2018c). *National Center for Health Statistics. Health, United States, 2017: With special feature on mortality. National Center for Health Statistics. Health, United States, 2017: With special feature on mortality.* Retrieved from www.cdc.gov/nchs/data/hus/hus17.pdf

CDC. (2018d). *Social determinants of health: Know what affects health.* Accessible at www.cdc.gov/socialdeterminants/index.htm

CDC. (2019). *Health and economic costs of chronic disease.* Retrieved from www.cdc.gov/chronicdisease/about/costs/index.htm

CDC. (2010). *Nursing home care.* Retrieved from www.cdc.gov/nchs/fastats/nuringh.htm

Centers for Medicare and Medicaid Services (CMS). (2006a). *2006 Annual report of the boards of trustees of the federal hospital insurance and federal supplementary medical insurance trust funds.* Retrieved from www.cms.hhs.gov/ReportsTrustFunds/downloads/tr2006.pdf

Centers for Medicare and Medicaid Services, Office of the Actuary, National Health Statistics Group. (2006b). Retrieved from www.cms.hhs.gov/NationalHealthExpendData/downloads/PieChartSourcesExpenditures2004.pdf

Centers for Medicare and Medicaid Services, Office of the Actuary, National Health Statistics Group. (2006c). Retrieved from www.cms.hhs.gov/NationalHealthExpendData

Centers for Medicare and Medicaid Services (CMS). (2006d). *Historical national health expenditure data.* Retrieved from www.cms.hhs.gov/NationalHealthExpendData/02_NationalHealthAccountsHistorical.asp#TopOfPage

Centers for Medicare and Medicaid Services (CMS). (2010). Retrieved from www.cms.gov/NationalHealthExpendData/downloads/proj2009.pdf

Cooper, R. A., Getzen, T. E., McKee, H. M., & Laud, P. (2002). Economic and demographic trends signal an impending physician shortage. *Health Affairs, 21*(1), 140–154.

Department of Defense (DOD). (2003). *TRICARE: The basics.* Retrieved from www.tricare.mil/Factsheets/viewfactsheet.cfm?id=127.

Diagnosis-Related Group. (2009). Available at en.wikipedia.org/wiki/Diagnosis-related_group#References

Donabedian, A. (1966). Evaluating the quality of medical care. *Milbank Quarterly, 20*(1), 137–141.

Dracup, K., Cronenwett, L., Meleis, A. I., & Benner, P. E. (2005). Reflections on the doctorate of nursing practice. *Nursing Outlook, 53*(4), 177–182.

Draye, M. A., Acker, M., & Zimmer, P. A. (2006). The practice doctorate in nursing: Approaches to transform nurse practitioner education and practice. *Nursing Outlook, 54*(3), 123–129.

Frogner, B. & Anderson, G. (2006). *Multinational comparisons of health systems data, 2005.* The Commonwealth Fund. Retrieved from www.commonwealthfund.org/~/media/Files/Publications/Chartbook/2006/Apr/Multinational%20Comparisons%20of%20Health%20Systems%20Data%20%202005/825_Frogner_multinational_complhtsysdata%20pdf.pdf

Ginsburg, P. B. (2003). Can hospitals and physicians shift the effects of cuts in Medicare reimbursement to private payers? *Health Affairs, W3,* 472–479.

GovTrack. (2010). *Health care and education reconciliation act of 2010. GovTrack.* Available at www.govtrack.us/congress/bill.xpd?bill=h111-4872

IOM. (2003a). *Priority areas for national action: Transforming health care quality.* Available at www.iom.edu/?id=35961

IOM. (2003c). *Keeping patients safe: Transforming the work environment of nurses.* Available at www.iom.edu/?id=35961

IOM. (2003d). *Patient safety: Achieving a new standard for care.* Available at www.iom.edu/?id=35961

IOM. (2005). *Performance measurement: Accelerating improvement.* Available at www.iom.edu/CMS/2955.aspx?show=0;3#LP3

IOM. (2006). *Preventing medication errors: Quality chasm series.* Available at www.iom.edu/?id=35961

Jha, A. K., Li, Z., Orav, E. J., & Epstein, A. M. (2005). Care in U.S. hospitals—The Hospital Quality Alliance program. *New England Journal of Medicine, 353*(3), 265–274.

Kahn, C. N., Ault, T., Isenstein, H., Potetz, L., & Van Gelder, S. (2006). Snapshot of hospital quality reporting and pay-for-performance under Medicare. *Health Affairs, 25*(1), 148–162.

Kaiser Family Foundation (KFF) and Health Research and Education Trust. (2007). *Employer health benefits: 2007 annual survey.* Publication number 7672. Retrieved from www.kff.org

Kaiser Family Foundation (KFF) and Health Research and Education Trust. (2009). *Employer health benefits: 2009 annual survey.* Publication number 7936. Retrieved from www.kff.org

Kaiser Family Foundation (KFF). (2006). *The uninsured: A primer. Key facts about Americans without health insurance.* Publication number 7451-02. Retrieved from www.kff.org

Kaiser Family Foundation (KFF). (2007a). *Trends in health care costs and spending*. Menlo Park: Kaiser Family Foundation. Retrieved from www.kff.org/insurance/upload/7692.pdf

Kaiser Family Foundation (KFF). (2007b). *Health care spending in the United States and Organisation for Economic Co-operation and Development (OECD) countries*. Retrieved from www.kff.org/insurance/snapshot/chcm010307oth.cfm

Kaiser Family Foundation (KFF). (2008). *Addressing the nursing shortage*. Retrieved from www.kaiseredu.org/topics_im.asp?imID=1&parentID=61&id=138

Kaiser Family Foundation (KFF). (2010). *Summary of new health reform law*. Publication Number 8061. Retrieved from www.kff.org

Kaiser Family Foundation (KFF). (2005). *Navigating Medicare and Medicaid, 2005: Medicaid*. Washington, DC: Kaiser Family Foundation. Accessible at www.kff.org/medicare/7240/medicaid.cfm

Kaiser Family Foundation (KFF). (2006). *The uninsured: Key facts about Americans without health insurance*. Washington, DC: Kaiser Family Foundation. Accessible at www.kff.org/uninsured/upload/7451-021.pdf

Mundinger, M. O. (2005). Who's who in nursing: Bringing clarity to the doctor of nursing practice. *Nursing Outlook, 53*, 173–176.

National Bureau of Economic Research. (2006). *Healthcare expenditures in the OECD*. Retrieved from www.nber.org/aginghealth/winter06/w11833.html

National Healthcare Disparities Report (NHDR). (2008). Rockville, MD: Agency for Healthcare, Research and Quality. Retrieved from www.ahrq.gov/qual/nhdr08/nhdr08.htm

National Healthcare Quality Report (NHQR). (2009). Rockville, MD: Agency for Healthcare, Research and Quality. Retrieved from www.ahrq.gov/qual/nhqr09/nhqr09.htm

Organisation for Economic Co-operation and Development. (2008). *OECD health data 2008: How does Japan compare*. Paris: Organisation for Economic Co-operation and Development. Retrieved from www.oecd.org/document/46/0,3343,en_2649_33929_34971438_1_1_1_1,00.html

The Commonwealth Fund. (2017, July 13). *New 11-country study: U.S. Health Care System Has Widest Gap Between People with Higher and Lower Incomes*. Retrieved from www.commonwealthfund.org/press-release/2017/new-11-country-study-us-health-care-system-has-widest-gap-between-people-higher

U.S. Department of Health and Human Services. (2000). *Healthy people 2010: Understanding and improving health* (2nd ed.). Washington, DC: U.S. Government Printing Office. Retrieved from www.usnews.com/news/best-countries/quality-of-life-rankings

U.S. Department of Health and Human Services. (2006). *Annual update of the HHS poverty guidelines*. Accessible at http://aspe.hhs.gov/poverty/06fedreg.pdf

Ware, J. E., & Sherbourne, C. D. (1992). The MOS 36-item short form health survey I: Conceptual framework and item selection. *Medical Care, 30*, 473–478.

WHO & UNICEF. (2018). *A vision for primary health care in the 21st century: towards universal health coverage and the Sustainable Development Goals*. Retrieved from https://apps.who.int/iris/handle/10665/328065

World Health Organization (WHO). (2000). *The world health report 2000—Health systems: Improving performance* (pp. 27–35). Geneva: World Health Organization.

WHO. (2008). Cuba's primary care revolution: 30 years on. *Bulletin of the World Health Organization, 86*(5), 321–416. Retrieved from www.who.int/bulletin/volumes/86/5/08-030508/en/index.html

World Population Review. (2019). *Best healthcare in the World population*. Retrieved from http://worldpopulationreview.com/countries/best-healthcare-in-the-world

Yong, P., Saunders, R., & Olsen, L. (2010). *Healthcare imperative: Lowering costs and improving outcomes: Workshop series summary* [National Institutes of Health]. doi: www.nap.edu/catalog/12750.html

3

Nursing Leadership and Management in a Historical Context

Brigid Lusk, PhD, RN, FAAN

Midwest Nursing History Research Center, University of Illinois at Chicago, College of Nursing, Chicago, IL, USA

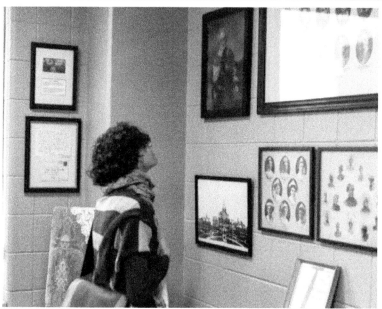

Rebecca Singer, new doctoral graduate, examines historical artifacts.
Source: Midwest Nursing History Research Center, University of Illinois at Chicago College of Nursing.

Why study nursing history? The answer lies in the work we do every day with the patients, families, and communities we serve. Understanding how early twentieth-century nursing leaders sought educational advancement in higher education, advocated health care policy reforms, supported immigrant populations, and developed innovative models of care offers much for the profession today.

Sandra Lewenson, PhD, RN, FAAN

OBJECTIVES

Upon completion of this chapter, the reader should be able to:

1. Discuss the founding of nursing.

2. Review the dawn of professional nursing.

3. Discuss visiting nurses and the birth of public health nursing.

4. Review the development of professional nursing organizations

5. Discuss evolving hospital nursing in the 1920s and 1930s.

6. Review evolving of professional nursing in the 1920s and 1930s.

Kelly Vana's Nursing Leadership and Management, Fourth Edition. Edited by Patricia Kelly Vana and Janice Tazbir
© 2021 John Wiley & Sons Ltd. Published 2021 by John Wiley & Sons Ltd.
Companion Website: www.wiley.com/go/kelly-Nursing-Leadership

7. Discuss collegiate education in nursing.

8. Review the development of nursing research in the 1950s to the 1970s.

9. Discuss emerging nursing specializations in the 1980s and 1990s.

10. Review historic contributions and future nursing challenges.

OPENING SCENARIO

You graduated about a year ago, as one of 10 male nurses in your class, and now work in the critical care unit of a major teaching hospital. Most of your work has been on the night shift. One evening, with a few nights off duty coming up, you go out with some friends from college. Talking with them, you realize that they don't have a clue about what you do. They joke that you must have entered nursing because of the numbers of eligible women. They have no idea of your responsibilities or your stress when at work. They don't know that a few nights back you diagnosed a probable pulmonary embolism and thus saved a young woman's life. They don't know that you calmed a hysterical man in the waiting room whose wife had just unexpectedly died. Most aggravating is their response when you tell them that you're planning to return to college for your doctorate—a PhD or a DNP, you're not sure yet—and they look amazed and exclaim "A nursing Dr.! Who knew?"

1. *Aside from wishing that your friends would be subjected to a nurse's care sooner rather than later, how can you succinctly describe the knowledge base of nursing to them?*

2. *What would you say to them about the need for nurses with doctorates?*

3. *Discuss the history of men and other minorities in nursing.*

Nursing history is the story of nursing care given through antiquity to the present day. The history of nurses and nursing can be fascinating but, with a nursing curriculum that is positively bursting at the seams, is history relevant and important enough to be included in all nursing educational programs? The answer is a resounding YES! Here's why: knowledge of nursing's history: (a) positively impacts patient care, (b) generates professional identity by reflecting the profession's history as well as the profession's current status, and thus contributing to career stability, (c) demands critical thinking, and (d) supports effective writing, a skill that is essential in nursing leadership. Additionally, the sheer fascination of reading nurses' notes written long ago or touching worn student nurses' uniforms—with patients' blood and students' sweat still visible on them—may be added to these reasons for studying the history of nursing.

Let's tackle these four reasons one by one, bearing in mind that they can't really be looked at separately. First, how can knowledge of nursing history positively impact patient care? One reason is that the patients' voices we "hear" through historic documents such as nurses' notes, or case studies, or in the meeting minutes of patient care committees, remind us that our patients are the *raison d'etre* of our work. In today's technological world this is sometimes forgotten. Another reason is that history is the basis for nursing practice research. For example, with current outbreaks of infectious diseases such as measles, nurses want to study ways to increase the percentage of childhood immunization. Yet any research on immunization rates would be flawed if nurses ignored the history of why parents had refused immunization for their children in the past. Historical research, such as that conducted by Lusk, Keeling, and Lewenson (2016), identified the critical interconnected variables of poverty, social class, ignorance, and fear of authority that was demonstrated during the forced smallpox vaccinations at the turn of the last century. Historical research provides the foundation for current nursing investigations

Second, nursing history generates **professional identity,** that is the public's understanding of what a nurse does, by reflecting the profession's history as well as the profession's current status, and thus career stability. Satisfying careers, whether in the arts or the sciences, usually have a history. Think of some familiar careers. Today's chemists or biologists or mathematicians proudly follow famed predecessors and carry part of their mystique. Likewise, artists of every stripe add to the acknowledged body of art that came before them. Knowing that nurses, too, have a long and rich history provides professional identity and commitment, thus leading to career stability. However, nursing history hasn't been adequately acknowledged, either within or outside the profession. Today's nurses and members of the public are not aware of nursing's rich and important past. That needs to change for everyone's benefit—including the patients. If nurses leave nursing because work that doesn't have a history isn't worth fighting for, then the nursing shortage continues and the patients suffer.

The third claim, that nursing history demands critical thinking, is based on the complexity of nursing's past. The history of nursing is not a linear progression from simple to advanced. For example, Florence Nightingale is revered as being the founder of modern nursing, but she was vehemently against registration for nurses. Taken at face value, that is probably shocking to most nurses today. Yet closer analysis of this issue by nurse historian Carol Helmstadter suggests that Nightingale had good reasons for objecting to nurse registration. Registration, Nightingale thought, would create an elite class of nurses who had the financial means to afford the requisite nursing education. Working-class nurses, the vast majority of nurses at the time, would be excluded. Further, Nightingale wisely understood that registration would legally place nurses under the authority of physicians, typically male, and thus limit nursing's female empowerment. Lastly, Nightingale found the state registration proposals for credentialing inadequate. She believed that registration, if attempted, should be more rigorous (Helmstadter, 2007). The registration issue, as are most issues, was nuanced, requiring critical thinking. Attempting to understand historical complexities serves as excellent preparation for understanding the intricacies of our patients and their care.

Finally, the last claim, that nursing history supports effective writing that is clear and convincing, was made because history requires reading—history is not a series of numbers or bullet points. With longer reading comes better analysis and writing skills. It is that simple. So that when you need to develop and fight for a plan, or you need to argue that person A is right for a position and person B is not, or when you are on a board promoting a health care initiative, reasoning and writing skills are imperative. Indeed, the need for effective writing is more relevant today, in this electronic age, than ever.

This chapter will give you selected highlights of the history of professional nursing in the United States. Other parts of the world have their own historical stories. Nurses who have excelled in leadership and management covering a range of workplaces will be featured as case studies. Critical thinking boxes will pose overtly nuanced scenarios chosen to illustrate that nursing practice is complex. The chapter will start with a discussion of the founding of nursing in the years before nurses received any kind of specialized training and close with a review of nursing's historic contributions and future nursing challenges. Nursing's history was affected by the role of women and women's place in society, social forces, industrialization, scientific awakening, and discrimination toward race and gender (negatively impacting minorities, women, and men). As former nursing dean Helen Grace wrote: "The struggles reflected in the development of nursing as a profession. . .mirror the struggles of women through the ages in defining a position of equality and worth" (Grace, 1978, p. 17).

The Founding of Nursing

Women and men practiced nursing whenever human beings gathered. Nurses helped people through illness, childbirth, and death. These nurses were often friends or family members or local women and men who were known for their healing and consoling skills. The past few hundred years have provided more evidence of these nurses' work as they gained in specialized knowledge. Military religious nursing orders, known as Hospitallers, were men who undertook nursing in the Crusades of the Middle Ages (Donahue, 2011). English midwives in the seventeenth century trained in unofficial midwifery apprenticeships and were licensed by the church (Evenden, 2000). Historian Nina Rattner Gelbart (1998) relays the fascinating history of Madame du Coudray who, on the orders of the King, traveled all over France educating midwives in the eighteenth century. For her teaching demonstrations, Du Coudray invented a model doll and pelvis, her "obstetrical machine," made of wicker, fabric, leather, stuffing, and sponges. From du Coudray's time through to the start of the nineteenth century, when medicine in Europe had become increasingly based on science, more educated nurses were needed (Helmstadter & Godden, 2011).

In the United States (U.S.), Native Americans had a long history of nursing their ill with natural remedies, rituals, and prayer when the European settlers arrived in the seventeenth century (Keeling, Hehman, & Kirchgessner, 2018). Unfortunately for these settlers, they chose to fight the Native Americans rather than learn from them. As the decades progressed and thousands of settlers had died through famine and/or disease, rudimentary order began to surface. The diary of Maine midwife, Martha Ballard, written from 1785 to 1812, offers a detailed and intimate picture of her work as meticulously presented by historian Laurel Thatcher Ulrich (1991). We learn that Ballard was a highly skilled midwife who delivered 816 babies over the 27-year period of her diary. She was also a wife, the mother of nine, and an accomplished nurse. Ulrich notes that Ballard "knew how to manufacture salves, syrups, pills, teas, and ointments, how to prepare an oil emulsion, how to poultice wounds, dress burns, treat dysentery, sore throat, frostbite, measles, colic, "Whooping Cough," [sic] "chin cough," "St. Vitus dance," "flying pains," the salt rhume," and "the itch," how to cut an infant's tongue, administer a "clyster" (enema), lance an abscessed breast, apply a "blister" or a "back plaster," induce vomiting, assuage bleeding, reduce swelling, and relieve a toothache, as well as deliver babies (Ulrich, 1991, p. 11).

We have less information about most other nurses' work, but there are some things to be elicited from surviving records. For example, Susanna Emlen's letters describing her breast amputation because of a tumor in 1814, without anesthesia of course, note that a nurse came with the surgeon, as well as his sister and his daughter. Four other doctors also attended. "About one o'clock," Emlen wrote, "Nurse Hooke came into the chamber I was in to tell me the Doctors waited my coming in my own room. She covered my head with a handkerchief, as she led me in, hoping it might save me the sight of the preparations—I however saw Dr. Dorsey with his sleeves tucked up and his cloaths [sic] covered with a large apron . . . .. My suffering was severe beyond expression" (Garfinkel, 1990, p. 21). We may extrapolate from this that Nurse Hooke was an experienced nurse. She was brought by the lead doctor to attend Susanna Emlen, and she had the skill to try and protect her patient from the visual impact of the impending surgery.

Sadly, it was wartime, in this period we are thinking of the U.S. Civil War, lasting from 1861 to 1865, which publicized and even romanticized nurses' work. Thousands of women volunteered as nurses during the Civil War. In all, the Union Army's hospital records alone listed approximately 5,600 women as nurses. However, historian Mary Holland notes that no African American women were recorded as nurses. They were listed as "laundress" or "cook." Of course, these women were actually nurses (Holland, 1998). Most Northern nurses worked in the Army hospitals and their work was primarily concerned with the patient's diet, his physical needs such as laundry, and his emotional and spiritual care. From these nurses came the impetus for the first U.S. Training Schools. Matilda Morris, one Union Army nurse, recalled the scene after the second battle of Bull Run. "A sadder sight one could not imagine than those loads of wounded men. That day my life as a hospital nurse began. Our hearts and hands were full, tending to so many. Some died before they reached the building. Each ward had 50 beds and two nurses. . .first we gave each a drink of cold water, as that was their only cry. I shall never forget one who was lying near an old building. He looked as if he were dead, but I stopped to make sure, and I thought I saw his lips move. The man who was carrying the pail cried: "Come along! He is dead, fast enough." "No, wait a minute," I replied, and began to wet his lips. Very soon I had him revived enough, so much that he could drink out of my cup" (Holland, 1998, p. 187).

Further, as historian Christopher Maggs has pointed out, in times of war, nurses could and did substitute for doctors (Maggs, 1996). For example, Civil War nurses, just years after the discovery of ether and chloroform anesthesia, administered anesthesia on the battlefield before surgery (Lusk, Cockerham, & Keeling, 2019). At that time, administering anesthesia was typically a physician's responsibility.

These Civil War nurses were exemplars of nursing management and leadership. Note that Matilda Morris had the charge of 50 patients, along with one other nurse, and note that she overruled the man accompanying her who wanted her to leave a dying man. Imagine having the care of 50 wounded men in need of food and dressings and sanitation. Thus, modern nursing began in the United States.

The Dawn of Professional Nursing

Florence Nightingale did not invent the training of nurses all by herself—it took a "village" of scientific advances in knowledge, nineteenth century social forces including rapid industrialization, women's desire for greater independence, and the work of many other strong and smart women and men. But let's start with Nightingale because she is an integral part of nursing's heritage.

Florence Nightingale first attracted international attention because of her work for the British army during the Crimean War, 1853 to 1856, when Britain allied with France and Turkey to prevent Russian expansionism. A key factor in this war was that newspaper reporters, for the first time, came out and witnessed the fighting and destruction. Among other war news, the English were horrified to read about the terrible state of their wounded men. They demanded action. Thus Nightingale, accompanied by 38 nurses, went to the large British military hospital at Scutari, a Turkish army barracks near what is now Istanbul. Conditions were ghastly. Most of the men were dying from typhus, typhoid, cholera, and dysentery rather than from their wounds. The place was filthy. "There was no clean linen; the clothes of the soldiers were swarming with bugs, lice, and fleas; the floors, walls, and ceilings were filthy; and rats were hiding under the beds" (Fee & Garofalo, 2010, p. 1591). Nightingale rose to the challenge—through sound management, political understanding, firm leadership, and good use of her society connections back in England. Mortality among the soldiers plummeted and the British public revered Nightingale as the "Lady with the Lamp." In Nightingale's honor, the public collected the enormous sum of £45,000 (almost two million dollars U.S. today). In 1860, Nightingale used this money to set up a nurses' training school at St. Thomas's Hospital in London. In 1873, three training schools were founded in the United States, in Connecticut, Massachusetts, and New York, using Nightingale's principles. Nurse training schools were based in hospitals where students typically worked full time while hearing lectures in their off duty hours.

Nurse Training Was Inevitable

Nightingale believed in good nutrition, cleanliness, and fresh air. These, she was sure, would put the body in the strongest position to recover. But later nineteenth century scientific advances further necessitated specialized training for nurses. Important early discoveries included anesthesia and, later, antisepsis. Anesthesia for patients undergoing surgery had been known since the 1840s and enabled patients to tolerate complex surgeries. Under anesthesia the muscles were relaxed, the patient wasn't in danger of neurogenic shock from pain, and there was time for delicacy and skill.

Likewise, use of antiseptic techniques during and after surgery hugely increased the likelihood that patients would survive surgery. Hungarian obstetrician Ignaz Semmelweis is rightly honored for discovering that, somehow, washing hands with a chlorinated lime solution before assisting at childbirth drastically reduced the incidence of puerperal fever. But this was in the mid-nineteenth century and the germ theory of disease had not yet gained widespread scientific support. Even Nightingale was not a believer in microorganisms until her later years. Joseph Lister was the Scottish surgeon who, apprised of Louis Pasteur's assertions that "tiny little organisms floating in the air and settling on organic matter caused its decay" (cited in Goldman, 1987, p. 8), took action. Lister instituted a process he termed "antisepsis"—that is, warding off sepsis before it started—using carbolic acid. In 1869, Lister was appointed Chair of Clinical Surgery at Edinburgh

Evidence from the Literature

Source: Adapted from Holme, A. (2015). Big ideas. Why history matters to nursing. *Nurse Education Today, 35,* 635–637.

Discussion: Holme cites a media and public complaint that nurses today, possibly because of a higher level of education, are not as compassionate as they were 50 years ago. Nursing history contradicts this. Just like today, in years past, some nurses were compassionate and others were not. Higher education has not made nurses less compassionate. However, without historical awareness, nurses are not prepared to rebut this perception. Holme argues that it is imperative that nurses know their history.

Implications for Practice: Policy makers might act on this incorrect assumption about level of compassion as they respond to their constituents. Nursing education may then be forced to recede, through funding cuts and other policy initiatives, to the detriment of patients.

University and his methods, with the resultant drop in patient mortality, gained international acceptance (Goldman, 1987).

Additional factors that demanded trained nurses included the rapid industrialization of the nineteenth century, which caused immense social upheaval. Work environments changed and became increasingly dangerous. Many women had to work outside the home, leaving children, the elderly, and the sick to manage as best they could. Meanwhile, enhanced communication through newspapers, telegrams, and even the telephone informed society of scientific and medical advances.

Nineteenth-Century Nurse Training Schools in the United States

By 1873, when the first U.S. nurse training schools were established, science was starting to exponentially expand medical understanding and treatment. Skilled and knowledgeable nursing was necessary. That said, as historian Christopher Maggs reminds us, a lot of nursing was still the work that women traditionally had done but now it was "professional." Maggs writes: "Only by strict interpretation of discipline, the routinization of rituals and tasks and discussions in textbooks and training about ventilation and sewage disposal could cleaning be inculcated as the 'science of hygiene'" (1996, p. 23).

In 1880, the Illinois Training School for Nurses was founded by a group of prominent Chicago women along the lines of Nightingale's school in London. The school was not part of a hospital but its students provided care to patients in some wards of the sprawling Cook County Hospital—the city's only public hospital. Cook County paid the Illinois Training School for the students' work through using money saved by dismissing the untrained nurses—"many of them men" (Brainard, 1922).

That last point, that many of the untrained nurses who were dismissed from Cook County Hospital were men, is worthy of discussion. Before the later nineteenth century, there were many men in nursing but early nursing leaders, including Nightingale, considered nursing solely as a women's profession. Nursing, like teaching, was a professional field that women could own and develop just for women. And it wasn't just nursing leaders who wanted only female nurses—a glance through the *Journal of the American Medical Association* in the 1880s and 1890s indicated that many doctors also only wanted women as nurses (Lusk & Robertson, 2005). For male physicians during this period, female nurses were viewed as having the qualities of good women; they were submissive, obedient, and good housekeepers.

To return to the Illinois Training School for Nurses. In 1905, the first student, Isabella Lauver, remembered her arrival: "Twenty-five years ago trained skirts were in vogue. My dress was of that style." The superintendent "having viewed me over she found some pins and shortened my skirt, took a ribbon bow from my hair, and I was ready to go to work. . . Then the third night it was thought best to take charge of the night work as well as the day, and I was chosen for the first night nurse. What a responsibility!" (Schryver, 1930, p. 23) Figure 3.1.

The Illinois Training School for Nurses at that time was responsible for just two wards in the sprawling Cook County Hospital—the female surgical and the male medical, each averaging 50 patients (Schryver, 1930). Apparently, Isabella Lauver did well—she graduated in 1882 after just over 2 years of nurse training. Her first year was spent working on the wards, her second year was spent either in the wards or being sent out as a private duty nurse in the homes of "the rich or the poor" (Schryver, 1930, p. 21). The only actual lectures were given in the evenings by the medical staff after the students had completed a 12-hr working day. This type of nursing education was typical of nurse training schools of this era Figure 3.2.

Let us dissect Nurse Lauver's work in terms of management and leadership. Her superintendent described her as a woman of "calmness and common sense sufficient to make up for lack of experience" (Schryver, 1930, p. 24). She had to be! Imagine this young woman as the only nurse for a ward of 50 sick and/or post-operative patients. And then imagine her as a young woman in 1882, nearly 40 years before women even had the right to vote, leaving her home to start training as a nurse. She was stepping out into the unknown into this new opening for women who wanted something meaningful out of their lives other than being a housewife or a teacher—the only other respected occupations open to women. For the next 47 years, Isabella Lauver worked as a nurse in private duty and in institutions (Schryver, 1930).

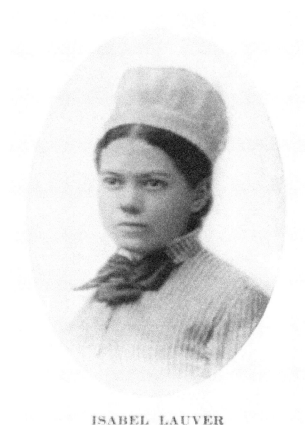

ISABEL LAUVER

FIGURE 3.1 Isabella Lauver.
Source: Illinois Training School Collection, Midwest Nursing History Research Center, University of Illinois at Chicago, College of Nursing.

Visiting Nurses and the Birth of Public Health Nursing

Other young nursing graduates opened up the field of public health nursing during these early years of the nursing profession as **Visiting Nurses**. These Visiting Nurses went to the homes of the poor to provide free nursing care and coordinate support services. Wealthier patients hired nurses to stay with them. The 1890s were years of severe economic need in the U.S.; an economic depression as severe as that of the more infamous 1930s Great Depression occurred. In addition, U.S. cities became home to thousands of immigrants who were new to the American language and customs. Some nursing organizations, staffed by a small cadre of trained nurses in the late nineteenth century, responded to the people adversely affected by these conditions. It is worthwhile noting that these nurses often connected with their patients through the use of the newly invented telephone. Patients and doctors typically called the local pharmacy and left messages for the nurse. The nurse, in turn, visited the pharmacy at a set time each day to review the messages and then plan her work Figure 3.3.

One of the foremost nurse leaders and activists at this time was Lillian Wald, who is regarded as the founder of U.S. public health nursing. After her nurse's training in New York, and disenchanted with her first job in a children's home, Wald entered medical school. During her first semester, in 1893, she was told of a need for a teacher to conduct a home nursing course for immigrants on the lower East Side of the city. Wald volunteered and thus changed her life and the lives of countless others. She described making her way to a student's home "... through crowded 'evil-smelling' streets, past open courtyard

Case Study 3.1

M. Helena McMillan, an 1894 graduate of the Illinois Training School, founded Chicago's Presbyterian Hospital School of Nursing in 1903. McMillan, who had a college degree from Montreal's McGill University, planned a curriculum that focused on education rather than service. The first class attracted women from across the U.S. for the three and a half-year program, which included a six-month period with no clinical duties. Students needed a high school diploma to enter and one or more years of college were preferred. The school was affiliated with Rush Medical College. In 1903, McMillan wrote: "a special feature of the school is that the pupils will not be overworked." McMillan was active in professional organizations including being a founding member of the International Council of Nurses in 1899. In Illinois, she spearheaded the passage of the state's first Nurse Practice Act in 1907. Upon her retirement in 1938, the *American Journal of Nursing* editors wrote that she had been "Associated with practically every progressive movement in nursing" (Lusk, 2001, p. 575).

Compare McMillan's plan for nursing education, as Director of Chicago's Presbyterian Hospital School of Nursing, to the experience of Isabella Lauver at the Illinois Training School for Nurses 30 years earlier.

Early nurse leaders such as McMillan would have objected to physicians who wanted nurses to be submissive and obedient. McMillan wanted well-educated nurses who were legally protected by the state's Nurse Practice Act. Can you give some reasons, from the perspective of patient safety, why nurses today should continue to follow McMillan's lead and resist policy makers or others who want nurses to be submissive and obedient?

Discuss the founding of nursing through the lenses of gender, society, science and place.

1. Use the history of professional nursing to inform and guide decision making in nursing practice.

2. Interpret the founding of professional nursing through the lenses of gender, society, science, and place.

3. Appreciate nursing's important contributions to society's health.

4. Articulate future challenges for nursing based on a critical analysis of nursing's past.

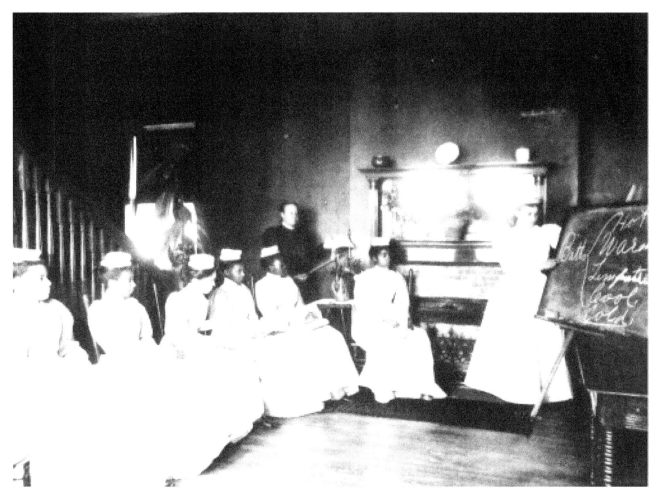

FIGURE 3.2   Student nurses listening to a lecture after work. This photograph is from Chicago's Provident Hospital—a hospital founded in 1891 by African Americans to train African American nurses and physicians because they were not admitted to "White" hospitals.
Source: Chicago Medical Society (1922). *History of medicine and surgery and physicians and surgeons in Chicago.* Chicago: Biographical Publishing Corp.

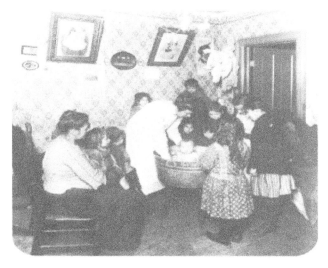

FIGURE 3.3   Chicago VNA nurse in patient's home, c. 1890s.
Source: Chicago VNA Collection, Midwest Nursing History Research Center, University of Illinois at Chicago, College of Nursing.

'closets', up slimy settlement steps, and finally into the sickroom" (Buhler-Wilkerson, 2001, p. 99). That same year, 1893, Wald and her friend Mary Brewster founded New York City's Visiting Nurse Service and Wald founded the **Henry Street Settlement House**, a site for poor and immigrant children and families to receive social services and health care.

In 1889, 4 years before the Henry Street Settlement House, a group of society women in Chicago founded the Chicago **Visiting Nurse Association** (VNA). The Chicago VNA aimed to provide nursing care to the poor, many of them immigrants, in their homes. Remember, in these days before antibiotics became available in the 1940s, most invalids required long periods of nursing to recover from an illness or surgery. The Chicago VNA nurses were assigned to all parts of the city and cared for patients suffering from multiple diseases including tuberculosis, smallpox, and polio, as well as giving maternity and chronic disease care. Jane Addams, the Nobel Prize winner and founder of Chicago's Hull House Settlement, was a charter member of the Chicago VNA. One of the VNA nurses was based in Hull House. In 1892 her supervisor wrote: "No one could conceive the dirt and ignorance that the Hull House nurse has to contend with. She has often had to care for a typhoid fever patient in a small room crowded with a dozen or more chattering and gesticulating Italian men and women, not one of whom could speak a word of English. Pigeons underfoot or flying on the bed" (VNA Annual Report, 1892, pp. 14–15, cited in Lusk et al. 2016). We can reflect on the difficulties these families endured, in a strange city with a very ill loved one, enduring the dangers, the dirt, and the overcrowding. And one can admire the intrepid and hardworking nurses visiting these homes.

In addition, the Chicago VNA was an early provider of school nursing, industrial nursing, and social services. In 1893/4, the city's last major smallpox epidemic occurred. Chicago had 3,726 smallpox cases and 1,210 deaths. The city's smallpox hospital was so crowded that tents had to be set up to accommodate the overflow of disease victims. Chicago VNA nurses staffed a temporary isolation hospital and cared for 265 patients. Twenty-six VNA nurses volunteered to work in this hospital and 4 contracted smallpox. In 1903, the VNA also formally recognized the high incidence and dreadful toll of tuberculosis and established a Tuberculosis Committee that became the Chicago Tuberculosis Institute in 1906 (Burgess, 1990).

Reflect on this. Over a hundred years ago, nurses exposed themselves to dangerous diseases such as smallpox, were active in public health such as forming a tuberculosis committee or initiating school nursing, and were responsible for skilled hospital work. Thus, nurses such as Harriett Fulmer, an early superintendent of the Chicago VNA and the founder of the Illinois State Association of Graduate Nurses, realized that trained nurses needed to organize in order to protect the name of "nurse" and thus the new profession of nursing.

The Development of Professional Nursing Organizations

Early on, nurse leaders saw the need for nurses to unite. Isabel Adams Hampton, a superintendent of the Illinois Training School for Nurses, who then founded the Johns Hopkins Training School for Nurses, attended the World's Columbian Exposition in Chicago in 1893. During the Exposition, multiple talks were presented, including talks by nurses in a nursing section chaired by Hampton. Edith Draper, superintendent of the Illinois Training School for Nurses, stated: "I know that to every thinking woman among us, the needs for a national organization are becoming more and more strongly realized, until now our success for the future depends on our unity" (Draper, 1894, p. 569). Hampton and others proposed forming an association. The 18 women present at the Chicago Exposition meeting, superintendents of nurse training schools across the country, founded the American Society of Superintendents of Training Schools for Nurses, now known as the **National League for Nursing** (NLN).

But these nurse leaders knew of the need for regular working nurses, not just superintendents, to have an association

of their own. In 1896, 3 years after the American Society of Superintendents of Training Schools for Nurses was formed, 12 representatives from the society met with 12 members of nurse training school alumnae associations in Brooklyn, New York. There they formed the Nurses Associated Alumnae of the United States and Canada, now the **American Nurses Association** ANA. Isabel Adams Hampton was elected the first President (Keeling, Hehman, & Kirchgessner, 2018).

African American women during these times did not have the opportunities open to Whites. Nurses' training was rarely open to Black women in White hospitals and, likewise, the fledgling professional nursing organizations were not open to Blacks in all parts of the U.S. Thus, the leadership of such women as Martha Franklin, who graduated as a nurse in 1897, is all the more impressive. In 1907, Franklin, an African American graduate of the nurse training school of the Women's Hospital of Philadelphia, personally wrote 1,500 letters to Black nurses throughout the United States asking about forming a society. In 1908, 52 Black nurses met in New York and founded the National Association of Colored Graduate Nurses. Franklin was the first president. At the close of the first meeting, Lillian Wald invited the women to the Henry Street Settlement House for lunch and to offer support and mentorship (Keeling et al., 2018).

Lillian Wald was among those nurses who established another significant nursing organization, the National Organization of Public Health Nurses. In 1911, a committee, formed of members of the American Society of Superintendents of Training Schools for Nurses and the Nurses Associated Alumnae of the United States and Canada, met to standardize the field of public health nursing. They wrote to over a thousand organizations that employed public health nurses and, at the 1912 meetings of the two organizations held in Chicago, the public health organization was formed (Kandel, 1920). Wald, considered to be the founder of public health nursing, became the first president (Keeling, et al., 2018). It is instructive to appreciate how important public health nursing was at this time. We might think that nurses mainly worked in hospitals prior to quite recently—but they didn't. Nurses have been actively involved with public health, working to promote health and support home care, for centuries. In terms of leadership, these pioneers who founded early nursing organizations deserve our respect for their imagination and sense of purpose. Today, nursing organizations present a rich source of support for all nurses. Many nurses join a general national organization, such as the ANA, as well as one that is specific to their nursing specialty.

The following Table 3.1 lists just a few of the scores of national nursing professional organizations, beginning with the oldest, the American Society of Superintendents of Training Schools for Nurses.

Professional Nursing Matures

Nursing education was, in some respects, a victim of its own success. Nursing students were both superior to untrained

Table 3.1 Professional Nursing Organizations Compiled by B. Lusk

Year founded	Organization
1893	American Society of Superintendents of Training Schools for Nurses—now the National League for Nursing
1896	Nurses' Associated Alumnae of the United States and Canada—now the American Nurses Association
1908	National Association of Colored Graduate Nurses—merged with the American Nurses Association in 1951
1912	National Organization of Public Health Nurses—merged with the National League for Nursing in 1951
1922	Sigma Theta Tau International Honor Society of Nursing—now Sigma
1931	American Association of Nurse Anesthetists
1941	American Association of Nurse Midwives—merged with the American College of Nurse Midwives in 1969
1952	National Student Nurses Association
1955	American College of Nurse-Midwives
1967	American Organization of Nurse Executives
1969	American Association of Colleges of Nursing
1971	American Assembly for Men in Nursing
1971	National Black Nurses Association, Inc.
1978	American Association for the History of Nursing
1985	American Association of Nurse Practitioners
1995	National Association of Clinical Nurse Specialists

Real World Interview

The possibilities and the problems we confront in our daily work raise new questions that we look to documents in our archives to answer. Our generation wonders how groups of nurses influenced broader movements of social change, transforming their lives as well as those of their patients and communities, and created opportunities and aspirations that took them beyond the health care system itself.

Patricia D'Antonio, PhD, RN, FAAN
Carol E. Ware Professor in Mental Health Nursing
Director, Barbara Bates Center for the Study of the History of Nursing
University of Pennsylvania School of Nursing
Philadelphia, Pennsylvania.

Case Study 3.2

Adah Belle Thoms graduated from the Lincoln Hospital School of Nursing in 1905, a New York City school only for Black students, although under White administration. During the First World War, nurses volunteering for war service joined the American Red Cross but Black nurses were rarely accepted. Only during the last month of the war, in the fall of 1918, were 24 Black nurses called up. Meanwhile, 22,000 White nurses had been accepted. Seeing the futility of trying to volunteer, Thoms set up an organization of Black nurses called the Blue Circle Nurses, which was associated with the recently founded Circle for Negro War Relief. These nurses functioned as public health nurses for needy Black families. In 1929, Thoms was appointed the first Black Assistant Superintendent of Nurses at Lincoln Hospital. That same year, Thoms' book, *Pathfinders*, the first account of prominent Black nurses, was published (Clark Hine, 1989).

Consider why Black patients, nurses, medical, and ancillary staff needed Black hospitals during the late nineteenth and early twentieth centuries.

Thoms was a remarkable early nurse leader, as evidenced by her organization of the Blue Circle Nurses, her administrative work, and her book, all accomplished within the context of rampant racism. Can you identify some leadership qualities she might have possessed to support her in accomplishing all this?

women and cheaper than graduate nurses. Nursing students were highly disciplined and compliant young women who could work longer and harder than nursing employees at a fraction of the cost. Nursing students were expected to work at least 8 hr a day and then spend time preparing for classes. In most schools, students worked more than 48 hr a week on day duty and, in about 40% of schools, they worked over 70 hr a week on night duty (Committee, 1934, p. 166). Disturbingly, most of the nursing superintendents in the mid-1920s preferred student nurses rather than graduate nurses to give patient care. Some of their reasons were: "The student nurse is less apt to be careless in technique, gives better cooperation in regard to hospital regulations, is less extravagant with hospital linen and supplies, and with the help and advice of an experienced supervisor, gives her patients care equal to that of the graduate". . . "Graduates on general duty are demanding, exacting, and shifting" (Burgess, 1928, p. 412).

The 1920s and 1930s: Evolving Hospital Nursing

The nurse training period in the 1920s was typically 3 years. This time was mainly spent working within different wards of the hospital and attending lectures after work. But this was not an apprenticeship. The students were the nurses for the hospital patients. They were not practicing under the direction of graduate nurses. A national study by the Committee on the Grading of Nursing Schools in the early 1930s found that two-thirds of the schools did not have even one graduate nurse employed for bedside nursing (Committee, 1934, p. 180). Upon graduation, the new crop of nurses were given

a diploma and left the hospital, mainly to work as nurses in private homes, while the hospital nurse training school admitted a new batch of students. Hospital administrators could not ignore the advantage of an unpaid nursing workforce and the number of nurse training schools mushroomed. In 1880, there had been 15 schools. In 1920, there were 2,155 schools (Burgess, 1928, p. 35). However, many of these new nurse training schools were situated in small or specialist hospitals, entirely unsuited to general nursing education. Furthermore, as noted earlier, African Americans were rarely accepted as students or nurses at White hospitals, while men were rarely accepted at any hospital or nurse training school. A few male only and African American only nurse training schools were founded; the latter also served as training and practice sites for African American physicians and other health care workers.

Nurse leaders were concerned at the direction nursing education was taking. Some university schools of nursing were opening and the large teaching hospitals still gave a broad education and attracted well-educated nursing students. But these nurse training schools were in the minority. The Committee on the Grading of Nursing Schools, cited earlier, publicized this issue but did not correct it. The correction came from the financial collapse of the Great Depression. In essence, people

Case Study 3.3

Anne Larson Zimmerman, born in 1914, graduated with her diploma in nursing in 1935. Later she remembered a nursing school instructor whom she had greatly admired, who told Zimmerman that she, "had been promised when she came that if her work was satisfactory after the first year, she would be given a raise in salary," and then the superintendent said to her, "Well, we're doing so much charity and we are so poor that we really won't be able to give you a raise," and she said, "Well, but sister, I am doing your charity, not you . . . and I don't think I should subsidize what you call your charity" (Fitzpatrick, 1985, p. 2). Zimmerman's nursing school instructor's words remained with her as she worked as a single mother in Montana, California, and finally in Illinois. As the Executive Director of the Illinois Nurses Association, Zimmerman encouraged nurses to stand up for their rights. At Chicago's Cook County Hospital, where the conditions for nurses and patients were awful, a colleague remembered that Zimmerman "was excellent. There on every picket line. Always there. She would never ask you to do something she had not done herself" (Stafford, 2016). As President of the ANA from 1976 to 1978, Zimmerman advocated for economic welfare for nurses, nationalized health care, and passage of the equal rights amendment. Not surprisingly, Zimmerman successfully argued that the ANA president deserved a salary.

With some insight into nursing history, what do you think about nurses unionizing today?

Zimmerman remembered a former nursing instructor who would not accept the superintendent's denial of her raise. What is your opinion of the nursing instructor's argument that she should not have to subsidize "what you call your charity"? Figure 3.4

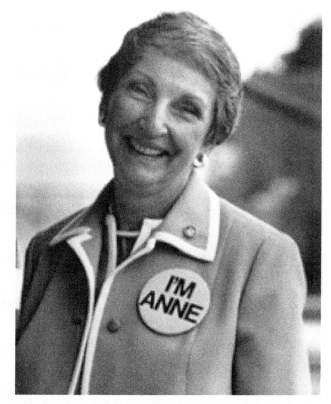

FIGURE 3.4 Anne Zimmerman. *Source:* Anne Zimmerman Collection, Midwest Nursing History Research Center, University of Illinois at Chicago, College of Nursing.

could not afford to hire nurse training school graduates as private duty nurses. Thus, the graduate nurses were desperate for work and accepted positions in hospitals for just their room and board. This being even cheaper for hospitals than operating training schools, the smaller, poorer schools rapidly began to close. From 1926 to 1936, there was a drop in the number of hospital-based diploma nursing schools nationwide, from 2,155 schools in 1926 to 1,478 schools in 1936 (JAMA, 1937).

Collegiate Education in Nursing

Mary Adelaide Nutting, a renowned nurse educator and activist, declared in 1908, "There is no place in its (the hospital) strenuous scheme of life for the machinery of a school. All the space, the effort, the means which the hospital can provide are needed to carry out its immediate purpose, which is the care of the sick, and any scheme of education must, of necessity, take a secondary and insignificant place" (Nutting cited in Grace, 1978, p. 20). In other words, nursing education had to get out from under hospital control. But, until the mid-1950s, most nursing programs continued in the 3-year diploma, hospital-based training model.

University programs for nurses had been around since 1909, but their development was accelerated by a study, commissioned in 1948 by the National Nursing Council, to examine who should organize, administer, and finance schools of nursing. The National Nursing Council was composed of multiple constituent nursing organizations. The study's Director, Esther Lucille Brown, an anthropologist, strongly recommended that nursing education move out of hospitals and into colleges and universities (Brown, 1948). Starting in the mid-1950s, the number of 3-year diploma, hospital-based nurse training schools went down and the number of baccalaureate and associate degree programs increased.

In the early 1950s, after World War II, there occurred, as has happened quite regularly over the years, a nursing shortage. Nurses leaving the profession, many of whom wanted to get married or to start a family after the war, exacerbated this shortage. Other nurses, who had served in the armed forces, didn't want to return to the constraints and rules of civilian nursing and, possibly, wanted to utilize the G.I. Bill of Rights to gain a college education. In addition, the Hill-Burton Act of 1946 supported extensive new hospital construction, which required more nurses. Mildred Montag, a nurse who was pursuing a doctorate in education at Teachers College, Columbia University, in New York, proposed a novel educational solution. Her dissertation, titled "Education for Nursing Technicians," proposed a 2-year Community College program for nurses. **Nursing technicians** could, as conceived by Montag, perform the technical rather than the professional components of nursing (Montag, 1963). A later grant enabled Montag to put her proposal into action in seven Community Colleges in six states, New York, New Jersey, Michigan, Utah, California, and Virginia (Montag, 1959). Montag's study showed that the 2-year nursing program, and

at this time it was just 2 years, with 1 year of general studies and 1 year of nursing, attracted non-traditional students. Furthermore, graduates of the 2-year program compared favorably with 3-year diploma graduates in terms of test scores and satisfaction from all parties. Montag's plan was for the 2-year associate degree program to develop a technical nurse—not a "professional" one (Montag, 1963). She thought that associate degree and baccalaureate degree programs should not blend with each other because they were just too different (Orsolini-Hain & Waters, 2009). Supported by the Nurse Training Act of 1964, associate degree nursing programs grew exponentially. By 1980, approximately 80% of new graduates were from associate degree programs (Orsolini-Hain & Waters, 2009).

Meanwhile, back in 1899, Teacher's College at Columbia University in New York had established the first graduate education program for nurses in the fields of hospital economics and educational administration (Grace, 1978). However, the bulk of nursing graduate education was developed in the 1950s and 1960s, as the need for nurse educators in the college programs expanded (Gerard, Kazer, Babington, & Quell, 2014). The early nursing graduate programs focused mainly on education and administration. Later, in the 1960s, graduate degrees for clinical nursing roles came to the forefront (Gerard et al., 2014).

The Development of Nursing Research in the 1950s to the 1970s

Early nursing research focused on the education of nurses. This was understandable because graduate degrees for nurses had been based on theories of education. But as nursing education started to shift away from hospital-based schools to colleges and universities, a separate and independent body of nursing knowledge was needed. That is, nursing needed to clarify the scientific knowledge behind nursing practice.

Essential to an independent body of nursing knowledge was the development of independent theories of nursing. In 1959, nurse Dorothy Johnson wrote: ". . .the question of the existence of a body of substantive knowledge which can be called the science of nursing. . .is a question of considerable significance for nursing's continued development as a recognized professional discipline" (Johnson, 1959, cited in Tobbell, 2018, p. 65). Historian Dominique Tobbell (2018) has outlined three reasons why theories of nursing were developed during the 1960s and the following decades.

- First, most doctorates that nurses had obtained were in education or, to a smaller degree, in the social and behavioral sciences. These disciplines all had their own theoretical orientations.

- Second, nursing wanted to show that it was separate from medicine. Thus, nurses did not want to use the biomedical sciences as their theoretical base since they were in use as the base for medical science,

- Third, distinctive nursing theories differentiated nursing science from other disciplines.

In 1972, the NLN required that a nursing conceptual model should frame nursing curricula. Within the 1950s, 1960s, and 1970s, many nurse theorists developed theories of nursing science based on a functional view of nursing and health (Im & Chang, 2012). Table 3.2 details several prominent nurse theorists and their work.

Emerging Nursing Specialization in the 1980s and 1990s

With the introduction of Diagnosis Related Groups in 1983 as an attempt by the U.S Federal Government to rein in Medicare costs, the number of hospitalized patients decreased, but their acuity (level of illness) went up. Around the same time, the **Human Immunodeficiency Virus** (HIV), the cause of **Acquired Immunodeficiency Syndrome** (AIDS), emerged as a new and terrifying disease. Caring for patients infected with HIV caused nurses to examine their courage and their ethical beliefs in a way that was new in modern nursing. Modern scientific treatments, such as vaccines and antibiotics, had lulled nurses and others into a false sense of safety in their work. HIV was different because it was fatal. Barbara Fassbinder was a Wisconsin nurse who looked after a very ill patient admitted to the emergency room on a busy night in 1986. Because of that care, Fassbinder was later identified as the first nurse to contract AIDS from a patient. Fassbinder died in 1994 (Lusk, 1997).

Increased patient acuity, exacerbated by shorter hospital stays, demanded that nurses have further education in specialized fields. Of the currently accepted Advanced Practice Nursing Roles (Nurse Midwife, Nurse Anesthetist, Clinical Nurse Specialist, and **Nurse Practitioner** (NP)), nurse midwifery and nurse anesthetist have the longest history. In the U.S., many nurses at the start of the twentieth century frowned upon nurse midwives. Clara Noyes, a noted nurse leader, wrote in 1912: "The word 'midwife', in America, at least, is one to which considerable odium is attached and immediately creates a mental picture of illiteracy, carelessness and general filth" (Noyes, 1912, p. 466). At the same time, in the early twentieth century, the medical profession in the U.S. was growing in prestige and flaunted its expertise. Physicians were eager to join with early nurse leaders in disparaging midwives as ignorant and dangerous. Childbirth evolved as a medically lucrative pathology rather than a natural event. Yet many women were unable, due to geographical location or cost, to obtain medical care and relied upon the local untrained but experienced midwife. Within a few decades, during the 1930s and 1940s, nurse midwifery schools opened. The public's interest in natural childbirth during the 1970s supported further growth in nurse midwifery (Lusk, Cockerham, & Keeling, 2019).

The story for nurse anesthetists started more abruptly with the discovery in the mid-nineteenth century of gases that induced anesthesia. Isabel Adams Hampton, in her 1893 nursing textbook, gives instructions to nurses on how to administer both ether and chloroform (Hampton, 1893). However, in these early days, nurses primarily gave anesthesia in situations where no physicians were present except for the surgeon. The first specific nurse anesthesia training was probably given by Dr. William Worrell Mayo during his surgeries in the late 1890s at St. Mary's Hospital in Rochester, Minnesota. Nurse Alice Magaw, sometimes referred to as the "mother of anesthesia," worked for Dr. Mayo and wrote of her anesthesia "observations" of over a thousand cases in 1900 (Lusk et al., 2019).

The Clinical Nurse Specialist role had its foundation in psychiatric nursing. Indeed, the woman known as the first trained nurse in the U.S., Linda Richards, an 1870s graduate, organized a nursing school for the preparation of nurse specialists in psychiatric nursing (Richards, 1911). NPs, the fourth type of Advanced Practice Nursing role, include diagnosis and treatment in their nursing care. Forerunners of today's NPs were

Table 3.2 Prominent Nurse Theorists and Their Work

Nurse theorist	Theory	Brief description
Helen Erickson	Modeling and Role Modeling	Recognizes the unique perspective of each patient; accepts that the patients are experts in their own care.
Virginia Henderson	Need Theory	Supports patients to become as independent as possible.
Imogene King	Theory of Goal Attainment	Describes a dynamic, interpersonal relationship in which a patient grows and develops to attain certain life goals.
Madeleine Leininger	Culture Care Theory	States that Nursing is informed by patient's culture and cultural background.
Betty Neuman	Neuman Systems Model	Has a holistic view of patients; patients are seen as people and not merely a pathology.
Dorothea E. Orem	Self-Care Deficit Theory	Helps patients become more independent by recognizing that people want to care for themselves.
Hildegard Peplau	Theory of Interpersonal Relations	Describes 7 roles of nursing, which are applied selectively to optimize care.
Callista Roy	Adaptation Model of Nursing	Promotes adaptation of patient to health and to illness.
Jean Watson	Philosophy and Science of Caring.	Uses caring as a generalized framework for nursing.

Source: Compiled with information from *Nursing Theory* at www.nursing-theory.org. Retrieved on October 3, 2019.

nurses who treated patients who were often too poor to obtain medical care. Such a nurse was Rose Hawthorne.

Teacher's College, Columbia University, instituted the first doctoral degree for nurse educators, granting the education doctorate in 1924 (Robb, 2005). By 1949, there were 24 doctoral programs open to nurses in the U.S., 75% of which were in education. Twenty years later, this number had grown to over 300

with 10% of these doctoral programs in nursing and 21% in the social sciences and the remainder in education (Grace, 1978). Over the ensuing years, doctoral nursing education acquired such titles as Doctor of Nursing Science (DNSc) and the Doctor of Science in Nursing (DSN). Today we have primarily the titles of Doctor of Philosophy (PhD), a research doctorate, and the Doctorate in Nursing Practice (DNP), a clinical doctorate.

Case Study 3.4

Rose Hawthorne was born in 1851 and, after the death of her only child from diphtheria, she left her husband and took a short course in cancer nursing at the New York Cancer Hospital, now Memorial Sloane-Kettering Cancer Center. Her aim was to nurse poor people with cancer. Hawthorne ran a dispensary and then a home for people dying of cancer, without attracting questions from the medical establishment about encroachment on their medical practice. Hawthorne applied different types of salves (ointments) to the open wounds of her patients, depending on her judgment of the wound's condition and the type of dressing needed. For Mary Watson, her first patient, Hawthorne cleansed the wound with either water or a weak creolin (tar) solution, or with peroxide. She

then applied the type of ointment she thought appropriate. Hawthorne also gave Watson one to three tablets of morphine a day (Hawthorne, 1896). Hawthorne's patients were poor and that is probably why she was allowed to diagnose and prescribe without complaints from physicians. Hawthorne was indeed practicing as a NP back in the nineteenth century.

Has the knowledge that NPs have a long history, as demonstrated by Hawthorne, changed your perspective, as a consumer and as an undergraduate nurse, of the NP role today?

Based on your knowledge of nursing at this time, do you think you could set up a nursing practice that included diagnosis and treatment, such as Hawthorne's practice, today? Why or why not?

Real World Interview

I'll admit, when I started my doctoral program, I had no interest in the history of nursing. Nor did I understand its value within the profession. When I took a required historical research methods course, I realized I could use history to answer my research questions instead of the more traditional methods of research I had always known. Now as a new faculty member, I continue to pursue historical scholarship, promote historical methods among the doctoral students, and host a historical

book club among faculty and students to discuss important events of the past and how they inform our present profession and society.

Gwyneth Milbrath, PhD, RN
Clinical Assistant Professor
University of Illinois at Chicago College of Nursing
Chicago, Illinois

Critical Thinking 3.1

Historically, the public appears to hold nurses in higher esteem during wartime. The media's image of nurses both reflects and influences nurses' professional identity. Lusk, the author of this chapter, has conducted two studies assessing: (a) how nurses were portrayed in the general literature, 1880–1928, and (b) how nurses were portrayed in hospital management journals, 1930–1950 (Lusk, 2000, 2002). Lusk found that nurses were indeed portrayed as more knowledgeable and autonomous in these media during war years. As the First World War started, images of nurses and articles about them burgeoned in the popular press. Reporters were sent over to Europe to write about hospital work. The reporters stressed that only trained nurses, not volunteers, were needed. Nursing was portrayed as a highly patriotic occupation in which female nurses had a significant presence near the front lines. The Second World War was similarly covered. In marked contrast to the 1930s and the 1950s, when nurses were depicted as minimally skilled and subservient to physicians, nurses in advertisements during the war years of the 1940s showed nurses engaged in more complex and independent procedures, for example, adjusting nasogastric suction and setting up oxygen delivery systems. These changes may be correlated with peace time perceptions of nurses' work as lower skilled physicians' helpers as opposed to war time perceptions of nurses' work as skilled, autonomous providers of care who would help the country "win the war." What do you think of the fact that nurses' professionally benefit from positive portrayals during times of war? There are many reasons we can speculate about why nurses were portrayed less positively after the war, during the 1950s. Some of these affect the image of nurses today. What reasons can you think of?

Critical Thinking 3.2

In 2018 the Gallup Organization found, for the 17th year in a row, that the public consider nursing to be the most ethical profession. By ethics, we mean the study of morality from a range of perspectives (American Nurses Association (ANA), 2015). In 2016 the Hastings Center produced a Report titled: *Nurses at the Table: Nursing, Ethics, and Health Policy* (Ulrich, Grady, Hamric, & Berlinger, 2016), sponsored by the American Academy of Nursing. The Report implied that nurses were uniformly ethical. In contrast to this, historian Lynn Dunphy (2001) wrote about nurses who cared for children with polio who were in external pressure ventilators, "iron lungs," during the polio outbreaks of the mid-twentieth century. These ventilators were metal tubes in which the patient's body was placed, and only the patient's head was outside the tube. Dunphy quoted a former patient: ". . .she [the nurse] told me to stop crying. She said she would turn my respirator off if I didn't stop crying. When she did, I passed out immediately" (p. 20). Dunphy wrote that stories like that abounded in her interviews.

Do you think that this was unusual nursing behavior?

Have you ever seen nurses behave with questionable ethics?

What would you do if you saw such behavior today?

In 2016, there were just under 5,000 nursing students enrolled in research focused doctoral programs compared with over 25,000 nursing students in DNP programs (American Association of Colleges of Nursing (AACN), 2017).

Historical Contributions and Future Challenges

This chapter has skimmed over some of the key events in nursing's history. It has told some stories in depth, for example, that of nursing student Isabella Lauver's early experiences at Cook County Hospital in the 1880s and Madame du Coudray's work in France in the 1700s. The point is to alert you to the complexity of history. There was no golden age of nursing when nurses were always wise and had plenty of time for hands-on patient care. That is a product of wishful thinking on the part of today's public and public policy makers. Likewise, nursing education didn't start with Florence Nightingale, as demonstrated by Madame du Coudray and her "obstetrical machine" of the century before Nightingale. The past was both worse and better than we might imagine and it cannot be judged with today's lens. Furthermore, we cannot consider nursing's past in isolation from its contextual issues of gender, society, science, and place. Society in the nineteenth and early twentieth centuries lacked today's social safety nets, such as Medicaid, Medicare, and Social Security, but medical science was advancing rapidly. Nurses thus witnessed extraordinary patient need alongside the new realities of, for example, effective drugs and newly developed vaccines. The concept of place in nursing's past means that nurses' education and practice was affected by the geographical setting—urban or rural, southern state or northern state, general hospital or tuberculosis hospital.

The rise of public health nursing came from late nineteenth, early twentieth century concerns about great income disparities and lack of health care for immigrants and the poor. Some nurses addressed these concerns at the policy level, while thousands of public health nurses went from door to door doing the actual work of nursing. The work of these public health nurses of the past has influenced health care administration today with the current shift to outpatient care wherever possible (McDermott, Elixhauser, & Sun, 2017). Additionally, nursing has a history of giving care to the poor, who in these days are the uninsured. Witness the work of Rose Hawthorne discussed in Case Study 3.4.

The checkered story of formal education in nursing, briefly covered in this chapter, must be placed in the context of society in the nineteenth century, particularly the role of women at that time. In the nineteenth century and the early decades of the twentieth century, women's education was not a priority. Women were expected to become mothers and housewives. But the scientific advances of the nineteenth and twentieth centuries required that nurses, even though they were predominantly women, become appropriately educated. The importance of professional organizations over the decades, and their leadership, cannot be overemphasized in the history of nursing. From the NLN's early nursing curricula, starting in 1917, to the Advanced Practice Nurse organizations' recent moves in clarifying and publicizing the advanced practice roles, professional organizations have led the way forward.

Appreciation of nurses' current ethical responsibilities must be guided by awareness of nursing's complex past, as described in Dunphy's (2001) story of the iron lung nurses in the 1950s and 1960s. History has shown us that nursing is not exempt from ethical wrongdoing; to state that nurses are always ethical is naïve. Critical thinking, strengthened by historical analysis, will support nurses' understanding of complex issues and ethical questions. Table 3.3 summarizes key events in the history of nursing in order to expose you to thought-provoking elements of your profession and pique your interest for further study.

Table 3.3   Historically Significant Events in the History of Nursing Compiled by B. Lusk

1846	First public use of anesthesia during surgery: allowed more complex surgeries and thus required more skilled nursing.
1851–1854	Crimean War: English aware of poor nursing care for troops. Nightingale and 38 volunteer nurses sent to English army hospitals in Turkey, near the Crimean peninsula.
1860	Nightingale establishes first training school for nurses in London, England
1863	International Red Cross established in Geneva, Switzerland.
1873	First "Nightingale Type" Nurse Training Schools opened in the U.S.
1880s	Germ theory of disease developed
1899	International Council of Nurses founded.
1893	National League for Nursing (NLN) founded. Lillian Wald founds the Visiting Nurse Service of New York.
1896	American Nurses Association (ANA) founded.
1902	Lina Rogers Struthers hired, in New York, as the first U.S. school nurse.
1908	National Association of Colored Graduate Nurses founded; merged with the ANA in 1951.
1909	First university-based school of nursing opened at the University of Minnesota.
1912	Public Health Nurses Association founded; merged with the NLN in 1951.
1917	Standardized curriculum for nursing developed by NLN.
1920	Women gained the vote.
1922	Sigma Theta Tau founded at Indiana University.
1923	Goldmark Report on Nursing Education. Mary Breckenridge founds the Frontier Nursing Service.
1924	First doctoral program for nurses, in education, opened at Teacher's College, Columbia University, New York.
1930s	Great Depression: Graduate nurses began staffing hospitals; closure of some hospital-based training schools; start of hospital insurance programs.
1934	Grading Committee Report on Nursing Education.
1942	Penicillin (discovered in 1928) starts to be used to treat infections.
1945	Cadet Corps nursing program initiated.
1946	Hill-Burton Act. Infusion of money into hospital construction.
1948	Brown Report on Nursing Education.
1950s	Beginning of associate degree education for nurses, closure of some hospital diploma training schools.
1953	National Student Nurses Association founded.
1960s	Development of specialized hospital patient units for coronary and critical care. Growth of nursing specialization.
1964	Nurse Training Act. Infuses Federal money into nursing and nursing education.
1965	First Nurse Practitioner program established at University of Colorado; Development of Medicaid and Medicare programs—expands insured health care.
1970s	Clinical Nurse Specialist role developed.
1971	American Assembly for Men in Nursing founded.
1974	Florence Wald founds first U.S. Hospice in Connecticut.
1986	National Center for Nursing Research founded.
1993	National Institute of Nursing Research, one of the National Institutes of Health, founded.
2004	Doctorate in Nursing Practice endorsed by member schools of the American Association of Colleges of Nursing.
2008	Consensus model for Advance Practice Registered Nurses developed by the National Council of State Boards of Nursing and the APN Consensus Work Group. The roles are: Certified Nurse Midwife, Certified Registered Nurse Anesthetist, Clinical Nurse Specialist, and Certified Nurse Practitioner.
2010	Affordable Care Act—expands health insurance.

KEY CONCEPTS

1. Nursing history must be interpreted through the contexts of gender, society, science, and place.

2. In 1873, three nurse training schools, using Nightingale's principles for nursing education, were founded in the U.S.

3. Scientific progress required nurses' more extensive education.

4. Early nursing contributions to society's health included nursing knowledge-based care within hospitals and nursing public health initiatives in the wider community.

5. Public health nursing was central to the early professional development of nursing.

6. Nursing professional organizations were initiated soon after formal nursing education began.

7. During the Great Depression of the 1930s, nursing practice moved from private duty nursing to hospital staff nursing.

8. The move from hospital training schools for nurses to collegiate nursing education accelerated in the 1950s and 1960s.

9. Nursing theories were foundational to nursing science research.

10. Advanced Practice Nursing roles have had a long history.

KEY TERMS

Nursing history	Visiting Nurses	Image of nurses
Professional identity	Henry Street Settlement	Ethics
Nurse Training Schools	Nursing technicians	

REVIEW QUESTIONS

1. Nurses who had graduated from nurse training schools largely moved from private duty nursing to hospital staff nursing during the 1930s because of which of the following?
   a. Medical care was becoming increasingly complex and more graduate nurses were needed.
   b. Student nurses' liability insurance would not cover student nurses in the role of primary caregivers.
   c. Graduate nurses were cheaper for hospitals than running their own nurse training schools.
   d. Student nurses' education was moving away from hospital training schools to colleges and universities.

2. The public views nurses more favorably during which of the following times?
   a. Complimentary television shows.
   b. War.
   c. Infectious disease outbreaks.
   d. When the results of the Gallop Poll, which showed nurses rate highest in ethics, is released.

3. The movement toward formal education for nurses in the 1870s came about for all the following reasons EXCEPT for which of the following?
   a. Rapid industrialization.
   b. Expansion of scientific knowledge, such as anesthesia and antisepsis.
   c. Expansion of hospital building.
   d. Women's desire for more independence.

4. In the nineteenth century, during the early years of nurse training schools, student nurses usually had classes during which of the following times?
   a. In 3 month blocks every year.
   b. After their 12 hr shift on the wards.
   c. On their day off from clinical work.
   d. After their 6 hr shift on the wards.

5. Which of the following professional nursing organizations was NOT one of the first nursing organizations
   a. American Society of Superintendents of Training Schools for Nurses—now the NLN.
   b. Sigma Theta Tau International Honor Society of Nursing—now Sigma.
   c. National Organization of Public Health Nurses.
   d. Nurses' Associated Alumnae of the United States and Canada—now the ANA.

6. Which scientific discovery came first?
   a. Anesthesia.
   b. X-Rays.
   c. Antisepsis.
   d. Penicillin.

7. What was one outcome of the Hill-Burton Act of 1946?
   a. More nurses were needed.
   b. More acute care patients were admitted to hospitals.
   c. Hospital insurance could be more readily obtained.
   d. Fewer Medicaid recipients were admitted to hospitals.

8. After World War II, several factors converged to worsen the nursing shortage. Which of the following was NOT a factor?
   a. Nurses wanted to leave nursing to get married.
   b. Military nurses didn't wish to return to the constraints and rules of civilian nursing.
   c. Nurses wanted to have children and start a family that had been delayed by the war.
   d. The military wounded required an infusion of nurses to care for them.

9. The early associate degree programs in nursing took about how long to complete?
   a. Two years to complete.

b. Three years, like the length of the diploma programs, to complete.
   c. Two years plus however long the general education courses took to complete.
   d. One year to complete.

10. Lillian Wald was primarily considered to be which of the following?
   a. Nurse educator.
   b. Nurse midwife.
   c. Public health nurse.
   d. Nurse administrator.

REVIEW QUESTION ANSWERS

1. Answer: C is correct.
   Rationale: During the Great Depression of the 1930s graduate nurses were unable to obtain private duty work. It was cheaper for hospitals to employ trained nurses rather than run a nurse training school. Medical care was becoming more complex but this was not the direct cause of the change from private duty to hospital nursing (A). Student nurses did not carry liability insurance at this time (B) and this was before the move of most nursing education to colleges and universities (D).

2. Answer: B is correct.
   Rationale: The text explains that nurses are more highly thought of in times of war. Perhaps surprisingly, complimentary television shows (A) and infectious disease outbreaks (C), such as the 1918 flu pandemic, do not alter the public's view of nurses. The Gallop Poll shows that the public considers nurses highly ethical (D).

3. Answer: C is correct.
   Rationale: There was not a hospital expansion during the late nineteenth century. The other answers (A, B, D) all influenced the need for formal nursing education.

4. Answer: B is correct.
   Rationale: Most student nurses at this time worked 12 hr shifts, although in some more progressive schools the students just worked 8 hr a day. Lectures were given in the evening after work (B). They did not have blocks of classroom time (A), days off (C), or 6 hr shifts (D).

5. Answer: B is correct.
   Rationale: Sigma Theta Tau International Honor Society of Nursing was founded in 1922. The American Society of Superintendents of Training Schools for Nurses—now the National League for Nursing was founded first in 1893 (A), the Nurses Associated

Alumnae followed in 1896 (D), and the National Organization for Public Health Nurses was founded in 1912(C).

6. Answer: A is correct.
   Rationale: Anesthesia was first publicly used for the purpose of painless surgery in the 1840s. When antisepsis was developed in the 1880s (C) the two necessary factors for complex yet relatively safe surgeries were in place. X-rays were developed in the late 1890s (B) and penicillin in the 1940s (D).

7. Answer: A is correct.
   Rationale: More nurses were needed, which exacerbated an already severe post war nursing shortage. The Act didn't have an impact on patient acuity (B), or hospital insurance (C), and Medicaid was not initiated until the 1960s (D).

8. Answer: D is correct.
   Rationale: While the wounded doubtless needed more nurses , the other three reasons given (A, B, C) also significantly exacerbated the shortage.

9. Answer: A is correct.
   Rationale: The early programs really did just take two years—one of general education and one of nursing. More recently, the AD nursing curriculum has expanded and more general education courses may be required and these programs typically take longer. Answers B, C, and D are incorrect.

10. Answer: C is correct.
   Rationale: Wald is considered to be the founder of public health nursing. She was not in education (A) and she was not a midwife (B). Some could consider her an administrator (D)—she ran the Henry Street Settlement—but her primary role was in public health.

REVIEW ACTIVITIES

1. Explore the images on the National Library of Medicine's images website. www.nlm.nih.gov/hmd/ihm, Accessed May 30, 2019.

2. Identify a content area you are interested in from the National Library of Medicine Images website (e.g., WWI, WWII, 1950s

health care, magic lantern slides, or public domain images) and pull out about six images for discussion.

3. Explore one of the traveling exhibits on the National Library of Medicine website at www.nlm.nih.gov/hmd/about/exhibition/index.html Accessed May 30, 2019.

4. Click on the "digital gallery" tab found on the National Library of Medicine traveling exhibits website. Find an image that is particularly meaningful to you and describe why it is significant.

5. This chapter has mentioned scores of nurses. There are millions more. Contact or identify a nurse who practiced 50 or more years ago and discover her or his history.

6. Identify a nursing intervention, such as assessing blood pressure or giving an enema, and explore the Internet, journals, textbooks for historical use of that intervention and the changes over time related to that intervention (This question taken from Lewenson, 2004).

DISCUSSION POINTS

1. In the chapter's opening paragraph, Dr. Sandra Lewenson states that studying history provides us with opportunity. A nursing student was inspired by the story of Mary Breckinridge, who in 1925 founded the Frontier Nursing Service in Kentucky. The history of Breckinridge gave that student her opportunity. She traveled to Kentucky to personally find out about the Frontier Nursing Service as soon as she could. How can the knowledge of nursing's past provide you with an opportunity?

2. Most nurses in the late nineteenth century wanted nurses to be licensed by the state before they could practice nursing. However, Florence Nightingale disagreed with the concept of nurse licensure. What are some of the benefits of licensure for nurses? Why didn't Nightingale want nurses to be licensed?

3. Before the later nineteenth century, there were many men in nursing. Why do you think Nightingale and many doctors preferred women as nurses? How do you think this early opposition toward men in nursing has affected the nursing profession today?

4. Mildred Montag's dissertation work introduced the concept of community college education for, what she termed, nursing technicians. Do you think that the separation of nurses' roles into technical roles and professional roles was ever a workable model?

DISCUSSION OF OPENING SCENARIO

1. Nursing's knowledge base has expanded in the same way that medical science has expanded over the last 150 years. Historically, nurses have taken the lead in public health and practiced autonomously for many years, particularly among the indigent.

2. Doctorally prepared nurses are necessary to maintain and develop nursing's knowledge base for practice, health care policy, and health care administration. Consider the extent of scientific knowledge on one hand and the inadequate quality of U.S. health care on the other. Well-educated nurses are needed to redress this inequity. As more nursing education is necessary so more research-based faculty are needed to teach nurses. Other clinical health care fields (e.g., dentistry, pharmacy, physical therapy, and medicine) require a doctoral level of education. Nurses should not, considering their high level of responsibility, be less well prepared.

3. There have always been males and other minorities within nursing. During the late nineteenth century, the development of professional nursing resulted in males and other minorities being excluded. White women were seen as entitled to have professional nursing as their own profession. Few training schools and professional organizations accepted males and other minorities. Male only and African American only training schools were founded; the latter also served as training and practice sites for African American physicians and other health care workers.

EXPLORING THE WEB

- North Carolina nursing history, accessed November 11, 2018:
  http://nursinghistory.appstate.edu
- Nursing Clio, accessed November 11, 2018:
  https://nursingclio.org
- Florida nursing history, accessed November 11, 2018:
  https://fnhxp.nursingnetwork.com
- American Association for the History of Nursing, accessed November 27, 2018:
  www.aahn.org
- National Library of Medicine, History of Medicine, accessed November 27, 2018:
  www.nlm.nih.gov/hmd
- Rush University Medical Center Archives, accessed November 27, 2018:
  https://rUShu.libguides.com/rUSharchives
- Midwest Nursing History Research Center, University of Illinois, accessed November 27, 2018:
  http://nursing.uic.edu/our-impact/research/centers-labs-interest-groups/midwest-nursing-history-research-center
- Barbara Bates Center for the Study of the History of Nursing, University of Pennsylvania, accessed November 27, 2018:
  www.nursing.upenn.edu/history
- Eleanor Crowder Bjoring Center for Nursing Historical Inquiry, University of Virginia, accessed November 27, 2018:
  www.nursing.virginia.edu/nursing-history

INFORMATICS

1. Visit the Nursing Clio website at https://nursingcleo.org and review an article related to nursing.

LEAN BACK

- How has nursing's image influenced nurses' ability to practice to the full extent of their education today?

- One could argue that nurses practiced more autonomously at the turn of the last century and one could argue the opposite, that nurses are more autonomous today. What are justifications for both positions?

- Understanding context is essential for attempting to accurately interpret historical events. Think of a few instances where knowledge of context is imperative. For example, nurses administered anesthesia during the American Civil War. The context of war is necessary to appreciate that nurses did not usually administer anesthetics during the 1860s.

- How will knowing some nursing history impact your patient care, including your future career choices?

REFERENCES

American Association of Colleges of Nursing. (2017). *Annual report.* Retrieved from www.aacnnursing.org/Portals/42/Publications/Annual-Reports/AnnualReport17.pdf

American Medical Assocation. (1937). Hospital service in the United States sixteenth annual presentation of hospital data by the Council of Medicsa Education and Hospitals of the American Medical Association. *Journal of the American Medical Association, 108*(13), 1035–1059. doi:10.1001/jama.1937.02780130019007

American Nurses Association. (2015). *Code of ethics for nurses with interpretive statements.* Silver Spring, MD: Carter Lucas. http://babel.hathitrust.org/cgi/pt?id=uiuo.ark:/13960/t21c1w69m&view=1up&seq=6

Brainard, A. (1922). Evolution of public health nursing. In F. Billings & J. S. Hurd (Eds.), *Hospitals, dispensaries, and nursing.* New York: Carter Lucas. https://babel.hathitrust.org/cgi/pt?id=uiuo.ark:/13960/t21c1w69m&view=1up&seq=6

Brown, E. L. (1948). *Nursing for the future.* New York: Russell Sage.

Buhler-Wilkerson, K. (2001). *No place like home.* Baltimore, MD: Johns Hopkins.

Burgess, M. A. (1928). *Nurses, patients, and pocketbooks.* New York: The Committee.

Burgess, W. K. (1990). *This beautiful charity: Evolution of the Visiting Nurse Association of Chicago 1889–1920.* University of Wisconsin – Milwaukee, Milwaukee, WI Unpublished doctoral dissertation. (Filed with VNA Collection, Box 11).

Clark Hine, D. (1989). *Black women in white.* Bloomington & Indianapolis: Indiana University Press.

Committee on the Grading of Nursing Schools. (1934). *Nursing schools today and tomorrow.* New York: The Committee.

Donahue, M. P. (2011). *Nursing. The finest art* (3rd ed.). Maryland Heights, MO: Mosby.

Draper, E. (1894). The necessity of an American Nurses' Association. In J. Billings & H. M. Hurd (Eds.), *Hospitals, dispensaries, and nursing, international congress of charities, correction and philanthropy, section III, Chicago, 1893.* Baltimore, MD: Johns Hopkins Press.

Dunphy, L. M. (2001). "The steel cocoon". Tales of nurses and patients of the iron lung-1955. *Nursing History Review, 9,* 3–33.

Evenden, D. (2000). *The midwives of seventeenth-century London.* Cambridge, UK: Cambridge University Press.

Fee, E., & Garofalo, M. E. (2010). Florence Nightingale and the Crimean war. *American Journal of Public Health, 100,* 1591.

Fitzpatrick, L. (1985). *Oral history interview with Anne Zimmerman.* Midwest Nursing History Research Center Archives. Chicago, IL: University of Illinois at Chicago.

Garfinkel, S. (1990). "This trial was sent in love and mercy for my refinement": A Quaker woman's experience of breast cancer surgery in 1814. *New Jersey Folklife, 15,* 18–31.

Gelbart, N. R. (1998). *The king's midwife.* Berkeley, CA: University of California Press.

Gerard, S. O., Kazer, M. W., Babington, L., & Quell, T. T. (2014). Past, present, and future trends of master's education in nursing. *Journal of Professional Nursing, 30,* 326–332.

Goldman, M. (1987). *Lister ward.* Bristol & Boston: Hilger.

Grace, H. K. (1978). The development of doctoral education in nursing in historical perspective. *Journal of Nursing Education, 17*(4), 17–27.

Hampton, I. A. (1893). *Nursing. Its principles and practice.* Philadelphia: Saunders.

Hawthorne, R. (1896). Mrs. Mary Watson (Notes). Rose Hawthorne Lathrop Papers, Dominican Sisters of Hawthorne Archives, Hawthorne, New York.

Helmstadter, C. (2007). Florence Nightingale's opposition to state registration of nurses. *Nursing History Review, 15,* 155–166.

Helmstadter, C., & Godden, J. (2011). *Nursing before nightingale, 1815–1899.* Burlington, VT: Ashgate.

Holland, M. G. (1998). *Our army nurses.* Minnesota: Edinborough Press.

Holme, A. (2015). Big ideas. Why history matters to nursing. *Nurse Education Today, 35,* 635–637.

Im, E., & Chang, S. J. (2012). Current trends in nursing theories. *Journal of Nursing Scholarship, 44,* 156–164.

Johnson, D. E. (1959). A philosophy of nursing. *Nursing Outlook, 7,* 198–200.

Kandel, E. (1920). *Report, price series.* Letter from Gardner to Morgan. Retrieved from www.google.com/search?hl=en&tbm=bks&sxsrf=ALeKk03dhhh2daKEuLGeBK3yj1BxftGNQA%3A1590600122963&ei=uqHOXvK5OoLSsAWL4rGgBQ&q=gardner+1920+nursing&oq=gardner+1920+nursing&gs_l=psy-ab.3...2855.4367.0.4499.8.7.0.0.0.0.325.602.2-1j1.2.0....0...1c.1.64.psy-ab..6.0.0....0.KwHHl0RDFd0

Keeling, A. W., Hehman, M. C., & Kirchgessner, J. C. (2018). *History of professional nursing in the United States*. New York: Springer.

Lewenson, S. L. (2004). Integrating nursing history into the curriculum. *Journal of Professional Nursing, 20*, 374–380.

Lusk, B. (1997). What values drive nursing science? *Reflections, 23*(3), 46–47.

Lusk, B. (2000). Pretty and powerless: Nurses in advertisements, 1930-1950. *Research in Nursing and Health, 23*, 229–236.

Lusk, B. (2001). M. Helena McMillan. In R. L. Schultz & A. Hast (Eds.), *Women building Chicago, 1790-1990* (pp. 573–575). Indiana: Indiana University Press.

Lusk, B. (2002). The image of trained nursing in lay magazines. *Nursing History Review, 10*, 109–125.

Lusk, B., & Robertson, J. (2005). U.S. organized medicine's perspective of nursing: A review of JAMA, 1883-1935. In S. McGann & B. Mortimer's (Eds.), *New directions in the history of nursing* (pp. 86–108). New York: Routledge.

Lusk, B., Keeling, A. W., & Lewenson, S. B. (2016). Using nursing history to inform decision making: Infectious diseases at the turn of the twentieth century. *Nursing Outlook, 64*, 170–178.

Lusk, B., Cockerham, A. Z., & Keeling, A. W. (2019). Highlights from the history of advanced practice nursing in the United States. In M. F. Tracy & E. T. O'Grady (Eds.), *Hamric and Hanson's advanced practice nursing* (pp. 1–24). MO: Elsevier.

Maggs, C. (1996). A history of nursing: A history of caring? *Journal of Advanced Nursing, 23*, 630–635.

McDermott, K. W., Elixhauser, A., & Sun, R. (2017). Trends in hospital inpatient stays in the United States, 2005–2014. *Healthcare Cost and Utilization Project, AHRQ, Statistical Brief #225.*

Montag, M. L. (1959). *Community college education for nursing*. New York: McGraw Hill.

Montag, M. L. (1963). Technical education in nursing? *The American Journal of Nursing, 63*, 100–103.

Noyes, C. D. (1912). The midwifery problem. *American Journal of Nursing, 12*, 466–471.

Orsolini-Hain, L., & Waters, V. (2009). Education evolution: A historical perspective of associate degree nursing. *Journal of Nursing Education, 48*, 266–271.

Richards, L. (1911). *Reminiscences of America's first trained nurse*. Boston, MA: Whitcomb & Barrows.

Robb, W. J. W. (2005). The ABCs of nursing doctoral degrees. *Dimensions of Critical Care Nursing, 24*(2), 89–96.

Schryver, G. F. (1930). *A history of the Illinois training school for nurses*. Chicago, IL: Illinois Training School.

Stafford, M. (2016). *Interview for the Anne Zimmerman project*. Midwest Nursing History Research Center Archives. University of Illinois at Chicago.

Thatcher Ulrich, L. (1991). *A midwife's tale: The life of Martha Ballard, based on her diary, 1785-1812*. New York: Random House.

Tobbell, D. (2018). Nursing's boundary work. Theory development and the making of nursing science, 1950-1980. *Nursing Research, 67*(2), 63–73.

Ulrich, C. M., Grady, C., Hamric, A. B., & Berlinger, N. (2016). Nurses at the table: Nursing, ethics, and health policy. *Hastings Center Report, 46*(S 1), S2. -outside back cover

SUGGESTED READINGS

Brenan, M. (2018). Nurses again outpace other professions for honesty, ethics. *Gallop News*. Retrieved from https://news.gallup.com/poll/245597/nurses-again-outpace-professions-honesty-ethics.aspx

D'Antonio, P., Connolly, C., Mann Wall, B., Whelan, J., & Fairman, J. (2010). Histories of nursing: The power and the possibilities. *Nursing Outlook, 58*(4), 207–213.

Fairman, J., & D'Antonio, P. (2013). History counts: How history can shape our understanding of health policy. *Nursing Outlook, 61*, 346–352.

Foth, T. (2012). Nurses, medical records and the killing of sick persons before, during, and after the Nazi regime in Germany. *Nursing Inquiry, 20*(2), 93–100.

Lagerwey, M. D. (2010). Ethical vulnerabilities in nursing history: Conflicting loyalties and the patient as "other." *Nursing Ethics, 17*, 590–602.

Nelson, S., & Gordon, S. (2004). The rhetoric of rupture: Nursing as a practice with a history? *Nursing Outlook, 53*, 53–54.

Pollitt, P. (2018). Nurses fight for the right to vote. *American Journal of Nursing, 118*(11), 46–54.

Price, S. L., & McGillis Hall, L. (2013). The history of nurse imagery and the implications for recruitment: A discussion paper. *Journal of Advanced Nursing, 70*, 1502–1509.

4

Organization of Patient Care in High Reliability Care Organizations

Patti Ludwig-Beymer
Purdue University Northwest, College of Nursing, Hammond, IN, USA

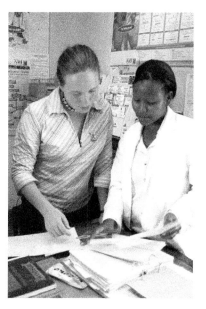

A strong safety culture requires skillful leaders with exceptional communication abilities.
Source: Used with permission from the U.S.A. Government.

A strong safety culture begins with leadership; their behaviors and actions set the bar. I urge all health care leaders to make safety culture a top priority at their health care organization. Establishing and improving safety culture is just as critical as the time and resources devoted to revenue and financial stability, system integration and productivity—because a lack of safety culture can have serious consequences for patients, staff and other stakeholders.

> Ana Pujols McKee, MD, Executive Vice President and Chief Medical Officer, The Joint Commission (TJC, 27 December 2017, para. 6).

OBJECTIVES

Upon completion of this chapter, the reader should be able to:

1. Describe the current state of quality and safety in health care organizations.

2. Define High Reliability within healthcare settings.

3. Evaluate the characteristics of **high reliability organizations** (HROs).

4. Analyze the impact of **Quality and Safety Education for Nurses** (QSEN) competencies on high reliability.

5. Discuss nursing's role in high reliability organizations.

6. Identify resources nurse leaders can use to foster a culture of high reliability.

Kelly Vana's Nursing Leadership and Management, Fourth Edition. Edited by Patricia Kelly Vana and Janice Tazbir
© 2021 John Wiley & Sons Ltd. Published 2021 by John Wiley & Sons Ltd.
Companion Website: www.wiley.com/go/kelly-Nursing-Leadership

OPENING SCENARIO

Ms. Smith's daughter Kali is a patient in the Neonatal Intensive Care Unit (ICU). Ms. Smith diligently pumps her breasts to provide nourishment to her newborn. After pumping, Ms. Smith gives the milk to the nurse, who labels it and places it in the refrigerator. The next day, the nurse prepares a feeding for Kali. After administering the feeding, the nurse notices that the milk is labeled with Ms. Brown's name.

By definition, this is a serious safety event. The organization takes immediate action: it notifies both Ms. Smith and Ms. Brown, and tests Ms. Brown for a variety of infectious diseases. In addition, the error is thoroughly investigated by a team that includes nurses, nursing assistants, physicians, and staff from infection prevention, risk management, quality, information technology, and administration. The team conducts a root cause analysis to determine the underlying cause of the breast milk mis-administration and creates a corrective action plan. The executive leadership team and board of directors review the information and approve the corrective action plan. Everyone at the hospital expresses confidence that the processes put into place will prevent this event from happening again. Unfortunately, within a few months, the incorrect breast milk is administered to a baby in the pediatric department.

The **Institute of Medicine** (IOM, 1999) described the safety of U.S. health care in *To Err is Human*. They suggested that 44,000–98,000 people die in hospitals each year from medical errors that could have been prevented and provided a roadmap to safety. The IOM outlined strategies to prevent errors, including enhancing knowledge about safety; identifying and learning from errors; raising expectations for improving safety; and implementing safety systems in health care organizations to ensure safe practices at the patient care delivery level. Seventeen years later, Makary and Daniel (2016) estimated that medical errors cause 251,000 deaths each year. This makes medical errors the third leading cause of death in the Unites States (U.S.) after heart disease and cancer.

Safety is the responsibility of every nurse and each member of the interprofessional team. Despite the heavy focus on quality and safety, errors continue to occur. Nursing managers and leaders are in a unique position to foster a culture of high reliability. This chapter will describe the current state of quality and safety in health care organizations. After defining and evaluating the characteristics of HRO s, the chapter will analyze the impact of QSEN competencies on high reliability. Last, the chapter will describe the role of the nurse in creating a culture of safety and identify resources nurse leaders can use in a journey toward high reliability.

Definitions of Error

Health care is dangerous, and mistakes or errors can have devastating consequences for patients and staff. Nurses and other health care professionals do not come to work intending to harm patients. However, humans make mistakes. It is part of the nature of being human. Most medical errors do not result from individual recklessness. Instead, many medical errors are caused by faulty health care systems, processes, and conditions that lead people to make mistakes or fail to prevent them. This means that health systems can best prevent mistakes by creating processes that make it easier to do the right thing and harder to do the incorrect thing.

Internal Standards

An **error** is defined as a deviation from generally acceptable performance standards. Performance standards may be found within a health care organization or may exist external to the organization. **Internal standards** include policies, procedures, protocols, and order sets.

External Standards

External standards include professional practice standards and practice requirements imposed by accreditation.

Near Miss Safety Events

An error may cause varying levels of harm to a patient. A **near miss safety event** occurs when the safety event doesn't reach the patient because it is caught by chance or because the process was engineered with a detection barrier. For example, Ms. Johnston and Ms. Johnsen may both be hospitalized on the same nursing unit. The nurse may accidently bring Ms. Johnston's medications to Ms. Johnsen. By properly identifying the patient using two unique identifiers, this error can be identified before causing harm to the patient. Nurses often fail to report Near Misses, rationalizing that no one was hurt. However, near miss safety events serve as an early warning system of something that could go wrong. By reporting near miss safety events, health care organizations can work on improving processes so that no one else makes the same error.

Precursor Safety Events

Precursor safety events occur when the health care error reaches the patient and results in no harm or minimal detectable harm. For example, the nurse may do a finger stick to check a blood sugar for Ms. Johnston when it was ordered for Ms. Johnsen. The error has reached the patient but has resulted in minimal harm, in this case a finger stick. Like near miss safety events, precursor safety events should be reported so that they can be used to improve care.

Adverse Events and Serious Events

Adverse events or serious safety events occur when the error reaches the patient and results in moderate to severe harm or even death.

Sentinal Events

Sentinel events are a subcategory of adverse events. A sentinel event is a patient safety event *that is not primarily related to the natural course of the patient's illness or underlying condition*, reaches the patient, and results in death, permanent harm, or severe temporary harm (TJC, January 2018). For example, imagine that the nurse administered a unit of packed red blood cells intended for Ms. Johnston to Ms. Johnsen. The results could be catastrophic, and the health care team would need to take immediate action to save Ms. Johnsen's life. After the immediate crisis is handled, sentinel events must be carefully investigated. Corrective action plans must be created to reduce risk and prevent harm for future patients.

TJC is an independent, not-for-profit group in the United States that provides accreditation for many hospitals and other health care organizations. TJC publishes a list of the most frequently occurring sentinel events, summarized in Table 4.1. The reporting of sentinel events is voluntary and represents only a small proportion of actual sentinel events.

The Anatomy of an Error

Active Errors

Errors are often noticed at the point of care, where nurses and other clinicians interact with patients. This is considered the "sharp end" of a triangle (Cook & Woods, 1994). These errors are considered **active errors** because they occur at the point of interface between humans and a complex system. Clinicians often blame themselves when errors happen. However, their work with patients is influenced by many factors and decisions made before an actual error occurs. These factors and decisions are considered the "blunt end" of the triangle.

Latent Errors

Latent errors are hidden problems within health care systems that contribute to adverse events (**Agency for Healthcare Research and Quality [AHRQ], 2018a, 2018b**). For example, policies and procedures within an organization may be inaccessible, difficult to understand, or inaccurate. Work processes might be confusing and patient handoffs may be rushed and inadequate. The environment may be cramped and noisy, making it difficult to concentrate. Technology may fail or be cumbersome to use. Individuals may blame others rather than taking personal responsibility. The culture of the hospital might hinder a nurse's ability to speak up about safety concerns. All of these "blunt end" factors may contribute to an error at the "sharp end," where clinicians interact with the patient.

James Reason (1997) proposed the *Swiss Cheese model*, shown in Figure 4.1, to illustrate how errors occur. The model suggests that every step in a process has the potential for error.

Table 4.1   Five Most Frequent Sentinel Events, 2014 through 2017 (TJC, January 2018)

Event	Definition	Number of Reported Events
Unintended Retention of a Foreign Body	An unintended retention of a foreign body is defined as the retention of a foreign object in a patient after surgery or other procedure.	481
Wrong-patient, wrong-site, wrong-procedure	A wrong-patient procedure occurs when the procedure is performed on the incorrect patient. A wrong-site procedure involves operating on the wrong side of a patient. A wrong procedure occurs when an incorrect procedure is performed on a patient.	409
Fall	A fall sentinel event is defined as an unplanned descent to the floor resulting in death, permanent harm, or severe temporary harm.	404
Suicide	A suicide sentinel event is defined as intentionally killing oneself in a healthcare setting.	361
Delay in treatment	A delay in treatment sentinel event is when a patient does not get any type of treatment (medication, lab test, etc.) that was ordered for them in the time frame in which it was supposed to be delivered, and the delay results in death, permanent harm, or severe temporary harm.	290
Total number of reported sentinel events	A subcategory of Adverse Events, a Sentinel Event is a patient safety event (not primarily related to the natural course of the patient's illness or underlying condition) that reaches a patient and results in any of the following: Death; Permanent harm; or Severe temporary harm.	3,326

Source: The Joint Commission (January 2018). Patient Safety Systems. Retrieved from https://www.jointcommission.org/assets/1/6/PS_chapter_HAP_2018.pdf.

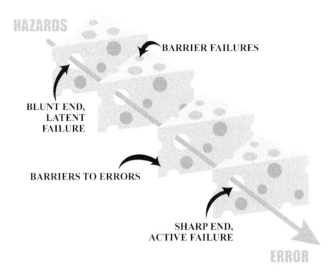

HAZARDS

BARRIER FAILURES

BLUNT END,
LATENT
FAILURE

BARRIERS TO ERRORS

SHARP END,
ACTIVE FAILURE

ERROR

FIGURE 4.1 Swiss cheese model.
Source: © Used with permission granted from Patti Ludwig-Beymer.

The holes in the Swiss cheese represent opportunities for a process to fail, and each slice is a defensive layer to prevent an error in the process. An error may pass through a hole in one layer but in the next layer, the hole is in a different spot and the layer catches the error before it reaches the patient. More layers of cheese and smaller holes allow more errors to be stopped or caught. When the holes in the Swiss cheese line up, an error occurs.

High Reliability Organizations

Building an HRO is a cultural transformation designed to ensure safe practices and reduce errors and sentinel events in health care. Health care is complex and involves the risk of significant and potentially catastrophic consequences when failures occur. HROs operate under these trying conditions and have fewer accidents. They have the ability to provide consistent health care at a high level of excellence over a long period of time. HROs in health care establish and maintain high quality and safety expectations for patient care. Quality and safety error rates are near zero in HROs (Weick & Sutcliffe, 2007).

The risk of health care error is a function of both probability and consequence. For example, consider the care needed for a dehydrated patient with renal failure. Administering fluids too slowly can result in prolonged hypotension. Administering fluids too rapidly can result in fluid retention and heart failure. An IV pump is used to assist the nurse in providing accurate amounts of fluid. The IV pump decreases the probability of error. However, if the pump is programmed incorrectly or fails completely, the consequences can be catastrophic. By decreasing the probability of an error, HROs operate to make health care systems safer.

Origins of HRO

HROs operate in complex, high-hazard situations for extended periods without serious accidents or catastrophic failures.

HROs relentlessly prioritize safety over other performance pressures. An example is a military aircraft carrier. The carrier operates under significant production pressures with aircrafts taking off and landing every 48–60 seconds; constantly changing conditions; and a hierarchical (military) organizational structure. However, personnel consistently prioritize safety and have both the authority and the responsibility to make real-time operational adjustments to maintain safe operations as the top priority (AHRQ, 2018a, 2018b).

In the 1970s, research conducted by the National Aeronautics and Space Administration suggested that most commercial airplane crashes were caused by communication failures among pilots and crew, not by mechanical failures. In some cases, co-pilots were aware that pilots were making unsafe decisions but did not verbalize their concerns because of authority gradient. Authority gradient refers to one's position within a group or profession. It was defined first in aviation when it was noted that pilots and copilots did not always communicate effectively in stressful situations if there was a significant difference in their perceived authority. Multiple aviation, aerospace, and industrial incidents have been attributed to authority gradients. This information was used to develop and implement the **Crew Resource Management** (CRM) training program. The training program focuses on interpersonal communication, leadership, and decision making in the cockpit, with the informal motto "see it, say it, fix it." CRM is credited with the dramatic safety improvements in the airline industry (Helmreich, Merritt & Wilhelm, 1999) and has been adapted for use in health care and many other industries.

Similarly, the nuclear power industry has worked for many years to improve safety. The Institute of Nuclear Power Operations defines safety culture characteristics, some that are adaptable to the health care environment, and include: everyone is responsible for safety, leaders demonstrate commitment to safety, trust permeates the organization, decision making reflects safety first, a questioning attitude is cultivated, organizational learning is embraced and safety needs constant examination (Institute of Nuclear Power Operations, 2004). The American College of Healthcare Executives and **Institute for Healthcare Improvement** (IHI) published a blueprint for safety (2014) and is summarized in Table 4.2. These characteristics are essential for cultural transformation and are as applicable for all health care organizations.

HRO Characteristics

Weick and Sutcliffe (2007) identified five key principles of HROs that are used to this day, summarized in Table 4.3. These characteristics, when present, help an organization to achieve high reliability. Each characteristic is described in detail below.

Preoccupation with Failure

In **preoccupation with failure,** nurses and other health care providers are aware that the risk of error is always present.

Table 4.2   Safety Culture Characteristics

1. Establish a vision for safety
2. Build trust, respect, and inclusion
3. Select, develop, and engage your Board
4. Prioritize safety in the selection and development of leaders
5. Lead and reward a just culture
6. Establish organization behavior expectations

Source: Based on American College of Healthcare Executives and Institute for Healthcare Improvement. (2017). Leading a Culture of Safety: A Blueprint for Success. Retrieved from www.osha.gov/shpguidelines/docs/Leading_a_Culture_of_Safety-A_Blueprint_for_Success.pdf

Table 4.3   HRO Characteristics

Characteristic	Activities
Preoccupation with failure	Pay attention to near-miss events Look for weaknesses in the delivery of care
Reluctance to simplify	Acknowledge the complex nature of health care delivery Focus on the root (true) cause of errors
Sensitivity to operations	Develop awareness of how the environment, resources, and supplies impact safety Acknowledge the effect of relationships on safety
Commitment to resilience	Anticipate and alleviate errors Work to decrease risk of harm Develop recovery strategies when adverse events occur
Deference to expertise	Recognize individuals' knowledge, skill, and expertise Employ teamwork Foster active participation by healthcare providers Eliminate hierarchical thinking Share information

Source: Patti Ludwig-Beymer.

An HRO recognizes that failures can occur and deploys processes to diminish harm. An HRO proactively identifies high risk activities and analyzes all the potential error points in the process. This analysis can be performed as a **Failure Modes and Effect Analysis** (FMEA), a rigorous process in which a team of clinicians identify and eliminate known and potential failures, errors, or problems before they occur (Hughes, 2008). Failures are prioritized according to the seriousness of the consequences, how frequently they occur, and how easily they can be detected. An FMEA example is provided in Figure 4.2.

Preoccupation with failure requires that critical information be communicated across time, across the health care team, and across sites of care. For example, a patient may be seen in the **Emergency Department** (ED) and require admission to the acute care hospital. Prior to transferring the patient, the ED nurse provides a thorough report to the nurse on the receiving unit.

In preoccupation with failure, nurses report questionable or unsafe practices. They notice and learn from near miss safety events and precursor safety events. These events are viewed as early warnings that something is wrong. Nurses recognize when an error can or has occurred, feel confident in stopping unsafe practices, and assume the responsibility for reporting errors or near misses. The organization then uses the reports to correct unsafe processes through rigorous process improvement activities.

Reluctance to Simplify

Reluctance to simplify motivates an organization to understand errors. Nurses in HRO health care facilities focus on drilling down to determine the true cause of error. They challenge the current situation to make health care processes and structures safer. For example, a nurse may fail to check a patient's blood sugar as ordered. Initially, the nurse may just indicate "I forgot." However, analyzing the situation for contributing factors to this failure helps the organization to find real, root cause, and develop solutions. Multiple factors could have contributed to the failure to check a patient's blood sugar. The patient may have been off the unit for a test. The information may not have been shared at change of shift, or a reminder prompt in the **electronic health record** (EHR) may have been missing. The necessary supplies and equipment may not have been available. An examination of each of these factors allows an HRO to determine ways to prevent this error.

Reluctance to simplify also requires taking action to eliminate work=arounds, the use of short cuts to streamline care without realizing the potential impact on safety. For example, a national patient safety goal requires the use of hand cleaning guidelines from the Centers for Disease Control and Prevention or the World Health Organization. Nurses may save time by rinsing rather than thoroughly washing their hands. Unfortunately, this increases risk to patients and staff. Leaders in HROs identify and extinguish these types of work-arounds.

Sensitivity to Operations

Sensitivity to operations acknowledges the complex nature of health care. Factors such as fatigue, distractions, and workload can contribute to unsafe conditions. In HROs, nursing leaders make rounds and talk to staff to look for weaknesses in the care delivery system that allow errors to occur. When weaknesses are identified, leaders allocate resources to prevent harm. For example, the automated medication dispensing system may be in a hallway on a medical surgical unit. When making rounds, the nurse leader may see that the nurse is interrupted by physicians, patients, visitors, and other staff while obtaining medications from the dispensing system. Nurses on the unit may express concern about this process, which interferes with their ability to concentrate on preparing the medications. The nursing leader may resolve the problem by allocating funds to create a small medication room to house the automated medication dispensing system and minimize distractions.

Example Failure Modes Effect Analysis (FMEA)

Number	Failure Mode	Potential Causes	Scoring			Action Item	Responsible Person(s)	Targeted Completion Date
			Severity	Probability	Criticality			
1	Medication not ordered appropriately	Roles not clearly defined	4	10	40			
		Clinical condition not recognized	10	1	10			
		Provider orders wrong dose, route or concentration	10	10	100			
		3 way feedback not verbalized	7	10	70			
2	Medication not appropriately prepared	Wrong needle/syringe used	1	7	7			
		Wrong dose drawn into syringe	10	10	100			
		Needle not changed prior to administration	4	4	16			
3	not administered correctly	Second nurse not available	7	10	70			
		Second nurse not familiar with dosing	10	10	100			
		Medications not documented correctly	1	7	7			

Scoring Code:
Severity = How severe the consequences would be if this error occurred on a scale of 1-10
Probability = The likelihood this error will occur on a scale of 1 to 10
Criticality = Severity multiplied by Probability; higher numbers indicate higher criticality

Process Steps:
The team determines the failure modes, potential causes, severity, and criticality.
The team identifies action items based on causes with the highest criticality.
The team then assigns the work to a person or team and targets a completion date.

FIGURE 4.2   FMEA.
Source: Patti Ludwig-Beymer.

Commitment to Resilience

Commitment to resilience is the ability to overcome problems, learn from mistakes, and move forward. It allows nurses and clinicians to recover when a serious safety event occurs. Because we are humans, mistakes will happen. Rather than blaming others, nurses in HROs discuss how the error occurred and what can be done to prevent such an error in the future. Transparency is essential; errors are openly discussed and used to improve health care processes. In HROs, nurses learn to perform quick situational assessments when an error occurs, work as a team to contain or manage the error, and then take steps to reduce the harm.

In HROs, clinicians are offered support when they are involved in a safety event. Nurses and other clinicians feel guilty when they make an error that harms a patient. The term "Second Victim" is used to describe the pain and anguish experienced by the clinician (Wu, 2000). Programs have been developed to assist clinicians to build resilience and recover from these safety events. The forYOU program (Scott, 2015) is an evidence-based second victim intervention that provides immediate emotional and social support. Members of the forYOU team provide emotional support using three levels: local support from a colleague, support from specially trained peers, and support through a network of chaplains, social workers, and employee assistance programs. Resources that help build resilient nurses are also available through the Academy of Medical-Surgical Nurses (n.d.) and the American Association of Critical Care Nurses (2014).

Simulation learning is used in HROs to practice responses to errors or safety events. Drills for environmental disasters, active threats, rapid responses, and cardiopulmonary resuscitation allow nurses and other clinicians to practice as an interprofessional team and build resilience for emergency situations (Figure 4.3).

Deference to Expertise

Deference to expertise acknowledges that collective knowledge is better than the proficiency of one individual. This allows a team to recognize and use the unique skills of everyone involved. HROs minimize the authority gradient and

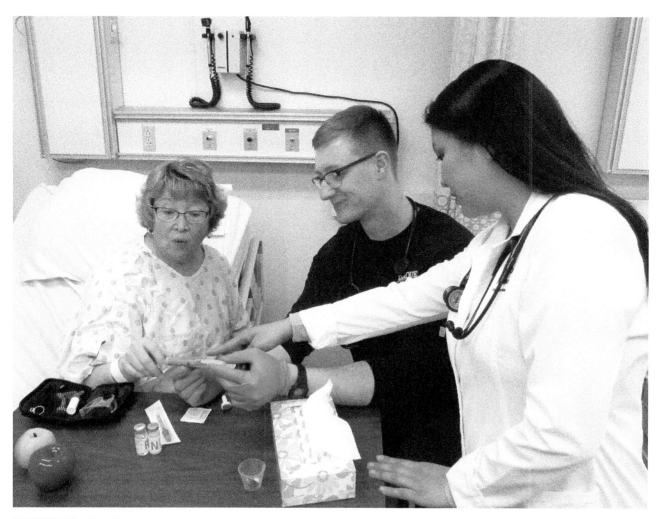

FIGURE 4.3 Simulation exercise.
Source: Used with permission.

hierarchy so that everyone feels comfortable about speaking up. Authority gradients exist in nursing and in other health care professions. Consider the difference in perceived authority between direct care nurses, nurse managers, nurse directors, and the **Chief Nursing Officer** (CNO). Hierarchy also exists in health care settings and refers to the perceived level of power across groups. Consider, for example, the perceived power for a housekeeper compared to a direct care nurse, or a direct care nurse and a physician. Health care has been and remains hierarchical. Physicians have been historically viewed as the "captain of the ship," with nurses and other clinicians viewed as less powerful.

Regardless of authority gradient, or hierarchy, deference to expertise stipulates that team members with the most expertise about the issue have the authority to make decisions. In an HRO, decisions about nursing practice are informed by and driven by practicing nurses rather than by the CNO or by physicians. Deference to expertise also requires open communication with information flowing in all directions among all team members.

Nursing's Role in High Reliability Organizations

Every nurse, at every level of the organization, plays a role in an organization's journey toward high reliability. Each nurse and each member of the interprofessional health care team must be committed to high reliability. Direct Care nurses are essential in HROs. While many contributing factors lead to errors, an actual error occurs when the nurse or another clinician interacts with the patient, at the "sharp end" of care. The nurse is often the last line of defense against health care errors. As such, the nurse must be cognizant of personal behaviors to enhance safety and communication techniques that can be helpful in preventing errors and patient harm.

However, individual actions are not sufficient. Committed nurse leaders are needed to implement system changes that are essential for becoming an HRO. In collaboration with other organizational leaders, nurse leaders are accountable for the provision of effective and efficient care while protecting the safety of patients, employees, and visitors. Leadership's failure to create an effective safety culture is a contributing factor for many types of adverse events (The Joint Commission, 2018a, 2018b, 2018c). Shaping an organization into a culture of safety and reliability is essential for enhancing safety and improving the "blunt end" or care.

To prepare nursing students to function in the complex health care environment. The QSEN project was established. The QSEN Institute is a collaborative of healthcare professionals focused on education, practice, and scholarship to improve the quality and safety of health care systems. Their goal is to prepare future nurses at the baccalaureate and graduate levels with the knowledge, skills, and attitudes necessary to continuously improve the quality and safety of the health care systems within which they work. Based on earlier work completed by the Institute of Medicine (2001), QSEN identified six core competencies for new graduates, as outlined in Table 4.4 (QSEN, 2018). Each core competency is described below. The competencies are used to frame this chapter's discussion of high reliability.

Real World Interview

When nursing staff is asked the question "what can leadership improve upon?", the answer is often related to communication and education with respect to change. While safe staffing ratios are vitally important, adverse safety events and job dissatisfaction may come from implementing a new process, device, or expectations without properly notifying or educating staff. Providing up-to-date information—even laying the framework to changes or potential concerns coming in the future, can help nurses adapt to and implement changes quickly.

We love our unit newsletter because it allows us to look at where we are and where we are going while always keeping safety in the front of our minds. It is a collaborative effort between the educators, management, infection control, and various other departments (like pharmacy and the vascular team). Fun articles celebrating employee birthdays, anniversaries, and humor segments along with unit pride pieces help make the newsletter fun to read as well as educational. Creating a graph of catheter-associated urinary tract infections (CAUTI) rates has been largely unsuccessful in convincing nurses of the importance of HAIs. Writing a short article on the number of CAUTIs the hospital has had for the month and on which units they occurred gets everybody talking about the problem. It's a different spin on the same material. The hope is that in combination with staff meetings, education sessions, huddle alerts, updated intranet splash pages, and other communication strategies, we are bombarding our staff with information to keep their patients—and themselves—SAFE. When we are consistently safe, we improve patient outcomes and nurses are more engaged in their work and their hospital.

Bonny Dieter, MS, RN, CMSRN
Clinical Leader and Creator of PMU Newsletter
Pulmonary Medicine Unit
Edward Hospital
Naperville, IL Figures 4.4 and 4.5

Table 4.4   QSEN Competencies

Patient-Centered Care

Teamwork and Collaboration

Evidence-based Practice (EBP)

Quality Improvement (QI)

Safety

Informatics

Source: QSEN.org.

Patient-Centered Care

In this competency, nurses recognize that the patient or designee is the source of control. Patients are full partners when the nurse is providing compassionate and coordinated care. Patients identify their designees, typically family members or close friends. Nurses respect the preferences, values, and needs of their patients and the way in which patients define family.

The relationship between direct patient care and patient-centered care is easy to understand. In addition, nurses and nurse leaders must consider patients and their designees in a broader context. Nurse leaders must create organizational cultures that assess and support patient and family preferences. They must use current evidence when designing patient care areas to promote patient-centered care. Nurse leaders must also work within their institutions to remove barriers to the presence of families and their designees. Establishing a Patient Family Advisory Committee can be helpful in providing input for nurse leaders and other organizational leadership. Patient-centered care is discussed in greater detail in Chapter 8.

Teamwork and Collaboration

In this competency, nurses function effectively within both nursing and interprofessional teams. They foster open communication, mutual respect, and shared decision-making to achieve quality patient care. This needs to happen at every level of the organization. Direct care nurses must function within their scope of practice and integrate the contributions of others to help patients achieve health outcomes. Nurses must communicate effectively with the nursing team and with many other clinicians to enhance patient care and minimize risks associated with handoffs. Nurse leaders must lead or participate in the design and implementation of systems that support effective teamwork. They must create an organization that appreciates and values clear communication. Several strategies for enhancing communication are described below.

Effective Communication

Improving the effectiveness of communication among caregivers is one of the National Patient Safety Goals (TJC, 2018a, 2018b, 2018c). Communication ensures that messages are heard correctly and accurately; prevents incorrect assumptions and misunderstandings that could lead to wrong decisions; and is essential within nursing and with other members of the interprofessional team.

TeamSTEPPS

TeamSTEPPS® (AHRQ, 2013a, 2013b) provides several tools for improving communication, including call-out and closed-loop (or three way) communication.

Call-Out

Call-Out is a tool used to communicate important information. It informs all team members simultaneously during an emergency and helps team members anticipate next steps. For example, during a code, the nurse uses a call-out to report "I've administered 1 mg Epinephrine IV."

Closed Loop Communication

Closed loop communication ensures that the message received is the same as what was intended by the sender. The sender initiates communication with a receiver by providing a

---

Case Study 4.1

Providing patient-centered care is an important part of building a high reliability culture. Chris, a nurse on the Pediatric ICU, is caring for a 3-month-old with a history of supraventricular tachycardia, cough, and congestion. Chris reviews the patient's EHR and finds an order for Propranolol 20 mg TID. As an experienced pediatric nurse, Chris realizes this dose is high. She knows pediatric doses are weight-based and consults a drug reference book to determine the appropriate dose. Chris also talks with the mother and learns that the infant was taking 2 mg of Propranolol three times a day at home. She then speaks to the physician, who changes the medication order and thanks Chris for her diligence.

1. Why did Chris consult a drug reference book?

2. Why did Chris talk with the patient's mother?

3. How might Chris best present this information to the physician?

4. How does Chris's diligence and the thank you from the physician help to build a culture of high reliability?

In this scenario, Chris took two positive safety actions: she demonstrated a questioning attitude while providing patient care, and she involved the patient's mother in his investigation. Chris carefully considered the patient care situation and asked herself some key questions. Is this what I expected to see? Does this fit with what I know? Does this make sense to me? She then investigated by checking with independent, expert sources, competent people, and written materials that could help resolve the question.

Case Study 4.2

Sam is a nurse on a medical-surgical unit. When he receives a telephone order from a physician, he enters it into the EHR and reads it back to the physician. Sam waits for the physician to verify the order before concluding the conversation. Sam also uses closed-loop communication when communicating with or delegating to a nursing assistant.

1. Why does Sam read back the telephone order to the physician?

2. What factors may tempt Sam to skip this important safety step?

3. How does closed-loop communication between Sam and a nursing assistant build strong teams and foster patient safety?

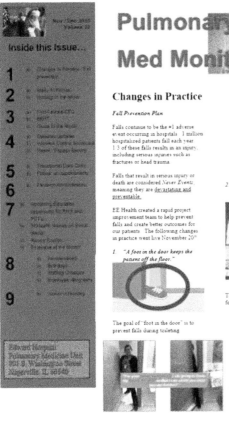

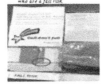

FIGURE 4.4   PMU Newsletter. Newsletter designed to increase communication on safety issues.
Source: **Bonny Dieter.**

request, information, or clinician order. The receiver acknowledges the communication with a repeat-back. The sender then confirms the accuracy of the acknowledgement by saying "that's correct." If communication isn't clear, the nurse must clear up the confusion. "Let me ask a clarifying question" is a helpful and non-threatening phrase to use when attempting to clarify communication.

I PASS THE BATON

Communication also includes the transfer of information during transitions of care, for example across units or sites of care, during shift changes, and during hospital discharge. These communication handoffs provide an opportunity to ask questions, clarify information, and confirm understanding. The tool **I PASS the BATON** can be used effectively in handoffs. The I PASS the BATON acronym for remembering the key components of the handoff is presented in Figure 4.6

SBAR

SBAR is another helpful tool for handoffs. The acronym **SBAR** stands for Situation, Background, Assessment and Recommendation. Kaiser Permanente originally adapted a United States Navy tool to enhance collaboration between nurses and physicians (Institute for Health Care Improvement, 2018c). *Situation* refers to a concise statement of the immediate problem. *Background* is a brief summary of pertinent information related to the situation. *Assessment* refers to analysis and consideration of action options. *Recommendation* addresses the actions requested.

Nursing and Interprofessional Teams

Health care delivery requires strong and supportive health care teams, where members monitor team function, share the workload, and support each other. TeamSTEPPS (AHRQ, 2013a, 2013b)

Case Study 4.3

Jean uses SBAR as a nurse in labor and delivery. When caring for Mrs. Jones, she calls the obstetrician to report, "Here's the situation. I have some concerns about Mrs. Jones' baby related to the fetal heart rate. For the past two hours the baby has had a rising baseline from 135 to 170. Now, the strip has minimal variability with no elicited fetal heart rate accelerations using vibroacoustic stimulation and position change. I need you to come and visualize this strip and assess the situation. When can I expect you?"

1. What critical information does Jean communicate with the physician?

2. How does this clear communication enhance patient safety?

3. How do you suppose the physician responded to Jean's telephone call?

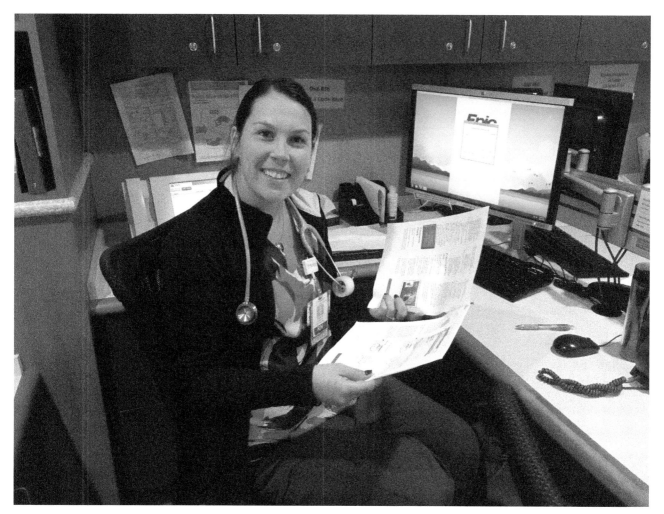

FIGURE 4.5   Registered nurse catches up on safety news by reading the PMU newsletterr.
Source: Kary Blaschak.

I	Introduction	Introduce yourself and your role
P	Patient	Patient's name, identifiers, gender , & location
A	Assessment	Diagnosis, chief complaint, vital signs, & symptoms
S	Situation	Current status or circumstances, including recent changes, response to treatment, code status & level of uncertainty
S	Safety	Critical lab values, allergies, alerts (isolation, fall, etc.(, & socio-economic factors

The

B	Background	Co-morbidities, previous episodes, current medications, family history
A	Actions	Actions that were taken or are required, brief rational for actions
T	Timing	Level of urgency and explicit timing, prioritization of actions
O	Ownership	Person(s) responsible (e.g. nurse, physician, team), patient & family responsibilities
N	Next	What will happen next? Anticipated changes? What is the plan? Contingency plan?

FIGURE 4.6   I PASS the BATON.
Source: Patti Ludwig-Beymer.

Evidence from the Literature

Source: Adapted from Leach, L.S. & Mayo, A.M. (2013). Rapid response teams: Qualitative analysis of their effectiveness. *American Journal of Critical Care*, 22(3), 198–210.

Discussion: The article describes the effectiveness of rapid response teams in a large teaching hospital using grounded theory methodology. Researchers found that effective team performance included the concepts of organizational culture, team structure, expertise, communication, and teamwork. Because of inconsistency in membership, team members had little opportunity to develop relationships or team skills.

provides team strategies and tools to enhance performance and patient safety. CRM, described earlier in this chapter, was adopted into health care from aviation to promote and reinforce the team behaviors of cooperation, coordination, and sharing regardless of formal position. It's been used to improve patient care in obstetrics, the operating room, the emergency department, and other settings (Kreiser, 2012).

To enhance patient safety and quality, many hospitals have implemented rapid response teams. These interprofessional teams are activated by a staff nurse or other clinician when a patient's condition deteriorates unexpectedly. A rapid response brings clinical experts quickly to the patient's bedside and can be implemented in a cost-effective manner (Mitchell, Schatz, & Francis, 2014). In recognition of patient-centered care, some facilities permit a rapid response team to be activated by patients and family members (Gerdik, Vallish, Miles, Godwin, Wludyka, & Panni, 2010).

Implications for Practice

Implications for Practice. Communication between team members and managing a crisis are critical aspects of an effective response team. Team training is needed to enhance the performance of teams that work together infrequently and experience time pressure to perform.

High team performance is facilitated when nurses and other staff members are expected to and comfortable with providing both positive and constructive feedback to team members. Positive feedback is essential for reinforcing safe behavior. Clinicians perform many safe actions every day and should be recognized for that. Constructive feedback is needed to discourage and change unsafe behaviors. People tend to avoid constructive feedback because they are uncomfortable providing it. However, a simple reminder is often all that is needed to correct behavior. Constructive feedback should always be met with a thank you, and a change in behavior.

Cross Monitoring

Cross-monitoring is a tool to assist in error reduction in teams and allows team members to monitor unusual situations or hazards, identify safety slips or lapses, and provide impromptu consultation and feedback. For example, many HROs use two-person patient identification when administering narcotics via a patient-controlled administration system. If the pump were set incorrectly, the patient could receive an inappropriate dose, have a respiratory arrest, and potentially die. The two-person process is an essential safety step and reinforces teamwork when providing care.

Mutual Support

Providing **mutual support** to team members is the ability to anticipate team members' needs and provide assistance as needed through accurate knowledge about their workloads and responsibilities. Team members are expected to advocate for the patient. Feedback should be timely, respectful, specific, and directed toward quality improvement.

Evidence-Based Practice

In this competency, nurses integrate best current evidence with clinical expertise and patient/family preferences and values to deliver optimal health care. Direct care nurses develop an individualized plan of care for each patient based on the evidence, patient values, and their clinical expertise. Nurse leaders design the work environment and organizational systems to support evidence-based practice and facilitate the integration of new evidence into standards of practice. They also translate knowledge into practice and generate new knowledge for nursing practice. Providing care based on the evidence is essential for an HRO and plays a key role in fostering both staff and patient safety. Evidence-based practice is discussed in greater detail in Chapter 10.

Quality Improvement (QI)

In this competency, nurses use data to monitor the outcomes of care processes. They also use improvement methods to design and test changes to continuously improve the quality and safety of health care systems. As part of the nursing process, direct care nurses evaluate the care they deliver to each patient. In addition, direct care nurses work together to improve the outcomes of care for the populations served in the care setting. Clinical nurses and nurse leaders identify gaps between local outcomes and best practice outcomes. Nurse leaders lead and provide resources for quality improvement efforts, including access to quality data, quality improvement tools, and quality experts.

An HRO has a strong commitment to health care process improvement. Becoming an HRO requires that the organization systematically review the complexity of health care processes, identify the root causes of failures, implement

Case Study 4.4

Nurses who work on an Orthopedic Unit notice that their patients have a longer length of stay after hip replacement surgery than the national average. They use QI tools to understand this variation and determine that an underlying cause is inconsistent patient preparation prior to surgery. Some patients anticipate a speedy recovery and have not identified the help they will need after discharge. Other patients expect to be admitted to a rehabilitation unit to recover after surgery, which may not be indicated for the procedure. These situations result in discharge delays while the unit's nurse case manager arranges for family help, home care services, or rehabilitation services. The nurses work with other members of the interprofessional team, including physicians, physical therapists, and occupational therapists, to design a test of change. They create a patient education video that clearly outlines recovery expectations and guides patients in establishing a post-discharge plan of care.

After implementing the intervention, they note that length of stay has decreased and there are still opportunities for improvement. The team designs another test of change. In addition to the video, each patient also receives a call from the nurse case manager to answer questions and discuss and document the plan of care. Again, the team sees a decrease in length of stay and continued opportunities. The team designs a third test of change. The day before the surgery, a nurse from the Preadmission Testing Unit (PAT) calls the patient and verifies the plan of care that the patient developed with the nurse case manager. If the plan is still in place

and appropriate, the surgery is performed as scheduled. If the plan needs to be changed, the PAT nurse notifies the surgeon and nurse case manager and they work together to resolve the issues. After implementing this test of change, length of stay for patients having total hip replacement surgery is lower on the orthopedic Unit than the benchmark, and the team also sees a decrease in 30-day readmission rates.

1. What was the original opportunity that the nurses wanted to improve?

2. Why was it important for the nurses to work with the interprofessional team to address this opportunity?

3. Why did the team elect to conduct three tests of change rather than implementing everything at once?

4. Why was the use of a patient video partially effective in reducing length of stay for patients after total hip replacement surgery?

5. Why did the conversation with the nurse case manager improve the length of stay for patients after total hip replacement surgery?

6. Why did the call from the PAT nurse further improve length of stay?

7. What factors may have resulted in the decrease in the 30-day readmission rate?

solutions, measure and monitor outcomes, and sustain the improvement. In some cases, an entirely new process may be required to enhance safety. Increasingly, patients and their families are being engaged to assist in health care process improvements. Quality improvement is described in greater detail in Chapter 18.

Safety

In this competency, nurses minimize risk of harm to patients and providers through both system effectiveness and individual performance. Direct care nurses incorporate human factors and other safety design principles into their care. They use effec-

tive strategies to decrease reliance on memory to reduce risk of harm to self and others. Direct care nurses identify and report concerns about safety and participate in analyzing errors and designing system improvements. They participate in root cause analyzes and use national patient safety resources in their professional development. Nurse leaders strategically plan to improve practice and reduce risk of harm to patients, staff, and others. They create HROs based on human factors research and foster a safe and reliable culture where safe design principles are developed and implemented. Nurse leaders anticipate and mitigate system failures and hazards and design and implement changes in response to identified hazards and errors.

Real World Interview with Karen Zaehler – Edward Quality Council

The purpose of the Nursing Quality Council is to review house-wide quality data and share unit-based quality improvement projects. As chair of the council, my role was to support staff nurses working on quality improvement projects by helping to provide data, research evidence, and other resources needed. Working with patients directly at the bedside gives staff nurses a unique insight on what positively affects quality of care. Having staff nurses involved in quality and safety improvement is vital, as it not only

broadens the staff nurse's knowledge related to performance data, but also empowers them to offer their perspective on improvement projects that will directly affect patient care.

Karen Zaehler, BSN, RN, CMSRN
Staff Nurse, Surgical Care Unit, Edward Hospital
Naperville, IL

Incorporate Human Factors

Incorporate Human Factors. Humans function primarily in three performance modes: skill-based, rule-based, and knowledge-based. Errors occur in each performance mode. By understanding the way humans function, nurses can decrease the number of errors that occur in each performance mode.

Skill-Based Performance

Individuals use **skill-based performance** for routine, familiar tasks that can be done without thinking about them. The drive home, for example, may be so familiar that drivers arrive without knowing how they got there. Nurses often function in this mode because of the repetitive nature of some nursing tasks. Consider, for example, Jerry who is completing his documentation in the EHR. Jerry logs onto the EHR many times each day and he doesn't need to think about his user identification or his password. He's on auto-pilot. He pulls up his assigned patients in the EHR and begins to document.

Generally, skill-based performance is accurate, but there is still risk for error. *Slips* occur when, without intending to, the individual does the wrong thing. Jerry could open a patient's record and document care that was delivered to a different patient. *Lapses* occur when, without intending to, the individual fails to do what he meant to do. Jerry could document on the correct patient but forget to save or file his work before closing the record. *Fumbles* occur when, without intending to, an individual mishandles a word or action. Jerry might notice that his patient was visited by a "dear friend" and accidently document that the patient was visited by a "dead friend."

Several strategies help nurses to stop and think before acting to prevent skill-based errors. Nurses may use *PAR* (Pause-Act-Review). With this technique, nurses pause for 1 or 2 s to focus their attention on the task; act by concentrating and performing the task; and review their actions to check for the desired result. This self-checking takes only a few seconds but greatly reduces the probability of making an error. *Double checking* one's own work also helps to prevent these errors. Nurses learn to check, re-check, and check a third time before administering medications. Determining that the right drug in the right dose is being given by the right route, at the right time, and to the right patient involves checking the medication label against the medication order or medication administration record three times. In addition, two unique patient identifiers are verified prior to administering the medication. Health care facilities typically define which two patient identifiers are to be used, most often full name and date of birth. High risk medications, such as insulin, may require independent verification by another nurse. The independence of this double-check helps to prevent skill-based errors.

Rule-Based Performance

In **rule-based performance**, the clinician applies a learned rule to an appropriate situation. The delivery of health care is largely based on rules, often called protocols. Rules may be learned in nursing school or through life experience, clinical experience, or continuing education. Errors may occur when functioning in a rule-based performance mode. Leaders need to track data on staff compliance with rule-based clinical performance and continually look for ways to improve practice. Errors occur in three ways: using the wrong rule; misapplying the rule; and disregarding the rule.

Sometimes, clinicians use the wrong rule. They may have been taught or somehow learned the wrong response for a situation. For example, Donna graduated many years ago and learned to treat patients for hypoglycemia if the glucose was 60 mg/dl or less. If Donna has not kept current with more recent diabetes and hypoglycemia guidelines, she will fail to treat a patient with a glucose of 70. The solution to this type of error is to educate clinicians with the right rule.

A rule-based error also occurs if the clinician misapplies the rule. The nurse may know the right response but select another response instead. For example, Donna's patient has a blood sugar of 64 mg/dl. Donna knows it needs to be treated. Rather than rely on her memory, she quickly consults the hypoglycemia algorithm—an excellent safety practice. The algorithm indicates treatment with 15 g of glucose. Donna misreads the algorithm and gives 30 g of carbohydrates instead. This could over-correct the low blood sugar, causing the blood sugar to spike and creating another patient safety event. This type of error may be prevented by pausing and thinking or reviewing a second time.

Rule-based performance errors may also be caused by disregarding the rule, as when the clinician knows the rule but chooses not to follow it. For example, Donna's patient has a hypoglycemic event and she treats it appropriately. Donna knows that she should recheck her patient's glucose level 15 to 30 minutes after treating hypoglycemia. She sees that the patient is alert and oriented and looks fine. Donna tells the patient to put on her call light if she runs into any problems and does not recheck the blood sugar. Non-compliance with rules can be prevented in several ways. First, Donna needs to understand the risks involved in not following the rules. In addition, organizations need to reduce the burden or difficulty of following the rules. Nurse leaders need to consider if there are adequate numbers of bedside glucose monitors so that a glucose recheck can be easily accomplished. They need to examine staffing to ensure it is enough to allow time for the glucose recheck. Last, Donna may need to be coached by her manager to make better decisions. If this is a repeated behavior, Donna will need to be counseled and disciplined by a nurse manager.

Knowledge-Based Performance

In **knowledge-based performance**, a clinician is solving problems in a new and unfamiliar situation. Clinicians may try to figure out how to perform based on what they already know, using trial and error, or even guessing at the solution. This is very dangerous. For example, Cindy is an experienced nurse who has been working in critical care for 15 years. When she arrives on her shift, her patient is receiving Continuous Renal Replacement Therapy. Cindy has not previously managed

---

Critical Thinking 4.1

Donna, RN is caring for Mrs. Miller. Nursing Assistant Carly tells Donna that Mrs. Miller's routine bedside glucometer reading was 63 mg/dL. Donna appropriately treats Mrs. Miller with 15 g of glucose and asks Carly to recheck the blood sugar for the patient in room 532 in a half hour or so. Forty-five minutes later, Carly tells Donna that she checked Mrs. Martin's blood sugar and it was 97 mg/dL. The nurse enters Mrs. Miller's room an hour later and finds her pale, diaphoretic, and confused.

Answer these questions:

1. What communication errors occurred in this scenario?
2. How did Carly confuse Mrs. Miller and Mrs. Martin?
3. What has happened to Mrs. Miller?
4. How could Donna have prevented the confusion and miscommunication?

---

this therapy and is not familiar with the supplies and fluids used. Rather than proceeding independently, Cindy needs to stop and consider requesting a safer assignment. Alternatively, Cindy may work with an expert and consult a written resource such as an evidence-based protocol while providing care.

Nurses and nurse leaders need to understand skill, rule, and knowledge-based performance when investigating errors. Nurses who have been involved in an error should focus on how they made the decision they did. Did they develop a short cut or work-around to save time? Did they fail to do a double check of their own work? Did they proceed even though they were not familiar with the procedure? Each type of error requires a different solution. The three performance modes are critical to keep in mind when designing error prevention strategies.

Root Cause Analyses

Root cause analysis (RCA) is an error analysis tool used in health care to investigate serious adverse events. TJC has mandated the use of RCAs to analyze sentinel events since 1997. RCAs identify underlying problems that increase the likelihood of errors rather than focusing on mistakes made by individuals. An RCA uses a systems approach to identify both active and latent errors. The goal of an RCA is to prevent future harm by eliminating the latent errors that often underlie adverse events.

RCAs begin with data collection and reconstruction of the event through record review and participant interviews. An interprofessional team then analyzes the sequence of events leading to the error, with two main goals: identify how the event occurred through identification of active errors; and identify why the event occurred through systematic identification and analysis of latent errors (AHRQ, 2018a, 2018b). Action plans are developed, implemented, and evaluated based on RCA findings.

Nurse leaders striving for high reliability must facilitate RCA investigations into how and why errors occur. These investigations make errors visible, encourage learning from events, and help prevent errors in the future. Direct care nurse involvement in RCAs is critical to their success. As part of the RCA investigation, nurses need to be comfortable while recounting the actions they took and the rationale for their actions. In addition, direct care nurses are crucial for the development of action plans to help mitigate future risk.

Creating a Culture of High Reliability

This is a critical role for the CNO and other nurse leaders within an organization. Patients are counting on health care organizations for help and do not expect to be injured as part of that care. Nurse leaders must take many actions to achieve this culture. It begins with strategic planning.

Strategic Planning

Strategic planning is a continuous, systematic process of making decisions today with the greatest possible knowledge of their effects on the future (Drucker, 1974). The final product of the strategic planning process is the creation of a strategic plan. A strategic plan has several purposes. First, it clearly defines the mission of the organization and establishes realistic goals and objectives consistent with that mission. Next, it communicates the mission, goals, and objectives to the organization and the community. Third, a strategic plan helps to ensure that the needed resources are available to carry out the initiatives that have been identified as important to the organization. Next, it provides a method to track progress and a mechanism for making changes when needed in the future. Last, a strategic plan allows nurse leaders to select among seemingly equal alternatives based on each alternatives' potential to move the organization toward the desired end goal.

Strategic planning may be conducted for an entire organization, a unit or division, or a major initiative. This chapter will focus on creating a strategic plan to embark on a journey toward high reliability.

Large strategic planning projects benefit from the formation of an advisory board selected from various constituencies what will be affected by the plan. The advisory board does not have formal authority over a program but is instrumental in reviewing the plan and making recommendations and suggestions. Because the advisory board is deliberately selected to reflect representation from various areas, the board will be able to identify potential concerns and provide sound guidance for the plan.

Various strategic planning approaches or models exist. Because they are both based on the scientific method, strategic planning steps are similar to the steps in the nursing process. In strategic planning, the organization analyzes the environment, reviews the literature, formulates goals, develops strategies and action plans, implements the plan, and evaluates the plan. Table 4.5 lists more detailed steps in the strategic planning process.

Environmental Assessment

An **environmental assessment** requires a broad view of the organization's current environment. Both the external and the internal environment are carefully appraised. The external environmental assessment is broad based and attempts to view trends and future issues and needs that could impact the

Table 4.5 Steps in the Strategic Planning Process

- Perform environmental assessment
  - SWOT analysis
  - Stakeholder analysis
- Review literature for evidence-based best practices
- Determine congruence with organizational mission, vision, and values
- Identify planning goals and objectives
- Design strategies or programs to achieve goals
  - Estimate resources required for the plan
  - Prioritize according to available resources
- Establish action plans
  - Identify timelines, resources, and responsibilities
- Develop a marketing plan
  - Write and communicate the business plan/strategic plan
- Implement the strategic plan
- Evaluate the plan

Source: Patti Ludwig-Beymer.

organization. The internal assessment seeks to inventory the organization's assets and liabilities.

SWOT Analysis

A **SWOT analysis** is frequently used to conduct environmental assessments. SWOT is an acronym for strengths, weaknesses, opportunities, and threats. A SWOT analysis identifies strengths and weaknesses in the internal environment and opportunities and threats in the external environment. The SWOT analysis is useful both for initial brainstorming and for a more formal planning document. Table 4.6 provides a hypothetical SWOT analysis focused on creating an HRO in a community hospital.

Stakeholder Assessment

Stakeholder assessment is an important part of an environmental assessment. A stakeholder is any person, group, or organization that has a vested interest in the program or project under review. A stakeholder assessment is a systematic consideration of all potential stakeholders to ensure that the needs of each of these stakeholders are incorporated in the planning phase. For an organization or program to be successful, the involvement of those who will be affected is essential. This is true whether the stakeholders are in the community or are unit staff who will be affected by a proposed strategic plan. When stakeholders are not involved in the project planning, they do not gain a sense of ownership and may not enthusiastically accept a program or strategic goal.

Other Methods of Assessment may be used to support involvement in the strategic planning process. Thoughtful planning is required to determine the method and when to use the method.

Frequently, surveys or questionnaires are used when there are many stakeholders. For example, staff might be polled to see whether they would attend continuing education on safety and high reliability and which days and times would be most desirable.

Table 4.6 SWOT Analysis for a Hypothetical Hospital

Internal	
Strengths	**Weaknesses**
Board of Directors and Physician Leadership Team supportive of HRO	Variable levels of knowledge about high reliability
Organization has cultivated an open culture and has been recognizing staff for speaking up for 10 years	Competing priorities include patient experience and staff satisfaction
Organization has been recognized as a Magnet hospital for 14 years	Quality improvement department has limited resources
Chief nursing officer and chief medical officer work well together and share a passion for safety	Direct care staff are jaded and ask if this will be the "flavor of the month"

External	
Opportunities	**Threats**
A state collaborative is focusing on patient safety	After years of growth, patient volumes are stable
Several HRO experts are available for consultation at a reasonable cost	Financial pressures are increasing
A local university has a robust aviation program with expertise in high reliability	State and federal quality databases suggest that other area hospitals are outperforming this hospital

Source: Patti Ludwig-Beymer.

Critical Thinking 4.2

Think about a health care organization with which you are familiar.
- What is the mission of that organization?
- Is it clearly communicated to the stakeholders?
  What activities of the organization are reflective of its mission?

Focus Groups

Focus groups are small group meetings composed of individuals selected because of a common characteristic. Members are invited to meet in a group and respond to questions about a topic in which they are expected to have an interest or expertise. For example, a group of patients who recently had experiences with childbirth might be asked to come together to discuss their obstetric experiences at the institution in the hope that the discussion will lead to insights or information that could be used for enhancing safety. Focus groups are usually more time consuming and expensive to conduct than questionnaires or surveys. They work best when the topic is broad and qualitative input is being sought by the organization.

Review of the Literature

A **review of the literature** should be completed early in the strategic planning process. This allows the project team to identify similar organizations or programs, their structures and processes, successes, and potential problems and challenges. It helps to make the plan evidence-based. The literature review is an ongoing process that includes tentatively identifying programs, searching the literature for successes and issues, and then refining the program ideas. Identifying best practices or evidence-based innovations that have been adopted with success by other organizations can facilitate strategic planning. Nurse leaders need to carefully examine the existing evidence and practices prior to beginning planning.

Determining the Congruence of the Project or Program

Determining the congruence of the project or program with the organizational mission is another step in the strategic planning process. Early in the planning process, the project or program must be considered within the context of the organizational mission to ensure that the project or program is congruent with organization's main mission. Typically, the overall mission and vision of the organization is reviewed as part of strategic planning. At times, the mission of the organization needs to be modified. For example, to become an HRO, the central theme of safety needs to be a part of the organization's mission.

Goals and Objectives

Next, the Strategic Planning team next identifies **goals and objectives.**

Strategies or Programs

Then the Strategiv Planning team designs **strategies or programs** to achieve their goals and objectives. After the goals, objectives, and strategies have been identified, they are prioritized according to strategic importance, resources required, and time and effort involved.

Action Plans

Action plans are established based on this prioritization. Action plans identify timelines, financial resources, and individuals responsible for the implementation. A realistic timeline allows an organization to evaluate each goal and objective and the degree to which each can be implemented in the specified time frame and with the available resources. Setting a timeline for completing a strategic plan is similar to the prioritization process in that the strategic importance, resources, and effort required are major considerations. Realistic timelines and individual responsibilities must be developed, specified, clarified, and communicated to all stakeholders. This will help to avoid misunderstandings and unmet expectations.

Marketing Plan

A plan for communicating the strategic plan, often called a **marketing plan**, is required for all strategic plans. This holds true whether the strategic planning involves new programming for external audiences or only internal redesign or restructuring. All constituents need to understand the strategic plan, goals, and objectives. This communication is essential when building a culture of high reliability. Designing, implementing, and evaluating new safety strategies will require substantive changes in work flow and in the way that nurses and other staff members carry out their day-to-day work processes. Clearly communicating education requirements will help to ensure proper preparation for nurses, physicians, and other staff members. Without adequate thought to communication across the organization about the project, there is less chance of success and a greater risk of poor cooperation. A marketing plan ensures that all stakeholders have the needed information.

Implementation and Evaluation

Implementation and **evaluation** of the strategic plan are the final two steps in the process. The action plans must be put into place, and outcomes associated with the plan need to be evaluated. For organizations on the journey toward high reliability, it is expected that safety events will initially rise as nurses and other staff begin to feel more comfortable reporting errors. However, over time, those safety events decrease as the organization begins to practice in new and safer ways.

When implementing a strategic plan with a focus on creating an HRO, nurse leaders must make their *commitment to safety* clear. This may be achieved by including safety stories at each meeting. A safety story can review a tool for preventing error, provide an example of using the tool, explain why safety is important, summarize a harmful event, or thank a staff member for being committed to patient or employee safety. Many hospitals use safety stories to keep safety at the top of everyone's mind.

Fostering a Fair and Just Culture

Nurse leaders are responsible for creating a fair and just culture to minimize blame and punishment and encourage individuals to report errors so that the system problems can be corrected. In the past, health care took a punitive approach toward errors, viewing those who made errors as "bad apples" (Institute of Medicine, 1999). This approach served as a disincentive to reporting errors and mistakes and resulted in missed opportunities to uncover and correct problems that impacted safety. The approach also over-simplified safety by overlooking the impact of the system on safety care. More recently, the concept of a just culture has been embraced within health care.

A just culture creates an atmosphere of trust, encouraging and rewarding people for providing essential safety-related information (Reason, 1997). It views errors as opportunities to improve the understanding of both health care system risk and individual behavioral risk. It changes staff expectations and behaviors so that everyone looks for risks in the environment, reports errors, helps to design safe health care systems, and makes safe choices. A just culture also identifies what constitutes acceptable and unacceptable behavior. The American Nurses Association (2010) has endorsed the just culture model.

Learning Organization

Ultimately, the just culture model creates a learning culture that is open and fair; manages behavioral choices; and designs safe health care systems. An HRO cannot exist in the absence of learning. The **learning organization** is an organization where people continuously learn and enhance their capabilities to create (Senge, 1990). Nurse leaders in HROs view each failure as an opportunity to learn from mistakes. They readily admit weaknesses and commit to learning from its mistakes. They take a systems approach to safety and improving the culture of safety. Nurse leaders in these organizations create a supportive learning environment by putting processes in place to facilitate learning and encourage creativity among employees. Such a learning environment requires transparency related to safety, so that everyone is aware of opportunities for improvement.

Reporting errors and near miss safety events can assist in understanding a problem rather than hiding that a problem exists. As a result, nurse leaders must put tactics in place to *increase error reporting*. Speaking up for safety may appear to be easy. Health care providers come into health care to do the right thing, help patients, and cause no harm. However, errors happen. In an HRO, all health care providers are responsible for reporting safety events, including near misses, adverse events, and sentinel events. This type of reporting has its limitations, as it depends on both the recognition of the safety event and the completion of a safety event report. When using voluntary reporting and error tracking, only around 10 to 20 % of all errors are reported in health care organizations (Classen, et al., 2008). A study of Medicare beneficiaries found that only 14 % of patient harm events were captured in hospital incident reporting systems (Health and Human Services, 2012). Nurse leaders must encourage and reward staff who report safety events and decrease the fear inherent in error reporting.

This starts with a robust error-reporting system which can be easily accessed and completed by direct-care nurses and other clinicians. Next, nurse leaders need to thank staff for reporting errors, mistakes, events, and near misses. The Good Catch award, implemented in many hospitals across the country, is one way to recognize staff who report near misses or close calls. Edward Hospital in Naperville Illinois implemented the Good Catch award in 2008. Each month, Risk Managers compile a list of safety events that have been identified by staff and have not reached the patient to cause harm. Members of the senior leadership team vote on the most significant event. The person or team is recognized at a Management Team meeting and receives a certificate, a lapel pin, and a Good Catch trophy. The program recognizes those who speak up and fosters a culture of transparency and safety.

Speaking up for safety requires more than reporting actual or potential errors. It also involves clinicians stopping a care process whenever a member of the care team has a safety concern. This may be uncomfortable for clinicians who have historically viewed health care as hierarchical. As a result, nurse leaders must clearly communicate that everyone has the authority to stop for a safety concern at any time. Nurses are expected to voice their concern and "stop the line" if they sense or discover a safety issue. The acronym *CUS* may be used. The letters represent "I am Concerned;" "I am Uncomfortable;" and "This is a Safety Issue." Consider this powerful and effective way of speaking up: "I am concerned with Mr. Lopez's sudden hemiparesis and am concerned with your choice of not implementing the stroke protocol. I believe this is a safety issue."

Managing Behavioral Choices

The just culture model requires leadership competencies to **manage behavioral choices.** The Just Culture recognizes that many errors result from interactions between humans and the systems in which they work. Nurses and other clinicians should not be held accountable for system failings over which they have no control. Discipline should be tied to the behavior of individuals and the riskiness of their behavior, not only to the actual outcome of their actions (Marx, 2001). Nurse leaders must appropriately hold individuals accountable for their behaviors and investigate the behaviors that led to the error.

Building and reinforcing accountability is part of managing behavioral choices. Nurse leaders must set clear behavioral expectations, educate staff, and build staff skills. Everyone within the organization must be educated on these expectations. Nurse leaders must recognize that three types of accountability exist: vertical, horizontal, and intrinsic accountability.

Vertical and Horizontal Accountability

Vertical accountability occurs when humans perform in a certain way because someone, like a manager, is watching. **Horizontal accountability** occurs when humans perform in a certain way because of peers, teamwork, or the desire to function as effectively as others.

Intrinsic Accountability

Intrinsic accountability exists within the individual. Nurse leaders need to expect accountability and enhance the intrinsic motivation of the nurse to meet performance expectations. In addition, nurses need to hold their peers accountable for safety. While each type of accountability is important, the ultimate goal is for staff to practice in a safe manner even when nobody's watching.

A *Performance Management Decision Guide* is available to guide management decisions when human error occurs (Reason, 1997). The first step is a deliberate act test. If the individual acted with malicious intent, disciplinary action and a report to a professional group, regulatory body, and/or law enforcement is warranted. If there is confirmed ill health and the individual was unaware, a leave of absence and physician referral is appropriate. If substance abuse is suspected, testing, disciplinary action, and treatment are warranted. If the individual chose to take an unacceptable risk based on policies, procedures, and protocols commonly used within the organization, disciplinary action may be warranted. However, if the individual adhered to generally accepted performance expectations and simply made an unintended error, the individual needs to be consoled and coached. In every case, leadership is also responsible for correcting safety problems that contributed to the error.

The just culture model acknowledges that humans make mistakes. As a result, no system can be designed to produce perfect results. However, health care systems can be designed to decrease risk. Consistent with creating a Just Culture and demonstrating sensitivity toward operations, nurse leaders must *identify and correct system problems*.

Daily Safety Huddle

Many system problems can be discovered at a **daily safety huddle**, a short meeting at the beginning of the day that includes senior and operational leaders. This meeting allows the organization to address safety issues for patients or staff quickly and efficiently. Operational leaders review actual or potential safety issues from the past 24 hours and anticipate issues that may occur over the next 24 hours. They identify how the safety issues may impact other departments. They discuss any barriers to safe care, such as inadequate staffing, supplies, medications, or technology. They describe any high-risk or non-routine situations, such as a planned surgery for an incarcerated individual. Appropriate experts are mobilized and empowered to solve the problem. For example, leaders from several clinical areas may report a needle stick injury to a nurse. Without a daily safety huddle, leaders may not be aware of this increase until monthly or quarterly data are tabulated. Because of the safety huddle, however, the information may be used to quickly launch a system-wide task force to determine the causes of the injuries and develop strategies to decrease the needle stick injuries.

Frequent and regular *leader rounding* in clinical practice areas allows nurse leaders to see the conditions under which care is delivered and to talk with staff about safety concerns for themselves and their patients. Nurse leaders can also provide feedback and reinforcement to staff. Both positive and constructive feedback is needed to decrease human errors, and the majority should be positive. Immediate and specific feedback helps to reinforce positive behaviors. Thanking nurses for practicing safely helps to reinforce safe behaviors. If nurse leaders observe unsafe behaviors, they should immediately correct the behavior and offer a practice tip to extinguish the unsafe behavior. For example, a nurse leader may see a nurse enter a room and provide care without sanitizing her hands. The nurse leader should correct the nurse, tie hand hygiene to the core value of safety, and ask the nurse to commit to performing hand hygiene and helping others to do the same in the future.

Assessing Organizational Culture

Nurse leaders must also assess the organizational culture to determine the shared values and beliefs of individuals in a group or organization. This chapter will consider culture as it relates to safety and high reliability.

Culture is sometimes described as the way people act when no one is looking. For example, consider Beth, a patient care technician caring for a patient in isolation. Beth entered the patient's room without wearing appropriate personal protective equipment. By deviating from policy, she put herself, her family, her patients, other staff, and everyone she encountered at risk for infection. When asked about her behavior, Beth stated that she knew the patient was in isolation and that she should put on a gown and gloves. She further explained that she did not think anyone was watching. This illustrates an employee who has not yet internalized a culture of safety.

On the other hand, consider Bill, a housekeeper who informed his supervisor that he found a sharp metal edge on a door handle on the Adolescent Behavioral Health Unit. Bill and his supervisor were concerned that someone could get hurt and alerted the unit manager. The manager asked Joe from facilities to fix the handle as quickly as possible. Joe noticed that two screws were missing from the metal plate. The manager of the unit was notified, and staff members searched the unit including each patient's room. The missing screws were eventually located in a patient's tooth brush holder. Because Bill and Joe paid attention to detail and spoke up, the patient was kept safe from harming himself. This scenario exemplifies employees who are living a culture of safety.

Many organizations use a culture of safety survey tool to capture the perspectives of health care providers. Two commonly used tools are the Survey on Patient Safety Culture (AHRQ, 2017) and the Safety Attitudes Questionnaire (Sexton et al., 2006). Organizations may also choose to assess their stage of organizational maturity toward becoming an HRO using a model proposed by Chassin and Loeb (2013).

The AHRQ sponsored the development of separate patient safety culture surveys for hospitals, nursing homes, medical offices, community pharmacies, and ambulatory surgery centers. Each survey measures multiple dimensions of safety culture. For example, the hospital survey measures teamwork within units; supervisor/manager expectations and actions promoting patient safety; organizational learning; management support for patient safety; overall perceptions of patient safety; feedback and communication about error; communication openness; frequency of event reporting; teamwork across units; staffing; handoffs and transitions; nonpunitive response to errors; number of events reported; and asks the participant to assign a patient safety grade to the organization. The Patient Safety Culture surveys are available in English and Spanish and are publicly available at no cost on the AHRQ website.

AHRQ also created databases for Patient Safety Culture survey data from organizations that administer the surveys. The databases allow health care organizations to compare their patient safety culture survey results to similar sites in support of patient safety culture improvement. Survey results are used by organizations to raise staff awareness about patient safety; assess and diagnose the current status of the patient safety culture; identify strengths and areas of opportunity for patient safety culture improvement; examine trends in patient safety culture changes over time; evaluate the impact of patient safety initiatives and interventions on the culture; and conduct internal and external evaluations the culture of safety. AHRQ provides an Action Planning Tool to assist an organization in analyzing and improving their patient safety culture.

The Safety Attitudes Questionnaire was developed with funding from the Robert Wood Johnson Foundation and the AHRQ. The 36-item survey obtain frontline staff perspectives about specific patient care areas. The key factors that are measured include teamwork climate; safety climate; perceptions of management; job satisfaction; working conditions; and stress recognition. The survey is used by health care organizations to compare themselves to other organizations; identify interventions needed to improve safety attitudes; and measure the effectiveness of the interventions.

Chassin and Loeb (2013) developed a grid to allow health care organizations to assess their stage of organizational maturity toward becoming an HRO: beginning, developing, advancing, and approaching. Chassin and Loeb identified performance based on Position (Board, CEO/Management, Physicians); Initiatives (quality strategy, quality measures, and information technology); Safety Culture (trust, accountability, identifying unsafe conditions, strengthening systems, and assessment); and Robust Process Improvement (methods, training, and spread). Their grid may be used by leaders to assess their journey toward becoming an HRO.

Informatics

In this final QSEN competency, nurses use information and technology to communicate, manage knowledge, mitigate errors, and support decision making. Direct care nurses apply technology and information management tools to support safe processes of care. They effectively navigate the EHR and respond appropriately to clinical decision-making supports and alerts. They use information management tools to monitor outcomes of care and they use high quality electronic sources of health information. Nurse leaders ensure that nurses participate in the selection, design, implementation, and evaluation of information technology. They also anticipate unintended consequences of new technology and participate in the design of clinical decision support systems.

Intravenous pumps with built-in limits for medication doses serve as an example of technology that assists in preventing catastrophic medication errors.

In an HRO, health information technologies help facilitate and sustain quality improvement efforts to improve patient safety. Using health information systems to document care and gather quality and safety information is essential. Additionally, health care information systems provide a method for reporting errors and near misses. The lack of health information systems can impede progress to an HRO. Health care organizations are challenged to devote scarce resources to implement information systems that require significant capital expense and ongoing maintenance costs. In addition, hospital leaders sometimes apply technology to faulty health care processes. Technology can only help improve health care processes when applied appropriately. As part of technology implementation, safe health care processes must be designed and technology must be used to support and sustain the improvements. As seen below, telehealth technology can also be used to make resources available to patients and clinicians remotely (Figure 4.7).

Informatics can also help organizations to identify events that cause harm to patients in order to select and test changes to reduce harm. The Institute for Healthcare Improvement

Critical Thinking 4.3

Tina is caring for a patient with pulmonary emboli. She reviews the medication orders to administer 80 units of heparin per kilogram by intravenous bolus, followed by 18 units per kilogram as an hourly infusion. Tina knows her patient weighs 161 pounds, or 73 kg. She correctly calculates and administers the initial dose of 5,840 units. Tina calculates the continuous infusion rate at 1,314 units per hour. When programming the pump, however, her finger slips and she enters the numbers 11,314 into the pump. Because the programmed dose is beyond the normal range for heparin, the pump does not administer the drug, and Tina receives an error message from the pump. She quickly identifies and corrects the programming error. An independent double check from a peer for this high-risk medication would also catch this programming error before it reaches the patient.

Answer these questions:

1. What factors may have contributed to this programing error?

In this scenario, the IV pump caught the error because the dose was excessive. What other strategies could Tina use to catch a programming error before it reaches the patient?

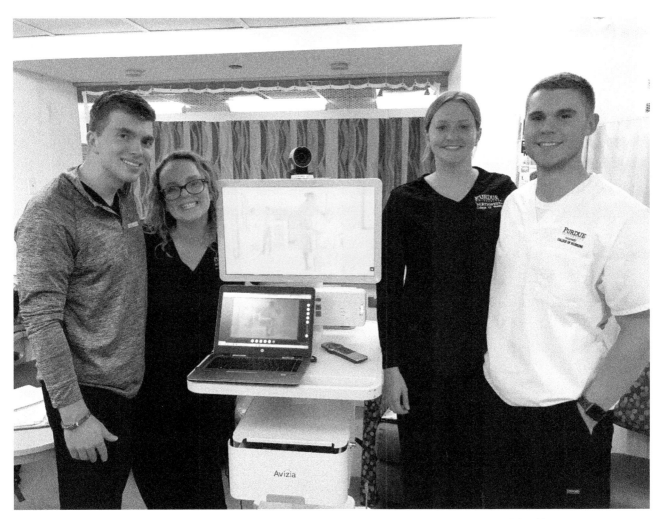

FIGURE 4.7   Four senior nursing students at Purdue University Northwest demonstrate how to use a Telehealth cart.
Sources: Joshua Kocoj, Amber Mills, Jonathan Miskus and Riley Wayco.

Global Trigger Tool (IHI, 2017) helps health care organizations get a clearer understanding of the safety of care by measuring risk and harm at the hospital level. The **Global Trigger Tool** (GTT) uses specific patient care triggers as indicators that an adverse event may have occurred. Using GGT to identify **adverse events** (AEs) is an effective method for measuring the overall level of harm from patient care in a health care organization. GTT provides an easy-to-use method for accurately identifying AEs (harm) and measuring the rate of AEs over time. Tracking AEs over time is a useful way to tell if changes being made are improving the safety of the patient care processes.

More than 50 triggers are consolidated into categories on the GTT related to the provision of surgical, ICU, perinatal, medication, and emergency department care (Institute for Healthcare Improvement, 2018). For example, transfer to a higher level of care is one of the Global Triggers. Consider a situation where a patient is transferred from a medical–surgical unit to the ICU due to a rapid drop in blood pressure and decreased level of consciousness. This event would activate a trigger. The patient's EHR would be reviewed to determine what happened to the patient, when it happened, and if it could have been avoided. In an HRO, investigation results and the GTT results are shared with health care providers and process improvement changes are put into protocols, policies, and procedures to reduce the chance of future safety problems occurring. In an HRO, a multifaceted reporting approach is needed that is comprehensive and provides accurate measurements of errors and near misses.

Resources for the Journey toward High Reliability

Increasingly, the government is mandating public reporting for healthcare safety, quality, and financial indicators. This transparency holds health care providers and organizations accountable for quality care and is designed to help the consumer make informed choices about selecting health care providers. Public awareness of medical errors, poor quality outcomes, and perceived low value are driving changes in health care. Multiple groups are now focused on safety in health care. Many resources are available to nurses in the journey toward high reliability. Resources include nursing associations, interprofessional organizations, government agencies, accreditation agencies, and consumer organizations.

Nursing Organizations

Many nursing associations addresses safety, high reliability, or one or more of the five components of HROs. For example, the American Nurses Association identified the Culture of Safety as their focus for 2016. They focused on a different theme each month to explore the benefits of a collaborative commitment to safety, and how to achieve it (ANA, 2016). The American

Association of periOperative Nurses (2018) uses "Safe Surgeries Together" as their tagline. Their website includes publications on many topics, including patient and worker safety, perioperative safety, medication safety, radiation safety, surgical smoke safety, sharps safety, and product and equipment safety. The Association of Women's Health, Obstetric and Neonatal Nurses' website (2018) includes a variety of educational modules designed to improve safety for obstetric and neonatal patients.

Magnet® Designation

Designation by the **American Nurse's Credentialing Center** (ANCC) as a Magnet™ organization denotes nursing excellence and is factored into payer reimbursement and recognition (ANCC, 2017). The components of the Magnet Recognition Program® are congruent with the HRO concepts. The Magnet components include Transformational Leadership; Structural Empowerment; Exemplary Professional Practice; New Knowledge, Innovations and Improvements; and Empirical Outcomes. The original Forces of Magnetism emphasized structure and process. The current Magnet Model recognizes that an excellent infrastructure must result in positive outcomes in order to create a culture of excellence and innovation. Safety is a main component of a culture of excellence.

The Transformational Leadership component of the Magnet Model requires strong advocacy and support for staff and patients by all nursing leaders. The CNO must be positioned to effectively influence other executive stakeholders, including the board of directors. In a Magnet-designated hospital, the CNO is an active leader in creating an HRO by working with the hospital's executive team to establish a strategic plan for quality and safety. These strategic goals support the organization's commitment to zero major quality failures.

The Structural Empowerment component of Magnet addresses the need to create structures and processes that allow nurses to practice safely and effectively. For example, one source of evidence related to Structural Empowerment calls for clinical nurse involvement in interprofessional decision-making groups at the organizational level. Five of the 13 Structural Empowerment sources of evidence address nursing's role related to quality and safety. Both the Transformational Leadership and Structural Empowerment components of Magnet require the active engagement of nurses.

Evidence from the Literature

Source: Adapted from Jeffs, L., Baker, G. R., Taggar, R., Hubley, P., Richards, J. et al. (2018). Attributes and actions required to advance quality and safety in hospitals: Insights from nurse executives. *Nursing Leadership*, *31*(2), 20-31. doi:10.12927/cjnl.2018.25606

Discussion: The article describes qualitative research conducted to explore nurse executives' understanding of and engagement with patient safety and quality improvement. Three themes

emerged: 1) being a strategic and system thinker while possessing emotional intelligence and influencing staff; 2) building credibility and relationships with point-of-care staff, board of directors, and the leadership team; and 3) creating a culture of safety and high reliability.

Implications for Practice. Study findings are helpful for nurse leaders at all levels to enhance their knowledge, attitudes, and skills in quality and safety.

The Exemplary Professional Practice component of Magnet indicates that "achievement of exemplary professional practice is grounded in a culture of safety, quality monitoring, and quality improvement" (ANCC, 2017, p. 40) and that "[n] urses participate in safety initiatives that incorporate national best practices" (ANCC, 2017, p. 41). Many of the Exemplary Professional Practice sources of evidence require documentation of safe nursing practices. For example, all organizations that provide inpatient care are required to report on two nurse-sensitive clinical indicators: patient falls with injury and hospital-acquired pressure injury, stages 2 and above. The hospitals must report two additional measures from a list that includes: central line-associated blood stream infection, catheter-associated urinary tract infection, *Clostridium difficile*, Methicillin-resistant *Staphylococcus aureus*, venous thromboembolism, peripheral intravenous infiltrations, physical and sexual assault, and device-related hospital-acquired pressure injury. Two ambulatory indicators must also be reported. The performance on each of the six indicators must exceed the mean or median value for the majority of units the majority of the time to meet Magnet standards. Other sources of evidence require examples of nurse partnership with patients and/or families to influence change in the organization; and improved outcomes related to the professional practice model, interprofessional collaborative plan of care, interprofessional quality improvement activity, interprofessional education, and clinical nurse involvement in the evaluation of patient safety data at the unit level. Last, nurse safety is also addressed within the Exemplary Professional Practice component. Organizations must provide an example of an improved workplace safety outcome for nurses specific to workplace violence.

The New Knowledge, Innovations and Improvements component of Magnet requires nurses to use evidence and innovation for safe, high-quality care. Last, the Empirical Outcomes component of Magnet requires the organization to continually assess and monitor a variety of indicators for nursing leadership and clinical practice. Sustained quality performance on empirical outcomes will move an organization on the journey to becoming an HRO.

Interprofessional Organizations

Participation in interprofessional organizations can also assist nurse leaders in their quest to become HROs. Organizations include the IHI, The **Institute for Safe Medication Practices** (ISMP), National Patient Safety Foundation, **National Quality Forum** (NQF), and Patient Safety Organizations.

Institute for Healthcare Improvement

The work of the **IHI** began as part of a demonstration project to redesign health care into a system without errors, waste, delay, and unsustainable costs. IHI works with health systems, countries, and other organizations on improving quality, safety, and value in health care. They use a science of improvement approach, characterized by combining expert subject knowledge with improvement methods and tools. This interprofessional approach draws on clinical science, systems theory, psychology, statistics, and other fields. IHI's methodology is based on the work of W. Edwards Deming, who taught that organizations can increase quality and simultaneously reduce costs (Institute for Healthcare Improvement, 2018). The IHI Model for Improvement asks three questions: 1) What are we trying to accomplish; 2) How will we know that a change is an improvement; and 3) What changes can we make that will result in improvement? As seen in Figure 4.8, the model then employs **Plan-Do-Study-Act** (PDSA) cycles for small, rapid-cycle tests of change (Institute for Healthcare Improvement, 2018).

Institute of Safe Medication Practices

The **ISMP** is a nonprofit organization devoted to medication error prevention and safe medication use. It provides impartial, timely, and accurate medication safety information. ISMP's initiatives are built on non-punitive approaches and system-based solutions. It focuses on knowledge, analysis, education, cooperation, and communication. ISMP reviews all medication error reports submitted by health care facilities and health care professionals. In addition, it works directly and confidentially with the pharmaceutical industry to prevent errors that stem from confusing or misleading naming, labeling, packaging, and device design (Institute for Safe Medication Practices, 2018).

ISMP publishes monthly newsletters to educate the health care community about safe medication practices (Figures 4.4 and 4.5). They suggest that nursing students have a key role to play in a culture of safety. ISMP analyzed nursing student-associated medication incidents and created the following practice tips to enhance the culture of safety: (a) students bring a new

---

Real World Interview

Magnet is a continuous journey that creates a culture that strives to improve outcomes centered on safety, quality, and service for patients and nurses. As nurses lead the care delivery environment, they are at the sharp point of creating a healthy environment and delivering safe quality care which are the pillars of a Magnet organization.

Wendy Tuzik Micek, PhD, RN, NEA-BC
Director Nursing Science and Magnet Program Director
Advocate Children's Hospital
Oak Lawn, IL

Find an opportunity to improve

Organize a team with members who understand the process

Clarify the current knowledge of the process

Uncover the root cause of the poor outcome and/or the variation

Start the PDSA cycle

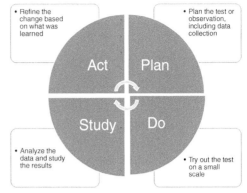

- Refine the change based on what was learned
- Plan the test or observation, including data collection
- Analyze the data and study the results
- Try out the test on a small scale

Act   Plan

Study   Do

FIGURE 4.8   PDSA Quality Improvement Model.
Source: Institute for Healthcare Improvement, 2018.

perspective to the medication-use system and should be encouraged to question, identify, and report errors or gaps; (b) be sure that the preceptor's workload accounts for the level of supervision each student needs to optimize her of his learning in a safe environment; and (c) review organizational challenges impacting students to identify opportunities to improve the culture of safety (Institute for Safe Medication Practices, September 2018).

National Patient Safety Foundation

The National Patient Safety Foundation (NPSF) partners with patients and families, the health care community, and key stakeholders to create a world where patients and those who care for them are free from harm. They work collaboratively to advance patient safety, promote health care workforce safety, and disseminate strategies to prevent harm. NPSF offers a portfolio of programs targeted to diverse stakeholders across the health care industry. The American Society of Professionals in Patient Safety (ASPPS) is part of NPSF. It provides education and oversees professional certification in patient safety and quality. The Institute for Healthcare Improvement and the National Patient Safety Foundation began working together as one organization in May 2017. The merged entity uses its combined knowledge and resources to focus and energize the patient safety agenda in order to build systems of safety across the continuum of care (National Patient Safety Foundation, 2018).

National Quality Forum

The National Quality (NQF) focuses on improving the quality of health care, with patient safety central to achieving the goal. About 100 of the 600 NQF endorsed quality measures are patient-safety focused. NQF has endorsed 34 Safe Practices for Better Health Care and 28 Serious Reportable Events. There are still significant gaps in the measurement of patient safety. By convening panels and other educational forums, NQF works with quality measure developers and others in health care to help understand measurement gaps and encourage strategies to fill them. A list of 28 adverse events, also called Never Events because they should never occur in health care, are grouped into six categories; surgical, product

or device related, patient protection, care management, environmental, radiologic, and potential criminal events (National Quality Forum, 2018).

Patient Safety Organization

A **Patient Safety Organization (PSO)** is a group, institution, or association that improves patient care by reducing errors. PSOs exist to allow organizations to learn from their own safety events and the safety events of others. The Patient Safety and Quality Improvement Act of 2005 was enacted in response to the publication *To Err is Human* (Institute of Medicine, 1999) and growing patient safety concerns in the United States. The law provides confidentiality and privilege protections, which means the information cannot be included in a law suit. A complete list of federally-approved PSOs may be found on the AHRQ website (AHRQ, n.d.).

Government Agencies

Government agencies also focus on safety and provide resources for organizations on a journey toward high reliability. Key agencies include the Agency for Healthcare Research and Quality; Centers for Disease Control and Prevention; and the Centers for Medicare and Medicaid.

Agency for Healthcare Research and Quality

The **Agency for Healthcare Research and Quality (AHRQ)**'s mission is to produce evidence to make health care safer; of higher quality; more accessible, equitable, and affordable; and to work with the U.S. Department of Health and Human Services and with other partners to make sure that research findings are understood and used. AHRQ funds a variety of research and demonstration initiatives and creates materials to teach and train health care providers and health care system professionals to put the results of research into practice. In addition to the AHRQ initiatives already discussed in this chapter, AHRQ safety innovations include:

- The Comprehensive Unit-based Safety Program (CUSP) – this strategy for preventing health care-associated infections (HAIs) combines improvement in safety culture, teamwork, and communication.

- EvidenceNOW – this initiative aligned with Million Hearts® provides clinical practice support to over 5,000 primary care physicians with the goal of improving the heart health of millions of patients and improving the capacity of the practices to incorporate new research findings and information into practice.

- Healthcare Cost and Utilization Project – this initiative highlighted the opioid overdose epidemic and contributed to Health and Human Services' launch of a major multipronged initiative to reduce opioid abuse.

- Re-Engineered Discharge (RED) – this structured protocol and assortment of implementation tools help hospitals rework their discharge processes to reduce readmissions by determining patients' needs and designing and communicating discharge plans.

Centers for Disease Control and Prevention

The **Centers for Disease Control and Prevention (CDC)** provides tools and data to assist organizations on their journey toward high reliability. Their website includes information on diseases and conditions; healthy living; travelers' health; emergency preparedness; injury, violence and safety; environmental health; and workplace safety and health (CDC, 2019). CDC provides educational material for both consumers and health care workers. For example, the website includes a variety of tools and promotional materials available at no cost to enhance the performance of hand hygiene (Figure 4.9) (Centers for Disease Control and Prevention, 2019).

Centers for Medicare and Medicaid

As a major financial reimbursor for health care services in the United States, the **Centers for Medicare and Medicaid (CMS)**, recognizes the escalation of health care costs, poor patient outcomes, health care errors, and waste. As such, CMS posts safety, quality, and patient experience data on the CMS website (www.medicare.gov/hospitalcompare/search.html). CMS created the Centers for Medicare and Medicaid Innovation as part of the Affordable Care Act to enhance the quality of health care and reduce costs through innovative approaches to health care delivery.

CMS ties financial incentives to reliability through pay for performance programs focused on care provided in hospitals, home care, physician practices, and skilled nursing settings (Centers for Medicare and Medicaid Services, 2018a, 2018b, 2018c, 2018d). The three hospital-based pay for performance programs are the **value-based purchasing** (VBP) program, the readmission reduction penalty program, and the **hospital-acquired conditions (HAC)** reduction program. Hospitals with better than expected outcomes receive higher reimbursement for patients insured under Medicare, while those with worse than expected outcomes receive lower reimbursements.

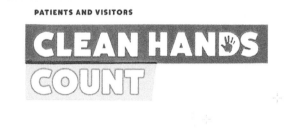

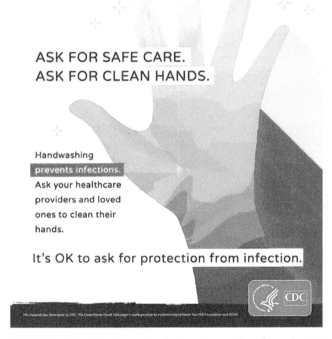

FIGURE 4.9 This Clean Hands Flyer Count Flyer from the CDC increases patients' and visitors' involvement in safe care.
Source: Clean Hands Campaign, Centers for Disease and Control (2019). Retrieved August 29, 2019. Retrieved from: from www.cdc.gov/handhygiene/campaign/index.html

Value-Based purchasing

In value-based purchasing (**VBP**), hospitals earn scores based on achievement of or improvement in their safety, quality, patient experience, and financial performance (Centers for Medicare and Medicaid Services, 2018a, 2018b, 2018c, 2018d). VBP evaluates a hospital on five domains: patient and caregiver centered experience of care and care coordination; clinical care outcomes; efficiency and cost reductions; safety; and clinical care processes.

Hospital Readmission Reduction Penalty Program

The **hospital readmission reduction penalty program** focuses on patients being readmitted to hospitals for six specific conditions: acute myocardial infarction, coronary artery bypass graft surgery, chronic obstructive pulmonary disease, heart failure, pneumonia, and total hip and knee arthroplasty. The hospital's actual readmission rate is compared to the expected rate of readmissions given the patient's comorbidities (Centers for Medicare and Medicaid Services, 2018a, 2018b, 2018c, 2018d). Comorbidities are two or more coexisting medical conditions or disease processes that are additional to an initial diagnosis. For example, a patient may be admitted for pneumonia. If the patient also has diabetes and heart failure, these coexisting conditions must be documented because they make patient care more complex.

HAC Reduction Program

The **HAC reduction program** examines hospitals' performance on safety indicators and hospital-acquired infections. Safety indicators are based on physician, advanced practice registered nurse, and physician assistant documentation. The coded data are then analyzed as part of the Agency for Healthcare Research and Quality Patient Safety Indicators (PSI-90). For hospital-acquired infections, hospitals are required to submit their data on central line-associated bloodstream infections, CAUTI, surgical site infections for colon and hysterectomy surgeries; methicillin-resistant *Staphylococcus aureus bacteremia, and Clostridium difficile* infections to the Center for Disease Control and Prevention **National Healthcare Safety Network** (NHSN) databases. Each hospital's performance is compared to the mean. Poor performing hospitals receive a 1 % penalty (Centers for Medicare and Medicaid, 2018).

CMS publicly reports each hospital's performance on these measures. In addition, many states require health care organizations to report specific adverse events and safety, quality, and staffing indicators. These indicators are available to the public at state websites.

Medical Product Safety Network

The **Medical Product Safety Network (MedSun)** is an adverse event reporting program within the U.S. Food and Drug Administration's Center for Devices and Radiological Health (FDA, 2018). MedSun's goal is to work collaboratively with the clinical community to identify, understand, and solve problems with the use of medical devices.

The Safe Medical Devices Act requires hospitals and other health care organizations to report medical device problems that result in serious illness, injury, or death. Once a problem is identified, MedSun clarifies the problem and shares information with the clinical community and the public, without facility and patient identification, so that other clinicians can take preventive actions. MedSun participants are also highly encouraged to voluntarily report problems with devices that resulted in actual or potential harm. By monitoring reports about problems and concerns before a more serious event occurs, the FDA, manufacturers, and clinicians can work together to prevent serious injuries and death. Sometimes, this results in a product redesign.

Current Educator, Clinical Educator, Novasyte Health representing Hill-Rom Figure 4.10

Baldrige Award

The Baldrige Award is conveyed by the **National Institute of Standards and Technology** (NIST), which is part of the U.S. Department of Commerce. NIST recognizes organizations that have improved and sustained quality results. The Baldrige Award in health care is designed to challenge organizations to improve their effectiveness of care and health care outcomes to pursue excellence, which moves organizations toward becoming an HRO. The Baldrige framework is built on core values and concepts and requires measurement, analysis, and knowledge management. The framework embraces integration between leadership, strategy, customers, workforce, operations, and results (National Institute of Standards and Technology (NIST), n.d.).

Accreditation Agencies

The three hospital accrediting agencies address patient safety. These agencies include Det Norske Veritas Healthcare, Inc. (DNV), **Healthcare Facilities Accreditation Program (HFAP)**, and TJC.

Real World Interview

Nancy Withers

I was providing care for a patient who had just been transferred into ICU after a rapid response. I saw what appeared to be a purple band on the patient. At my hospital, like at many hospitals across the country, a purple band designates a DNR (Do Not Resuscitate) code status. There was no indication of a DNR order for this patient, so I asked the patient about the purple band. The patient told me she was wearing it because she'd had an implantable port placed, and the band was part of the kit provided by the vendor. Staff at the surgical center suggested that the patient wear the band to remind health care providers of her port. When I looked at the band closely, I noticed it was actually a gradation of colors, purple fading to gray. I clarified the patient's code status with her and removed the band for patient safety.

I also completed an unusual occurrence, which brought the situation to the attention of our risk manager. The risk manager reported the event to the FDA through a MedSun report as a near miss. MedSun told us later that they worked with the manufacturing company to change their practices. The company was not aware of the national efforts underway to standardize arm band colors and has now stopped including the purple band in their port kits.

Nancy Withers, BSN, RN
Former Clinical Leader, ICU, Edward Hospital
Current Educator, Clinical Educator,
Novasyte Health representing Hill-Rom.

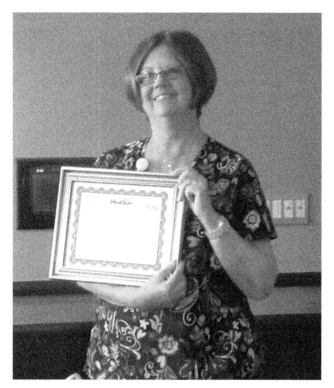

FIGURE 4.10   Nancy Withers, BSN, RN, displaying her MedSun recognition certificate.
Source: Nancy Withers.

Det Norske Veritas Healthcare, Inc.

Det Norske Veritas Healthcare, Inc. (DNV) empowers quality and patient safety through an outcomes-based accreditation program. They received authority from the **Centers for Medicare and Medicaid (CMS)** to provide accreditation to hospitals in 2008, and integrate the CMS Conditions of Participation with the ISO 9001 Quality Management Program. The ISO 9001 quality system is a structured way of delivering a better service or product, supported by detailed procedures such as work instructions, quality manuals, and written quality

policies to provide all employees with detailed, understandable, and workable instructions that define expectations and actions to achieve the stated quality goals. DNV's goal is to enable a broader culture change toward high performance and continual improvement by combining the mandatory CMS evaluation with a quality management system into one seamless program (DNV, 2018).

Healthcare Facilities Accreditation Program

Healthcare Facilities Accreditation Program (HFAP) was originally created in 1945 to conduct an objective review of services provided by osteopathic hospitals. In 1965, HFAP received authority from the Centers for Medicare and Medicaid to provide accreditation to hospitals, ambulatory care/surgical facilities, mental health facilities, physical rehabilitation facilities, clinical laboratories, and critical access hospitals. HFAP adopted the 34 Safe Practices set forth by the National Quality Forum (NQF) in 2009 (HFAP, 2017).

The Joint Commission

The mission of **TJC** is to continuously improve health care for the public, in collaboration with other stakeholders, by evaluating health care organizations and inspiring them to excel in providing safe and effective care of the highest quality and value (TJC, 2018a, 2018b, 2018c). Founded in 1951, TJC uses the Donabedian conceptual framework of structure, process, and outcomes to assess an organization. TJC (March 1, 2017) identified 11 leader expectations for developing a safety culture, as outlined in Table 4.7. These expectations are very appropriate for nurse leaders in every level of an organization.

Summary

The journey toward high reliability is complex and involves every aspect of an organization. The role of the governance or the board of directors is essential. Table 4.8 identifies questions board members should ask to ensure that the health

---

Table 4.7   **Joint Commission Expectations for Leaders in Developing a Safety Culture**

1. Create a transparent, non-punitive approach to reporting and learning from adverse events, close calls, and unsafe conditions.
2. Establish clear, just, and transparent risk-based processes for recognizing and separating human error and error arising from poorly designed systems from unsafe or reckless actions that are blameworthy.
3. Adopt and model appropriate behaviors and champion efforts to eradicate intimidating behaviors.
4. Establish, enforce, and communicate to all team members the policies that support safety culture and the reporting of adverse events, close calls, and unsafe conditions.
5. Recognize team members who report adverse events and close calls, who identify unsafe conditions, or have good suggestions for safety improvements.
6. Establish an organizational baseline measure on safety culture performance using the Agency for Healthcare Research and Quality (AHRQ) Hospital Survey on Patient Safety Culture or another tool, such as the Safety Attitudes Questionnaire.
7. Analyze safety culture survey results from across the organization to find opportunities for quality and safety improvement.
8. Develop and implement unit-based quality and safety improvement initiatives designed to improve the culture of safety.
9. Embed safety culture team training into quality improvement projects and organizational processes to strengthen safety systems.
10. Proactively assess system strength and vulnerabilities and prioritize them for enhancement or improvement.
11. Repeat organizational assessment of safety culture every 18 to 24 months to review progress and sustain improvement.

Source: The Joint Commission. (2018b). *2019 Hospital National Patient Safety Goals.* Retrieved from www.jointcommission.org/assets/1/6/2019_HAP_NPSGs_final.pdf.

Table 4.8   Questions to Confirm a Healthcare Organization's Focus on Safety

1. Is safety positioned as an uncompromising core value?
2. Is there a comprehensive plan for improving patient and workplace safety and for monitoring progress?
3. Is transparency embraced for sharing adverse patient safety events and lessons learned across the system?
4. Is there a healthy reporting environment and a fair and just culture?
5. Is respect expected for patients, co-workers, and physicians within the organization?
6. Are patient stories heard regularly?
7. Are quality and safety implications considered for every major organizational decision?
8. Does the board of directors or governance structure devote sufficient time to safety, quality, and the patient experience of care?

Source: Patti Ludwig-Beymer.

care organization is focused on safety (American College of Healthcare Executive, 2017). Nurse leaders must put resources in place and create a culture so that these questions can be answered affirmatively.

Becoming an HRO involves creating a culture of safety and reliability. This type of culture improves safety, an important element for an effective, efficient health care system. Similarly, a culture of high reliability enhances quality. In addition, a culture of reliability enhances the patient experience. Afterall, what patients or family member is pleased if their care is unsafe or of poor quality? Last, a culture of safety and reliability improves the financial performance of a health care organization.

Much of the early work on safety and high reliability was done in other industries, like commercial aviation and nuclear power. These industries experienced major safety improvements because of their focus on high reliability principles. Health care organizations can apply what has been learned in other safety-focused industries to improve patient safety.

Regardless of role and setting, nurses must apply the six QSEN competencies to enhance safety. Nursing organizations, interprofessional organizations, government agencies, and accreditation agencies serve as valuable resources when building a culture of safety and high reliability. Nurses are in a strong position to advocate for patient safety and lead interprofessional efforts to achieve high reliability.

KEY CONCEPTS

- Errors occur because we are human.

- HROs operate under trying conditions but have fewer than expected safety events.

- Healthcare has learned a great deal about high reliability from other industries, such as commercial aviation and nuclear power.

- Health care organizations on a journey toward high reliability share five characteristics: preoccupation with failure, reluctance to simplify, sensitivity to operations, commitment to resilience, and deference to expertise.

- The six QSEN core competencies help nurses create a culture of safety and reliability.

- Strategic planning is an important step in developing a HRO.

- A fair and just culture minimizes blame and punishment and creates a learning environment where errors are reported so that system problems can be corrected.

- Organizational culture can be assessed with valid and reliable tools to support a journey toward becoming an HRO.

- Professional, governmental, and accreditation organizations provide resources to support the journey toward high reliability.

- The components of the Magnet Recognition Program are congruent with HRO concepts.

KEY TERMS

Action plans	Financial performance	Organizational culture
Adverse event	FMEA	Patient-centered care
Authority gradient	Hierarchy	Precursor safety event
Blunt end	HRO	QSEN
Call-out communication	Human factors	Quality
Closed loop communication	Interprofessional	Reliability
Comorbidities	Knowledge-based performance	Root cause analysis
Culture of safety	Latent errors	Rule-based performance
Daily safety huddle	Learning organization	Safety
Error	Marketing plan	SBAR
Fair and just culture	Near miss safety event	Sentinel event

Serious safety event	Strategic planning	Transparency
Sharp end	Swiss Cheese model	Work-around
Skill-based performance	Teamwork	

REVIEW QUESTIONS

1. The nurse administers insulin to the wrong patient. The nurse should (select all that apply):
   a. Monitor the patient closely
   b. Report the error to the patient's physician
   c. Resign from the hospital
   d. Complete an error report

2. A nurse leader makes frequent and regular rounds to nursing units and talks to staff about patient safety. The nurse leader is most likely rounding to:
   a. Criticize the safety practices of nurses and other clinicians
   b. Look for weaknesses in the care delivery system that allow errors to occur
   c. Conduct an FMEA
   d. Rally the troops for the next strategic initiative

3. The delivery of health care is largely based on rules, often called protocol. Nurse leaders need to track data on staff compliance with rule-based performance because:
   a. Nurses frequently experience slips, lapses, and fumbles
   b. This will help them to punish nurses who make errors
   c. Nurses forget to double check each other's work
   d. This will help them to look for ways to improve practice

4. The continuous, systematic process of making decisions today with the greatest possible knowledge of their effects on the future is the definition of:
   a. Mission, vision, and values
   b. Strategic planning
   c. Root cause analysis
   d. SWOT analysis

5. A just culture creates an atmosphere of trust because it (select all that apply):
   a. Never punishes clinicians for their behaviors
   b. Encourages and rewards people for providing essential safety-related information
   c. Views errors as opportunities to improve health care system risks
   d. Views errors as opportunities to improve individual behavioral risk
   e. Makes only managers responsible for reporting errors

f. Makes everyone responsible for identifying safety risks

6. The nurse behaves in one way when her manager and peers are watching and another way when she believes she is not being observed. She is demonstrating:
   a. Intrinsic accountability
   b. Horizontal and vertical accountability
   c. Intrinsic and horizontal accountability
   d. Vertical accountability

7. An organization may regularly administer a culture of safety survey to (select all that apply):
   a. Identify areas of patient safety strengths
   b. Increase staff awareness about patient safety
   c. Highlight areas of opportunity for patient safety culture improvement
   d. Examine trends in patient safety culture over time
   e. Evaluate the impact of specific interventions

8. Key components of the Magnet Model include (select all that apply):
   a. Transformational leadership
   b. Exemplary Professional Practice
   c. Information Technology
   d. Structural Empowerment
   e. Teamwork and Collaboration
   f. New Knowledge, Innovations, and Improvements
   g. Empirical outcomes

9. 9. The Institute for Healthcare Improvement uses the PDSA cycle for small, rapid-cycle tests of change. PDSA is an acronym for:
   a. Plan-Develop-Start-Act
   b. Plan-Do-Study-Act
   c. Prepare-Do-Select-Acquire
   d. Prepare-Develop-Stop-Ask

10. The Centers for Medicare and Medicaid tie financial incentives to reliability through pay for performance programs. These programs include (select all that apply):
    a. Value-based purchasing
    b. Hospital report card act
    c. Hospital readmission reduction penalty
    d. Hospital-acquired conditions reduction

REVIEW QUESTION ANSWERS

1. The correct response is: A, B, C
   Rationale:
   a. Monitor the patient closely—*Correct. It's important to monitor this patient for signs and symptoms of hypoglycemia.*

   b. Report the error to the patient's physician—*Correct. The physician needs to be aware of this error so that the medical treatment plan can be appropriately adjusted.*
   c. Resign from the hospital—*No. Errors happen and need to be addressed and prevented in the future. However,*

resignation from the hospital because of an error is not appropriate.

   d. Complete an error report—*Correct. An error report should be completed. This allows the error to be investigated and optimizes the chances of preventing similar errors in the future.*

2. The correct response is: B
Rationale:
   a. Criticize the safety practices of nurses and other clinicians—*No. The nurse leader rounds to look for safety opportunities, not to criticize clinicians.*
   b. Look for weaknesses in the care delivery system that allow errors to occur *Correct. Nurse leaders are looking for opportunities to improve the systems of care to enhance patient safety.*
   c. Conduct an FMEA—*No. An FMEA is conducted with an interprofessional team to proactively identify potential safety issues.*
   d. Rally the troops for the next strategic initiative—*No. The nurse leader is focusing on patient safety.*

3. The correct response is: D
Rationale:
   a. Nurses frequently experience slips, lapses, and fumbles—No. These errors occur with skill-based performance, not rule based performance.
   b. This will help them to punish nurses who make errors—No. Rather than punishing nurses who make errors, nurse leaders strive to create a fair and just culture.
   c. Nurses forget to double check each other's work—No. Double checking each other's work is an important tool used to prevent skill-based errors.
   d. This will help them to look for ways to improve practice—Correct. Collecting and analyzing data on protocol compliance will help the nurse leader identify improvement opportunities.

4. The correct response is: B
   a. Rationale:
   b. Mission, vision, and values—*No. Mission, vision, and values guide an organization and are part of strategic planning.*
   c. Strategic planning—*Correct. Strategic planning is an ongoing effort to position an organization for the future.*
   d. Root cause analysis—*No. A Root Cause Analysis is an in-depth investigation of a serious or sentinel safety event.*
   e. SWOT analysis—*No. A SWOT analysis examines strengths, weaknesses, opportunities, and threats as part of strategic planning.*

5. The correct response is: B, C, D, F
Rationale:
   a. Never punishes clinicians for their behaviors—*No. While a just culture minimizes blame and punishment, it holds people accountable for their actions. Blatant disregard for the rules is punished.*
   b. Encourages and rewards people for providing essential safety-related information—*Correct. People are recognized and praised for speaking up about safety concerns.*

   c. Views errors as opportunities to improve health care system risks—*Correct. Errors are analyzed to determine what went wrong and corrections are made to improve the system.*
   d. Views errors as opportunities to improve individual behavioral risk—*Correct Errors are examined for human factors and processes are modified accordingly.*
   e. Makes only managers responsible for reporting errors—*No. Everyone is responsible for reporting errors.*
   f. Makes everyone responsible for identifying safety risks—*Correct. A just culture sets the expectation that everyone looks for risks in the environment, reports errors, helps design safe systems, and makes safe choices.*

6. The correct response is: A
   a. Horizontal and vertical accountability—Yes. Horizontal accountability occurs when the nurse performs a certain way because her peers are watching and vertical accountability occurs when she performs a certain way because her manager is watching.
   b. Intrinsic and horizontal accountability—No. This nurse is not demonstrating intrinsic accountability within herself.
   c. Vertical accountability—No. Vertical accountability applies only to the manager, not to the nurse's peers.

7. The correct response is: A, B, C, D, E
   a. Identify areas of patient safety strengths—*Correct. It is important to recognize and celebrate areas of strength.*
   b. Increase staff awareness about patient safety—*Correct. Administering the survey helps to reinforce the importance of safety in the minds of nurses and other members of the interprofessional team.*
   c. Highlight areas of opportunity for patient safety culture improvement—*Correct. The survey helps to identify where effort is needed to improve safety.*
   d. Examine trends in patient safety culture over time—*Correct. It's important to track changes in the culture of safety over time.*
   e. Evaluate the impact of specific interventions—*Correct. As the organization implements safety initiatives, the survey can be used to measure changes.*

8. The correct response is: A, B, D, F, G
Rationale:
   a. Transformational leadership—Correct. This is one of the five key components of the Magnet® model.
   b. Exemplary Professional Practice—Correct. This is one of the five key components of the Magnet® model.
   c. Information Technology—No. This is one of the six QSEN competencies for nurses. While this is important to Magnet®, it is subsumed under New Knowledge, Innovations and Improvements.
   d. Structural Empowerment—Correct. This is one of the five key components of the Magnet® model.
   e. Teamwork and Collaboration—No. This is one of the six QSEN competencies for nurses. While this is important to Magnet®, it is subsumed under Exemplary Practice.
   f. New Knowledge, Innovations and Improvements–Correct. This is one of the five key components of the Magnet® model.

g. Empirical outcomes—Correct. This is one of the five key components of the Magnet® model.

9. The correct response is: B
   Rationale:
   a. Plan-Develop-Start-Act—*No*
   b. Plan-Do-Study-Act—*Correct. PDSA means plan-do-study-act. Some people refer to it as "plan-do-check-act" instead.*
   c. Prepare-Do-Select-Acquire—*No*
   d. Prepare-Develop-Stop-Ask—No

10. The correct response is: A, C, D
    Rationale:

a. Value-based purchasing—*Correct. This program rewards hospitals based on safety, quality, patient experience, and financial performance.*
b. Hospital report card act—*No. The Hospital Report Care Act is a state program that provides consumers access to information about the quality of health care in their state.*
c. Hospital readmission reduction penalty—*Correct. This program penalizes the hospital if its actual readmission rate for patients with six conditions is higher than expected readmissions adjusted for patient comorbidities.*
d. Hospital-acquired conditions reduction—*Correct. This program examines safety indicators and hospital-acquired infections and penalizes poor performing hospitals.*

REVIEW ACTIVITIES

1. Review the mission, vision, and values of a health care organization, either at the facility or on the facility's website. How do the documents address concern for high reliability and patient safety?

2. While you're at a health care facility, ask a nurse to describe the process in place to report an error, and what happens when an error is reported. Based on what you've learned, is the reporting method focused on learning or blame?

3. Leaders are responsible for creating a culture of high reliability. Review the QSEN competencies outlined in this chapter. During your next clinical rotations, assess the culture of the health care organization. Are the leaders visibly committed to safety? Are nurses involved in process improvements? Is technology used to enhance safety?

4. Review the chapter content related to the Science of Human Error. Why is it important to know if the error is skill-based, rule-based, or knowledge-based? Which types of errors have you made, in your personal or professional life? What tools would help prevent these errors?

5. Review the chapter content related to the I PASS the BATON and SBAR communication tools. The next time you are providing care, try using one of these tools in your handoff to another provider. Did the tool help you to organize your thoughts more concisely? Did it prompt you to share the most pertinent information?

6. The government and other organizations are mandating public reporting for health care safety, quality, and financial indicators. How does this transparency influence quality and safety? What nursing resources are available to assist a health care organization on the road to high reliability? What interprofessional resources are available?

DISCUSSION POINTS

1. During your last clinical experience, how was quality nursing care visible?

2. What types of quality initiatives were visible on the nursing unit?

3. What quality improvement models were used in the institution?

4. How does the culture of a hospital affect nurse involvement with quality improvement projects?

5. How can you improve quality and safety as a direct care nurse?

DISCUSSION OF OPENING SCENARIO

1. What factors may have contributed to the original error?

2. Why was an interprofessional team convened for the root cause analysis?

3. What factors may have contributed to a second error in the pediatric department?

4. Both human factors and organizational factors may have contributed to this error. The nurse may have been fatigued or rushed. She may not have treated the breast milk like a medication, and may not have checked the table three times. The nurse may have experienced confirmation bias, seeing what she expected to see. The nurse may have read the label correctly but reached for the wrong container. The label may have been handwritten and difficult to read. The room may have been poorly lit, making it difficult to read the label. Breast milk storage may not have been individualized for each patient, making it easy to grab the wrong container. The organization may not have invested in bar code scanning technology.

5. Although on the surface this appears to be a simple nursing error, as seen above, many factors may have contributed to the error. All stakeholders should be involved in a root cause analysis to provide a broad perspective and create the most effective plan for preventing the error in the future.

6. Organizational culture, communication, and human factors may allow the same error to occur in different areas within the same organization. If an organization lacks transparency, lessons learned from errors in one area are not shared with other areas. They are kept "secret." Even if an organization aspires to transparency, communication must be clear, concise, and targeted so that the information is received and perceived to be important by the clinicians who may be affected. Nurses and other clinicians must realize they, too, are vulnerable to making errors. The attitude of "I would never make that mistake" needs to be expunged.

EXPLORING THE WEB

1. www.ahrq.gov, to review an Agency for Healthcare Improvement Patient Safety Survey tool, Accessed August 28, 2019.

2. www.medicare.gov/hospitalcompare/search.html, to compare hospital quality performance, Accessed August 28, 2019.

3. https://ww2.mc.vanderbilt.edu/crew_training for Vanderbilt Crew Training information, Accessed August 28, 2019.

4. http://qsen.org to review QSEN competencies for undergraduate and graduate nurses, Accessed August 28, 2019.

5. https://nursingworld.org to see nursing's position on culture of safety and just culture, Accessed August 28, 2019.

INFORMATICS

Go to the website for the Centers for Medicare and Medicaid Hospital Compare, www.medicare.gov/hospitalcompare/search.html. Accessed August 28, 2019. Enter several hospitals located close to your zip code. Review the ratings. What are their strengths? Where do they have opportunities to improve their safety?

LEAN BACK

• What do you see in practice that is different from what you read in this chapter? Why do you think these differences exist?

• How does the information from this chapter influence you as a nursing student?

• How do you think you will use this chapter's information to change practice as a nurse?

• How much or how little do you think this chapter's information will matter to you as a nurse leader?

REFERENCES

Academy of Medical-Surgical Nurses. (2019). *Nurse resiliency.* Retrieved from www.amsn.org/practice-resources/healthy-practice-environment/nurse-resiliency

Agency for Healthcare Research and Quality. (2013a). *Agency for Healthcare Research and Quality (AHRQ).* www.ahrq.gov

Agency for Healthcare Research and Quality. (2013b). *TeamSTEPPS pocket guide.* Retrieved from www.ahrq.gov/sites/default/files/wysiwyg/professionals/education/curriculum-tools/teamstepps/instructor/essentials/pocketguide.pdf

Agency for Healthcare Research and Quality. (2017). *Surveys on patient safety culture™.* Retrieved from www.ahrq.gov/professionals/quality-patient-safety/patientsafetyculture/index.html

Agency for Healthcare Research and Quality. (2018a). *Patient Safety Network. Root cause analysis.* Retrieved from https://psnet.ahrq.gov/primers/primer/10/root-cause-analysis

Agency for Healthcare Research and Quality. (2018b). *Patient Safety Network: High reliability.* Retrieved from https://psnet.ahrq.gov/primers/primer/31/high-reliability

Agency for Healthcare Research and Quality. (n.d.). *Patient safety organization (PSO) program: Federally-listed PSOs.* Retrieved from www.pso.ahrq.gov/listed

American Association of Critical Care Nurses. (2014). *ICU nurses benefit from resilience training.* Retrieved from www.aacn.org/newsroom/ajcc-resilience-research

American Association of periOperative Nurses. (2018). *AORN: Safe surgery together.* Retrieved from www.aorn.org

American College of Healthcare Executives and Institute for Healthcare Improvement. (2017). Leading a Culture of Safety: A Blueprint for Success. Retrieved from https://www.osha.gov/shpguidelines/docs/Leading_a_Culture_of_Safety-A_Blueprint_for_Success.pdf

American Nurses Association. (2010). *Position statement: Just culture.* Retrieved from https://nursingworld.org/psjustculture

American Nurses Association. (2016). *Culture of Safety.* Retrieved from www.nursingworld.org/practice-policy/work-environment/health-safety/culture-of-safety

American Nurses Credentialing Center (ANCC). (2017). *2019 magnet application manual.* Silver Springs, MD: American Nurses Credentialing Center.

CDC. (2019, June 26). *Promotional materials: clean hands count.* Retrieved from www.cdc.gov/handhygiene/campaign/promotional.html

CDC. (2019). *Centers for Disease Control and Prevention.* Retrieved from www.cdc.gov

Centers for Disease Control and Prevention (CDC). (2019). *Hand hygiene in health care settings.* Retrieved from www.cdc.gov/handhygiene

Centers for Medicare and Medicaid Services. (2018a). *Hospital-acquired condition reduction program (HACRP).* Retrieved from www.cms.gov/Medicare/Medicare-Fee-for-Service-Payment/AcuteInpatientPPS/HAC-Reduction-Program.html

Centers for Medicare and Medicaid Services. (2018b). *The hospital value-based purchasing (VBP) program*. Retrieved from www.cms.gov/Medicare/Quality-Initiatives-Patient-Assessment-Instruments/Value-Based-Programs/HVBP/Hospital-Value-Based-Purchasing.html

Centers for Medicare and Medicaid Services. (2018c). *Readmissions Reduction Program (HRRP)*. Retrieved from www.cms.gov/Medicare/Medicare-Fee-for-Service-Payment/AcuteInpatientPPS/Readmissions-Reduction-Program.html

Centers for Medicare and Medicaid Services. (2018d). *What are the value-based programs?* Retrieved from www.cms.gov/Medicare/Quality-Initiatives-Patient-Assessment-Instruments/Value-Based-Programs/Value-Based-Programs.html

Chassin, M. R., & Loeb, J. M. (2013). High-reliability health care: Getting there from here. *The Milbank Quarterly, 91*(3), 459–490.

Classen, D. C., Lloyd, R. C., Provost, L., Griffin, F. A., & Resar, R. (2008). Development and evaluation of the Institute for Health care improvement global trigger tool. *Journal of Patient Safety, 4*(3), 169–177.

Cook, R., & Woods, D. (1994). Operating at the sharp end: The complexity of human error. In M. S. Bogner (Ed.), *Human error in medicine* (pp. 255–310). Hillsdale, NJ: Erlbaum and Associates.

DNV. (2018). *Hospital Accreditation*. Retrieved from http://dnvglhealth http://care.com/accreditations/hospital-accreditation

Drucker, P. F. (1974). *Management: Tasks, responsibilities, practices.* New York: Harper & Row.

FDA. (2018). *MedSun: Medical Product Safety Network*. Retrieved from www.fda.gov/MedicalDevices/Safety/MedSunMedicalProductSafetyNetwork/default.htm

Gerdik, C., Vallish, R. O., Miles, K., Godwin, S. A., Wludyka, P. S., & Panni, M. K. (2010). Successful implementation of a family and patient activated rapid response team in an adult level 1 trauma center. *Resuscitation, 81*(12), 1676–1681.

Health and Human Services Office of Inspector General. (2012). *Hospital incident reporting systems do not capture most patient harm*. Retrieved from https://oig.hhs.gov/oei/reports/oei-06-09-00091.asp

Healthcare Facilities Accreditation Program. (2017). *About HFAP*. Retrieved from www.hfap.org/about-hfap/

Helmreich, R. L., Merritt, A. C., & Wilhelm, J. A. (1999). The evolution of crew resource management training in commercial aviation. *The International Journal of Aviation Psychology, 9*(1), 19–32.

Hughes, R. G. Tools and Strategies for Quality Improvement and Patient Safety. In R. G. Hughes (Ed.), *Patient Safety and Quality: An Evidence-Based Handbook for Nurses*. Rockville, MD: Agency for Healthcare Research and Quality (US); 2008 Apr. Chapter 44. Available from: https://www.ncbi.nlm.nih.gov/books/NBK2682/

Institute for Healthcare Improvement. (2018). *IHI global trigger tool for measuring adverse events*. Retrieved from www.ihi.org/Topics/TriggerTools/Pages/default.aspx

Institute for Safe Medication Practices. (2018). *Institute for Safe Medication Practices*. Retrieved from www.ismp.org/about/default.aspx

Institute of Medicine. (1999). *To err is human*. Washington, DC: National Academy of Sciences.

Institute of Medicine. (2001). *Crossing the quality chasm*. Washington, DC: National Academy of Sciences.

Institute of Nuclear Power Operations. (November 2004). *Principles for a Strong Nuclear Safety Culture*. Retrieved from www.emcbc.doe.gov/Content/Office/inpo_principles_for_a_strong_nuclear_safety_culture.pdf

Jeffs, L., Baker, G. R., Taggar, R., Hubley, P., Richards, J., Merkley, J., Shearer, J., Webster, H., Dizon, M. & Fong, J. H. (2018). Attributes and actions required to advance quality and safety in hospitals: Insights from nurse executives. *Nursing Leadership, 31*(2), 20–31. doi:10.12927/cjnl.2018.25606

Kreiser, S. (2012). High reliability health care: Applying CRM to high-performing teams, Part 5. *PSQH – Patient Safety and Quality Health care*. Retrieved from www.psqh.com/news/high-reliability-health care-applying-crm-to-high-performing-teams-part-5.

Makary, M. A., & Daniel, M. (2016). Medical error – The third leading cause of death in the U.S. *BMJ, 353*, i2139.

Marx, D. (2001). *Patient safety and the "just culture": A primer for health care executives* (pp. 1–28, Rep). Edinburgh, UK: David Marx Consulting. Prepared by David Marx, JD, for Columbia University under a grant provided by the National Heart, Lung, and Blood Institute. (Grant RO1 HL53772, Harold S. Kaplan, MD, Principal Investigator)

Mitchell, A., Schatz, M., & Francis, H. (2014). Designing a critical care nurse–led rapid response team using only available resources: 6 years later. *Critical Care Nursing, 34*(3), 41–56. doi:10.4037/ccn2014412

National Institute of Standards and Technology (NIST). (n.d.). *Baldrige performance excellence program*. Retrieved from www.nist.gov/baldrige

National Patient Safety Foundation. (2018). *National patient safety foundation*. Retrieved from www.npsf.org/default.aspx

National Quality Forum. (2018). *National quality forum*. Retrieved from www.qualityforum.org

QSEN Institute. (2018). *Quality and safety education for nurses*. Retrieved from http://qsen.org

Reason, J. (1997). *Managing the risks of organizational accidents*. Burlington, VT: Ashgate.

Scott, S. D. (2015). Second victim support: Implications for patient safety attitudes and perceptions. *Patient Safety and Quality Healthcare*, 26–31.

Senge, P. (1990). *The fifth discipline. The art and practice of the learning organization*. New York City: Doubleday.

Sexton, J. B., Helmreich, R. L., Neilands, T. B., Rowan, K., Vella, K., Boyden, J., Roberts, P. R. & Thomas, E. J. (April 3, 2006). The safety attitudes questionnaire: Psychometric properties, benchmarking data, and emerging research. *BMC Health Services Research, 6*, 44.

The Joint Commission. (2018a). *About the Joint Commission*. Retrieved from www.jointcommission.org

The Joint Commission. (2018b). *2019 Hospital National Patient Safety Goals*. Retrieved from www.jointcommission.org/assets/1/6/2019_HAP_NPSGs_final.pdf

The Joint Commission. (2018c). *Patient safety systems*. Retrieved from www.jointcommission.org/assets/1/6/PS_chapter_HAP_2018.pdf

Weick, K. E., & Sutcliffe, K. M. (2007). *Managing the unexpected: Resilient performance in an age of uncertainty* (2nd ed.). San Francisco, CA: Jossey-Bass.

Wu, A. (2000). The second victim: The doctor who makes the mistake needs help too. *British Medical Journal, 320*, 726–727.

SUGGESTED READINGS

ASPPS. (2017). *American Society of Professionals in Patient Safety.* Retrieved from www.npsf.org/default.asp?page=aspps&DGPCrPg=1&DGPCrSrt=7A.

Gawande, A. (2009). *The checklist manifesto: How to get things right.* New York: Metropolitan Books.

Health Research & Educational Trust. (2016). *Preventing patient falls: A systematic approach from the joint Commission Center for Transforming Healthcare project.* Chicago, IL: Health Research & Educational Trust. Retrieved from www.hpoe.org/Reports-HPOE/2016/preventing-patient-falls.pdf

HFAP. (2018). *Overview.* Retrieved from www.hfap.org/about/overview.aspx

Institute for Healthcare Improvement. (2018a). *Institute for Healthcare Improvement.* Retrieved from www.ihi.org

Institute for Healthcare Improvement. (2018b). *SBAR communication technique.* Retrieved from www.ihi.org/Topics/SBARCommunicationTechnique/Pages/default.aspx

Institute of Medicine. (2001). *Crossing the quality chasm.* Washington, DC: National Academy of Sciences.

Kelly, O., Vottero, B. A., & Christie-McAulifee, C. A.. (Eds.). (2018). *Introduction to quality and safety education for nurses* (2nd ed.). New York: Springer Publishing Company.

Patterson, K., Grenny, J., McMillan, R., & Switzler, A. (2002). *Crucial conversations: Tools for talking when stakes are high.* New York: McGraw Hill.

Stolzer, A. J., Halford, C. D., & Goglia, J. J. (2011). *Implementing safety management systems in aviation.* Burlington, VT: Ashgate Publishing.

The Joint Commission. (December 27, 2017). *Top quality improvement quotes from 2017.* Retrieved from www.jointcommission.org/dateline_tjc/top_quality_improvement_quotes_from_2017

Wakefield, M. K. (2008). The quality chasm series: Implications for nursing. In R. Hughes (Ed.), *Patient safety and quality: An evidence-based handbook for nurses.* Chapter 4. AHRQ Publication No. (pp. 08–0043). Rockville, MD: Agency for Healthcare Research and Quality.

5

Organization and Staffing of Patient Care at the Unit Level

Diane Spoljoric[1], Marsha M. King[2]
[1] Purdue University Northwest, Westville, IN, USA
[2] University of Saint Francis, Crown Point, IN, USA

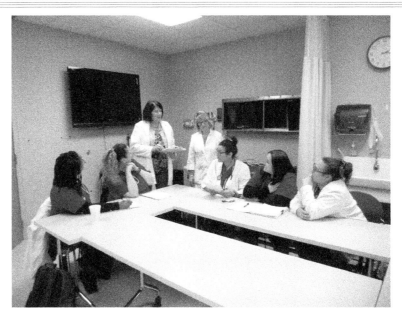

Nursing Unit Team Members Discussing Staffing. Used with permission by Lisa Young and Kim Ziegler.

Rejoice in your work; never lose sight of the nursing leader you are now and the nursing leader you will become.

(Fitzsimon, 2016)

OBJECTIVES

Upon completion of this chapter, the reader should be able to:

1. Understand the importance of an organization's mission, vision, values, or philosophy, and the impact of these on the organization of patient care at the department and unit level.

2. Define the purpose and identify the steps in the strategic planning process as it relates to patient care and staffing.

3. Understand the structure of professional practice at the organization, department, and unit level.

4. Understand the components of developing a staffing plan.

5. Analyze scheduling practices that impact the matching of nursing resources to patient needs.

6. Differentiate models of care delivery and their impact on patient outcomes.

7. Identify the impact of organizational, staff, and patient dynamics on patient and nursing outcomes.

Kelly Vana's Nursing Leadership and Management, Fourth Edition. Edited by Patricia Kelly Vana and Janice Tazbir
© 2021 John Wiley & Sons Ltd. Published 2021 by John Wiley & Sons Ltd.
Companion Website: www.wiley.com/go/kelly-Nursing-Leadership

OPENING SCENARIO

A nursing colleague is telling you she is planning to resign as unit coordinator. She accepted the position a few months ago and was really excited when she started. She is responsible for the overall organization of patient care and coordinates the staffing for the unit. But she tells you of her frustration with never feeling that she has the information she needs for decision making. She feels that this puts her in a poor position to be a staff and patient advocate for her unit. She states, "I feel as if my manager has so many areas that are taking up her time, she really can't concentrate on our unit's needs. It seems as if we are always putting out fires. We never have a chance to step back and actually plan programs and operational processes that could make a big improvement on the unit. The organization's mission statement says that we value education, but I continually have to turn down requests from staff to go to educational programs because of inadequate staffing. We are not recruiting and hiring nurses for all our budgeted positions. There are plenty of nurses routinely scheduled on days and not nearly enough on evenings when most patients are now discharged. Consequently, we have our major needs for discharge planning and patient education in the evening, and there is no plan for providing this necessary information in a consistent manner. The result is dissatisfied patients, staff, and physicians."

1. *What are your thoughts about this situation?*
2. *What advice do you have for your colleague?*
3. *Is this situation unusual?*
4. *Can it be improved? What would you recommend for improvement?*

There are increasing opportunities for nurses to become involved in the organization of patient care and strategic planning for the delivery of health care services in their organizations. Workers in today's health care systems are considered knowledge workers—professionals hired for their knowledge, skills, and expertise. They need a system that supports their ability to practice to the full extent of their professional accountability. Yet, to be effective in leadership roles, nurses need a basic understanding of the way in which organizations are structured, how organizational systems function, and how to engage in the strategic planning process.

Leadership in the health care organizations of the twenty-first century demands competent nurses with different skill sets than in the past. That is because performance in a leadership role in today's highly complex health care environment requires a good understanding of how systems function and how to improve health care delivery. Yet health care providers, including professional nurses, have been slow to integrate this information into their clinical practice. Planning for continuous improvement of quality, service, and cost-effectiveness is a critical competency for nurses in twenty-first century health care organizations.

In its seminal report *To Err Is Human: Building a Safer Health System*, the **Institute of Medicine** (IOM) spoke to the patient safety problems in health care. They estimated that as many as 98,000 hospitalized Americans die each year, not due to their illness or disease, but as a result of preventable errors in their care (IOM, 2000). The initial IOM report was soon followed by the 2001 IOM report, *Crossing the Quality Chasm: A New Health System for the twenty-first century* (IOM, 2001). This report focused on how the health care system can be reinvented to be innovative and to ultimately improve the delivery of health care. The IOM believes any and all advances in health care must begin with a commitment from all health professionals, federal and state policy makers, public and private purchasers of care, regulators, governing boards, and consumers to continually reduce the burden of illness, injury, and disability, and improve the health and functioning of people in the United States. There are six aims recommended for the improvement of health care. These aims are that health care be **Safe, Timely, Effective, Efficient, Equitable, and Patient-centered** (STEEEP). If we focus on these six STEEEP aims, we would be far better at meeting patient needs (IOM, 2001).

The way a nurse's work is organized is a major determinant of patient safety and overall welfare. It is now generally understood that quality and patient safety is dependent on the implementation of care by interprofessional collaborative teams that address the realities of practice and patient care. In 2011, the IOM published *The Future of Nursing: Leading Change, Advancing Health* and stated that nursing has the potential to have a major effect on the current health care system. Nurses have the opportunity to be full partners with other health care professionals to improve and redesign the health care system. The **American Nurses Association** (ANA) states that errors occur as a result of system failure rather than human failure (ANA, 2018a). Consequently, nurses in leadership positions must be educationally prepared to be able to develop and implement organized systems for the effective delivery of patient care. Although many health care organizations collect large sets of data and use scientific methods to improve the services they render, these activities are typically fragmented, isolated from nurses at the bedside and nurses in formal leadership positions, lack alignment with organizational strategy, and can lead to errors in patient care delivery.

This chapter will discuss how the health care organization's mission, vision, values or philosophy, and strategic plan impact both the nursing department, and the individual nursing unit's development of their own mission, vision, values or philosophy, and strategic plan. This lays the foundation for decision making and the ability to deliver effective, safe patient care. Understanding the impact of this foundation on patient outcomes and nursing practice and satisfaction is imperative. The ability to delivery safe and effective care is dependent on many variables, including shared decision making, acuity of patients, and the knowledge, skill level, and experience of staff. These variables include planning, staffing, scheduling, and receiving organizational support and ultimately affects both patient outcomes and nursing satisfaction. By the end of this chapter, you will understand how the nursing department and unit is guided by the organization's mission, vision, and values or philosophy to develop a strategic plan and how to plan and measure the effectiveness of a staffing plan. You will also be able to differentiate models of care delivery and how they impact patient outcomes.

Organizational Mission, Vision, and Values or Philosophy

Generally, the parent organization starts with a guiding mission and vision. Many organizations may also articulate their values or philosophy. These documents guide the development of a strategic plan and allows the organization to scan the environment and develop strategic goals based on changes in the rapidly changing health care environment.

Mission Statement

The **mission statement** is a formal expression of the primary purpose or reason for the existence of the organization, department, or unit. An organization's mission statement defines how it is unique and different from other organizations that provide a similar service. Mission statements are formed based on the organization's core values and beliefs. The mission statement guides the development of the strategic plan and the day-to-day operations and decision making of the organization (Williams, 2008). When a mission is formally stated, quality can be measured. See Table 5.1 for an example of how a mission drives the goals and quality measures. Mission statements with phrases such as, "without consideration for ability to pay," or "with respect for the dignity of every person," or "a healthy and bright future for all children," provide clues to the type of service that you can expect from an organization.

Vision Statement

In addition to the mission statement, there is a need clarify the vision statement of the organization, department, and the unit. While a mission statement describes what an organization, department, or unit wants to do now, a vision statement outlines what an organization, department, or unit wants to be in the near future, for example the next three to five years. A **vision statement** commonly provides a declaration of a "destination" or outlines long-term objectives and is intended to guide its internal decision making. It is the thought of as a road map, indicating what the organization, department, and unit wants to become (Swayne, Duncan, & Ginter, 2012). A vision statement informs us of how the mission will be actualized. Even though it is future-oriented, a vision statement is written in the present tense, using action words as if the vision had already been achieved. In health care, a vision statement describes a balance of addressing the needs of the providers, the patients, and the environment.

Values or Philosophy

As you research different health care organizations, you will commonly find that the guiding mission and the vision statement are easy to locate and are clearly stated. In addition, some organizations have a statement of their values and others have a philosophy. Conceptually, both are similar in meaning. **Values** define the organization's basic philosophy, principles, and ideals. Values also set the ethical tone for the institution. A **philosophy** is a statement of an organization's beliefs or assumptions based on their core values—the inner forces that gives purpose to their work (Burkhardt & Nathaniel, 2013). An organization's values or philosophy are evident in the statements that define the organization and the processes used to achieve its mission and vision. In the best of worlds, there is congruence among the stated mission, vision, values or philosophy, and the behavior of the organization. Sometimes, this congruence is not the case. For example, does the mission statement read, "Our patients are our highest priority," only to organize the environment and services in such a manner that there are inadequate directional signs and registration staff? The result is that these "highest priority" patients are often not able to find their way around the health care organization and have unduly long waits for registration. See Table 5.2 for an example of the Mission, Vision, Values or Philosophy of **Riverview Regional Health Systems** (RRHS).

Developing a Nursing Department's and Nursing Unit's Mission Statement

Building from the organization's mission statement, the nursing department's and nursing unit's mission statement reflects why the unit exists and provides a clear view of what the unit is trying to accomplish. A mission statement will be most valued if it is developed based on the core values or beliefs of those involved. It is the nursing department's and nursing unit's chance to articulate their primary purpose within the organization. It will determine how it is different from other departments and units of care within the organization. For the department and unit mission statements to have the greatest effect, all members of the department and unit staff should

Table 5.1   Mission, Goals, and Quality Measures

Mission

The People's Choice Health Care Center provides excellent patient-centered care to all through partnerships with patients, families, the interprofessional team, and the community in collaboration with nursing and medical practitioners as well as with other health care staff. We believe in evidence-based practice and continuous education for patients, health care staff, and future health care providers. We are committed to patient quality and patient safety to promote optimal health care and the prevention of disease and disability.

Goals

1. Collaborate with the interprofessional health care team to improve patient care
2. Increase patient satisfaction scores
3. Increase number of emergency room visits
4. Increase patient visits
5. Increase use of informatics and computers by all staff
6. Increase funding for staff's continuous education
7. Encourage all staff to attend a minimum of two education programs yearly
8. Increase number of nurses certified in ACLS[a], PALS[a], as CENs[a], and other specialties.
9. Monitor nurse-sensitive patient outcomes such as incidence of cardiac arrest, urinary tract infections (UTI), gastrointestinal (GI) bleeding, thrombophlebitis, failure to rescue, suicide, etc.
10. Decrease medication errors
11. Increase patient safety and quality
12. Monitor hospital readmissions

The National Quality Forum (NQF) 2017.

www.qualityindicators.ahrq.gov, accessed May 3, 2019.
Falls prevalence
1. Falls with injury
2. Restraint prevalence (vest and limb only)
3. Skill mix (RN, LPN, UAP[b], and contract)
4. Nursing care hours per patient day (RN, LPN, and UAP[b])
5. Practice Environment Scale—Nursing Work Index (composite and five subscales)
6. Voluntary turnover

Quality Measures for Emergency Department (ED)

Patient
1. Increase in patient satisfaction
2. Increase in patient return
3. Decrease in patient complaints
4. Increase in market share
5. Decrease in repeat asthma patient visits
6. Develop patient education materials for emergency department visits
7. Develop evidence-based standards for care of patients with cardiac arrest, urinary tract infections (UTI), upper gastrointestinal (GI) bleeding, CVA, trauma, attempted suicide, thrombophlebitis, and those that are ventilator dependent.
8. Decrease door to treatment time for potential stroke patients
9. Decrease door to treatment time for myocardial infarction (MI) patients
10. Review all emergency department deaths

Financial
1. Increase use of informatics and computers on all units
2. Monitor budget compliance
3. Improve nurse staffing ratios
4. Improve computerized order-entry system for medications.
5. Improve electronic health records

Internal Processes
1. Achieve 90% on key performance improvement measures
2. Decrease sick time and overtime by 10 %
3. Increase number of nursing evidence-based projects
4. Achieve Magnet status
5. Increase use of evidenced-based practice educational materials by all patients and staff
6. Increase participation of nursing, medicine, and UAP[b], as well as pharmacy staff in quality improvement activities
7. Set up interprofessional committee on medication administration safety

Employee Growth and Learning
1. 50% of the nursing department join a nursing professional association
2. All nurses working in the ED are certified in ACLS[a] and PALS[a]
3. All nurses working in ED are CENs[a]
4. One-third of nurses are continuing their nursing education
5. 50% of all staff are cross-trained and can work in an ICU[c]
6. 90% of employees are very satisfied
7. 90% of staff are retained
8. All nurses are able to use the computer for patient information, to search literature, and so forth
9. 20% of nursing staff present a community program on pertinent topics annually

Source: The National Quality Forum (NQF), (2016). Patient Safety 2015: Final Technical Report; The National Quality Strategy (NQS), (2017). www.qualityforum.org/Projects/n-r/Patient_Safety_2015-2017/Patient_Safety_2015-2017.aspx, accessed June 15, 2019. Agency for Healthcare Research and Quality and the National Quality Forum (NQF). Endorsed Individual and Composite Measures (2017) www.qualityindicators.ahrq.gov, accessed May 3, 2019.

[a] Advanced Cardiac Life Support (ACLS), Pediatric Advanced Life Support (PALS), Certified Emergency Nurse (CEN).

[b] RN, LPN, and unlicensed assistive personnel (UAP).

[c] Intensive Care Unit (ICU).

Table 5.2   Mission, Vision, Values or Philosophy of Riverview Regional Health Systems (RRHS)

RRHS Mission: To provide the highest quality of personalized patient-centered care. To use excellent interprofessional staff members who value teamwork and collaboration. To always provide the latest technology and informatics. To incorporate evidence-based practice while maintaining high safety standards in the delivery of patient care.
RRHS Vision: To be the trusted leader in providing high-quality patient-centered health care to our communities of service.
RRHS Values or Philosophy: We strive to deliver the best care to every patient every day. A positive patient and family experience is our number one priority. We strive to make sure that our patient's needs and expectations are always met.

Source: https://www.myriverviewmedical.com/for-patients-and-visitors/about-us/mission-vision-and-values

Critical Thinking 5.1

Examine these two examples of an organization's mission statements and then respond to the questions that follow.

Hospital A: "Our mission is to ensure the highest quality of care for the patients in our community. We believe that each patient has the right to the most innovative care that current science and technology can provide. To that end, we have assembled a world-renowned medical staff who will strive to ensure that the latest developments in medical science are used to combat disease."

Hospital B: "Our mission is to provide quality patient-centered health care to all. Our interprofessional health care team of physicians, nurses, practitioners, and other health care professionals believe that evidence-based, patient-centered care can best be provided in an atmosphere of safety, teamwork, collaboration, and partnership with our patients and community. We believe in education and the efficient use of informatics for our patients, for our interprofessional team members, and for our future health care providers. At all times, we strive for optimal health promotion and the prevention of disease and disability."

1. Which hospital values the contributions of nursing?
2. Which hospital would be more likely to offer low cost or free annual physical exams for uninsured patients?
3. Which of these hospitals do you think would be more likely to have a patient lecture series on "Living with Heart Disease?"
4. Which hospital is more likely to provide experimental therapy for the treatment of cancer?
5. Which hospital utilizes informatics to improve care delivery for patients and staff?

participate in their development. Questions to be answered by these groups as they develop both the department's and unit's mission statements include the following:

- What do we stand for?
- What principles or values are we willing to defend?
- Who are we here to help?

Mission statements are often so broad that many nursing departments and nursing units adopt the same mission statement, as shown in Table 5.3, which is also based on the overall organization's mission statement.

Creating a Vision Statement for the Nursing Department and Unit

The nursing department and nursing unit's vision statements reflect what they want to be in the future. They are based on the governing organization's vision of what the organization wants to be and need to reflect the nursing department's and the nursing unit's long-term objectives. The nursing department and nursing unit will develop their visions and use them as a guide map. The nursing department's and nursing unit's vision statements are written in present tense and use action words, as though they were already accomplished.

Developing a Nursing Department's and Nursing Unit's Values or Philosophy

Building on the organization's values or philosophy, the nursing department and nursing units within an organization craft and create their own specific philosophy statements. A nursing department's and nursing unit's core beliefs may be guided by the Quality and Safety in Nursing Education (QSEN) competencies. These six QSEN competencies include patient-centered care, quality improvement, evidence-based practice, safety, teamwork and collaboration, and informatics (QSEN, 2019). They can be complex or they can be short statements developed from a staff brainstorming session, such as "patient-centered," "evidence-based," "quality healing environment," "safety," "interprofessional teamwork," and the like. The Patient-Centered Nursing Practice Model developed by Patricia Kelly Vana (2019) illustrates how the QSEN competency of patient-centered care is the center of what we do in nursing (Figure 5.1). A nursing department's core beliefs or values are incorporated into the nursing unit's mission and vision statements.

Organization of Patient Care at the Unit Level

Organization of patient care occurs at the unit level and is related to the coordination of the organization's and the

---

Table 5.3 **IMCU South Nursing Unit Mission Example provided by D. Spoljoric and M. King.**

The IMCU South Nursing Unit is a group of autonomous, professional nurses committed to patient-centered care, patients' families, the hospital, community, and each other. We strive for nursing and patient care quality and safety excellence based on a solid foundation of professional standards, interprofessional teamwork and collaboration, ongoing education, and evidence-based practice. We continuously strive for excellence and leadership in building our knowledge of informatics to improve patient care.

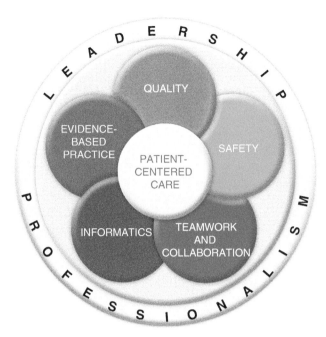

FIGURE 5.1   Patient-centered nursing practice model.
Created by Vana-Kelly 2019.

nursing department's resources and clinical processes to promote patient care delivery. An organization is driven by the organization's mission, vision, and values or philosophy. Coordination of resources, clinical processes, and care delivery is led and managed by senior, middle, and frontline nurses. All nurses utilize the nursing process to assess, plan, implement, and evaluate the outcomes of care for populations of patients.

Strategic Planning

Strategic planning is a management activity that is often used to bring focus to how an organization's energy will be utilized, to establish priorities, and to strengthen operations to achieve targeted goals. Drucker (1973) defines strategic planning as "a continuous, systematic process of making risk-taking decisions today with the greatest possible knowledge of their effects on the future" (p. 125). A health care organization needs to have a good idea of where it fits into its environment and what types of programs and services are needed and demanded by its patients and other stakeholders. A **stakeholder** is any person, group, or organization that has a vested interest in a program or project under review, for example, the community, physicians, nurses, insurance companies, etc. Employers, employees, and stakeholders all play a pivotal role in the strategic planning process. A frequently overlooked but highly important area for analysis is a stakeholder assessment. A **stakeholder assessment** is a systematic consideration of all potential stakeholders on a project to ensure that the needs of each of these stakeholders are incorporated in the planning phase of the project.

It is important that everyone have the same vision for where the organization is headed. A good strategic plan can help to ensure that the needed resources and budget are available to carry out the mission and vision that has been identified as important to the organization. In addition, a clear strategic plan allows the organization, the nursing department, and the unit to select among seemingly equal alternatives based on the alternative's potential to move the organization toward a desired end goal.

While there is no particular timeline that a strategic plan must follow, it is an ongoing process and many organizations strive to look forward two to three years in the future, while others create a fresh strategic plan annually. Strategic planning is especially needed whenever the organization is experiencing problems, including internal/external quality and safety review problems.

The purpose of a strategic plan at the nursing department or unit level is to enable nurses to have an understanding of which programs and services are valued by a patient population. A strategic plan also allows for the planning of high quality, evidence-based, safe patient care and impacts the staffing plan of the unit.

Steps in Strategic Planning Process

In any strategic planning process, there are steps to be followed (Table 5.4). The strategic planning process is similar to the nursing process. You assess and plan before implementing a nursing treatment, and then it is important to evaluate the outcome of the treatment and whether it is working or not. And then the process starts over again. This is equally important when developing an organizational, department, or unit strategic plan.

Perform an Environmental Assessment

It is important that both the external health care environment as well as the internal health care environment be carefully appraised. Whereas the external environmental assessment is broad based and attempts to view community trends, future issues, and needs that could impact the organization, the internal assessment seeks to inventory the organization's assets and liabilities. One method frequently utilized to assess the external and internal environment is a SWOT analysis. A **SWOT Analysis** identifies Strengths, Weaknesses, Opportunities and Threats in the external and internal environment. The SWOT analysis is useful both for initial brainstorming and for developing a more formal strategic planning document.

**Table 5.4   Steps in Strategic Planning Process
Table complied by D. Spoljoric and M. King.**

1. Perform an environmental assessment.
2. Conduct stakeholder assessment.
3. Review and prioritize goals and objectives.
4. Identify timelines and responsibilities.
5. Develop a marketing plan.
6. Evaluate.

Conduct Stakeholder Assessment

For a program to be successful, the involvement of those who will be affected is essential. This is true whether the stakeholders are in the community or they are the hospital, department, or unit staff who will be affected by a proposed strategic plan. Frequently, surveys or questionnaires are used when there is a large number of stakeholders and only a general idea of the options available. For example, staff might be polled to see whether they would attend continuing education and which days and times would be most desirable. **Focus groups** are small groups of individuals who are invited to meet in a group and respond to questions about a topic in which they have interest or expertise. An example of a focus group would be a group of patients who have recently had experiences with childbirth. They might be asked to come together to discuss their obstetric experiences at the organization in the hope that the discussion will lead to insights or information that could be used for improving care or development of marketing strategies in the future. Focus groups are usually more time consuming and expensive to conduct than questionnaires or surveys. Focus groups work best when the topic is broad and the options are not clear. For example, an organization might conduct patient focus groups to determine what programs would be of most interest to a community. When stakeholders are not involved in the project planning, they do not gain a sense of ownership and may accept a program or strategic goals only with limited enthusiasm, or not at all.

Review and Prioritize Goals and Objectives

After the strategic plan has been developed, goals and objectives need to be reviewed and prioritized according to strategic importance, resources required, and time and effort involved. Whether a strategic plan includes programs for external audiences, like a health and wellness fair, or if it only includes programs for internal redesign or restructuring, for example, opening a new chest pain clinic, the strategic plan will need to be communicated to all stakeholders involved.

Identify Timelines and Responsibilities

A timeline should be set for the strategic plan. Realistic timelines and responsibilities must be developed, specified, clarified, and communicated to all stakeholders. This will help to avoid misunderstandings and unmet expectations. This will also allow a thoughtful evaluation of the strategic plan and the degree to which it can be implemented in the specified time frame and with the available resources. Such communication will be needed, for example, when an organization is planning to implement a new computer system to ensure that it remains competitive in the market. Designing, implementing, training, and evaluating a new computer system will require substantive changes in work flow and in the way that employees carry out their day-to-day work processes. If there has not been adequate thought given to the communication about project timelines and individual responsibilities across the organization, there is less chance of success and a greater risk of poor cooperation.

Develop a Marketing Plan

A marketing plan ensures that all stakeholders have the needed information about the project or service under development. **Marketing** is the process of creating a product or health care service for patients, and it uses the four Ps of marketing—Patient, Product, Price, and Placement, to Place desirable health care services or Products in desirable locations at a Price that benefits both Patients and the health care facility. In this way, the health care organization, the patient, and the community all benefit. Marketing of services does have a price tag, such as the cost of advertising campaigns on television and radio. Using printed and electronic materials, mailing and emailing information to patient residences, and advertising on the internet, in journals, magazines, and newspapers, are all examples of ways to market, educate, and stimulate the public for future referrals for health care services.

Evaluate

Once marketing strategies are implemented, most organizations attempt to evaluate their effectiveness and their return on investment. Continuous evaluation of the strategic plan is important to assess whether the plan is working or whether revisions are required.

Professional Nursing Practice at the Unit Level

Professional Nursing Practice at the unit level requires nursing leadership; organizational, department, and shared decision making or shared governance structures; effective patient care delivery processes; and measurement of the outcomes of patient care delivery. Shared Governance is a participatory decision-making model that allows nurses to make decisions regarding their professional practice, quality improvement, staff and professional development, and research (ANCC, 2015). The organization of patient care is built on professional nursing practice and requires a structure of shared decision making or shared governance between nursing leadership and nursing staff at the organizational department, and unit level. Nurses are at the forefront of patient care, incorporating quality and safety for patients within their professional nursing practice.

When organizing patient care at the unit level, quality and safety need to be the driving forces. Quality and Safety Education for Nurses (QSEN) competencies have been integrated into nursing undergraduate and graduate curricula across the country, yet are not widely incorporated into the practice setting (Burke, Johnson, & Sites, 2017). There should be seamless integration from the education of nurses to the actual practice of nursing and the continuum of care (Massachusetts Department of Higher Education Nursing Initiative, 2016).

The Patient-Centered Nursing Practice Model created by (Kelly Vana, 2019), illustrated earlier in Figure 5.1, identifies the QSEN competency of patient- centered care at the core of the Model. The other QSEN competencies of quality improvement, evidence-based practice, safety, interprofessional teamwork and collaboration, and informatics are also part of the foundation of contemporary nursing practice at the organizational, departmental, and unit level, along with nursing leadership and professionalism, both now and in the future.

Shared Governance

Shared governance is an organizational model grounded in a philosophy of decentralized leadership that fosters autonomous decision making and professional nursing practice (Porter-O'Grady, Hawkins, & Parker, 1997). Shared Governance incorporates those QSEN competencies noted earlier in the Patient-Centered Nursing Practice Model shown in Figure 5.1 (Kelly Vana, 2019). Data supports there is a reduction in nurse turnover and increased levels of nursing satisfaction with a shared governance process (Danna, 2013). Shared Governance incorporates leadership, professionalism, and interprofessional collaboration. Further delineation of shared governance in action encompasses patient-centered care, safety, quality improvement, teamwork and collaboration. Therefore, implementation of shared governance helps to incorporate the QSEN competencies at the organization, department, and unit level.

In a shared governance nursing environment, nurses are leaders of patient care. In most health care organizations, nurses fall into two distinct categories: (a) nurses demonstrating leadership in giving direct patient care such as frontline staff nurses, and (b) nurses demonstrating leadership in managing the overall provision of patient care, such as nursing department or nursing unit managers. These nursing department unit or unit managers relinquish overt control over issues related to clinical practice. In return, staff nurses accept responsibility and accountability for professional clinical practice at the bedside.

Shared governance decentralizes decision making, allows for participative management, and expands the span of control of patient care. Staff can be involved in management, education, quality, practice, and research issues (Danna, 2013). This ultimately affects patient outcomes. Shared governance can be hospital organization based, nursing department based, or nursing unit based.

Murray et al. (2016) notes that implementation of a shared governance model can positively affect nurse retention and job satisfaction. These benefits can include lower rates of nurse burnout and fewer patient adverse events. Nurse empowerment through a professional shared governance model can be associated with a greater intent to stay on the job and greater opportunities for nurses to be involved in leadership activities. Shared governance is instrumental in transformational change at the organizational, department, and unit level. Nursing shared governance generally focuses on these areas:

accountability, practice, quality, education, research, and management. The shared governance model encourages nurses at the unit level to demonstrate leadership and professionalism (Porter-O'Grady, 2009; Porter-O'Grady et al., 1997). Figure 5.2 illustrates a Shared Governance Model. Each nursing organization develops its own shared governance model based on the needs of the organization, size of the organization, and the number of councils needed. Larger organizations may need a higher number of councils to implement shared governance versus a smaller organization. A shared governance councilor model generally addresses the following areas of professional practice: clinical practice, quality, education, research, and management.

Coordinating Council

Shared governance models include an overarching coordinating council. The purpose of the coordinating council is to facilitate and integrate the activities of the other councils. This council is usually composed of the nurse managers and the chair people of the other councils.

Clinical Practice Council

The purpose of the clinical practice council is to establish practice standards for the nursing department. This council is accountable for determining policy and procedures related to clinical practice. Evidence-based practices fostered by research utilization initiatives ensure that clinical practice standards are developed based on the state of the science of clinical practice and not merely on tradition.

Quality Council

The purpose of the quality council is to monitor the appropriateness and effectiveness of the care provided by nursing staff. The quality council can review and analyze data to measure and monitor nursing-sensitive patient outcomes. The council may recommend an action plan based on data analysis. This council can also assist in the dissemination of nursing qual-

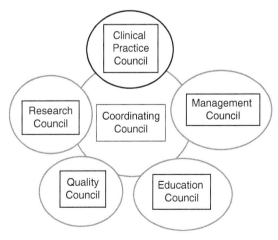

FIGURE 5.2 Shared governance model. Figure created by D. Spoljoric and M. King.

ity information and quality improvement initiatives across the organization.

Education Council

The purpose of the education council is to assess the learning needs of the nursing staff and develop and implement programs to meet these needs. The education council usually works closely with the organization's education and training departments. Unit orientation programs and training programs related to new clinical techniques and new equipment are examples of programs sponsored by the education council.

Research Council

The research council advances evidence-based practice with the intent of staff incorporating research-based findings into the clinical standards of unit practice. Evidence-based practice involves staff critiquing the available research literature and then making recommendations to the clinical practice council so that clinical policies and procedures can be based on evidence-based research findings. The research council may also coordinate any nursing research projects.

Management Council

The purpose of the management council is to ensure that the standards of practice and governance agreed upon by unit staff are upheld and that there are adequate resources to deliver patient care. The unit's patient care manager is a standing member of this council.

Unit-Based Councils

Unit-based shared governance structures are most successful if there is an organization-wide structure of nursing shared governance in place that unit-based functions can articulate with. In most health care organizations, nursing shared governance is adopted first, as nursing is the largest professional work group and practices closest to the point of service delivery (Porter-O'Grady et al., 1997). Unit-based shared governance councils can assist with decision making and autonomy at the unit level and point of care. Jordan (2016) indicates that to achieve best practice in the formulation of unit councils, clinical nurses, nurse leaders, and executive nursing leadership need to be in harmony for successful implementation and sustainability of unit council activity.

Ensuring Competence and Professional Staff Development

Professional practice through the vehicle of shared governance requires competent staff. **Competence** as defined by the ANA (2016) is the "expected level of performance that integrates knowledge, skills, abilities, and judgment." Competence of professional staff can be ensured through credentialing processes developed around a career ladder staff promotion framework. A career ladder can indicate vertical job promo-

tion. Gokenbach and Thomas (2020) point out that a **Career Ladder** demonstrates progression within an organization from an entry level position to increasing levels of pay, skills, and responsibility. A career ladder acknowledges that staff members have varying skill sets based on their education and experience. The partnering of shared governance and career laddering can ensure empowerment of nurses that leads to positive patient outcomes that are measurable and sustainable.

Career ladders should be optional as not all staff may be interested in career ladder advancement. Employees may function at a lower level of unit responsibility yet contribute to overall patient outcomes and successfully meet the criteria for the job (Gokenbach & Thomas, 2020). Career ladders may be varied in structure according to organizational needs, goals, and fiscal resources.

As the health care environment changes with expectations for quality outcomes, nursing career ladders need to be reviewed and revised from a manager-led process to a peer-led process (DeMarco & Pasadino, 2018). As clinical practice evolves and involves multiple generations of nurses, career ladders must continue to support professional practice, growth, and autonomy. Models that were relevant in the past may not meet the needs of new generations in the changing face of nursing growth, emphasis on quality and safety, and motivational factors of different generations. Quality and safety at the organizational, departmental, and unit level are of the highest priority for nursing practice. Burke, Johnson, and Sites (2017) discusses the incorporation of QSEN competencies into job descriptions and career ladder levels that will meet both patient and family needs in the current health care environment. Models of competency validation are changing to reflect moving from a task driven model to a competency process that focuses on quality and safety (Coxe & Llewellyn, 2016). Newer models of competency validation are incorporating the original six QSEN competencies into their framework and guiding principles to encompass a competency-based education and a practice partnership model. The Nurse of the Future Nursing Core Competency Model (Massachusetts Department of Higher Education Nursing Initiative, 2016) places nursing knowledge at the core of their model with 10 competencies based on QSEN, which guide nursing curricula and practice providing for a seamless transition from student to nursing practice. These 10 competencies surrounding nursing knowledge are: patient-centered care, professionalism, informatics and technology, evidence-based practice, leadership, system-based practice, safety, communication, teamwork and collaboration, and quality improvement.

Benner's Novice to Expert Model

Benner's Novice to Expert Model (Benner, 1984) provides a framework that, when developed into a career ladder, facilitates professional staff development by building on the skill sets and experience of each practitioner. Benner's model acknowledges that there are tasks, competencies, and outcomes that practitioners

Real World Interview

The University of Pennsylvania Health System, an urban academic health system, recognized the need to revise their clinical advancement program to promote the contemporary practice of nurses and to better meet the needs of their increasing complex patients. Using an evidence-based practice approach and building on the competencies identified in the Institute of Medicine Report and the Quality and Safety in Nursing Education (QSEN) competencies, the frontline nursing staff and leadership developed eight competency domains and 186 Knowledge, **Skills and Attitudes** (KSAs) that formed the foundation for new Nursing Position Descriptions, Performance Appraisals, and the four level competency-based Clinical Advancement program. Using the Delphi technique, they validated the newly defined competencies and KSAs as essential for nursing practice and the developmental progression of the KSAs through the competency-based clinical advancement program (Burke, Johnson, & Sites, 2017). The eight competency domains include Continuous Quality Improvement*, Evidence-Based Practice* and Research*, Leadership*, Person and Family Centered Care, * Professionalism*, Safety*, Teamwork*, and Technology and Informatics*. These competencies define practice expectations and identify the variety of competencies that frontline nurses need to care for patients in a complex health care system. With the specific KSAs, nurses can clearly identify any practice gaps and learning needs. In addition, nurses can drive quality and safety on their units as frontline staff participate in quality improvement initiatives and identify safety issues. Incorporation of the eight competency domains and the 186 KSAs into a framework for the clinical advancement program clearly defines role expectations, enhances accountability, elevates nursing practice, and can improve clinical outcomes and quality of care. The eight competency domains also form the building blocks for ongoing competency assessments, orientation, and residency programs.

*QSEN Competencies

Kathleen G. Burke, Ph.D., RN-BC, CENP, FAAN
Corporate Director, Nursing Professional Development
and Innovation
Co-Director, Continuing Interprofessional Education
University of Pennsylvania Health System
Advanced Senior Lecturer, School of Nursing
Senior Fellow, Leonard Davis Institute of
Health Economics
University of Pennsylvania
Philadelphia, Pennsylvania

Case Study 5.1

You are a staff nurse who is a member of the credentialing committee of the quality council. A fellow nurse has presented his packet of credentials for review in hope of being promoted to the next level on the career ladder. You review the packet and make the recommendation that he be promoted. However, at the credentialing committee meeting, it is revealed that the patient care manager and the individual's preceptor, another member of the committee, have not recommended promotion. You wonder if your fellow nursing colleague is aware that there are concerns about his performance.

1. Are there performance guidelines that you are not aware of that have not been met?
2. What is the next course of action for the credentialing committee?
3. What should your response be at this meeting?
4. What steps can be discussed with the nurse to enable his promotion in the future?

can be expected to have acquired based on five stages of experience, that is novice, advanced beginner, competent, proficient, and expert. Table 5.5 discusses Benner's model and shows the appropriate application to nursing practice that a professional nurse would be expected to demonstrate at each stage. Proficiency in completion of each stage demonstrates readiness for promotion along a career ladder. Note that all nurses who care for patients must meet basic criteria for safe care.

Nurse Residency Orientation Programs

As the health care environment has become increasingly complex related to the acuity level of patients, advanced technology, quality and safety expectations, and coordination of care across practice settings, the need for the development of nurse residency orientation programs has increased. These nurse residency orientation programs address progression of the newly licensed nurse through the novice nurse and advanced beginner stages in the development of skills, competence, and the confidence required to be successful in their career (Goode, Ponte, & Havens, 2016). Nurse Residency orientation programs can successfully increase the retention and satisfaction level of new nurses, and improve patient outcomes and patient safety. Nurse Residency orientation programs typically last for a period of 12 months, depending on the organization (Norris, 2019) (Figure 5.3).

Table 5.5 Benner's Model of Novice to Expert

Stage of Model	Application to Nursing Practice
Novice nurses are recognized as being task oriented and focused on the rules. They need direction and coaching from a mentor. They tend to see nursing as a list of tasks to do rather than seeing the big picture of patient care needed to meet patient care goals. After novices have mastered most tasks required to perform their ascribed roles, they move on to the stage of advanced beginner.	The novice nurse is educated in techniques associated with delegation. The novice nurse is new to the direct patient care setting and may have been educated in principles of delegation, but he or she has not used them in the clinical setting. These nurses are very task oriented and focused and are often still in orientation. They may delegate tasks clearly outlined by the hospital, for example, they may ask an Unlicensed Assistive Personnel (UAP) to pass water. They often cannot decide what else to delegate. Novices often tend to do all tasks themselves and need direction and coaching from mentors.
Advanced beginner nurses demonstrate marginally acceptable independent performance. They are learning to apply newly acquired knowledge and skills to many situations. They have enough experience to grasp many aspects of the situation. This nurse still focuses on the rules but is more experienced and just needs some coaching. This nurse still needs help identifying priorities.	Advanced beginner nurses are out of orientation, have worked for a short while on the unit, and are able to perform most nursing tasks that are required for patient care. This nurse is becoming more comfortable independently delegating simple tasks to UAP, such as bathing, running errands, assisting in positioning of patients, and taking vital signs. This nurse is often reluctant to delegate to staff whose personality is resistant to delegation. This nurse still needs coaching from a mentor.
Competent nurses have one to three years' experience and have developed the ability to see their actions as part of the long-range goals set for their patients. They lack the speed of the proficient nurse, but they are able to manage most aspects of clinical care. Competent nurses can cope with the contingencies of clinical nursing. They use conscious planning to help achieve efficiency and organization skills. They recognize patterns and use this knowledge to make decisions. They can personalize care for each patient. They are gaining perspective but are not yet able to select out the most important patient care elements in the overall picture.	One to three years in the same role has allowed competent nurses to develop the ability to delegate to the Licensed Practical Nurses (LPNs) and Unlicensed Assistive Personnel (UAPs). They have developed a higher level of ability to apply the nursing process and use nursing skills. The competent nurse is more able to assess the LPN and UAP's abilities, communicate expectations effectively, and gather clinical information from them. The competent nurse is more comfortable communicating and delegating to staff, even in the presence of personality conflicts. This nurse expects that all staff must work to meet the requirements of their job description.
Proficient nurses usually have three to five years' experience and characteristically perceive the whole patient care situation rather than just perceiving a series of tasks. They have often been on the job fof several years and have been delegated total responsibility for their patients' care. They develop a plan of care and then guide the patient from Point A to Point B. These nurses need minimal guidance and control and only occasional support from a mentor. They draw on their past experiences and know that in a typical situation, a patient must exhibit specific behaviors to meet specific goals. They realize that if those behaviors are not demonstrated within a certain time frame, then the plan of care needs to change.	These nurses are often charge nurses developing plans of care for the whole unit. They can see delegation of tasks as an important part of guiding patients from Point A to Point B. They are able to use past experiences with the patients, LPNs and UAPs to guide the delegation process. They may need a little occasional support from their mentors.
Expert nurses usually have five years' experience or more and intuitively know what is going on with their patients. Their expertise is so embedded in their practice that they have been heard to say to the physician, "There is something wrong with this patient. I'm not sure what is going on, but you need to come and evaluate them." Not heeding the call derived from the intuitive sense of an expert nurse can result in a patient's condition deteriorating, with subsequent development of the nurse-sensitive outcome of cardiac arrest. These expert nurses usually seek continuing education.	Expert nurses intuitively know what is going on with patients and their needs. They can quickly assess what needs to be delegated. They evaluate the situation continuously and adjust the plan of care accordingly.

Source: Developed with information from Benner, P. (1984). From novice to expert. Menlo Park, CA: Addison-Wesley.

The Process of Professional Practice

Ongoing professional staff development is part of the regular performance feedback that staff can expect to receive from their patient care manager. However, all patient care managers provide ongoing professional development of staff in their daily interactions on the unit by identifying projects and activities that enhance a staff member's readiness for leadership development and advancement.

Nursing leaders are instrumental in conjunction with a shared governance model in creating the enthusiasm and vision necessary to create a healthy work environment at the

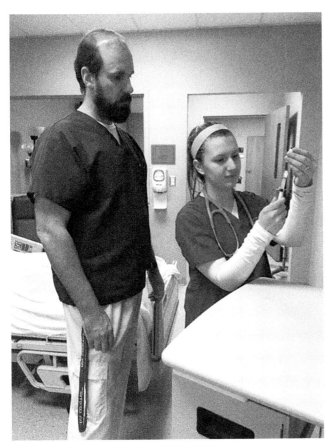

FIGURE 5.3 Photo of novice nurse guided by expert.
Source: Patricia Kelly.

Directing ⟷ coaching ⟷ supporting ⟷ delegating

Novice ⟷ Advanced Beginner ⟷ Competent ⟷ Proficient ⟷ Expert

Novice will require more directing from leadership and will do less delegating, while an expert will do more delegating and will require less directing

FIGURE 5.4 Leadership Continuum. Created by D. Spoljoric and M. King.

leadership behavior through styles along the leadership continuum including: directing, coaching, supporting, and delegating (Figure 5.4).

Leadership styles in the current health care environment are used to promote goal attainment and empowerment of patient care at the unit level. Contemporary leadership styles in addition to situational leadership, include transformational and transactional. **Transformational leaders** inspire and promote the mission and goals of the organization, create a vision, empower others to achieve the vision, and create engagement among the staff (Cherry & Jacob, 2019). Those leaders promote leadership and professionalism among their staff. **Transactional leaders** are concerned with day-to-day operations. They reward staff for desired work, monitor work performance, and correct as needed. These transactional leaders may wait until problems occur and then will address at that time (Cherry & Jacob, 2019). Nurses who demonstrate transformational leadership achieve increased levels of staff satisfaction and effectiveness of their work groups (Burke, Flanagan, Ditomassi, & Hickey, 2017). Transformational leaders coach and mentor their staff and have a passion for excellence. Combining shared governance, empowerment of staff, career ladders, and transformational leadership creates the foundation and framework for the organization of patient care at the unit level.

Scheduling

As the consideration of building a staffing plan at the unit level begins, the scheduling of staff requires attention to placing the appropriate staff on each day and shift for safe, effective patient care. There are many factors to consider as you schedule staff: the patient type and acuity, the number of patients, the experience of your staff, and the supports available to the staff. The combination of these factors should guide the number of staff scheduled on each day and shift. These factors must be reviewed on an ongoing basis as changing patient types and patient acuity drive different patient needs and staff expertise requirements.

Development of a Staffing Plan

The ability of a nurse to provide safe and effective care to a patient is dependent on many variables. These variables include the knowledge and experience of the staff, the severity of illness of the patients, patient dependency needs for daily activities, complexity of care, amount of nursing time available, care delivery model, care management tools, and the organizational supports in place to facilitate care. When planning for staffing needs, these factors and how they affect planning for scheduling staff, and achieving patient outcomes,

organizational, departmental, and unit level that translates into exemplary patient care. Their leadership sets the guidelines and is essential for the quality and safety of patient care at the organizational, departmental, and unit level.

Leadership at the Unit Level

The leadership framework developed by Hersey and Blanchard (1993), when combined with an individual's position on a career ladder, is useful to a patient care manager in discerning the best approach to take in developing the potential of staff members.

Situational leadership is an adaptive style of leadership. Situational leadership focuses on developing people and workgroups and bringing out the best in people (St. Thomas University, 2018). Situational leadership is considered flexible and encourages leaders to choose the leadership style that best fits the needs of the situation in an organization and the needs of the unit. Effective leadership lies in matching the appropriate leadership style to the individual's or group's level of readiness. A basic assumption of situational leadership is the idea that a leader should help staff grow in their readiness to perform new tasks as far as they are able and willing to go. This development of staff is accomplished by adjusting

Case Study 5.2

You are a new nurse manager of a 30-bed medical unit that uses a team-based nursing care model. You have 40 employees who work full and part time, with vacancies for eight additional full-time staff. The current schedule includes all 12-hour shifts. The research on health worker fatigue and patient safety clearly demonstrates that extended work hours contribute to high levels of worker fatigue, decreased productivity, and increased risk of adverse events (The Joint Commission Sentinel Event Alert 48, Addendum, May 2018).

As a new manager who wants to exemplify transformational leadership qualities, how would you want to re-introduce the concept of eight-hour shifts to your staff?

1. How would you introduce this potential change to staff?
2. How can the concept of shared governance at the unit level contribute to the staff's buy-in and acceptance of change?
3. How can you accommodate the needs of all staff if some staff would do 8-hour shifts and others would do 12-hour shifts?
4. What effect would varied shifts have on your care delivery?

need to be focused on. In any organization, the cost of staffing will significantly impact the financial resources available. Creating an effective staffing plan is viewed as challenging because it is necessary to find the right balance between being fiscally responsible and achieving quality, safety, patient outcomes, and staff satisfaction (Hunt, 2018).

Determination of Staffing Needs

Historically, patient census was used to determine staffing needs. This resulted in fixed nurse-to-patient care ratios. This method of patient census staffing proved to be highly inaccurate because of the variability of patient care needs (Gran-Moravec & Hughes, 2005). Staffing is much more complex that just meeting a "ratio," a certain number of nurses for a certain number of patients. The ANA (2018b) supports that all nurses are providers of care; however, individual nursing characteristics directly impact patient care outcomes. Nurse's knowledge, experience, professional judgment, and skills sets need to be taken into account when planning and addressing staffing needs. The American Nurses Association (ANA, 2012) supports taking into consideration the following variables when determining staffing: patient characteristics, intensity of nursing care, context of the unit (size, layout, work flow, technology, arrangement of the unit, etc.), and staff expertise. Nursing characteristics related to staff expertise should include: licensure, experience with population served, level of experience (novice to expert), competency with technology, professional certification, educational preparation, language capabilities, and organizational experience (ANA, 2012). In this complex and ever-changing health care environment, these nursing characteristics are considered in determining nurse staffing requirements. The effectiveness of the staffing pattern is only as good as the planning that goes into its preparation.

Key Terms of Staffing

Gaining knowledge of key terms of staffing—**full-time equivalents** (FTEs), productive time, nonproductive time, direct and indirect care, nursing workload, and units of service—is necessary for understanding staffing patterns. In today's health care environment, nursing works in an interprofessional collaborative relationship with the finance department to create a staffing plan. Staffing plans can be created on anything from simple spread sheets to algorithmic interdepartmental budgeting software. The use of budgeting software is useful and can remove the need for manual calculation of staffing needs. A **full-time equivalent (FTE)** is a measure of the work commitment of an employee who works 40 hours per week for 52 weeks a year. This amounts to 2,080 hours of work time yearly. A full-time employee who works 40 hours a week is referred to as a 1.0 FTE. An employee who works 36 hours (three 12-hour shifts) is considered to be a full-time employee for benefit purposes in many organizations but is assigned 0.9 FTE for budgeting purposes (36/40 = 0.9 FTE). A part-time employee who works five eight-hour days in a two-week period is considered a 0.5 FTE. FTE calculation is used to mathematically describe how much an employee works.

FTE hours are a total of all paid time. This includes worked time as well as non-worked time. Hours worked and available for patient care are designated as **productive hours**. Benefit time such as vacation, sick time, and education time is considered **nonproductive hours**. When considering the number of FTEs needed to staff a unit, count only the productive hours available for each staff member, because this represents the amount of time required to direct patient care needs. Available productive time can be easily calculated by subtracting benefit time from the time a full-time employee would work (Figure 5.5). These figures vary greatly depending on institutional policy and availability of human resource benefits

Employees who work with patients can be classified into two categories: those who provide direct care and those who provide indirect care. **Direct care** is time spent providing hands-on care to patients. **Indirect care** is time spent on activities that support patient care but are not done directly with the patient. Documentation, order entry, time consulting with members of the interprofessional team, and time spent following up on outstanding patient care issues are good examples of indirect care hours. Even though RNs, **licensed practical nurses** (LPNs), and **unlicensed assistive personnel** (UAP)

Vacation time	15 days or 120 hours
Sick time	5 days or 40 hours
Holiday time	6 days or 48 hours
Education time	3 days or 24 hours

Total nonproductive time = 232 hours

2,080 − 232 = 1,848 hours of productive work time available for each staff member with these benefits.

FIGURE 5.5   Calculation of productive and nonproductive time. Example provided by D. Spoljoric and M. King.

engage in indirect care activities, the majority of their time is spent providing direct care; therefore, they are classified as direct care providers. Nurse Managers, clinical specialists, unit secretaries, and other support staff are considered indirect care providers, because the majority of their work supports the work of the direct care providers and is indirect in nature.

One of the most important questions to ask when scheduling nurses to work is, how many actual FTEs does the unit need to cover the needs of the department and the patients the majority of the time? Staffing plans should reflect the needs of the unit, but not to the extent of overstaffing the unit. Overstaffing can lead to nurses being not needed to work based on the unit census and then being sent home. Staffing plans do not want to create a situation where there are too many low census situations (Hunt, 2018). A low census situation occurs when the number of patients on a unit drops and nurses are sent home or put on call while at home. Complexity of the variables in staffing include units of service and the impact on the intensity of service needs. Nurses working with members of the finance team can create models of staffing plans with various calculations created in a software program versus manual calculations. Different models can be explored to take into account the complexity of staffing at the unit level.

Units of Service

Nursing workload is dependent on the nursing care needs of patients. Both patient volume and work intensity—that is, severity of illness, patient dependency for activities of daily living, complexity of care, and amount of time needed for care—contribute to nursing workload. **Units of service** include a variety of volume measures that are used on various types of patient care units that reflect different types of patient encounters as indicators of nursing workload (Figure 5.6). Units of service will vary depending on the unit type. Units of service are used in budget negotiations to project nursing needs of patients and to assure adequate resources for safe patient care.

Nursing Hours Per Patient Day

Nursing hours per patient day (NHPPD) is the amount of nursing care required per patient in a 24-hour period and it is usually based on midnight census and past unit needs, expected

Unit Type	Units of Service
Inpatient unit	Nursing hours per patient day (NHPPD)
Labor and delivery	Births
Operating room	Surgeries/procedures
Home care	Patient visits
Emergency services	Patient visits

FIGURE 5.6   Units of service—volume measures by unit type. Example provided by D. Spoljoric and M. King.

unit practice trends, national benchmarks, professional staffing standards, and budget negotiations. NHPPD reflects only productive hours (hours available for patient care) of nursing time needed. Calculation of NHPPD is displayed in Figure 5.7. Since the majority of nurses practice on inpatient units, the calculations in Figure 5.7 reflect nursing hours on an inpatient unit. The midnight census can be an ongoing challenge as it does not always accurately reflect the activity on a unit during the day. These unit activities include all the patient admissions, discharges, and transfers which involve additional workload (Hunt, 2018). NHPPD are variable due to many factors affecting the need for patient care hours. Variables include patient care unit related variances, patient physical and psychological variances, variances that affect the unit function, staff related variances, unit hour variances, and organization related variances (Hunt, 2018).

Patient turnover is a measure reflecting patient admission, transfer, and discharge, all of which are time consuming activities for the RN. As the health care industry pushes to reduce costs through shorter lengths of stay, this time commitment related to patient turnover consumes an increasing proportion of the RN's shift. As **length of stay** (LOS) shortens, the intensity and need for NHPPD increases. When only looking at the midnight census or **average daily census** (ADC), these numbers do not always take into account the true number of patients cared for when factoring in admissions and discharges.

Patient Classification Systems

A **patient classification system (PCS)** is a measurement tool used to articulate the nursing workload for a specific patient

This example is based on an Inpatient 24-bed Medical Unit where the ADC is 20 and NHPPD is targeted at 8 (The budgeted target of 8 is determined in collaboration with the nursing department, the finance department and benchmarking with outside hospitals or organizations such as NDNQI).

Step 1: Formula: Number of patients (ADC) × NHPPD/care hours per day = shifts needed per 24 hours staff productive time per shift divided by 8 = number of 8 hour shifts needed per 24 hours.

$$\text{Example: } 20 \times 8 = \frac{160 \text{ care hours per 24 hour day}}{8} = 20 \text{ 8-hours shifts needed per 24 hours}$$

Step 2: Allocate 20 total staff to the unit based on 8-hour shift and skill mix

	% of Staff per Shift	# of Staff	RN	Tech/Unit Clerk
Days	40 %	8	4	4
Evenings	35%	7	4	3
Nights	25%	5	4	1
			12	**8**
				(Total 20 staff needed per day)

Step 3: Calculate FTE to cover staff days off. (Calculations are in parentheses in the matrix below.)

$$\text{Formula: } \frac{\text{number of staff needed per shift} \times \text{Days of needed coverage}}{\text{Number of shifts each FTE works}}$$

$$\text{Example: } \frac{4 \times 7}{5} = 5.6 \quad \text{FTE's to cover days off}$$

	% of Staff per Shift	# of Staff	RN	Tech/UnitClerk
Days	40%	8	4 (5.6)	4 (5.6)
Evenings	35%		7	4 (5.6)	3 (4.2)
Nights	25%		5	4 (5.6)	1 (1.4)
			12 **(16.8)**	8 **(11.2)** = 20 (**28** FTE's includes covering for days off)

Step 4: Provide coverage for benefits

$$\text{Formula : } \frac{\text{budgeted nonproductive hours}}{\text{Productive hours}} = \text{percent of nonproductive hours} \times \text{total FTE} = \text{additionalFTE needed to cover benefits}$$

Productive + nonproductive FTE to cover each week = Grand Total FTE to staff the unit

Example:

232 (non-productivehours) / 2080 (productive hours) = 0.11(% of non-productive hours) × 28

(Total FTE's from Step 3) = 3.08(FTE's to cover benefit time)

3.08 + 28 = **31.08 Grand Total FTEto staff the unit**

FIGURE 5.7   Calculation of nursing hours per patient day (NHPPD). Example provided by D. Spoljoric and M. King.

or group of patients over a specific period of time. The measure of nursing workload that is generated for each patient is called the patient acuity. Patient classification data can be used to predict the amount of nursing time needed based on the patient's acuity. **Acuity** is reflective of the clinical condition of the patient, care and time spent on both direct, indirect, and support care activities (The Nash Group, 2018). As a patient becomes sicker, their acuity level rises, meaning the patient requires more nursing care. As a patient acuity level decreases, the patient requires less nursing care. In most PCSs, each patient is classified once a day using weighted criteria that then predict the nursing care hours needed for the next 24 hours. The weighted criteria reflect care needed for patients, for example bathing, mobilizing, eating, supervising, assessing, observing, treating, and so on. Because patient care is dynamic and changing, it is impossible to capture future patient care needs using a one-time measure (Gran-Moravec & Hughes, 2005).

With the increased patient acuity at the unit level, nursing leaders are faced with the continual challenge of staffing for safe patient care, nursing satisfaction, and clinical and organizational excellence (American Nurse Today, 2016). In today's environment of optimizing high quality care and fiscal responsibility, acuity-based staffing is another model. **Acuity-based staffing** is a model that looks at a variety of factors influencing the assignment of each patient and each nurse (Trepanier, Lee, & Kerfoot, 2017). The expected nursing needs of individual patients is taken into consideration when making the staffing assignment. Patient diagnosis, care plan, co-morbidities, physical and mental function, and other potential factors are part of the staffing assignment decision making process. Acuity-based staffing has been linked to improved clinical and operational outcomes (American Nurse Today, 2016).

There has been a recent increase in acuity assessment software. This software can apply a mathematical value to the acuity and bedside care needs of a patient and generate assignments based on the identification of this value. This software can be costly, and many organizations have developed their own software utilizing the electronic medical health record data (Thomas & Roussel, 2020).

Acuity-based staffing has been linked to decreases in mortality, adverse outcomes, falls, pressure ulcers, and lengths of stay (American Nurse Today, 2016). Moving from the older model of PCSs to acuity-based staffing with the use of sophisticated technology can improve the staffing process for nurse leaders and improve accuracy and improve patient outcomes (Trepanier et al., 2017).

Considerations in Developing a Staffing Plan

Developing a staffing plan is a science and an art. The following sections will consider other areas of staffing in addition to the acuity data and NHPPD just discussed. Each of these areas should be reviewed and the findings incorporated into development of the staffing plan.

Benchmarking focuses on best practices and works toward a goal of continuous quality improvement. It is a comparison and measurement of a health care organization's services against that of other national competitors, who are considered industry leaders. It allows for the sharing of best practices and evidence-based practices at a national level (Davis, 2015). Often, benchmarking data provides only data about comparable units of service and does not provides data about quality of care indicators that can link quality patient care outcomes to units of service. Data may only be related to staffing numbers and not associated with quality outcomes, such as falls with injuries, or development of pressure ulcers, etc. In developing a staffing pattern, it is important to benchmark your planned NHPPD against other organizations with similar patient populations as part of evidence-based decision making.

The **National Database of Nursing Quality Indicators** (NDNQI) can serve as a benchmarking option. NDNQI is a repository for data that can be used to aid in the delivery of high-quality care (Roussel, 2020). The NHPPD measurements were developed by the American Nurses Association for the NDNQI to better assist organizations nationwide to be able to benchmark against one another to compare the effectiveness of their nursing model. The NDNQI values for average NHPPD are set at the 25th percentile, median, and 75th percentile (Thomas & Roussel, 2020). If your unit is staffing at the 25th percentile, that means that 75% of hospitals with similar units are staffing better than your unit. Those percentiles represent hospitals staffing at varying levels, best practice would be at the 75th percentile.

A **balanced scorecard** in health care is a tool to continually display benchmarking data and quality performance. It monitors an organization's or a unit's goals associated with the overall mission and vision. A nursing balanced scorecard may also monitor a variety of staffing and quality indicators specific to nursing nationally, within a hospital system, hospital's nursing department or unit.

Regulatory Requirements

Historically, few regulatory requirements have prescribed nurse staffing. This changed when the **Health Services Research Administration** (HRSA) released a 2002 study on over 5 million patient discharges. The study found a consistently strong relationship between nurse staffing and patient care outcomes (Needleman, Buerhaus, Mattke, Stewart, & Zelevinsky, 2002). This landmark study's findings supported changes in staffing models at the national, state, and local hospital levels. The 42 *Code of Federal Regulations* (Centers for Medicare and Medicaid Services, 2007) requires Medicare-Certified hospitals to have adequate numbers of direct care providers, leaving it up to the states to determine appropriate staffing. The American Nurses Association (2018b) has endorsed *The Safe Staffing for Nurse and Patient Safety Act of 2018* but Congress has failed to enact it. Therefore, some states have taken action at the state level to ensure that staffing is appropriate for patient needs. Following the American Nurses Association

Real World Interview

The purpose of the Trinity Health System Nursing Balanced Scorecard is to look for success across the system and benchmark across all 94 hospitals. Internal comparison of hospitals allows for identification of opportunities for improvement and learning from best practices. We look for best practices within the 94 hospitals and benchmark with the National Database for Nursing Quality Indicators (NDNQI) to compare ourselves with other organizations across the country. A Balanced Scorecard will look at a variety of outcomes generated by our clinical microsystems. A clinical microsystem is the dynamics of the team within a clinical area that are regularly working together in health care to achieve optimum patient care. On an inpatient nursing unit, the clinical microsystem would be everyone on that unit, including staff, patients, and families. The culture of the clinical microsystem and evidence-based practice principles drive areas of improvement in employee satisfaction, patient experiences, falls with injuries, hospital acquired infections, prevention of harm, tenure and turnover, etc. The Nursing Balanced Scorecard can drive improvements at the system, hospital, department, and unit level. Comparison within an individual hospital should include similar Balanced Scorecards of outcomes within units. Units can compare performance and nursing leaders can recognize opportunities for improvement. Balanced Scorecards also allows recognition of units doing well and exploration of how can we learn from them. A unit can post and share their unit-specific Balanced Scorecard related to patient care outcomes and patient satisfaction, so that staff can readily visualize their performance and work for improvements. Organizations within the Trinity Health System are recognized when their performance is in the top quartile. Those organizations share their journey in Trinity Health System conferences with other organizations. As a system, we lift them up and ask them to teach and share, so others can learn and replicate. The implementation of a Nursing Balanced Scorecard can improve practice. Studies have shown that both staffing and nursing satisfaction impact positive patient outcomes. When nursing staff know the results of their Balanced Scorecard and own it, staff engage and drive improved performance. Engagement includes knowing the standards, interventions, and strategies that will accelerate improvement at the system, hospital, department, and unit level.

Gay Landstrom PhD, RN, NEA-BC, FACHE
Senior Vice President and Chief Nursing Officer
Trinity Health System
Livonia, Michigan

recommendations, state staffing laws should include language that addresses the following:

1. Require hospitals to have a staffing committee

2. Mandate specific nurse-to-patient ratios in legislation or regulation

3. Require facilities to disclose staffing levels to the public and/or regulatory body (ANA, 2018b).

To date, 14 states have enacted legislation to address nurse staffing. Seven states require hospitals to have a staffing committee; these include Connecticut, Illinois, Nevada, Ohio, Oregon, Texas, and Washington. California is the only state that mandates the minimum nurse-to-patient ratio to be maintained at all times including lunches, breaks, etc. Massachusetts passed a law that is **Intensive Care Unit** (ICU) specific, requiring a 1 : 1 or 1 : 2 nurse/patient ratio dependent on patient stability. Minnesota requires a Chief Nursing Officer or designee to develop a core staffing plan with input from others. Five states (Illinois, New Jersey, New York, Rhode Island, and Vermont) require mandatory public reporting of staffing levels (ANA, 2018b).

The Joint Commission (JC) surveys hospitals on the quality of care provided. The JC does not mandate staffing levels but it does assess staffing effectiveness. Staffing effectiveness is the appropriate level of nurse staffing that will provide the best possible outcome of individual patients throughout a particular facility (The Joint Commission, 2018). The Joint Commission standards on staffing require organizations to monitor a correlation between two clinical and two human resource indicators—for example, NHPPD against hospital-acquired pressure ulcer occurrence or NHPPD against patient falls. Findings must then be used to adjust staffing levels, for example, if patient falls are high and NHPPD are low, then staffing should be increased.

Skill Mix

Skill mix is another critical element in nurse staffing. **Skill mix** is the percentage of Registered Nurse (RN) staff compared to other direct care staff (LPNs, UAPs, etc.). For example, in a unit that has 40 FTEs budgeted, with 20 of the FTEs being RNs and 20 FTEs of other skill types, the RN skill mix would be 50%. If the unit had 40 FTEs, with 30 of them being RNs, the RN skill mix would be 75%. The skill mix of a unit should vary according to the patient care workload or patient acuity and the care delivery model utilized. For example, in a **Critical Care Unit** (CCU), the RN skill mix will be much higher in CCU than in a nursing home where the skills of an RN are required to a much lesser degree. It is important to note that RN hours of care are costlier than those of less skilled workers, but there is evidence that RNs are a very productive and efficient type of labor. A higher number of RNs has been associated in evidence-based research with improved patient outcomes, which includes patient falls, infection rates,

Case Study 5.3

You are the manager of a 16-bed Intensive Care Unit (ICU) with a nurse-to-patient ratio of one nurse to every two patients. At this time, the unit is full with 16 patients. The nurses identify four patients who have improved enough for transfer to a medical-surgical unit. The nurse-to-patient ratio on the medical-surgical unit is one nurse to four patients. The hospital census (number of patients in the hospital) is high and no medical-surgical beds are available for the ICU patient transfers. Because of this, the patients will have to stay in ICU for the next two shifts. In planning staffing for the next two shifts for your ICU unit, you need to adjust staffing based on the patient information.

1. What factors should be considered?
2. What is your plan for staffing the next two shifts?
3. How will you communicate the staffing plan to the staff?

Real World Interview

Here is my typical daily work schedule as an RN

0700 Huddle.

During a huddle, the oncoming shift of nurses and Unlicensed Assistive Personnel (UAP) gather with the supervisor and charge nurse as well as with the previous shift of nurses. A UAP may be called a nurse aide or a patient care assistant in other hospitals. Staffing, policy updates, and any adverse events that occurred during the previous shift are quickly discussed and the huddle usually ends with a prayer.

0710–0800 Shift or Staff Handoff Report.

The oncoming RN and the previous shift RN go into the assigned patient rooms together. The oncoming nurse is introduced to the patient by the previous shift nurse. An exchange of the events from the previous shift is communicated. The patient is included in the report. If they have any comments or questions, they are addressed at this time. The oncoming RN puts their identification picture card, portable phone number, and current date in the patient's room in the designated area.

0800–0820 Communication, Delegation, Blood Sugars, Hourly Rounding, UAP Report Guidelines

- The RN signs in and puts their portable phone number in the computer so all the team can easily see which nurse is taking care of which patient. The team communicates throughout the day in person, on the computer, and with portable phones. The RN reviews all patient vital signs and enters them into computer.
- The RN gives report and delegates care to the UAPs. UAPs do not have access to the same patient information as the RN, so the RN must make sure the UAP assisting them in caring for their patient knows all of the pertinent information they need to know to safely meet the patient's needs. The UAP is given guidelines of what and when to report patient information back to RN.
- An RN or UAP performs blood sugar checks on the diabetic patients, and if necessary, they help the patient place their breakfast order.
- Hourly rounding begins and continues throughout the shift—The RN assesses certain specific items regularly on each patient, e.g.,
  - Does the patient need help with bathing? Eating? Assistance to bathroom? Dressing change?
  - Is the patient's IV running well? Are they having pain? Do they need to be medicated?

  - Is the patient comfortable in bed or in the chair? Would they like to be repositioned?
  - Is it time to turn bedbound patients on Q2H schedule to prevent pressure ulcers?
  - Is it time to ambulate patient? Make sure that the patient, if able, is up and moving and/or is in the recliner for two meals a day unless contraindicated.
  - Are the patient's personal belongings, e.g., call light, cell phone, glasses, tissues, dentures, and hearing aids, etc. in their reach?

0820–0945 Vital Signs, Medications, Nutrition

- The RN must obtain vital signs on each patient and records them in the computer before morning medications are given.
- The RN administers medications to their patients. Insulin is administered when the diabetic patient's breakfast tray arrives. The RN is responsible for verifying this breakfast tray is available and at the patient's bedside. In addition, the RN or UAP may also assist or help prepare the patient to eat by cutting up food, removing lids, and assisting the patient with denture care.

0945–1045 Ongoing Patient Assessment

- The RN works to finish all their initial physical assessments in order to be up to date on the patient's overall condition and plan of care before rounding with the physicians. Some nurses do their assessments at the same time as they administer medications. Some nurses prefer to do it as a separate step.

1045–1130 Documentation

- The RN completes as much computer charting on each patient as possible before moving on to the next task. Sometimes you can accomplish a lot, but it is not uncommon that you will be interrupted every five minutes by phone calls, family members, patient needs, and other staff member needs.

1130–1200 Rounding Huddle with Interprofessional Team, Vital Signs

- Rounding huddle with physicians. The nurse and physician, along with the UAP, dietician, respiratory therapist, case manager, supervisor, and unit manager, as needed, visit each patient for about one to two minutes to briefly discuss the plan of care and address any anticipated needs of the patient, including discharge planning. The nurse leads this huddle with current information about the patient and the plan of care.

- Obtain 1,130 vital signs

  1200–1300 Blood Sugars, Medications, New Orders, New Labs

- Perform blood sugar checks on the diabetic patients in preparation for lunch to arrive.
- Administer 1,200–1,300 medications.
- Check computer to see if there are any new orders written on each patient. If there are changes to ambulation status, diet, or upcoming testing, this needs to be communicated to your UAP also. Any new orders should always be communicated to patient and family. Also check for any lab or test results that may have been completed.

  1300–1400 Medications, New Orders

- Administer 1,300–1,400 medications.
- Review charts again for new patient orders. Sometimes a doctor will enter orders into the computer while on another floor and these orders are easy to miss.

  1400–1500 Medications, Documentation, Lunch

- Administer 1,400–1,500 medications.
- Catch up on charting, or take lunch break, if there is time!!

  1500–1600 Medications, Vital Signs, Blood Sugars, Nutrition

- Administer 1,500–1,600 medications.
- Review 1,600 vital signs
- Do blood sugars on diabetic patients and if necessary, assist with ordering dinner

  1600–1700 Medications, Nutrition

- Administer 1,630–1,700 medications
- Administer insulin as dinner trays arrive and help prepare patient to eat

  1700–1800 Documentation, Ambulation, Medications, Handoff

- Finish up charting, if not complete
- Ambulate your patient a second time if they are able.
- Administer any med that is due between 1,700–1,800
- Prepare a brief written handoff shift form for the oncoming nurse. This does not replace the verbal handoff shift report. It is another tool to prevent important information from slipping through the cracks. The form contains anticipated tests, procedures, and any abnormal findings, as well as any patient needs or complaints.

  1800–1900 Final Hourly Rounding, Documentation, Check Orders

- Hourly rounding—with this last hourly rounding of the shift, the room should be checked for cleanliness. Any extra linens should be put away, trash emptied, tables cleared of clutter. Make sure that the patient's needs have been met, patient has been taken to bathroom and has been medicated for pain, if needed.
- Sign off all of the computer orders from your shift. Signing off the orders means you are the RN responsible for initiating all the orders correctly to assure they will be completed.
- Put away all supplies that you have had out and been using during your shift. Make sure areas are clean and restocked with supplies. Check and refill medication cart with supplies.

  1900 Huddle.

- This huddle is for the oncoming shift. Your job is to cover the call lights and monitor the patients until the oncoming shift huddle is over.

  1900–1945 Shift or Staff Handoff Report.

- Report is done between you and the oncoming RN. Report is done in the room. You will introduce the oncoming RN, say goodbye to the patient and thank them for choosing your institution for their health care needs. Remove your picture from the room and erase your portable phone number.

  1945 Finish Your Shift

- Once report is finished, you must go into the computer system and remove your name from your team of patients and remove your phone number from the system. Finish charting and sign off any remaining orders. Clock out. You will get out on time some days and late on other days. It all depends on the day, how busy you are, and how you manage your time. Do it again tomorrow!!

Robyn L. White, BSN, RN, CMSRN, MJ, CLNC
Utilization Review RN
Mishawaka, Indiana

medication errors, family complaints, and death (Hunt, 2018). However, it is essential to critically evaluate patient care requirements and identify who can perform necessary functions. Each staff member should work within their full scope of practice, which can result in fiscal accountability and positive patient outcomes. (Hunt, 2018).

Staff Support

Another important factor to consider in determining staffing needs is the supports in place for the operations of the department or unit. For instance, does the organization have a systematic process to deliver medications to the unit, or do unit personnel have to pick up patient medications? Does the organization have staff to transport patients to and from ancillary departments? An additional important unit-based need is secretarial support. If the unit has many admissions, discharges, and transfers, it makes sense to provide unit secretarial support for the peak periods of the day. This kind of support for nursing staff allows them to spend their available time with patients. The less support available to nursing staff, the more nursing hours have to be built into the staffing pattern to provide care to patients.

Considering the many variables that affect staffing, it helps to ask the following questions: What has worked in the past? Were the staff able to provide the care that was needed? How many patients were cared for? What kind of patients were they? How many staff were utilized? What was the skill mix of the staff? These questions can help to identify staffing issues that would not be apparent otherwise. For example, an older part of a facility may not have a pneumatic delivery tube system, which is available in the newer parts of the facility. Because the tube system is generally available, you may overlook its absence, but the lack of a tube system means that a significant amount of time will be required to collect needed items, thus affecting the staffing plan you develop.

As older hospitals are being replaced with new structures, workflow redesign will need to be taken into account when developing a staffing plan. Transformational change can occur in patient unit design and construction that can impact staffing, efficient workflow, removal of wasteful work processes and work-arounds, and create safe, efficient, effective, and ergonomically-correct patient care environments. When new construction is designed, the following are focused on to create new health care flows: flow of staff, flow of patients, flow of families and care partners, flow of information, flow of supplies, flow of equipment, and flow of output (Cardon, 2015). Improved health care redesign can positively impact staffing needs.

Creating the Staffing Plan

A staffing plan articulates how many and what kind of staff are needed by shift and day to staff a unit or department. There are basically two types of developing a staffing plan. One is generated by determining the required ratio of staff-to-patients and then calculating nursing hours and total FTEs. It can also be generated by determining the number of nursing care hours needed for a specific patient or patients and then generating the FTEs and staff-to-patient needed to provide that care. In most cases, a combination of methods to develop a staffing plan is utilized. Below is an example of a staffing plan needed to determine the required ratio of staff-to-patients on a Medical Inpatient Unit.

Inpatient Unit

An **inpatient unit** is a hospital unit that provides care to patients 24 hours a day, seven days a week. Establishing a staffing plan for this kind of unit utilizes all the data discussed in the previous areas. To illustrate the concept of calculating a staffing plan, a typical Medical Inpatient Unit will be used with 24 beds and an average daily census of 20. **Average Daily Census (ADC)** is calculated by taking the total numbers of patients at census time, usually midnight, over a period of time—for example, weekly, monthly, or yearly—and dividing by the number of days in the time period. Many institutions budget their staffing based on ADC and then adjust for patient census and acuity changes. Utilizing Figure 5.7, Calculation of NHPPD, we will identify the number and type of staff needed during the week and on weekends for 24 hours a day for the number of patients on the Medical Inpatient Unit.

Development of a Medical Inpatient Unit Staffing Plan

Step 1: To develop a staffing plan using NHPPD, start with a target NHPPD (Figure 5.7). If the target NHPPD were 8, for example, and there were 20 patients on the 24-bed unit, multiply 8 NHPPD times 20 patients to get 160 productive hours needed every day. Generally, the NHPPD are an agreed upon target derived from variables such as acuity of patients, benchmarking, and discussion with the Finance Department related to budget. The NHPPD of 8 will then be part of the unit nursing budget. Dividing 160 productive hours by the 8-hour shifts worked by each staff member calculates to 20 staff members needed per 24-hour day.

Step 2: Once the determination has been made of how many 8-hour shifts are needed in 24 hours, the next step is to allocate staff to the plan, based on how care is delivered on the unit. To fully understand the complexity of decisions involved in this step, review the Models of Care Delivery section later in the chapter. Allocating FTEs cannot be separated from an intelligent understanding of how patient care is delivered and how to use the right mix of staff to accomplish that patient care. The example in Figure 5.7 is a medical unit.

Taking the 20 shifts that are needed for patient care in our example, the nurse manager must determine the mix of staff, the weighting of staff per shift, and whether this staffing changes by day of the week. The census on this unit does not lower on the weekends, so calculate the staffing for the entire week. If the unit had reduced census on specific days of the week, those days would be calculated separately. The result of step 2 is a snapshot of the staffing plan for 24 hours (Figure 5.7). This staffing plan has now been determined on a unit. The staffing plan calculates the number of FTEs needed per day.

Step 3: The next calculation is the amount of additional staff that will be needed to provide for days off. Direct caregivers will need to be replaced, but some other support staff may not need to be replaced for days off or benefited time off. Managers typically are not replaced on days off. The formula for calculating coverage for staff days off is the number of staff needed per shift multiplied by the number of days of needed coverage, usually seven, divided by the number of shifts each FTE works per week. For each 8-hour staff member needed in the daily plan, the unit must hire 1.4 FTEs ($1 \times 7/5 = 1.4$). In a 12-hour staffing model, the manager must hire 2.3 FTEs for each 12-hour staff member needed in the daily plan ($1 \times 7/3 = 2.3$). This is true because each 12-hour staff member works only three days per week.

In this example for step 3, the calculations for seven-day coverage are in parentheses in the staffing plan. To have four RNs on day shift, for example, you need to hire 5.6 FTEs. In total, there will be a need to hire 28 FTEs to have 20 staff working seven days per week.

Step 4: The next step is to provide additional FTEs for coverage for benefit time away from work. Benefit time includes vacations, educational time, orientation time, and so on. The amount of benefit time away from work varies by organization. If every employee receives the benefit time outlined in Figure 5.5, 232 benefit hours are needed per employee. Continuing the need to determine what percent of each FTE's productive time the benefits represent. In the example, 232 is 11% of 2,080. Take the total FTEs from step 3 and multiply by 0.11 ($28 \times 0.11 = 3.08$). Thus, an additional 3.08 FTEs is needed to work when other staff are taking benefit time. This figure is then added to our total from step 3 to get our grand total FTEs for the budget to staff the medical unit ($28 + 3.08 = 31.08$ FTE).

Staffing for Patient Needs

PCSs do not tell you when the nursing activity will take place over the next 24 hours for patient needs. Acuity-based staffing takes into account the scope of nursing and the time needed to maintain standards of practice. In planning for the acuity of patients, the staffing plan must support having staff working when the work needs to be done. A good example of this would be an oncology unit on which chemotherapy and blood transfusions typically occur on the evening shift. On this unit, staffing on the evening shift may need to be higher than for other shifts to support these nurse-intensive activities. As patient acuity changes, so do patients' needs and staffing requirements. Adding a population of step-down patients from the ICU would likely require additional FTEs on a medical-surgical unit. Anytime patient populations change, staffing and NHPPD should be reassessed. A general rule is that the higher the patient acuity, the more consistent the staffing needs are across shifts. A CCU is continuously monitoring patients around the clock, whereas a surgical unit has activities concentrated before and after surgeries each day, with somewhat less activity on the late evening and night shifts.

Experience and Scheduling of Staff

Each nurse differs regarding their knowledge base, experience level, and critical thinking skills. A novice nurse takes longer than a proficient nurse requires to accomplish the same task. A proficient RN can handle more in terms of the workload and the acuity of the patients (Benner, 1984). If your unit requires special staff skills and competencies, you would want to schedule staff with special skills and competencies when the patient care needs arise. Note, the underlying principle of good staffing is that, those you serve come first. This may dictate some undesirable shifts and overtime, but your responsibility is to ensure that there are appropriate numbers and types of staff on hand to care for the patients you serve. A careful staffing plan should help to avoid problems.

Staff members should be scheduled for the number of days for which they are committed, such as five days a week for a full-time, eight-hour employee, and less time for part-time employees, as determined by their hiring commitment. When staff are hired, there is an agreement between the manager and the employee as to the shift, schedule, and work commitment. If the unit workload is consistent, the scheduled days should be assigned so that there are equal numbers of staff available through all shifts. Typically, the spread of FTEs across the 24-hour period falls within the following guidelines: days 33–50% FTEs, evenings 30–40% FTEs, and nights 20–33% FTEs. Remember though, the distribution of FTEs should be based on patient need!

Fixed and Flexible Staffing Schedules

To attract and retain employees, organizations offer both fixed and flexible staffing schedules to meet organizational and employee needs. Flexibility should be utilized to ensure staffing needs are met in real time and to enhance nursing satisfaction (American Nurses Association, 2015). Staffing models and staffing plans in the beginning phase should have input from direct clinical staff to ensure that aspects of the unit's environment, patient care needs, staff skill mix and skill level, and education of the staff are taken into consideration. A Shared Governance structure or participative decision-making model will allow front line caregivers the ability to be part of these decisions (American Nurses Association, 2015).

Fixed staffing schedules are a rigid type of staffing model that utilizes fixed staffing ratios and staffing grids. This can include a set number of nurses for a particular unit or shifts and unalterable nurse-to-patient ratios (American Nurses Association, 2015). Fixed or rigid staffing ratios don't recognize the potential hourly changes that are the norm in a patient care environment. There are many variables that impact staffing such changes in patient acuity, nursing skill mix, change in census, etc. For example, a surge in admissions or discharges, a high number of post-op patients, or patients undergoing procedures will have an effect on staffing. Increased Emergency Department admissions can also quickly affect the workflow of a unit in a rigid staffing model (American Nurses Association, 2015).

Flexible staffing schedules approach staffing by reviewing the number of nurses and/or the nurse-to-patient ratio and adjusting staffing based on changing factors. Staffing is based on patient's condition, acuity of care, nursing skill level required, and changes in patient census (American Nurses Association, 2015).

California is the only state that stipulates by law and regulations a minimum nurse-to-patient ratio to be maintained at all times on a unit. There are two national bills being considered regarding safer staffing ratios, patient staffing, and patient outcomes (Blitchok, 2018). They are the Nurse Staffing Standards for Hospital Patient Safety and Quality Act and the Safe Staffing for Nurse and Patient Safety Act of 2018 (ANA, 2018b).

New Options in Staffing Plans

In recent years, new options in staffing plans have emerged that take into consideration both the health care worker and the patient's needs. Twelve-hour shifts have become prevalent across the country. In many organizations, employees can work 36 hours per week and get full-time benefits. In this situation, a nurse could work three 12-hour shifts per week, have four days off, and still be full time. Advantages to 12-hour shifts include: increased productivity, fewer handoffs, increased continuity of patient care, and increased nursing morale. Disadvantages include longer working hours, less breaks during the workday, inability to have sufficient rest between consecutive work shifts, and increased fatigue (Emergency Nurses Association, 2013). The Joint Commission issued an addendum in 2018 to their Sentinel Event Alert Issue 48 regarding health care worker fatigue and patient safety. This addendum indicates that extended work hours contribute to higher levels of worker fatigue and reduced productivity. This Sentinel Event Alert indicates that fatigue increased the risk of adverse events, can affect patient safety, and impacts risk to personal safety and well-being (The Joint Commission, 2018).

The increasing use of overtime has become a global concern related to the impact on patient well-being, nurse's overall health and retention, and the fiscal implications (Lobo et al., 2018). When scheduling 12-hour shifts, it may be viewed as easier to pick up additional shifts when the nurse is scheduled three 12-hour shifts a week. Considering the factors that contribute to overtime, which include: staffing shortages, increasing patient acuity, increasing patient volumes, hiring freezes and fiscal restraints, nurses may feel pressure to work additional shifts to help alleviate heavier workloads and fewer staff at the unit level (Lobo et al., 2018).

Another popular staffing option is a weekend program. Weekend programs with varying degrees of commitment can be part time or full time. Some of these weekend programs include full-time benefits as well. The purpose of this kind of program is to improve weekend staffing for staff retention purposes and allow full-time staff members who usually work 26 weekends a year to work fewer weekends.

In some hospitals or units, flexibility of scheduling may expand the use of varying hours of shifts that correlate with census, patient care needs, patient safety, or procedures, etc. Shift lengths can vary including 4, 6, 8, 10, or 12-hour shifts. In the Emergency Department, the flow of patients may be significantly different than a medical surgical unit, requiring different length of shifts. This type of flexibility can be a nurse satisfier based on meeting the needs of personal/family life, and giving greater periods of time off (Emergency Nurses Association, 2013).

Any time there is an implementation of a scheduling plan, it is critical to assess what the effect will be on the care of patients. For example, work weeks made up of three 12-hour shifts have in many units disrupted continuity of care. **Continuity of care** is generally defined as the follow-through in patient care that is inherent in having the same nurse return to care for patients on subsequent shifts on sequential days of the week. Disruptions in continuity of care are especially the case when 12-hour shifts are not scheduled on sequential days. To mediate this disruption, 12-hour staff can be paired so that the patient has the same pair of nurses every day for three days, and then the patient can be transitioned to a new pair of 12-hour staff. Units that have short patient lengths of stay may

have fewer continuity problems than units with longer lengths of stay. The number of staff or shift handoff reports per day also affects continuity of care. A **handoff** according to the Joint Commission (2017) is a transfer and acceptance of patient care responsibility that is directly affected by appropriate and accurate information. A handoff occurs in real time when patient-specific information is passed from one caregiver to another. The purpose of a staff or shift handoff is to ensure continuity of care and patient safety. Inadequate handoff communication is a significant problem that leads to adverse events including sentinel events (The Joint Commission, 2017). A handoff report is an opportunity for missed communication and errors in patient care. In 8-hour shifts, there are three shift handoffs per 24 hours, whereas in 12-hour shifts, there are only two shift handoffs. This is a type of continuity of care staffing that promotes patient safety and must be balanced with the number of shifts per week that each nurse can safely work. When implementing staffing plans, one must ensure that there are always staff members scheduled who are familiar with the patients and the events that have transpired previously.

Financial Implications of Staffing Plans

New staffing plans may have significant financial implications. A number of new staffing plans are being put into place to recruit staff and encourage staff to work more hours.

There may be incentive plans that will encourage nurses to pick up additional shifts for a monetary bonus. Weekend programs are a recruitment and retention tool, but they are more expensive than traditional staffing plans because of the higher rate of hourly pay. To implement a new staffing program or other new programs, collaboration with the finance and human resources departments of the organization is necessary. This collaboration must be used to develop a financial analysis to measure the dollar and human resource impact of the staffing program.

Self-Scheduling

Inflexible work schedules and other staffing issues can be a major deterrent for nursing satisfaction. Staffing conflicts can result in increased nurse turnover, job dissatisfaction, and eventually leaving the organization (Wright, McCartt,

Evidence from the Literature

Source: Adapted from Shin, S., Park, J., & Bae, S. (2018). Nurse staffing and nurse outcomes: A systematic review and meta-analysis, *Nursing Outlook*, 66, 273–282.

Discussion: Hospital nursing staff provide holistic care for patients and families 24 hours a day. There have been a number of studies that examine the relationship between nurse staffing and patient outcomes. However, none of the reviews examined the relationship between nurse staffing and nursing outcomes through meta-analysis. The meta-analysis showed that staffing with less

nurses to more patients was consistently associated with a higher degree of burnout among nurses, decreased job satisfaction, and higher intent to leave their place of employment.

Implications for Practice: Studies indicate that nurse staffing is related to patient outcomes. In addition, optimal nurse staffing is also directly related to nursing outcomes. Optimal nurse-to-patient ratio levels are needed, to not only improve patient outcomes but also to reduce negative nursing outcomes and retain nurses in hospital settings.

Raines, & Oermann, 2017). Self-scheduling gives the nurse the opportunity to have more independence with their personal and professional schedules. Increasing autonomy and educational opportunity can ultimately contribute to overall nurse retention (Wright et al., 2017). **Self-scheduling** is a process in which unit staff take leadership in creating and monitoring the work schedule while working within defined guidelines. Often, there is a staffing committee that is part of shared governance on a unit, where staff manage their professional practice through unit committees. Increasing staff control over scheduling is a major factor in nurse job satisfaction and retention and has been associated with reductions in sick time usage. The nurse manager retains an important role in self-scheduling through mentoring, providing open communication, and holding everyone to equal expectations.

Boundaries of Self-Scheduling

To implement self-scheduling, responsibilities and boundaries need to be established that clearly state expectations of staff. This ties into leadership, teamwork and collaboration, and professionalism identified earlier as part of nursing practice. Self-scheduling is best done by a committee made up of staff. It is important to spell out the roles and responsibilities of those involved. The creation of healthy work schedules should be the goal. Health care organizations also need to promote staffing practices and strategies that support sleep health in nurses, which results in a healthier nurse workforce and increasing patient safety. Fatigued nurses are at risk for fatigue-related patient care errors and their own personal risks (Caruso et al., 2017). Long shifts, overtime, mandatory overtime, excessive consecutive shifts, and rotating shifts can have a direct bearing on absenteeism, patient safety, and related costs (Jeffery, Borum, & Englebright, 2017).

Self-scheduling guidelines need to be established regarding fairness, fiscal responsibility, evaluation of self-scheduling, and the staffing approval process. Table 5.6 spells out specific issues that must be addressed. During the self-scheduling process, the unit staff should participate and be educated about the self-scheduling staffing they are helping to develop. For this self-scheduling process to be successful, all staff members must understand self-scheduling guidelines, their responsibilities, and the effect of their decisions on staffing. All staff must also be committed to providing safe staffing on all shifts for their patients.

Informatics Support for Evidence-Based Staffing

Information technology is poised to provide innovative solutions to support evidence-based nurse staffing. Informatics is a QSEN competency that is being incorporated into the hospital setting. Hospitals currently capture data electronically from a variety of sources, such as admissions, discharges, transfers, bar-coding, call light timing, computerized charting of risk assessments, nurse profiles, and so forth. Some hospitals even use infrared signals to identify the nurse's location on the unit. When all of this data is combined, it provides meaningful information on nursing care needs, supply of qualified nurses, and quality of care outcomes (Hyun, Bakken, Douglas, & Stone, 2008). Similar to a puzzle, pieces of data can be found throughout a hospital. Separately, they provide small glimpses of the picture. To see the entire picture, it requires a computer program that is able to take each piece of data and put it together to create meaning.

Real World Interview

We implemented self-scheduling on many of our nursing units years ago. This is a huge staff satisfier. The staff has the autonomy to manage their work-life balance. Our general process is: an open schedule is put out; staff have a specific amount of time to fill in their requests; the manager or supervisor reviews the schedule and then posts it. Many staff understand that some changes will be made. We have had to implement some work rules such as: work at least two Fridays in six weeks or only one four-day weekend in six weeks, etc. We prefill staffing for any holidays and the weekends. We have found that the staff has more initiative to find self-coverage and plan vacations around each other with the new self-scheduling.

We then implemented Kronos computerized scheduling. This took our self-scheduling process electronic. The same self-scheduling process applies, but the staff can log on at home, on their phone, basically anywhere they have the Internet. Kronos allows even more flexibility in staff's ability to plan and balance their life. Some managers and nurses were hesitant and did not want to use the computer scheduling program. They would still do the schedule on paper and then transfer it. The departments that took self-scheduling on from the beginning and implemented the process by using the concept, "*NO PAPER*," have been the most successful. The other departments are still struggling to this day. The Kronos program is in real time and helps prevent errors. The majority of the nurses love self-scheduling and computerized scheduling. Newer nurses are pros at it. Some of the older nurses struggle and just want to use paper. Overall, it has been a positive experience and was very well received.

Elaine Flemming RN, MSN
Administrative Director, Care Management AND UTI-
Lization Review Acute Inpatient Rehabilitation, Nursing
Administration and Language Resources
Saint Joseph Health System
Mishawaka/Plymouth Indiana

Table 5.6   Issues to Be Spelled Out in Self-Scheduling Guidelines Created by D. Spoljoric and M. King.

- Scheduling period: Is the scheduling period for two-, four-, or six-week intervals?
- Schedule timeline: What are the time frames for staff to sign up for regular work commitment, special requests, overtime, and as-needed workers?
- Staffing pattern: Will eight- or twelve-hour shifts be used? A combination?
- Weekends: Are staff expected to work every other weekend? If there are extra weekends available, how are they distributed?
- Holidays: How are they allocated?
- Vacation time: Are there restrictions on the amount of vacation time during certain periods?
- Unit vacation practices: How many staff from one shift can be on vacation at any time?
- Requests for time off: What is the process for requesting time off?
- Short-staffed shifts: How are short-staffed shifts handled?
- On call, if applicable: How do staff get assigned to or sign up for on-call time?
- Cancelation guidelines: How and when do staff get canceled for scheduled time if they are not needed?
- Sick calls: What are the expectations for calling in sick, and how are these shifts then covered?
- Military/National Guard leave: What kind of advance notice is required?
- Schedule changes: What is the process for changing one's schedule after the schedule has been approved?
- Shifts defined: What are the beginnings and endings of available shifts?
- Committee time: When does the self-scheduling committee meet and for how long?
- Seniority: How does seniority play into staffing and request decisions?
- Staffing plan for crisis/emergency situations: What is the plan when staffing is needed quickly?

Standardizing how computer programs collect and represent data allows different computer programs to work together. For example, data is collected and reported from a variety of sources such as pagers, laboratory, nurse charting, glucometers, call light timing, medication bar-code and administration, etc. The ability of each source to interact with the other sources and provide data on real-time care provision by nurses provides information on the actual workload of nurses. Think of the vast amount of data continuously flowing on a clinical unit. The ability to capture and consistently gather data regarding real-time staffing needs is critical. Computer systems can pull the pieces of data together in real time and combine it with historical trends to help inform staffing decisions. For example, a medical-surgical unit experiences multiple patient admissions, discharges, and transfers during a Monday shift. In the morning, the 30-bed unit has 26 beds occupied. Computerized staffing data identifies six potential discharges and seven surgical admissions. In addition, the average number of call light signals is 67.3 per shift, with the length of time spent with the patient being 8.9 minutes per call. The computerized staffing program also alerts that there are four experienced nurses and one new nurse scheduled for the day shift. Another computerized alert shows that a surgeon is back from vacation, the emergency department is full, and historically Mondays have an emergency department admission rate of 4.2 patients. The ability to access this real-time information on variables that impact staffing during a shift from a variety of sources assists in determining appropriate staffing needs.

Computerized programs that support staffing allow for automated staff scheduling, online staff bidding for shifts, and prompt notification of open shifts. Computerized scheduling in conjunction with self-scheduling can generate staff schedules based on workload information, staff skills, staffing ratios, availability, seniority, shift preferences, polices, and labor regulations. Over the past decade, computerized programs have advanced to include sophisticated patient tracking through the hospital and identification of appropriate extended care placement for patient case management. The future of informatics promises to bring even more innovative solutions to support staffing and improve quality patient care outcomes.

Models of Patient Care Delivery

To ensure that nursing care is provided to patients, the work must be organized. A patient care delivery model organizes the work of caring for patients. Over the history of nursing, there have been many models of patient care delivery. Patient care delivery models outline task assignments, responsibilities, and authority to be able to deliver patient care. When considering a patient care delivery model, the objective is to match the patient care needs to the number and types of caregivers. The goal is to provide safe quality care to ensure positive patient outcomes matched with fiscal accountability (Cherry & Jacob, 2019). Different departments and patient care units may need a particular type of patient care delivery model based on the type of patients, patient needs, and acuity levels. Nursing Managers have the responsibility to implement patient care delivery models and evaluate the outcomes in their area. Staff have the responsibility to engage in the implementation and evaluation process. Each patient care delivery model has strengths and weaknesses that should be considered when deciding which to implement. Several different patient care delivery models are explored in the following sections.

There are four types of classic nursing models of patient care delivery that have been used to provide staff for patient care for many decades: total patient care, functional nursing, team nursing, and primary nursing. Newer models for the future will inevitably need to be developed with the nursing shortage, technology advances, patient acuity, rapidity of admissions and discharges, and the emphasis on patient safety and clinical outcomes (Cherry & Jacob, 2019).

Critical Thinking 5.2

Recently, you have been able to access data on your unit's rates of pressure ulcers. In researching further, you discover that your unit's rates are significantly higher than those of other units. Your staffing has been stable and in accordance with your staffing plan.

Your staff are experienced, and, in fact, you have the longest tenured staff in the hospital.

1. What are possible explanations for why your pressure ulcer rates are higher than those on other units?
2. How would your unit develop an action plan?

Total Patient Care

In **total patient care**, the nurse is responsible for the total patient care delivery of assigned patients for the shift worked. It is one of the oldest patient care delivery models. Units that are most likely to engage in this total patient care model would be ICUs or post anesthesia units, where continuous assessment and highly skilled clinical expertise is necessary (Cherry & Jacob, 2019). The RN has one to two patients for whom he or she is responsible. The nurse may have some support from LPN or UAP, when needed but those staff are not assigned to a specific group of patients. They are assigned to help with all patient care.

Advantages and Disadvantages

The advantage of the total patient care model for the patient is the consistency of one individual caring for patients for an entire shift. This enables the patient, nurse, and family to develop a relationship based on trust and holistic care. This model provides a higher number of RN hours of care than do other models. The nurse has more opportunity to observe and monitor the progress of the patient. A disadvantage is that this model utilizes a high level of RN hours to deliver care and is costlier than other models of patient care delivery. This model works well in specialized units with high patient acuity.

Functional Nursing

The functional nursing model of patient care delivery became popular during World War II when there was a significant shortage of nurses in the United States. This model allows staff members to take on specific functions for a group of patients. LPAs and UAPs are key components of this model. **Functional nursing** divides the nursing work into functional roles that are then assigned to one of the team members. In this model, each care provider has specific duties or tasks for which they are responsible. For instance, a typical division of labor for RNs is medication nurse, admission/assessment nurse, etc.; LPNs change dressings, etc.; and UAPs obtain vital signs and give bed baths, etc. Decision making is usually at the level of the charge nurse (Figure 5.8).

Advantages and Disadvantages

In the functional nursing model of patient care delivery, care can be delivered to a large number of patients. This model utilizes other types of health care workers when there is a shortage of RNs. Advantages include cost efficiency and the fact that tasks may be completed quickly. Patients are likely to have care delivered to them in one shift by several staff members. A risk of this model of care is that patients may feel their care is disjointed. Patients receive pieces of their care from different people rather than receiving care as an integrated whole. This may alter communication and may also alter the patient's overall perceptions of their care. In the current health care environment, this is especially problematic as patient perception of care and patient satisfaction are directly tied to financial reimbursement for organizations.

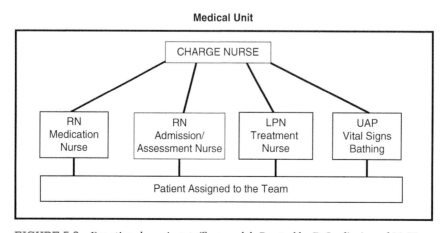

FIGURE 5.8   Functional nursing staffing model. Created by D. Spoljoric and M. King.

Team Nursing

Team nursing is a patient care delivery model that assigns staff to teams that then are responsible for a group of patients. A patient care unit may be divided into two or more teams. Each team is led by an RN. The team leader supervises and coordinates all the care provided by those on the team. The team is most commonly made up of LPAs and UAPs. The team leader is responsible for safely delegating specific duties to the team. The larger the team, the more the RN is stretched to safely monitor and care for the patients (Figure 5.9). Newer models of team nursing are being developed to improve the care experience and clinical outcomes. The goal is to maximize the skill mix and collaborative practice to begin transformational change in the current health care environment (Hastings, Suter, Bloom, & Sharma, 2016).

A **modular nursing** staffing system is a kind of team nursing that divides a geographical space into modules of patients, with each module cared for by a team of staff led by an RN. It is a modification of team nursing. The modules may vary in size but center in a geographical location and may be associated with a decentralized nursing station. Nursing stations are close to patients to meet the needs of the patients and enhance workflow.

Advantages and Disadvantages

The advantage of team nursing is that this model allows each team member to participate in decision making and contribute their expertise to patients (Cherry & Jacob, 2019). In team nursing and modular nursing, the RN is able to get work done through others, but patients may receive fragmented, depersonalized care. Communication in these models is complex. The shared responsibility and accountability can cause confusion and a lack of accountability. These factors contribute to RN dissatisfaction with these models. The team nursing and modular staffing models require the RN to have very good delegation and supervision skills.

Primary Nursing

Primary nursing is a patient care delivery model that clearly delineates the responsibility and accountability of the RN and designates the RN as the primary provider of care to patients. This primary nurse retains 24-hour accountability for care coordination for a set of patients throughout the patients' hospital stay. Patients are assigned a primary nurse, who is responsible for developing a plan of care with the patient that is followed by all other nurses caring for the patient. Nurses and patients are matched according to needs and abilities. Patients are assigned to their primary nurse regardless of unit geographical considerations. Daily care is provided by the primary nurse or by the associate nurses who deliver the plan of care in collaboration with the primary nurse when the primary nurse is not working (Figure 5.10).

Advantages and Disadvantages

An advantage of the primary nursing patient care delivery model is that patients and families are able to develop a trusting relationship with the primary nurse. There is defined accountability and responsibility for the primary nurse to develop a plan of care with the patient and family. A holistic primary nursing approach to care facilitates continuity of care rather than a shift-to-shift focus. Nurses, when they have adequate time to provide necessary care, find this model professionally rewarding, because it gives the authority for decision making to the nurse at the bedside. Disadvantages include a high cost, because there is a higher RN skill mix. The person making out the assignments needs to be knowledgeable about all the patients and the staff to ensure appropriate matching of nurses to patients. With no geographical boundaries within the unit, nursing staff may be required to travel long distances at the unit level to care for their primary patients. Nurses often perform functions that could be completed by other staff. Finally, nurse-to-patient ratios in the primary nursing patient care delivery model must be realistic to ensure that enough nursing time is available to meet the patient care needs.

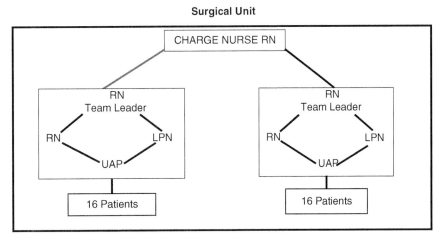

FIGURE 5.9   Team nursing staffing model. Created by D. Spoljoric and M. King.

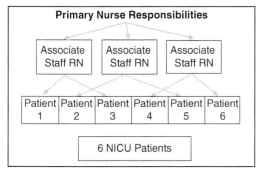

FIGURE 5.10   Primary nursing staffing model. Created by D. Spoljoric and M. King.

Patient-Centered Care or Patient-Focused Care

Patient-centered care or patient-focused care is a patient care delivery model designed to focus on patient needs rather than staff needs. The Institute of Medicine (IOM, 2011) defines patient-centered care as "providing care that is respectful of, and responsive to, individual preferences, needs and value, and ensuring that patient values guide all clinical decisions." **QSEN Patient Centered Care** (QSEN, 2019) is defined as recognizing the patient or designee as the source of control and full partner in providing compassionate and coordinated care based on respect for the patient's preferences, values, and needs.

In a Patient-Centered Care model, required care and services are brought to the patient. In the highest evolution of this model, all patient services are decentralized to the patient area, including radiology and pharmacy services. Staffing is based on patient needs. In this model, there is an effort to have the right person doing the right thing. Care teams are established for a group of patients. The patient care teams may include other disciplines such as respiratory or physical therapists. In these patient care teams, disciplines collaborate to ensure that patients receive the care they need. Staff are kept close to the patients in decentralized work stations. For example, on a rehabilitation unit, physical therapists may be members of the patient care team and work at the unit level rather than in a centralized physical therapy department. Consider patient-centered care as more of a philosophy versus a patient care delivery model. In today's health care environment, patient-centered care has become foundational. Patient-centered care should be incorporated into any nursing care delivery model to ensure engagement from patient and family members. Some hospital organizations have instituted patient and/or family advisory councils to help facilitate their being part of the decision-making process (Cherry & Jacob, 2019).

Advantages and Disadvantages

The pros of the patient-centered care or patient-focused care models are that they are most convenient for patients and expedite services to patients. But it can be extremely costly to decentralize major services in an organization. A second disadvantage is that some staff have perceived these models as a way of reducing RNs and cutting costs in hospitals. In fact, this has been true in some organizations, but many other organizations have successfully used the patient-centered care staffing model to have the right staff available for the needs of the patient population.

Care Delivery Management Tools

In 1983, the Centers for Medicare and Medicaid Services (CMS) established **diagnostic-related groups** (DRGs) as part of a payment system for hospitals. In DRGs, the national average of a typical LOS for a specific patient group is used to determine payment for that grouping within the Medicare (CMS) patients. **Length of stay (LOS)** refers to the average number of days a patient is hospitalized from the day of admission to the day of discharge. In DRGs, hospitals are paid the same amount for caring for a patient from a DRG patient group regardless of the actual LOS of the specific patient. These prompted initiatives in hospitals to reduce LOS and reduce hospital costs. There have been further adjustments to DRG hospital payments based on patient co-morbidities, that is, additional health care conditions that add to the complexity of care needed by a patient with other health care conditions, for example, heart disease, diabetes, or hypertension. With DRGs, hospitals were able to benchmark their LOS for specific patient populations against a national database published through the Medicare DRG system. As hospitals looked for opportunities to reduce costs through reduction in the LOS, clinical pathways and case management surfaced as significant strategies.

Another Federal Government initiative is Hospital **Value-Based Purchasing** (VBP). This is a program that was implemented by the Centers for Medicare and Medicare Services (CMS) that rewards acute care hospitals with incentive payments for the quality of care provided to Medicare beneficiaries. Hospital Value-Based Purchasing Programs support better care for individuals, better health for patient populations, and lower cost, for example, by eliminating or reducing adverse events (health care errors resulting in patient harm). Hospital Value-Based Purchasing payments are based on quality rather than quantity of care (CMS, 2017). Staff nurses at the unit level in addition to case managers are key drivers of success in VBP.

Clinical Pathways

Clinical pathways were a major initiative to come out of the efforts to reduce LOS and are widely used to enhance patient outcomes and contain costs. **Clinical pathways** are care management tools that outline the expected clinical course and outcomes for a specific patient type. Clinical pathways should be evidence-based, reflecting the best knowledge to date for patient care. Typically, clinical pathways outline the normal course of care for a patient. For each day, expected outcomes are articulated. Patient progress is measured against expected outcomes. Clinical pathways are composed of physical assessment guidelines, lab tests, diagnostics tests, medications, procedures, patient and family education, nutrition needs, and discharge planning from the day of admission. For example, a patient is admitted to the hospital with heart failure. From the day of admission to the day of discharge, the specific clinical pathway for heart failure identifies milestones that a patient should achieve during the progression of patient care (Cherry & Jacob, 2019). This serves as a road map throughout the patient's care episode. Any variance in achieving the clinical pathway milestones can be noted and acted upon to get the patient back on track. In some facilities, clinical pathways have practitioner orders incorporated into the clinical pathway to facilitate care. Clinical pathways can be comprised of all interprofessional orders for care, including orders from nursing, medicine, and allied health professionals, such as physical therapy and dietary services.

Advantages and Disadvantages

By articulating the normal course of care for a patient population, clinical pathways are a powerful tool for managing care. In most cases, the implementation of a clinical pathway will improve care, reduce variability, and shorten the LOS for the patient population on the clinical pathway. Clinical pathways also allow for data collection of variances to the clinical pathway. The data can then be used to continuously improve hospital systems and clinical practice. Some practitioners perceive clinical pathways to be cookbook medicine and are reluctant to participate in their development. Practitioner participation is critical. Development of interprofessional clinical pathways requires a significant amount of work to gain consensus from the various disciplines on the expected plan of care. For patient populations that are nonstandard, clinical pathways are less effective, because the clinical pathway is constantly being modified to reflect the individual patient's needs.

Case Management

Case management is a second initiative to reduce LOS, enhance patient outcomes, and contain costs. **Case Management** is a collaborative process of assessment, planning, facilitation, care coordination, evaluation, and advocacy for options and services to meet an individual's and family's comprehensive health needs through communication and available resources to promote patient safety, quality of care, and cost-effective outcomes (Case Management Society of America, 2019). Typically, a nurse case manager is responsible for coordinating care and establishing patient goals from preadmission through discharge. In the typical model of case management, a nurse case manager is assigned to a specific high-risk patient population or service, such as cardiac surgery patients. The nurse case manager has the responsibility to collaborate with all member of the interprofessional team to facilitate care. For example, if a postsurgical hospitalized patient has not met ambulation goals according to the clinical pathway, the case manager would work with the practitioner and nurse to determine what

is preventing the patient from achieving this goal. If it turns out that the patient is elderly and is slow to recover, they may agree that physical therapy would be beneficial to assist the patient in ambulating. In other case management models, the case management function is provided by the staff nurse at the bedside. If the patient population requires significant case management services, there needs to be enough RN time allocated for this activity. In addition to facilitating care, the case manager usually has the responsibility to monitor and improve care. In this role, the case manager collects aggregate data on patient variances from the clinical pathway. The data are shared with the responsible practitioners and other disciplines that participated in the clinical pathway and are then used to explore opportunities for improvement in the clinical pathway or in hospital patient care delivery.

Care Delivery Management Tools of the Future

As the complexity of the health care environment continues to grow, the delivery of patient care in both inpatient and outpatient settings will change dramatically in the future. The following factors will greatly affect the need for this dramatic change. that is technological advances, increasing rapidity of admissions and discharges, and a strong focus on the nurse's impact on patient safety and quality of care. Increasing demand for high-quality outcomes of care and consumers demand for immediate access to care and information will drive the need for new delivery models (Cherry & Jacob, 2019). As inpatient care focuses on the highest acuity patients, outpatient and community-based settings will also face unprecedented challenges to provide positive patient outcomes with early hospital discharges and emphasis on reducing readmissions t.o acute care settings. Nurses need to be at the forefront of these changes. Nurses, because of their roles, educational background, and being in a well-respected profession, can lead these changes. A leading factor that will contribute to needed change is the move from episodic patient care to team based patient-centered care across the continuum while providing the highest quality care, even beginning at the unit level (Salmond & Echevarria, 2017).

Evaluation of Staffing Effectiveness

Many patient outcomes are driven by the available hours of care delivered and the competence of staff delivering the care. For example, the nurse manager and the Chief Nursing Officer have the ongoing responsibility to monitor the effectiveness of the staffing plan. To ensure objectivity, staffing outcomes must be identified, measured, and revaluated.

Patient Outcomes and Nurse Staffing

The American Nurses Association (ANA) commissioned an integrative review of research on nurse staffing and the effects on patient outcomes. The ANA looked at optimal staffing to improve quality of care and patient outcomes. The published studies show that appropriate nurse staffing has a measurable impact on patient satisfaction, reduction in medical and medication errors, patient mortality, hospital readmissions, and LOS. Optimal staffing reflected a decrease in the number of preventable events, such as falls, pressure ulcers, central line infections, health-associated infections, and other potential complications related to hospitalizations. Appropriate staffing also affects nurse fatigue, nurse safety, and nurse job satisfaction within their unit and the overall organization. Additionally, these findings suggest that nurse-patient ratios are important and that they must be modified with the level of experience of the nurse, the characteristics of the organization, and the quality of interprofessional interactions (ANA, 2015). For instance, a new nurse should be assigned less-critical patients or have a lower nurse-to-patient ratio to allow for learning, whereas a proficient or expert nurse would be expected to handle the standard nurse-to-patient ratio for the unit. Characteristics of a high-quality organization include appropriate staffing based on the selected care delivery model, presence of a charge nurse or team leader without assigned patients, availability of resources such as advanced practice nurses to assist with care, and an environment of autonomy over nursing practice. The quality of interprofessional interactions involves the presence and availability of ancillary departments (respiratory, physical therapy, etc.) as well as the utilization of hospital physician intensivists (physicians whose primary responsibility is the care of hospitalized patients) and case managers.

In addition, to the association of staffing with increased mortality and patient errors etc. there is also recent evidence that indicates staffing is related to "missed nursing care." **Missed nursing care** is defined as any aspect of standard and required nursing care that is delayed, partially completed, or not completed at all (Duffy, Culp, & Padrutt, 2018).

Other professional organizations are weighing in on staffing and patient outcomes. For example, the **American Association of Critical Care Nurses** (AACN) considers appropriate staffing to be one of six key standards of sustaining healthy work environments for nurses. According to the AACN, six key nursing standards create a healthy work environment, that is, skilled communication, true collaboration, effective decision making, appropriate staffing, meaningful recognition, and authentic leadership (2016).

Nurse Staffing and Nurse Outcomes

In addition to patient outcomes, nurse outcomes should also be measured. Nursing perception of the effectiveness of staffing should be tracked along with measures of acceptable staffing levels. Nurses' perception of staffing effectiveness, for example, must be monitored by hospitals seeking Magnet Status. Initiating such review of staffing effectiveness can lead to comparisons for benchmarking best practice in the future and linking RN staffing levels to patient outcomes.

The Magnet Recognition Program of the American Nurses Credentialing Center is an initiative that was designed to recognize health care organizations that demonstrated a commitment to quality improvement focused on nursing care delivery (ANCC, 2015). In today's current environment, creating a healthy work environment including staffing can enhance patient safety, nursing satisfaction, and quality outcomes (Graystone, 2018). Nursing units with a higher rating of satisfaction with staffing have lower overall rates of nursing turnover. However, an environment where nurses perceive staffing and resources as adequate, experience an even lower nursing turnover rate (Nelson-Brantley, Hye Park, & Berquist-Beringer, 2018). In Magnet recognized hospitals, there are significant improvements in the quality of the work environment and patient outcomes than those in non-Magnet hospitals (Kutney-Lee et al., 2015). There should be an avenue for staff to communicate to nursing leadership, both in written and verbal form regarding staffing concerns. Nurses have an obligation to report to their supervisor any concerns regarding staffing, and every manager has the responsibility to follow up on staffing issues identified by staff.

Organization of patient care at the unit level is carefully orchestrated through nurse leadership, shared governance, appropriate nursing care delivery models, and the creation of healthy work environments. These concepts, in conjunction with fiscal responsibility and a commitment to appropriate staffing, will ensure safe, quality care, promote nursing satisfaction, and lead to positive patient care outcomes. Organization and staffing at the unit level is variable and complex. Decisions that drive organization and staffing at the unit level are based on the mission, vision, and values of the organization. Many factors impact the delivery of patient care at the unit level. Each of these factors are taken into account when establishing the patient care delivery on that designated unit. Ultimately, the goal is to establish an organizational staffing plan congruent with a patient care delivery model that will result in patient safety, quality patient outcomes, and nursing satisfaction.

KEY CONCEPTS

- The mission statement is a formal expression of the primary purpose or reason for the existence of the organization, department, or unit. An organization's mission statement defines how it is unique and different from other organizations that provide a similar service. Mission statements are formed based on the organization's core values and beliefs. The mission statement guides the development of the strategic plan and the day-to-day operations and decision-making of the organization.

- A vision statement outlines what an organization, department, or unit wants to be in the near future, for example the next three to five years. A vision statement commonly provides a declaration of a "destination" or outlines long-term objectives and is intended to guide its internal decision making. It is the thought of as a road map, indicating what the organization, department, and unit wants to become.

- Values define the organization's basic philosophy, principles, and ideals. Values also set the ethical tone for the institution. A philosophy is a statement of an organization's beliefs or assumptions based on their core values—the inner forces that gives purpose to their work.

- Strategic planning is a management activity that is often used to bring focus to how an organization's energy will be utilized, to establish priorities, and to strengthen operations to achieve targeted goals.

- A health care organization needs to have a good idea of where it fits into its environment and what types of programs and services are needed and demanded by its patients and other stakeholders.

- A stakeholder is any person, group, or organization that has a vested interest in a program or project under review, for example, the community, physicians, nurses, insurance companies, etc.

- A stakeholder assessment is a systematic consideration of all potential stakeholders on a project to ensure that the needs of each of these stakeholders are incorporated in the planning phase of the project.

- A good strategic plan can help to ensure that the needed resources and budget are available to carry out the mission and vision that has been identified as important to the organization. In addition, a clear strategic plan allows the organization, the nursing department, and the unit to select among seemingly equal alternatives based on the alternative's potential to move the organization toward a desired end goal.

- A SWOT Analysis identifies Strengths, Weaknesses, Opportunities, and Threats in the external and internal environment. The SWOT analysis is useful both for initial brainstorming and for developing a more formal strategic planning document.

- A marketing plan ensures that all stakeholders have the needed information about the project or service under development. Marketing is the process of creating a product or health care service for patients, and it uses the four Ps of marketing—Patient, Product, Price, and Placement, to Place desirable health care services or Products in desirable locations at a Price that benefits both Patients and the health care facility.

- Organizations are structured or organized in a manner that is designed to facilitate the execution of their mission, vision, and values or philosophy and their strategic plans.

- Organization of patient care management is the coordination of resources and clinical processes that promote service delivery to patients.

- Shared governance is an organizational framework grounded in a philosophy of decentralized leadership that fosters autonomous decision making and professional nursing practice.

- Successful orchestration of patient care in today's health care environment is achieved through shared governance and QSEN competencies for nursing practice.

- Benner's model of novice to expert provides a framework that facilitates professional staff development.

- Situational leadership, transactional, and transformational leadership are leadership styles necessary in this current health care environment.

- To plan nurse staffing, you must understand and apply the concepts of full-time equivalents (FTEs) and units of service such as nursing hours per patient day (NHPPD).

- Patient classification systems or acuity-based systems predict nursing time and workload required for groups of patients; the data can then be utilized for staffing, budgeting, and benchmarking.

- Units of service, regulatory requirements, delivery systems, skill mix, staff support, historical information, and the physical environment of the unit impact, creating a staffing plan.

- In developing a staffing plan, additional FTEs must be added to a nursing unit budget to provide coverage for days off and benefited time off.

- Scheduling of staff is ultimately the responsibility of the nurse manager, who must take into consideration patient need and intensity, volume of patients, and the needs and experience of the staff.

- Appropriate staffing and resources impact patient outcomes, nursing satisfaction and financial resources.

- Different type of patient care delivery models impact developing a staffing plan and achieving patient outcomes.

- Case management and clinical pathways are care management tools that have been developed to improve patient care and reduce hospital costs; they should be evidence-based.

KEY TERMS

Acuity	Clinical Pathways	Functional Nursing
Acuity Based Staffing	Continuity of Care	Handoff
Balanced Scorecard	Competence	Indirect Care
Benchmarking	Direct Care	Inpatient Unit
Career Ladder	Focus Groups	Length of Stay (LOS)
Case Management	Full-time Equivalent (FTE)	Marketing

Mission statement	Primary Nursing	SWOT Analysis
Modular Nursing	Productive Hours	Team Nursing
Nonproductive Hours	QSEN Competencies	Total Patient Care
Novice to Expert Model	Shared Governance	Transactional Leaders
Nursing Hours per Patient Day (NHPPD)	Self-Scheduling	Transformational Leaders
Patient Acuity	Situational Leadership	Units of Service
Patient-Centered Care	Skill Mix	Values
Patient Classification System (PCS)	Stakeholder	Vision statement
Patient Turnover	Stakeholder Assessment	
Philosophy	Strategic Planning	

REVIEW QUESTIONS

1. Patient outcomes are the result of variables, including the model of care delivery that is utilized. Which of the following care delivery models would be the least conducive to meeting patient's needs?
   a. Oncology patients cared for in a primary nursing model
   b. Outpatient surgery patients being cared for using a functional nursing model
   c. Rehabilitation Unit patients being cared for in a patient-centered nursing model
   d. Medical Intensive Care Patients being care for in team nursing model

2. When creating staffing plans and schedules, the most important driving focus should be which of the following?
   a. Personnel policies regarding vacation time, shift, and holiday rotation
   b. Organizational mission and vision
   c. Budget allocations and financial resources
   d. Delivering safe, high-quality patient care

3. Which of the following would need to be taken into account when developing a staff schedule for an 8-week period of time? Select all that apply.
   a. Two full-time RNs will be starting Family Medical Leave during that schedule
   b. One RN and two Unlicensed Assistive Personnel are scheduled for vacation during that time period
   c. The majority of the nurses on the unit have 5–10 years of experience
   d. A new nursing graduate will be off orientation during this 8-week period
   e. Painting of the patient rooms on this unit has begun and 4 rooms per week will be closed for this work during this period

4. In developing a staffing plan for your unit, which of the following should be considerations? Select all that apply.
   a. The nursing department has an active Shared Governance Model
   b. The nursing unit is located in a hospital in San Francisco, California
   c. The data for census trends should be reviewed for the past year

   d. The benchmarking data on staffing from the National Database of Quality Indicators (NDNQI) should be reviewed
   e. The geographical layout of the nursing unit

5. Appropriate staffing is associated with quality patient outcomes and nursing satisfaction. Which of the following would be positive indicators representing these two areas? Select all that apply.
   a. A decrease in nursing turnover
   b. Benchmarking demonstrates staffing at the 75th percentile
   c. Reduction of medication errors
   d. Improvement in nursing satisfaction scores
   e. Recent implementation of hourly rounding

6. Shared Governance is best described as which of the following?
   a. A career ladder based on Quality and Safety in Nursing Education (QSEN)
   b. A tested framework of organizational development
   c. A nursing delivery care model
   d. A model that focuses on decentralized leadership, autonomous decision making, and promotion of professional nursing practice

7. If your full-time staff members receive four weeks of vacation and 10 days of sick time per year, how many productive hours would each FTE work in that year if they utilized all of their benefited time?
   a. 2,080 productive hours
   b. 1,840 productive hours
   c. 1,920 productive hours
   d. 1,780 productive hours

8. A Mission statement defines the uniqueness of an organization, a nursing department, or unit from others that provide similar services. What is a mission statement based on?
   a. The organizations, nursing department, or unit's strategic plan
   b. What an organization, nursing department, or unit wants to be in the near future, for example the next three to five years
   c. The core values and beliefs of the organization, nursing department, or unit
   d. The long-term goals and objectives of an organization, nursing department, or unit.

9. When calculating paid nonproductive time, the nurse manager considers which of the following?
   a. Overtime pay and evening and night shift differentials
   b. Total hours available to work
   c. Vacation time, sick time, and educational hours
   d. All hours that are paid but not worked on the assigned unit

10. The medical-surgical unit provides 200 hours of care daily to 20 patients. Their NHPPD is which of the following?
    a. 1
    b. 10
    c. 20
    d. 200

REVIEW QUESTION ANSWERS

1. Answer: D is correct.
   Rationale: In a Medical Intensive Unit continuous assessment and highly skilled expertise is necessary. In this type of unit, the RN has 1–2 patients that allow for total care of the patient, not a team nursing mode (D). (A) Oncology patients and their families need to develop a trusting relationship with the nurse. Primary care facilitates 24-hour care coordination during the patient's entire hospital stay. (B) Functional nursing allows staff members to take on specific functions for a group of patients. LPNs and UAPs are key components of this model. Outpatient surgery patients who are admitted and discharged on the same day with lower acuity is a unit that could allow for a functional nursing model. (C) Patient-centered care is designed to focus on patient needs versus staff needs. In this model, required care and services are brought to the patient. These services may include disciplines such as physical therapy, occupational therapy, etc. A Rehabilitation Unit requires different disciplines for patient care needs.

2. Answer D: is correct.
   Rationale: When creating staffing plans, the most basic foundation is developing a plan that delivers safe quality patient care (D). (A) Policies regarding vacation time, shift, and holiday rotation need to be taken into account but only if they allow for the delivery of safe and quality patient care. (B) Organizational philosophy is not direct consideration when creating a staffing plan. (C) Budget allocations and financial resources must be taken into consideration, but are not the most important driving focus to creating a staffing plan.

3. Answers A, B, D, and E are correct.
   Rationale: When developing a staffing schedule for an 8-week time period, all potential events that could alter the need for staffing or consideration of staff available to meet safety and quality care for patient care need to be addressed. (A) Two full-time nurses taking Family Medical Need will create a definite gap in their shifts that need to be filled. In addition, (B) 1 RN and 2 UAPs are scheduled for vacation during that time, which will intensify the need for filling shifts. (C) Having the majority of nurses on the unit with 5 to 10 years' experience is a positive factor for safe quality care, but does not alter the number of staff that the unit needs to safely take care of patients. It will assist in mentoring the new graduate off orientation. (D) A new nursing graduate will be off orientation and will assist in filling those gaps; however, the new nurse immediately off orientation will need assistance from experienced nurses. (E) Painting of the patient rooms and blocking off 4 rooms at a time for a period of 10 weeks, will also alter the number of staff you will need during this time frame, since there will be less patients on the unit.

4. Answers A, B, C, D, and E are correct.
   Rationale: (A) fosters decentralized leadership and professional nursing practice, that should be taken into account when developing a staffing plan. (B) The nursing unit is in California; this state has mandated nursing ratios, that also require coverage for lunch and breaks. (C) Reviewing census trends for the past year can shed light on time frames of high census and unit activity, which can assist in creating a staffing plan. (D) Reviewing benchmarking data on staffing from NDNQI can assist in comparing other similar units with staffing trends. (E) Geographical layout of the unit can affect staffing plans, based on location of key services for staff, supplies, computer access, medication dispensing equipment, and all private rooms versus semi private rooms.

5. Answers A, B, C, and D are correct.
   Rationale: Quality outcomes is linked to overall nursing satisfaction and staffing. (A) When nurses are satisfied with their work settings, there will be a decreased number of nurses leaving the organization. (B) Benchmarking demonstrates staffing at the 75th percentile; this is a high percentile. That indicates that only 25% of hospitals have staff higher than this organization. (C) Appropriate nursing staffing has a measurable impact on reduction of medication errors. (D) Appropriate staffing also affects nurse job satisfaction at the unit level and with the overall organization. (E) The implementation of hourly rounding was to impact patient satisfaction, but would not have an impact on nursing satisfaction.

6. Answer: D is correct.
   Rationale: Shared Governance is an organizational model that is grounded in the philosophy of decentralized leadership, and fosters nurses be able to be autonomous in decision making and their professional nursing practice (D). (A) A QSEN-based career ladder is not dependent on a Shared Governance Model. (B) Shared Governance is not a tested framework of organizational development. (C) Shared Governance is not a delivery model of care.

7. Answer: B is correct.
   Rationale: Full-time Equivalent (FTE) is 2,080 hours a year – 160 hours of vacation – 80 of sick time = 1,840 productive hours.

8. Answer: C is correct.
   Rationale: Mission statements are formed based on the organization's core values and beliefs. The mission statement is a formal expression of the primary purpose or reason for the existence of the organization, department, or unit. An organization's mission statement defines how it is unique and different from other organizations that provide a similar service (C). (A) A mission statement guides the strategic plan. (B) While a mission statement

describes what an organization, department, or unit wants to do now, a vision statement outlines what an organization, department, or unit wants to be in the near future, for example the next three to five years. (D) A vision statement commonly provides a declaration of a "destination" or outlines long-term objectives and is intended to guide its internal decision-making. It is the thought of as a road map, indicating what the organization, department, and unit wants to become.

9. Answer: C is correct.
    Rationale: Non-productive time of an employee considers the vacation time, the sick time, and any educational hours. Non-patient care time – hours worked and available for patient care are designated as productive hours. Benefit time such as vacation, sick time, and education time is considered nonproductive hours. When considering the number of FTEs needed to staff a unit, count only the productive hours available for each staff member, because this represents the amount of time required to direct patient care needs. Available productive time can be easily calculated by subtracting benefit time from the time a full-time employee would work (C). (A) Overtime hours, evening and night shift differential, include patient care, and would be considered productive time. (B) Total number of hours available to work is the scheduled hours, if patient care during those hours would be productive. (D) Each unit is responsible for the budget and hours worked by their unit-based staff; if a person floats to another unit and is doing patient care, it is productive hours.

10. Answer: B is correct.
    Number of patients X NHPPD/care hours per day = shifts needed per 24 hours staff productive time per shift divided by 8 = number of 8-hour shifts needed per 24 hours.

REVIEW ACTIVITIES

1. You are part of the planning for a new Maternal-Child Clinic. Develop a mission, vision, and values or philosophy for the new clinic.

2. Using the steps of the strategic planning process, determine who your target audience will be, and how you will solicit them for input.

3. It has been determined that the new Maternal-Child Clinic will house 15 beds. Develop a staffing plan based on the Team Nursing approach to assignments. How would that change if there is Functional Nursing approach?

4. How do you know whether the outcomes of your staffing plan are positive? What measures can you use in your organization to indicate that your staffing is adequate or inadequate?

5. You are the nurse manager for the Mother-Baby Unit of the new clinic. What would you consider in planning for FTEs and staffing for this unit?

6. You are a new nurse and you have increasing concerns regarding the staffing levels on your unit. You are becoming increasingly anxious each time you go to work. What would you do?

DISCUSSION POINTS

- Did you read the mission statement of the last hospital you were assigned to? Did it provide you with any insight into the hospital's commitment to the community?

- In your last clinical experience, did you feel staffing was adequate for quality patient care?

- Was self-scheduling implemented on the unit of your last clinical experience?

- Was there any evidence on that unit of the association between staffing and patient and nursing satisfaction?

- What type of patient care delivery system was evident on the unit of your last clinical experience?

- How will knowledge of Benner's Novice to Expert Nurse impact you as a new nursing graduate?

DISCUSSION OF OPENING SCENARIO

1. What are your thoughts about this situation?
    a. **Discussion:** Has your colleague, the unit coordinator, talked to her manager? There are many unanswered questions that need to be addressed. Perhaps her manager is unaware of the staffing concerns and difficulty in getting employees to educational opportunities. Are there other indications that the organization is not living up to their mission? If the underlying problem is scheduling of the nurses that are on the unit, who is in charge of the scheduling? It also seems like there is a staffing need and a budget for new hires, but there is not an active recruitment effort in place. Is everyone aware of this? What is the marketing plan?

2. What advice do you have for your colleague?
    a. **Discussion:** You can suggest that your colleague, the unit coordinator, identify her concerns and schedule a meeting with the nursing manager where she can determine what is happening from the nursing manager's point of view. Encourage communication, and suggest your colleague goes to the meeting well prepared, well informed, and with possible solutions to some of the issues. It sounds like both the unit coordinator and her manager are very busy and have many challenges to meeting the unit's needs.

3. Is this situation unusual?
   a. **Discussion:** Not at all. Many times each person in an organization is struggling to find the time to address everything in their domain. Often, it seems like one "is putting out fires." But doing that is critical to the overall operation of the unit, and the organization. The new unit coordinator needs to have open and in regular communication with her manager.

4. Can it be improved? What would you recommend for improvement?
   a. **Discussion: Yes,** it can be improved. The first step is to review what exactly the concerns are that the unit

coordinator has. She needs to assess and evaluate the work flow of the unit, the staffing, and the acuity of the patients. Regarding scheduling, she needs to consider a staffing model that will allow staff input and follow the guidelines of the amount of staff for each shift. The unit coordinator should schedule regular weekly meetings with the nursing manager. With scheduled meeting times, there is more likelihood that issues can be addressed and follow-up can begin. The unit coordinator should hang in there and try different strategies to help the unit live up to the mission and vision of the organization and be the best it can be before she considers resigning as unit coordinator.

EXPLORING THE WEB

Preparing for an Interview
Upon completion of your nursing degree, you are planning to interview for a position at an area hospital. In preparation for your interview, you want to understand the mission as well as other information about that hospital. Today, that information is readily available on the Web. For example, if you were planning to apply at Loyola University Chicago, you would go to /www.loyolamedicine.org, accessed May 3, 2019. Another example is Lurie Children's Memorial Hospital in Chicago at /www.luriechildrens.org, accessed May 3, 2019. Look at these hospitals' home pages, paying particular attention to the descriptions they provide of their organizations' mission.

- What impressions do you form about these organizations and their missions?
- Does the stated mission seem to fit with the general "feel" that you get from the website?
- Could you easily find information about positions available? About the institution?
- Try this same exercise with your local hospital or health care center.

Considering Safe Staffing
Look to nursing organizations and the literature to determine what others are saying about staffing issues. Are nurse-patient ratios important as you consider safe and effective nursing care?

- Read about Nurse staffing measures, American Nurses Association, www.nursingworld.org/practice-policy/health-policy/regulatory/nurse-staffing-measures, accessed February 35, 2019.
- Compare opinions regarding staffing as you search a website regarding Nurse-Patient Ratios and Safe Staffing, https://nurse.org/articles/nurse-patient-ratios-and-safe-staffing, accessed February 25, 2019.
- What are patient outcomes regarding staffing? Review nurse staffing and patient experience outcomes, American Nurse Today, www.americannursetoday.com/nurse-staffing-and-patient-experience-outcomes, accessed March 1, 2019.
- Review quality as a main staffing concern and search for, Staffing and quality from the Agency for Healthcare Research and Quality, go to www.ahrq.gov/research/findings/nhqrdr/nhqdr17/index.html, accessed March 1, 2019.

Thinking about Worker Fatigue and Patient Safety
Safety is impacted by many factors. Go to the Joint Commission website and read about health care worker fatigue and patient safety, Joint Commission, www.jointcommission.org/sea_issue_48, accessed 2 March 2019.

INFORMATICS

1. Go to the 2017 National Healthcare Quality and Disparities Report at www.ahrq.gov/research/findings/nhqrdr/nhqdr17/index.html (accessed February 27, 2019). Review the impact of staffing on nursing and patient outcomes. Type in, staffing, in the search bar. Click on, State-Mandated Nurse Staffing Levels Alleviate Workloads, Lead to Lower Patient Mortality.

2. Go to http://qsen.org (accessed March 2, 2019) and enter the term, safe staffing. Click on, The Quality-Safety Project Poster. Explore the website to: (a) identify a quality-safety problem in the clinical area; (b) use quality tools to analyze issues; and (c) determine an action plan to address the issues.

LEAN BACK

- In your clinical rotations, do you see the mission and vision of the organization at the nursing unit level?
- Do you see Shared Governance implemented at the unit level?
- Do you see that patient acuity is taken into account when staffing?
- Do you see staffing practices that are different than what you read about in this chapter?
- What information in this chapter will affect your future practice? Why?

REFERENCES

American Association of Critical Care Nurses. (2016). *AACN standards for establishing and sustaining health work environments a journey to excellence* (2nd ed.). Retrieved from www.aacn.org/~/media/aacn-website/nursing-excellence/healthy-work-environment/execsum.pdf?la=en

American Nurse Today. (2016). Practical steps for applying acuity-based staffing. *American Nurse Today, 11*(9). Retrieved from www.american-nursetoday.com/practical-steps-for-applying-acuity-based-staffing

American Nurses Association. (2012). *ANA's principles for nurse staffing* (2nd ed.). Retrieved from www.nursingworld.org/~4af4f2/globalassets/docs/ana/ethics/principles-of-nurse--staffing--2nd-edition.pdf

American Nurses Association. (2015). *Optimal nurse staffing to improve quality of care and patient outcomes: Executive summary.* Retrieved from www.indiananurses.org/index.php?option=com_content&view=article&id=52:policy&catid=20:site-content&Itemid=130

American Nurses Association. (2016). Professional competencies can ease your transition into a new specialty. *American Nurse Today, 11*(3).

American Nurses Association. (2018a). *Nurse staffing plans and ratios. Nursing World.* Retrieved from www.nursingworld.org/practice-policy/advocacy/state/nurse-staffing

American Nurses Association. (2018b). *Principles of staffing and workforce management: The future of nursing as holistic providers and advocates of care.* Retrieved from www.nursingworld.org/~49fbb4/globalassets/practiceandpolicy/call-for-public-

American Nurses Credentialing Center (ANCC). (2015). *The importance of shared governance in achieving nursing excellence.* Retrieved from https://consultqd.clevelandclinic.org/the-importance-of-shared-governance-in-achieving-nursing-excellence and www.qualityindicators.ahrq.gov/

Benner, P. (1984). *From novice to expert.* Menlo Park, CA: Addison-Wesley.

Blitchok, A. (2018). *Proposed federal RN ratios—what you can do about it.* Retrieved from https://nurse.org/articles/federal-staffing-ratios

Burke, D., Flanagan, J., Ditomassi, M., & Hickey, P. A. (2017). Characteristics of nurse directors that contribute to registered nurse satisfaction. *The Journal of Nursing Administration, 47*(4), 219–225.

Burke, K. G., Johnson, T., & Sites, C. (2017). Creating an evidence-based progression for clinical advancement programs. *American Journal of Nursing, 17*(5), 22–36.

Burkhardt, M. A., & Nathaniel, A. (2013). *Ethics and issues in contemporary nursing* (4th ed., pp. 32–35). Stamford, CT: Cengage Learning.

Cardon, K. (2015). Designing for hospital efficiency. *Health Facilities Management, 16.*

Caruso, C., Baldwin, C. M., Berger, A., Chasens, E. R., Landis, C., Redeker, N., et al. (2017). Position statement: Reducing fatigue associated with sleep deficiency and work hours in nurses. *Nursing Outlook, 65*(6), 766–758.

Case Management Society of America. (2019). Retrieved from www.cmsa.org/who-we-are/what-is-a-case-manager

Centers for Medicare & Medicaid Services. (2007). *Conditions for coverage (CfCs) & conditions of participations (CoPs).* Retrieved from http://edocket.access.gpo.gov/cfr_2007/octqtr/pdf/42cfr482.23.pdf.

Centers for Medicare and Medicaid Services (CMS). (2017). *What are value-based programs?* Retrieved from www.cms.gov/Medicare/Quality-Initiatives-Patient-Assessment-Instruments/Value-Based-Programs/Value-Based-Programs.html

Cherry, B., & Jacob, S. R. (2019). Staffing and nursing care delivery models. In B. Cherry & S. R. Jacobs (Eds.), *Contemporary nursing issues, trends, and management* (pp. 359–371). St. Louis, MI: Elsevier.

Coxe, D. N. & Llewellyn, A. (2016). *Quality and safety education for nurses (QSEN) competencies in initial nursing staff competencies: The shift from a task driven competency model to a dynamic competency process that focuses on quality and safety.* QSEN Poster Presentation, ANA Annual Conference.

Danna, D. (2013). Organizational structure and analysis. In L. Roussel (Ed.), *Management and leadership for nurse administrators* (6th ed., pp. 237–239). Burlington, MA: Jones & Bartlett Learning.

Davis, C. (2015). Let's talk about benchmarking. *Nursing Made Incredibly Easy, 13*(2), 4.

DeMarco, K., & Pasadino, F. (2018). Transforming a nurse practice advancement program for the new millennium. *Nurse Leader, 16*(4), 234–239.

Drucker, P. (1973). *Management tasks, responsibilities, and practices.* New York, NY: Harper & Row.

Duffy, J. R., Culp, S., & Padrutt, T. (2018). Description and factors associated with missed nursing care in an acute care community hospital. *Journal of Nursing Administration, 48*(7), 361–367.

Emergency Nurses Association. (2013). *Nurse fatigue.* Retrieved from www.ena.org/docs/default-source/resource-library/practice-resources/white-papers/nurse-fatigue.pdf

Fitzsimon, S. (2016). *10 Inspiring nursing quotes.* Retrieved from www.aanac.org/Information/AANAC-Blog/Blog-Detail/post/10-inspiring-nursing-quotes/2016-05-03

Gokenbach, V., & Thomas, P. L. (2020). Maximizing human capital. In L. Roussel, P. L. Thomas, & J. L. Harris (Eds.), *Management and leadership for nurse administrators* (8th ed., pp. 220–222). Burlington, MA: Jones & Bartlett Learning.

Goode, C. J., Ponte, P. R., & Havens, D. S. (2016). Residency for transition into practice. *The Journal of Nursing Administration, 46*(2), 82–86.

Gran-Moravec, M. B., & Hughes, C. M. (2005). Nursing time allocation and other considerations for staffing. *Nursing & Health Sciences, 7*(2), 126–133.

Graystone, R. (2018). Creating the framework for a healthy practice environment. *The Journal of Nursing Administration, 48*(10), 469–470.

Hastings, S. E., Suter, E., Bloom, J., & Sharma, K. (2016). Introduction of a team-based care model in a general medical unit. *BMC Health Service Research, 16,* 245.

Hersey, R. E., & Blanchard, T. (1993). *Management of organizational behavior.* Riverside, NJ: Simon & Schuster.

Hunt, P. (2018). Developing a staffing plan to meet inpatient unit needs. *Nursing Management, 49*(5), 24–31.

Hyun, S., Bakken, S., Douglas, K., & Stone, P. W. (2008). Evidence-based staffing: Potential roles for informatics. *Nursing Economics, 26*(3), 151–173.

Institute of Medicine. (2000). *To err is human: Building a safer health system.* Washington, DC: National Academy Press.

Institute of Medicine. (2001). *Crossing the quality chasm: A new health system for the 21st century.* Washington, DC: National Academy Press.

Institute of Medicine. (2011). *The future of nursing: Leading change, advancing health.* Washington, DC: National Academy Press.

Jeffery, A. D., Borum, C., & Englebright, J. (2017). Healthy schedules, healthy nurses. *American Nurse Today, 12*(10), 1–2.

Jordan, B. A. (2016). Designing a unit practice council structure. *Nursing Management, 47*(1), 15–18.

Kutney-Lee, A., Witkowski Stimpfel, A., Sloane, D. M., Cimiotti, J. P., Quinn, L. W., & Aiken, L. H. (2015). Changes in patient and nurse outcomes associated with magnet hospital recognition. *Medical Care, 53*(6), 550–557.

Lobo, V. M., Ploeg, J., Fisher, A., Peachey, G., & Akhat-Danesh, N. (2018). Critical care nurses' reasons for working or not working overtime. *Critical Care Nurse, 38*(6), 47–57.

Massachusetts Department of Higher Education Nursing Initiative. (2016). *Massachusetts nurse of the future nursing core competencies.*

Murray, K., Yasso, S., Schomberg, R., Terhaune, M., Beidelschies, M., et al. (2016). Journey of excellence: Implementing a shared decision-making model. *American Journal of Nursing, 116*(4), 50–56.

National Quality Forum. (2016). *Patient safety 2015: Final technical report.* Retrieved from www.qualityforum.org/field_guide/

National Quality Forum. (2020). *Field guide to NQF resources.* Retrieved from www.qualityforum.org/field_guide/

Needleman, J., Buerhaus, P., Mattke, S., Stewart, M., & Zelevinsky, K. (2002). Nurse-staffing levels and the quality of care in hospitals. *New England Journal of Medicine, 346*(22), 1715–1722.

Nelson-Brantley, H. V., Hye Park, S., & Berquist-Beringer, S. (2018). Characteristics of the nursing practice environment associated with lower unit-level RN turnover. *Journal of Nursing Administration, 48*(1), 31–37.

Norris, T. (2019). Making the transition from student to professional nurse. In B. Cherry & S. R. Jacobs (Eds.), *Contemporary nursing issues, trends, and management* (8th ed., pp. 409–430). St. Louis, MI: Elsevier.

Porter-O'Grady, T. (2009). *Interdisciplinary shared governance.* Sudbury, MA: Jones & Bartlett Publishers.

Porter-O'Grady, T., Hawkins, M. A., & Parker, M. L. (1997). *Whole-systems shared governance: Architecture for integration.* Gaithersburg, MD: Aspen.

QSEN. (2019). *QSEN definitions: Patient-centered care.* Retrieved from http://qsen.org/competencies/pre-licensure-ksas/#patient-centered_care

Roussel, L. (2020). Forces influencing nursing leadership. In L. Roussel, P. L. Thomas, & J. L. Harris (Eds.), *Management and leadership for nurse administrators* (8th ed., pp. 220–222). Burlington, MA: Jones and Bartlett Learning.

Salmond, S., & Echevarria, M. (2017). Healthcare transformation and changing roles for nursing. *Orthopedic Nursing, 36*(1), 12–25.

St. Thomas University. (2018). *What is situational leadership? How flexibility leads to success.* Retrieved from https://online.stu.edu/articles/education/what-is-situational-leadership.aspx

Swayne, L. E., Duncan, J. W., & Ginter, M. P. (2012). *Strategic management of health care organizations* (6th ed.). San Francisco, CA: Jossey-Bass.

The Joint Commission. (2018). *Sentinel event alert issue 48: Health care worker fatigue and patient safety.* Retrieved from www.jointcommission.org/sea_issue_48

The Joint Commission. (2017). *Sentinel event alert inadequate hand-off communication.* Retrieved from www.jointcommission.org/assets/1/18/SEA_58_Hand_off_Comms_9_6_17FINAL_(1).pdf

The Nash Group. (2018). *Leading healthcare practices for workforce management: Aligning care requirements with proper workloads (PowerPoint slides).*

Thomas, P. L., & Roussel, L. (2020). Procuring and sustaining resources: The budgeting process. In L. Roussel, P. L. Thomas, & J. L. Harris (Eds.), *Management and leadership for nurse administrators* (8th ed., pp. 220–222). Burlington, MA: Jones and Bartlett Learning.

Trepanier, S., Lee, D. W., & Kerfoot, K. K. (2017). Interoperable acuity-based staffing solutions: Lessons learned from a multi-hospital system. *Nursing Economics, 35*(4), 184–188.

Williams, L. S. (2008). The mission statement: A corporate reporting tool with a past, present, and future. *International Journal of Business Communication, 45*(2), 94–119.

Wright, C., McCartt, P., Raines, D., & Oermann, M. H. (2017). Implementation and evaluation of self-scheduling in a hospital system. *Journal for Nurses in Professional Development, 11*(33), 19–24.

SUGGESTED READINGS

Agency for Healthcare Research and Quality (AHRQ). (2015). *Patient safety network: Glossary.* Retrieved from www.psnet.ahrq.gov/glossary.aspx

Agency for Healthcare Research and Quality (AHRQ). (2017). *National quality strategy: About the national quality strategy.* Rockville, MD: U.S. Department of Health & Human Services. Retrieved from www.ahrq.gov/workingforquality/about/index.html

Aiken, L. H., Sloane, D. M., Barnes, H., Cimiotti, J. P., Jarrín, O. F., & McHugh, M. D. (2018). Nurses' and patients' appraisals show patient safety in hospitals remains a concern. *Health Affairs, 37*(11), 1744–1751.

Bates, D. W., & Singh, H. (2018). Two decades since to err is human: An assessment of progress and emerging priorities in patient safety. *Health Affairs, 37*(11), 1736–1743.

Brown, N. (2015). How the American Heart Association helped change women's heart health. *Circulation: Cardiovascular Quality and Outcomes, 8*, 60–62.

Covey, S. R. (1997). *The seven habits of highly effective people.* New York, NY: Simon & Schuster.

Creative Care Management. (2017). *A quick guide to relationship-based care.* Minneapolis, MN: Creative Health Care Management, Inc.

Faber, K. (2013). Relationship-based care in the neonatal intensive care unit. *Creative Nursing, 19*(4), 214–218.

Gulati, R., Mikhail, O., Morgan, R., & Sittig, D. (2016). Vision statement quality and organizational performance in U.S. hospitals. *Journal of Healthcare Management, 61*(5), 335–351.

Institute of Medicine. (2010). *The healthcare imperative: Lowering costs and improving outcomes: Workshop series summary.* Washington, DC: The National Academies Press. doi:10.17226/12750

Kowalski, S. L., & Anthony, M. (2017). Nursing's evolving role in patient safety. *American Journal of Nursing, 117*(2), 34–48.

Melnyk, B. M., Gallagher, F. L., Thomas, B. K., Troseth, M., Wyngarden, K., & Szalacha, L. (2016). A study of chief nurse executives indicates low prioritization of evidence-based practice and shortcomings in hospital performance metrics across the United States. *Worldviews on Evidence-Based Nursing, 13*(1), 6–14.

Melnyk, B. M., Gallagher, F. L., Zellefrow, C., Tucker, S., Thomas, B., et al. (2018). The first U.S. study on nurses' evidence-based practice competencies indicates major deficits that threaten healthcare quality, safety, and patient outcomes. *Worldviews on Evidence-Based Nursing, 15*(1), 16–25.

Shin, S., Park, J., & Bae, S. (2018). Nurse staffing and nurse outcomes: A systematic review and meta-analysis. *Nursing Outlook, 66,* 273–282.

Sigma Theta Tau International. (2010). In N. Rollins-Gantz (Ed.), *101 global leadership lessons for nurses: Shared legacies from leaders and their mentors.* Indianapolis, IN: Sigma Theta Tau International.

Wesorick, B., & Shaha, S. (2015). Guiding health care transformation: A next-generation, diagnostic remediation tool for leveraging polarities. *Nursing Outlook, 63*(6), 691–702.

Health Care Economics

Lanette Stuckey[1], Debra A. Cherubini[2], Samuel A. Sacco[2]
[1] Lakeview College of Nursing, Danville, IL, USA
[2] Salve Regina University, Newport, RI, USA

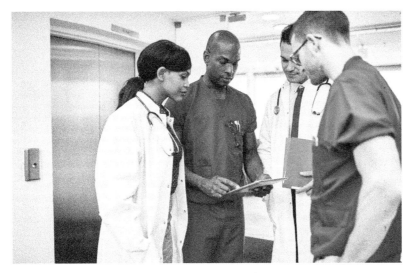

Health care team collaboration. *Source:* langstrup/123 RF.

The purpose of creating and analyzing records of what transpires in hospitals is to know how the money is being spent; whether it is, in fact, doing good, or whether it is doing mischief.

(*Florence Nightingale,* 1859)

OBJECTIVES

Upon completion of this chapter, the reader should be able to:

1. Analyze economic principles related care to nursing and health care.

2. Distinguish why health care must be managed as a business.

3. Discover factors affecting access to health services.

4. Analyze the role of state and federal government and third-party payers in health care financing.

5. Differentiate economic principles of nursing and health care.

6. Review factors that influence health care spending and affect health care outcomes.

7. Analyze the impact of health care reform, e.g., value-based purchasing and hospital-acquired conditions payment adjustments on the health care industry.

8. Discover how a health care enterprise is balancing quality and profit by assigning its satisfaction rating and margin to an appropriate square on the **Nosek-Androwich Profit: Quality** (NAPQ) Matrix.

Kelly Vana's Nursing Leadership and Management, Fourth Edition. Edited by Patricia Kelly Vana and Janice Tazbir
© 2021 John Wiley & Sons Ltd. Published 2021 by John Wiley & Sons Ltd.
Companion Website: www.wiley.com/go/kelly-Nursing-Leadership

OPENING SCENARIO

You and your spouse are vacationing in a foreign country. You rent small hand-held aqua scooters that pull you through the saltwater lagoon, and you gleefully romp in the quiet water. As you make a turn near the island of dead coral in the center of the lagoon, you lose your balance and are dragged along the sharp coral, lacerating both thighs. A lifeguard hears your screams and dashes to your aid. Hotel personnel put you in a taxi and send you to a nearby hospital emergency room. There, with your limited local language and the help of one person who speaks limited English, you discover that all health care is government run and provided free to all citizens. You
are told that you cannot be treated, because there is no provision for accepting your American insurance and no provision for paying cash.

1. *What do you think the issue is with the hospital?*

2. *Do you see the problem the same way the hospital does?*

3. *When cost is removed from the equation, what drives the decision to provide or not provide health care?*

4. *If cost were not a driving consideration in providing health care in the United States, what would the health care system be like?*

Regardless of how expert, creative, collaborative, and altruistic a health care system may be, it cannot function without money. Over the ages, depending on the culture and country, the government or citizens have often provided the resources to keep the community healthy. The funding can vary, including philanthropy, volunteerism, fee for services, insurance, and government subsidies. Balancing cost with revenue is key to achieving the mission of providing health care and is now viewed by many as the shared responsibility of humans around the world.

This chapter will discuss the importance of analyzing economic principles related to nursing and health care. It will distinguish why health care must be managed as a business and discover factors that affect access to health services. Additionally, the role of federal government and third-party payers will be analyzed along with the economic principles of nursing and health care. Factors that influence health care spending and affect health care outcomes will be discussed along with the impact of health care reform, form example value-based purchasing and hospital-acquired conditions payment adjustments on the health care industry. Finally, the chapter will discuss how health care enterprises are balancing quality and profit by assigning a satisfaction rating and margin to an appropriate square on the Nosek-Androwich Profit: Quality (NAPQ) Matrix.

Health Care Economics

Education programs focus on building knowledge, the application of clinical and procedural skills, critical thinking, interprofessional communication, and problem solving. Today nurses are broadly educated and may work in a variety of roles. Examples include critical care, case management, home and long-term care, school and occupational nursing, public health, and disaster preparedness. Nurses must be aware of the specific health needs of the community they serve and today's nurses also need to be educated on the business aspects of

patient care delivery. Increased knowledge of the budgetary needs of a patient care organization, patient access to health insurance, and state and federal funding is necessary to support optimal health outcomes and sustain the daily operations of health care organizations and programs.

The Institute of Medicine progress report on the Future of Nursing 2020 goals (2018) focused on the importance of nurses advancing their education and expanding their practice to care for the present needs of an aging population. The patient population in the twenty-first century is changing, living longer, and requires more complex health care due to chronic illness, ethnic diversity, and variations in socioeconomic status (IOM, 2015). These changes support the need for nurses to expand their leadership competencies, such as in policy development, evidence-based research, health care delivery, and reimbursement payment systems (IOM, 2015).

The 2010 Patient Protection and **Affordable Care Act** (ACA 2010) legislated broad health care overhauls in insurance company policy, funding of nursing education, and primary care provider support. In addition, for the first time, it rewarded providers that do a good job providing quality care. Conversely, if mistakes are made or a hospital-acquired infection occurs, payment may be withheld (The Patient Protection and Affordable Care Act, 2010). Nightingale's early search for the "good" versus "mischievous" outcomes of the money spent on health care may have initiated an unspoken commitment to financial stewardship among nurses. All nurses need to be aware of new health care legislation so that they can provide quality health care to patients and families in a manner consistent with their insurance benefits and rights to health care coverage.

Economic Principles Related to Nursing and Health Care

Every nurse today needs to have a basic understanding of health care economics. Health care economics studies effectiveness and efficiency in the delivery of health care and the operational use of health care systems (Johns Hopkins Bloomberg School of Public Health, 2019). The study of economics is based on the analysis of the distribution, production, and consumption of goods and services (Public Health Action Team, 2017). This analysis of these economic activities is based on certain related principles.

Economic principles are founded on how reasonable individuals would act given a situation where goods and or services were limited. If a Family Practice Clinic knew that every summer they would need to provide an increased number of physical exam appointments for patients, then it would behoove them to plan based on this historical patient data. The plan would include providing the structures, such as appointment times, office space, supplies, etc., and processes, such as staffing, etc. to achieve optimal high quality, safe patient care outcomes (Figure 6.1).

Mediating Factors affecting the Structure + Process = Outcomes process of health care may or may not be controlled, such as the needs of the patient population, access to health care, health insurance, availability of specialty providers and nursing staff, equipment, and supplies. Not every patient has the same level of health insurance and not every provider will take every type of health insurance. Patients may need services that are not covered by their insurance and they may not have the income or resources to pay for needed services, thus placing their health in danger.

Health care costs may increase without a clear improvement in the outcomes of health care. For example, consider the economic concept of price elasticity, which is related to the price that an individual is willing to pay for a given item. Normally, as the price goes up, the demand goes down. When the purchase is health care, however, the price may be viewed as irrelevant to the decision or need to purchase. Think of a wristwatch that you might readily purchase for $5, would likely not buy at $50, and would never consider at $500. Now, imagine that instead of a wristwatch, the item in question is a medication or therapy needed to save your sick child. Now the consideration of price in the decision-making process is different. Thus, health care is much less "elastic" with reference to price than are many other consumer goods.

Management of Health Care as a Business

The health care system is more complex than the seller of a product such as a wristwatch would be. A wristwatch would be paid for by the buyer. Health care is a product that is often paid for by a third-party payer, a government program such as

Medicaid or Medicare or a health insurance company, not by the patient. This alters the financial impact of the purchase and alters the power of both the patient and the third-party payer, that is the government program or health insurance company that pays the health care provider.

Traditional Perspective: Health Care Helps People

The long-standing tradition of health care is to help people achieve their optimal level of health so that they can enjoy their maximum quality of life. **Health care reform** refers to major changes in health care policy or the development of a new health care policy or program (O'Rourke, 2017). An example of health care reform is the ACA. The ACA Act has three primary goals (ACA, 2010): They are to:

1. Make health insurance more affordable to all individuals

2. Increase the Medicaid program to provide access to care for individuals with incomes below the poverty level, and

3. Support new medical treatments, programs, and technology that will lower health care costs and improve patient outcomes.

Change from Chronic Care to Preventive Care

The ACA put an emphasis on preventative care. Prior to the 1980s, the focus of health care was on the treatment of chronic conditions such as diabetes, heart disease, and cancer. This method of health care delivery is very costly due to possible patient needs of maintenance medications, cancer treatments, and evaluation using expensive medical equipment. Because individuals are currently living longer and often working longer, new efforts are being placed on prevention and preventive care. Healthy People 2020 (2015) lists four overarching Goals for the Future:

- Attain high-quality, longer lives free of preventable disease, disability, injury, and premature death

- Achieve health equity, eliminate disparities, and improve the health of all groups

- Create social and physical environments that promote good health for all

- Promote quality of life, healthy development, and healthy behaviors across all life stages (www.cdc.gov/oralhealth/healthy_people/index.htm, 2015, paragraph 1, accessed July 6, 2019).

Furthermore, it is the goal of Healthy People 2020 to improve access to health care for all. The Institute of Medicine (2010) notes the ACA of 2010 increased access to patient care and expanded services for both Medicare and Medicaid.

```
Structure + Process = Outcome
```

FIGURE 6.1   Structure + Process = Outcome.

However, access to care does not mean that every patient can afford the extra insurance co-pays that come with the level of insurance coverage they purchase, thus limiting patient access to health care, including prevention screenings and preventive care.

Right to Health Care at Any Cost

The cost of health care was not considered, let alone questioned, until the early 1960s. The American belief system firmly held that every individual was entitled to all the knowledge, skill, and technology related to health care at any cost. Health care was claimed to be a "Right"; it was the "American Way," although certain factors such as race, location, and income had some effect on the availability of health care. In an attempt to ease the burden of health care costs, the United States Government, in 1965, enacted Titles XVIII and XIX, Amendments to the Social Security Act. These Amendments include the Medicare and Medicaid programs, which provide health care services for the elderly and the indigent. Payment for these health care services rely heavily on strong documentation of the type and amount of patient services and treatment provided. It was anticipated that by requiring health care providers to account for the cost of Medicare and Medicaid patients' care, spending would be curbed. Other insurers soon followed with their own requirements for documentation of care.

Factors Affecting Access to Health Services

Possibly the most common reason given for entering a health care profession is "to help people." Virginia Henderson, viewed by some as the contemporary Florence Nightingale, defined nursing as:

> *. . .primarily helping people (sick or well) in the performance of those activities contributing to health, or its recovery (or to peaceful death) that they would perform unaided if they had the necessary strength, will, or knowledge. It is likewise the unique contribution of nursing to help people to be independent of such assistance as soon as possible. (Henderson & Nite, 1978)*

Nurses often have believed that this altruistic nursing definition applies irrespective of the site where nursing care is given. Yet nurses also have begun to recognize that the cost of providing care in the traditional altruistic way is prohibitive and that achieving patient independence from nursing care as quickly as possible conserves scarce nursing resources.

Out with altruism, when patients and providers had to recognize that health care was a business requiring payment, in came a completely new language, that of business and consumers and profit and margin and competition and cost, *cost,* COST. The bottom line (cost) became the focus, of not only managers and administrators, but also of all employees at all levels of all health care entities. Everyone needed to question what they did, how they did it, and how many it took to do it in order to determine whether it was required for safe care and quality outcomes and whether there was a less costly way of attaining a safe, quality outcome. In 1960, Abdellah had challenged health care providers to determine the care that was needed and to provide no more, no less (Abdellah, Beland, Martin, & Matheney, 1960). Nearly 60 years later, health care providers are still trying to come to grips with just that.

Need for Health Care Determined by the Consumer

Consumer attention has shifted toward the need for measurable safe, high-quality outcomes. **Total quality improvement** (TQI) and **continuous quality improvement** (CQI) programs have been initiated to assure health care consumers that cost management was not compromising safety or quality. These programs require all stakeholders, including patients, to work together to evaluate and improve outcomes. The expertise of allied health care providers has been recognized, and through the growing access to information technology, consumers have been empowered to better understand their own health, the complex technologies available, their options for managing decisions about their care, and the cost implications of those decisions. No longer is health care the exclusive realm of the health care practitioner and other professionals. Despite such attempts at improving quality, there remains cause for concern. Hospital-acquired infections, uncontrolled bleeding during surgery, medication errors, and patient falls remain a primary risk for patients in hospitals. Furthermore, breakdown in communication, judgment errors, incompetent skills, and diagnostic errors can directly affect patient harm and death. If medical error was a disease, it would rank as the third leading cause of death in the U.S. (Makary & Daniel, 2016). Bouldin (2013) and a team of researchers developed a comprehensive study using data from the **National Database of Nursing Quality Indicators** (NDNQI) collected between July 1, 2006 and September 30, 2008, to estimate prevalence and trends of falls occurring in adult medical, medical-surgical, and surgical nursing units. More than 88 million patient days (pd) of observation were contributed from 6,100 medical, surgical, and medical-surgical nursing units in 1,263 hospitals across the United States. The study identified a total of 315,817 falls had occurred (rate = 3.56 falls/1,000 patient days (pd)), of which 82,332 (26.1%) resulted in an injury (rate = 0.93/1,000 pd). Both total falls and falls with injury rates were highest in medical units (fall rate = 4.03/1,000 pd.; fall with injury rate = 1.08/1,000 pd) and lowest in surgery units (fall rate = 2.76/1,000 pd.; injurious fall rate = 0.67/1,000 pd).

Serb (2006) points out that many years ago, Harvard Business School Professor Regina Herzlinger predicted a revolution in health care toward a consumer-based model with greater choice, that is, focused factories of provider teams, flexible insurance products, and widely available information on quality and cost. Many dismissed her ideas, and Herzlinger herself delayed publication of her award-winning book, *Market-Driven Health Care*, until after the heyday of the **Health Maintenance Organizations** (HMOs)—whose gatekeepers, top-down managements, and tight networks seemed the opposite of consumerism. Since Herzlinger's predictions, access to reliable, extensive health care information, as well as cost and quality data, have become ever more available on the Internet. In addition, the 2010 Patient Protection and ACA provides more-affordable health care insurance and accessibility through state-administered High Risk Pool insurance plans. These High Risk Pool insurance plans are for patients previously refused insurance due to preexisting health care conditions, and they provide affordable health care insurance for 45 million uninsured Americans. These uninsured persons can either choose a government-run insurance plan or they can choose from private insurance plans (Affordable Health Care for Americans, 2010).

Right to Health Care at a Reasonable Cost

The contemporary value system holds that individuals have the right to health care at a reasonable cost. Reasonable cost is currently determined by insurers. When it refers to fees charged for services, a reasonable cost is the usual and customary fee charged in the region. When referring to fees charged for technology, complex and expensive procedures, or expensive, extensive pharmacologic therapies, there is no established standard for how much it should cost to provide someone with enhanced quality of life over time. Clearly, the lack of consensus on what constitutes reasonable cost is at the heart of the controversies among insurers, patients, and their professional health care providers.

Managed Care

In the 1980s, Managed Care was created to control health care costs and determine reasonable costs for specific diagnoses and treatments, while factoring in geographical location variations. This effort to control cost extended through the Medicare and Medicaid programs and marked the beginning of health care reform. The method of paying doctors and hospitals 100% of their billing stopped in the 1980s. There was keen anticipation that if the care of the neediest—the elderly and the poor—was managed centrally from one location, access, cost, and quality would be optimally controlled. When it became evident that the Medicare and Medicaid program costs had been woefully underestimated, (HMOs), or managed care, emerged as the answer to cost-efficient and quality care.

Managed care is not easily defined and categorized. It is the product of a series of efforts to establish an effective program for all **stakeholders** (providers, employers, customers, patients, and payers who may have an interest in, and seek to influence, the decisions and actions of an organization). Managed care has resulted in a complex, still-evolving array of structures and processes to deliver health care.

Managed care emphasizes delivery of a coordinated continuum of services across the care spectrum from wellness to death, using financial incentives to achieve cost efficiency. Figure 6.2 shows **national health expenditures** (NHE) as a share of Gross Domestic Product, 2013–2023. Note that the U. S. National Health Expenditures (NHE) as a share of Gross Domestic Product are expected to grow from 17.2% in 2013 to 19.3% by 2023. Additionally, Kamal, Sawyer, and McDermott (2018) report that "per capita expenditures are projected to grow from $10,724 in 2017 to $16,168 in 2026, which is an average annual growth of 4.7%" (p. 5).

Preapproval by a health care insurance company for payment of health care is required under managed care, and health care coverage is selective, effectively rationing care. Choice of health care practitioner or other provider and choice of site for health care are restricted, which are additional methods of rationing care. An added incentive to health care rationing is a copayment for care requirement that must be paid by the patient at the time that care is received. Despite insurance industry assurances that health care is not rationed, rationing is the undergirding concept of managed care. Managed care is not about providing health care; it is about being a for-profit business in which the managed care company acts as an agent who negotiates the contract about how the provision of health care will be accomplished.

There are a variety of models of managed care companies. Included are staff, group, network, **Preferred Provider Organizations** (PPOs), **Point Of Service** (POS), and mixed models, each model having its own unique structure and risks. The most common form of a managed care company is the PPO. A PPO generally consists of a hospital and a number of health care practitioner providers. The PPO contracts with the hospitals and health care practitioner providers (both practitioners and hospitals) and payers (self-insured employers, insurance companies, or managed care organizations) to provide health care services to a defined population for predetermined fixed fees. Discount rates may be negotiated with the health care providers in return for expedited patient claims payment and a somewhat predictable market share of patients. In the PPO model, patients have a choice of using PPO or non-PPO health care providers; however, financial incentives are built in to encourage utilization of PPO health care providers.

Nongovernmental health insurance has predominantly been accessed in the U.S. through employment. Employers provide health coverage to employees as a benefit for working for their company. Therefore, the employer chooses the coverage with cost in mind and negotiates an acceptable package of benefits on behalf of the employees. If the employer offers a selection of benefit packages, the employee may choose the package that is most suitable. Many benefit packages available through employers are currently HMOs.

Managed care has become the focus for the anger of many health care providers and much of American society. Because care decisions are driven, in significant part, by the care options for which insurance coverage will pay rather than by the free choice of the patient in consultation with a professional health

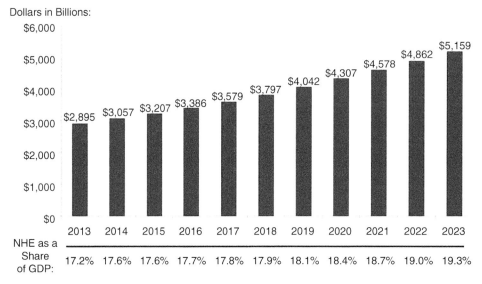

Projections of National Health Expenditures and Their Share
of Gross Domestic Product, 2013–2023

Dollars in Billions:

Year	2013	2014	2015	2016	2017	2018	2019	2020	2021	2022	2023
	$2,895	$3,057	$3,207	$3,386	$3,579	$3,797	$4,042	$4,307	$4,578	$4,862	$5,159

NHE as a Share of GDP: 17.2% 17.6% 17.6% 17.7% 17.8% 17.9% 18.1% 18.4% 18.7% 19.0% 19.3%

FIGURE 6.2   National health expenditures (NHE) as a share of gross domestic product, 2013–2017.
Source: Kaiser Family Foundation calculations using NHE data from Centers for Medicare & Medicaid Services, Office of the Actuary, National Health Statistics Group, at www.cms.hhs.gov/NationalHealthExpendData/ see Projected; NHE Historical and projections, 1965–2023, file nhe-23 zip, accessed 7 September 2019.

care provider, feelings of distrust and anger about necessary compromises in care are often strongly held by both patients and health care providers. As the public becomes more knowledgeable, it also becomes more demanding.

To ease the pressure from health care practitioners, patients, consumer advocates, and employers, many HMO programs recently dropped the requirement for managed care preapproval prior to hospitalization or consultation with a specialist. In response to the patient demand for greater choice of provider, care plans were adapted to permit those who can afford to pay higher premiums and insurance copayments to have broader choices. Efforts to salvage the reputation of managed care have spawned another name. Coordinated care is replacing the term, managed care, *to* better describe a system of mutual decision making among insurers, providers, and patients. In 2001, a patient's bill of rights was introduced into Congress to, among other things, allow patients to sue their coordinated care providers. Although passed by the House of Representatives, a revised version failed to gain Senate approval.

Such proposed or legislated changes diminished the insurance company clout and with it the ability to contain costs. Nationally renowned health care economist, Uwe Reinhardt of Princeton University, stated that "health plans can no longer bully and threaten the providers of care." Dr. David Lawrence, Chief Executive of the Kaiser Foundation Health Plan and Hospitals, noted, "When one uses financial tools to try to change

the delivery of care, A, they are not very powerful, and B, they make people mad." (accessed www.nytimes.com/2001/07/02/business/a-changing-world-is-forcing-changes-on-managed-care.html July 10, 2019).

Universal Health Care

Universal health care systems provide health care to all the citizens in a community, district, or nation, regardless of the person's ability to pay. Health care that uses a lot of high technology or that does a lot of elective surgery, for example plastic surgery, is usually not covered in a universal health care system.

Many industrialized countries around the world provide a basic health care plan for all citizens. The differences in the health care plans depend on the type of priorities set by the citizens and the nation. In the United States, Oregon has had a prioritized medical care services list for Medicaid recipients since 1989. The list emphasizes prevention and patient education. (www.oregon.gov/oha/hpa/dsi-herc/Pages/index.aspx, accessed March 30, 2019)

Health care programs in Sweden and the United Kingdom are funded from income taxes and selected other taxes. Germany and the Netherlands rely on payroll taxes for funding. Canada's health care is funded through taxes and covers most patient needs, with a few exceptions—e.g., dental care, eye care, prescription drugs. Canada provides the same level of care to all of its citizens, has lower overall costs, much lower drug prices, and supplies education funds for health care professionals. The U.S. system has shorter waits for seeing health care providers; allows greater choice in health care provider selection; provides higher wages and salaries for health care professionals; and invests more in health care technology, research, and development.

Canada has better outcomes in infant mortality and life expectancy than does the United States but pays less than half the amount for health care. Direct comparisons of health statistics across nations are complex. The Commonwealth Fund, in its annual survey, "Mirror, Mirror on the Wall," compares the performance of the health care systems in Australia, New Zealand, the United Kingdom, Germany, Canada, and the United States. Its 2017 study found that although the U.S. system is the most expensive, it consistently underperforms compared to the other countries. As shown in Table 6.1, the United States ranks last in health care system performance among the 11 countries included in this study. The U.S. ranks last in Access, Equity, and Health Care Outcomes, and next to last in Administrative Efficiency, as reported by patients and providers. Only in Care Process, based on performance across the four subdomains of prevention, safe care, coordination, and patient engagement, does the U.S. perform better, ranking fifth among the 11 countries (Commonwealth Fund, 2017).

A major difference between the United States and the other countries in the study is that the United States is the only country without universal health care. Especially note in Table 6.2, the poor performance of the United States on infant mortality,

Table 6.1   Health Care System Performance Rankings–2017

	AUS	CAN	FRA	GER	NETH	NZ	NOR	SWE	SWIZ	UK	US
Overall Ranking	2	9	10	8	3	4	4	6	6	1	11
Care Process	2	6	9	8	4	3	10	11	7	1	5
Access	4	10	9	2	1	7	5	6	8	3	11
Administrative Efficiency	1	6	11	6	9	2	4	5	8	3	10
Equity	7	9	10	6	2	8	5	3	4	1	11
Health Care Outcomes	1	9	5	8	6	7	3	2	4	10	11

Source: Commonwealth Fund Analysis, 2017 (https://interactives.commonwealthfund.org/2017/july/mirror-mirror, accessed June 30, 2019)

Table 6.2   Life Expectancy vs. Health Care Spending in 2016 for The Organization for Economic Co-operation and Development (OECD) Countries

Country	Life expectancy	Infant mortality rate	Physicians per 1,000 people	Nurses per 1,000 people	Per capita expenditure on health (USD)	Health care costs As a % of GDP	% of government revenue spent on health	% of health costs paid by government
Australia	82.5	3.1	3.6	11.6	3,109	9.45	34.9	36.2
Canada	81.9	4.7	2.7	9.9	3,382	10.44	40.6	69.8
France	82.4	3.7	3.4	10.5	4,068	11.07	53.2	56.6
Germany	81.1	3.4	4.2	12.8	4,869	11.15	17.6	44.5
Japan	84.1	2.0	2.4	11.3	3,971	10.90	35.7	39.4
Norway	82.5	2.2	4.7	17.7	5,339	9.98	54.9	48.8
Sweden	82.4	2.5	3.6	4.3	4,606	11.01	49.8	49.6
UK	81.2	3.8	2.8	7.9	3,341	9.88	38.0	42.2
USA	78.6	8.2	2.8	11.6	8,047	16.84	33.3	37.4

Life Expectancy vs. Health Care Spending in 2016 for OECD Countries, compiled with information from www.oecd.org./home; OECD Health Data 2017—Frequently Requested Data, available at (2017) https://data.oecd.org/healthres/doctors.htm#indicator-chart (2017); https://data.oecd.org/healthres/nurses.htm#indicator-chart (2017); https://data.oecd.org/healthstat/infant-mortality-rates.htm (2017); https://data.oecd.org/healthstat/life-expectancy-at-birth.htm#indicator-chart (2017); https://data.oecd.org/healthres/health-spending.htm (2017); https://data.worldbank.org/indicator/SH.XPD.CHEX.GD.ZS (% of GDP dollars spent on healthcare) (2015); https://data.oecd.org/gga/general-government-spending.htm#indicator-chart (2015); https://data.oecd.org/gga/general-government-revenue.htm#indicator-chart (2015). The World Bank. *Sources:* OECD and World Bank.

per capita expenditure on health, and life expectancy. Many countries in the world face similar challenges of aging populations with chronic disease, the need to ration costly technology, and severe budget shortfalls.

As reflected in Table 6.2, U.S. life expectancy was 78.6 years in 2017, the benefits reaped in the U.S. health care system seem to be those of enhanced quality of life rather than enhanced longevity. Quality of life must be defined within the specific cultures and value systems of each country. In the United States, qualities of life highly valued by Americans include prompt access to diagnostic and treatment services, even when health problems are not life threatening; ready availability of cutting-edge technology and pharmaceuticals; the ability to choose among health care practitioners and sites for care; and participation in health care decisions. All these contribute to the cost of health care in the U.S. Is that enough to justify spending more than any other country in the world and nearly twice as much as European countries with similar health and financial circumstances?

Medicare Hospital Value-Based Purchasing (VBP) Program

Medicare Hospital Value-Based Purchasing (VBP) programs are an emerging movement in health care. The Hospital VBP Program encourages hospitals to improve the quality and safety of acute inpatient care for Medicare beneficiaries and all patients by:

- Eliminating or reducing adverse events (health care errors resulting in patient harm)

- Adopting evidence-based care standards and protocols that make the best outcomes for the most patients

- Changing hospital processes to make patients' care experiences better

- Increasing care transparency for consumers

- Recognizing hospitals that give high-quality care at a lower cost to Medicare.
  Hospitals are gauged on measures of outcome such as:

- Mortality and complications

- Healthcare-associated infections

- Patient safety

- Patient experience

- Process

- Efficiency and cost reduction, available at www.cms.gov/Medicare/Quality-Initiatives-Patient-Assessment-Instruments/Value-Based-Programs/HVBP/Hospital-Value-Based-Purchasing.html, Accessed July 31, 2019.

VBP encourage hospitals to follow established best clinical practices and improve patient satisfaction scores via HCAHPS (the Hospital Consumer Assessment of Healthcare Providers and Systems Survey). A "value pool" of funds is generated by reducing all Medicare payments to acute-care hospitals by 2%. These funds are then redistributed to the hospitals as determined by their performance on measures that are divided into four quality domains: (a) safety, (b) clinical care, (c) efficiency and cost reduction, and (iv) patient and caregiver-centered experience. Hospitals are scored on the various measures based on "improvement" and "achievement" where improvement compares them to their own scores during a baseline period, and achievement compares them to the scores of other hospitals. CMS uses the higher of the two scores to determine financial awards, available at https://catalyst.nejm.org/pay-for-performance-in-healthcare, accessed July 31, 2019.

VBP programs are a fundamental change from fee-for-service payment. Payment disincentives, such as eliminating payments for negative consequences of care (e.g., medical

Evidence from the Literature

Source: Adapted from The Economist (2018). Land of the Free-for-All: America is a healthcare outlier in the developed world. Retrieved from www.economist.com/special-report/2018/04/26/america-is-a-health-care-outlier-in-the-developed-world, July 30, 2019.

Discussion: America has some of the best hospitals in the world but it is also the only large rich country without universal health care coverage. About half of Americans have their health insurance provided by their employers. Health care costs can be financially ruinous for others. In 2016, Americans spent $10,348 per person on health care, roughly twice as much as the average for comparably rich countries. On average, both hospital cost and drug prices can be 60% higher in the United States than in Europe.

The American Affordable Care Act expanded the health insurance system and cut the number of insured people from 44 million to 28 million, but still left a gap among people not poor enough to qualify for Medicaid but not rich enough to buy private insurance.

In the United States, prices for the same service can vary enormously. Having your appendix removed, for example, can cost anywhere from between $1,500 to $183,000, depending on the insurer. Add to this the fact that 9 of the 10 best paid occupations in the United States involve medicine and we can see that people in medicine have little incentive to change the system.

Implications for practice: Nurses must participate in and lead some of the discussion about the improvement of health care. Americans need to realize that better health care can be developed, perhaps a combination of universal health care and private health care. Let's examine all similar countries' systems and develop the best system in the world.

errors, hospital readmissions, and increased costs), have also been proposed. Table 6.3 provides a full list of negative **Hospital Acquired Conditions** (HAC) that affect payments through Medicare and Medicaid services. Although many programs originate from CMS, commercial insurers are just as committed to performance-based payment models. In 2017, almost 50% of insurer's reimbursements were in the form of value-based care models.

It is important to note that the United States and Canadian health care models differ. As noted, in the U.S., we have a private health care system. Residents of Canadian provinces are covered by public insurance. In Canada, physicians are private health care providers rather than government employees. These health care providers see patients and charge insurance plans, just as they do in the U.S. In this instance, "Obamacare" vs. the Canada Health Act have some similarities as they are both reimbursed by the Government (American Institute of Medical Sciences and Education, March 29, 2018). Review Table 6.4. While the United States and Canadian health care models differ, the top leading causes of death are similar. This is reflective of health care systems where health care costs are paid publicly and or supplemented by private insurance.

Future Perspectives on the Cost of Health Care

Future perspectives on the cost of health care are needed to guide health care to organize for success. Health care providers have been thrashing in chaos for many years, reinventing their health care structures and processes, right-sizing their health care enterprises, outsourcing to better focus on their core health care business, and merging to share scarce or expensive health care resources. Although there have been some short-term cost savings, and the rise in health care spending has slowed, several evolving trends keep the overall costs growing. Although the health care market landscape

Table 6.3 Categories of Hospital Acquired Conditions (HAC) that affect Payment by U.S. Centers for Medicare & Medicaid Services (CMS)

These 14 categories of hospital acquired conditions affect payment by CMS:

- Foreign Object Retained After Surgery
- Air Embolism
- Blood Incompatibility
- Stage III and IV Pressure Ulcers
- Falls and Trauma
  - Fractures
  - Dislocations
  - Intracranial Injuries
  - Crushing Injuries
  - Burn
  - Other Injuries
- Manifestations of Poor Glycemic Control
  - Diabetic Ketoacidosis
  - Nonketotic Hyperosmolar Coma
  - Hypoglycemic Coma
  - Secondary Diabetes with Ketoacidosis
  - Secondary Diabetes with Hyperosmolarity
- Catheter-Associated Urinary Tract Infection (UTI)
- Vascular Catheter-Associated Infection
- Surgical Site Infection, Mediastinitis, Following Coronary Artery Bypass Graft (CABG):
- Surgical Site Infection Following Bariatric Surgery for Obesity
  - Laparoscopic Gastric Bypass
  - Gastroenterostomy
  - Laparoscopic Gastric Restrictive Surgery
- Surgical Site Infection Following Certain Orthopedic Procedures
  - Spine
  - Neck
  - Shoulder
  - Elbow
- Surgical Site Infection Following Cardiac Implantable Electronic Device (CIED)
- Deep Vein Thrombosis (DVT)/Pulmonary Embolism (PE) Following Certain Orthopedic Procedures:
  - Total Knee Replacement
  - Hip Replacement
- Iatrogenic Pneumothorax with Venous Catheterization

Source: Hospital-Acquired Conditions. Centers for Medicare & Medicaid Services. Public Domain.www.cms.gov/Medicare/Medicare-Fee-for-Service-Payment/HospitalAcqCond/Hospital-Acquired_Conditions.html, retrieved August 1, 2019

Real World Interview

During my many experiences over the past years with the Ontario, Canada, health care system and the **Ontario Health Insurance Program** (OHIP), I have had annual visits to my **General Practitioner** (GP) with referrals to specialists for various tests, including X-rays, blood work, and hospital stays, as needed. All my medical expenses while in these doctors' care is covered completely by the OHIP funds. Medications, glasses, and dental work are not covered unless one's gross annual income is a very minimal amount, in which case some medications, dental, and hospitalizations are covered.

My husband was a diabetic, and he had a stroke 20 years ago at the age of 53. His GP met us at the hospital and assessed him through triage. My husband lost the use of his right arm and leg and his ability to comprehend language. The supreme care and compassion of his doctors and nurses helped my husband and family cope with the severity of this horrific disease. We paid for an upgrade to a semiprivate room. All other expenses while he was in the hospital were covered by OHIP. His rehabilitation began two weeks after his stroke, and he was transferred to the rehabilitation center, where he stayed for three months. All expenses while he was there were funded by OHIP.

After his acute illness, my husband saw a specialist every three months to monitor his blood sugar levels. He saw his GP every three months for his hypertension and saw his optometrist every year. He went for speech therapy once a week, to physical therapy three times a week, and to a nutritionist twice a year. This was all covered by OHIP.

He had several episodes of congestive heart failure through the years. Each time, I called 911, and the fire department came within minutes, administered oxygen, and inquired about his medical problems and medications while waiting for the ambulance medics to arrive. The medics took his vitals, gave him nitro, and called the admitting hospital.

We have four hospitals in Hamilton, Ontario, where I live. In the **Emergency Department** (ED), my husband was always processed immediately. When a heart specialist was called in, it took about an hour for him to arrive. Then the heart specialist would decide whether my husband was to be admitted to Intensive Care or a ward. There were times when a bed was not available until the next day, and we had to wait in the ED.

All emergencies in our ED are taken care of fairly promptly, the most severe first. Elective surgery, such as knee or hip replacements, eye cataracts, etc., require a longer waiting period, sometimes up to six months. Hospital and emergency patients are on the priority list for **Magnetic Resonance Imaging** (MRI) and CT scans. Other patients may have to wait for a couple of months for these tests. I also have the option, if I can afford it, of visiting the Buffalo, New York, area clinics for MRIs, etc., if it is not an emergency and I want to do it quicker. I would have to pay for these visits and tests out of pocket. All in all, I have been fairly pleased with our Canadian health system.

Flo Paradisi
Hamilton, Ontario, Canada

Table 6.4   Leading Causes of Death in U.S. and Canada (2016)

Leading causes of deaths in Canada	Leading causes of deaths In U.S. (2016)
Malignant neoplasms	Heart disease
Diseases of heart	Cancer
Cerebrovascular diseases	Accidents (unintentional injuries)
Chronic lower respiratory diseases	Chronic lower respiratory diseases
Accidents (unintentional injuries)	Stroke (cerebrovascular diseases)

Source: Statistics Canada, available at www150.statcan.gc.ca/t1/tbl1/en/tv.action?pid=1310039401 Accessed July 2, 2019, and National Center for Health Statistics, available at www.cdc.gov/nchs/fastats/leading-causes-of-death.htm Accessed July 2, 2019.

---

remains unchanged from a legislative perspective, continuing health care market evolution has resulted in health care providers facing decreased reimbursement and consumers with limited access to health plans by metropolitan statistical area across the country. This has resulted in decreased availability of commercial health insurance through traditional carriers and self-funded employers driving health care market change (Vogenberg & Santilli, 2018, Health Care Trends for 2018,

www.ncbi.nlm.nih.gov/pmc/articles/PMC5902765, accessed July 10, 2019)

Highly complex and expensive technology, including surgery, continue to develop (Table 6.5). Diseases that require expensive or long-term treatment, such as Type 2 Diabetes, Obesity, Acquired Immune Deficiency Syndrome, and other infectious diseases, continue to be a problem. With the eradication or successful management of selected diseases such

Table 6.5 Selected Costs of Common Surgeries

Heart valve replacement: $170,000
Heart bypass: $123,000
Spinal fusion: $110,000
Hip replacement: $40,364
Knee replacement: $35,000
Angioplasty: $28,2000
Hip resurfacing: $28,000
Gastric bypass: $25,000
Cornea: $17,500
Gastric sleeve: $16,000

Source: Data from Fay, B. (2018) Hospital and Surgery Costs: 2018 Average Costs for Common Surgeries, available at, https://www.debt.org/medical/hospital-surgery-costs/, accessed March 18 2020.

as tuberculosis, populations are surviving longer. With that lengthened survival come the debilitating diseases of aging.

We look to futurists to help us make decisions about what health care services we ought to be prepared to provide. Current questions include: Will 45 million uninsured Americans find comprehensive primary care that is accessible? Is competition between health care providers a positive influence on health care delivery? Will a few strategically located hospitals provide only an intensive level of care, while acute care is managed on an ambulatory basis without invasive procedures? Will preventive, primary, and restorative care be the purview of advanced nurse practitioners practicing at community sites? Will unselfish concern for the welfare of others no longer be the basis for caring health care careers? Will nurses still be "asked to care" in a society that no longer values caring? Will the United States adopt a health care delivery system similar to those in European countries and Canada?

Economic Principles of Health Care

The mission statement of any health care business describes the purpose for existence of the business and the rationale that justifies that existence. The mission statement directs decision making about what is or is not within the purview of the health care business. The health care vision statement is a logical extension of the mission into the future, establishing long-range goals for the health care vision. After the health care vision is established and the business can articulate its health care goals and where it wants to go, a strategic plan for how to achieve the vision, or how to reach the goals, is developed. There must be cohesion and consistency across the mission, vision, and strategic plan for the business to successfully achieve its mission. There must also be money, for without it no mission can be accomplished. Therefore, the economic cost equation becomes: MONEY = MISSION = MONEY.

Health Care Provider Economics

Economic risk is borne by individuals, as well as by organizations. Both individuals and organizations may experience actual or perceived pressure to provide less health care service than is optimal, in order to contain costs. Individual professionals risk what can be referred to as the "dumbing down" of their respective professions. "Dumbing down" occurs when cost-saving strategies include using individuals with less knowledge to perform health care services usually performed by people with advanced knowledge. When this happens, the quality of the services delivered may decrease without actual harm occurring to patients and without patient recognition that the services are not optimal. If the enterprise is willing to provide less-than-optimal services by less qualified people to save money, those with advanced knowledge may face loss of job security. Eventually, if care is judged to be inadequate or inappropriate, there may be risk of expensive litigation that can threaten both individuals and the organization with loss of licensure and livelihood.

Organizations' attempts to provide more economical care by changing the mix of caregivers is ultimately regulated by the respective state's practice acts (laws), along with their accompanying rules. State nursing and medical practice acts define the scope of nursing and medical practitioner practice. Both state nursing and state medical practice acts regulate the practice components that can be delegated and the accountability that follows delegation of care. The state nursing and medical practice acts determine the extent to which an organization can stipulate that medical care or nursing care will be managed by delegation of that care in order to capture fiscal economies.

Individual providers such as nursing and medical practitioners and therapists receiving direct payment from insurers bear risk when they must lower their usual fees to a flat rate in order to be eligible for payment by the HMO. A catch-22 exists for individual providers. If the provider agrees to participate in an HMO as a preferred provider, a lower payment rate may be part of the agreement. If the provider chooses not to participate in an HMO as a preferred provider, there is risk of attracting only the limited number of patients willing and able to pay out-of-pocket fee-for-service rates. To minimize their own expenses for providing services, individual providers regulate the amount and selection of services they provide, as well as the time spent with each patient. As a result, patients may be dissatisfied with the services and choose an alternate provider.

Patients bear the risk of being unable to access services they regard as optimal or services regarded as representing the least possibility of harm. Clearly, frivolous services are not available under the managed care philosophy, but patients may find themselves co-opted or moved away from their preferences for health care services by incentives to accept less expensive levels of service. Patients' out-of-pocket expense, or copayment, is usually considerably lower if they accept care from a member of a PPO than if they choose to obtain care from a provider that is not a member of a PPO.

With the cost of employer-sponsored health care benefits approaching $15,000 per employee in 2019, large U.S. employers continue to make changes, new research reveals. Many want to hold down cost increases and are steering employees toward cost-effective health care providers.

(SHRM – Miller, 2018 www.shrm.org/resourcesandtools/hr-topics/benefits/pages/employers-adjust-health-benefits-for-2019.aspx, accessed July 10, 2019).

Business Profit

Revenue (income) minus cost (expense) equals profit. Profit is not restricted to for-profit businesses. Profit is not a dirty word. All businesses must realize a profit to remain in business. In for-profit businesses, a portion of the profit is distributed to stockholders in appreciation for their investing in the business, and the remainder is used to maintain and grow the organization. In nonprofit businesses, there are no stockholders to share the profit, so all of it is fed back into the business for maintenance and growth.

Nonprofit organizations desiring a purer image than the term *profit* engenders refer to their profit as contribution to margin, with the rule of thumb being to secure 4–5% of the total budget as profit or margin. **Margin** is defined as the amount by which revenue from sales or services exceeds costs in a business. Mission and margin are strategically and operationally linked by the reality that margin is resources required to carry out the organization's strategic plan and achieve its mission. Without margin, or with limited margin, there would be a lack of money to replace infrastructure such as worn-out equipment, maintain existing buildings or undertake new construction, purchase state-of-the-art technology, replace heating and lighting systems, and establish new services or enlarge existing services in response to changing community needs for health care. Failure to maintain infrastructure can impair the organization's ability to be competitive, resulting in failure to meet its mission and eventual organizational failure. Profit or margin is the elasticity that accommodates improvements in patient and staff education, recruitment and hiring of expert staff, and special programming that yields personal and professional growth. Profit or Margin is a critical requirement for doing business. A truism of business: no margin, no mission. Achieving and sustaining margin is a constant challenge for health care enterprises. The 2010 Patient Protection and ACA was implemented with unique pricing and budget structures in each state. Each state has its own philosophy of how to generate health care dollars for citizens who do not have private insurance.

Fundamental Costs of Care

There are many ways to examine or classify the costs of care. One fundamental method is to view costs as direct or indirect. A **direct cost** is a cost directly related to patient care within a manager's unit, such as the cost of nurses' wages and the cost of patient care supplies. An **indirect cost** is a cost not explicitly related to care within a manager's unit but it is a cost necessary to support care. The costs of electricity, heat, air conditioning, and maintenance of the facility are all considered indirect costs.

Those same costs may also be considered either fixed or variable costs. These distinctions are somewhat artificial and are related to the volume of services that are provided. A **fixed cost** is a cost that exists irrespective of the number of patients for whom care is provided. Examples of fixed costs are the cost of the rent or the monthly mortgage for the space in which the care is provided and the cost of salaried (but not hourly) wage earners, such as the nurse manager or nurse administrator. These fixed costs would be the same whether one or 1,000 patients were served. A **variable cost**, on the other hand, is a cost that varies with volume and it will increase or decrease depending on the number of patients. Medical supplies, laundry for the linens used in patient care, and patient meals are variable costs that increase or decrease in proportion to the number of patients served.

Some costs are step variable, that is, they vary with volume, but not smoothly. The key to step variable costs is that they are fixed over volume intervals, but they vary within the relevant range. For instance, a fixed number of nurses may be able to care for 11–21 patients. However, if even one additional patient beyond 21 patients requires care, additional nurses are required.

Cost Analysis

There is an old saying that numbers do not lie. There is also an old saying that statistics can be manipulated to show whatever is desired. Both sayings are true, and therein is the challenge, the frustration, and occasionally the glory of clinical cost management. The health care industry commonly embraces the position that the past is a prologue for forecasting its future. The ability to predict the behavior of cost in the future based on its past behavior, then, is considered requisite to successful cost management and thereby the achievement of the mission and vision. A **budget** is a plan that provides formal quantitative expression for acquiring and distributing funds over the ensuing time period (generally one year). A budget is based on what is known about how much was spent in the past and how that will inevitably change in the coming year. A cost prediction is simply a tool for developing a budget. The three most common methods of cost prediction are high-low cost estimation, bivariate regression analysis, and break-even analysis.

High-Low Cost Estimation

High-Low Cost Estimation is not the tool to choose for cost prediction if a sophisticated, statistically rigorous cost prediction is needed, but it does surpass just guessing at costs. Examining both fixed and variable cost information from the most recent five years for each category of expense provides a "good enough" cost projection for many items that remain relatively constant in volume of consumption and cost. Both fixed and variable dollars need to be adjusted upward to account for inflation, and the total projected cost needs to be adjusted upward to cover anticipated or other wage increases and to cover bad debt when services are rendered but payment does not occur.

The following is an example that clarifies High-Low Cost Estimation:

Highest wage cost = $500,000

Lowest wage cost = $300,500

Difference in cost = $199,500

Highest number of patient days = 9,000 days

Lowest number of patient days = 7,500 days

Difference in Volume = 1,500 days

Difference in cost ($199,500)/Difference in volume (1,500) = $133 per patient day of variable cost

Variable cost ($133) × Lowest number of patient days (7,500) = $997,500 = Total annual variable cost

Total annual labor cost for the unit from this year's fiscal department records ($1,100,000)–Total annual variable cost ($997,500) = $102,500 Fixed cost

If 1,000 additional patient days are anticipated in the ensuing year, there would be an additional cost as follows:

$133 per patient day variable cost × 1,000 additional days = $133,000

Fixed cost (regardless of the number of patient days) = $102,500

Total additional cost = $235,500

Thus, the total cost for this unit next year, using high-low cost prediction, will be this year's cost of $1,100,000 plus $235,500 in new costs, or $1,335,500.

Bivariate Regression Analysis

A more precise method of cost prediction can be realized using the statistical tool, bivariate regression analysis. Whereas the high-low method prediction method relies on only two data points—the highest and the lowest—for historical cost behavior, bivariate regression analysis examines all available past cost information over a specific time period.

Bivariate regression analysis assumes that there is only one dependent variable (cost), with only one independent variable (volume) causing change in that dependent variable (cost). Bivariate regression analysis also assumes that, mathematically, cost behavior can be shown in a linear fashion by drawing a straight line through a scatter diagram showing all fixed and variable costs at all volumes of use. When all the cost information is plotted as a dot on a vertical axis and all volume information is plotted as a dot on the horizontal axis, a scatter diagram results. The straight line through the scatter diagram that best approximates all the points is used to predict

cost at a specific volume of use. This line that approximates the points is also known as "the Best Fit" line. Selecting a volume on the horizontal axis of the scatter diagram and examining where a vertical line from that point intersects the straight regression line, then moving horizontally to the vertical cost axis, provides the cost prediction for that specific volume, as shown by the dotted lines in the scatter diagram in Figure 6.3. The analysis is carried out for each item for which cost needs to be predicted.

Break-even Analysis

The business goal of health care organizations is accruing profit to enhance the quality of services provided and to achieve optimal competitive market position. Thus, projecting whether and when profitability will be achieved is necessary for both proposed and well-established programs and services. The third most common method of cost prediction is break-even analysis. Break-Even Analysis assists the provider in predicting the volume of services that must be provided (and for which payment must be received) for the "total variable cost" of providing the services plus the "total fixed costs" to be equally matched by the payment received, yielding neither a profit or loss. The formula for computing a break-even analysis (Zaichkin, 2018) is as follows:

$$\text{Total Revenue} - \text{Total Variable Cost} - \text{Total Fixed Cost} = 0 = \text{Break} - \text{Even}$$

A common application of the break-even analysis is the determination of how many procedures must be completed using a new piece of equipment before the payments for the procedure cover the cost of the equipment and other resources consumed while doing the procedure (the break-even point at which income and expenses are equal), with all additional procedures generating profit.

To make the use of the break-even analysis clearer, consider that the purchase of a new piece of radiology equipment is proposed. The underlying question is, would the purchase generate a profit or a loss, or would the organization just break even?

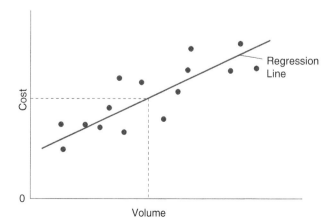

FIGURE 6.3 Regression Analysis on a scatter diagram.
Source: Created by L. Stuckey, D. A. Cherubini & S. A. Sacco.

Applying the break-even analysis formula, if the new procedure costs $50,000, the wages of the technician operating the equipment for one hour for each use is $20 per use. Therefore, the payment for each procedure is $50, so it would take 1,667 procedures to pay for the new equipment and technician's wages before a profit would begin to accrue.

$$\text{Volume} = \$50,000 / (\$50 - \$20) = 1,667 \text{ procedures}$$

If the payment for the procedure were $100, a profit would begin to accrue after only 625 procedures.

$$\text{Volume} = \$50,000 / (\$100 - \$20) = 625 \text{ procedures}$$

Thus, a projection can be made about how long it will take before the new equipment would be a profitable venture, guided by the decision about how much cost the purchaser of the procedure is likely to tolerate.

Relative Value Unit

A **relative value unit (RVU)** is a measure of value used by The Centers for Medicare And Medicaid Services (CMS) to calculate reimbursement fees for three types of provider resources, that is provider work RVUs, practice expense RVUs, and professional liability insurance RVUs. Provider work RVUs account for the time, technical skill and effort, mental effort and judgment, and stress to provide a service. Practice expense RVUs account for the nonprovider clinical and nonclinical labor of the practice, as well as expenses for building space, equipment, and office supplies. Professional liability insurance RVUs account for the cost of malpractice insurance premiums.

Current Procedural Terminology (CPT) Code Sets and the **Healthcare Common Procedure Coding System** (HCPCS) determine standardized fees for provider services, such as same-day surgery procedures, post-op follow-up assessment, and outpatient office visits (Table 6.6).

Nurse managers can use RVUs to assess the complexity of care for scheduled appointments and procedures. This information assists in the planning for length of appointment and procedure times, supplies, equipment, and the number of providers and staff required to complete the delivery of care. A high number of RVUs would indicate a higher complexity of care and the need for more resources, versus a lower RVU number which would indicate a lesser complexity of care and a need for less resources.

As mentioned above, a **relative value unit (RVU)** is a measure used to calculate reimbursement fees for three types of provider resources: provider work RVUs, practice expense RVUs, and professional liability insurance RVUs. Patient acuity is rated on a scale of 1–5 and it is the measurement of the intensity of nursing care required. A patient with an acuity of 1 requires the least care and a patient with an acuity level of 5 requires the most care. The actual consumption of nursing resources is not linear; that is, caring for an acuity level 2 patient does not consume twice as many nursing resources as caring for an acuity level 1 patient. RVUs provide a proportional comparison between the resources required by patients with level 1 acuity (always a value of 1) and any other acuity level. For example, only 20% (1.2 RVUs) more resources may be consumed by an acuity level 2 patient than an acuity level 1 patient, but twice as many resources may be consumed by a level 3 patient acuity (2.0 RVUs), and more than three times as many resources may be consumed by a level 4 patient acuity (3.33 RVUs), and so forth, as shown in Table 6.7.

As you review Table 6.7, note as the RVU weight increases, so does the acuity of care and the number of care hours. This indicates increased complexity of care. Nurse managers use complexity of care information to determine the number of nurses, providers, and other staff required to provide quality care and ensure optimal patient outcomes. This information can also be used to track and report staff productivity. Productivity reports help nurse managers support the current

Table 6.6   Relative Value Units for Selected Services, 2014

Service (HCPCS[a])	Total RVU's	Provider's work	Practice expenses	Professional liability insurance
Intermediate Office Visit (99214)[b]	3.01	1.50	1.41	0.10
Diagnostic Colonoscopy (45378)[b]	11.03	3.69	6.78	0.56
Total Hip Replacement (27130)[c]	38.94	20.72	14.32	3.90

Source: Centers for Medicare and Medicaid (CMS), public domain. Retrieved from www.cms.gov/apps/physician-fee-schedule/overview.aspx Accessed August 8, 2019.
[a] Healthcare Common Procedure Coding System (**HCPCS**).
[b] Service delivered in a provider's office.
[c] Service provided in a facility.

Table 6.7   Comparative Values of Patient Acuity, Patient Care Hours, and Relative Value Units

Acuity	Care hours*		RVU weight		Total RVUs
1	125	×	1.00	=	125.00
2	200	×	1.20	=	240.00
3	500	×	2.00	=	1,000.00
4	550	×	3.33	=	1,831.50
5	400	×	5.00	=	2,000.00
Total	1,775				5,196.50

*Care hours in nursing is the number of indirect and direct care requited by a patient (Giannasi & Rudman, 2018). The RVUs captured will determine the complexity of the patient care provided.

Dividing the total cost of nursing wages by the total RVUs yields the cost per RVU.

$1,250,000/5,196.50 = $240.55 per RVU.

staffing levels or the need to request additional staffing. Over time, there may be an increase in workload as indicated by the RVUs. This workload increase would support a budgetary request to hire additional staff.

The RVUs can be used to calculate the relative costs of nursing care, using the following reasoning:

For the time period of interest, the total cost of nursing wages = $1,250,000 (Table 6.7). Consider that also, for the time period of interest, the Comparative Values of Patient Acuity, Patient Care Hours, and Relative Value Units are as follows (Table 6.8):

Patients' acuity varies, even within the same day, as patients experience invasive procedures, intensive treatments and medication, complications, or progress toward wellness. As patient acuity varies, consumption of nursing resources also varies. It follows that the cost for direct nursing care would be consistent with nursing resource consumption and could be determined using RVU calculations.

This approach provides a reasonably accurate per-patient costing approach. It does not, however, account for the

Table 6.8   Comparative Values of Patient Acuity, Patient Care Hours, and Relative Value Units for the Time Period of Interest

Acuity	Care hours	Relative value weight
1	3.00	1.00
2	3.60	1.20
3	6.00	2.00
4	9.99	3.33
5	15.00	5.00

difference in cost based on the category of worker providing the care. For example, an RN's salary is more than that of a nurse aide's salary. Indirect fixed costs that do not vary dependent on patient classification, such as salaried wages, overhead, service contracts, and noncapital equipment purchases, must be added to arrive at the full cost of nursing care.

Critical Thinking 6.1

Reducing costs and improving quality at the same time is a very realistic goal. Frequently, quality problems are very costly. Examples of this are found in Kliger, Lacey, Olney, Cox, and ONeil (2010) article on Nurse-driven programs to improve patient outcomes in the Journal of Nursing Administration. The article describes a **Transforming Care at the Bedside** (TCAB) project funded by the Robert Wood Johnson Foundation and the Institute for Healthcare Improvement. The main focus of their TCAB project was to implement staff nurse identified solutions to quality or safety concerns. The identified solutions were adopted for two weeks and the solutions were evaluated for effectiveness. If the staff nurse identified the solution worked, it was adopted. If not, the solution was scrapped. One example given was the staff

nurse identified the need for a shelf to place items on outside the patient rooms in order to facilitate handwashing. With this simple added shelf, handwashing improved and the innovation was a success. Moreover, Kliger's (2018) article in the Journal of Nursing Administration emphasizes that as the national quality agenda continues to be a key driver in health care, more programs are being developed to teach staff nurses how to lead quality and safety change projects. Nurses are in a unique position to do this work.

Identify some ways in which nurses can participate in reducing waste, influencing best practices, and improving quality and safety in these areas.

Is keeping current with the literature in your specialty necessary to be effective in improving quality and safety?

Critical Thinking 6.2

Nursing is a collaborative profession existing in a complex health care system. At one time it was influenced by three factors: cost, access, and quality. Today there are five influencing factors: cost, access, cost, quality, and cost (John M. Lantz, RN, PhD, Dean and Professor, School of Nursing, University of San Francisco).

Is this an accurate description of the factors that influence contemporary nursing practice today?

What do these five influencing factors suggest may be an organization's focus as you interview for a staff nurse position?

You notice that a colleague frequently does not record patient charge items for elderly patients. When you inquire about it, you are told that your colleague feels sorry for those on fixed incomes and wants to save them money. Who pays when your colleague does this?

The Role of State and Federal Government and Third-Party Payers in the Financing of Health Care

The Federal Government plays an important role in controlling the financing of the health care system by mandating health insurance and other social insurance, ensuring the quality and safety of treatment, managing public health projects, and promoting research and development. Similarly, the States shape the health care system in many ways, influencing key components, such as insurance coverage, quality of care, and information and provider infrastructures.

State Payment and Health Care Delivery System Reform Initiatives

In several States, innovative state payment and health care delivery system reforms have been implemented, aimed at improving value in Medicaid for a long enough period of time to generate a track record of results that can be evaluated. A report on state payment and health care delivery system reform initiatives in 2014 showed promising results in Medicare savings of major payment and delivery system reforms in Maryland, Massachusetts, Oregon, and Arkansas (Paying for value in Medicaid, 2014). These States launched ambitious reforms in an attempt to reduce health care costs while maintaining or improving health care quality. This is in stark contrast to recent waiver proposals by some states to roll back Medicaid eligibility and benefits through policies such as work requirements and lock-out periods. Lock-out periods are a predetermined amount of time that you are unable to change your insurance coverage. While the lock-out periods merely shift costs to low-income individuals and families, the state reforms reviewed attempt to tackle the actual underlying costs of health care (Huelskoetter, 2018, Evaluating State Innovations to Reduce Health Care Costs, www.americanprogress.org/issues/health-care/reports/2018/04/06/448912/evaluating-state-innovations-reduce-health-care-costs, accessed June 25, 2019).

Medicare Medication Costs

Medicare Part D was adopted in 2005 to provide a prescription drug benefit to enrollees with low incomes and high drug costs.

Rules for membership and eligibility and a gap in coverage that has come to be called the "doughnut hole" have Americans confused and disappointed. The doughnut hole from Medicare is a coverage gap. This means that after you have spent a certain amount of money for covered medications, you have to pay all costs out-of-pocket for your prescriptions up to a yearly limit.

The ACA signed into law on March 23, 2010 (available at http://healthinsurance.about.com/od/reform/a/Affordable-Care-Act-What-You-Should-Know-About-The-Affordable-Care-Act.htm, accessed June 25, 2019) made several changes to Medicare Part D to reduce out-of-pocket costs when you reach the donut hole, including:

- In 2019, if you reach the donut hole, you will be given a 75% discount on most of the total cost of brand name drugs and 63% discount for generic drugs while in the donut hole gap. The donut hole continues until your total out-of-pocket cost reaches $5,100, (www.medicareinteractive.org/get-answers/medicare-prescription-drug-coverage-part-d/medicare-part-d-costs/phases-of-part-d-coverage, accessed July 10, 2019)

- By 2020, the above changes will effectively close the donut hole, and, rather than paying 100% of medication costs while in the donut hole, patient responsibility will be 25% of medication costs.

The annual out-of-pocket spending amount for health care services includes the yearly **deductible** (money paid for health care services yearly by an insurance policy holder before an insurance company will pay for any expenses), **copayment** (money paid for health care services by an insurance policy holder each time they receive a health care service), and **coinsurance amounts** (fixed percentage of money a patient must pay for a health care services bill after the deductible is satisfied).

Factors that Influence Health Care Spending and Their Effect on Health Care Outcomes

Medications are a significant item in the overall health care budget and are subject to annual increases (see Table 6.9). Approximately 397 drugs increased in price in 2018 and 32 drugs decreased in price (www.goodrx.com/blog/2018-

Table 6.9 Drug List Price Percentage Increase from January 1, 2018 to November 30, 2018

WP thyroid	55.8%
Gleostine	30.8%
Zomig	20.8%
Onzetra	15.1%
Prenatal Vitamins	14.7%
Amicar	9.9%
Oralair	9.9%
Rexulti	9.9%
Talz	8%
Victoza	7.9%

Source: Adapted from 2018 in Review: The Good(Rx) and the Bad in Prescription Drug Prices. www.goodrx.com/blog/2018-in-review-goodrx-prescription-drug-rices Accessed June 25, 2019. Originally published GoodRX blog, www.goodrx.com.blog

in-review-goodrx-prescription-drug-rices, accessed June 25, 2019). These prices are based on the list price of a drug, which is the official price set by the manufacturer. While few people actually pay the list price for their drugs, as patients are protected by their insurance, the list price is a good measure for the cost of a drug.

Of the approximately 397 drugs that saw price increases, most saw an increase above 6%. As the conversation regarding drug prices has heated up over the past couple of years, manufacturers have slowly taken a pledge to keep price increases below 10% annually—but they continue to push the limit. In 2018, 62 drugs increased in price by 9.9%.

Health Care Salaries

Health care salaries have enjoyed a steady uphill climb since the recession period of 2008–2010, a trend that experts predict will continue (Table 6.10). This salary trend is likely to persist despite the current political climate that is making it difficult to predict what might happen to the ACA and its impact on health care employment and salaries (https://hiring.monster.com/hr/hr-best-practices/recruiting-hiring-advice/managing-hiring-costs/2017-healthcare-job-salaries.aspx, accessed June 25, 2019). "The demand for talent will continue to grow as the Baby Boomer generation retires, and as more individuals have insurance, demand for services will grow," says Dana Cates, a health care human resources consultant at Lean Human Capital by Health CareSource, a talent-management resource company based in Woburn, Massachusetts (from https://hiring.monster.com/employer-resources/recruiting-strategies/compensation/2017-healthcare-job-salaries, accessed June 25, 2019)

An Aging Population and the Affordable Care Act (ACA)

The one-two punch of an aging population and expanded coverage under the ACA has increased demand for health care, pushing wages up, says Katie Bardaro, Vice President of data analytics at PayScale. "Since 2016, health care wages have grown by 4.2%, compared to national wages growth at 3.2%. If current patterns hold, we can likely expect wages to continue growing by another 2–4% in health care," Bardaro says. (from www.payscale.com, accessed June 25, 2019) Front-line primary care providers in particular have seen high demand. Cates, the health care human resources consultant mentioned above, says physician assistants and nurse practitioners saw job growth after the implementation of the ACA. Behavio-

Table 6.10 Health Care 2018 Median Pay/Compensation

Occupation	2018 median pay/compensation
Physicians and surgeons	Equal to or greater than $208,000
Dentist	$156,240
Pharmacist	$126,120
Nurse anesthetists, nurse midwives, and nurse practitioners	$113,930
Physician assistants	$108,610
Healthcare administrators in Illinois	$96,770
Physical therapists	$87,930
Dietician	$60,370
Registered nurses	$71,730
Licensed practical nurse/licensed vocational nurse	$46,240
Nursing assistants and orderlies	$28,530

Sources: U.S. Bureau of Labor Statistics, Occupational Outlook Handbook and HealthcareAdministration EDU.org. available at, www.healthcareadministrationedu.org/salaries accessed July 2, 2019.

ral health and clinical informatics also have expanded under the ACA, Cates says, as more people have gained access to mental health services and organizations have turned to technology to manage information more efficiently. (from https://hiring.monster.com/employer-resources/recruiting-strategies/compensation/2017-healthcare-job-salaries/,accessed June 25, 2019)

Political Uncertainty Will Make Long-Term Planning a Challenge

Medical facilities that are already dealing with an influx of patients due to more people having health coverage are finding it difficult to plan for the long term. In addition, changes in international visa policies could make it difficult to fill positions with people from overseas. This will drive salaries up for those unfilled positions. www.urban.org/sites/default/files/publication/94396/2001576-how-have-providers-responded-to-the-increased-demand-for-health-care-under-the-affordble-care-act_0.pdf, accessed July 10, 2019. Also, some health care roles will require special attention in regards to compensation, Bardaro says, requiring employers to pay a premium to attract and retain top talent (from www.payscale.com, accessed June 25, 2019)

Meanwhile, demand for some health care positions may decline if there are major changes in the ACA. "While we saw an increase in health development and community health employment opportunities last year, we have seen a sharp downturn after the elections and in the first few weeks of the new presidency," says Olivia

Jaras, founder and CEO of Salary Coaching for Women in Hanover, New Hampshire. Most of the community-based health initiatives have slowed or frozen new hiring until further notice. (from https://hiring.monster.com/employer-resources/recruiting-strategies/compensation/2017-healthcare-job-salaries/, accessed June 25, 2019)

Hospital Costs, Patient Charges, Nursing Costs, and Room Charges

Hospital costs are different from patient charges in hospitals. Hospital costs are the "wholesale" version of how much hospitals pay for supplies, staffing, new equipment, and maintaining the physical plant of the hospital. Patient charges are what is billed to patients once they have received care, for example the hospital cost of acetaminophen may be 10 cents for one 500 mg tablet. The patient charge may be $20.00 for that one tablet because of the indirect cost of staff processing and administering the medication.

Presently, nursing in most hospitals is not a separate cost center for patient charges; nursing is included in the overall room charge. Room charges for one day in a hospital room may be $1,000, and a certain percentage of that room charge is due to the cost of nursing care.

Fiscally, most organizations view nursing as a cost center that does not independently generate revenue. Although some

deviation from that fiscal philosophy may occur when nurse practitioners are permitted by law to bill directly for their unique professional services, the cost of providing nursing care (wages, benefits, supplies and equipment, overheads) is commonly bundled into a catchall room or per diem room charge that assumes that every patient consumes identical nursing resources each day. Such a view is not only antiquated, it is incorrect. Nursing care is not an identical product delivered in assembly line fashion. Nursing care varies remarkably in intensity, in depth, and in breadth across patients, consistent with patients' unique, individual needs.

The cost of providing nursing care varies by patient acuity, type of surgical procedure, primary diagnosis, secondary diagnosis, etc. Depending on the type of patient, nurses and hospitals need to know the cost of providing nursing care per patient day; per acuity-adjusted patient day; per hour; per visit; per **diagnosis-related group** (DRG); or even, per minute. Nursing costs can vary for the same patient during their hospital stay as the patient's needs change. A clear understanding of nursing costs is important so that nurses and hospitals have an improved understanding of the contribution that nursing makes to the organization as a whole. The information generated by improved cost information can be used to help nurses make effective decisions and to better control the cost of providing nursing services. Periodic nursing shortages make it even more important to understand the nursing resources needed by patients. Cost information is also useful for examining changes in the way nursing care is provided, for example the cost of Primary Nursing versus Team Nursing. When access to both nursing care and medical technology is needed, hospitalization is unquestionably appropriate. Consequently, the revenue generated from hospitalization is, in fact, payment primarily for consumption of medical technology and nursing services and should be recognized as such. The revenue generated from consumption of nursing resources should also be accurately assigned to each patient and charged at a rate consistent with the volume, acuity, and complexity of care consumed by that patient.

Ongoing efforts to measure and establish the cost of the diverse, yet related, components of nursing care are disappointing. Nursing care includes direct hands-on care, teaching, and coordinating discharge, as well as documentation, consultation, critical problem solving and decision making, and supervision of multiple levels of workers. These nursing care components contribute to the long-established cost of other practitioner and therapist services, yet the value, and thus the cost, of nursing care has eluded measurement and agreement. If all nurses became a part of practice teams or groups as physical therapists do, nurses could contract out nursing services to hospitals and then charge per patient. This would prevent nursing charges from being bundled with the room charge and other hospital charges. Nurses would no longer be hospital employees. They would be contracted professionals, just like physical therapists.

The efficiency and effectiveness of work flow and the way work is accomplished affects nursing workload also. This may involve something as simple as the nurse making multiple trips back and forth to access supplies in an awkward physical room arrangement and configuration of the work environment. It may also involve something as complex as making innovative adjustments to a familiar work pattern to accommodate physical, cognitive, behavioral, or sociocultural challenges presented by a "difficult" patient.

Diagnostic, Therapeutic, and Information Technology Cost

A common perception held by both society and the health care industry is that payroll costs constitute the largest expense item in organizational budgets and that the most expensive health care personnel are **registered nurses** (RNs). Therein lies the rush to downsize the number of RNs when a determination is made that costs need to be cut and better managed. Livanos (2018) describe a clear link between nurse-patient ratios and the size of the nurse's patient assignment and how well the nurse can do the job. With more patients to care for and higher patient acuity, patient morbidity and mortality increases. In recent years, patient safety has entered the nurse-to-patient ratio debate. For example, with mandated ratios for nursing in California, morbidity and mortality has decreased (Livanos, 2018).

Close examination of the entire hospital budget is likely to reveal that although the nursing payroll is the most expensive payroll item and the most expensive operating budget item, the most expensive item on the total budget is diagnostic, therapeutic, and information technology. This technology is required to meet society's demand for state-of-the-art care; professionals' demand for quicker, keener ways to work; and the organization's need to maintain a competitive business edge. Technology items characteristically appear in the capital budget because of their considerable cost. With cost management generally focused on the operating budget, the cost of diagnostic, therapeutic, and information technology is often conveniently overlooked because it is deemed "strategic" and therefore untouchable during cost-cutting initiatives.

Moreover, despite a rise in nursing payroll costs over the past 20 years, that rise has proportionately been considerably more gradual than that of diagnostic, therapeutic, and information technology, resulting in a widening gap in costs that suggests that nursing is a cost bargain.

Recently, managed health care programs have exerted oversight of the use of complex, expensive technology by requiring justification and approval prior to its use for payment to occur. Only when less costly approaches had been exhausted would the possibility of using highly specialized technology be considered. Diagnostically, movement has been away from "fishing expeditions" such as ordering the **Comprehensive Metabolic Panel** (CMP) and routine chest X-rays on all patients and toward completing only that diagnostic testing which is minimally required to reach a reasonable diagnosis based on overt signs and symptoms. The question that arises is whether assurance of correct diagnosis has been critically compromised or whether sharper clinical skill have resulted.

Use of the Computer to Capture Nursing Costs

Many hospitals are beginning to examine the use of computers to capture nursing costs. Computers will be much better at assisting in measuring the nursing resources expended on each patient when algorithms are developed that account for the cognitive and assessment work of nurses, as well as the physical care. At that point, the computer should be able to track sophisticated data on nursing resource usage by patient. With computers, nurses record not only when they are with each patient but also what they are doing for each patient. The specific cost of the nurse's care can be calculated by having the computer multiply the time spent with the patient by the salary of the nurse providing the care. When nurses are doing some indirect activities, such as documentation, the computer can also assign that cost to the appropriate patient, because the documentation is being done on the computer.

The computer system will need a fast way to record data so that it does not greatly increase the documentation work

---

Real World Interview

The ongoing and escalating shortage of nurses and other health care professionals may be the major health care issue well into the twenty-first century and at least for the next 20 years. There must be valid and reliable mechanisms for calculating the requirement for nursing care time and intensity.

Models of care delivery that maximize the use of **Nursing Assistive Personnel** (NAP) and provide for sufficient professional nursing expertise and time for both care delivery and supervision are a necessity. The number of nursing hours provided to each patient over a 24-hour period (nursing hours per patient day) that is commonly used to project staffing needs provides insufficient

and inadequate information for planning and staffing decisions that can best assure quality clinical outcomes for patients. Mechanisms used to track or predict nursing workload must be able to differentiate between the care that requires professional nurses and the care that can safely and effectively be done by NAP. Definitions and measurements of nursing workload must be standardized so that comparative data can be collected and analyzed.

Sheila Haas, PhD, RN
Dean and Professor
Loyola University, Chicago, Illinois

Evidence from the Literature

CITATION: Audet, L.-A., Bourgault, P., Rochefort, & Christian M. (2018, April). Association between nurse education and experience and the risk of mortality and adverse events in acute care hospitals: A systematic review of observational studies. *International Journal of Nursing Studies,* 80, 128–146.

Discussion: The aim of this study was to provide knowledge from the summarization of evidence on the relationships between RN education and experience and the occurrence of mortality and adverse events in acute care hospitals.

Prior studies have provided evidence that better nurse staffing (e.g., low nurse-to-patient ratios, higher nursing hours per patient per day, richer RN skill mixes) and supportive work environments are associated with lower risks of patient mortality and adverse events in acute care hospitals. There is mounting evidence that the characteristics of registered nurses, namely higher levels of education and more experience, are also associated with lower risks

of mortality and adverse events, but existing evidence remains scattered.

Higher levels of RN education were associated with lower risks of failure to rescue and mortality in 75% and 61.1% of the reviewed studies pertaining to these adverse events, respectively. There is emerging evidence that the 80% Bachelor of Science in Nursing degree threshold proposed by the Institute of Medicine is associated with shorter hospital stays and reduced risk of hospital readmissions.

Nursing Implications: This study further demonstrates the need to increase the overall BSN-prepared workforce. The research suggests that a more highly educated nurse workforce is needed and associated with better patient outcomes. Furthermore, policies are needed to help hospitals transition toward BSN staffing. These policies could include compensating hospitals for the nursing care required to produce better outcomes.

Evidence from the Literature

Citation: Marsa, L. (2017, September). Take charge of your health care: Surgeries and side effects (page 20). Accessed at aarp.org/health/conditions-treatments/info-2017/choose-a surgeon-doctor-surgeries.html.

Discussion: These are among the most common surgeries for Americans over 50 and the most common complications. In 2–4% of all cases, complications happen, and the patient needs to be readmitted to the hospital within 30 days.

Surgery	Complication	Occurrence
cataract removal	posterior capsule opacity	20%
pacemaker implant	hematoma	2.2% in patients over 70
colectomy	infection	12.4%
coronary artery bypass	atrial fibrillation	24%
hip replacement	dislocation	2%

Surgery	Complication	Occurrence
knee replacement	blood clot	1%
prostate removal	bleeding	5.3%
inguinal hernia	infection	0.3% open surgery 0.2% laparoscopic surgery
cholecystectomy	infection	7.6% open surgery 1% laparoscopic surgery
appendectomy	infection	4.3% open surgery 1.9% laparoscopic surgery

Implications for nursing:

Nurses must be aware of the higher incidence of complications in patients over 50 and work to implement health care strategies with the interprofessional team to limit the incidence of complications.

of the nurse. **Radio Frequency IDentification (RFID)** chips may eventually assist with that task. An RFID chip embedded in the nurse's name tag can be detected by a sensor in the door frame. The sensor is a data receiver that transmits information to the computer. It records the times of the nurse's entry into and exit from the patient's room and links that information with the patient's hospital identification (ID) number (Paaske, Bauer, Moser, & Seckman, 2017).

Impact of Health Care Reform Legislation on the Health Care Industry

Evidence-based concepts of quality are grounded on scientific evidence that a diagnostic or therapeutic approach improves patient outcomes. This concept exploded into the health care industry in the early 1990s with evidence-based clinical practices. The four core components of quality measurement are:

Increased quality > Increased volume > Increased profit > Enhanced programs/services > Increased quality

Decreased quality > Decreased volume > Decreased profit > Cutting corners > Decreased quality

FIGURE 6.4   Increased quality vs. decreased quality. *Source:* Created by L. Stuckey, D. A. Cherubini & S. A. Sacco.

1. A mechanism that establishes local or regional consensus about what constitutes the best practices based on scientific research findings,

2. Strong feasible processes to accomplish such practices,

3. A deliberate program of outreach to the community on disease prevention and health promotion, and

4. A rigorous system to review actual performance and clinical outcomes, as well as identification and implementation of improvement methodologies that achieve a dynamic balance between economy and quality.

Regardless of its particular size or mission, every contemporary health care **enterprise** (an organization of any size, established as a business venture) must commit to cost improvement and quality improvement as core goals for strategic business and clinical success. Clearly, this is not a new notion, but the recent intensification of the focus on cost and quality improvement and its expansion from hospitals to diverse ambulatory and home care sites is startling (Moyer, 2018). The more critical cost containment and cost improvement become, the more critical attention to quality improvement becomes. Quality and cost are inextricably linked.

Logic suggests that increased quality could lead to an increased volume of use of the organization by patients and providers who have the flexibility to make choices about where they seek health care. Increased volume generally leads to increased profits, which, in turn, may be directed toward enhanced programs/services, thus achieving increased quality, a very positive spiral that can result in the organization's thriving. An obverse spiral is more likely when quality is shoddy, a very negative and potentially fatal spiral (Figure 6.4).

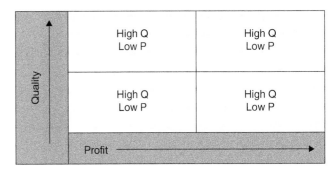

FIGURE 6.5   Nosek-Androwich profit quality (NAPQ) matrix. *Source:* Created by L. Stuckey, D. A. Cherubini & S. A. Sacco.

Nosek-Androwich Profit Quality (NAPQ) Matrix

Securing a profit might suggest that high quality is also secured, because it facilitates purchase of state-of-the-art equipment and the hiring of expert practitioners. Quality and profit do not necessarily go together, however. The Nosek-Androwich Profit Quality (NAPQ) Matrix (Figure 6.5) identifies four possible relationships between high or low profit and high or low quality that may exist in a health care organization. Any organization can fit into any quadrant, and a single organization may shift among quadrants from time to time in response to market forces. The challenge for the organization is to maintain its place in the high-profit, high-quality quadrant to be best positioned for both clinical success and business success, the mission of the organization. A common mission, consistent vision, collaboration, and constant vigilance to the elements of quality and profit by all employees and stakeholders together are keys to maintaining organizational positioning and achieving economic and quality success.

Critical Thinking 6.3

Access the annual report published by any health care enterprise. Based on the profit margin reported by the finance department, as compared to the rule of thumb of the 3–5% margin required for business success, would you rate that organization as high profit or as low profit? Based on the overall satisfaction score reported for all services of that organization, would you rate it as high quality or as low quality? (Hint: If the satisfaction score is not published, it may be because that score is relatively low.) In which quadrant of the NAPQ Matrix (Figure 6.5) does the health care enterprise fit?

Customer Satisfaction

Regardless of how superior an organization may perceive its product or service to be, if customers fail to perceive it as a needed or wanted service provided conveniently by skilled and knowledgeable people in a caring manner at a reasonable cost and consistent with their own culture and value system, the organization may fail. Perception, accurate or not, is the key. Therefore, organizations use a variety of indices to measure both internal and external customer satisfaction.

Commercial surveys, such as Press-Ganey, measure how satisfied patients are with their care, food, physical environment, emotional ambiance, and interactions with various health care workers, and then provide comparison rankings across similar organizations and populations nationally. The Veterans Affairs system of hospitals conducts its own unique patient satisfaction survey after patient discharge. Hospital Consumer Assessment of Healthcare Providers and Systems (HCAHPS) surveys are also becoming increasingly important for organizations to maintain market share

---

Real World Interview

The Joint Commission (TJC) is a nonprofit organization that is committed to continuously improve the safety and quality of health care provided to the public. TJC accomplishes this mission primarily through regular inspection and survey of health care organizations by a multidisciplinary professional team using extensive standardized measures of facility, clinical care, and material standards that support improvement in quality. A health care organization is assigned a numeric score that must meet a minimum level for the enterprise to be accredited. TJC currently accredits nearly 21,000 health care organizations in the United States, including burn hospitals and home care organizations, and more than 8,000 organizations that provide long-term care or behavioral health care, as well as laboratory and ambulatory services. Extensive

education about the nature of quality and how to best achieve it is also provided to health care enterprises by TJC.

Health care organizations commit a great deal of time and energy to preparing for both prescheduled and "surprise" on-site surveys, in order to successfully comply with TJC standards and receive a favorable accreditation status. TJC standards are developed through a definitive process of input from the field, expert consultation, and research to validate each standard as a measure of quality.

Sally A. Sample, RN, MN, ND, DSc, FAAN
Nurse at Large, Board of Governors, Joint Commission
Tucson, Arizona

Real World Interview

One generally does not associate nurse practice acts with nursing economics. However, a connection can be formulated. Nurse practice acts delineate scope of practice and define the educational preparation necessary to perform nursing care. These nurse practice acts restrict the health care agencies from unilaterally determining that an RN, practical nurse, or nursing assistant may work beyond their scope of practice. The health care agencies must

conform to the law and employ qualified nurses, which invariably impacts health care costs.

ANITA RISTAU, RN, MS
Executive Director, Vermont State Board of Nursing
Montpelier, Vermont

Case Study 6.1

You have just been hired as a nurse in a home care agency. One of the first things you noticed when you took a tour of the agency during your interview process was the disarray of the supply area. In fact, as you peered into the area, you overheard a staff member letting off frustration at once again not being able to find the supplies he needed for his day's assignments. Although he looked a bit sheepish, your tour guide quickly dismissed the incident, stating that a STAT delivery of the supplies could easily and promptly be arranged. Now that you are an employee, you too are having difficulty locating things in that supply area. Broken and outdated

supplies take up significant space and new supplies sit unopened in stacks around the room. No one seems to have the time or interest to change the situation. You volunteer to lead a team effort to improve both the quality and the cost impact of the lack of organization in the supply area.

What method will you use to identify the issues?

What are some of the issues the staff might identify?

What are some of the options the staff might identify to address the issues?

How will you implement the options chosen?

and avoid losing reimbursement. Under VBP programs, hospitals with lower HCAHPS scores can be financially penalized. Many organizations use instruments developed internally to measure attributes of unique interest to that organization. Research protocols use a variety of statistical methods to test satisfaction. Results of such surveys are analyzed as part of the organization's quality improvement program.

KEY CONCEPTS

- Health care economics is grounded in past values and culture. Nearly 150 years ago, Florence Nightingale recognized that the resources being used to care for sick people ought to be tracked and analyzed to improve clinical and business outcomes.

- Nurses at all levels of all health care organizations are responsible for basic economic processes.

- Contemporary health care is characterized as a business struggling to balance cost and quality. Patients are fearful that health care is rapidly becoming unaffordable and they are demanding care at a reasonable cost.

- In the United States, multiple programs exist to pay for health care. Managed care is a common nongovernmental structure for health care payment, with a variety of Health Maintenance Organizations (HMOs) operating independently and offering a variety of health insurance packages.

- The Medicare Hospital Value-Based Purchasing (VBP) Program is working to improve patient care quality and decrease costs.

- Government programs for eligible individuals are tax supported. Other industrialized countries around the world offer tax-supported socialized universal health care to every citizen, through centralized or decentralized programs, at about half of the U.S. per capita cost.

- An economic break-even formula can be used to compute the cost of health care equipment.

- The ability to track and manage both cost and quality is critical. To achieve the organization's economic and quality goals, administrators and clinicians at all levels and in diverse health care organizations must focus on a common mission and consistent vision to improve health care.

- Futurists agree that significant change will occur in the health care industry. They predict that the mechanism of change will be tumultuous. Futurists believe the focus on value received for dollars spent, the inextricable link of cost and quality, will grow.

- Quality measurement in organizations is supplemented by external regulatory bodies that oversee safety and quality on behalf of society. Satisfaction indices may be measured both internally and externally and then compared to the performance of similar organizations.

- The Nosek-Androwich Profit Quality Matrix identifies the balance between quality and profit.

KEY TERMS

Break-even point	Economics	Payer
Budget	Enterprise	Preferred provider organization (PPO)
Coinsurance amounts	Fixed cost	Reengineering
Copayment	Indirect cost	Relative value unit (RVU)
Deductible	Margin	Stakeholder
Direct cost	Patient classification system (PCS)	Variable cost

---

REVIEW QUESTIONS

1. The study of Economics is based on which of the following?
   a. Analysis of the distribution, production, and consumption of good and services.
   b. Maximizing profit.
   c. Interpreting health care legislation.
   d. Expediting billing and payment systems in a clinical setting.

2. Prior to the 1980s, the focus of health care was on which of the following?
   a. Limiting patient readmissions.
   b. Treatment of chronic conditions.
   c. Managing health care plan reimbursement requirements.
   d. Creating preventative health plans.

3. Total Quality Improvement (TQI) and Continuous Quality Improvement (CQI) programs were initiated to do which of the following?
   a. Assure society that cost management was not compromising safety or quality.
   b. Maximize cost reduction.
   c. Reduce hospital-acquired infections.
   d. Identify the most important stakeholders, including the practitioner and other professionals.

4. Which of the following is required under managed care?
   a. Quick discharge of patients.
   b. Extensive testing of patients.
   c. Rationing of care.
   d. Preapproval of care.

5. Nongovernmental health care has been predominantly accessed through which of the following sources?
   a. Doctor's offices and other clinical settings.
   b. Employment.
   c. HMOs.
   d. Preferred Provider Networks.

6. Canada has better outcomes in life expectancy than does the United States, but pays what amount for health care compared to the United States?
   a. The same.
   b. Much less.
   c. Much more.
   d. Less than half.

7. The only industrialized country(ies) without universal health care is (are) which of the following?
   a. Canada and the United States.

   b. United States.
   c. United Kingdom and the United States.
   d. Canada, United States, and France.

8. Providers under the Medicare Pay-for-Performance (P4P) program are which of the following?
   a. Paid based on results of patient outcomes.
   b. Paid the same way as fee-for-service
   c. Paid based on patient volume.
   d. Paid based on quality of care, but not efficiency.

9. The economic cost equation of businesses is which of the following?
   a. Mission = Quality = Training
   b. Money = Technology = Efficiency
   c. Money = Mission = Money
   d. Money = Margin = Profits

10. A direct cost is which of the following?
   a. Not explicitly related to patient care within a manager's unit.
   b. Varies with volume and depends on the number of patients.
   c. Amount by which revenue from sales exceeds costs.
   d. Directly related to patient care within a manager's unit.

REVIEW QUESTION ANSWERS

1. Answer: A is correct.
   Rationale: Health care economics studies effectiveness and efficiency in the delivery of health care and the operational use of health care systems. The study of economics is based on the (A) analysis of the distribution, production, and consumption of goods and services. This analysis of these economic activities is based on certain related principles. (B) maximizing profit, (C) interpreting health care legislation, or (D) expediting billing and payment systems in a clinical setting is not the study of economics.

2. Answer: B is correct.
   Rationale: Prior to the 1980s, the focus of health care was on the (B) treatment of chronic conditions such as diabetes, heart disease, and cancer. This method of health care delivery is very costly due to possible patient needs of maintenance medications, cancer treatments, and evaluation using expensive medical equipment. (A) Limiting patient readmissions was not the focus of health care prior to the 1980s. After the 1980s, the focus was on (C) managing health care plan reimbursement requirements and (D) creating preventative health plans.

3. Answer: A is correct.
   Rationale: Total quality improvement (TQI) and continuous quality improvement (CQI) programs were initiated (A) to assure society that cost management was not compromising safety or quality. These programs required all stakeholders, including patients, to work together to evaluate and improve outcomes. The expertise of allied health care providers was recognized, and through the growing access to information technology, consumers were empowered to better understand their own health, the complex technologies available, their options for choosing to manage the decisions about their care, and the cost implications

of those decisions. TQI and CQI were not initiated to (B) maximize cost reduction, (C) reduce hospital-acquired infections, or (D) identify the most important stakeholders including the practitioner and other professionals.

4. Answer: D is correct.
   Rationale: Managed care is the product of a series of efforts to establish an effective program for all stakeholders. Managed care has resulted in a complex, still-evolving array of structures and processes to deliver health care. (D) Preapproval of health care for insurance is required under managed care, and health care coverage is selective, effectively rationing care. Managed care does not require (A) quick discharge of patients, (B) extensive testing of patients, or (C) rationing of care.

5. Answer: B is correct.
   Rationale: Nongovernmental health insurance has predominantly been accessed in the U.S. through (B) employment. Employers provide coverage to employees as a benefit for working for their company. Therefore, the employer chooses the coverage with cost in mind and negotiates an acceptable package of benefits on behalf of the employees. If the employer offers a selection of benefit packages, the employee may choose the package that is most suitable. Nongovernmental health insurance is not accessed through (A) Doctor's offices and other clinical settings. The range of benefit packages available through employers has narrowed to being nearly exclusively HMOs but (C) they are not accessed through HMOs, or (D) Preferred Provider Networks.

6. Answer: D is correct.
   Rationale: Canada has better outcomes in infant mortality and life expectancy than the United States but pays (D) less than half the amount for health care. Canada does not pay (A) the same, (B) much less, or (C) much more for health care compared to the United States.

7. Answer: B is correct.
   Rationale: A major difference between the United States and the other countries in the study is that the (B) United States is the only industrialized country without universal health care. (A) Canada has universal health care but the United States does not. (C) The United Kingdom has universal health care but the United States does not. (D) Canada and France all have universal health care but the United States does not.

8. Answer: A is correct.
   Rationale: Medicare Pay-for-Performance are rewarded (A) based on results of patient outcomes. Based on the results of patient outcomes, health care providers under this P4P arrangement are rewarded based on the results of improved patient outcomes, efficacy of care, and long-term outcomes related to improved patient outcomes and health care costs. P4P programs are not (B) paid the same way as fee-for-service, or (C) paid based on patient volume, or (D) based on quality of care, but not efficiency.

9. Answer: C is correct.
   Rationale: The economic cost equation is: (C) MONEY = MISSION = MONEY. The equation is not (A) Mission = Quality = Training, (B) Money = Technology = Efficiency, or (D) Money = Margin = Profits.

10. Answer: D is correct.
    Rationale: A **direct cost** is (D) directly related to patient care within a manager's unit, such as the cost of nurses' wages and the cost of patient care supplies. Indirect costs are (A) not explicitly related to patient care within a manager's unit. Variable costs (B) varies with volume and depends on the number of patients. Margin is the (C) amount by which revenue from sales exceeds costs.

REVIEW ACTIVITIES

1. Using the formula provided in this chapter, determine the cost of nursing care for the past 24 hours for a unit where you have had recent clinical experience.

2. With your nursing faculty's permission, invite the head nurse of a unit where you have your current clinical experiences to your post-conference to gain an understanding of how various costs are managed. Use the following questions to guide the interview:

   • What method is used to measure nursing cost?

   • What percentage of profit did the organization make last year, and how was it allocated after profit was made? How typical is this?

   • Which therapists' services are billed directly?

3. With your nursing faculty's permission, invite the head nurse of a unit where you have your current clinical experiences to your post-conference to explore what the most challenging clinical economic issue currently is for nursing in the organization and how it is being addressed.

4. Consult a seasoned member of the medical staff for a personal perspective on the adjustments in practice that person made, if any, related to cost and quality issues in practice as his or her career unfolded. Compare and contrast what you discover to be the experiences of a second member of the medical staff you consult who has been in practice for only the past 10 years. What level of passion about the discussion was demonstrated by each interviewee? What did they view as their greatest challenge?

DISCUSSION POINTS

1. What appeals to you about any of the health care economics in this chapter?

2. During your last clinical experience, were there any insurance or Medicare questions brought forth by patients?

3. What suggestions do you have for how health care enterprises can balance quality and profit?

DISCUSSION OF OPENING SCENARIO

1. What do you think the perceived issue is with the hospital?
   a. Answer. You certainly perceive the problem differently from the hospital. Your injury requires immediate medical attention. That is your sole interest. The hospital's perceived issue is with payment for their services.

2. Do you see the problem the same way the hospital does?
   a. Answer. The hospital views your injury and treatment in a more business-like manner and is considering cost and reimbursement issues related to your situation. As a patient, you would not see the problem in the same way as the hospital does. Your focus is on your injuries and receiving treatment.

3. When cost is removed from the equation, what drives the decision to provide or not provide health care?
   a. Answer. When cost is removed from the situation, both patient and health care provider are similarly focused on adequate treatment and a favorable patient outcome.

4. If cost were not a driving consideration in providing health care in the United States, what would the health care system be like?
   a. Answer. In the United States, if cost was not a primary consideration in providing health care, coverage might be more universal for its citizens and potentially improve overall quality and efficiency. More people would have access to health care and be able to receive treatment.

EXPLORING THE WEB

- Centers for Medicare & Medicaid Services, www.cms.hhs.gov, accessed July 10, 2019.

- Bureau of Labor Statistics, www.stats.bls.gov, accessed July 10, 2019.

- Health Catalyst, www.healthcatalyst.com/insights/top-7-health-care-outcome-measures, accessed July 10, 2019.

- Medicare Rights, www.medicarerights.org, accessed July 10, 2019.

INFORMATICS

1. Go to the Commonwealth Fund site, www.commonwealthfund. org/publications/newsletter-article/using-patient-reported-outcomes-improve-health-care-quality (accessed 6/28/2019). Search for the article "Using Patient-Reported Outcomes to Improve Health Care Quality" for ways that patient-reported outcome measures can help improve the health of patients.

2. Review the article at www.ncbi.nlm.nih.gov/pmc/articles/ PMC5242136 (accessed June 28, 2019). Identify ways that health care outcomes can be improved through patient education and partnerships.

3. Review the Medicare links at http://qsen.org/faculty-resources/ practice/miscellaneousmedicare (accessed July 15, 2019). Identify what Medicare will and will not cover for home health services. Discuss who is eligible for Medicare and how much it will cost the patient.

LEAN BACK

- How does this information about health care economics impact you today as a student nurse?

- How do you see this impacting you as you start your career as a nurse?

REFERENCES

Abdellah, F., Beland, I., Martin, A., & Matheney, R. (1960). *Patient centered approaches to nursing*. New York: Macmillan.

Affordable Care Act. (2010). *Patient protection and affordable care act*. Retrieved from www.healthcare.gov/glossary/patient-protection-and-affordable-care-act/

Affordable Health Care for Americans. (2010, March 20). *The health insurance exchanges, house committees on ways and means, energy and commerce, and education and labor*. Retrieved from http://docs.house.gov/energycommerce/EXCHANGE.pdf

Commonwealth Fund. (2017). *Mirror, mirror 2017: International comparison reflects flaws and opportunities for better U.S. health care*. Retrieved from https://interactives.commonwealthfund.org/2017/july/mirror-mirror

Erin, D., Bouldin, E. M., Andresen, N. E., Dunton, M., Simon, T. M., Waters, T.M., Liu, M., Daniels, M., Mion, L., & Shorr, R. (2013). *Falls among Adult Patients Hospitalized in the United States: Prevalence and Trends*. *Journal of Patient Safety, 9*, 13–17.

Fay, B. (2018). *Hospital and Surgery Costs, 2018. Average Costs for Common Surgeries*. Retrieved from www.debt.org/medical/hospital-surgery-costs

Giannasi, A., & Rudman, J. (2018). Using the care hours per patient day tool: One hospital's experience. British Journal of Nursing, 27(3), 156–160. doi:10.12968/bjon.2018.27.3.156

Henderson, V., & Nite, G. (1978). *Principles and practice of nursing* (6th ed.). New York: Macmillan.

Huelskoetter, T. (2018). *Evaluating State Innovations to Reduce Health Care*. Retrieved from www.americanprogress.org/issues/healthcare/reports/2018/04/06/448912/evaluating-state-innovations-reduce-health-care-costs

Institute of Medicine of the National Academies. (2010). *The future of nursing: leading change, advancing health*. Report Brief. Retrieved from www.iom.edu/nursing

Institute of Medicine of the National Academies. (2015). *The future of nursing: leading change, advancing health*. Report Brief. Retrieved from www.annanurse.org/article/iom-releases-report-assessing-progress-future-nursing-report-december-04-15

Johns Hopkins Bloomberg School of Public Health. (2019). *What is public health*. Retrieved from www.jhsph.edu/admissions/how-to-apply/prospectus-request/_pdf/2018-2019_prospectus.pdf

Kamal, R., Sawyer, B., & McDermott, D. (2018). *How much is health spending expected to grow?* Retrieved from www.healthsystemtracker.org/chart-collection/much-health-spending-expected-grow/#item-start

Kliger, J., Lacey, S. R., Olney, A., Cox, K. S., & O'Neil, E. (2010). Nurse-driven programs to improve patient outcomes: Transforming care at the bedside, integrated nurse leadership program, and the clinical scene investigator academy. *Journal of Nursing Administration, 40*(3), 109–114.

Life Expectancy. (2006). Retrieved from www.en.Wikipedia.org

Livanos, N. (2018). A broadening coalition: Patient safety enters the nurse-to-patient ratio debate. *Journal of Nursing Regulation, 9*(1), 68–70.

Makary, M. A., & Daniel, M. (2016). Medical error—The third leading cause of death in the US. *British Medical Journal, 353*. doi:10.1136/bmj.i2139

Moyer, A. (2018). A quality improvement project for understanding work-based need in ambulatory care. *Nursing Economics, 36*(6), 276–290. Retrieved from www.nursingeconomics.net/cgi-bin/WebObjects/NECJournal.woa

Nightingale, F. (1859). Notes on hospitals; being two papers read before the National Association for the Promotion of Social Science, at Liverpool in October, 1858. With evidence given to the Royal Commissioners on the State of the Army in 1857 (2). London: Parker.

Nosek, L. J. & Androwich, I. M. (2012). Basic Clinical Health Care Economics in Kelly, P., (2012) Nursing Leadership and Management (2nd ed.). Clifton Park, NY. Delmar Cengage Learning.

O'Rourke, T. W. (2017). Lost in the Health Care Reform Discussion: Health Care as a Right or Privilege. *American Journal of Health Education, 48*(3), 138-141.doi:10.1080/19325037.2017.1292879

Paaske, S., Bauer, A., Moser, T., & Seckman, C. (2017). The benefits and barriers to RFID technology in healthcare. *Online Journal of Nursing Informatics, 21*(2), 10–11. Retrieved from www.himss.org/ojni

State Health Access Data Assistance Center. (2014). *Paying for value in medicaid: A synthesis of advanced payment models in four states.* Retrieved from www.macpac.gov/wp-content/uploads/2015/01/MACPAC_Visits_Final-Report-Feb-2014.pdf

Public Health Action Team. (2017). Available at https://sph.umich.edu/practice/centers-and-programs/phast/

Serb, C. (2006). Financial fitness test: 10 ways to get in shape for a new payment era. *Hospitals & Health Networks,* 34–36, 38, 40, 49

Society for Human Resource Management – Stephen Miller. (2018). *For 2019, employers adjust health benefits as costs near $15,000 per employee.* Retrieved from www.shrm.org/resourcesandtools/hrtopics/benefits/pages/employers-adjust-health-benefits-for-2019.aspx

The 2010 Patient Protection and Affordable Care Act. (2010). Retrieved from www.gpo.gov/fdsys/pkg/PLAW-111publ148/pdf/PLAW-111publ148.pdf

Vogenberg, F. R., & Santilli, J. (2018). Healthcare trends for 2018. *American Health Drug Benefits, 11,* 48–54.

Zaichkin, D. L. (2018). Financial principles for nurse leaders. In *Essential knowledge for CNL and APRN nurse leaders.* Springer Publishing (pp. 197).

SUGGESTED READINGS

Elton, J. (2016). *Healthcare disrupted: Next generation business models and strategies*

Gawande, A. (2015). *Being mortal: Medicine and what matters in the end.*

Goran, R., Gleason, S., & Ridic, O. (2012). *Comparisons of health care systems in the United States, Germany and Canada.* Retrieved from www.ncbi.nlm.nih.gov/pmc/articles/PMC3633404

Jones, B. (2018). *Healthcare is in "an economic boom," and that means it's time to plan for disruption.* Retrieved from www.healthcarefinancenews.com/news/healthcare-economic-boom-and-means-its-time-time-plan-disruption

Kamal, R. & Cox, C. (2018). *How has U.S. spending on healthcare changed over time?.* Retrieved from www.healthsystemtracker.org/chart-collection/u-s-spending-healthcare-changed-time

Pauley, M. & Field, R. (2018). *Beyond Obamacare: What's ahead for U.S. health care in 2018.* Wharton School of the University of Pennsylvania. Retrieved from http://knowledge.wharton.upenn.edu/article/the-future-of-the-aca

Rosenthal, E. (2018). *An American sickness: How healthcare became big business and how you can take it back New York, NY: Penguin Books.*

Sahadi, J. (2018). *Warren buffet is right. Health care costs are swallowing the economy.* CNN Business. Retrieved from https://money.cnn.com/2018/01/30/news/economy/health-care-costs-eating-the-economy/index.html

Sisko, A., & Keehan, S. (2019). *National health expenditure projections, 2018–2027: Economic and demographic trends drive spending and enrollment growth.* Retrieved from www.healthaffairs.org/doi/10.1377/hlthaff.2018.05499

7 Hospital Department and Unit Budgets

Isabelle Clarke Garibaldi
LifePoint-Sumner Regional Medical Center, Gallatin, TN, USA

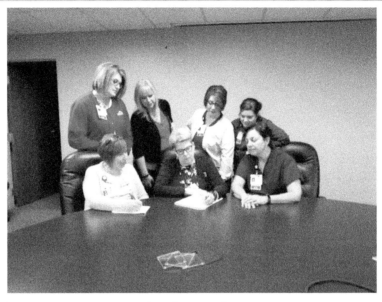

Nursing Team Budget Meeting: L-R FRONT: Gail Gerth, RN; Cathy Batzner, RN; Rose Burns, RN; L-R BACK: Katie Kerwin, RN; Nicole Salas, RN; Jessica Pech, RN; Leanne Seifert, RN.

By getting involved in the management of budgets, you will have the ability to convert what could be merely an academic interest in cost and value into practical activities and subsequent results.

(*Walsh*, 2016)

The nurse work environment, defined as characteristics of a practice setting that facilitate or constrain professional nursing practice, has been linked to patient outcomes. Interventions to improve nurse engagement, and adequate staffing serve as strategies to improve patient safety.

(*Brooks Carthon et al.*, 2019)

OBJECTIVES

Upon completion of this chapter, the reader should be able to:

1. Comprehend commonly used types of budgets for planning and management.
2. Identify the budget preparation process for health care organizations.
3. Comprehend key elements that influence budget preparation and monitoring.
4. Identify revenue opportunities associated with patient care delivery.
5. Identify expense liabilities associated with organizational management and patient care delivery.
6. Discuss components of the budgeting process and roles that the health care team have in that process.
7. Understand and discuss factors that influence reimbursement.

Kelly Vana's Nursing Leadership and Management, Fourth Edition. Edited by Patricia Kelly Vana and Janice Tazbir
© 2021 John Wiley & Sons Ltd. Published 2021 by John Wiley & Sons Ltd.
Companion Website: www.wiley.com/go/kelly-Nursing-Leadership

You are a nursing student assigned to a medical/surgical inpatient unit at an acute care hospital for one of your clinical experiences. As you interact with the nursing unit manager, you wish to determine what types of services are provided to patients on this unit and how the costs for these services are controlled. Activities to engage in with your instructor and the nursing unit manager include a review the organization's strategic plan, the departmental budget, and the unit's scope of service. Questions to ask the instructor and nurse manager may include:

- What types of patients are cared for on this unit?
- Is the unit's scope of service limited to specific patient diagnosis types or age groups?
- How does the staffing model help ensure provision of care for patients on this unit?
- How would staffing fluctuations or shortages affect the staffing model?
- What are the productivity targets for this unit?

Introduction

The role of the nurse is not limited to bedside patient care. Nurses are also an integral part of decision-making processes by which patient care is delivered. A key component of those processes is the cost involved in the delivery of services. Both human and material resources are required to support patient care delivered by nurses and clinical support staff. These resources cost money. The overall economic success of a health care organization depends on those who appropriately manage care and resources on the unit and at the bedside. The decline in health care reimbursement, rising patient care costs, and aggressive interfacility competition for patient volume growth and cash flow requires hospitals to improve operational efficiency and make sound economic decisions (Phelps & Madhavan, 2018). Despite these challenges, the challenge for health care leaders must also ensure that the quality of care and the quality of staff competence are not compromised in our heavily monitored health care environment.

Nurses need to understand how to manage the cost of patient care as it relates to their own clinical practice. Nurses are uniquely accountable for the distribution and utilization of organizational resources. Therefore, it is essential that appropriate decisions be made regarding cost-effective practices. Cost containment affects nursing department finances, the patient bill, and ultimately the organization itself. Nurses must be informed and collaborate with their management team to deliver quality care while controlling expenses in an accountable and responsible manner. Regulatory and accrediting health care organizations, such as **The Joint Commission** (TJC) and the Centers for Medicare and Medicaid Services (CMS), assert that departmental budgets should be developed as a collaborative effort between an organization's leadership and its frontline staff.

The purpose of this chapter is to provide an overview of budget preparation and development, introduce commonly used types of budgets for planning and management, and to provide a framework for further discussion about the budgeting process as it applies in health care organizations. Common financial language is discussed so novice nurses can understand the processes involved in high-quality, cost-effective patient care delivery.

Types of Budgets

Health care organizations use several types of budget frameworks to facilitate operational management and future business planning. These types of budgets include operational, capital, and construction budgets. A budget's scope can be large (system level) or small (unit level); and serves as a standard to plan, monitor, and evaluate the performance of a health care system, an individual facility, a department, or a unit over a specified period of time.

Operational Budget

An **operational budget** accounts for the daily activity associated with revenue and expenses, generated from patient care and operational functions. Revenue generation in a health care organization is based upon billable services and costs associated with equipment, supplies, staffing, and indirect expenses. Revenue can be generated from the time spent on care delivery, such as the number of days that a patient stays on an inpatient unit or the number and frequency of visits in an outpatient setting. Revenue may be also be generated from procedural activities such as the type, intensity, and length of services delivered to a patient in an operating room.

Controlling expenses is equally as important as revenue generation. Labor costs, supply costs, and variable daily operating expenses need to be monitored and analyzed frequently. Supply utilization and expense control can be influenced by front-line caregivers, and nurses in particular. Depending on reimbursement rates and requirements, expenses are sometimes "bundled" together or included in procedure costs or room charges. An example of bundled expenses are inpatient admission supplies. These supplies are provided to patients by the health care organization, and normally include a wash-basin, water bottle, non-skid socks, and a toothbrush/toothpaste. It is also important to note that some departments within organizations charge separately for supply items. This is particularly true in procedural areas such as operating rooms, interventional radiology/cardiology suites, and emergency departments. Examples of unbundled, individually billed items include intravenous (IV) tubing, leukocyte removal filters, nasogastric tubes, ventilator set-up kits, wound care items, and specialized dressings.

Hospitals and other health care facilities will have a variety of charge capture methods to ensure that both bundled and unbundled items are charged appropriately, and then correctly applied to the patient's bill. These methods include barcode scanning and computer-based charge set-up programs. Some less automated organizations may use a charge method requiring a manual "sticker" system in order to capture patient charges. Using this manual system, staff remove stickers from packaged items, which are then placed on a patient-specific tracking log or materials management charging card. The log is eventually sent to either the facility's materials management or finance department for computerized application to the patient bill.

Operational budgets are typically adjusted annually to meet the every-changing health care environment. Adjustments to planned budgets are made for a variety of reasons, including fluctuating product and services costs, supply variations, and the use of group purchasing /vendor contracts. Group purchasing/vendor contracts are an area often scrutinized very closely regarding expense control. These contracts are negotiated/ renegotiated so that:

- Predetermined reduced rates can be realized when organizations purchase large quantities of supplies.

- An organization realizes **economies of scale,** which are cost advantages that organizations obtain due to the quantity of item(s) used. This occurs when the cost per item decreases as its widespread use increases, i.e., the more a product is used, the more an organization can negotiate a lower cost-per-item rate.

- The organization can benefit financially from being a part of a multi-facility purchasing group.

For example, if a hospital purchases a large quantity of one product, the vendor may reduce the price below the list price as an incentive for the organization to remain a loyal customer. Additionally, if a hospital can demonstrate that a particular product is used at a certain percentage level across its enterprise (e.g., 90% of all facilities within a health care corporation use the same antibacterial soap), then a reduced rate may also be offered by the vendor.

Capital Budget

Capital budgets account for the purchase or replacement of major equipment. Equipment is usually purchased or replaced when:

- New technology becomes available.

- Older equipment becomes too expensive to maintain.

- Equipment is no longer contractually or operationally supported by the original vendor.

- Accreditation and regulatory bodies require equipment or technology updates for patient safety standard(s) compliance.

- Age-related inefficiencies and interface issues make it more practical to replace equipment.

Significant expense is associated with equipment acquisition; therefore, organizations want to make informed, fiscally responsible decisions. Staff members who are stakeholders in the acquisition of capital equipment and the budgeting process have diverse, specialized input in the decisional process. For these reasons, staff members from a variety of areas, including materials management, clinical units, legal counsel, biomedical engineering, information technology services, the board of directors, the finance department, and executive administration, often participate in planning for capital purchases. A substantial analysis of a capital purchases is required because equipment features, interdepartmental integration, benefits, and limitations must be understood as they relate to a department and/or institutional needs and goals. Often, multiple vendors or companies sell similar products with variable features, contract terms and conditions, warranties, and maintenance agreements. These variables can have short- and long-term effects on a facility's budget over time. For example, a thorough analysis of capital purchase variables may help avoid purchase decisions that may not integrate with other facility systems or may be too expensive to maintain over time. Thinking globally regarding capital purchases will prevent operationalization mistakes once purchases have been initiated (Sussman, 2017).

Organizations differ greatly regarding the dollar amount that is considered a capital acquisition. Small, stand-alone organizations may set capital expense thresholds beginning at $1,000.00 USD. Larger, integrated organizations may consider capital expense items at purchase prices beyond $100,000.00 USD. Capital expense thresholds vary, and are generally set by the Board of Directors, corporate partners, and the organization's finance department. Capital acquisition purchases will generally meet certain criteria. These criteria include:

- A dollar expenditure threshold
- The ability to be applied or utilized across the facility (not single-patient use), and
- Vendor-supported lifespan greater than two years.

A multi-patient use item such as a CT scanner is an example of capital budget item. The CT scanner is a capital item because its expected cost is greater than $500,000 USD, its use is not directly tied to one specific patient, and its vendor-supported useful life expectancy is seven to 10 years. Intracoronary stents and conductivity devices, such as pacemakers and implantable defibrillators, are used routinely in the **cardiac catheterization laboratory** (CCL). Costs for these items can range from $2,000.00 USD to $65,000.00 USD or more, with costs fluctuating widely by vendor. Stents, pacemakers, and implantable defibrillators are examples of equipment which are direct patient care/direct patient cost items. They are not considered a capital expense because they are single-use items for one specific patient.

Construction Budget

A **construction budget** is developed when an organization plans renovation or when new structures are needed. It typically includes construction labor, materials, building permits, inspections, equipment for the renovation or new structure, architectural planning, and legal costs. If it is anticipated that a unit or department will need to close or limit services during construction, any projected lost revenue is also accounted for in the construction budget. In order to avoid closing units or limiting services during the construction period, organizations may shift revenue and expenses to a secondary department. The secondary department will, of course, absorb costs and gain revenue from the delivery of services on this temporary basis.

Budgeting Process Overview

The budgeting process refers to the manner through which organizations create and approve a budget. During this process, organizations use financial data that outline anticipated revenue and expenses over a specified period. The budget process translates operational plans into financial and statistical terms. Budgeting requires forward thinking so operational tactics, capital expenditures, and construction projects are appropriately planned, integrated, and designed. The budgeting process helps the organization analyze items and services by projecting how **revenue** and **expenses** are generated. Revenue is simply the income generated from doing business. Expenses are costs incurred to do that business. The budget and budgeting processes also serve as a

yardstick to measure whether the planning expectations were realistic and if revenue and expense reduction benchmarks can actually be met. Typically, budgets are monitored daily and reviewed monthly at the unit level so that if variances occur, corrective action plans can be instituted early. Corrective action plans are often initiated to prevent long-term effects in a particular area such as unintended waste, low productivity, or supply loss. Finally, high-functioning organizations use budgets as tools to foster collaboration and function between departments so organization goals can be achieved.

The budget and budgeting processes are also used to project and document **profit** or **loss.** Profit results when revenue exceeds expenses and conversely, loss results when expenses exceed revenue. Organizational profitability results when overall revenue is higher than expenses over time. Budgets also connect operational planning with the allocation of resources. This is especially important because health care organizations measure multiple performance, or "key" indicators of performance over time. All these indicators are intertwined and hold value in terms of patient care and operational excellence. A performance scorecard**, or **dashboard,** is a documentation tool which uses a snapshot image in time of pertinent operational information and activities. The purpose of dashboard is to provide a visual pulse of how a unit, department, or facility is achieving its goals. Dashboards visually illustrate a variety of **key performance indicators** that demonstrate the connectivity between two or more data points, such as financial performance and quality outcomes. These key performance indicators usually consider financial performance, customer satisfaction, patient outcomes, internal operating efficiency (productivity), and organizational growth. For example, along with financial performance, organizations routinely evaluate quality patient outcomes indicators, patient satisfaction with care, and departmental productivity. Dashboards gage monthly progress and culminate with **year-to-date** (YTD) statistics. Scorecards and dashboards may also give rise to the creation of organization-specific dynamic reports that help health care managers consistently measure performance, detect outliers, analyze causes of performance, communicate performance to staff, and plan for the future (Ghazisaeidi et al., 2015). A scorecard or dashboard can also help the nurse manager quickly identify key performance indicators which require organizational focus and action.

Table 7.1 displays the measurable activity for a perioperative care department using a dashboard platform. It includes the specific patient care units of surgery, post-anesthesia recovery, and sterile processing. The dashboard reports and analyzes actual results in relation to specific quality or financial goals for each area of performance. Any **variance** is the difference between what was expected and the actual result. Overall performance is monitored through the identification of key activities. These activities are depicted on the dashboard (Table 7.1) and reflect service excellence (quality and service), customer approval for care provided (patient satisfaction),

Table 7.1   Perioperative Services Dashboard

Perioperative Services Dashboard					
Quality and Service	**Goal/Tool**	**Year**	**January**	**February**	**YTD**
Operating Room Turnaround Time	GOAL: <20 min TOOL: EMR data	Goal	20 min	20 min	20 min
		Actual	21 min	18 min	19.5 min
Sterile Processing of Instrumentation: Immediate Use Sterilization (I US) Rate	GOAL: <3% TOOL: EMR data	Goal	3.00%	3.00%	3.00%
		Actual	2.20%	5.17%	3.69%
First Case/On-Time Start	GOAL: >95% TOOL: EMR data	Goal	95.00%	95.00%	95.00%
		Actual	91.20%	96.23%	93.72%
Patient Satisfaction	**Goal/Tool**	**2018**	**January**	**February**	**YTD**
Overall Satisfaction with Care: Hospital-wide	GOAL: >85% TOOL: Press Ganey/ HCAHPS	Goal	85.00%	85.00%	85.00%
		Actual	85.20%	88.00%	86.60%
Surgery/PACU - Satisfaction Re: Communication with Nurses	GOAL: >85% TOOL: Press Ganey/ HCAHPS	Goal	90.00%	90.00%	90.00%
		Actual	94.81%	91.88%	91.36%
Surgery/PACU - Pain: Communication and Attention to Needs	GOAL: >85% TOOL: Press Ganey/ HCAHPS	Goal	65.00%	65.00%	65.00%
		Actual	57.92%	66.42%	62.17%
High Performing Workforce	**Goal/Tool**	**2018**	**January**	**February**	**YTD**
RN Voluntary Turnover	GOAL: <15% Annually	Goal	15.00%	15.00%	15.00%
		Actual (cumulative)	6.25%	1.67%	7.92%
Percentage of RNs Surgery and PACU certified in specialty	GOAL: 75% certified	Goal	75.00%	75.00%	75.00%
		Actual	50.00%	62.00%	56.00%
Surgery: Total Man Hours/ Stat (Surgical Minutes)	GOAL: Stat met TOOL: Operational Budget	Goal	0.25	0.25	0.25
		Actual	0.24	0.22	0.23
		Variance	0.01	0.03	0.02
Operational Excellence	**Goal/Tool**	**2018**	**January**	**February**	**YTD**
Procedure Activity (# of cases)	GOAL: > Projection by 5% TOOL: Operational Budget	Goal	187	236	423
		Actual	172	257	429
		Variance	(0.025)	8.90%	1.014%
Total Revenue	GOAL: > Projection by 5% TOOL: Operational Budget	Goal	$ 1,749,680.00	$ 2,086,543.00	$ 3,836,223.00

Table 7.1 (Continued)

		Perioperative Services Dashboard			
		Variance	$ 1,658,696.64	$ 2,343,187.79	$ 4,308,078.43
		Actual	−5.20%	11.23%	11.23%
Total Expenses	GOAL: < Projection by 5% TOOL: Operational Budget	Goal	$ 44,879.00	$ 86,154.00	$ 131,033.00
		Actual	$ 39,493.52	$ 92,357.09	$ 131,850.61
		Variance	(0.12)	7.20%	0.00162%

Year-to-Date (YTD) Improvement Plan for areas not meeting goal: Revised monthly

1. Improvement plan to address IUS rate
2. Improvement plan to address On-Time Starts
3. Improvement plan to address Pain Communication and Attention to Needs
4. Improvement plan for RN certification Rate
5. Improvement plan statement addressing Operational Excellence Statistics

Note. Values do not reflect proprietary organizational information. (Chapter Author Created for instructional purposes by Isabelle Clarke Garibaldi, Chapter Author.)

employee engagement (high performing workforce), and the number of surgeries performed (operational excellence) in relation to revenue and expenses.

Budget Preparation

Formulating a budget begins with preparation and planning. Organizational leaders gather fundamental information about a variety of elements that will influence the organizational budget, including demographic and marketing information, competitive and competitor analysis, regulatory influences, and strategic plan elements that relate to budget preparation. Additionally, it is helpful to review unit level scopes of service, goals, and the financial history for each department in order to align budgets with the organization's overarching quality and financial goals. Prior to the beginning of the budget year, most organizations devote at least six months to preparing and developing their budgets. Once completed, budgets usually cover a 12-month time period. This 12-month time period can be based on a fiscal year as determined by the organization (e.g., September 1 through August 31) or a calendar year (e.g., January 1 through December 31). Shorter- or longer-term budgets may also be developed based on specific strategic planning goals.

Organizing the Budgeting Process

Organizations typically use one of two methods to organize and develop a budget. One method is called **historical-based budgeting** (HBB), and the other method is called **zero-based budgeting** (ZBB). **Historical-based budgeting** (HBB) examines past performance data as a retrospective baseline to better understand and plan for future activities on a unit, within a department, and for the entire organization. These data are used as a starting point, to assist in interpreting potential revenue and common expenses associated with past productivity and performance. **Zero-based budgeting** (ZBB) projects expected performance without referencing current or past performance. As new procedures are introduced or when a manager wants to ascertain the actual supply expenses associated with a procedure or activity, ZBB may be used. The ZBB philosophy is that the budgeting process will start from "zero," and that all revenue and expenses will be justified or re-justified annually. For practical purposes, health care organizations generally use the HBB method when planning an annual operational budget, and a ZBB when new services or revenue streams are planned.

ZBB is also the process used to drill down and identify expenses by detailing every supply item and the quantity of items typically used for a particular procedure or patient care event. A list of all supplies is developed, along with the itemized expense of each. Supplies are often packaged in bulk and sold in quantity. Therefore, the expense of single items has to be calculated and backed out of the bulk figure to accurately depict the expense. This can be a time-consuming exercise that requires attention to detail and accurate cost quantification. See Table 7.2, which outlines ZBB for a new endoscopy suite.

Key Budgeting Elements and Influences

During the budget-preparation phase, it is important to examine individual hospital department operations thoroughly. Large

Table 7.2 Zero Based Budgeting: Endoscopy Suite Labor and Supply

Zero-Based Budgeting for Endoscopy Suite: Labor & Supply Costs Per Case

General Supplies	Cost Per Item	Quanity Used/Procedure	Cost	Forms and Clerical Supplies	Cost Per Item	Quanity Used/ Procedure	Cost
Masks	$0.30	2	$0.60	Consent to treat (Scanned)	$0.26	1	$0.26
Gloves	$0.17	4	$0.68	Consent for Anesthesia (Scanned)	$0.26	1	$0.26
Disposable Gowns	$5.51	2	$11.02	Patient Procedure Education Forms	$3.18	1	$3.18
Disposable Head Covers	$0.38	2	$0.76	Patient Discharge Education Forms	$3.18	1	$3.18
Disposable Shoe Covers	$0.49	4	$1.96	**TOTAL**			**$6.88**
Disposable Patient Underpad (Chux - Pkg of 4)	$0.07	1	$0.07				
Yankauer Suction	$2.87	1	$2.87	**Pharmacy**	Cost Per Item	Quanity Used/ Procedure	Cost
Suction Tubing	$1.20	1	$1.20	Propofol 50 mcg/ml	$5.50	1	$5.50
Emesis Bag	$0.05	1	$0.05	Versed 2 mg	$0.66	1	$0.66
Bite Block	$3.14	1	$3.14	Fentanyl 50 mcg/ml	$0.22	1	$0.22
O2 Nasal Cannula	$0.38	1	$0.38	Cetacaine Spray Bottle 20 Gm	$2.60	1	$2.60
Denture Cup	$0.22	1	$0.22	Atropine 0.4 mg/ml vial	$3.53	1	$3.53
Non-Skid Slippers	$1.80	1	$1.80	Normal Saline 10 cc vial	$0.65	1	$0.65
Patient Belongings Bag	$1.36	1	$1.36	Normal Saline or D5LR 1,000 cc	$3.38	1	$3.38
Disposable Electrodes	$0.03	5	$0.15	Sterile Water 1,000 cc	$1.83	1	$1.83
Surgi-Lube (30 cc packet)	$0.46	3	$1.38	**TOTAL**			**$18.37**
CDs (Patient Downloads)	$0.90	1	$0.90				
Gauze 4 × 4 (2 per pkg)	$0.62	5	$3.10	Labor	Avg. Hourly Salary	Case Minutes	Cost
Gauze 6 × 6 (2 per pkg)	$0.82	5	$4.10	(1) Preadmit/ Admitting Staff	$18.00	25	$7.50
Syringe 10 cc	$0.33	1	$0.33	(2) Staff RN (Intra-Procedure)	$36.52	35	$21.30
Syringe 30 cc	$0.57	1	$0.57	(3) Ambulatory Care Staff (Pre/Post)	$28.15	140	$65.68
Syringe Toomey 60 cc	$1.17	1	$1.17	**TOTAL**			**$94.48**
Alcohol Wipes (2 × 2)	$0.02	2	$0.04				
Angiocath 20 g	$2.26	1	$2.26				
IV Start kit	$4.83	1	$4.83				
IV Tubing	$6.28	1	$6.28				
IV J-Loop	$2.19	1	$2.19				

Table 7.2   **(Continued)**

Zero-Based Budgeting for Endoscopy Suite: Labor & Supply Costs Per Case							
General Supplies	**Cost Per Item**	**Quanity Used/Procedure**	**Cost**	**Forms and Clerical Supplies**	**Cost Per Item**	**Quanity Used/ Procedure**	**Cost**
Bandaid	$0.18	1	$0.18				
Scope Cleaning Brush	$4.220	1	$4.22				
TOTAL			**$57.81**				
						Grand Total	**$148.74**

Note. Values are for instructional purposes only and reflect mean industry standards for pricing. Created for instructional purposes by Isabelle Clarke Garibaldi.

hospital divisions are frequently divided into departments comprised of multiple units for budgeting purposes. An example of a nursing department with multiple units is a perioperative services department, which may include surgery, central sterile processing, the **post-anesthesia care unit** (PACU), and ambulatory care/day surgery that report up through that perioperative department. Units within a department can further be classified as a **cost center** or (income-generating) **revenue centers**. The difference between a cost center and a revenue center is that a cost center primarily generates expenses, with limited direct responsibility to generate revenue (Linton, 2018). An example of a clinical cost center is a medical/surgical unit because it primarily incurs expenses in the form of nursing labor and supplies as opposed to the income it generates in the form of reimbursement from inpatient census. An example of a clinical revenue center is a radiology department, because of its direct responsibility of generating revenue from the performance of procedures as opposed to the amount of labor and supplies needed to perform those procedures.

Obtaining Reimbursement

If new or enhanced services are offered, a method for recouping expenditures must be established to ensure that the organization receives appropriate payment for costs incurred from the delivery of care. Charges are dollar amounts that the organization bills the patient from the provision of goods or services. Payments on the patient's behalf can be made in the form of an out-of-pocket payment (cash from the patient) or through payment from a third-party source /guarantor, such as an insurance company or governmental payer source, such as Medicare/Medicaid.

Demographic Information and Marketing

Community demographics and the ability to market services will have a direct impact on potential reimbursement. By pulling together demographic information relative to the population that the organization serves is most helpful, because it identifies unique market characteristics such as age, race, sex, income, and so on that influence patient behavior, service needs, and organizational preferences. Demographics and capture rate (the percent of the population who use the organization as a consumer) of the immediate and secondary market regions helps paint a clear picture regarding patient population demographics and the type of patient who may choose a particular organization for health care.

Marketing is the process of creating interest and providing information regarding products and services. It is important to understand demographics as it relates to the type of patients that organizations wish to target as their customer base. Marketing strategies are built around the population types that an organization is attempting to attract. For example, if a hospital is constructing an open-heart patient care unit, marketing and outreach activities would be developed to attract those patients who can benefit from cardiovascular screening, prevention modalities, and/or treatment services. Another example is marketing for an obstetrical practice. It is expected that marketing efforts would a target population of childbearing women, rather than a geriatric male population. Therefore, it is important to understand that health care facilities sometimes use the "four P's of marketing" which address product, place, price, and patient. This allows the organization to place desirable health care services and products in convenient locations, and at a price that benefits both patients and the health care facility. In this way the health care facility, the patient, and the community benefit. Using printed materials, social media, search-engine positioning and paid advertising, direct-mailing information, and advertising in journals, magazines, and newspapers, are all examples of ways to educate and stimulate the public for future referrals for health care services. However, marketing of services does have a price tag. The cost of advertising campaigns on television and radio are exponentially more costly than distributing organizationally generated printed materials. Once marketing strategies are implemented, most organizations attempt to measure the effectiveness or the return on investment from marketing strategies. A real-life example of measuring marketing effectiveness is a hospital's inquiry into the effectiveness of advertising for a new cardiovascular patient care unit on social media. By surveying new patient referrals who responded that their service choice was a direct result from the hospitals' social media exposure, the effectiveness of that marketing initiative can be discerned.

Competitive Analysis

An analysis of an organization's geographical competition, called a **competitive analysis,** is important because it examines the extent to which one organization is performing as compared to other health care organizations within the same physical location. Being a successful competitor within a market increases reimbursement potential by increasing the likelihood that consumers will use an organization's services. A competitive analysis also examines organizational strengths and weaknesses in addition to other details such as the convenience of a location, planned services, existing services, and technology. Having this knowledge can influence decisions regarding the implementation or continuance of new services or programs, hiring of specialty staff, and the purchasing of equipment. Table 7.3 represents a competitive analysis of two different hospitals for an oncology service line.

Regulatory Influences

Organizational reimbursement is heavily affected by regulatory requirements, which therefore influences the budgeting process. Regulatory requirements come from a multitude of

governing bodies. One such regulatory body is the Centers for Medicare & Medicaid Services (CMS), whose mission is to ensure health care quality and security for its beneficiaries. CMS (www.cms.hhs.gov) administers federal controls, quality assurance, and fraud and abuse prevention for Medicare/Medicaid, and the **State Children's Health Insurance Program** (SCHIP). Under the auspice of the Department of Health and Human Services, CMS is also responsible for coordinating health care policy, planning, and legislation. Another example of a regulatory body is The Food and Drug Administration (www.fda.gov), which controls the approval and use of drugs, food products, and medical devices in the United States.

Other regulatory bodies influence organizational reimbursement by ensuring that federal and state laws are followed through an approval or accreditation process. Obtaining accreditation is viewed as a desirable process, allowing organizations to establish that they meet minimum standards of consumer quality and service excellence. Accreditation is also important because it is required in order for an organization to receive payment from federally funded programs such as Medicare and Medicaid. One such accrediting body is TJC, formerly known as the **Joint Commission on Accreditation of Healthcare Organizations** (JCAHO) (www.jointcommission.org). TJC accredits hospitals, behavioral health care entities, medical laboratories, home health, rehabilitation, and ambulatory care centers to ensure those organizations meet specific quality standards.

Strategic Plans

Generally, health care organizations use strategic plans to map out business direction. Strategic plans guide organization

Table 7.3   Oncology Services Competitive Analysis Created for instructional purposes by Isabelle Clarke Garibaldi.

Oncology services competitive analysis		
	Hospital A	**Hosptial B**
Location	Metropolitan City: Northwest Suburb	Metropolitan City: Urban / Inner City Limits
Primary Service Area Population	265,000	1,128,000
Affiliation	36-Hospital Affiliated System	Single Entity University Hospital
Financial Designation	For-Profit	Not-For-Profit
Clinical Description	Focused Oncology Services	Hospital and Clinic: Integrated Oncology Services
Support Services	Trauma Level 3 Linear Accelerator Home Infusion Services High Dose Rate intraoperative Radiation Therapy Stereotactic Surgery Comprehensive Breast Center Ambulatory Infusion Center Dedicated Oncology Unit Brachytherapy	Trauma Level 1 Linear Accelerator Home Infusion Services Hospice Care and Palliative Care Programs High Dose Rate Center Intraoperative Radiation Therapy Stereotactic Surgery Hyperthermia Management Comprehensive Breast Center Ambulatory Infusion Center 4 Dedicated Oncology Units Pain Clinic Brachytherapy Therapeutic Pheresis Transplant Services/Unit
Miscellaneous	Tumor Registry Tumor Board Radiosurgery Conferences Home Health Cancer Advisory Council Integrated and Holistic Medical Council General Cancer Support Group Annual Cancer Awareness Fair	Community Cancer Screening Events Tumor Registry Tumor Board Radiosurgery Conferences Home Health Cancer Advisory Council Integrated and Holistic Medical Council Tumor-Specific Survivors and Family Support Group

leaders, managers, and front-line staff, so that the entire organization has shared mission, vision, and value structure, with clearly defined steps to meet their goals. A **mission statement** describes an organization's purpose. A **vision statement** provides direction, perseverance, and focus, so that organizations can effectively carry out operational goals. A **values statement** describes core priorities within an organization's culture that drive its strategic plan.

While organizations as a whole develop an overall strategic plan, individual departments develop specific goals which should feed up into the organization's overall strategic plan. A strategic planning initiative, for example, may be to become the preferred provider of outpatient orthopedic care the organization's primary service market. A department plan to support this organizational initiative may be to focus on increasing patient satisfaction and decreasing procedure room turnaround time in order to increase volume.

Scope of Service and Goals

A departmental or unit scope of service(s) supports the mission/vision/values of the organization as well as the overall strategic plan. Each department or unit defines its own operational **scope of service** (see Table 7.4: Perioperative Scope of Service.). The scope of service document is helpful because it provides information related to service types and location(s), where services are offered, usual treatments and procedures,

hours of operation, practice guidelines, and parameters for appropriate clientele. The department of unit scope of service should include a scope of practice statement with role definitions for staff. Any changes in a department or unit scope of service should correlate with clinicians' scope of practice, competence, clinical experience, and professional developmental planning (AONE, 2015).

Unit professional and developmental goals may include the introduction of new technology or treatments, patient education, and creation of a special patient care environment. Staff members should be engaged to determine whether they have any proposed quality and operational goals or initiatives which should be included in an organization's strategic plan. Any new quality and operational initiatives must identify costs related to their operationalization. New initiatives can add both revenue and costs from the early induction phase through full implementation of the initiative. Be aware that additional treatment modalities, patient care items, equipment, and documentation tools may require different types and/or amounts of supplies and technology integration, which may come at significant cost.

Creating the Budget

Once foundational data related to costs and revenue for goods and services is gathered, the work of creating a budget can begin. This process includes projecting gains/losses for a revenue or cost center. Revenue gains are income generated

---

Real World Interview

Marie Duval Macke DNP, RN, MBA, NEA-BC
  Systems Director of Behavior Health Services; St. Catherine's Hospital, East Chicago, IN

  Health care is an ever-changing dynamic industry that requires large sums of support and resources, such as staff, equipment, and supplies; but has a difficult time sustaining itself financially without cutting those resources. One of the most challenging aspects of the budgeting process is balancing between estimating a realistic revenue, purchasing expensive equipment and supplies while reducing non-essential expenditures. Coordinating each of these three important but separate aspects of the budgeting process is difficult, as each aspect has its own unique characteristics.

  Revenue comes from multiple sources such as government dollars, research, philanthropy, and patient care; however, reimbursement from patient care is the largest and the least predictable source of income for the hospital. Value-based reimbursement is increasing while fee for service is reducing. Reimbursement is no longer based on volume. Instead, reimbursement is based on quality and value such as patient care quality metrics, and treatment outcomes, and patient satisfaction is slowly emerging and changing workflows and documentation by health care practitioners.

  New equipment and highlighted patient care programs are essential but they come with a high cost ticket to purchase and implement. This can be a dilemma as hospital revenue decreases but there is still a need to remain competitive with other health care organizations. To balance an increase in programs and equipment, health care managers are asked to be more efficient, buy less supplies, and eliminate unproductive patient care programs. It is very difficult and detrimental to morale when patient care programs are dismantled and staff are reassigned. Also, there can be a general perception that quality of care is reduced when programs or staff are reduced.

  As health care administrators, we need to be able to balance all of these components and increase efficiencies for staff and providers to deliver high-quality care, while reducing unnecessary expenses. The budget process helps administrators find this balance and should not be considered a once-a-year activity. Rather, year-long dynamic processes toward estimating, forecasting, proposing, evaluating, and eliminating unnecessary steps must be employed.

Marie Duval Macke DNP, RN, MBA, NEA- BC
Systems Director of Behavior Health Services
St. Catherine's Hospital, East Chicago, Indiana

Table 7.4   Perioperative Services Department: Sample Scope of Services

Perioperative Department: Scope of Services
GOAL: In collaboration with the hospital's leadership team, the perioperative services department employees care for surgical and/or invasive procedural patients from pediatric, adult, obstetrical, behavioral health, and geriatric populations. The Perioperative Department provides compassionate, patient-centered care by meeting the holistic needs of the patient and family. This comprehensive approach will meet the surgical patients' health needs in the acute care practice setting by having each patient receive an individualized plan of care that meets his/her specific physical, spiritual, psychological, education, and social needs. Eleven (11) surgical suites and four (4) endoscopy suites are located on the second floor of the acute care hospital and are designed to services, which require surgical and/or procedural intervention. The Perioperative Department works with other hospital departments to ensure an appropriate, timely, and safe care environment and positive patient outcomes.
Perioperative Services Leadership includes the Director of Perioperative Services, the Manager of Ambulatory Care Services, the Manager of Central Sterile Processing and Materials Management, the Surgery Manager, and the Surgery/Endoscopy Scheduling Lead. In collaboration with the Perioperative Clinical Nurse Educator, the Chief Nursing Officer, and the hospital's shared governance council, clinical practice guidelines are developed, evaluated, and executed.
The attending Surgeon, in conjunction with the Anesthesia Care Provider, will direct patient based on his or her preoperative and intraoperative assessments and will document such care in the electronic medical record. Nursing care in perioperative services will be directed and supervised by a Registered Nurse, specializing or certified in surgical care. The Registered Nurse is assisted by support clinicians who are either licensed or demonstrate competence through certification, education, or annual objective-based assessment(s).
Hours of Operation:

* 0500 – 2,100 Monday – Friday for all Perioperative Specialties
* After hours 24/7 on-call General Surgery Services
* After hours 24/7 on-call Neurosurgery Services
* After hours 24/7 on-call Cardiac Surgery Services
* Sub-Specialty Services on-call as per recommendations from the Medical Executive Committee and Department of Surgical Services. The Perioperative Services sub-specialty on-call schedule is posted on the hospital's intranet, in the OR, in the Emergency Department, and at the switchboard desk.

Services Provided within Surgical Services
Orthopedics
Urology
Gynecology/Obstetrics
Ear/Nose/Throat
Podiatry
Ophthalmology
Thoracic/Vascular
Plastic Surgery
General Surgery
Endoscopy and Colonoscopy
Surgical Oncology
Tissue and Organ Procurement
Dental and Oral Surgery
Neurosurgery
Catheter-Based and Open Cardiothoracic Surgeries
Practice and Standards Guidelines:
The Perioperative Department will utilize the following guidelines when caring for patients and shaping the clinical environment:

* Joint Commission
* OSHA
* The Organization's Operating Room specific policies and procedures, developed based on the standards from the American College of Surgeons (ACS), the Association for Operating Room Nurses (AORN), the Association of Surgical Technologists (AST), Association for the Advancement of Medical Instrumentation (AAMI), and the American Society of PeriAnesthesia Nurses (ASPAN).

All Registered Nursing positions require Basic Life Support (BLS), Advanced Cardiac Life Support (ACLS), and Pediatric Advanced Life Support (PALS) training. All other perioperative clinical support staff positions require Basic Life Support (CPR). Staff compliance with mandatory education and competencies is required. The Manager of Surgical Services, along with inter-professional team monitors patient outcomes, standards for continuing education, and adherence to current, evidence-based practice standards. Created for instructional purposes by Isabelle Clarke Garibaldi.

through a variety of means, including billable patient services, investments, grants, endowments, and donations to the organization. Procedural departments typically generate specific, fee-based revenue by billing for services such as X-rays, invasive diagnostic or therapeutic procedures, drug therapy, surgical procedures, physical therapy, laboratory services, devices, and so on. Revenue in procedural areas can also be generated through the delivery of multiple episodes of a service over time, such as hourly rates for chemotherapy administration or outpatient antibiotic infusions. An anticipated number and type(s) of services and procedures should be projected annually for each department or unit budget. Each type of service may have varying volume associated with it. For example, projecting volume from the type of procedures conducted in a cardiac catheterization unit ("Cath Lab") is based upon historical budgeting data, conclusions from referring physicians and technical staff, marketing projections, and projected growth based on the organization's strategic plan.

Similarly, the same types of projections occur for other units, which are primarily cost centers. An example of a cost center is an inpatient unit. Inpatient unit projections should include the number of patients anticipated to be admitted (based on previous years' census), the average length of stay (e.g., one to four days for hip replacement surgery) and the unit's projected daily occupancy rate. The type and amount of services and patient days can also be measured. The number of patient days or the services delivered are commonly called service units or primary statistics, and are measured so that productivity and efficiency can be tracked.

It is important to note that the reimbursement rates from third-party payers affect revenue and can change from year to year (Johnston, 2017). Medicare, Medicaid, managed care companies, and insurance companies dictate or negotiate rates with health care organizations and they may include negotiated rates or discounts on charges. Health care organizations determine charges based on their costs and mark-up practices. Health care payers determine which specific costs they will pay for related to admissions, procedures, visits, or services. Payment rates vary from State to State and between individual and employer-based health care insurance plans. Additionally, these payment rates can change monthly, such as with the **Ambulatory Payment Classification** (APC) system from Medicare, which applies to the outpatient setting (American Hospital Association, 2018; Centers for Medicare & Medicaid Services, 2018). The reimbursement rates or payments received by hospitals often do not equal the actual hospital or unit charges for the services rendered. For example, there may be a fixed reimbursement rate per procedure or diagnosis, regardless of how long the patient stays in the hospital or how much the hospital pays for the supplies and labor attached to that encounter. If an organization's costs exceed the reimbursement rate, the service provider (the organization) absorbs any remaining costs.

Reimbursement can also be paid in the form of a payment classification system. **Diagnosis Related Groups** (DRGs) are used to group or classify inpatients into categories based upon an algorithmic reimbursement formula which accounts for factors such as severity of illness, prognosis, treatment difficulty, the need for intervention, and resource intensity (Centers for Medicare & Medicaid Services, 2016). DRG reimbursement for inpatient diagnoses are all-encompassing; meaning that reimbursement covers all care received, regardless of type. Examples of items covered in a DRG payment during an inpatient stay include the patient's room and meals, lab and radiology testing, physical/occupational/speech therapy, and nursing care hours. Typically, actual dollars reimbursed through the DRG model are 30–60% of actual charges.

Organizations review their anticipated patient population mix and payer mix to ascertain the percentage of patients carrying different types of health care coverage and the third-party payer (Medicare, Medicaid, Commercial Insurance Payer) reimbursement potential. These proportions help measure the anticipated dollars to be received and expenditures incurred for services delivered. It also helps the organization make projections for the coming year. It is difficult to predict third-party payer reimbursement due to continually fluctuating reimbursement rates. It remains unclear what the future holds relating to third-party payer reimbursement as well as the continuing impact of the Affordable Care Act and Reconciliation Act (2010). In addition, some patients do not have health care insurance or the ability to pay for their health care. This results in zero payment for services. Costs incurred for these patients often end up being the sole-responsibility of the hospital or health care organization. The facility will then account for these costs as charity care or uncollectable debt in its accounting structure.

If charges for patient care reimbursement are negotiated with third-party payers such as insurance companies and managed care corporations, payment rates are generally not re-negotiable after the patient has received care. Third-party payers often impose a penalty fee as a disincentive, should a health care organization change a charge amount already under contract. The penalty often exceeds the charge amount and will usually create a loss for the organization. Let's look at the differences in reimbursement related to a specific procedure:

Typical hospital charges for a cardiac pacemaker or defibrillator implantation procedure can range between $25,000–$65,000 or more, depending on the device type and the patient's severity of illness. In this example, we will assume that the charge for implantation of a cardiac defibrillator is $60,000. These charges include the use of the fluoroscopy equipment, supplies, the actual pacemaker device, nursing time during an inpatient unit stay, and cardiac catheterization laboratory (Cath Lab) technical staff time. If a hospital places 100 pacemakers per year, the anticipated annual revenue from cardiac pacemaker implantation charges can be calculated at $6,000,000. The breakdown of third-party payers becomes important, because the total revenue from charges does not mean that the hospital will be reimbursed for the full amount of $6,000,000. Third-party payers typically contract with health care organizations for a portion of the total charges amount that the third-party payer is willing to pay. Demonstrate the potential reimbursement rates based upon varying third-party payers. What are the organizational implications? How can you apply this analysis to your own unit or department? (Table 7.5)

Expenses

Expenses are determined by identifying the costs associated with the delivery of service. Expenses are resources used by a health care organization to deliver patient care services, and

Table 7.5   Third-Party Payer: Reimbursement for a Cardiac Pacemaker Created for instructional purposes by Isabelle Clarke Garibaldi.

Third-party payer	Percent of charges	Expected reimbursement per case @ $60,000 in charges
Managed Care Contractor "A"	52% of Charges	$31,200 ($60,000 × 0.52)
Medicare	45% of Charges	$27,000 ($60,000 × 0.45)
Private Insurance Company "B"	55% of Charges	$33,000 ($60,000 × 0.55)

Critical Thinking 7.1   The Budget and Daily Operations

Front-line staff are uniquely qualified to identify best practices which impact efficiency and cost-effectiveness. Managers can learn from staff and organize processes to assist with unit-based improvement. Think back on nursing actions during a shift as they complete tasks and deliver care. Reflect on handoff communication and how information is received. Examine the amount of time spent in patient care versus other activities. What problems may include supplies, labor, equipment, utilities, and miscellaneous items. Rising costs over time has outpaced revenue gains, leading to unprecedented cost pressures for all health care organizations (Advisory Board, 2017). As clinical leaders strive to anticipate expenses, the appropriate charges will be put in place to cover services rendered. Expenses are commonly broken down into line items that represent specific categories which contribute to the cost of the procedure or activity. These line items include such items as office supplies, medical supplies, drugs, medical devices, etc. This breakdown of line-items helps identify where significant expenses lie in relation to a service or in relation to a specific nursing unit.

in the flow of activity and gaps in communication or efficiency did you find? Does communication affect care quality, revenue generation, and expense control? If so, how? How could you improve your team's functioning? How would you communicate your findings to management and executive leadership to improve nursing care delivery and care quality? Discuss your observations with your co-workers and manager.

Labor as Expense

Labor is significant expense associated with medical and nursing care. Health care services are very labor intensive and require a workforce with specialized training and knowledge. The accepted, classical standard that organizations use to esti-

mate labor costs is somewhere between 50% and 60% of their overall operational costs (Berman & Weeks, 1982). It is very important to analyze and calculate the amount of time that staff members are involved with direct (bedside) and indirect patient care (support services) care, because labor is such a large, disproportionate part of the operating budget.

Labor costs are not solely tied to direct patient care. Indirect patient care time is time needed to prepare and facilitate direct patient care. Examples of indirect care include appointment scheduling, registering a patient, transporting patients to a procedure room, and using the **electronic medical record** (EMR) for charting and other documentation purposes. This indirect time must be calculated into the overall cost of patient care when preparing the budget.

For example, in an ambulatory care area, staff time is calculated relative to the delivery of specific procedures, including pre-procedure care, intra-procedure care, and post-procedure care. Pre-procedure care includes gathering supplies, assembling equipment, and preparing the environment. It may

---

Case Study 7.1   Ambulatory Care Unit

The nurse manager of the ambulatory care unit asks for staff participation in order to identify ways to increase the accuracy of charging single-patient use medical supply items. The cost of these items has risen in excess of the budget by 20% in the last two months. This is the first time that the staff members have been involved in helping with expense containment and improving charging accuracy. Novice nurses, experienced nurses, nursing assistants, and unit-based secretarial assistants have been invited

to participate in this expense reduction endeavor. When beginning an analysis of supply use and charging accuracy, what might be the first step in the process? If you were to break the staff into work groups, which members should be chosen to analyze the process of supply charging accuracy? How would you proceed if you were leading this initiative? Can you identify an innovative way to improve charging processes in your work environment?

Real World Interview

Nicole Salas, BSN RN, Director, Acute Care Services, Watertown Regional Medical Center, Watertown, WI

The nurse staffing model not only plays a role in patient care quality outcomes, but it also critically impacts how patient care units plan their budgets. Health care organizational structures vary widely and therefore use different staffing models to provide high-quality care to patients while ensuring fiscal responsibility. Certainly, an acute care hospital will staff and budget differently from a long-term care facility or an outpatient surgery center.

When discussing staffing models, it's important to recognize that staffing and scheduling models are not the same. Staffing models are concerned with aligning direct-care nurses' skills with the needs and demands of the patient population; while scheduling models are primarily focused on assigning the number and type of staff needed to a certain number of patients to meet potential patient care needs. Typically, staffing and scheduling models are used in conjunction with each other to find a balance between budgeted, nurse-patient ratios, and patient acuity.

There are three predominant staffing models used by health care organizations: budget-based, nurse-patient ratios, and patient acuity. All three staffing models have unique strengths and weaknesses, and all three models' success are incumbent upon input from front-line staff who providing patient care. Direct-care nurses are just as responsible as managers and directors when establishing and implementing a staffing model. Direct-care nurses must provide input on the staffing model and patient acuity to ensure that fiscal responsibility for staffing costs is balanced with the need to ensure the provision of high-quality patient care. Decreasing variability of patient care while simultaneously accounting for patient acuity increases the nurse's ability to provide quality patient care and helps the unit manager plan the unit's labor budget

It has become best practice to create staffing committees, consisting of members of the organization that focus on creating unit-specific and shift-specific staffing guidelines. Flexibility within one's staffing model is necessary to meet patient needs and budget plans. Many organizations have low census guidelines, to help them plan to decrease staff as the unit census decreases. Conversely, patient influx guidelines help the nurse manager to up-staff in order to ensure appropriate patient care based on volumes and to ensure patient care needs are being met.

Nicole Salas, BSN RN
Director, Acute Care Services, Watertown Regional Medical Center, Watertown, WI

Critical Thinking 7.2   Unit Census Growth Projection

Background: Due to the organization's activities around growth and service-line development, the Chief Nurse Executive, Chief Operating Officer, and the Medical/Surgical Unit Nurse Manager expect an increase in the unit's census over the next two years. This expectation is based on an analysis of growth activities on the organization's strategic plan. The nurse manager must plan for this growth by ensuring there are enough Registered Nurses (RNs) available to care for the project patient census growth. It has been calculated that the unit will need five more RNs over the next two years. The plan is to hire 2 RNs the first year and 3 RNs the second year.

Calculate the added expense that a nurse manager will need to add to his/her budget over the next two years based on the addition of two registered nurses in future next year one and three registered nurses in future year two. A total gain of five full-time equivalents (FTE)* will be added. For this exercise, annual hours for one FTE = 2,080 (annual hours budgeted).

Multiply the RN average hourly rate by the annual hours for an FTE (2080), and then by the total paid number of nurses needed per year to get the unit's annual RN salary expense. (e.g., $30.00×2,080 hr annually per FTE×5 FTEs = $312,000.00) (Table 7.6).

Table 7.6   Growth Unit Salary Expense Projection Created for instructional purposes by Isabelle Clarke Garibaldi.

	Present year	Future year one (Additional 2 FTEs)	Future year two (Additional 3 FTEs)
Average Hourly Rate*	$31.25	$32.18* *Accounts for 3% annual salary increase	$33.15* *Accounts for 3% annual salary increase
Total FTEs (2080 hr Annually)	40	42	45
Salary Expense	2,600,000.00 $31.25 × 2080 × 40 = $ 2,600,000.00	2,811,244.80 $32. 18 × 2080 × 42 = $2,600,000.00	3,102,840 $33.15 × 2080 × 45 = $ 2,600,000.00
Salary Expense Increase	–	$211,244.80 Increase over present year	$291,595.20 Increase over year one

Evidence from the Literature

Source: Adapted from Brooks Carthon, J. M., Hatfield, L., Plover, C., Dierkes, A., Davis, L., Hedgeland, T., Sanders, A. M., Visco, F., Holland, S., Ballinghoff, J., Del Guidice, M., & Aiken, L. H. (2019). Association of Nurse Engagement and Nurse Staffing on Patient Safety. *Journal of Nursing Care Quality. Jan/Mar, 34*(1): 40–46.

Discussion: More than 20 years ago, the institute of Medicine (IOM) released its groundbreaking publication, *To Err is Human: Building a Safer Health System.* Subsequent to that publication, which highlighted many health care problems, many programs and ideas have been initiated to reduce patient harm at health care organizations. Unfortunately, safety concerns and adverse patient care events persist (Bates & Singh, 2018). One major recommendation from the IOM's publication was that changes in nurse work environments must be considered in order to increase patient safety. Brooks Carthon et al., (2019) describe optimal nurse work environments as those having the attributes of safe staffing levels, and nurses who are highly engaged in shared governance and decision making, good communication between caregivers, teamwork with physicians, and competent, supportive management.

The literature has well established that lower patient mortality, fewer patient falls, and lower rates of infection correlate to optimized, foundational nursing practice environment features. These features include appropriate staffing ratios and operational systems aligned toward patient care. The purpose of the Brooks Carthon, et al., study (2019) was to examine whether nurses' assessments of patient safety differ under varying levels of nurse engagement and staffing.

Data Analysis: Hospital and nursing characteristics, including frequency distributions, measures of central tendency, and bivariate correlations, were evaluated. Logistic regression models were then used to determine the association of nurse engagement and nurse staffing on our outcome of unfavorable patient safety ratings and patient safety climate before and after controlling for nurse and hospital characteristics. All analyses were completed using STATA (version 14.2; College Station, Texas). The level of significance was set at $P < .05$. All tests were two-tailed, and the analyses also accounted for the clustering of nurses within hospitals.

Implications for Practice: The authors' findings revealed that higher levels of nurse engagement in unit activities and governance as well as lower nurse-to-patient staffing ratios were consistently associated with positive ratings of patient safety. There was a relationship between nurse staffing and patient safety, which was consistent with the work of others who noted increased medical errors and threats to patient safety when staffing is inadequate, Nurses consistently reported patient safety concerns, including patient information "falling through the cracks" when nurses assumed high patient workloads, suggesting that further investments in nurse staffing may increase nurses' ability to detect patient safety threats and intervene when they occur. Increased staffing appeared to be closely tied to improved patient safety efforts. The findings of a relationship between nurse engagement in unit activities and governance and reports of patient safety, even after accounting for staffing, suggest that an additional opportunity to improve assessments of patient safety may lie in increasing the opportunities for nurses to engage in decision-making bodies in hospital settings. A number of health care systems have now initiated efforts to incorporate nurse engagement efforts in patient safety initiatives. Nurse engagement in unit activities and governance coupled with adequate staffing promote improved patient safety.

---

involve taking a history, completing a physical examination, administering medication, taking specimens, placing tubes or establishing an intravenous line, and positioning the patient. Intra-procedure care is the actual care delivered as a procedure is being performed. Post-procedure care may require activity such as educating and discharging a patient, or delivering extensive recovery activities requiring several hours of direct nursing care and removal of equipment and supply items.

Staffing

The amount and type of labor needed to deliver quality patient care is accounted for in the budget. However, the way labor is utilized is actually accounted for in a staffing model. The staffing model outlines the number **full time equivalent personnel** (FTEs) and skill level of those FTEs required for patient care based upon a primary statistic such as procedural minutes, or direct care hours per patient day. An FTE is defined as the equivalent number of employees working full time, or 2,080 hr per year. One FTE is 'equivalent' to one employee working 2,080 hr per year. An outpatient staffing model may focus on the number of procedure minutes and rooms that require staff. An inpatient staffing model may focus on the patient load per nurse based on the amount of direct nursing care needed and accounting for the acuity of (patients') illness and direct care activities during certain times of the day. Inpatient nurses are generally assigned a fixed number of patients plus new patient admissions during their shifts. The nurse-to-patient ratio on a medical telemetry nursing unit may be appropriately set at one nurse to six (1:6) patients during the day and evening shift; whereas it may be 1:8 during the night shift. By comparison, nurse-to-patient ratios in a cardiovascular intensive care unit may be 1:2 for all shifts.

Staffing ratios and salary data are particularly important because of the high cost to recruit and retain nurses and other clinical staff. In order to combat staff attrition, some organizations offer higher salaries in turnover-prone patient care units, which can vary from organization to organization, depending upon supply and demand. For example, if a hospital is experiencing challenges in recruiting and retaining obstetrical/labor and delivery nursing staff, the hospital *may* choose to offer sign-on bonuses or increase salaries on that unit to alleviate the staffing deficit. Additionally, a health care organization may change its benefits, offering more attractive benefit packages that include continuing education, more **paid time off** (PTO), or professional membership expense reimbursement. Organizations may also look for alternative ways to supplement their workforce during staff shortages or during times of higher census. This means that supplemental staff—such as contracted agency nurses or nurses from a hospital's in-house registry (i.e., float pool) may be hired at a different/higher salary rate.

It is important to note whether a unit has had historical difficulty retaining or recruiting staff. Recruitment and retention—especially marketing, interviewing, hiring, and orienting staff—require dollars. The Lewing Group's (2009) ground-breaking study, *Evaluation of The Robert Wood Johnson Wisdom at Work: Retaining Experienced Nurses Research Initiative*, found that RN replacement costs can range from $22,000 to over $64,000; with an average cost to replace a full-time RN being $36,657. A Consumer Price Index cost assessment, after inflation adjustments, correlated total nursing turnovers costs to be between $7.9 and $8.5 million annually (Kurnat-Thoma, Ganger, Peterson, & Channell, 2017). Turnover costs include the orientation of replacement RN employees, orientation time, salary, benefits, back-filling open position working hours, using overtime or supplemental staffing, and other departmental labor costs related to hiring new employees such as human resource and finance department employee time.

Productive and Non-Productive Time

Productive time is a measure of how much work is done in a given amount of time, tied directly to the performance of a job or task and accounted for on a budget. The Fair Labor Standards Act (2018) defines **non-productive time** working hours as working hours spent on the job, not associated with the direct or indirect operations or direct performance of a job or a job task which also must be accounted for in the budget process. This time is associated with sick, vacation, bereavement, personal, holiday, and education hours. Most employees in health care organizations accrue non-productive time through employer benefit plans. These non-productive hours can be accrued as individual line items (e.g., 40 hr of vacation and 24 hr of education time annually); while some organizations grant nonproductive hours as lump-sum of *"Paid Time Off"* (PTO) hours. The lump-sum method allows the employee to flex their PTO hours at their discretion to account for their individual desire for more sick time, education time, or vacation time during the course of a year, instead of facility-allocated sick time or vacation time. PTO benefit hours are calculated at a greater percentage for employees with longer tenure, meaning a 20-year employee will accrue more PTO than the three-year employee. Organizations generally calculate non-productive time and costs at a rate between 15% and 25% of the employee's base annual salary. For example, if a new employee is paid a base salary of $75,000 annually, the organization would calculate the total employee salary expense to be $75,000 × 115% (100% of direct/indirect care salary + another 15% to cover nonproductive time). The final, annual labor cost of productive and non-productive time for

Table 7.7 Nonproductive Time Calculations Created for instructional purposes by Isabelle Clarke Garibaldi.

Registered Nurse "A" = 2 years of employment at County Hospital Pay Rate = $25.00/hr: 12 hr Shifts			Registered Nurse "B" = 22 years of employment at County Hospital Pay Rate = $40.00/hr: 12 hr Shifts		
	Annual Hours Per Organization Benefit Structure	Salary Costs		Annual Hours Per Organization Benefit Structure	Salary Costs
PTO Hours (Includes Vacation, Sick, Personal Time)	240 ($25.00 × 240)	$6,000	PTO Hours (Includes Vacation, Sick, Personal Time)	300 ($40.00 × 300)	$12,000
Education Hours (2 Days)	16 ($25.00 × 16)	$400	Education Hours (3 Days)	24 ($40.00 × 24)	$960
Holiday Hours (7 Days)	84 ($25.00 × 84)	$2,100	Holiday Hours (7 Days)	84 ($40.00 × 84)	$3,360
TOTALS[a]	340	$8,500	TOTALS	408	$16,320
Percentage of Salary Costs[b]	16.34%		Percentage of Salary Costs	19.62%	

[a] Salary dollars change depending on pay rate and shift length (8-, 10-, 12-hr shifts).

[b] Increased costs are relative to tenure and benefit structure by organization.

Critical Thinking 7.3   Metrics and Operations

As you walk onto your assigned patient care unit, ask a staff member what key initiatives the unit is working on that reflect patient-focused process improvement and revenue/expense metrics. Are the metrics posted on the unit and displayed in a manner that staff, patients, families, visitors, and leadership can easily understand? What are the quality goals for the unit that correlate to these metrics and how are staff participating in decisions so that the goals may be achieved? Think about how these initiatives may also increase productivity, staff, and patient satisfaction, and decrease potential patient harm. Is the impact of these initiatives self-evident?

In this chapter, the budget process and commonly used budget types were discussed in detail. Key elements of budget preparation process were outlined; including the roles of health care team members, budget development/scope of services offered, operationalization of the budget, and budget/goal monitoring for health care organizations. Revenue opportunities, factors that influence reimbursement, and expense liabilities were discussed relative to patient care. Please review how these objectives can be applied in your organization.

this employee would then be $86,250.00. It is important to understand this concept because the amount of PTO for a long-term employed staff member will be considerably higher than for newly hired staff. Table 7.7 illustrates the average number of PTO benefit hours, which two nurses at a fictional institution may accrue in a 12-month period. It is also important for the nurse leader to remember that this time off may require coverage by another nurse or contract labor to back fill the open hours.

Fixed and Variable Costs

Like labor expenses, the costs of care delivery can be further broken down as either direct or indirect costs. **Fixed costs** are those expenses that are constant and are not related to productivity or volume. Examples of these fixed costs are building and equipment depreciation, and administrative salaries. **Variable costs** fluctuate, depending upon the patient census and types of care required. Medical supplies, drugs, laundry, and food costs often increase with the patient census.

Budget Approval and Monitoring

Once developed by hospital managers and leaders, budgets are submitted to executive team leaders for review, revision, and final approval. Although exact titles can vary, the makeup of a health care organization executive team is typically the **Chief Executive Officer** (CEO), the **Chief Nursing Officer** (CNO), the **Chief Operating Officer** (COO), and the **Chief Financial Officer** (CFO). Additional officer positions at larger organizations may include a **Chief Information Officer** (CIO) and a Chief Administrative and Human Resources Officer. The final budget approval process may take several months in order to integrate the overall budget, with operational budget, capital budget, and construction budgets. The executive management, in conjunction with the organization's Board of Directors and possibly corporate owner entities, usually make final decisions regarding acceptance of a finalized budget.

Once accepted, the unit or department manager is responsible for monitoring and controlling their budget. Budget monitoring is generally carried out on a daily, weekly, and monthly basis. The purpose of budgetary monitoring is to ensure that revenue is generated and expenses are controlled in correlation with projected productivity and standards. Organizations often utilize a flexible, or "range" budget guidelines that allows for acceptable variances and adjustments if the patient census increases or decreases. If the patient census increases, it is likely that expenses will increase proportionately. If the patient census decreases and expenses increase, then the manager needs to determine what actions are necessary to control or bring down costs. Many organizations require managers to complete a budget variance report, which is a tool used to identify when budget categories are out of line and to identify the need for corrective action.

Team Roles and Responsibilities in the Budgeting Process

The entire health care team has a role in the budgeting process and is responsible for ensuring that revenue is captured, expenses are controlled, and that volume or census is maintained. The manner in which this is accomplished depends on the organization. Most institutions request that monthly budget variance reports be developed and submitted, reflecting interdepartmental activity at a glance. Variance reports may be posted so that all staff members have an opportunity to review them and participate in quality improvement activities. The root cause of the variance needs to be identified so that effective action plans for improvement can be developed.

Staff often meet with management to discuss implementation and enforcement of strategies that can positively affect the budget. Staff engagement regarding these strategies is key to long-term budgeting success and expense containment. Examples of such strategies are as follows:

- Analyze efficiency of staff and overall performance related to patient care.

- Educate staff regarding the process for entering patient charges and other expense reduction opportunities.

- Plan for supplies needed per every patient encounter and consciously eliminate unnecessary items.

- Share how your department is reimbursed for services delivered, identifying covered and excluded expenses.

- Utilize automated technology such as barcode scanning.

- Discuss quality and cost differences in supplies with staff and management.

- Analyze cause of schedule delays, canceled cases, and extended procedure times.

- Explore new products with vendor representatives, and network with colleagues who have tried both new and older products.

- Reduce patient length of stay through the early engagement of case managers.

- Enhance staff productivity through rigorous process improvement activities.

- Post overtime and productivity analyses.

- Explore how efficiency studies may increase identify care gaps or duplications.

- Analyze patient supplies and review cost-per-patient encounter (e.g., chemotherapy administration, dialysis, insertion of indwelling or peripheral catheter).

- Track various steps in patient care that are time consuming or problematic for a unit (e.g., communication from front desk to recovery room, staff response to patient call lights, number of staff responding to an emergency code).

- Acquire a working knowledge of how a department/unit monitor both financial and quality indicators.

- Participate in the development of action plans to increase patient satisfaction efforts.

KEY CONCEPTS

- Nurses play an integral role in the preparation, implementation, and evaluation of a unit or department budget.

- If nurse leaders and front-line staff are not conscious of revenue and expenses, deviation from the expected financial performance will occur.

- Organizational performance outcomes are dependent upon the skills and critical thinking of staff members.

- Health care organizations use several types of budgets to help with future planning and management. These include operational, capital, and construction budgets.

- The budget preparation phase consists of data gathering related to a variety of elements that influence an organization. These elements include demographic information, competitive analysis, regulatory influences, and strategic initiatives. Additionally, it is helpful to understand the department's scope of service, goals, and history.

- During the budget preparation phase, it is important to examine the individual nursing or department or section thoroughly. Hospital systems are frequently divided into sections, departments, or units for organizational and cost-accounting purposes. These subsections or units are commonly called cost centers or revenue centers. Cost center or revenue center data are used to track financial data.

- Organizations typically use past performance as a baseline of experience and data to better understand activity in a department or unit.

- Expenses are determined by identifying the costs associated with the delivery of service.

- Expenditures are any resources used to deliver services. They may include direct or indirect expenses.

- Once developed, budgets are submitted to an organization's executive team for review and final approval. The approval process may take several months as the unit budgets are combined to determine the global budget for the health care organization.

KEY TERMS

Capital budget	Full time equivalent (FTE)	Profit
Competitive analysis	Historical-based budgeting	Revenue
Construction budget	Key performance indicators	Scope of service
Cost centers	Loss	Values statement
Dashboard	Mission statement	Variable costs
Diagnosis-related groups	Non-productive time	Variance
Economies of scale	Operational budget	Vision statement
Fixed costs	Productive time	Zero-based budgeting

REVIEW QUESTIONS

1. An operational budget accounts for which of the following?
   a. The purchase of major equipment
   b. Construction and renovation
   c. Income and expenses associated with an organization's daily activity
   d. Acquisition of new technology

2. Revenue can be generated through which of the following?
   a. Billable patient care services
   b. Expanding fixed costs
   c. Use of generic drugs
   d. An electronic medical record (EMR)

3. The purchase of a new piece of equipment with a cost >$650,000.00 would be accounted for by which type of document?
   a. Operational budget
   b. Staffing grid
   c. Construction budget
   d. Capital budget

4. An expense that is associated with patient care is a:
   a. Fixed
   b. Direct
   c. Indirect
   d. Variable

5. You are a new manager for an ambulatory surgical facility. Part of your job is to develop and maintain the facility's budgets and track expenses. Medical and surgical supplies, drugs, laundry, and food are considered _____?
   a. Fixed
   b. Variable Costs
   c. Direct Expenses
   d. Indirect Expenses

6. A payment classification system used for reimbursement of health care cost by Medicare is:
   a. Managed Care Contract
   b. Penetration Rate Revenue
   c. Diagnosis-Related Groups (DRGs)
   d. Length of Stay reports

7. A(n) _____ budget is created when an organization is planning to renovate and expand the number of operating rooms in its patient tower to accommodate a new cardiovascular service line.
   a. Capital
   b. Operational
   c. Construction
   d. Balanced

8. Identify which of the following are indirect expenses. Select all that apply.
   a. Salary for staff providing care to ICU patients
   b. Gas, electric, telecommunication
   c. Patient-chargeable medical supplies
   d. Office supplies
   e. The cost of patient admission kits
   f. The cost of a cardiac pacemaker

9. A _____ is important because it examines the extent to which one organization is performing as compared to other health care organizations within the same physical location.
   a. _____ Competitive Analysis
   b. _____ Dashboard
   c. _____ Scope of Service
   d. _____ Diagnosis-Related Group

10. Sick time, vacation time, and holiday time are not considered to be which of the following? Select all that apply.
    a. Productive time
    b. Non-productive time
    c. Direct expenses
    d. Variable costs
    e. PTO

REVIEW QUESTION ANSWERS

1. Answer: C is correct.
   Rational: An operational budget accounts for the daily activity associated with revenue and expenses, generated from patient care and operational functions (C). The purchase of major equipment (A), construction or renovation facilities (B), and (D) the acquisition of a new health record are generally capital acquisitions due to the magnitude of costs.

2. Answer: A is correct.
   Rational: Revenue generation in a health care organization is based upon billable services (A) and costs associated with equipment, supplies, staffing, and indirect expenses. Revenue can be generated from procedural activities such as the type, intensity, and length of services delivered to a patient in an operating room. Expanding fixed costs (B), and the use of generic drugs (C), and/or EMR (D) alone do not generate revenue.

3. Answer: D is correct.
   Rational: Capital budgets account for the purchase or replacement of major equipment and usually involve considerable expense

(D). Operational budgets (A) account for daily activity associated with revenue and expenses, generated from patient care and operational functions. Construction budgets (C) are used when an organization plans renovation or new structures. Staffing grids (D) do not directly correlate with the accounting of equipment purchases.

4. Answer: B is correct.
   Rational: Direct expenses are those expenses that can be directly associated with patient care (B). Fixed costs are expenses that are constant and are not related to productivity or volume (A). Indirect expenses are expenses not directly related to patient care (C). Variable costs fluctuate depending on the volume or census and types of care required (D).

5. Answer: B is correct.
   Rational: Variable costs tend to fluctuate depending on the volume, census, or types of care required. Medical and surgical supplies, laundry, and food costs often increase with volume (B). Direct expenses are those expenses that can be directly associated

with patient care (C). Indirect expenses are expenses not directly associated with patient care (D).

6. Answer: C is correct.
   Rational: Diagnosis-related groups, or DRGs, are used by Medicare to group patients into predetermined categories for reimbursement purposes (C). The other responses: Penetration Rate Revenue (A), Diagnosis-Related Groups (DRGs) (B), and Length of Stay reports (D) are not classification systems.

7. Answer: A is correct.
   Rational: A capital budget accounts for the purchase of major new or replacement equipment (A). An operational budget accounts for the income and expenses associated with day-to-day activities (B). A construction budget is developed when renovations or new structures are planned (C). A balanced budget (D) is not covered in this text.

8. Answers B, D, and E are correct.
   Rational: Utilities (B), office supplies (D), and electronic medical records (E) cannot be directly tied to one patient's record and therefore cannot be a direct patient charge. Salaries and wages

(A), patient-chargables (C), and medical supplies (pacemakers) (F) are direct care costs.

9. Answer: A is correct.
   Rational: A competitive analysis examines the extent to which one organization is performing as compared to other health care organizations within the same physical location or geographical region (A). Dashboards (B) and scopes of service (C) help the manager with an analysis of (unit) performance; while DRGs (D) are payment classification systems used for reimbursement of health care cost by Medicare.

10. Answers A and E are correct.
    Rational: Productive time is when staff are engaged in direct patient care (A). Non-productive time is when staff are not working, such as during sick time, vacation time, and holiday time (B). Direct expenses are those expenses that can be directly associated with patient care and its related costs (C). Variable costs are influenced by fluctuating employee accrual and discretional disbursement protocol by pay period and census, and fluctuate depending on the volume or census and types of care required (D) and non-productive hours as lump-sum of "Paid Time Off" (PTO) hours (E) that include sick time, vacation time, and holiday time.

REVIEW ACTIVITIES

- Physically tour your organization. Do you see any dashboard displays of quality and economic measures? What does the dashboard prevalence (or lack thereof) reveal about your agency?

- Using the tables in this chapter as a guideline, construct a competitive analysis of one or more of the agencies or health care facilities in your community. Do they have more than a physical presence in the community? Do they have a technology or social media presence as well?

- Using the zero-based budgeting figures in this chapter, construct an analysis of one of the clinical procedures in your organization.

DISCUSSION POINTS

- During your last clinical experience, how was quality nursing care tied to the budgeting process?

- Does your clinical site or employer post quality and financial goals and outcomes? If so, it is easily accessible to, and understood by, front-line staff?

- Which aspects of the budgeting process are you currently utilizing in your current role? Will you be comfortable using budgeting processes in the health care setting/as a direct care clinical nurse?

- How do you expect to improve quality as a direct care clinical nurse, using your newly acquired knowledge of the budgeting process?

- How does your facility's culture affect the budgeting process?

DISCUSSION OF OPENING SCENARIO

An opening scenario was introduced at the beginning of this chapter. Utilization of the budgeting process with a thorough understanding of relevant terms, coupled with detailed review of your facility's strategic plan, will help the nurse optimally function within the scope of patient care and services, the staffing model, and productivity goals. Collegial relationships between organizational leadership and front-line staff are imperatives in order to make these goals a reality.

EXPLORING THE WEB

(All Sites Accessed December 15, 2018)

- Review the Joint Commission web site. What information do you find there relating to budgets? www.jointcommission.org

- Visit Advisory Board Company: www.advisory.com. What is an advisory board and how can you become a member?

- Visit the American College of Healthcare Executives: www.ache.org and see how current executives deal with budgets.

- Visit the American Nurses Association: www.nursingworld.org and see what the ANA thinks about our current US budget.

- Visit the Centers for Medicare & Medicaid Services: http://www.cms.hhs.gov and see how innovative models are spending smarter.

- Go to Healthcare Financial Management Association: www.hfma. org and listen to current podcasts on current financial challenges.

Informatics

- Go to the Agency for Healthcare Research and Quality: www.ahrq. gov and search budget. How is their mission tied to budgeting?

- Review the site for the American Organization of Nurse Executives. What are the resources available for the novice nursing leader? www.aone.org

Lean Back

- What have you learned from this chapter that you will take forward into your practice?

- Does this chapter make you realize the incredible costs associated with health care in a clearer way?

- Do you see yourself as a manager some day dealing with budgeting issues?

REFERENCES

Advisory Board. (2017). *Rebuild the Foundation for a Resilient Workforce. Best practices to repair the cracks in the care environment.* Washington, DC: Advisory Board Publishing.

Affordable Care Act and Reconciliation Act. (2010). Retrieved from www. hhs.gov/sites/default/files/ppacacon.pdf

American Hospital Association. (2018). *2018 AHA guide*. Chicago, IL: AHA.

American Organization of Nurse Executives. (2015). *AONE nurse manage competencies.* Chicago, IL: American Organization of Nurse Executives. Retrieved from: www.aone.org/resources/nurse-manager-competencies. pdf and www.aone.org

Bates, D. W., & Singh, H. (2018). Two decades since to err is human: An assessment of progress and emerging priorities in patient safety. *Health Affairs*, *37*(11), 1736–1743. https://doi-org.ezproxy.rush.edu/10.1377/ hlthaff.2018.0738. Retrieved from: http://www.aone.org/resources/nurse-manager-competencies.pdfwww.aone.org

Berman, H. J., & Weeks, L. E. (1982). *The financial management of hospitals.* Chicago, IL: Health Administration Press.

Brooks Carthon, J. M., Hatfield, L., Plover, C., Dierkes, A., Davis, L., Hedgeland, T., Sanders, A. M., Visco, F., Holland, S., Ballinghoff, J., Guidice, M. D. & Aiken, L. H. (2019). Association of Nurse Engagement and Nurse Staffing on patient safety. *Journal of Nursing Care Quality*, *34*(1), 40–46.

Centers for Medicare & Medicaid Services. (2016). *Design and development of the diagnosis related group.* Retrieved from www.cms.gov/ICD10Manual/version34-fullcode-cms/fullcode_cms/Design_and_development_ of_the_Diagnosis_Related_Group_(DRGs)_PBL-038.pdf.

Centers for Medicare & Medicaid Services. (2018). *Regulations & guidance.* Retrieved from www.cms.gov/Regulations-and-Guidance/Regulations-and-Guidance.html

Fair Labor Standards Act. 2018). *Employment law handbook.* Retrieved from www. employmentlawhandbook.com/federal-employment-and- labor-laws/flsa/

Ghazisaeidi, M., Safdari, R., Torabi, M., Mirsaee, M., Farzi, J., & Goodini, A. (2015). Development of performance dashboards in healthcare sector: Key practical issues. US National Library of medicine National Institutes of Health. *Acta Informatica Medica : AIM : journal of the Society for Medical Informatics of Bosnia & Herzegovina : casopis Drustva za medicinsku informatiku BiH*, *23*(5), 317–321. Retrieved from https://doi.org/10.5455/ aim.2015.23.317-321

Johnston, J. (2017). *With so much uncertainty, how do you build your hospital's budget?* Healthcare Financial Management. Retrieved from www. hfma.org/Content.aspx?id=51828

Kurnat-Thoma, E., Ganger, M., Peterson, K., & Channell, L. 2017). *Reducing annual hospital and registered nurse staff turnover: A 10 element onboarding program intervention.* SAGE Publication Journals: SAGE Open Nursing. https://doi.org/10.1177%2F2377960817697712 Retrieved from https://journals.sagepub.com/doi/full/10.1177/2377960817697712.

Lewing Group. (2009). *Evaluation of the Robert Wood Johnson wisdom at work.* Robert Wood Johnson Foundation. Retrieved from https://www. rwjf.org/en/library/research/2009/01/evaluation-of-the-robert-wood-johnson-wisdom-at-work.html

Linton, I. 2018). *What is the difference between a revenue center & an expense center?* Small Business. http://Chron.com. Retrieved from http:// smallbusiness.chron.com/difference-between-revenue-center-expense-center-37418.html

Phelps, C., & Madhavan, G. (2018). Resource allocation in decision support frameworks. *Cost Effectiveness & Resource Allocation*, *16*(1). Retrieved from https://doiorg.ezproxy.rush.edu/10.1186/s12962-018-0128-5

Sussman, J. H. (2017). *Strategic allocation and management of capital in healthcare.* Chicago, IL: American College of Healthcare Executives.

Walsh, K. (2016). *Managing a budget in healthcare professional education. Annals of Medical & Health Sciences Research*, *6*(2), 71–73.

SUGGESTED READINGS

Advisory Board. (2018). *Rising above the bottom line: Nurse-led opportunities to achieve sustainable cost savings.* Retrieved from www.advisory.com/research/nursing-executive-center/studies/2017/rising-above-bottom-line

Advisory Board Nurse Executive Center. (2018). *Rebuild the Foundation for a Resilient Workforce. Best practices to repair the cracks in the care environment.* Washington, DC: Advisory Board Publishing.

Antwi, Y. A., & Bowblis, J. R. (2016). *The impact of nurse turnover on quality of care and mortality in nursing homes: Evidence from the*

great recession. Upjohn Institute Working Paper 16–249. W.E. Upjohn Institute for Employment Research, Kalamazoo, MI. https://doi. org/10.17848/wp15-249

Fitz, T., & Shaikh, M. (2018). *4 Tactics of effective strategic technology planning for the digital future.* Healthcare Financial Management, 1–10. Retrieved from http://ezproxy.rush.edu/login?url=http://search.ebscohost. com/login.aspx?direct=true&db=ccm&AN=132859159&site=ehost-live

Joint Commission. (2018). *Comprehensive accreditation manual for hospitals (CAMH): The official handbook.* Oakbrook Terrace, IL: Joint Commission.

Jones, C., Finkler, S. A., Kovner, C. T., & Mose, J. N. (2019). *Financial management for nurse managers and executives.* St. Louis, MO: Elsevier.

Khan, B. P., Quinn Griffin, M. T., & Fitzpatrick, J. J. (2018). Staff nurses' perceptions of their nurse managers' transformational leadership Behaviors and their own structural empowerment. *Journal of Nursing Administration, 48*(12), 609–614.

Kohn, L. T., Corrigan, J. M., & Donaldson, M. S. (1999). To err is human: Building a safer health system. Washington, DC: National Academy Press.

Knickman, J. R., & Kovner, A. R. (2015). *Jonas & Kovner's health care delivery in the United States.* New York, NY: Springer Publishing Company.

Lindley, L. C., & Cozad, M. J. (2016). Nurse knowledge, work environment, and turnover in highly specialized Pediatric end-of-life care. *The American Journal of Hospice & Palliative Care, 34*(6), 577–583.

Ma, C., Shang, J., & Bott, M. J. (2015). Linking unit collaboration and nursing leadership to nurse outcomes and quality care. *Journal of Nursing Administration, 45*(9), 435–442.

Sammer, C., Miller, S., Jones, C., Nelson, A., Garrett, P., et al. (2017). Developing and evaluating an automated all-cause harm trigger system. Joint commission. *Journal of Quality and Patient Safety, 43*(4), 155–165.

Wisconsin Employment Law Updates. (2018). Retrieved from www.employmentlawhandbook.com/employment-law-updates/2018-2/wisconsin.

8

Patient-Centered Care

Tom Blodgett, PhD, RN, GCNS, AGACNP-BC and Nicole Petsas Blodgett, PhD, RN
Duke University, Durham, NC, USA

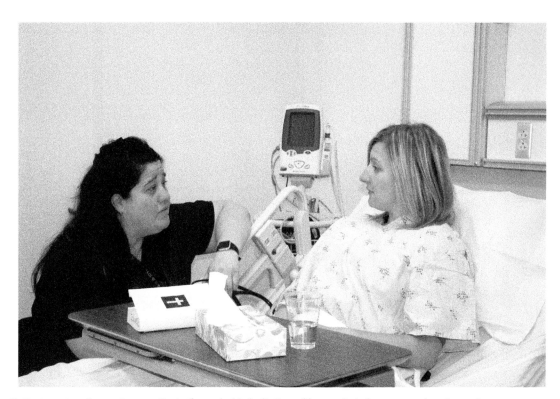

Patient-centered care views patients through this holistic and humanistic lens respecting the patient as a human being.
Source: Photo used with permission.

> Brave leaders are never silent around hard things.
>
> *Brené Brown (2019). The Call to Courage (2019).*

OBJECTIVES

Upon completion of this chapter, the reader should be able to:

1. Define **patient-centered care** (**PCC**) and similar terms.

2. Explain historical, political, cultural, and economic influences on PCC.

3. Describe PCC competencies for nurses.

4. Describe the potential impact of PCC on health outcomes.

5. Compare and contrast between episodes of care that are patient-centered and that are not patient-centered.

Kelly Vana's Nursing Leadership and Management, Fourth Edition. Edited by Patricia Kelly Vana and Janice Tazbir
© 2021 John Wiley & Sons Ltd. Published 2021 by John Wiley & Sons Ltd.
Companion Website: www.wiley.com/go/kelly-Nursing-Leadership

OPENING SCENARIO

You received report from the night nurse that your new patient needs pain medication, education about their diagnosis and having a difficult time coping with their acute pancreatitis. You know that managing pain is a priority and quickly head into the patient's room. When you enter, you notice the patient is solemn and resting comfortably. During your assessment she begins to share her fears about having pancreatitis.

You are faced with a decision: do you stop and listen to the patient or do you teach her about pain management?

Patients and families entrust nurses and other health care professionals with their most private information and often at the most vulnerable times in their lives. The relationship between patient and nurse is rooted in our shared humanity, and it should be the goal of every nurse to see each of their patients as the patient sees themselves—as holistic beings with their own priorities, goals, resources, and life experiences. **PCC** occurs when members of the health care team view their patients through this holistic and humanistic lens, respect the patient's input as being equally important to their own, and allow patients to guide how their care is delivered. Although PCC is not a new concept, it can easily be misunderstood or misused. Furthermore, failure to deliver care in a patient-centered manner can have unintended and unfortunate health outcomes.

The purpose of this chapter is to provide an overview of PCC, how this approach to care developed over time, and how it can be used to guide nurses in their care of patients in a variety of settings and circumstances. This chapter will define PCC and similar terms; explain historical, political, cultural, and economic influences on PCC; describe PCC competencies for nurses; describe the potential impact of PCC on health outcomes; and compare and contrast between episodes of care that are patient-centered and that are not patient-centered.

Definitions of Patient-Centered Care

The **National Academy of Medicine** (**NAM**; formerly the Institute of Medicine) defined PCC in its landmark report, *Crossing the Quality Chasm* (2001), as, "providing care that is respectful of and responsive to individual patient preferences, needs, and values and ensuring that patient values guide all clinician decisions." Numerous professional organizations have adopted this definition of PCC, including the **Institute for Healthcare Improvement** (**IHI**). Although succinct, this definition encompasses the three major philosophical underpinnings of PCC. First, that care should be designed around the patient's own priorities—not those of the health care team. Second, that these priorities must represent all of the various domains of health (i.e., it must be holistic). Lastly, that the views of the patient have no less value than those of the providers—the patient and the providers are indeed an equally balanced team.

These three combined features distinguish PCC from similar concepts, such as **holistic care**, **shared decision-making**, and **patient satisfaction**. Holistic care is a foundational feature of nursing in which healing involves a mind-body-spirit-emotion-environment approach. While PCC relies upon this holistic perspective, holistic care does not necessarily address how clinicians use the patient's input to make health care decisions. Holistic care is therefore only one piece, albeit an important one, of PCC.

Similarly, shared decision-making is closely related to PCC, but they are not one and the same. Shared decision-making originated around the same time as PCC, and some would argue to achieve the same purpose—to give patients greater autonomy to make decisions that affect their own health. However, shared decision-making is more conditional than PCC. To participate in shared decision-making, the patient must be empowered by the clinician with knowledge so that they and their health care provider are making decisions together with the same information. This implies, but does not always guarantee, that the patient's decision will be guided not only by their own priorities and values, but also by the same scientific knowledge that their health care provider possesses.

While this seems almost identical to PCC, shared decision-making has two important shortcomings. First, PCC has, by definition, a deliberately holistic approach, whereas shared decision-making does not. Second, with PCC, the patient's input is recognized as equally important to their provider's, regardless of the patient's baseline knowledge about their health conditions, whereas with shared decision making, having a full understanding of their health condition is a prerequisite to having input in making decisions. These shortcomings of shared decision-making are indeed subtle, but together, they distinguish shared decision-making from true PCC.

The third similar concept is patient satisfaction. When the Patient Protection and Affordable Care Act was passed in 2010, the federal government adopted a system of reimbursement for health care services based on the quality of care that a facility provided. This new reimbursement structure, known as value-based purchasing, penalized facilities where patients were consistently dissatisfied with their care. As a quality measure, patient satisfaction is measured using surveys that are distributed to patients after they are discharged from the hospital. These surveys ask patients to rate how satisfied they were with various aspects of the care they received, including: responsiveness of their nursing staff, how well their pain was managed, cleanliness of the environment, and other topics (see Table 8.1).

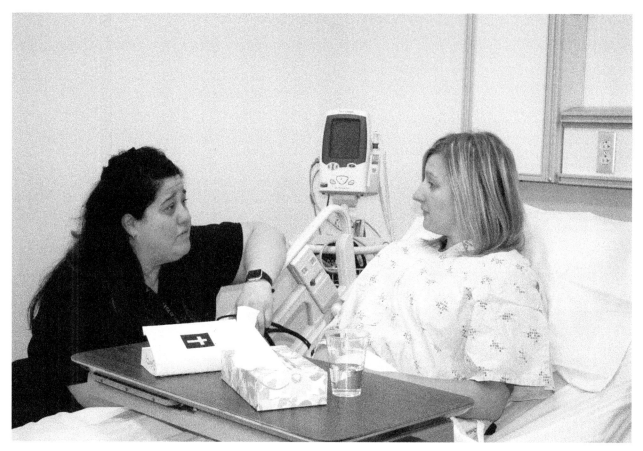

PHOTO 8.1 Patient-centered care views patients through this holistic and humanistic lens respecting the patient as a human being. *Source:* Photo used with permission.

Table 8.1 The HCAHPS Patient Satisfaction Survey (Hospital Version)

Your Care From Nurses	
During this hospital stay, how often did nurses treat you with <u>courtesy and respect</u>?	Never
During this hospital stay, how often did nurses <u>listen carefully to you</u>?	Sometimes
	Usually
During this hospital stay, how often did nurses <u>explain things</u> in a way that you could understand?	Always
During this hospital stay, after you pressed the call button, how often did you get help as soon as you wanted it?	Never
	Sometimes
	Usually
	Always
	I never pressed the call button
Your care from doctors	
During this hospital stay, how often did doctors treat you with <u>courtesy and respect</u>?	Never
During this hospital stay, how often did doctors <u>listen carefully to you</u>?	Sometimes
	Usually
During this hospital stay, how often did doctors <u>explain things</u> in a way that you could understand?	Always
The hospital environment	
During this hospital stay, how often were your room and bathroom kept clean?	Never
During this hospital stay, how often was the area around your room quiet at night?	Sometimes
	Usually
	Always

Table 8.1   (Continued)

Your Care From Nurses

Your experiences in this hospital

During this hospital stay, did you need help from nurses or other hospital staff in getting to the bathroom or in using a bedpan?	Yes No (if no, skip next question)
How often did you get help in getting to the bathroom or in using a bedpan as soon as you wanted?	Never Sometimes Usually Always
During this hospital stay, did you have any pain?	Yes No (if no, skip next 2 questions)
During this hospital stay, how often did hospital staff talk with you about how much pain you had?	Never Sometimes Usually Always
During this hospital stay, how often did hospital staff talk with you about how to treat your pain?	
During this hospital stay, were you given any medicine that you had not taken before?	Yes No (if no, skip next 2 questions)
Before giving you any new medicine, how often did hospital staff tell you what the medicine was for?	Never Sometimes Usually Always
Before giving you any new medicine, how often did hospital staff describe possible side effects in a way that you could understand?	

When you left the hospital

After you left the hospital, did you go directly to your own home, to someone else's home, or to another health facility?	Own home Someone else's home Another health facility
During this hospital stay, did doctors, nurses, or other hospital staff talk with you about whether you would have the help you needed when you left the hospital?	Yes No
During this hospital stay, did you get information in writing about what symptoms or health problems t look out for after you left the hospital?	

Overall rating of hospital

Using any number from 0 to 10, where 0 is the worst hospital possible and 10 is the best hospital possible, what number would you use to rate this hospital during your stay?	0 (WORST) 6 1 7 2 8 3 9 4 10 (BEST) 5
Would you recommend this hospital to your friends and family?	Definitely no Probably no Probably yes Definitely yes

Understanding your care when you left the hospital

During this hospital stay, staff took my preferences and those of my family and caregiver into account in deciding what my health care needs would be when I left.	Strongly disagree Disagree Agree Strongly agree
When I left the hospital, I had a good understanding of the things I was responsible for in managing my health.	
When I left the hospital, I clearly understood the purpose for taking each of my medications.	Strongly disagree Disagree Agree Strongly agree I was not given any medication when I left the hospital

Note. Health Consumer Assessment of Healthcare Providers and Systems. (2019). *HCAHPS Hospital Survey.* Retrieved on Friday, September 6, 2019, from www.hcahpsonline.org/globalassets/hcahps/survey-instruments/mail/april-1-2019-and-forward-discharges/2018-2019_survey-instruments_english_mail_omb-expiration.pdf.

Source: HCAHPS Survey.Centers for Medicare and Medicaid Services.Public Domain

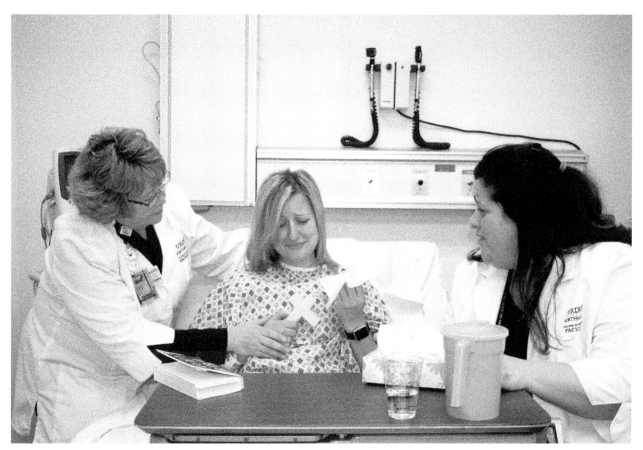

PHOTO 8.2 Holistic care is a foundational feature of nursing in which healing involves a mind–body-spirit-emotion-environment approach. Patient centered care combines holistic care, shared decision-making and patient satisfaction.
Source: Photo used with permission.

Scores for each question, as well as a global score representing how satisfied the patient was overall, are aggregated across patient surveys over a period of time and compared to a national benchmark. Depending upon how well the facility performed compared to other facilities, and if there was improvement in satisfaction from previous years, the reimbursement rates might be penalized by as much as 3%.

Patient satisfaction reflects the feelings a patient has about how well they were cared for while at a particular health care facility. It is an inherently subjective measure, and it relies on a complex interplay between health care professionals (e.g., technical skills, interpersonal skills), patients (e.g., expectations about care, needs, priorities), and resources at the facility (e.g., staff availability, institutional policies, access to equipment and supplies). Some patients, despite the best efforts of their health care team, will not be satisfied with their care for reasons unrelated to how their care was delivered (e.g., receiving news of a poor prognosis, an underlying mental illness, misunderstandings, perceived unfair treatment). Because it is subjective, highly complicated, and for a variety of other reasons, patient satisfaction is a notoriously controversial measure of health care

Real World Interview

We have a multidisciplinary team that focuses on quality and safety at my Midwest hospital, which includes patient satisfaction. In the quality world, patient satisfaction is how we objectively measure PCC, but we also go out on the units and meet with patients and their families to make sure their personal goals and priorities are being met.

Our team consists of a director of **quality improvement** (**QI**), two data specialists, two nurses that track **Center for Medicare** and **Medicaid Services** (**CMS**) core measures, and a performance improvement medical staff specialist who works directly with the physicians and other providers to help them deliver quality care. We also have two transitional care nurses that meet with our patients who have hard-to-control chronic diseases before they are discharged home. These nurses work closely with the inpatient team and with the home care team to make sure their patients are set up for success given their unique situations so they are not re-admitted to the hospital. A team member from the QI department is on every committee throughout the hospital, including Nursing Shared Governance, the Critical Care Committee, and the Trauma Committee, to make sure that we are looking at ways to improve the quality of care we provide our patients every day. The QI department also provides updates to the chief nursing officer and chief executive officer of the hospital.

Every morning, the QI team leads interprofessional safety huddles with departments throughout the hospital, including Nursing, Surgery, Nutrition, Radiology, and Environmental Services, to discuss safety concerns. In our safety huddles, we discuss patients that have wounds, patients with the same names, high fall risk, the need for sitters, and equipment issues. Even though these huddles are focused on safety, we almost always have safety issues coming up that also deal with PCC, especially when it comes to preventing falls and infections.

One of our most important QI initiatives is improving the patient's experience at our hospital. We want them to feel like they are well taken care of and their needs matter to us. We see that patients are satisfied with their care when we look at their patient satisfaction, or **Hospital Consumer Assessment of Healthcare Providers and Systems** (**HCAHPS**) survey scores.

Reporting our hospital's quality data to the nurses is a critical part of what we do. The QI data specialist presents a monthly "score card" at unit meetings that display their progress on our quality initiatives, such as CAUTI reduction, CLABSI reduction, preventing re-admissions, improving hand hygiene compliance, and reducing surgical site infections. During these meetings, it is common for staff nurses to advocate for their patients' needs by telling our department how a certain QI project needs to be modified to allow the patients some room to make choices. We rely so much on our nurses to move these QI initiatives to the bedside and to make us aware when they aren't working for our patients.

Andrea Petsas, RN
Performance Improvement Medical Staff Specialist
Quality Improvement Department, Methodist Hospitals
Gary, Indiana

quality. The major strength of patient satisfaction is that it serves as a proxy measure of the "patient-centeredness" of care within a facility. With the move to systematically collect data about patient satisfaction, the federal government has issued a clear message to health care facilities that the patient's expectations, feelings, and priorities have meaning and must be considered when delivering health care services. In other words, PCC is not a luxury or an option—it is a bare necessity.

In summary, while holistic care and shared decision-making might both be considered essential elements of PCC, they are not by themselves interchangeable with PCC. Likewise, while patient satisfaction reflects "patient-centeredness" to some extent, it depends almost completely on the patient's willingness and ability to judge that their care met their expectations. Examples of PCC, holistic care, shared decision-making, and patient satisfaction are provided in Table 8.2.

Table 8.2   Examples of holistic care, shared decision making, patient-centered care, and patient satisfaction

N.K. is an 84-year-old female resident in the long-term care facility where you work as a Registered Nurse. It is time to administer N.K.'s morning medications, which include digoxin (Lanoxin), memantine (Namenda), aspirin, donepezil (Aricept), a multi-vitamin, calcium with vitamin D (Os-Cal), and polyethylene glycol (Miralax). She has recently been diagnosed with liver cancer that has metastasized to several ribs, so she is also taking continuous release oxycodone (Oxycontin), immediate-release morphine as needed, and acetaminophen (Tylenol) as needed. Due to end-stage Alzheimer's disease, she cannot communicate verbally, but her nonverbal pain scale score indicates that she is in severe pain. You know that N.K. s husband, daughter, son-in-law, and grandson met with the Director of Nursing and Social Worker at the facility yesterday, and they requested that N.K. receive "comfort care" only. However, N.K.'s nurse practitioner has not yet discontinued any of her regular medications, so now you must decide which (if any) to administer or hold.

Example of holistic care

Since all of these medications still have active orders, you administer the scheduled medications that are due now: digoxin, memantine, aspirin, donepezil, multi-vitamin, calcium with vitamin D, polyethylene glycol, and continuous-release oxycontin. However, since she is currently experiencing severe pain, you also administer a dose of immediate-release morphine and provide nonpharmacological pain relief.

Example of shared decision-making

Again, all of these medications still have active orders, so you cannot discontinue any without an order. Instead, you ask N.K. if there are any that she would like to take first. When she does not answer, you call N.K.'s husband (surrogate decision-maker) and you work together to prioritize her analgesic medications above the others. You give her the continuous-release oxycodone and immediate-release morphine first, and then wait to give the rest of her scheduled medications when her pain is under better control.

(Continued)

Table 8.2   (Continued)

Example of patient-centered care

An appropriate patient-centered approach to this case would be to focus on what N.K. and her family feel should be the highest priority—her pain relief. Although you ask N.K. if she feels up to taking the rest of her medications (giving her the opportunity to respond), she cannot verbalize an answer. Therefore, you contact her husband to verify the plan they created yesterday. You explain to him that N.K.'s provider has not been to the facility yet to discontinue her regularly scheduled medications, but that you would like to know which of these medications he thinks N.K. should still take. Based on his response, you call the nurse practitioner and receive a verbal order to discontinue any non-essential medications (memantine, aspirin, donepezil, and vitamins and minerals). For now, you will only administer N.K.'s continuous-release oxycodone and immediate-release morphine, and when her pain is under control, you will give the remaining scheduled medications with active orders (digoxin, aspirin, and polyethylene glycol).

Example of patient satisfaction

When N.K.'s husband comes to visit later that afternoon, he thanks you for seeking his input and for taking their wishes about pain control seriously. He gives you some feedback that "not all nurses would have done that," and that he can tell N.K. feels more comfortable than she has in weeks.

Source: T. Blodgett and N. Petsas Blodgett.

Case Study 8.1

A.S. is a 29-year-old male with a history of generalized anxiety disorder, seasonal affective disorder, and hyperthyroidism. You are working in the Emergency Department when A.S. arrives, accompanied by his roommate who states that A.S. "just started freaking out" when he learned that his paycheck would not cover the rent that month. A.S. shouts loudly that he doesn't want to "mooch off him again," and that he will have to find a quick way to make some more money.

His physical examination reveals a rapid and irregular heart rate, high blood pressure, diaphoresis, extreme agitation, rapid breathing, and a desire to pace back and forth. In addition, his eyes are darting around the room, he makes poor eye contact, and he refuses to answer questions about his health. You notice that he has a fine tremor and that his skin feels very warm.

His roommate provides you with the name of the pharmacy that A.S. uses to get his prescriptions filled. When the pharmacist in the Emergency Department calls to verify his prescriptions, the pharmacy technician reports that he has not picked up any of his medications in over 6 months (which include propylthiouracil for his hyperthyroidism, and citalopram and venlafaxine for his

depression and anxiety). When you go back in the room to ask A.S. when he last took his medications, he becomes extremely aggressive and punches a hole through the drywall in his room. He threatens to "tear this place apart" unless he gets discharged immediately.

Hearing the commotion, the physician's assistant in the ED runs to the room and tells you to give A.S. lorazepam 4 mg IM STAT to "calm him down." While you acknowledge that A.S. may need medications to help him manage his severe acute anxiety, the patient is on the verge of tears and is now sitting on the floor, rocking back and forth.

1. What might be causing this patient's agitation, changes in vital signs, tremor, and other symptoms? (HINT: Always remember to "rule out" physiological causes first!)

2. How can you use principles of PCC and therapeutic communication to help A.S. calm down?

3. How might this situation have been handled throughout American history? What has changed about this approach over the last 50 years?

Origin and Evolution of Patient-Centered Care

One of the central tenets of health care is that a "patient" (whether an individual, a family, or a population), who has either an actual or potential need for health care, receives health care services from a team of licensed and unlicensed health care personnel. Many health professions textbooks illustrate this relationship as a set of concentric circles (Figure 8.1), with the patient in the most central circle and various levels of health care personnel in surrounding circles. The purpose of this sort of diagram is to make it clear that the patient is "at the center" of health care decision-making and health care delivery; if not the patient, then whom? However, it is apparent through research, news stories, legal cases, and social media reports that the patient's expectations, prefer-

ences, and values are not always incorporated into their care. The purpose of this section is to provide a brief description of the history of PCC, how it has evolved over time, and the various forces that have shaped its evolution.

Origin of Patient-Centered Care

The first published description of PCC came from the world of psychoanalysis (Tanenbaum, 2015). Originally, PCC was intended to be used as an alternative approach to primary care medicine. Whereas illness-oriented medicine focused on treating a disease process involving one or more organ systems, "patient-oriented medicine" focused on treating the overall patient. For example, Katie is a patient visiting her primary care physician about chronic headaches. The physician who uses an illness-oriented approach might focus on

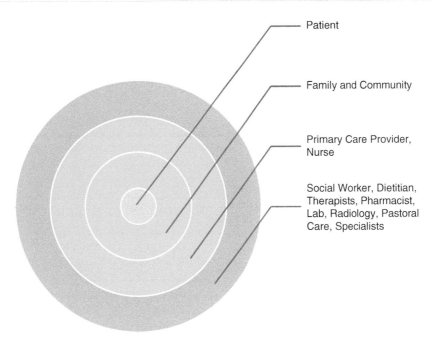

FIGURE 8.1 The Traditional Model of Patient-Centered Care diagram makes clear that the patient is "at the center" of health care decision making and health care delivery.
Source: Created by T. Blodgett, 2019.

Evidence from the Literature

Source: Bailoor et al. (2018). How acceptable is paternalism? A survey-based study of clinician and non-clinician opinions on paternalistic decision making. *AJOB Empirical Bioethics, 9,* 2, 91–98.10.1080/23294515.2018.1462273

Background: Although PCC is an important value in health care, certain medical circumstances may require others to interpret what the patient's values and priorities would be. Taking on this responsibility has consequences for those surrogate decision-makers, who may include family members and providers. When providers take on this responsibility in an attempt to help the family members, this is called "protective paternalism," which may or may not challenge the patient's autonomy. The authors hypothesized that certain circumstances may make protective paternalism more acceptable than others. The purpose of this article was to explore which, if any, types of health care situations make protective paternalism acceptable, from the viewpoint of clinicians and non-clinicians.

Methods: A mixed methods survey approach was used. Clinicians (physicians, nurses, nurse practitioners, and physician assistants) were recruited from an academic medical center in the Midwest. Non-clinicians were recruited from the public using a university-run research volunteer recruitment service. In both groups, participants must have been English-speaking adults with access to the Internet. The survey presented a case vignette of a patient who had an acute intracerebral hemorrhage, and the provider was asking the patient's daughter whether or not they should take the patient to have brain surgery. Each vignette was created using random degrees of "certainty" about the prognosis and despair from the daughter. For example, the provider may have told the patient's daughter that the patient "will not walk again" (high certainty) and that the daughter reacted by sobbing and saying that she felt overwhelmed (high surrogate distress). Both groups of respondents marked on 4-point Likert scales how acceptable paternalistic decision-making would have been in their vignette.

Results: 163 clinicians and 638 non-clinicians completed the survey. Respondents were predominantly female and non-Hispanic white. Overall, 15.3% reported that the paternalistic approach of withholding surgery for this patient was acceptable (30.2% clinicians, 11.4% non-clinicians). Among clinicians, more found this decision to be acceptable when there was higher prognostic certainty, regardless of the level of surrogate distress. Among non-clinicians, more found this decision to be acceptable when there was more prognostic uncertainty and lower surrogate distress.

Implications: Clinicians were more likely to find protective paternalism acceptable than non-clinicians. These groups also differed in which circumstances protective paternalism was acceptable. Clinicians tended to find it acceptable when there was more prognostic certainty, whereas non-clinicians did so when the prognosis was less certain. More research is needed before evidence-based recommendations about protective paternalism and PCC can be made.

neurological or cardiovascular causes of chronic headaches, order diagnostic tests to investigate these causes, and then treat Katie's headache with a non-steroidal anti-inflammatory drug, a triptan, acetaminophen, or another medication. If the physician used a patient-oriented approach, they might do the same but would also work with Katie to investigate psychosocial factors that could be contributing to her chronic headaches (e.g., stress, lack of sleep, occupational exposures).

Developing in parallel to patient-oriented medicine, although for slightly different reasons, was an educational movement in medical colleges toward the practice of biopsychosocial medicine. Once again, this approach to medical care sought to treat the whole patient rather than a specific organ system. An early pioneer of the biopsychosocial model was George Engel, a physician. He argued that biopsychosocial care would not distract the physician from delivering illness-oriented treatment, but rather that it would enhance and complement the treatment plan by extending medical science into the realms of psychology and sociology. For over three decades, the biopsychosocial model has been at the cornerstone of family medicine, and of course, it forms the foundation of the modern nursing.

These early efforts to practice patient-oriented biopsychosocial medicine are more similar to what we now call holistic care than PCC, but until this point in the 1960s and 1970s, medical and nursing care had been strictly illness-oriented; patient-oriented care was truly revolutionary in its own right. Neither the patient-oriented nor biopsychosocial approaches met the current defining characteristics of PCC—that care should be both holistic *and* guided by the patient's own values and preferences. To understand how and why the modern definition of PCC includes decision-making input from the patient, it is necessary to review some of the social and political changes that were happening in the United States while the modern definition of PCC was evolving.

Evolution of Patient-Centered Care

Rather than review all of the sociopolitical changes that happened during the 1960s through the 2000s, which is a topic so expansive that it could fill several books, the focus here will be much more limited. Instead, this section will draw upon specific examples of social movements and health policy changes that served as catalysts for PCC. To begin, it is important to understand how health care decisions were often made before these social movements and political initiatives began.

Prior to the 1960s, health care decisions were generally made by the physician, carried out by the nurse or a family caregiver, and largely unopposed by the patient. This relationship was based on **paternalism**, or the practice of a person in authority making decisions for a subordinate in the subordinate's supposed best interest. Essentially, the physician decided on the plan of care based on their professional expertise with minimal, if any, input from their patients. This was accepted as the social norm at that time (Kilbride & Joffe, 2018), and it still is in some circumstances (Bailoor, et al., 2018; Miller, Morris, Files, Gower & Young, 2016) and in some cultures (Cole, Kirlaev, Malpas, & Cheung, 2017; Muaygil, 2018). Paternalism was also, and in some populations continues to be, pervasive within the nurse-patient relationship (Bladon, 2019). Through analyzing conversations between nurses and patients with cancer, Siouta and colleagues (2016) found that the vast majority of communication from nurses to patients focused on biomedical issues; very little discourse reflected PCC. See Table 8.3 for examples of nurse-patient scenarios that highlight paternalistic nursing care.

The cultural revolution took full swing in the 1960s and has continued into the twenty-first century. During this era of social, cultural, and political reform, members of oppressed groups—women, African Americans, people with mental illness, and many others—used their collective voices to demand change. Social advocacy groups, including the **American Association of Retired Persons** (**AARP**) and the Patient Safety Movement, have also emerged as strong champions for PCC. Those

---

Table 8.3   Examples of Potential Paternalism in Health Care with Alternative Approaches

Examples of potential paternalism in health care

Withdrawing mechanical ventilation in a critically ill patient who is not improving.
An alternative approach would be to review the patient's advance directives or meet with the patient's family to determine or revise the goals of care.

Starting a patient with advanced dementia or Parkinson's disease on tube feedings.
An alternative approach would be to discuss this decision with the patient's family, a dietitian, a speech-language pathologist, a neurologist, a spiritual care provider, and/or a geriatrics clinical nurse specialist. The ultimate decision should lie with the surrogate decision-maker with support from the interprofessional team.

Advising the parent of a 13-year-old with severe anxiety not to let them attend summer camp.
An alternative approach would be to help the parent and child identify their goals for the summer camp experience, anticipate potential concerns and barriers, and help equip them to handle these if they arise. The child may also want to meet with an occupational therapist or mental health counselor to develop problem-solving and stress management strategies.

Source: T. Blodgett and N. Petsas Blodgett.

in positions of power—legislators, physicians, and hospital administrators—began to listen, but changes that would improve health care for these oppressed groups were slow to develop.

Rights of Women

Beginning in 1960, women won the fight to access birth control through their physician. While some physicians were initially reluctant to prescribe birth control, the demand for it grew. Eventually, other reproductive therapies and procedures, including elective abortion and assisted reproduction (e.g., *in vitro* fertilization), became available.

Rights of People with Mental Illness

The rights of people with mental illness also advanced in the second half of the twentieth century. The focus of care for this population shifted from the widespread use of powerful psychotropic drugs, physical restraints, and institutionalization to a more holistic and therapeutic approach that involved mental health counseling, selective use of medications, and a variety of self-care strategies (e.g., meditation, physical exercise, sleep hygiene). In addition, research activity in the specialty fields of psychiatric medicine and nursing increased exponentially so that these more holistic mental health interventions could become further refined and more widely adopted.

Health Policy Initiatives

Changes in health policy have revolutionized how health care is delivered, paid for, and evaluated. Examples include the development of managed care, bundled payments and prospective payment systems, meaningful use of the electronic health record, and value-based purchasing. Collectively, the overarching goals of these changes were to reduce the cost of health care, increase access to health care services, reduce health **disparities** (inequalities) across populations, and to improve health outcomes. As health policy changes became the new reality, PCC has become increasingly important in order to meet these goals. For example, to reduce health disparities across populations, providers and hospital administrators must be able to apply their knowledge about various payer systems and clinical practice guidelines to ensure that each patient receives equitable care.

Several health policy initiatives have stimulated the evolution of PCC, particularly in the late 1990s through the early 2010s. Recognizing that health care in the United States has been designed to meet the needs of health care providers rather than patients, leading to fragmented care, numerous attempts to redesign the health care system around the needs of patients have been made. A complete description of these important health policy changes is beyond the scope of this chapter, but a summary of key initiatives that affected health care delivery is provided in Table 8.4.

Table 8.4 U.S. Health Care Policies Affecting Patient-Centered Care

Health policy	Year passed	Impact on patient-centered care
New York v. Sanger	1917	Margaret Sanger, a proponent of women's birth control access, wins her lawsuit in New York that allows physicians to discuss birth control with their married patients.
19th Amendment to the U.S. Constitution	1920	Authorizes the right for women to vote.
Community Mental Health Act	1963	Led to the development of community-based mental health care centers, which essentially "deinstitutionalized" those with mental illnesses, developmental disabilities, and learning disabilities and allowed them to move back into their communities.
Griswold v. Connecticut	1965	By now, most states have overturned laws that prohibit the prescription use of contraceptives by married couples.
Eisenstadt v. Baird	1972	U.S. Supreme Court ruled that the right to use contraceptives applies to both married and unmarried persons.
Roe v. Wade Doe v. Bolton	1973	U.S. Supreme Court ruled that the Constitution protects a woman's right to terminate an early pregnancy.
Omnibus Budget Reconciliation Act	1987	Improved the quality of care in nursing homes, with an emphasis on: • Respect for resident's rights • Requirements for staffing and ongoing education of caregivers • Enforcement of minimum standards of care
Patient Self-Determination Act	1990	Requires health care facilities that accept Medicare and Medicaid funds to inform patients of their right to make decisions about their medical care and advance directives.
Family and Medical Leave Act	1993	Protects a person's job in the event of a medical or family-related leave of absence.
Patient Protection and Affordable Care Act	2019	Increases access to health insurance and health care, regardless of pre-existing conditions. Increases quality of care through a value-based purchasing system, which incorporates patient satisfaction as a measure of quality.

Case Study 8.2

M.T. is a 34-year-old female who presents to the Women's Health Clinic at 12-weeks gestation with her second pregnancy. After the ultrasonographer takes images and measures landmarks of the fetus, she takes M.T. and her husband back to the exam room so she can go over the results with her nurse midwife. After about 10 min, the nurse midwife enters the exam room and reveals that the fetus appears to have some ultrasonographic features of Down's syndrome. She offers to schedule M.T. for an amniocentesis to confirm the diagnosis, and M.T. and her husband agree to have this more invasive, though confirmatory, procedure performed the following week.

After the amniocentesis, M.T.'s nurse midwife calls her with the results—the fetus does indeed have three copies of chromosome 21. The Women's Health Clinic requires that M.T.'s care be transferred to an obstetrician at this point, though the nurse midwife may stay on the case to assist as needed. M.T. and her husband, who both work full time and are raising a 4-year-old daughter, are saddened by the news that their baby is going to be born with Down's syndrome. They reveal to you, their nurse, that they are not sure what to do with this pregnancy.

What concerns might M.T. and her husband have?

What options do M.T. and her husband have? What are the pros and cons of each?

How could you provide PCC in this situation?

Nurse Midwife, Obstetrician, Pharmacist. Or Social Worker?

What role might other members of the health care team play in M.T.'s care?

After 28 more weeks, M.T. delivers a baby boy with Down's syndrome who is otherwise completely healthy. M.T. and her husband name him Gavin. Over the first couple of years of Gavin's life, M.T. experiences postpartum depression, a job loss, and a divorce. In addition, Gavin is starting to develop dysphagia and frequent lower respiratory infections, most likely due to aspiration. Gavin's pediatrician is concerned and recommends that he have a feeding tube placed until he can develop a more reliable cough reflex. Although M.T. is initially hesitant, the pediatrician insists that this is the "only option" to keep Gavin healthy.

If you were the nurse working in this pediatrics clinic, what options might you discuss with Gavin's pediatrician to ensure PCC for Gavin and his mother?

Patient Advocacy Groups

In the 1980s, health care consumers started to unite in their dissatisfaction with the health care system. Of particular concern was the lack of humanity within the health care system. Based on personal experiences, Jean and Harvey Picker joined forces with the Commonwealth Fund and the Beth Israel Hospital in the late 1980s to start The Picker Institute—an organization that sought "to foster a broader understanding of the practical and theoretical implications of PCC by approaching healthcare with a focus on the concerns of patients and other healthcare consumers" (The Picker Institute, 2012). In order to achieve this vision, eight principles of PCC were developed along with specific behavioral competencies for each (see Table 8.5).

In addition, reports of abuse and neglect in nursing homes, medical errors, and miscommunication between health care professionals were becoming more common, as were medical malpractice lawsuits. In 1999, the NAM (then, the Institute of Medicine (IOM)) provided the megaphone that these small consumer-led advocacy groups needed by releasing the landmark report, *Crossing the Quality Chasm* (IOM, 2001). Among other important achievements, this report catapulted the health care quality problem into the forefront of our consciousness as health care professionals. It also provided details about the enormous scope of the health care quality problem and introduced the six domains of quality in health care that are still used today—safety, effectiveness, accessibility, equitability, timeliness, and patient-centeredness (IOM, 2001).

Table 8.5   Picker Principles of Patient-Centered Care

Respect for patient's values, preferences, and expressed needs

- Care should be provided in an atmosphere that is respectful of the individual patient and focused on quality of life issues.
- Informed and shared decision-making is a central component of patient-centered care.
- Provide the patient with dignity, respect, and sensitivity to his/her cultural values.

Coordination and integration of care

- Coordination and integration of clinical care
- Coordination and integration of ancillary and support services
- Coordination and integration of front-line patient care

Information, communication, and education

- Information on clinical status, progress, and prognosis
- Information on processes of care
- Information and education to facilitate autonomy, self-care, and health promotion

Table 8.5   (Continued)

Physical comfort

- Pain management
- Assistance with activities of daily living needs
- Hospital surroundings and environment kept in focus, including that the patient's needs for privacy are accommodated and that patient areas are kept clean and comfortable, with appropriate accessibility for visits by family and friends.

Emotional support and alleviation of fear and anxiety

- Anxiety over clinical status, treatment, and prognosis
- Anxiety over the impact of the illness on themselves and family
- Anxiety over the financial impact of illness

Involvement of family and friends

- Accommodation, by clinicians and caregivers, of family and friends on whom the patient relies for social and emotional support
- Respect for and recognition of the patient advocate's role in decision-making
- Support for family members as caregivers
- Recognition of the needs of family and friends

Continuity and transition

- Provide understandable, detailed information about medications, physical limitations, dietary needs, etc.
- Coordinate and plan ongoing treatment and services after discharge and ensure that patients and family understand this information
- Provide information regarding access to clinical, social, physical, and financial support on a continuing basis

Access to Care

- Access to the location of hospitals, clinics, and physician offices
- Availability of transportation
- Ease of scheduling appointments
- Availability of appointments when needed
- Accessibility to specialists or specialty services when a referral is made
- Clear instructions provided on when and how to get referrals

Source: The Picker Institute, 2012.

After *Crossing the Quality Chasm* was released, a variety of organizations emerged in response to concerns about health care quality and safety. These included organizations led by consumer advocacy groups, patients and families, health care professionals, and the federal and state governments (Table 8.6). The primary goal of many of these groups was, and continues to be, to improve health care quality.

Long-standing consumer advocacy groups, such as the AARP and the **National Association for the Advancement of Colored People (NAACP)**, formed committees, work groups, and task forces to find solutions to concerns about health care quality that affected their members. Individual health care consumers banded together to form organizations focused on telling their stories about illness, injuries, and deaths resulting

Table 8.6   Patient Advocacy Groups

Type of Group	Example Organization	Mission/Vision
Consumer Advocacy Group	American Association of Retired Persons (AARP) (https://www.aarp.org/politics-society/advocacy)	"To empower people to choose how they live as they age."
	National Association for the Advancement of Colored People (NAACP) (https://www.naacp.org/issues/health)	"To ensure equal political, educational, social, and economic rights for all persons and to eliminate race-based discrimination."
Health Care Consumers	Patient Safety Movement (https://patientsafetymovement.org)	"Our ultimate goal is to get to ZERO preventable deaths."
	Institute for Patient- and Family-Centered Care (IPFCC) (http://www.ipfcc.org/about/index.html)	"Advances the understanding and practice of patient- and family-centered care. In partnership with patients, families, and health care professionals, IPFCC seeks to integrate these concepts into all aspects of health care."
	The Josie King Foundation (http://josieking.org/home)	"Prevent others from dying or being harmed by medical errors. By uniting health care providers and consumers, and funding innovative safety programs, we hope to create a culture of patient safety, together."

(Continued)

Table 8.6   (Continued)

Type of Group	Example Organization	Mission/Vision
Health Care Professionals	Institute for Healthcare Improvement (IHI) (www.ihi.org)	
	National Association of Healthcare Advocacy (NAHAC) (https://www.nahac.com/#!event-list)	"The professional health care advocacy organization; we are dedicated to the improvement of patient outcomes through continuing education, promotion of national standards of practice, and active pursuit of policy changes, leading to a high standard of person-centered health care."
	National Academy of Medicine (NAM) (www.nam.org)	"To improve health for all by advancing science, accelerating health equity, and providing independent, authoritative, and trusted advice nationally and globally."
Government Agencies	Agency for Healthcare Research and Quality (AHRQ) (www.ahrq.gov)	"To produce evidence to make health care safer, higher quality, more accessible, equitable, and affordable, and to work within the U.S. Department of Health and Human Services and with other partners to make sure that the evidence is understood and used."
	VA National Center for Patient Safety (www.patientsafety.va.gov/index.asp)	"To develop and nurture a culture of patient safety throughout the Veterans Health Administration."

from encounters with the health care system. Many of these groups also provide free educational resources for patients, families, and health care professionals. Examples include the Patient Safety Movement, the Josie King Foundation, and Campaign Zero. Groups of health care professionals also joined forces to advocate for evidence-based practices that promote health care quality. Finally, several federal and state government agencies formed new organizations and departments dedicated to improving health care quality. Importantly, nurses were involved in the initial development and continued efforts of nearly all of these organizations—a fact that highlights the potential impact of nurse leaders on the United States health care system (Flynn, Scott, Rotter, & Hartfield, 2017).

Patient-Centered Care Today

After nearly 60 years of evolution, what does PCC look like today? Certainly, there is a desire and professional obligation to include patients and their families when making health care decisions. The demand for PCC is stronger than ever, and it has come from a variety of sources:

- National organizations, including the American Nurses Association, have strongly supported PCC as a core professional competency.

- Health policies that support PCC as a requirement for full health care reimbursement have been either approved or upheld in recent years.

- Evidence is emerging that demonstrates a strong connection between PCC and improved health and economic outcomes.

- Patients and families are using social media outlets to describe their encounters—both good and bad—with the health care system, creating a rapid exchange of information about providers and facilities that may influence where others seek care.

The reality is that PCC is not just "one way" to provide care—it is the "right way." Understanding the patient's values, expectations, resources, and challenges is vitally important in planning effective and compassionate care. From a nursing perspective, adhering to the domains of PCC ensures that our patients receive the services they need without being excessive or inadequate. For example, what good is it to discharge Mrs. Sanchez, a 74-year-old widowed female with glaucoma, severe osteoarthritis, and coronary artery disease to her home after she has had an acute myocardial infarction (AMI), if she does not feel that she can safely take care of herself at home without someone available to help her? Due to her low vision, she may not be able to adhere to her complicated medication regimen, drive to her appointments with the cardiologist, or read nutrition labels to monitor her sodium intake. Osteoarthritis may limit her mobility, resulting in deconditioning and the inability to participate in aerobic exercise. She may feel that her health-related quality of life is low, and that her goals should focus on relieving suffering rather than preventing another AMI. Perhaps she believes that, since she survived this AMI, it wouldn't be such a big deal if she had another one. After all, her children and grandchildren all visited her in the hospital—something that rarely happens at home; perhaps she believes that her AMI actually brought her family closer together.

Whether these limitations, beliefs, or expectations seem reasonable to us is irrelevant. When Mrs. Sanchez goes home, the choice to follow the care plan (or not) is ultimately up to her. Being able to anticipate how Mrs. Sanchez might choose to deviate from the care plan, and then addressing any potential barriers or challenges ahead of time, is a powerful way to design a care plan that she might actually be able to stick to.

Patient-Centered Care and Patient Safety

While holistic care and shared decision-making remain cornerstones of PCC, it is also vitally important to prevent harm whenever possible. Nurses must balance their obligation to deliver care that is patient-centered with their obligation to deliver care that is safe. This is a considerable challenge in populations that are particularly vulnerable to injury or illness (e.g., infants, elderly, immunocompromised). For example, a parent who believes that vaccines can cause autism might choose not to have their children vaccinated. While the parent could expect that their desire to abstain from vaccinations will be followed, the health care team has to consider this decision in light of current research showing that there is no empirical or theoretical link between vaccines and autism. Moreover, the health care team has to apply their knowledge that failure to vaccinate can result in harm to the child and to the community.

The challenge of delivering safe PCC is also readily apparent in managing pain. Nurses have a multitude of options—both pharmacological and non-pharmacological—at their disposal to help relieve pain. However, some of these options, particularly opioids, can lead to harm in the forms of addiction, respiratory and central nervous system depression, delirium, and many others. Furthermore, opioid pain medications can be sold or stolen for their high street-value, which makes opioids a potential threat to public health and safety. Mazurenko, Andraka-Christou, and Bair, (2019) interviewed nurses, hospital medicine physicians, and case managers to understand how they negotiated the need to control pain using a PCC approach with the need to maintain patient safety. They reported that safe pain management lies on a continuum based on the complexity of pain and the patient's prior experiences using opioids. For those with high pain complexity and/or an opioid use disorder, pain was more difficult to safely control. In these cases, clinicians needed to find a careful balance between PCC and safety by offering acceptable alternatives to opioids, helping the patient to set realistic pain goals and expectations, and involving pain specialists or other members of the health care team.

Critical Thinking 8.1

You are the nurse working in a family practice clinic, which employs physicians, nurse practitioners, a diabetes **clinical nurse specialist** (**CNS**), a part-time dietitian, social workers, medical assistants, medical lab technologists and phlebotomists, and registered nurses.

One of your patients today is M.B., a 44-year-old female with both type 1 diabetes mellitus and decreased insulin sensitivity. Recently, her fingerstick blood glucose levels have been in the 300's and 400's at home, and she has been experiencing a "buzzing" sensation in both of her feet. Your physical exam reveals that she is an obese but otherwise healthy-appearing female with decreased sensation to the plantar surfaces of both feet. She does not have any deformities or ulcerations on her feet, and she has good peripheral circulation (i.e., skin is warm, pulses 2+ and capillary refill less than 2 s bilaterally, no evidence of venous stasis or arterial insufficiency). The family practice physician places the following orders at this time:

- Fingerstick blood glucose STAT

- Labs—Basic Metabolic Panel (BMP; i.e., sodium, potassium, chloride, bicarbonate, **blood urea nitrogen** [**BUN**], creatinine, and glucose); **Complete Blood Count** (CBC; white blood cells, red blood cells, hemoglobin, hematocrit, and platelets); Hemoglobin A1c; Vitamin B$_{12}$; Folate; and **Thyroid Stimulating Hormone** (TSH).

In addition, M.B. says that she has not been sticking to her diabetic diet or exercise plan, and she cannot afford her insulin.

What can each of the following members of the interprofessional team do for M.B.?

- (a) Physician
- (b) Social Worker
- (c) Medical Assistant
- (d) Phlebotomist
- (e) Medical Lab Technologist
- (f) Dietitian
- (g) Diabetes CNS

What do you think explains the "buzzing" sensation she is having in her feet? Are there any tests you can do in the clinic to assess this problem further?

Lab results are back. Her fingerstick glucose is 436 mg/dL, serum glucose (part of the BMP) is 448 mg/dL, creatinine is 1.3, hemoglobin is 13.2 g/dL, and hemoglobin A1c is 11.2%; all other lab tests are within normal limits. The physician orders a change in her medications: (a) increase Lantus insulin from 34 units twice daily to 40 units twice daily, (b) increase pre-meal Humalog insulin from 10 units to 12 units; and (c) start metformin (Glucophage) 500 mg twice daily.

What is the patient's role in achieving high-quality care for managing her diabetes?

Patients as Health Care Consumers

A particularly disturbing trend in PCC is the shifting attitude toward viewing patients as consumers of health care. This is largely based on the supposition that patients will pay for services that they want from whichever providers and facilities they choose, and that if a patient/consumer is dissatisfied with either the service or the provider, they will go elsewhere for care in the future.

While it is true that patients "purchase" health care services (either directly or through a third-party payer), Gusmano, Maschke, and Solomon (2019) argue that patients are not true consumers; health care is not a commodity like orange juice, a new handbag, or an airline ticket because the price of health care services is not known before the "purchase" is made. Furthermore, they argue that health care is not subject to the same competitive market forces as in other industries. For example, if a shopper wants to find the best deal on a particular grocery item, they can freely go from store to store until they find the one that offers that item at the best price. Patients generally do not have this same opportunity to shop around for the best price for health care services. This is changing somewhat with recent legislation that requires hospitals to make the cost of services publicly available, and with direct-to-consumer online sources that compare the cost of medications at pharmacies within the patient's zip code (http://goodrx.com, 2019). However, there is still a very long way to go before the health care "market" resembles a marketplace designed for true consumerism.

Patient-Centered Care and Nursing Education

There is an increasing demand from employers of nurses (e.g., hospitals, ambulatory care settings) to make sure that new nurses are ready to use so-called "**soft skills**"—negotiation,

collaboration, problem-solving, and so forth—when they graduate from their nursing program (Peterson-Graziose & Bryer, 2017). These skills generally focus on interpersonal communication techniques or strategies that promote better performance within a team, which is vital within health care. The demand for strong interpersonal communication skills has been echoed by organizations that set the standards for nursing education and practice in the United States, such as the American Nurses Association, the **National Council of State Boards of Nursing (NCSBN)**, and the **American Association of Colleges of Nursing (AACN)**. However, exactly which of these skills are most important for the new nurse is unclear.

In 2007, a group of nurse educators, researchers, administrators, and clinicians developed a new initiative that helped give some structure to the soft skills that nurses would need to have to improve patient care. The purpose of this initiative, which they termed **Quality and Safety Education in Nursing (QSEN)**, was to better prepare new nurses to practice with quality and safety in mind (Cronenwett et al., 2007). To achieve this purpose, nurses would have to develop a wide range of interpersonal skills that they could call upon at any time when taking care of patients. For example, if the nurse received a physician's order that they believed might harm a patient, they would be able to use QSEN principles to share this concern with the ordering physician in a productive way.

QSEN provides a set of competencies that nurses must be able to demonstrate when caring for patients. These competencies center around six key areas: PCC, teamwork and collaboration, evidence-based practice, quality improvement, safety, and informatics (Cronenwett et al., 2007). As one of the six QSEN competency domains, PCC represents an essential and foundational area of knowledge, skills, and abilities for all nurses regardless of their educational achievement, length of time in nursing, or personal beliefs. For a list of specific knowledge, skills, and abilities within the competency area of PCC, see Table 8.7.

Table 8.7   QSEN Competencies for Patient-Centered Care

Patient-centered care
Definition: Recognize the patient or designee as the source of control and full partner in providing compassionate and coordinated care based on respect for patient's preferences, values, and needs.

Knowledge	Skills	Attitudes
Integrate understanding of multiple dimensions of patient-centered care: • Patient/family/community preferences and values • Coordination and integration of care • Information, communication, and education • Physical comfort and emotional support • Involvement of family and friends • Transition and continuity Describe how diverse cultural, ethnic, and social backgrounds function as sources of patient, family, and community values.	Elicit patient values, preferences, and expressed needs as part of the clinical interview, implementation of care plan, and evaluation of care. Communicate patient values, preferences, and expressed needs to other members of the health care team. Provide patient-centered care with sensitivity and respect for the diversity of human experience.	Value seeing health care situations "through patients' eyes." Respect and encourage individual expression of patient values, preferences, and expressed needs. Value the patient's expertise with own health and symptoms. Seek learning opportunities with patients who represent all aspects of human diversity. Recognize personally held attitudes about working with patients from different ethnic, cultural, and social backgrounds. Willingly support patient-centered care for individuals and groups whose value differ from own.

Table 8.7   **(Continued)**

Patient-centered care
Definition: Recognize the patient or designee as the source of control and full partner in providing compassionate and coordinated care based on respect for patient's preferences, values, and needs.

Knowledge	Skills	Attitudes
Demonstrate comprehensive understanding of the concepts of pain and suffering, including physiologic models of pain and comfort.	Assess presence and extent of pain and suffering.	Recognize personally held values and beliefs about the management of pain or suffering.
	Assess levels of physical and emotional comfort.	Appreciate the role of the nurse in relief of all types and sources of pain or suffering.
	Elicit expectations of patient and family for relief of pain, discomfort, or suffering.	Recognize that patient expectations influence outcomes in management of pain or suffering.
	Initiative effective treatments to relieve pain and suffering in light of patient values, preferences, and expressed needs.	
Examine how the safety, quality, and cost-effectiveness of health care can be improved through the active involvement of patients and families.	Remove barriers to presence of families and other designated surrogates based on patient preferences.	Value active partnership with patients or designated surrogates in planning, implementation, and evaluation of care.
Examine common barriers to active involvement of patients in their own health care processes.	Assess level of patient's decisional conflict and provide access to resources.	Respect patient preferences for degree of active engagement in care processes.
Describe strategies to empower patients or families in all aspects of the health care process.	Engage patients or designated surrogates in active partnerships that promote health, safety and well-being, and self-care management.	Respect patient's right to access personal health records.
Explore ethical and legal implications of patient-centered care.	Recognize the boundaries of therapeutic relationships.	Acknowledge the tension that may exist between patient rights and the organizational responsibility for professional, ethical care.
Describe the limits and boundaries of therapeutic patient-centered care.	Facilitate informed patient consent for care.	Appreciate shared decision-making with empowered patients and families, even when conflicts occur.
Discuss principles of effective communication.	Assess own level of communication skill in encounters with patients and families.	Value continuous improvement of own communication and conflict resolution skills.
Describe basic principles of consensus building and conflict resolution.	Participate in building consensus or resolving conflict in the context of patient care.	
Examine nursing roles in assuring coordination, integration, and continuity of care.	Communicate care provided and needed at each transition in care.	

Source: Cronenwett et al. (2007).

Many nursing education programs in the United States have successfully incorporated QSEN competencies into their curricula, particularly through simulation (Table 8.8) and clinical experiences (Forneris et al., 2012; Griffiths, 2018; Masters, 2016; Peterson-Graziose & Bryer, 2017; Schaar, Ostendorf, & Kinner, 2013). However, addressing PCC competencies during the initial academic preparation of nurses is only one part of the solution. Experienced nurses must model these competencies in their practice for them to be "real" to the new nurses they are mentoring or orienting. Health care facilities must adopt policies and procedures that support PCC in all areas of practice, and they should identify

Table 8.8   Simulation Scenario to Improve a QSEN Competency

	Using a simulation scenario to improve a QSEN competency: Teamwork and collaboration example		
Brief simulation scenario	**Knowledge**	**Skills**	**Attitudes**
A group nursing students enter a room to take care of an elderly woman. She needs a urinary catheter inserted and to update her health care provider with laboratory results.	During the simulation scenario, students will work together to insert a urinary catheter, gather assessment data, and laboratory results. The students will collaborate with each other to formulate a plan of care. After the simulation scenario, students will describe their own strengths, limitations, and values in functioning as a member of the team.	During the simulation scenario, students will act with integrity while inserting the urinary catheter and help each other to maintain sterility upon insertion. After the simulation, students will provide respect for those with differing views about sterile procedures.	During the simulation, the students will decide what their individual team role and contribute to the team as they care for an older adult. After the simulation, the students will explore the importance of working intra-professional communication and develop a plan for personal improvement.

Source: T. Blodgett and N. Petsas Blodgett.

ways to hardwire a Culture of Safety that encourages PCC as one strategy to create a safer environment.

Effectiveness of Patient-Centered Care

PCC has evolved into more of a method of providing care than an intervention by itself. Nevertheless, virtually any health care intervention can be delivered in a way that could be considered patient-centered. As such, the effectiveness of using a PCC approach to delivering health care services is testable through experimental and quasi-experimental research designs.

A cursory literature search on the CINAHL database using the terms "effectiveness" and "PCC" joined by the Boolean operator "AND," limited to the English language, and published between 2014 and 2019, found 496 sources. The quality and strength of each article was not appraised, so it is entirely possible that some of these are weak sources of evidence. Therefore, a random sample of these 496 articles ($n = 9$) was selected to provide an overview of the evidence to support or disprove PCC as being an effective strategy to deliver health care services to patients and their families. A brief description of each article is provided in Table 8.9.

Table 8.9   Effectiveness of Patient-Centered Care

Patient population (source)	Study description	Findings
People of any age with intellectual disabilities (Ratti et al., 2016)	Systematic review of 16 articles that evaluated the effectiveness of person-centered care on selected health and social outcomes.	PCC approaches have a positive moderate effect on community participation, participation in activities, and daily choice-making. The effect on other outcomes, such as employment, was inconsistent.
Adults with type 2 diabetes mellitus (Odgers-Jewell et al., 2017)	A single group pretest-posttest design was used to determine if a patient-centered group-based education program for adults with type 2 diabetes mellitus resulted in weight loss, decreased BMI, and decreased waist circumference, and to evaluate if this approach was feasible and acceptable to patients. The setting was a primary care clinic.	Participants lost an average of 0.72 kg (95% CI -1.44 to −0.01 [significant]). Their BMI decreased by 0.25 kg/m² (95% CI -0.49 to −0.01 [significant]). Waist circumference decreased by 1.04 cm (95% CI -4.52 to 2.44 [not significant]). Group education was acceptable and feasible.
Adults with chronic illnesses (Fredericks, Lapum, & Hui, 2015)	Systematic review of 40 articles that evaluated the effectiveness of PCC-based interventions on self-care behaviors in adults with chronic illness.	Overall, PCC interventions did not effectively improve self-care behaviors in this population.
Adults receiving care for head and neck cancer (Gyllensten, Koinberg, Carlstrom, Olsson, & Olofsson, 2019)	Randomized controlled trial comparing a patient-centered approach to cancer treatment (shared decision-making, availability of nurse coordinator, phone consultations, individualized care plan) to standard care (oncologist-directed treatment plan).	Costs of care and missed work tended to be lower in the PCC intervention group, but the differences were not statistically significant. Quality of life tended to be higher in the PCC intervention group, but the difference was not statistically significant.

Table 8.9 (Continued)

Patient population (source)	Study description	Findings
Children aged 3–17 years with complex medical problems who are undergoing MRI (Mastro et al., 2019)	Retrospective cohort study in which participants had an MRI under one of the following conditions: (1) anesthesia-free, PFC intervention with MRI; (2) anesthesia-free, no PFC intervention; (3) with anesthesia and child life specialist; or (4) with anesthesia but no PFC intervention or child life specialist.	Anesthesia-free MRI with a PFC intervention (group 1) resulted in significantly lower cost and shorter procedure times than the other 3 groups, and MRI images were of acceptable or better quality in group 1 than those in the other 3 groups.
Older adults living in the community (Zhang et al., 2018)	Randomized controlled trial in which participants were assigned to either a PCC intervention to control health-related risk factors or to routine clinical care.	Adherence to healthy lifestyle behaviors increased significantly over a 2-year period in the intervention group. Self-reported health indicators were also significantly improved in the intervention group. There were no significant changes in these outcomes in the control group.
Older adults living in the community (Uittenbroek et al., 2018)	Retrospective cohort study to determine the cost-effectiveness of a patient-centered integrated primary care service for older adults, compared to usual primary care.	Total average costs were significantly higher for patient-centered integrated primary care service with non-significant, though favorable, improvements in health-associated outcomes.
Adults being discharged from the hospital after a heart failure exacerbation (Gonzaga 2018)	Single-group pretest-posttest design was used to determine if a patient-centered educational program improved self-management of HF after discharge.	Patient-centered education enhances self-management and self-confidence in patients with heart failure.
Adults with coronary artery disease (Chiang, Choi, Ho, et al., 2018)	Systematic review and meta-analysis of pooled data from 15 articles (12 RCT's) that examined the effectiveness of patient-centered approaches for secondary prevention of cardiac disease. Several clinical outcomes were compared.	Methodological quality of studies was fair. Meta-analysis found significantly reduced smoking, improved adherence to exercise regimen, and reduced total cholesterol. Individual studies reported improved health-related quality of life, weight, and alcohol consumptions. There were no statistically significant differences in the following outcomes: dietary habits, mortality, certain cardiac physiological parameters, and self-efficacy.
Adults with multiple chronic comorbid conditions (Salisbury et al., 2018)	Randomized trial that compared a patient-centered approach that focused on managing individualized dimensions of health, depression, and drugs ("3D's"), compared to traditional primary care, to improve health-related quality of life over a 15-month period of time.	Health-related quality of life did not significantly improve in the "3D's" intervention group.

Source: Table compiled by T. Blodgett and N. Petsas Blodgett.

Evidence from the Literature

Source: Adapted from Vessey, J. A., Wendt, J., Glynn, D. M., & McVey, C. (2018). Teaching patient-centered care through the Veterans History Project. *Nurse Educator, 43*, 6, 322–325. doi: 10.1097/NNE.0000000000000506

Background: Nearly every nurse will care for a military veteran at some point in their career. However, learning how to interact with military veterans may not be discussed during undergraduate nursing education programs, which means that new nurses usually learn how to do this "on the job." The purpose of this article was to enhance the understanding of veteran culture among new nurses working in the Veterans Affairs (VA) health care system.

Methods: A qualitative approach was used. New nurses who were enrolled in the post-baccalaureate nurse residency program at a VA Medical Center in the Northeast United States participated in this project. Using the Veterans History Project (a program through the U.S. Library of Congress to collect first-person accounts of wartime service experiences) as a framework, nurse residents asked volunteer veterans who had served in a military conflict from World War II through Operation Enduring Freedom (Afghanistan) to describe their wartime service and share how their military experience has shaped their health, health behaviors, and health-seeking activities. Interviews were audio-recorded.

Nurse residents completed a brief evaluation instrument afterwards to gain feedback about their experience, knowledge about military culture, and comfort with talking to veterans.

Results: Nurse residents rated their interview experiences highly. They felt that this approach would help them provide more PCC to the veteran population, and that the interviews exposed them to the realities of military engagement that their future patients may also have experienced. Nurse residents reported that this experience helped them debunk stereotypes, understand intergenerational differences (e.g., slang, social norms), and develop a deeper understanding for the unique needs of military veterans.

Implications: Experiential learning opportunities, such as the Veterans History Project, can help new nurses (and perhaps undergraduate nursing students) to develop PCC competencies for working with military veterans.

Critical Thinking 8.2

Note the patient questions on the HCAHPS survey, www.advisory. com//-/media/Advisory-com/Research/PEC/Resources/2017/ HCAHPS%20Star%20Ratings.pdf. Questions include, for example, how often did nurses treat you with courtesy and respect? Does gathering information about nurses and other health care providers in this way improve PCC?

As the articles in Table 8.9 illustrate, patient-centered approaches to care tend to be at least as effective at improving health outcomes as the care that clinicians usually give. However, the effectiveness of PCC is inconsistent from population to population. Some studies found significant improvement in health outcomes while others found either no improvement or slight improvement that was not statistically significant. However, for a number of reasons, this should not necessarily prevent nurses from using patient-centered approaches when planning and delivering care. First, none of these studies found worse clinical outcomes in the group that received PCC. This means that PCC did not necessarily harm participants—only that they did not improve more than those who received traditional care. Second, it was unclear in several studies how the PCC interventions were substantially different than the "usual care" that patients in the comparison groups received. If the PCC interventions were not all that different than usual care, why should we expect the outcomes to be significantly different between these groups? Third, and probably most importantly, it is methodologically difficult to study patient-centeredness. If researchers cannot yet control or measure how patient-centered an intervention is, then the delivery of a purely patient-centered intervention cannot be guaranteed, nor the effect of its variability on health outcomes assessed. In other words, from a statistical perspective, the patient-centeredness is a messy variable to measure, and because it is messy, we don't know if the outcomes we are interested in changed because of how patient-centered the intervention was or because of something in the "messiness." Perhaps the outcome changed because the intervening nurse in the PCC group was simply more kind than the nurse in the non-PCC group. Kindness is not the same thing as patient-centeredness, but it can certainly impact how much a patient chooses to stick with an intervention.

In summary, patient-centered interventions tend to be at least as effective as the care that clinicians usually provide in terms of measurable health outcomes like weight, smoking status, and time to complete an MRI scan. However, there are myriad variables that are less measurable, such as the patient's perception of how much the nurse cares about them, feasibility and creativity of the care plan, and the patient's **self-efficacy** (belief that they have the power to change their own health behaviors and outcomes). These variables can all affect how likely the patient is to follow the plan of care—whether patient-centered or not. Therefore, nurses and other health care professionals should critically review the evidence that exists about the effectiveness of PCC within their population of interest, weigh this evidence against the patient's unique circumstances (e.g., resources, limitations, level of interest), and use their best clinical judgment to decide how best to intervene using a patient-centered approach to care.

Conclusion

In this chapter, we have provided an overview of PCC, how this approach to care developed over time, and how it can be used to guide nurses in their care of patients in a variety of settings and circumstances. We defined patient-centered care, and the explained historical, political, cultural, and economic influences on PCC; described PCC competencies for nurses; described the potential impact of PCC on health outcomes; and compared and contrasted between episodes of care that are patient-centered and that are not patient-centered.

Patients are entitled to receive health care services in a way that incorporates their own preferences and beliefs, respects their inherent right to choose what happens to their own body, and reinforces their dignity as holistic human beings. Nurses are uniquely positioned within the health care team to ensure that the voices of their patients—whether individuals, families, communities, or populations—are clearly heard by others on the team. While the definition and techniques of PCC has evolved over the past half-century since it was first described, the goal remains the same: To achieve the best possible health outcomes for our patients.

KEY CONCEPTS

- PCC is defined as providing care that is respectful of and responsive to individual patient preferences, needs, and values and ensuring that patient values guide all clinician decisions.

- Historical, political, cultural, and economic factors influenced PCC.

- There are PCC competencies for nurses.

- PCC has the potential to impact of health outcomes.

- There are episodes of care that are patient-centered and that are not patient-centered.

KEY TERMS

Health Care Consumers

Health disparities

Soft skills

Holistic care

Paternalism

PCC

Patient Satisfaction

Quality and Safety Education in
  Nursing (QSEN)

Self-efficacy

Shared decision making

REVIEW QUESTIONS

1. Patient-centered care (PCC) is defined as:
   a. when members of the health care team view their patients through this holistic and humanistic lens, respect the patient's input as being equally important to their own, and allow patients to guide how their care is delivered.
   b. when members of the health care team view their patients through this holistic and humanistic lens and allow patients to guide how their care is delivered.
   c. when members of the health care team view their patients through a narrow lens, the views of the healthcare provider are more important than the patient and allow patients to guide how their care is delivered.
   d. when patients view themselves as the leaders of the healthcare team.

2. Holistic care is a foundational feature of nursing in which healing involves a mind-body-spirit-emotion-environment approach. What is the relationship with holistic care and PCC?
   a. Holistic care and PCC are not related.
   b. Holistic care and PCC can be used interchangeably.
   c. PCC relies upon this holistic perspective; holistic care does not necessarily address how clinicians use the patient's input to make health care decisions. Holistic care is therefore only one piece of PCC.
   d. Holistic care address how clinicians use the patient's input to make health care decisions. PCC is a part of holistic care.

3. Which best describes an inherently subjective measure, and it relies on a complex interplay between health care professionals (e.g., technical skills, interpersonal skills), patients (e.g., expectations about care, needs, priorities), and resources at the facility (e.g., staff availability, institutional policies, access to equipment and supplies)?
   a. Patient satisfaction.
   b. Patient survey.
   c. Patient preferences.
   d. Patient consumers.

4. What cultural revolutions happened since 1960 that have helped draw attention to the importance of PCC? (Select all that apply.)

   a. Rights of Women.
   b. Rights of People with Mental Illness.
   c. Health Policy Initiatives.
   d. Social Security Act.

5. A parent who believes that vaccines can cause autism might choose not to have their children vaccinated. While the parent could expect that their desire to abstain from vaccinations will be followed, the health care team has to consider this decision in light of current research showing that there is no empirical or theoretical link between vaccines and autism. This is an example of:
   a. Patient-Centered Care and Patient Safety.
   b. Holistic Care and Patient Safety.
   c. Vaccination Programs and Patient Safety.
   d. Patient-Centered Care and Community Risk.

6. There is an increasing demand from employers of nurses (e.g., hospitals, ambulatory care settings) to make sure that new nurses are ready to use "soft skills" when they graduate from their nursing program. Which the following are considered "soft skills?"
   a. Negotiation, collaboration, and problem solving.
   b. Collaboration, following healthcare provider orders, and cooperation.
   c. Injections, urinary catheter insertion, and teamwork.
   d. Problem solving, self-scheduling, and management.

7. Which of the following is the most accurate statement about the effectiveness of PCC?
   a. Patient-centered interventions tend to be at least as effective as the care that clinicians usually provide in terms of measurable health outcomes like weight, smoking status, and time to complete an MRI scan.
   b. Patient-centered interventions are not effective as the care that clinicians usually provide in terms of measurable health outcomes like weight, smoking status, and time to complete an MRI scan.
   c. Patient-centered interventions tend to be more effective as the care that clinicians usually provide in terms of

measurable health outcomes like weight, smoking status, and time to complete an MRI scan.

d. There is little known about PCC interventions and effectiveness.

8. You are taking care of a 34-year-old pregnant mother who states, "I have the power to change my blood sugar by watching what I eat and start exercising." This is an example of:
   a. Self promotion.
   b. Inaccurate teaching.
   c. Self-Efficacy.
   d. Inaccurate information.

9. Which of these examples best describes paternalism?
   a. A male social worker and patient working together to get medications.

b. A female nurse and patient working on a plan of care.

c. A female physician making the decision that the patient should be in a nursing home.

d. A male physician and patient, with their family, decide to end dialysis.

10. QSEN provides a set of competencies that nurses must be able to demonstrate when caring for patients. These competencies center around which key areas (select all that apply):
    a. PCC.
    b. Teamwork and collaboration.
    c. Evidence-based practice.
    d. Quality improvement.
    e. Safety.
    f. Informatics.

REVIEW QUESTION ANSWERS

1. Answer: A is correct.
   Rationale: Patient-centered care (PCC) is defined as (A) when members of the health care team view their patients through this holistic and humanistic lens, respect the patient's input as being equally important to their own, and allow patients to guide how their care is delivered. (B) When members of the health care team view their patients through this holistic and humanistic lens and allow patients to guide how their care is delivered, (C) when members of the health care team view their patients through a narrow lens, and (D) when patients view themselves as the leaders of the health care team are incorrect.

2. Answer: C is correct.
   Rationale: PCC relies upon this holistic perspective; holistic care does not necessarily address how clinicians use the patient's input to make health care decisions. Holistic care is therefore only one piece of PCC (C). (A) Holistic care and PCC are not related, (B), holistic care and PCC can be used interchangeably, and (D) holistic care addresses how clinicians use the patient's input to make health care decisions, are correct.

3. Answer: A is correct.
   Rationale: (A) Patient satisfaction, PCC relies upon this holistic perspective; holistic care does not necessarily address how clinicians use the patient's input to make health care decisions. Holistic care is therefore only one piece of PCC. (B) Patient survey, (C) patient preferences, and (D) patient consumers are incorrect:

4. Answers A, B, and C are correct.
   Rationale: (A) Rights of Women, (B) Rights of People with Mental Illness, and (C) Health Policy Initiatives are correct. (D) The Social Security Act is incorrect.

5. Answer: A is correct.
   Rationale: (A) Patient-Centered Care and Patient Safety. This is an example of PCC and patient safety. (B) Holistic Care and Patient Safety, (C) Vaccination Programs and Patient Safety, and (D) Patient-Centered Care and Community Risk are incorrect.

6. Answer: A is correct.
   Rationale: (A) Negotiation, collaboration, and problem solving are "soft skills." (B) Collaboration, following health care provider orders, and cooperation, (C) injections, urinary catheter insertion, and teamwork, and (D) problem solving, self-scheduling, and management are incorrect.

7. Answer: A is correct.
   Rationale: (A) Patient-centered interventions tend to be at least as effective as the care that clinicians usually provide in terms of measurable health outcomes like weight, smoking status, and time to complete an MRI scan. (B) Patient-centered interventions are not effective as the care that clinicians usually provide in terms of measurable health outcomes like weight, smoking status, and time to complete an MRI scan, (C) patient-centered interventions tend to be more effective as the care that clinicians usually provide in terms of measurable health outcomes like weight, smoking status, and time to complete an MRI scan, and (D) there is little known about PCC interventions and effectiveness, are incorrect.

8. Answer: C is correct.
   Rationale: (C) This is an example of self-efficacy. (A) Self promotion, (B) inaccurate teaching, and (D) inaccurate information are incorrect.

9. Answer: C is correct.
   Rationale:(C) A female physician making the decision that the patient should be in a nursing home is an example of paternalism. (A) male social worker and patient working together to get medications, (B) a female nurse and patient working on a plan of care, and (D) a male physician and patient, with their family, decide to end dialysis, are incorrect.

10. Answers A, B, C, D, E, and F are correct.
    Rationale: QSEN competencies center around six key areas: (A) PCC, (B) teamwork and collaboration, (C) evidence-based practice, (D) quality improvement, (E) safety, and (F) informatics.

REVIEW ACTIVITIES

1. Compare and contrast the roles of healthcare team (nurse, physician, pharmacist, social work, physical therapy, etc.) to providing PCC. What are strengths of each profession? What are areas that need to be improved?

2. Analyze trends in PCC. How are these trends going to impact caring for patients in the future?

3. Create a plan to advocate for the use of PCC in a healthcare team.

4. Review the HCAHPS survey that measures patient satisfaction, and develop a plan to aimed at one of the patient measures.

DISCUSSION POINTS

1. During your last clinical experience; describe how you saw PCC modeled. Where there any historical, political, cultural, and economic influences on PCC?

2. How can you improve patient-centered care at your institution?

3. Why should your institution be motivated by the potential impact of patient-centered care on health outcomes?

4. During your last clinical experience, think of an experience that was not patient-centered. How was the patient, family, or healthcare team impacted?

DISCUSSION OF OPENING SCENARIO

In this scenario, we know how painful pancreatitis is and that your patient is having a difficult time coping with their illness. What would you do next?

- The PCC approach would be to stop and listen to the patient, answer any questions that arise, and provide health education about the re-occurrence of pancreatitis.

- What would happen if you treated the pain instead of listening to the patient? How would this effect his hospital stay and his prognosis?

- Since the patient is resting comfortably, pain isn't your first concern. If you were to treat his pain first, you may not be able to discuss his underlying fear related to his diagnosis. Once he can understand his diagnosis and cause of pain, he will be less anxious. Education about his diagnosis will help meet better health outcomes.

EXPLORING THE WEB

- National Academy of Medicine, https://nam.edu Accessed July 30, 2019.

- Patient Protection and Affordable Care Act, www.healthcare.gov/health-care-law-protections Accessed July 30, 2019.

- Agency for Healthcare Research & Quality, www.ahrq.gov Accessed on July 30, 2019.

- The U.S. Department of Veterans Affairs: VA Center for Patient Safety, www.patientsafety.va.gov,Accessed on July 30, 2019.

- American Nurses Association, www.nursingworld.org/ana Accessed on July 30, 2019.

- National Council of State Boards of Nursing, www.ncsbn.org/index.htm Accessed July 30, 2019.

- American Academy of Colleges of Nursing, www.aacnnursing.org Accessed July 30, 2019.

- Quality and Safety Education for Nurses, http://qsen.org, Accessed July 30, 2019.

INFORMATICS

Go to www.ahrq.gov Accessed on July 30, 2019. Click on Programs, and then click on, Quality & Patient Safety. Then click on CUSP Toolkit. Scroll down and find the role of the nurse manager. Watch

The Role of the Nurse Manager video. Download the CUSP toolkit. What did you learn from this activity?

LEAN BACK

- How to you think the information presented in this chapter will matter to you as a future nurse leader, nurse manager, or chief nurse officer?

- If I'm a patient, how would I expect to be treated by the health care team?

REFERENCES

Bailoor, K., Valley, T., Perumalswami, C., Shuman, A., DeVries, R., & Zahuranec, D. (2018). How acceptable is paternalism? A survey-based study of clinician and nonclinician opinions on paternalistic decision making. *AJOB Empirical Bioethics*, 9(2), 91–98. doi:10.1080/23294515.2018.1462273

Bladon, H. (2019). Avoiding paternalism. *Issues in Mental Health Nursing*. doi:10.1080/01612840.2019.1570405

Brown, B. (2019). *The Call to Courage*. Retrieved from https://thrivecounselingaustin.com/blog/2019/4/29/favorite-quotes-from-bren-browns-netflix-special-the-call-to-courage

Chiang, C., Choi, K., Ho, C., and Yu, S. (2018). Effectiveness of nurse-led patient-centered care behavioral risk modification on secondary prevention of coronary heart disease: A systematic review. International Journal of Nursing Studies, 84, 28–39. doi:10.1016/j.ijnurstu.2018.04.012

Cole, J., Kiriaev, O., Malpas, P., & Cheung, G. (2017). "Trust me, I'm a doctor:" A qualitative study of the role of paternalism and older people in decision-making when they have lost their capacity. *Australasian Psychiatry*, 25(6), 549–553. doi:10.1177/1039856217734741

Cronenwett, L., Sherwood, G., Barnsteiner, J., Disch, J., Johnson, J., et al. (2007). Quality and safety education for nurses. *Nursing Outlook*, 55(3), 122–131.

Flynn, R., Scott, S. D., Rotter, T., & Hartfield (2017). The potential for nurses to contribute to and lead process improvement science in health care. *Journal of Advanced Nursing*, 73(1), 97–107. doi:10.1111/jan.13164

Forneris, S. G., Crownover, J. G., Dorsey, L., Leahy, N., Maas, N. A., et al. (2012). Integrating QSEN and ACES: An NLN simulation leader project. *Nursing Education Perspectives*, 33, 184–187. doi:10.5480/1536-5026-33.3.18

Fredericks, S., Lapum, J., & Hui, G. (2015). Examining the effect of patient-centered care on outcomes. *British Journal of Nursing*, 24(7), 394–400. doi:10.12968/bjon.2015.24.7.394

Gonzaga, M. (2018). Enhanced patient-Centered educational program for HF self-care management in sub-acute settings. Applied Nursing Research, 42, 22–34. https://doi.org/10.1016/j.apnr.2018.

Griffiths, B. (2018). Preparing tomorrow's nurses for collaborative quality care through simulation. *Teaching & Learning in Nursing*, 13(1), 46–50. doi:10.1016/j.teln.2017.08.005

Gusmano, M., Maschke, K., & Solomon, M. (2019). Patient-centered care, yes; patients as consumers, no. *Health Affairs*, 38(3), 368–373. doi:10.1377/hlthaff.2018.05019

Gyllensten, H., Koinberg, I., Carlstrom, E., Olsson, L.-E., & Olofsson, E. (2019). Economic evaluation of a person-centred care intervention in head and neck oncology: Results from a randomized controlled trial. *Support Care Cancer*, 27(5), 1825–1834. doi:10.1007/s00520-018-4436-2

Health Consumer Assessment of Healthcare Providers and Systems. (2019). *HCAHPS Hospital Survey*. Retrieved from www.hcahpsonline.org/global-assets/hcahps/survey-instruments/mail/april-1-2019-and-forward-discharges/2018-2019_survey-instruments_english_mail_omb-expiration.pdf.

Institute of Medicine (IOM). (2001). *Crossing the quality chasm: A new health system for the 21st century.* Washington, DC: National Academy Press.

Kilbride, M. K., & Joffe, S. (2018). The new age of patient autonomy: Implications for the patient-physician relationship. *JAMA*, 320(19), 1973–1974. doi:10.1001/jama.2018.14382

Masters, K. (2016). Integrating quality and safety education into clinical nursing education through a dedicated education unit. *Nurse Education in Practice*, 17, 153–160. doi:10.1016/j.nepr.2015.12.002

Mastro, K., Flynn, L., Millar, T., DiMartino, T., Ryan, S., & Stein, M. (2019). Reducing anesthesia use for pediatric magnetic resonance imaging: The effects of a patient- and family-centered intervention on image quality, health-care costs, and operational efficiency. *Journal of Radiology Nursing*, 38(1), 21–27. doi:10.1016/j.jradnu.2018.12.003

Mazurenko, O., Andraka-Christou, B., & Bair, M. (2019). Balancing patient-centered and safe pain care for nonsurgical inpatients: Clinical and managerial perspectives. *The Joint Commission Journal on Quality and Patient Safety*, 45(4), 241–248. doi:10.1016/j.jcjq.2018.11.004

Miller, J., Morris, P., Files, D. C., Gower, E., & Young, M. (2016). Decision conflict and regret among surrogate decision makers in the medical intensive care unit. *Journal of Critical Care*, 32, 79–84. doi:10.1016/j.jcrc.2015.11.023

Muaygil, R. A. (2018). From paternalistic to patronizing: How cultural competence can be ethically problematic. *HEC Forum*, 30(1), 13–29. doi:10.1007/s10730-017-9336-1

Odgers-Jewell, K., Ball, L., Kelly, J., Isenring, E., Reidlinger, D., & Thomas, R. (2017). Effectiveness of group-based self-management education for individuals with type 2 diabetes: A systematic review with meta-analyses and meta-regression. *Diabetic Medicine*, 34(8), 1027–1039. doi:10.1111/dme.13340

Peterson-Graziose, V., & Bryer, J. (2017). Assessing student perceptions of quality and safety education for nurses competencies in a baccalaureate curriculum. *The Journal of Nursing Education*, 56(7), 435–438. doi:10.3928/01484834-20170619-09

Ratti, V., Hassiotis, A., Crabtree, J., Deb, S., Gallagher, P., & Unwin, G. (2016). The effectiveness of person-centred planning for people with intellectual disabilities: A systematic review. *Research in Developmental Disabilities*, 57, 63–84. doi:10.1016/j.ridd.2016.06.015

Salisbury, C., Man, M.-S., Bower, P., Guthrie, B., Chaplin, K., Gaunt, D. M., Brookes, S., Fitzpatrick, B., Gardner, C., Hollinghurst, S., Lee, V., McLeod, J., Mann, C., Moffat, K. R. & Mercer, S. W. (2018). Management of multimorbidity using a patient-centred care model: A pragmatic cluster-randomised trial of the 3D approach. *The Lancet*, 392(10141), 41–50. doi:10.1016/S0140-6736(18)31308-4

Schaar, G., Ostendorf, M., & Kinner, T. (2013). Simulation: Linking quality and safety education for nurses competencies to the observer role. *Clinical Simulation in Nursing*, 9(9), e40–e404. doi:10.1016/j.ecns.2012.07.209

Tanenbaum, S. J. (2015). What is patient-centered care? A typology of models and missions. *Health Care Analysis*, 23(3), 272–287. doi:10.1007/s10728-013-0257-0

The Picker Institute. (2013). www.picker.org

The Picker Institute. (2012). Patient- and Family-Centered Care. Retrieved October 22, 2020, from https://www.ipfcc.org/about/pfcc.htm

Uittenbroek, R., Asselt, A., Spoorenberg, S., Kremer, H., Wynia, K., & Reijneveld, S. (2018). Integrated and person centered care for community living older adults: A cost effectiveness study. *Health Services Research*, 53, 3471–3494. doi:10.1111/1475-6773.12853

Zhang, M., Chao, J., Li, D., Gu, J., Chen, W., Xu, H., Hussain, M., Wu, W., Deng, L., He, T. & Zhang, R. (2018). The effect of older-person centered and integrated health management model on multiple lifestyle behaviors: A randomized controlled trial from China. *Archives of Gerontology and Geriatrics*, 79, 45–51. doi:10.1016/j.archger.2018.07.012

SUGGESTED READINGS

Altmiller, G., & Hopkins-Pepe, L. (2019). Why quality and safety education for nurses (QSEN) matters in practice. *Journal of Continuing Education in Nursing*, *50*(5), 199–200. doi:10.3928/00220124-20190416-04

Fredericks, S., Lapum, J., & Hui, G. (2015). Examining the effect of patient-centered care on outcomes. *British Journal of Nursing*, *24*(7), 394–400. doi:10.12968/bjon.2015.24.7.394

Gonzaga, M. (2018). Enhanced patient-Centered educational program for HF self-care management in sub-acute settings. *Applied Nursing Research*, *42*, 22–34. doi:10.1016/j.apnr.2018.03.010 http://goodrx.com (2019). https://www.goodrx.com/?kw=price&utm_source=bing&utm_medium=cpc&utm_term=good.rx|p&utm_campaign=Brand&utm_content=Ad-Group_GoodRx&msclkid=146cc4745fcd1186b2c399622eae44ea

Gusmano, M., Maschke, K., & Solomon, M. (2019). Patient-centered care, yes; patients as consumers. *Health Affairs*, *38*(3), 368–373. doi:10.1377/hlthaff.2018.05019

Hack, S. M., Muralidharan, A., Brown, C. H., Lucksted, A. A., & Patterson, J. (2017). Provider and consumer behaviors and their interaction for measuring person-centered care. *International Journal of Person Centered Medicine*, *7*(1), 14–20.

Kilbride, M. K., & Joffe, S. (2018). The new age of patient autonomy: Implications for the patient-physician relationship. *JAMA*, *320*(19), 1973–1974. doi:10.1001/jama.2018.14382

Peterson-Graziose, V., & Bryer, J. (2017). Assessing student perceptions of quality and safety education for nurses competencies in a baccalaureate curriculum. *Journal of Nursing Education*, *56*(7), 435–438. doi:10.3928/01484834-20170619-09

Siouta, E., Muhli, U., Hedberg, B., Brostrom, A., Fossum, B., & Karlgren, K. (2016). Patients' experiences of communication and involvement in decision making about atrial fibrillation treatment in consultations with nurses and physicians. *Scandinavian Journal of Caring Sciences*, *30*, 535–546. doi:10.1111/scs.12276

9 Patient and Health Care Education

Rochelle R. Flayter[1], Lisa Kidin[2], Monika S. Schuler[3]

[1] US Health Southern Colorado, Colorado Springs, CO, USA
[2] Memorial Hospital-UCHealth, Colorado Springs, CO, USA
[3] College of Nursing, University of Massachusetts, Dartmouth, North Dartmouth, MA, USA

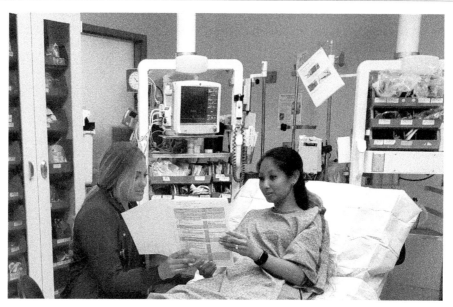

Picture of a patient sitting in bed, nurse with paperwork.
Source: Nicki Schroeder.

> Tell me and I forget, teach me and I remember, involve me and I learn.
>
> *(Chinese Proverb, 312–230 BCE, Goodreads (2019)). Public Domain.*

OBJECTIVES

Upon completion of this chapter, the reader should be able to:

1. Discuss the foundations of patient-centered and professional nursing education.

2. Analyze the role of the nurse in patient-centered education and professional development.

3. Identify the impact of reading and health literacy on patient-centered health care and patient outcomes.

4. Describe the desired **knowledge, skills, and attitudes** (KSAs) and their utility in designing learning experiences.

5. Utilize educational resources, patient-centered and professional development education.

6. Develop a lesson plan for a patient/family teaching session.

7. Evaluate the effectiveness of a patient-centered education experience.

8. Discuss strategies for professional development.

9. Develop a learning module/lesson plan for health care professionals based on adult learning principles.

10. Review nursing and health care related competencies.

11. Identify teaching strategies for the adult learner.

OPENING SCENARIO

*Your patient, Mr. DaPina is a 45-year old Portuguese immigrant who is ready to be discharged from your acute care setting following a new diagnosis of **chronic obstructive pulmonary disease** (COPD). You are preparing his discharge teaching.*

1. *How will you assess Mr. DaPina's learning needs?*

2. *How will you determine the best way to teach Mr. DaPina about his diagnosis?*

3. *What are some teaching strategies you will use to ensure Mr. DaPina has the knowledge he needs to manage his new diagnosis?*

This chapter will discuss both the patient and nurse perspective of education by focusing on the various domains of learning and how they impact learning experiences. At the end of the chapter the reader will be able to discuss the foundations of patient-centered care and professional nursing education with a focus on the adult learner. The reader will be able to analyze the role of the nurse in patient centered education, identify the impact of reading and health literacy on patient-centered education, describe the major learning domains and their use in designing learning experiences, and consider the utility of educational resources to develop educational programs including the development of lesson plans. The reader will also be able to develop learning modules for professional development and discuss effective teaching strategies for use in professional development.

Foundations for Patient-Centered and Professional Development Education

Education is an inherent part of nursing. Patient education has been a part of nursing care since the time of Florence Nightingale. As early as 1918, the National League of Nursing Education (now the **National League for Nursing** [NLN]) observed the value of patient education within the scope of nursing practice. In 1976, the Joint Commission on Accreditation of Health Care Organizations reinforced the value of patient education and identified that it was both a right and expectation of quality health care delivery. Today, patient education is both an expectation and a legal obligation of nursing in all states as part of Nurse Practice Acts. Patient-centered health care education has been associated with decreased hospitalizations, increased compliance with care plans, better self-management of disease processes and medications, decreased complications, and increased preventative screenings (Paterick, Patel, Tajik, & Chandrasekaran, 2017). **Patient-centered and staff health care education** is the communication of facts, ideas, and skills to change knowledge, attitudes, values, behaviors, and skills of patients, families, and fellow health care staff.

Quality patient care is linked to a well-educated nursing workforce that has continued their education beyond the completion of formal education in an academic setting. Current and future trends in health care require nurses to stay current in both emerging technologies and evidence-based practices. The purpose of staff education is to improve the quality of care delivered to patients by nurses who have developed enhanced competence in professional practices. Staff education may include formal orientation programs, inter-professional training, professional skill development, career and personal development, all of which play an important role in improving the quality of patient care. Further benefits of staff education include employee retention, enhanced morale, nursing practice efficiency, job competency, and subsequent improved patient satisfaction.

The Role of the Nurse in Patient-Centered Health Care Education

Today's health care environment is rapidly evolving and becoming increasingly more complex. This complex environment can be challenging to navigate and is even more challenging when one is compromised by an illness. Nurses play a key role in providing health care information to patients and their families. **Patient-centered care** recognizes the patient as the source of control and full partner in providing compassionate and coordinated care (Cronenwett et al., 2007). Patient-centered education is a set of planned learning activities in which nurses' work with patients and their families or caregivers to share information that will alter patient health behaviors with the goal of improving their health status and/or slowing the deterioration of their health. Patient-centered education is essential for helping the patient understand their diagnosis and condition, develop a realistic understanding of the prognosis and treatment options, assist in self-care, learn about available resources, and learn how to monitor for and prevent complications. This education is accomplished through a number of deliberate, chronological steps that, in many ways, parallels the nursing process: assessment of learning needs, planning of teaching methods to meet those needs, implementation of the teaching, and evaluation of the effectiveness of the teaching on patient outcomes.

Reading and Health Literacy

Before a nurse begins the patient education process, the nurse must have an understanding of and be able to assess the patient's reading and health literacy. There is a negative association between low literacy levels and health outcomes and health disparities (Rymer et al., 2018). In other words, a person with a low literacy level will have poorer health outcomes. **Reading literacy** is the ability to use printed and written information to function in society, to achieve one's goals, and to develop one's knowledge and potential (**National Assessment of Adult Literacy** (NAAL), 2019). In the United States, one in five adults and nearly two in five older adults read at or below the 5th grade level; however, much of printed patient education material is written at the 10th grade level or higher. An inability to use printed and written material can have a significant impact on patient health. When patients or their families are unable to read and understand written material provided to them, they rely on recall, leading to decreased comprehension. Many patients with poor or low literacy skills often are ashamed of their problem and are adept at hiding it from health care professionals (Fry-Bowers et al., 2014). While these patients are more likely to describe themselves as having poor health, they often avoid visiting primary care centers and instead have an over-reliance on visiting emergency departments for their health care. There is also a relationship between low literacy levels and negative patient outcomes, including decreased compliance with medication regimens and access to care (Huang, Shiyanbola, & Chan, 2018). Therefore, assessment of patient literacy is an essential nursing task.

Health literacy differs from reading literacy. The U.S. Department of Health and Human Services defines **health literacy** as "the degree to which individuals have the capacity to obtain, process, and understand basic health information and services needed to make appropriate health decisions" (U.S. Department of Health & Human Services, 2010). Health literacy requires a complex group of reading, listening, analytical, and decision-making skills, as well as the ability to apply these skills to health situations. The NAAL (2019) reported over 75 million adults had basic or below basic health literacy. Reading literacy is defined as being able to perform simple everyday reading activities and below basic literacy is defined as performing no more than the simplest and concrete reading skills (NAAL, 2019). Low health literacy is associated with increased hospitalizations, greater use of emergency services, decreased primary care screenings and vaccinations, poorer ability to understand and take medications as prescribed, poorer ability to interpret labels and health messages, and among elderly persons, poorer overall health status and higher mortality rates (Aboumatar, Carson, Beach, Roter, & Cooper, 2013). In addition to the health disparities associated with low reading and health literacy, the cost of low health literacy to the United States Economy is between \$106 and \$238 billion annually Berkman, et al., 2011). The elderly, those who did not complete high school, members of ethnic minorities, those with low income, immigrant populations, and people who spoke a language other than English at home, are at higher risks for low health literacy. Nurses are more likely to interact with these individuals in the hospital setting and thus must be prepared to address the challenges presented in the delivery of their care. In addition to assessing reading and health literacy, nurses must assess what type of learning is desired (e.g., what is the desired result in terms of doing, thinking, or behaving) and the style of learning that best meets the needs of the patient or staff nurse.

Assessment of Learning Styles

Every patient, family member, caregiver, and nurse learns differently. An individual's learning style refers to the way they interact with, take in, process, and retain information. An individual's learning style is related to cognitive, emotional, and environmental factors as well as one's previous experiences. Learning styles are generally categorized as one of three categories: visual, auditory, or kinesthetic learning. The **visual learner** learns best by seeing pictures, diagrams, or illustrations to help them understand information. Visual learners respond better to written instructions rather than verbal instructions as they can "see" the words. The **auditory learner** learns best by hearing the instructions and engaging in discussion. The auditory learner remembers things through verbal repetition. The nurse would do well to provide information to this learner rephrased in different ways to communicate the intended message. The **kinesthetic learner** learns best by performing tasks and getting physically involved. They want to touch, feel, and manipulate things, which helps them retain information. This learner tends to have good motor memory and often does well with return demonstrations, which reinforce the learning. Table 9.1 highlights these three learning styles, characteristics of the learner who prefer this style, and suggested teaching strategies.

Learning Domains

Whereas the style of learning refers to the way an individual prefers to learn, the **learning domain** refers to the specific knowledge, abilities, and values that result from the learning. There are three domains of thinking and performance used to describe learning and the intended outcome of that learning: affective, cognitive, and psychomotor (Bloom, 1956). The **affective domain** involves feelings, emotions, beliefs, values, and willingness to engage (or participate). Learning in the affective domain cannot be directly observed but is demonstrated through attitudes

Table 9.1   Learning Styles, Characteristics of the Learner, and Suggested Teaching Strategies

Learning style	Characteristics of the learner	Suggested teaching strategies
Visual learner	• Preference for information in pictures, diagrams, and charts to understand ideas and concepts • Remember what they read rather than what they hear • Will often take notes during instruction	• Provide instruction using pictures, diagrams, and charts • Use written instruction with various fonts that are appealing to the eye • Utilize visual technology, e.g. internet and videos.
Auditory learner	• Preference for information that is heard • Learns by rephrasing or explaining • Enjoys group discussion	• Read the instructions out loud while performing the task • Rephrase what was said in several different ways • Ensure learner can hear you clearly
Kinesthetic learner	• Preference for information that is experience based • Remember what was done, not what was seen or heard • Must be actively involved in a learning experience	• Use hands-on activities such as return demonstrations • Allow the patient to practice skills

Source: R. R. Flayter, L. Kidin & M. S. Schuler.

and behaviors. The affective domain is key to learner (e.g. patient or staff) motivation. The **cognitive domain** involves the development of intellectual/mental skills including, remembering, understanding, and the acquisition of knowledge. The cognitive domain results also cannot be directly observed but may be seen through behaviors. The **psychomotor domain** involves utilizing motor skills and performing a behavior or skills that are directly observable. This type of learning can also be thought of as learning by doing. According to Bloom's taxonomy of learning, the acquisition and adaptation of new information is broken down into six levels of understanding: knowledge, comprehension, application, analysis, synthesis, and evaluation. Each level of understanding is learned before moving to the next level.

Let us consider an instructional activity where the objective is for the learner to self-administer insulin safely. The affective domain is exemplified by the learner believing in the importance of safely self-administering insulin. The cognitive domain is exemplified by the learner's understanding of the importance of insulin self-administration, and the psychomotor domain is exemplified by the learner being able to demonstrate the ability to self-administer the insulin safely.

Each domain (affective, cognitive, and psychomotor) has multiple levels of learning that progress from basic, surface-level learning to more complex, deeper-level learning in an organized hierarchal manner (Table 9.2). In the affective domain, levels are organized according to the degree of internalization of attitudes, beliefs, or values. In the cognitive and psychomotor domains, learning is presented in the order of increasing complexity. These three domains are interdependent, though one may be more emphasized than the other in a teaching session depending on the desired outcomes of the learning experience. The identification of learning domains is an important first step in planning and designing patient education experiences. By understanding which domain a

---

Real World Interview

When I was in the hospital with a pulmonary embolism, it became clear that I needed to go home with Lovenox shots. The nurses gave me information on Lovenox and explained why I had to take shots and not a pill. Then they started showing me how to do the shots, explaining each step. After a few practice shots, they had me do the injection. With encouragement, I was able to give the shots to myself. The nurse repeated the instructions and made sure

I was comfortable. I was very nervous, but the nurse's patience with showing me each step and then letting me set the pace made it much easier for me to give my own shots at home.

Cynthia Hooker
Patient
Portsmouth, Virginia

Case Study 9.1

Mr. Cabelo, a 74-year-old married man, is admitted to your unit with a new diagnosis of heart failure. You are developing his education plan. His expected length of stay is 3–4 days. He will be adding carvedilol, furosemide, and potassium to his home medicine regimen.

1. Who else can you involve in the teaching plan?

2. How will you determine what topics to include in the teaching?

3. How will you determine if your teaching is understood prior to discharge?

Table 9.2   Learning Domains and Levels of Learning within Each Domain

Learning domain	Levels of learning	Action verbs for each level
Affective	Receiving—Being aware and willing to hear, having selected attention for the material being taught Responding—Participating in discussion about the topic Valuing—Attaching worth or value to a particular object, phenomenon, or behavior Organizing—Prioritizing what is important for care Characterizing - Having a value system that controls behavior	Ask, choose, select, locate Discuss, perform, follow Differentiate, justify Arrange, compare, relate, synthesize Revise, carry out, manage
Cognitive	Remembering—recalling information Understanding—grasping the meaning of the material Applying—utilizing the learned material in new situations Analyzing—breaking information into parts and detecting their interrelationship Evaluating—judging the value of the material Creating—putting parts together to form a new whole	Arrange, define, label, list Classify, describe, explain Apply, choose, practice, demonstrate Analyze, compare, differentiate Argue, assess, rate, support Design, create, develop
Psychomotor	Imitation—observing & copying an action or repeating the words of another Manipulation—reproducing an action/skill from instruction or memory Precision—accurately executing an action or skill independently Articulation—integrating multiple actions or skills and performing them consistently Naturalization—naturally and automatically performing skills or actions at a high level	Repeat, imitate, copy, show Build, execute, perform, recreate Demonstrate, show, complete Adapt, combine, connect, display Manage, create, revise, vary

Source: R. R. Flayter, L. Kidin & M. S. Schuler.

patient or staff nurse learns best, the nurse is able to determine which activities, assessments, and modes of instruction are optimal based on the learning outcome desired. The following table can be useful for the development of action verbs to direct the learning activity in each of the domains.

Developing Learning Objectives

Learning objectives are statements that define the expected outcomes or goals of the learning process. Well defined learning objectives provide the learner with a clear goal to focus their learning on, direct the choice of instructional activities, and guide assessment strategies. They clarify that which do you want the learner to be able to do? When developing learning objectives, one must consider who they want to perform the behavior and who is the audience. A second consideration is what do you want for a behavior outcome, what do you want the learner to be able to do? A third consideration is the conditions for the learning, that is, are there any restrictions or specific requirements involved in performing the behavior? Lastly, what is the degree of performance desired, for example how well should the person be able to perform the objective. One way to remember the components of an objective is to think of the ABCD method: A = Audience, B = Behavior, C = Condition, and D = Degree (see Table 9.3).

Learning objectives can be also based in the affective, cognitive, or psychomotor domains. Examples of learning objectives based on each of the domains include:

- Affective: The new-to-practice nurse will be able to reflect on the value of allowing family presence during resuscitation by the end of orientation.

  ○ Audience—New-to-practice nurse

  ○ Behavior—Reflect on value of family presence

  ○ Condition—During resuscitation

  ○ Degree—By end of orientation

- Cognitive: The new-to-practice nurse will be able to evaluate evidence-based practice guidelines for the early removal of catheters in clinical practice within the first 2 weeks of working on the medical-surgical floor.

  ○ Audience—New-to-practice nurse

  ○ Behavior—Evaluation of evidence-based practice guidelines for catheter removal

  ○ Condition—In clinical practice

  ○ Degree—Within the first 2 weeks of working on floor

- Psychomotor: The new-to-practice nurse will demonstrate competency in the insertion of an intravenous catheter in oncology patients with 100% accuracy by week 6 of orientation.

  ○ Audience—New-to-practice nurse

  ○ Behavior—Demonstrate competency in insertion of IV catheter

Table 9.3   Components of a Behavioral Objective

Audience	Behavior	Condition	Degree
Who will perform the behavior?	What will the performer do?	What limitations or other conditions will be placed on the performance?	What degree of measurement will be used to determine successful performance?
The patient	*Will identify the major valves of the heart*	*Using the anatomical heart chart provided by the teacher*	*With an accuracy of 100%*

Source: R. R. Flayter, L. Kidin & M. S. Schuler.

○ Condition—With oncology patients

○ Degree—100% accuracy by 6 weeks of orientation

Patient-centered education is an inherent part of nursing. Patient-centered education is a tool through which nurses bolster patients' self-care abilities by providing patients with information about specific disease processes, treatment methods, and health-promoting behaviors. Nurses have a responsibility to develop a personal understanding and awareness of their patient's learning needs. This can be accomplished, in part, through the nurse's empathetic traits inherent in the nursing process, including being authentically present and actively listening to the patient to understand needs. Patient-centered education occurs both informally and formally and in combination with almost all nursing interventions. Informal education can be as basic as exchanging information during a conversation with the patient, such as explaining a medication, procedure, or laboratory result. Formal education is planned, structured, and directed toward specific topics and goals. The first step in developing any type of individual or group educational session is to perform an analysis to define the type of education needed. The nurse should analyze three major elements:

- Context
- Learner
- Content

Context Analysis

The **context analysis** consists of a review of both the situation in which the educational need arises and the instructional environment in which the education will occur. It is essentially a review of the circumstances that created the need for the education. For example, is the patient who has a history of intermittent chest pain in need of a cardiac catheterization? Is this scheduled immediately which may limit some of the teaching or is it scheduled for later which gives the nurse and patient time to discuss the procedure and what the patient needs to know for subsequent self-care. Has the patient expressed concerns over an existing or a potential health care condition such as diabetes? Is the disease new to him/her? Is the patient receiving a new chemotherapy agent in an effort to ease some of the side effects the patient had been experiencing with the previous agent? When is the next

chemotherapy session scheduled? Is there a practitioner initiating a new neurosurgery procedure requiring staff education to support patient education?

The instructional environment refers to the conditions under which education will occur. Some potential questions the nurse may consider are: In what environment will the education be presented? Is the environment a health care facility, a home, a community environment, or some other setting? How will this environment affect the ability to provide and access teaching resources? How will the environment affect the nurse's ability to effectively control the education environment? How will it affect the learner's attention and motivation?

Other important considerations include the time for education. For example, when will the education occur? How long will the nurse have to teach? Is the amount of time planned for education adequate? Is the amount of time flexible or is it fixed, such as 1 hr allotted at a community center for giving a course on diabetes management?

Learner Analysis

The nurse should also conduct a learner analysis (Table 9.4). A **learner analysis** is the process of identifying not only who the learner is, but their unique characteristics and needs, and the ways their characteristics and needs can influence the education process. Understanding the learner's particular characteristics and needs is an important consideration when developing an individualized education plan that is relevant and effective. The first question facing the nurse is: Who is the learner? Is it the patient, family, nursing staff, ancillary staff, or someone else? In many cases, the learner will be the patient. However, in some cases, the patient may be unable or unwilling to participate in the learning process. In other cases, there may be other learners in addition to the patient, such as family members, legal guardians, or others, who make health care decisions for the patient. Learners may be caregivers who, whether related or not, will be participating in the patient's care. Other learners may not directly participate in the patient's care but may, with the patient's permission, require, or desire information.

The second component of the learner analysis is developing an understanding of the learner's characteristics and unique learning needs. Is the learner able to read? Does the learner have an illness that may impact learning? The learner's condition can be affected by physical factors, such as discomfort

Table 9.4   **Learner Analysis for Patient or Staff Education**

Education topic: _____

Target Audience (check all that apply):

_____Patient   _____Professional staff   _____Nonprofessional staff

_____Individual   _____Group   _____Adult (between 18 and 64 years)

_____Senior (> 64 years old) _____ Adolescent _____Child

Relationship of Group or Persons:

(Staff of same unit or multiple units, inter-professional team, family members)

_____

Purpose of Education:

_____Informational Patient Education   _____Introduction of new skill, procedure, technique

_____Professional development   _____Infection control

_____Introduction of new equipment   _____Quality improvement

Gender Preference: _____

Learner's primary language: _____   Translation assistance needed: _____

Limitations and barriers to patient/staff learning? Describe.

Affective: _____

Cognitive: _____

Psychomotor: _____

Physical: _____

Emotional: _____

Cultural/religious/lifestyle: _____

Motivational: _____

Language/literacy: _____

Other: _____

Literacy—level of educational material appropriate? _____

Previous health care experience with this topic? _____

Learning style assessment (visual, auditory, kinesthetic): _____

Source: R. R. Flayter, L. Kidin & M. S. Schuler.

or pain which may impact the patient's ability to concentrate. Additional considerations include psychological factors, such as depression or anxiety. Psychosocial factors such as cultural beliefs may also influence how patients view and react to the nurse during an education session. Culturally influenced suspicion of, or deference to, health care staff may prevent the patient from effectively responding to the education. Is the patient able to understand what you are saying? Are there language barriers? It is very important that patient education occurs in the language the patient prefers to learn in. Most health care organizations have trained translators or offer mobile devices for translation. Questions that the nurse might ask the patient to develop an understanding of the patient's unique learning characteristics and needs include:

1. What do you know about your condition/medications/treatment?

2. What are you most interested in learning about?

3. What are you most concerned about?

4. What are your goals for learning how to take care of yourself?

5. What do you feel you need to know to achieve your goals?

6. How will you manage your care at home?

When developing educational programs for nursing staff, it is important to remember they may present with unique learning characteristics depending in part on their experience, general preference, and education. For example, millennial nurses may prefer interactive technology rather than a traditional lecture for new learning. Visual rather than written materials may be preferred by nurses for whom English is a second language. Some nurse may feel more comfortable learning in an environment where they have an opportunity to engage and be part of a team, while others may prefer one-on-one instruction. Developing an understanding of the nurse's unique learning needs is very important. Questions that might be asked of the nurse include:

1. How do you learn best?

2. What is your current understanding of _____ (educational topic)?

3. What is your previous experience with _____?

4. How much time do you have for education and training?

The answers to any of these questions can seriously affect the learner's ability to learn. The nurse may not be able to identify all of the learner's characteristics prior to the education session. However, the more the nurse knows about the patient's or staff's unique learning characteristics and needs, the more the nurse can develop education that effectively incorporates strategies to address them.

Content Analysis

After the nurse has analyzed both the context in which the learning will take place and the learner, **content analysis** is the final element to consider. During content analysis, the nurse begins to pinpoint specific information that the education should address. For example, the practitioner has written an order for a medication you rarely administer on your unit. What specific information would you obtain to educate yourself and your co-workers on this medication? Could you use the same content information to educate the patient? Content information on this topic might include the following:

- Confirmation by pharmacy on the use of the medication for your unit

- Action of the medication

- Safe dose

- Side effects

- Route of administration

- Interactions with other medications or food

The nurse must also determine what information is essential to the education session. Although there may be a wealth of information available for a topic, all the available information may not be necessary information. Some of it may be irrelevant, redundant, or nonessential.

Educational Resources

It is important to consider resources that will be used during the education session. Educational resources consist of multimedia such as written, visual, audio, video, computer or internet-based resources, or combinations thereof. It has been noted that some patients may have low literacy skills. Nurses can assess patient education materials for readability through some common websites including:

- Plain http://language.gov, https://plainlanguage.gov/resources
- CDC health literacy, www.cdc.gov/healthliteracy/pdf/Simply_Put.pdf
- Readability analyzer, https://datayze.com/readability-analyzer.php

Nurses may choose to use a single multimedia resource or integrate more than one, depending on factors such as type of content, educational strategy, patient learning style, patient literacy level, teacher preference, limited resources available, etc. The nurse has several options but should seek to base their decisions on what would be best for the patient's learning style.

The nurse must consider two categories of multimedia for patient or staff development education—multimedia that will be used during the education session and multimedia that will be provided to the patient or staff as a reference to be used at a later time. Because the latter is likely to be used outside the presence and supervision of the nurse, it is especially important that it be appropriate for the patient or the staff nurse. When possible, the nurse should use multimedia resources that are up to date and readily available and reliable from government agencies, health care professionals, and researchers. Some common reputable multimedia resources are listed in Table 9.5.

Additional resources include some podcasts and social media platforms such as YouTube™, and pharmaceutical companies' or professional organizations' patient education webpages. The number of multimedia resources including social media sites and mobile apps that offer health information continues to grow every day. It is important to find out the patient's primary source for health information and it is incumbent the nurse educates patients and staff how to differentiate accurate from inaccurate or misleading multimedia sites. One option is to direct patients

---

Critical Thinking 9.1

Your patient has been given a new diagnosis of colon cancer. His brother died 3 months after being diagnosed with lung cancer. His physician wants to begin chemotherapy as soon as possible.

1. How do you evaluate the patient's readiness to learn about the disease and his treatment?

2. What physical and psychosocial factors would you think about before providing education to this patient?
3. Who else would you involve in the education?
4. What aspects regarding this patient's treatment would you consider in developing your teaching plan?

Table 9.5 **Multimedia Resources**

Source	Website (all accessed May 19, 2019)

Government Agencies

• National Institute of Health—Health Information	• www.nih.gov/health-information
• U.S. Department of Health and Human Services	• www.hhs.gov
• The Centers for Disease Control	• www.cdc.gov
• Agency for Healthcare Research and Quality	• wwsw.ahrq.gov
• Food and Drug Administration	• www.fda.gov/home

Nursing Societies

• National Institute of Nursing Research	• www.ninr.nih.gov
• American Nurses Association	• www.nursingworld.org/ana

Literature Resources/Searches

• PubMed	• www.ncbi.nlm.nih.gov/pubmed
• National Library of Medicine	• www.nlm.nih.gov
• Merck Manual of Diagnosis and Therapy	• www.merckmanuals.com/professional
• MedlinePlus	• medlineplus.gov
• WebMD	• www.webmd.com
• Mayo Clinic: Tools for Healthier Lives	• www.mayoclinic.org/healthy-lifestyle

Other

• The National Cancer Institute	• www.cancer.gov
• American Cancer Society	• www.cancer.org
• American College of Surgeons	• www.facs.org
• American Heart Association	• www.heart.org

to HealthWeb Navigator at https://healthwebnav.org. Health-Web Navigator publishes in-depth reviews of health-related websites and connects patients with accurate, easy-to-read, and up-to-date health information. Viewing content from reputable health care organizations or providers can prevent misinformation or conflicting messages (Stellefson et al., 2014). For patients for whom English is not their primary language, you might direct patients to the Ethnomed at https://ethnomed.org/patient-education for patient education resources. Ethnomed contains information about cultural beliefs, medical issues, and related topics pertinent to the health care of immigrants.

When assisting the patient or staff in the use of multimedia, the nurse should look at several factors. Things to consider include how accurate is the information these sites provide? How updated is the information? Additional questions include: Is the content presented within the material appropriate for the patient or staff's needs? Does the information come from a reputable and verifiable source? Is the material of suitable quality—for example, is the audio understandable, is the video of appropriate visual quality, are graphics understandable, is the text readable and at the appropriate reading level? A review of websites like WebMD and Med-Line Plus for readability and accuracy in medication education revealed that while the information was accurate, most was written at a higher than a 4th grade reading level (Kim, Metzger, Wigle, & Choe, 2011). Furthermore, many published patient educational materials are written at a 9th to 17th grade level (Hansberry et al., 2014; Kher, Johnson, & Griffith, 2017; Smith et al., 2014). To address this issue, there are a number of readability tools online that can be used to assess the educational material's reading level; however, there is no consensus on which tool should be used to analyze patient education literature. Once patient and staff begin to utilize multimedia, they often feel overwhelmed and confused with the information presented. The nurse can suggest that the patient or staff write down questions that they have from viewing these sites and bring them back to the nurse for discussion. The nurse will then have an opportunity to address any misconception and continue the learning process.

It is worth noting that patients newly diagnosed with an illness are often in a state of shock initially and may focus their learning on what is needed to survive. For these patients the nurse should consider focusing on what the patient may view as "survival skills." Survival skills-based patient-centered education occurs during the acute phase of the patient's newly diagnosed condition; this often occurs while the patient is still hospitalized. During this time, the education is focused on what is essential for the patient to know now for safe discharge home. Patient-centered education during this phase can include elements that ensure the patient has a general understanding of the key components of the disease and its treatment and is able to take medications accurately (Figure 9.1).

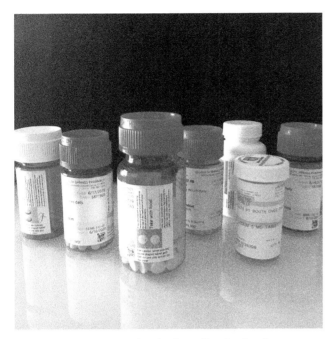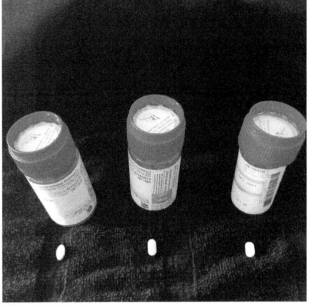

FIGURE 9.1   Picture of multiple medication bottles.
Source: Rochille R.Flayter.

Once the patient has a foundational understanding of his or her new illness, follow-up education is important. This allows further determination if discharge teaching was effective and to reinforce any educational gaps and address any new questions the patient may have. During follow-up education, patients often receive more comprehensive education about their illness in an outpatient setting.

Education in the outpatient setting is often accomplished in a clinic-like setting with classes or through self-paced online educational programs. Tele-management with the use of smart phones may also be used. It is important for nurses to follow up with patient's educational needs to ensure patients continue to learn about how to address their health care needs.

Therapeutic Patient Education Programs

As has been noted previously, when patients are diagnosed with a new illness, health care providers often provide basic information at an initial patient encounter to describe the diagnosis or the treatment required to manage it. However, for the management of many chronic illnesses, nurses work with patients to provide more comprehensive **therapeutic patient-centered education** (TPE) programs. TPE is education managed by health care providers trained in the education of patients, and designed to enable a patient (or a group of patients and families) to manage the treatment of their condition (Figure 9.2), support daily self-management, and prevent avoidable complications, while maintaining or improving quality of life. An additional goal is to avoid the need for repeated hospitalizations. TPE is often multi-dimensional and inter-professional and has been identified

as the most successful in behavior modification (Abu Abed, Himmel, Vormfelde, & Koschack, 2014; Beltran-Alacreu, López-de-Uralde-Villanueva, Fernández-Carnero, & La Touche, 2015). Studies have shown the benefits of these TPE programs to include a reduction in all-cause mortality and improved self-efficacy (Brown, Clark, Dalal, Welch, & Taylor, 2013; Julliere et al., 2013; Reif, deVries, Petermann, & Gorres, 2013).

Development of Lesson Plans

Once the nurse has assessment learner needs, considered the context and content for the material to be covered, and learning objectives developed, the next step is creating a lesson plan with learning objectives. A **lesson plan** is a formally developed document that provides a blueprint for an education session. A lesson plan typically has five components:

1. Objectives

2. Outline

3. Time frame

4. Teaching strategies

5. Evaluation.

The objectives guide the development of the content and design of both the teaching and evaluation strategies (Table 9.6). The outline of the lesson plan flows from the objectives. The use of an outline helps the nurse consider the organization and flow of ideas that will be presented to the patient or staff nurse. The third component of the lesson

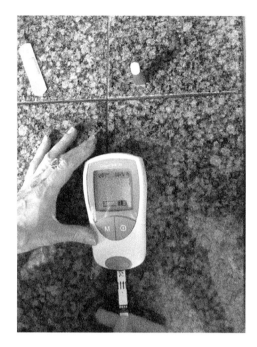
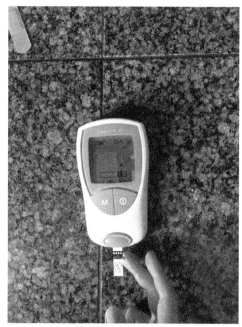
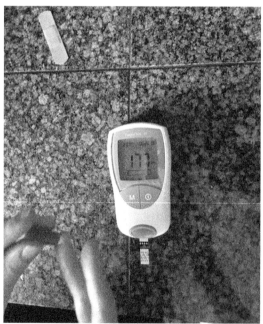

FIGURE 9.2   Photo of patient performing point of care testing with an INR machine for monitoring of warfarin.
Source: Rochille R. Flayter

plan is an estimation of the time frame needed to present the material. In general, the time frame is linked to the teaching strategies used to convey the material. Staff nurses may only have 15 min with which to deliver important patient-centered education. Nurses completing an in-service training session may be limited to 30-min sessions or less. By including a time frame in the lesson plan, nurses can ensure they cover all the topics they had planned within the allotted time frame.

The fourth component of a lesson plan includes identification of the teaching strategies planned for the educational activity. This component is often the most challenging aspect

to develop in the lesson plan. Identifying the most ideal teaching strategies that are appropriate for the content and learner can be difficult. These difficulties are often related to an incongruence between the way the nurse likes to learn and the way the patient or staff learns best. This can be mitigated by doing a comprehensive assessment of the patient or staff's learning styles beforehand.

The last component of the lesson plan describes how the patient or staff will be evaluated on the learning. How do you know the learner has received and processed the information you wished to impart? Evaluation of the learning

Table 9.6   Sample Lesson Plan

Lesson Plan Title: Diabetic Self-Management—Excerpt.

Patient	Juan Abado
Presenter	John Reilley, RN
Setting	Patient's hospital room
Brief patient/ learner summary	Patient is a 50-year-old English-speaking Hispanic male, college graduate, newly diagnosed with diabetes, and unfamiliar with the self-injection process. No other learners involved. No physical limitations to learning. Mild anxiety about self-injection, but high motivation. Initial interview suggests preference for learning through visual means.
Overall goal	The patient will understand and demonstrate diabetic self-care.
Objectives	After completing the session, the patient will be able to do the following: 1. Identify equipment for taking blood glucose reading 2. Demonstrate the procedure for taking a blood glucose reading 3. State the acceptable range of blood glucose level 4. Develop a diabetic behavior management plan 5. Identify symptoms of hypoglycemia and hyperglycemia 6. List foods that can raise blood glucose levels 7. Discuss the **American Diabetes Association** (ADA) diet plan 8. Develop a regular exercise plan 9. Identify equipment necessary for insulin self-injection 10. Discuss insulin and method for self-injection 11. Demonstrate correct procedure for insulin self-injection administration

Topic outline	Content

Time: 3 min	<u>Objective 1</u>. Identify equipment for taking a blood glucose reading
	
	 Topics:
	 1. Importance of taking a blood glucose reading
	 2. When/how often to take a blood glucose reading
	 3. Equipment for taking a blood glucose reading
	     a. Blood glucose monitoring machine
	     b. Interpretation strips
	
	 Strategy: Lecture and demonstration/return demonstration
	 Medium: Handout—*Monitoring Blood Sugar*

Evaluation	This segment can take the form of a behavioral checklist, in which the nurse checks off that the patient has acceptably performed the behavior, or specific evaluation items, such as questions or other forms of evaluation, e.g., Identifies equipment for taking blood glucose reading Yes__ No _
Time: 10 min	<u>Objective: 2.</u> Demonstrate the procedure for taking a blood glucose reading Topics: 1. How to put the glucose interpretation strip in the machine 2. How to disinfect the finger 3. How to stick the finger 4. How to apply the blood to the glucose interpretation strip 5. How to interpret the results Strategy: Presentation of video and discussion with patient; nurse demonstration followed by patient demonstration Medium: Equipment— blood glucose monitoring machine and interpretation strips; video segment— *Taking a Blood Glucose Reading;* handout—*Monitoring Your Blood Glucose* (Continue with this format for each objective in the session. Each segment lists the objective, the topics to be covered, the teaching strategy used, the presentation equipment and the amount of time needed to conduct each segment.
Evaluation	Demonstrates the procedure for taking a blood glucose reading Yes__ No ___ Blood glucose readings are taken using a blood glucose monitoring machine and _____. Before sticking the finger, you should: a. put the blood on the strip b. read the blood glucose results c. disinfect the finger d. close your eyes

Continued

Table 9.6 (Continued)

Lesson Plan Title: Diabetic Self-Management—Excerpt.

Patient	Juan Abado
Time: 3 min	Review In this segment, the nurse reviews the major objectives and topics covered in the session. This is also a useful time for asking the patient whether there are any topics he is unsure of or has further questions about. Strategies for retention/transfer In this segment, the nurse indicates any methods for helping the patient apply the teaching to future situations. Have patient perform their own blood glucose tests four times daily during remaining time in hospital.

Source: R. R. Flayter, L. Kidin & M. S. Schuler.

can be either formative or summative. Formative evaluation occurs when the nurse monitors patient or staff learning during a teaching session and uses this ongoing feedback to improve their teaching in real time. In summative evaluations, the patient or staff's understanding is assessed at the end of the teaching and compared to a desired standard or benchmark. Please see Tables 9.6 and 9.9 for excerpts from sample lesson plans.

Conducting the Education Session

During this time, the nurse actually conducts the education session. The lesson plan defines the objectives, provides an outline, and includes a time frame, teaching strategies to be utilized, and plans for evaluation. Other considerations include what equipment and materials may be needed for the session. Using this lesson plan, the nurse begins the education session. Various factors will affect the success of the session. Some of these factors are highly controllable, others less so. Some of the more influential factors are discussed below.

Environment

The environment in which the education will occur can have a major impact on the effectiveness of the education. Before beginning the education session, the nurse should evaluate physical environment factors such as lighting, temperature, and sound quality. The patient may have internal distractors or external distractors that need to be addressed, for example, internally the patient may be in pain or have anxiety. External distractors include a noisy room. The nurse must be aware of the learner's need for privacy. Also consider the learner's privacy needs. Some patients may not be comfortable discussing their illness in front of other patients, even if there is a curtain between them and the other patient. Patients may be easily distracted by alarm bells, television volume, or music in the background. If you plan on utilizing a white board or media to demonstrate something, you must consider if the resources you have in the patient's room will support the educational session. You may have to quickly adapt the education session in the case of unexpected situations.

An effective nurse educator must bring certain qualities to the patient-centered education experience. Although every nurse educator will have varying degrees of knowledge regarding the content being taught, nurse educators have an

Evidence from the Literature

Source: Barnason, S., White-Williams, C., Rossi, L., et al. (2017). Evidence for therapeutic patient education interventions to promote cardiovascular patient self-management. A scientific statement for health care professionals from the American Heart Association. *Circulation Cardiovascular Quality Outcomes, 10(6),* 1–23.

Discussion: An integrative review of published research on TPE for self-management of cardiovascular patients was analyzed. It included the categories: cardiovascular disease, atrial fibrillation, hypertension, acute coronary artery disease, and heart failure. The study assessed (a) the interventions used to promote

self-management, (b) the impact of TPE on patient outcomes, and (c) common barriers to the implementation of TPE.

Implications for Practice: Positive effects identified with TPE included tailoring the education to individual patient needs, use of an inter-professional approach to education, and utilizing multiple methods of instruction to improve self-management, for example, have a patient watch a video and then provide handouts to the patient regarding cardiovascular disease. Table 5 of the article highlights self-management TPE recommendations for clinical practice.

opportunity to make the most out of every educational session by demonstrating qualities that will facilitate an effective and engaging session. These qualities include having effective communication skills, and most importantly, being patient and flexible in the delivery of content to meet the learner's needs.

Communication

Communication is very important in developing successful education. Both verbal and nonverbal communication skills are essential to effective education. Create a welcoming and supportive environment for the patient. Assure privacy where the patient is free to ask questions and discuss concerns. Some simple communication skills to increase your patient's understanding are:

1. Be an active listener.

2. Use visual aids and illustrations.

3. Slow down the pace of your teaching.

4. Remember to be respectful, caring, and sensitive to the patient and family.

5. Limit the amount of information shared at each session and repeat, repeat, repeat.

6. Look for opportunities to clarify, support, encourage, and incorporate patient responses. This further involves the patient in the process and increases patient motivation.

7. Tell patients what their test results are and also give them the normal readings, such as: "Your cholesterol level is 290. A healthy cholesterol level is less than 200. We will be reviewing information with you on how to lower your cholesterol level."

8. Clarify and address any quizzical looks by the patient or family. Be aware that confused looks or blank stares by the patient or family may indicate a lack of understanding. If this occurs, rephrase the information, use simpler words, pause, and offer the education in smaller segments.

9. Avoid abbreviations and idioms. Avoid the use of "PRN," for instance; instead, say "as you need it." An idiom is a figure of speech that could be misunderstood. Avoid asking a patient if they are "under the weather." Instead, ask the patient to describe how they are feeling.

10. Use a "teach back" or "show me" approach with patients to confirm their understanding. **Teach back** is a method of confirming learner knowledge where the learner can teach back the new information in their own words and/or can demonstrate the correct way to perform a task. This teach back method allows the teacher to evaluate the learner's comprehension of the education. The patient should not view this as a test, but as a review of the instructions.

Patients will not only listen to what you say, they will also observe your body language during a teaching session. Body language says a lot about the nurse's level of interest and motivation. The nurse should maintain a professional appearance during the education event. Eye contact, use of hands, movement, and distance between the nurse and the patient all send messages about the nurse's attitude toward the education session.

Evaluating Effectiveness of Patient-Centered Education

Evaluation is the process of determining the effectiveness of education. The two major components of evaluation are learner evaluation and education evaluation:

- *Learner evaluation:* Did the learners understand what was intended to be learned?

- *Education evaluation:* Was the education presented in an effective manner?

Learner Evaluation

What to evaluate is determined by the learning objectives. There should be a direct correlation between the learning objectives established for the education session and the evaluation of the learning that occurs during the education. Learner evaluation can take many forms. Asking the learner to recall information, answer questions, perform procedures, solve relevant problems, analyze a situation, or construct a plan of action are all forms of learner evaluation. The nurse should choose learner evaluation methods based on how effectively they reflect learning objective, how realistically the learner can be expected to perform the evaluation, and how practically

---

Critical Thinking 9.2

You are caring for a patient with lung cancer. Smoking cessation has been difficult for her. Your preceptor would like you to identify resources that would assist the patient and staff in the plan of care for this patient utilizing internet-based patient-centered resources.

1. Identify one internet-based educational resource or social media platform that could be utilized to support this patient-centered education.

2. What are some other topics you can include in your education for this patient?

the nurse can observe and measure successful performance (Worral, 2019). If the learner is having trouble with certain topics, the nurse can revisit those topics or, if conditions make that approach impractical, the nurse can provide additional resources or referrals to the learner. Some patients or staff may feel a sense of anxiety when they realize they will be evaluated. The nurse educator can reduce learner anxiety by presenting evaluation in the context of a review of the education. The nurse must also remember that the purpose of evaluation is to validate that the patient has effectively processed and adopted the information. Often, communicating this purpose will ease the anxiety associated with the evaluation process.

An additional consideration in the evaluation process is assessing the effectiveness of a program in producing change. Some questions to consider include: what happened to program participants and how much of a difference did the program make for them? For example, evaluation for a smoking cessation program might include:

- Did the program succeed in helping patients stop smoking?

- Was the program more successful with certain groups of patients than others?

- What aspects of the program were most beneficial for patients?

Evaluation of the Educational Program Presentation

Education evaluation is concerned with whether the education event itself was effectively constructed and presented. It is useful for the nurse to examine the education session and identify areas for improvement as well as areas to reinforce the effective elements. Education evaluation can involve feedback from the nurse educator, the patient, and/or third-party observers. Measurement can be formal or informal and can involve verbal or written feedback. Table 9.7 identifies some of the elements that can be examined in education evaluation.

Evaluation of Materials

As has been discussed, when evaluating the content and materials, it is important to determine the context, relevance, and reading level of your audience. You can quickly determine your patient's literacy with the **Rapid Estimate of Adult Literacy in Medicine** (REALM) oral reading and recognition test (Davis, Crouch, & Long, 1993). This relatively quick test assesses a patient's ability to pronounce 66 common medical words and lay terms for body parts and illnesses. The test can differentiate if a patient reads at a 3rd grade or below reading level, between 4th and 6th grade, between 7th and 8th grade, or at a high school level. As a general rule, however, utilizing a 4th grade reading level as a guide helps ensure adequate comprehension of the materials and the ability to effectively influence behavior. The educator may use existing materials

when developing an education session. In many situations, the organization will have existing materials and encourage their use. In other situations, the nurse may have greater freedom in selecting education materials. In some situations, the educator or instructor may find that no materials exist or existing materials are not appropriate for the content to be taught. Therefore, materials may need to be created either to augment existing materials or to fill a gap.

Costs and Resources

It is important to consider the cost of resources used during the educational offering. Resources consist of various multimedia such as written, visual, audio, video, computer based or internet based, other material, or combinations of these materials. When selecting an education strategy, a single multimedia strategy may be used throughout the teaching event, or several may be used, depending on such factors as content type, education strategy, learning style, literacy level, teacher preference, or the limitations of what is available. Cost may be a constraint to consider when choosing the resources. Some resources may be free but not always appropriate to the actual teaching objectives. Many commercially produced teaching materials, for example, posters, booklets, and videos, are now available from pharmaceutical and equipment companies. Some of these materials may have inappropriate information, so use them with caution. Other material may be copyrighted and fees must be paid to use the material.

Accuracy and Appropriateness of Teaching Materials

Teaching materials, to be relevant, must be up-to-date, applicable, and cover the required scope of the subject. Health care practices are ever changing and new evidence-based research and technology is being developed. It is important that an expert or a team of health care providers specializing in a particular field has reviewed and approved the educational material to be provided to patients. The materials must be re-evaluated at a minimum of at least every 3 years or whenever new evidence emerges. Although evidence-based practice should be at the forefront of all patient educational material, differences in patient teaching and management do exist between health care institutions. Hopefully, they are all focused on the goal of evidence-based practice.

Strategies for Professional Development

Professional Development

Professional development is an important part of being a health care professional. Health care is a rapidly changing complex profession due to new technology and advancements in knowledge. Professional development allows nurses and other health care providers to remain current with evidence-based practice

Table 9.7   Education Evaluation

	Possible elements for education evaluation
Patient learning	**Did the patient learn the appropriate content, as indicated by such tools as learner evaluation results and follow-up observations? Were learner evaluation items appropriate and reliable?**
Patient satisfaction	Was the patient satisfied with the content presented? With the effectiveness of the presenter? Did the patient feel that questions were addressed appropriately?
Environment	Was the environment conducive to learning? Were there distractions from inside or outside the room? Was lighting appropriate? Room temperature?
Educational design	Were the objectives appropriate? The topics? The sequence?
Knowledge	Did the materials and/or teacher reflect adequate knowledge of the content?
Organization	Was the information well organized?
Accuracy	Was the information presented accurately?
Relevance	Was information presented relevant to the patient's situation? Was relevant information missing?
Delivery	Were education strategies effective? Were the educational materials effective?
Pacing	Did education move too fast or too slow? Were demonstrations given at a pace the patient could follow? If needed, was the patient given enough time for practice?
Variety	Was there too much of one type of activity or not enough variety in the education methods or presentation? Was there too much variety, creating a sense of confusion?
Involvement	Was there enough patient involvement? Was there a lack or shortage of activities and/or practice time?
Communication	Did the nurse communicate clearly and effectively with the patient?
Focus	Did the materials and/or educator stay on the topics?
Assistance	Did the educator provide enough assistance? Did the materials provide cues or explanations to assist the learners in completing activities?

Source: R. R. Flayter, L. Kidin & M. S. Schuler.

Case Study 9.2

A health care organization has recently transitioned its labor and delivery into two separate units. The current staff in the traditional labor and delivery unit has little experience with post-partum hemorrhages. A scenario was designed to target clinical skills, processes, and communication in a post-partum hemorrhage emergency (Figure 9.3).

1. What do you think would be an effective educational strategy to use for the nurses on this new unit? Discuss why.

2. What are some ways you would evaluate teaching effectiveness?

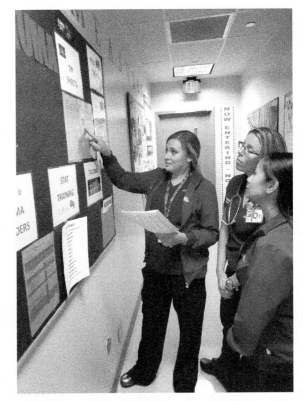

FIGURE 9.3   Picture of staff education in a patient care unit in the hospital setting.
Source: Nicki Schroeder.

and ensures that providers can give the highest quality care at the top of their licensure, scope of practice, and abilities. Professional development covers a wide range of activities from formal coursework or programs to formal or informal demonstration of skills that are purposefully acquired in the health care environment. Often, lifetime employment with one employer or remaining in one clinical area is no longer guaranteed and professionals must develop continually and go through additional orientation when changes in roles or settings occur (Spector et al., 2015). The changing workforce and nursing shortages increase the need for organizations to retain older workers, necessitating the need for a strong professional development plan across the span of a career continuum. A guide to this continuum of development plan is Patricia Benner's Novice to Expert Theory, which identifies the stages of competence in nurses. Benner's theory can be adapted to any health care provider but originally was designed for nurses (Benner, 1984). Benner described the five stages of her theory as: 1) Novice, 2) Advanced Beginner, 3) Competent, 4) Proficient, and 5) Expert. (Table 9.8).

Professional development is lifelong learning across a career continuum. During this career continuum, the nurse may fluctuate through various stages of Benner's theory based upon their specialty area. For example, a new nurse could begin as a Novice in labor and delivery and advance to the Proficient level after gaining additional knowledge and experience. Subsequently, if the nurse transfers to the **Intensive Care Unit** (ICU), they would become a Novice again. This highlights the importance of lifelong learning. Lifelong learning can be either formal or informal. An example of formal lifelong learning includes learning as part of the requirements for an advanced degree from a degree-granting college or university or that associated with becoming certified in your specialty area. Less formal lifelong learning includes learning that occurs through continuous education programs, orientations, or even attendance at seminars or workshops related to nursing practice.

Needs Assessment

When developing and implementing staff education, it is imperative to assess and understand the needs within a particular organization or unit. **Needs assessments** are processes conducted to identify strategic priorities, determine desired results, guide decisions based on gaps in knowledge skills and practices, and ensure that staff are competent and utilize evidence-based practice to the top of his/her scope of practice. The needs of an organization evolve over time and require an ongoing assessment process that allows for continued growth of the members in the organization. This process requires a commitment from the organization to support and develop staff members by providing adequate education and resources to ensure that staff are growing and adapting along with organizational changes.

Once particular needs are identified, it is important to determine who or what a particular group requires in order to customize an education plan to address the needs. For example, a new cardiac monitor is installed and the nurses and telemetry technicians need to be educated on how to operate the new technology. The first step is determining the best way to deliver this information so that is easy to understand and retain for the particular learners. Utilizing a tutorial and hands-on education may be the best methods to use based upon the needs assessment. It is important to time the education to maximize staff attendance. Factors such as holidays, weekends, and seasonal patterns of patient census can all affect the timing of delivery of new education.

Types of Needs Assessments

Needs assessments can be conducted in a variety of ways, including electronic needs assessments, learner or manager

---

Table 9.8   **Benner's Novice to Expert Theory**

Novice: A novice nurse is a beginner who has no practical experience of how to apply new knowledge and skills in unique situations. Performance is limited because strictly following the rules can impede the beginning nurse's ability to identify relevant tasks to perform in the situation.

Advanced Beginner: This stage begins when the nurse uses intuition based on previous experience and can recognize patterns and contexts of unique situations. At this stage, the advanced beginner is demonstrating some skill in parts of the practice areas and occasionally requiring support. Knowledge continues to develop.

Competent: The competent stage is marked by the nurse's ability to prioritize and utilize aspects of situations that are related. Thinking is more analytic and conscious. A sense of mastery and responsibility is developed as chosen actions and performance shortcomings are recognized by the competent nurse.

Proficient: The proficient nurse evaluates situations holistically and recognizes changing variables as a situation unfolds. Proficient nurses have mastered technical tasks and take less time to complete tasks. The proficient nurse knows what needs to be done and can modify care quickly based on changing circumstances.

Expert: Experience and intuition are highly developed in the expert nurse. The expert nurse operates from a deep understanding of the total situation and is able to combine the art and science of nursing. The expert nurse has able to draw on his/her analytical skills when faced with a new experience.

Benner, 1984.

Source: Benner, P. (1984). From novice to expert: Excellence and power in clinical nursing practice. . Menlo Park, CA: Addison-Wesley.

requested needs assessment, or quality-related or event-focused needs assessments. Electronic needs assessments include surveys of the staff, either by utilizing a questionnaire or gathering electronic information by direct observation. Learner or manager requested needs assessment based on new technology, process improvements, or organizational changes are also assessed, such as the previous example of the cardiac unit telemetry units. A quality-relater or event-focused needs assessment can be based on a quality improvement project or a particular patient safety event. Conducting needs assessments is crucial to development of all other professional development activities, including orientation/onboarding and development of both initial and ongoing nursing competencies. Needs assessments can often drive lesson plans targeting a specific topic identified in the needs assessment (see Table 9.9 for a sample staff lesson plan).

Continuing Education

Continuing education (CE) is an essential component of promoting and maintaining lifelong learning in nursing. **Continuing education** is defined as the systematic attempt to facilitate change in professional practice and ensure ongoing professional competence and increase employability to promote optimal patient outcomes (Wilson et al., 2017). In many states, health care practitioners are deemed by the state to have minimal competency standards during the initial licensure phase, but are required to maintain continuing education as a condition for license renewal (National Council of State Boards of Nursing, 2018, Spector, 2009). The goal of this requirement is to assure that health care practitioners remain competent during the duration of their practice. The U.S **Department**

Table 9.9 Sample Staff Lesson Plan for Management of the Patient with a CerebroVascular Accident (CVA)

Setting: 4th-floor Neurology Unit

Learner: 4th-floor unit staff

Overall Goal: The staff on the 4th floor will verbalize knowledge of management of the Patient with a CerebroVascular Accident (CVA)

Objectives: After completion of this session, the staff will:
1. Verbalize the definition of a CVA.
2. Identify the signs and symptoms of a CVA.
3. Discuss prevention and treatment of a CVA.

Topic: Management of a Patient with a CVA
In this lesson, the staff will receive the following information:

Definition of CVA: The sudden death of some brain cells due to lack of oxygen and nutrients. CVA occurs when the blood supply to part of the brain is interrupted or reduced due to a blocked artery (ischemic stroke) or due to a rupture of a blood vessel (hemorrhagic stroke). Within minutes, brain cells start to die

Signs and symptoms of CVA: SUDDEN difficulty walking, headaches, dizziness, numbness or tingling in the arms and legs, double vision or blindness in one or both eyes, confusion, faintness, loss of consciousness, slurred speech, or inability to talk, paralysis of one side of the body. The mnemonic BEFAST may help recognize signs, symptoms, and what to do in the event of a CVA.
    B = Balance
    E = Eyes, Vision
    F = Face drooping
    A = Arm weakness
    S = Slurred speech
    T = time to call
American Heart Association (2019)

Causes: CVA is caused the sudden death of brain cells due to lack of oxygen and nutrients.

Prevention: Exercise daily, do not smoke, check blood pressure regularly and maintain a normal blood pressure, follow a Dietary Approach to Stop Hypertension (DASH) diet, daily aspirin may be prescribed, limit alcohol, and avoid stress.

Treatment: Depends on the type of CVA—Thrombolytics such as tPA are given if the stroke has occurred within the previous four-and-a-half-hour time frame. Anticoagulants such as warfarin; and/or aspirin may be used in conjunction with physical, occupational, and speech therapy.

Strategy: PowerPoint presentation

Medium: Handout—CVA Management

Evaluation: Provide a five-question true or false quiz to staff members—Staff must obtain a score of 80% or better.

Evaluation tool for CVA management: Mark the correct answer.
____F____ 1. A CVA is a temporary increase in blood supply to the brain.
____T____ 2. Numbness and tingling are a symptom of a CVA.
____T____ 3. A CVA can be caused the sudden death of brain cells due to lack of oxygen and nutrients.
____T____ 4. One way to decrease the risk of a CVA is to avoid smoking.
____T____ 5. Two medications that may be prescribed for a CVA patient are aspirin and warfarin.

Source: Compiled with information from The American Heart Association at www.heart.org and The American Stroke Association www.strokeassociation.org Accessed in December, 2018.

of Health, Education, and Welfare (DHEW) recommended physicians undergo periodic re-examinations (DHEW publication, 71–11, 1971). In 1971, a similar report recommended that requirements to ensure continued education should be developed by professional nursing associations and state boards of nursing (NSCBN, 2018). As an alternative to re-examination, continuing education was deemed to be appropriate and has been adopted by several states. However, it remains controversial. Some states, such as Colorado, abolished the requirements, determining that continuing education did not ensure competence. Each state varies on the amount and whether or not they require continuing education for re-licensure.

The concept of continuing education goes back to Florence Nightingale who was one of the first advocates for continuing education. Nurses and other health care professionals can participate in CE activities for many reasons, including for general lifelong learning or to fulfill credits for licensure or specialty certification. Conferences, seminars, and web-based learning are an important component of continuing education. A conference is educational and allows for networking to learn from local, state, national, or international colleagues. Exhibition halls and educational presentations bring together the best and brightest nursing practice changes and ways to integrate new knowledge into current practice to ensure that the highest quality patient care is being provided. They often also expose the nurse to the latest technology and products (Figure 9.4).

Another component of continuing education which is becoming more and more important and recognized is professional certifications. **Certification** is a process by which a non-governmental agency or association certifies that an individual licensed to practice has met certain standards specified by a profession or specialty (ANCC, 2020). Certification increases the likelihood that nursing practice is consistent with national standards and often produces better patient outcomes (Straka et al., 2014). Some examples of advanced certifications for nursing include **Certified Pediatric Nurse (CPN)**, **Oncology Certified Nurse (OCN)**, and **Certified Registered Nurse Anesthetist (CRNA)**.

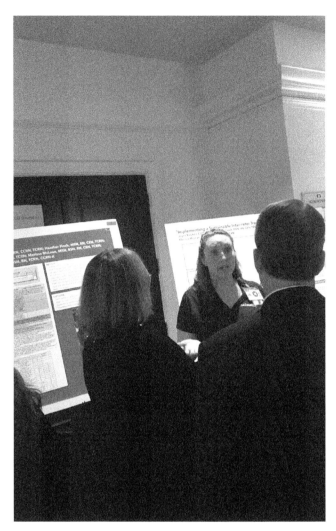

FIGURE 9.4   Professional poster presentation at a nursing conference. *Source:* Heather Estrada.

Orientation and Onboarding

There are various approaches to new employee orientation and onboarding based on each organization's structure, culture, resources available, and needs. While the terms onboarding and orientation are often used interchangeably, there are distinct differences. **Orientation** is a process that provides a big picture overview of the organization with the purpose of preparing the new employee for training. New employee orientation is the process in which employees are familiarized with the organization, staff roles, the inter-professional work team, and conditions of employment (Bowles, 2012)

Onboarding is a series of events that includes orientation but is much more in-depth to encompass the process of learning the employee's role and how that role contributes to the overall organization. The onboarding process focuses on what matters in that unit or department for that individual employee.

The goal of onboarding is to ensure that the new employee is ready to contribute to the organization. Managers and leaders play an integral role in onboarding by providing regular check-in meetings and goal setting with the new employee. The orientation and onboarding process can be assigned into four distinct roles: production, synergism, integration, and strategic planning (Kim, Chai, Kim, & Park, 2015).

Production suggests that the organization has production-based goals and employees are elements of this productivity (Kim et al., 2015). Because labor comprises a great deal of expense for any organization, the challenge is to ensure that new employees are able to be competent to carry out the required duties for the organization, yet this process must occur in the least amount of time to ensure that productivity goals are met. This has encouraged orientation programs to become more innovative and utilize various technologies to improve the experience for adult learners.

Synergism is the second component of the orientation and onboarding process, where the organization facilitates

Real World Interview

An Interview with a Nurse Educator

How did you begin your nursing career?

I started my career as a **certified nursing assistant** (CNA) in a local nursing home at the age of 16. I continued as a CNA through college. I started at Memorial Hospital in 1997 as a CNA on the Orthopedic floor. Five months later, I moved to the ICU. I am currently a Clinical Educator for critical care.

What made you interested in education?

I was an **assistant nurse manager** (ANM) in ICU for 5 years. During that time, my focus was building the neurology program in our unit. I enjoyed learning and sharing my knowledge with our team, building a core group of neuro champions. I developed the neuro education and supported growth and improvements toward both primary and comprehensive stroke accreditations. I was fortunate to have a manager that allowed me to focus on this direction and growth. I enjoy building teams and creating educational experiences with nurses, CNAs, and our doctors.

Was there something that helped prepare you for a leadership role in education?

I believe my years as an ICU charge nurse and ANM were beneficial in guiding me as a leader in our units.

What are some "pearls" you would like to share with the beginning bedside nurse who is interested in a role as an educator?

Health care is constantly changing and improving. There is always room to learn and grow in our profession. Join a national nursing organization. Absorb information from journals, books, webinars, podcasts, and everyone around you. Don't be afraid to share your knowledge and question everything. Being an educator isn't a title, it is who you are. You constantly are learning and sharing knowledge with those around you.

Nicole (Nicki) Seyller
August 26, 2019
Reproduced with permission of Nicole Seyller.

integration into a work group and the overall organizational culture to provide a sense of fit and belonging (Kim et al., 2015). This synergism is achieved often through the use of a preceptor and team-based learning. Synergism allows for new employees to meet various milestones in their training while socializing to the new environment and their role. Synergism is a key component in retention of new employees as it provides them with a sense of belonging and fit within the organization or unit.

Integration is the third component of orientation and onboarding where the culture and unit or organizational identity is transferred to a new person. Integration links the mission, vision, and values to the roles of the employee and their professional identity.

Finally, strategic planning is the fourth component and plays an integral part in orientation and onboarding. In this component, the relationship is established with the new employees and their contribution to the organization's strategy. A large component of strategic planning is the investment and encouragement of ongoing training and professional development. Ongoing training and professional development begin with the onboarding process and continues throughout the career of the employee at the organization.

A successful orientation and onboarding program should reflect the organizational strategies and considers the organization, the health care providers, and their needs. During the orientation and onboarding process, the employee is introduced to the mission, vision, and values of the organization and is socialized to the culture. Orientation and onboarding serve as key processes that facilitate the transition of a new employee to an advanced beginner based on Benner's "novice to expert" theory (Fitzpatrick & Gripshover, 2016).

Orientation is required by several hospital accreditation agencies, such as The Joint Commission or **Det Norske Veritas** (DNV), who may outline particular topics for Key Safety Content that must be completed before staff provides care, treatment, and services. This Key Safety Content often includes but is not limited to orientation to:

- Fire Safety and Response
- Infection Prevention and Control
- Emergency Response (Code Blue, Rapid Response, etc.)
- Active Shooters
- Bomb Threats
- Personal Safety
- Emergency Management (Internal/External Disaster Plans)
- Medical Equipment Failure and Reporting Process
- Utility System Disruptions and Reporting Process
- Additional content may include:
  - Work Schedule
  - Employee Attendance and Time and Resource Management Expectations
  - Employee Responsibilities in the Event of an Internal or External Disaster
  - Managing a Patient's Pain
  - Sensitivity to Cultural Diversity

- Patient Rights

- Code of Conduct Expectations

- Maintaining Privacy and Security of Protected Health Information; sometimes referred to as **Health Insurance Portability and Accountability Act** (HIPAA Training) (The Joint Commission Manual 2018).

Nursing and Health Care Competencies

Competency is the core functions and skills that are required to fulfill the role of a health care professional. Competency is a complex integration of knowledge, including professional judgment, skills, values, and attitudes (Fukada, 2018). Assessment and development of nursing competency is a dynamic ongoing iterative process. The goal of this process is to identify the skills needed to perform a role now, as well as in the future, and to reduce occurrences of adverse events (Liaw et al., 2015). Components of nursing assessment of competencies includes ensuring that all domains of skills are present, regardless of a particular role. The specific components of competencies include the technical, critical thinking, and interpersonal domains. Each of these domains interface to ensure that an individual will be able to perform the essential functions of the role selected. Competencies are assessed across a continuum: upon hire, during orientation, and throughout employment, flowing from population or organizational-based needs.

Competency upon hire is assessed through verification of licensure, education, and certification. Often competency is validated or demonstrated through the interview process to evaluate for particular knowledge, skills, or experience needed to be successful in the role. Initial competencies focus on the knowledge, skills, and abilities that are required in the first 6 months to a year of employment. During this time, the staff member will be in an orientation and onboarding phase with centralized orientation, onboarding on the unit, and working independently with close supervision.

Ongoing competencies throughout employment should build upon the competencies assessed during hire and orientation/onboarding. These competencies should also reflect the current environment and nature of the work expected in a specific role. In addition, ongoing competencies should reflect new, changing, high risk, and problematic issues of the role. Ongoing competencies are completed and documented periodically, as defined by organizational policies and the corresponding regulatory agency requirements.

The frequency or global premise behind the monitoring of ongoing competencies is required by external regulatory agencies. These include but are not limited to: The Joint Commission, DNV, **Occupational Safety and Health Administration** (OSHA), Centers for Medicare and Medicaid Services, as well as other state or federal agencies and licensure and certification boards. Many of these agencies and State Boards of Nursing require measurement of competence at various pre-defined

intervals. The primary objective for measuring competency is the demonstration or verification of a particular skill, knowledge, or ability. Education may be a component of the competency process but it is not a measure of competency. For example, attending an in-service on caring for pressure ulcers does not indicate competency in caring for pressure ulcers. However, it could be counted if there is documented demonstration or verification of competency of a particular knowledge, skill, or attitude built into the course.

Quality and Safety Education for Nurses

In 2003, the **Institute of Medicine** (IOM) challenged nursing faculty to mindfully transform learning experiences that shape the basis of professional nursing practice. The goal of this challenge was to create nursing educational experiences with an increased emphasis on quality and safety. The national initiative, **Quality and Safety Education for Nurses (QSEN),** was developed and focuses on preparing nurses with the KSAs required in six core competencies: patient-centered care, teamwork and collaboration, evidence-based practice, quality improvement, safety, and informatics (Table 9.10). The QSEN competencies, modeled after the IOM report, provide a tool for faculty and staff development educators to identify gaps in KSAs and then develop strategies to address these gaps. These QSEN competencies have been used extensively by national nursing organizations and are the central focus of the National Council of State Boards of Nursing and nurse residency programs (Dolansky & Moore, 2013), where the competencies are used to guide new hire orientation (James, Patrician, & Miltner, 2017). The ultimate goal of the QSEN competencies is to prepare nurses to ensure high-quality and safe patient care.

Academic-Practice Partnerships

Nursing professional organizations, such as the **American Association of Colleges of Nursing** (AACN) and the **American Organization of Nurse Executives** (AONE), recommended establishing partnerships with academia to develop best practices, drive realistic curriculums, establish joint faculty to educate nurses, and prepare graduate nurses to meet workforce needs and mitigate shortages (AONE, 2007). The IOM released a report on the Future of Nursing in 2010 that called for major initiatives to redesign nursing education to better prepare the nursing profession for the changing health care landscape (Institute of Medicine, 2011). **Academic-practice partnerships** are contractual agreements between hospitals or health care organizations and academic institutions to offer opportunities to improve health and health care by producing the educated workforce needed to transform health care. These opportunities include facilitating the transition to practice for new graduates, connecting nursing education, practice, and research to patient outcomes, and in enhancing education (Bakewell-Sachs, 2016).

Academic-practice partnerships allow academic institutions and health care organizations to create strategic relationships

Table 9.10   **QSEN Competencies and KSAs**

QSEN Competency	Definition	Knowledge, skills, and attitudes (KSA)
Patient-centered care	Recognize the patient or designee as the source of control and full partner in providing compassionate and coordinated care based on respect for patient's preferences, values, and needs.	**Knowledge:** Describe how diverse cultural, ethnic and social backgrounds function as sources of patient, family, and community values. **Skills:** Elicit patient values, preferences and expressed needs as part of clinical interview, implementation of care plan and evaluation of care **Attitudes:** Seek learning opportunities with patients who represent all aspects of human diversity
Teamwork and collaboration	Function effectively within nursing and inter-professional teams, fostering open communication, mutual respect, and shared decision-making to achieve quality patient care	**Knowledge:** Describe scope of practice and roles of health care team members **Skills:** Is able to communicate with and work effectively as part of health care team **Attitudes:** Respect the unique attributes that members bring to a team, including variations in professional orientation and accountabilities
Evidence-based practice	Integrate best current evidence with clinical expertise and patient/family preferences and values for delivery of optimal health care	**Knowledge:** Describe reliable sources for locating evidence reports and clinical practice guidelines **Skills:** Base individualized care plan on patient values, clinical expertise and evidence **Attitudes:** Value the need for continuous improvement in clinical practice based on new knowledge
Quality improvement	Use data to monitor the outcomes of care processes and use quality improvement methods to design and test changes to continuously improve the quality and safety of health care systems.	**Knowledge:** Describe strategies for learning about the outcomes of care in the setting in which one is engaged in clinical practice **Skills:** Seek information about outcomes of care for populations served in care setting**Attitudes:** Appreciate that continuous quality improvement is an essential part of the daily work of all health professionals
Safety	Minimize risk of harm to patients and providers through both system effectiveness and individual performance.	**Knowledge:** Examine human factors and other basic safety design principles as well as commonly used unsafe practices (such as, workarounds and dangerous abbreviations) **Skills:** Demonstrate effective use of technology and standardized practices that support safety and quality **Attitudes:** Value vigilance and monitoring (even of own performance of care activities) by patients, families, and other members of the health care team
Informatics	Use information and technology to communicate, manage knowledge, mitigate error, and support decision making.	**Knowledge:** Describe examples of how technology and information management are related to the quality and safety of patient care **Skills:** Seek education about how information is managed in care settings before providing care **Attitudes:** Appreciate the necessity for all health professionals to seek lifelong, continuous learning of information technology skills

Source: QSEN Institute. (2013). Competencies. Retrieved from http://qsen.org/competencies Accessed March 19, 2019.

based on the advancement of their mutual interests related to practice, education, and research (American Association of Colleges of Nursing, 2016). These strategic relationships can be informal or formally defined through contracts or memorandums of understanding between the organizations. These strategic relationships are important for increasing the pool of baccalaureate prepared nursing applicants, fostering the pursuit of Magnet designation, building a robust nursing workforce, developing excellent clinical leaders, and providing opportunities for continued professional development to support faculty, staff, and student nurse education programs. Continuing

to build these academic-practice partnerships should expand enrollment and enhance the overall nursing workforce.

Strategies for Engaging the Adult Learner

A goal for determining the delivery method and format of an educational offering is to develop strategies for engaging the adult learner that provide a supportive and engaging learning environment. These strategies will provide learners and instructors with a dynamic learning process and a positive

Table 9.11 Adult Learner Strategies.

Adult learning strategy	Description
Question and answer	The instructor asks open ended questions. The learners respond with answers.
Case studies	The instructor presents a realistic scenario that is analyzed to illustrate a key principle or concept. The case study often ends with questions for the learner.
Pre/post tests	The instructor provides a test prior to the educational event or experience. The same or similar test is provided after the educational event or experience to determine content retention.
Role playing	The instructor presents a realistic situation and learners explore the situation by interacting with other learners in a managed environment. This allows learners to experiment with different strategies in a safe, supporting environment.
Demonstration and return demonstration	The learner demonstrates what they have just been taught or had demonstrated to them.

Source: R. R. Flayter, L. Kidin & M. S. Schuler.

learning experience. To obtain this goal, there are several adult learning strategies that could be employed to meet the needs and preference of the learners. These are listed in Table 9.11.

E-Learning

E-learning is an umbrella term for various terms and concepts related to electronic learning such as digital, online, web-based, and mobile learning (De Caro, Marucci, & Lancia, 2016). E-learning provides content and instructional methods that can be tailored to the needs of individual learners. Advantages to e-learning include that it is cost-effective and can allow learners to learn at their own pace. It is not dependent on time or location. Studies have indicated that it has a positive impact on nurses' knowledge, skills, level of understanding, and self-satisfaction (Du et al., 2013; Lahti et al., 2014;). E-learning can be utilized to provide standardized information to a large number of learners that can be tested or reinforced by hands-on or testing. However, e-learning does provide barriers for some learners. For example, some learners have a low level of technology literacy and may not have the skills needed to utilize a particular device. These learners lose time when they encounter issues with the particular technology used in the delivery of the e-learning content.

When utilizing knowledge gained through e-learning, it is important to translate this knowledge into clinical practice. This process of knowledge translation can be complex and is often dependent upon the type of information provided, goals and objectives of the educational intervention, and the skill and composition of the target audience (Contandriopoulos & Brousselle, 2012). There are various educational technology methods of e-learning that can be used to enhance the classroom or nursing unit teaching methods, including simulation and virtual reality.

Simulation

Simulation provides a realistic environment that prepares learners to practice skills and knowledge in a testing environment that is similar to what will be encountered in a real-life situation (Liaw et al., 2015). It is a well-established tool in aviation and has recently been used in health care. Simulation is a tool that allows staff to practice clinical and communication skills in a realistic and safe environment (Figure 9.5). This can occur in a simulation laboratory or on a nursing unit. Simulation is part of an immersive learning strategy where a specific clinical scenario can be replicated. This method is often used to demonstrate high risk, low volume situations and allows the provider to maintain essential skills needed to adapt and respond to a specific scenario. During scenario-based simulation training,

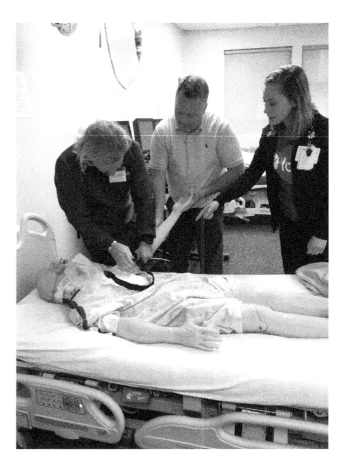

FIGURE 9.5 Simulation team picture.
Source: Siobhan Geraghty.

the learner can acquire such important skills as interpersonal communication, teamwork, leadership, decision-making, the ability to prioritize tasks under pressure, and stress management. Studies have supported the use of simulation to improve nurses' knowledge and self-confidence (Elder, 2017).

Debriefing after a scenario is an important component of simulation. Video recordings of the scenario are often used to initiate the debriefing discussion and to make sure that all learning objectives were covered. The debriefing process provides an opportunity for learners to improve performance with self-review and apply existing knowledge to acquire new knowledge (Ryoo & Ha, 2015). A systematic and structured debriefing process along with an instructor's active listening, non-judgmental demeanor can maximize the simulation experience for the learner. Using simulation technology can promote a positive experience and safe environment for learning. In addition, this methodology can be effective in the development of nursing competencies and continuing education. Simulation can be optimized when blended with other educational technologies as part of a blended learning strategy.

Virtual Reality

Virtual reality (VR) is a type of simulation using a three-dimensional computer environment that offers a variety of simulations to practice essential aspects of a clinical situation (Dubovi, Levy, & Dagan, 2017). The origin of VR used in skills validations in other industries such as aviation dates back to simulation-based training during the 1960s (Dubovi et al., 2017). VR has been used for skills training because it introduces the learner to the intricacy of clinical situations without exposure to harm. VR allows engagement of the operator via communication with the device using graphical displays, auditory indicators, and touch vibrations (Smith & Hamilton, 2015). VR serves as a mechanism to translate theoretical knowledge into practice. Initial studies have indicated that learners who use VR are more proficient with clinical skills (Smith & Hamilton, 2015).

The Role of Nursing Leadership in Professional Development

A key to success of any professional development program is an engaged and committed leadership team. Building and sustaining a successful professional development nursing program requires a strategic vision of excellence and innovation. Enabling nurses to build their clinical skills and grow profes-

sionally enhances quality patient care and ensures optimal patient outcomes by focusing on evidence-based practices. A strong commitment to investment in nursing professional development also has many additional benefits such as improved recruitment and retention of top talent, decreased turnover, improved competency, innovation, and a supportive environment for research and publication of outcomes.

Patient and staff education is an important component of clinical practice. The staff needs to be kept up to date on the latest nursing and health care research. Evidence-based nursing care is of the utmost importance to the bedside clinical nurse. Patient and staff education is a rewarding experience for the nurse. The nurse can provide a professional and gratifying learning situation through application of a structured approach to the design, development, and delivery of education. This begins when the nurse enters the organization through orientation/onboarding and continues with ongoing professional development. Ongoing professional development can be achieved through various methods including e-learning, simulation, and virtual reality. These are methods that are being used to deliver content in a meaningful way to the adult learner. By building affiliate agreements and partnerships between academia and nursing practice, organizations can offer new technologies and other methods to continuously enhance the knowledge and skills of the staff. Supporting a robust professional development program has many benefits including decreased turnover, improved recruitment and retention, and, most importantly, improved patient outcomes (D'Amato & Hertzfeldt, 2008).

In this chapter, we have discussed the foundations of patient-centered and professional nursing education, and analyzed the role of the nurse in patient-centered education and professional development. We have identified the impact of reading and health literacy on patient-centered health care and patient outcomes, described the desired KSAs and their utility in designing learning experiences, utilized educational resources and patient-centered and professional development education. We have also developed a lesson plan for a patient/family teaching session, evaluated the effectiveness of a patient-centered education experience, discussed strategies for professional development, developed a learning module/lesson plan for health care professionals based on adult learning principles, and reviewed nursing and health care related competencies. With the knowledge and skills developed in this chapter, you now have the tools to be a more effective teacher. Teaching is an integral part of nursing and a skill that must be continually developed as more resources and evidence become available.

KEY CONCEPTS

- A standard education methodology contains five major phases: analysis, design, development, implementation, and evaluation.

- Analysis consists of context analysis, learner analysis, and content analysis.

- The design phase of education consists of establishing objectives and sequencing content into an organized, structured framework.

- The development phase of education consists of establishing format, selecting strategies and media, and finalizing the lesson plan.

- The implementation phase of education consists of conducting education based on the lesson plan.

- The evaluation phase of education consists of learner evaluation, which measures how well the learner learned, and the education evaluation, which measures how well the education was conducted.

- Learners have individual learning styles and respond differently to specific educational methods.

- Health care literacy must be assessed when developing educational methods.

- All learning can be classified under three domains: cognitive, psychomotor, and affective. Each contains a hierarchy of behaviors.

- Behavioral objectives specify the Audience, Behavior, Condition, and Degree of measurement of the education session.

- Orientation is a key activity for a new employee to move from novice to advanced beginner.

- Onboarding is the process of learning the employee's role and how that role contributes to the overall organization. Onboarding focuses on what matters in that unit or department for that individual employee.

- Ongoing competencies should reflect new, changing, high risk, and problematic issues of a nursing role and should be assessed on a regular basis.

- Academic affiliations between health care entities and colleges develop best practices, drive realistic curriculums, establish joint faculty to educate nurses, and prepare graduate nurses to meet workforce needs and mitigate nursing shortages.

- A lesson plan documents the objectives, content, sequence, format, strategies, media, and evaluation methods of a teaching session.

- E-learning, simulation, and virtual reality are examples of types of learning that is tailored toward the needs of the adult learner in health care.

KEY TERMS

Patient-centered education	Learner analysis	Onboarding
Reading literacy	Content analysis	Competency
Health literacy	Therapeutic patient-centered education	Synergy
Learning domain	Lesson plan	Quality and Safety Education
Affective domain	Teach back	for Nurses (QSEN)
Cognitive domain	Education evaluation	Academic practice partnerships
Psychomotor domain	Continuing education	E-learning
Learning objectives	Needs assessment	Simulation
Context analysis	Orientation	Virtual reality

REVIEW QUESTIONS

1. A nurse manager of a unit with a large number of elderly patients just returned from a conference on a restraint-free environment. She wants to share this evidence-based practice with her staff and implement this practice change. The most effective way to introduce and implement this change to staff would be which of the following?

    a. Inform the unit charge nurses that restraint policies and current practice must be changed to integrate this new policy and that all staff must comply.
    b. Provide a lecture to the staff members about the new practice change during a shared governance meeting.
    c. Develop an e-learning module regarding the new restraint practice with a post-test to confirm the staff members comprehend the new practice.
    d. Distribute flyers on the unit with information on the new restraint practice.

2. A patient states he would like to use E-learning, and you recognize that E-learning includes all of the following methods except?

    a. Digital
    b. Online
    c. Mobile learning
    d. Classroom lecture

3. A young adult who is employed full-time as a factory worker has Type I diabetes mellitus. He has had an insulin pump for 3 years. The patient is now hospitalized for the second time in 4 months with an admitting diagnosis of Diabetic Ketoacidosis (DKA). He has had one prior emergency department admission for hypoglycemia. He is awake, alert, and oriented. The nurse considers which of the following to be the primary current issue and the focus for patient-centered education?

    a. Self-care behaviors and pump management
    b. Infusion set is malfunctioning because the tube is kinked
    c. Vacation and meal planning tips
    d. Working with his employer to ensure that his meal times are the same each day.

4. A nurse is developing a teaching plan for a patient with asthma. Which teaching point has the highest priority?
   a. Change filters on heating and air conditioning units frequently.
   b. Avoid goose down pillows.
   c. Avoid contact with fur-bearing animals.
   d. Take ordered medications as scheduled.

5. You are a nurse who works on a medical surgical unit and providing care for a woman who had surgery a few hours ago. Knowing that the woman is likely to experience pain, you plan to provide patient-centered education about pain. Which of the following considerations should be made when preparing to educate the post-operative client about pain management?
   a. A structured lesson plan would be beneficial.
   b. Identify an online pain management tool.
   c. Request the family be present before providing education.
   d. Review admission paperwork that identifies how your patient prefers learning.

6. A nurse is teaching an older adult at home about taking newly prescribed medications. Which of the following would be included?
   a. "You can identify your medications by their color."
   b. "I have written down the names of your drugs with times to take them."
   c. "You won't forget a medication if you count them every day."
   d. "Don't worry if the label comes off; just look at the shapes."

7. A patient informs the nurse that she would like to learn about her treatment options later when she is less tired and after her children have gone home. The nurse recognizes that honoring this request best reflects which QSEN competency?
   a. Teamwork and Collaboration
   b. Patient-centered Care
   c. Quality Improvement
   d. Evidence-based Practice

8. The nurse recognizes that purposeful hourly rounding in which health care providers check on their patients every hour and address the 4 P's: Potty, Possessions, Pain, and Position, is an example of which QSEN-based competency?
   a. Teamwork and Collaboration
   b. Informatics
   c. Community-centered Care
   d. Quality Improvement

9. A patient has been newly diagnosed with diabetes. As the nurse, you plan to provide patient-centered education. What is an important factor to consider before you begin teaching the patient about dietary restrictions?
   a. Determine who cooks the meals in the home.
   b. Confirm the name of the patient's primary care provider.
   c. Have pharmacy send an extra insulin pen for teaching purposes.
   d. Prepare the glucometer for quality testing.

10. An effective method for reducing hospital readmissions and in improving the quality of life for a patient with a chronic disease is:
    a. Have the family provide care for the patient.
    b. Therapeutic patient education.
    c. A scheduled follow-up appointment in 2 months.
    d. Provide the patient with a pamphlet about his disease process.

REVIEW QUESTION ANSWERS

1. Answer: C is correct.
   a. Rationale: (C) The use of e-learning can appeal to the adult learner to get information out to a large group that is tailored to that population. In this case, the group of nurses caring for the elderly. The nurses can also take the course at their own pace. The pre-posttest determines retention and critical thinking regarding if and how the information can be applied to the situation. It is important to vet the new practice to ensure staff will sustain and support the change. (A) Taking an authoritative approach does not allow time for teaching and learning of the new practice. (B) A lecture can be used but does not offer the most effective way to connect with all staff who need to learn the practice change. (D) Distributing flyers on the unit helps to reinforce education about the practice change, but will not be the most effective way to assess learning.

2. Answer: D is correct.
   a. Rationale: (D) E-learning is tailored to allow a person to learn at their own pace and can be tailored to the needs of the specific audience at the time and place that they choose. (A,B,C) Digital, online, and mobile learning are all considered e-learning methods.

3. Answer: A is correct.
   a. Rationale: (A) Self-care behaviors to determine the patient's willingness to manage the pump correctly need to be addressed. Some pump users get tired of managing the pump or forget to bolus, which can be evident if the patient has been hospitalized for episodes of unstable blood glucose, such as DKA or severe hypoglycemia. Also assess the infusion site. If the site is poor condition, this can also indicate lack of self-care. (B) Insulin pump clients are trained to assess if the infusion set is clogged or the tube is kinked. This issue would have been identified on the previous admission for DKA. The concern is that this is not a single occurrence. Additionally, if the tube was kinked or clogged, an episode of hypoglycemia would not occur. (C) Knowledge level or competency would not appear to be an immediate concern, since the client has had the insulin pump for 3 years. (D) Although exposure to influenza and other infections can trigger a DKA episode, the stem of the question provides no other information about a diagnosis of infection and the recent episodes that have occurred over the last 4 months.

4. Answer: D is correct.
   a. Rationale: (D) Take medications as prescribed is the highest priority to ensure prevention of an asthma exacerbation. (A, B, C) The other choices are similar in removing some potential triggers based on a patient's specific allergens, but may not be helpful to all asthmatic patients.

5. Answer: D is correct.
   a. Rationale: (D) Identifying how the patient prefers learning will provide the patient with the best opportunity to be prepared regarding post-operative pain management. (A) A structured lesson plan probably would not be required in this situation; a lesson plan is most often used for a chronic disease diagnosis. (B) Identifying an online pain management tool may be helpful in some cases, but is very patient dependent based on their learning preference. (C) Family may benefit from being present, but that should be discussed with the patient for her preference.

6. Answer: B is correct.
   a. Rationale: (B) The best way to identify newly prescribed medications when teaching a patient is by using the generic name, dose, and times per day to take them. (A, D) Manufacturers can provide the medication in various colors and shapes, so it is important to not teach a patient based on those characteristics. (C) Counting the number of medications may seem to be helpful for a patient, but should not be a tool used by the nurse when teaching about new medications.

7. Answer: B is correct.
   a. Rationale: (B) Focusing on the patient's needs and requests, or patient-centered care, is a crucial part of nursing competencies. The other QSEN competencies are also important, but in this scenario, the most important consideration is focusing on the patient. Patient-centered care involves recognizing the patient or designee as the source of control and full partner in providing compassionate and coordinated care based on respect for patient's preferences, values, and needs. (A) Teamwork and collaboration would focus on a nurse's ability to work effectively with peers and interdisciplinary teams. (C) Quality improvement specifically looks at opportunities to focus on improving outcomes of care processes, such as reducing hospital acquired injury or infection. (D) The

evidence-based practice competency is used to integrate best current evidence with clinical expertise and patient/family preferences and values for delivery of optimal health care.

8. Answer: D is correct.
   a. Rationale: (D) Using data to monitor the outcomes of care processes and using improvement methods to design and test changes to continuously improve the quality and safety of health care systems is the definition of Quality Improvement. Purposeful rounding is an example of a quality improvement initiative to ensure patient safety and satisfaction. (A) Teamwork and collaboration would focus on a nurse's ability to work effectively with peers and interdisciplinary teams. (B) Informatics uses technology to communicate, manage knowledge, mitigate error, and support decision making. (C) Community-centered Care is not a QSEN competency.

9. Answer: A iscorrect.
   a. Rationale: (A) When focusing on dietary restrictions for education, it is also important to consider who prepares the meals in the home in case a significant other may need to be included in the patient-centered teaching. (B, C, D) The other options may provide useful information or options to consider; however, the question asks about teaching related to dietary restrictions.

10. Answer: B is correct.
    a. Rationale: (B) Patient-centered education encompasses therapeutic patient education, which is most often employed with chronic conditions. This type of education focuses on chronic disease management, but also takes into consideration the patient's needs and learning preferences. (A) Having the family provide care for the patient may not prevent hospital readmissions if education has not been provided to the family on how to manage the chronic disease. (C) A scheduled follow-up appointment in 2 months is too long after hospital discharge to focus on prevention of readmission to the hospital; usually a patient should have an appointment to follow up within 7–10 days. (D) Providing the patient with a pamphlet does offer some educational material; however, it is not helping to ensure the patient reads, understands, and can follow specific disease management instructions.

REVIEW ACTIVITIES

1. Identify a patient education project that you can develop for one of your patients. Develop a lesson plan for this patient. Are your objectives in one, two, or three domains of learning?

2. Your patient is newly diagnosed with a venous thromboembolism and needs instruction in administering his enoxaparin injection. Using the A, B, C, D method in this chapter, develop one objective for this education. How would you evaluate if this patient met the objective?

3. You have developed a lesson plan for nursing staff on a new computer documentation system that is to take effect on all

the clinical units in your institution. Look at Table 9.9, which provides an exemplar for an evaluation of staff education. How would you develop an evaluation tool for your lesson plan by using all or some of these elements listed? Are there other areas you would want to include in the evaluation?

4. A patient comes to her outpatient appointment after she was discharged 1 week ago from the hospital with the diagnosis of myocardial infarction. She comes to the follow-up appointment with educational information from the internet. How would you help the patient evaluate the educational material, using the website at www.healthwebnav.org

DISCUSSION POINTS

During your last clinical experience:

- Did you have an opportunity to observe or perform any patient teaching?

- What did you identify as one of your patient's largest educational needs?

- Did you assist in a patient's discharge education? Who was present and what was provided to the patient/family? How did they receive the education?

- What patient education materials did you find on the unit?

- Did the unit have any staff education or updates that they received? Consider the examples presented in the chapter:

- Which examples would you feel the most comfortable using in the hospital setting as a direct care clinical nurse?

- How can you identify educational resources for your patient population as a direct care clinical nurse?

- As a nurse, if you have a question, where would you obtain the information needed to be more informed about a diagnosis or medication?

DISCUSSION OF OPENING SCENARIO

1. How will you assess Mr. DaPina's learning needs?

   Utilizing patient-centered education, as the nurse, you will determine a few things before discharge teaching Mr. DaPina. On the nursing admission assessment, specific learning related questions should have been asked of Mr. DaPina. Based on this information, you can determine if he can read in English or only in Portuguese. If only Portuguese, you will need to work with your hospital's translation service to assist you. If he can speak and read English, it is important that you provide it at a level for his best understanding. It will be best to ask him to repeat back information or ask him open-ended questions instead of ones that only require a yes/no response. Another consideration is, if Mr. DaPina has a relative who he would also like to have participate in the discharge teaching, does that individual speak/read in English?

2. How will you determine the best way to teach Mr. DaPina about his diagnosis?

   Determining what type of learner Mr. DaPina is will help you develop his teaching plan so he can have a better comprehension of the material being presented. Does he prefer visual, auditory, or kinesthetic learning? In regard to heart failure education, visual learning would be written instructions with pictures, such as a booklet or pamphlet. An auditory learner would prefer to hear the instructions and then teach back or repeat back. A kinesthetic learner will want to be physically involved, which could include demonstrating how to do pursed lip breathing, using the incentive spirometer, or the correct way to administer an inhaler.

3. What are some teaching strategies you will use to ensure Mr. DaPina has the knowledge he needs to manage his new diagnosis?

   You can use visual aids and illustrations, utilize the teach back method, or return demonstration. If he can repeat back or demonstrate the key pieces to manage his COPD upon discharge, you can feel comfortable that he can manage his care until his follow-up appointment where TPE can be provided on an outpatient basis.

EXPLORING THE WEB

Try these websites, all accessed on May 8, 2019, for quality online health care information:

- Center for Health Care Strategies www.chcs.org

- WebMD, www.webmd.com

- Up To Date Patient education, www.uptodate.com/contents/table-of-contents/patient-education

  Major United States and international health care websites:

- American Diabetes Association, www.diabetes.org

- American Heart Association, www.heart.org

- American Cancer Society, www.cancer.org

- American Dietetic Association, www.eatright.org

- Public Health Agency of Canada, www.canada.ca/en/public-health.html

- National Health Service, United Kingdom, www.nhs.uk

  Professional Development websites:
  Nursing Professional Development, www.anpd.org

- American Association of Colleges of Nursing (AACN), www.aacnnursing.org

- American Organization of Nurse Executives (AONE), www.aacnnursing.org

- Nurse Residency Programs, www.vizientinc.com/Our-solutions/Clinical-Solutions/Vizient-AACN-Nurse-Residency-Program

- Quality and Safety in Education for Nursing (QSEN) http://qsen.org/tag/staff-development

  Continuing Education, http://qsen.org/tag/continuing-education

INFORMATICS

All websites accessed May 18, 2019.

- Use https://medlineplus.gov Type in a search for, tutorial on evaluating websites. This connects to articles and to a tutorial by the National Library of Medicine on evaluating web-based health resources.

- Explore the Institute of Healthcare Improvement, www.npsf.org and search "health literacy." It provides resources to increase your patients' understanding of health information. This website has a basic overview of health literacy and teach back methodology with examples. There are connections to videos about health literacy. See also, http://hsl.lib.unc.edu/health-literacy, from the University of North Carolina and utilize a number of the resources listed on the left side of the website.

- Go to http://qsen.org/ten-minute-expert-evidence-based-bedside-teaching-bundle, review the 10 Minute Expert: Evidence Based Bedside Teaching Bundle from the QSEN website. Consider how you might integrate this teaching strategy as part of the professional development of new-to-practice staff nurses at your facility.

LEAN BACK

- What do you see in the clinical practice setting where patients are educated that is different from what you read in the text? Explain.

- How can this chapter's education information be directly applied to your NCLEX-RN knowledge and studying?

- If you have provided patient-centered education in your clinical rotations, how did the patient and/or family receive it? Would you do anything differently today?

- How can you apply this information directly to your practice as a staff nurse? In a nursing leadership role?

REFERENCES

Aboumatar, H., Carson, J., Beach, K., Roter, A., & Cooper, M. (2013). The impact of health literacy on desire for participation in healthcare, medical visit communication, and patient reported outcomes among patients with hypertension. *Journal of General Internal Medicine, 28*(11), 1469–1476.

Abu Abed, M., Himmel, W., Vormfelde, S., & Koschack, J. (2014). Video-assisted patient education to modify behavior: A systematic review. *Patient Education and Counseling, 97*(1), 16–22.

ANCC. (2020). *American Nurses Credentialing Center.* Retrieved from www.nursingworld.org/our-certifications/

American Association of Colleges of Nursing. (2016). *Advancing health care transformation: A new era for academic nursing.* Washington, DC: American Association of Colleges of Nursing. Accessible online at www.aacn.nche.edu/AACN-Manatt-Report.pdf

American Heart Association. (2019). *Stroke Symptoms.* Retrieved from www.strokeassociation.org/en/about-stroke/stroke-symptoms

American Organization of Nurse Executives (AONE). (2007). *AONE guiding principles for the role of the nurse executive in patient safety.* Chicago, IL: American Organization of Nurse Executives.

Bakewell-Sachs, S. (2016). Academic-practice partnerships; driving and supporting educational change. *Journal of Perinatal and Neonatal Nursing, 30*(3), 184–186.

Beltran-Alacreu, H., López-de-Uralde-Villanueva, I., Fernández-Carnero, J., & La Touche, R. (2015). Manual therapy, therapeutic patient education, and therapeutic exercise, an effective multimodal treatment of nonspecific chronic neck pain: A randomized controlled trial. *American Journal of Physical Medicine & Rehabilitation, 94*(10S), 887–897.

Benner, P. (1984). *From novice to expert: Excellence and power in clinical nursing practice.* Menlo Park, CA: Addison-Wesley.

Berkman, N. D., Sheridan, S. L., Donahue, K. E., Halpern, D. J., & Crotty, K. (2011). Low health literacy and health outcomes: An updated systematic review. *Annals of Internal Medicine, 155*(2), 97–107.

Bloom, B. S. (1956). *Taxonomy of educational objectives: The classification of educational goals.* New York: Longmans, Green.

Bowles, J. (2012). New employee orientation. In W. J. Rothwell. In *The encyclopedia of human resource management* (pp. 327–335). San Francisco, CA: Pfeiffer.

Brown, J. P., Clark, A. M., Dalal, H., Welch, K., & Taylor, R. S. (2013). Effect of patient education in the management of coronary heart disease: A systematic review and meta-analysis of randomized control trials. *European Journal of Preventative Cardiology, 20*(4), 701–714.

Contandriopoulos, D., & Brousselle, A. (2012). Evaluation models and evaluation use. *The Tavistock Institute, 18*(1), 61–77. doi:10.1177/1356389011430371

Cronenwett, L., Sherwood, G., Barnsteiner, J., Disch, J., Johnson, J., Mitchell, P., Sullivan, D. T., & Warren, J. (2007). Quality and safety education for nurses. *Nursing Outlook, 55*(3), 122–131.

D'Amato, A., & Hertzfeldt, R. (2008). Learning, orientation, organizational committment and talent retnation across generations. A study of European managers. *Journal of Management Psychology, 23*(8), 929–953.

Davis, T., Crouch, M., & Long, S. (1993). *Rapid estimate of adult literacy in medicine (REALM).* Shreveport, LA: Louisiana State University Medical Center.

De Caro, W., Marucci, A., & Lancia, L. (2016). Case study 2: E-learning in nursing education in Acedemic fields. Eysenbach, G., Editor. In *Umbrella reviews: Evidence synthesis overview of reviews and meta-Epidemographic studies* (pp. 290–303). Switzerland: Springer.

Dolansky, M. A., & Moore, S. M. (2013). Quality and safety education for nurses (QSEN): The key is systems thinking. *OJIN: The Online Journal of Issues in Nursing, 18*(3). doi:10.3912/OJIN.Vol18No03Man0

Du, S., Liu, Z., & Lui, S. (2013). Web based distance learning for nurse education: A systematic review. *International Nursing Review, 60,* 167–177.

Dubovi, I., Levy, S., & Dagan, E. (2017). Now I know how! The learning process of medicaiton administration among nursing students with non-immersive desktop virtual reality simulation. *Computers and Education, 113,* 16–27. doi:10.1016/j.compedu.2017.05.009

Elder, L. (2017). A tool to assist nursing professional development practitioners to help nurses to better recognize early signs of clinical deterioration of patients. *Journal for Nurses in Professional Development*, *33*(3), 127–130.

Fitzpatrick, S., & Gripshover, J. (2016). Expert nurse to novice nurse practitioner: The journey and how to improve the process. *The Journal of Nurse Practitioners*, *12*(10), 419–421.

Fry-Bowers, E. K., Maliski, S., Lewis, M., Macabasco-O, A., Connell, A., & Dimatteo, R. (2014). The Association of Health Literacy, social support, self-efficacy and interpersonal interactions with health care providers in low-income Latina mothers. *Journal of Pediatric Nursing*, *29*(4), 309–320.

Fukada, M. (2018). Nursing competency: Definition, structure and development. *Yonago Acta Medica*, *61*(1), 1–7.

Goodreads. (2019). Xun Kuang quote "Tell me and I forget, teach me and I may remember, involve me and I learn." Retrieved from www.goodreads.com/quotes/7565817-tell-me-and-i-forget-teach-me-and-i-may

Hansberry, D. R., Ramachund, T., Patel, S., Kraus, C., Jung, J., Agarwal, N., Gonzales, S. F., & Baker, S. R. (2014). Are we failing to communicate? Internet-based patient education materials and radiation safety. *European Journal of Radiology*, *83*(9), 1698–1702.

Huang, Y. N., Shiyanbola, O. O., & Chan, H. Y. (2018). A path model linking health literacy, medication self-efficacy, medication adherence, and glycemic control. *Patient Education and Counseling*, *101*(11), 1906–1913.

Institute of Medicine. (2011). *The future of nursing: Leading change, advancing health*. Washington, DC: The National Academy Press.

James, H. D., Patrician, A. P., & Miltner, S. R. (2017). Testing for quality and safety education for nurses (QSEN). *Journal for Nurses in Professional Development*, *33*(4), 180–184. doi:10.1097/NND.0000000000000365

Julliere, Y., Jourdain, P., Suty-Selton, C., Beard, T., Berder, V., Maître, B., Trochu, J. N., Drouet, E., Pace, B., Mulak, G., Danchin, N. & ODIN Cohort Participants. (2013). Therapeutic patient education and all-cause mortality in patients with chronic heart failure: A propensity analysis. *International Journal of Cardiology*, *168*(1), 388–395.

Kher, A., Johnson, S., & Griffith, R. (2017). Readability assessment of online patient education material on congestive heart failure. *Advances in Preventative Medicine*, 9780317, 8 pages. doi:10.1155/2017/9780317

Kim, K. Y., Metzger, A., Wigle, P. R., & Choe, P. J. (2011). Evaluation of online consumer medication information. *Research in Social and Administrative Pharmacy*, *7*(2), 202–207.

Kim, M., Chai, D., Kim, S., & Park, S. (2015). New employee orientation: Cases of Korean corporations. *Human Resource Development International*, *18*(5), 481–498.

Lahti, M., Hatonen, H., & Valimaki, M. (2014). Impact of e-learning on nurses' and student nurses knowledge, skills and satisfaction. *International Journal of Nursing Studies*, *51*, 136–149.

Liaw, S., Wong, L., Chan, S., Ho, J., Mordiffi, S., Leng Ang, S. B., Goh, P. S., & Kim Ang, E., N. (2015). Designing and evaluating an interactive multimedia web-based simulation for developing Nurses' competencies in acute nursing care: Randomized controlled trial. *Journal of Medical Internet Research*, *17*(1), e5.

NAAL. (2019). *National Assessment of Adult Literacy. United States Department of Education. National Center for Education Statistics.* Retrieved from https://nces.ed.gov/naal/

National Center for Education Statistic. (2003). National Assessment of Adult Literacy (NAAL). Retrieved October 23, 2020, from https://nces.ed.gov/naal

National Council of State Boards. (2018). Find Your Nurse Practice Act. Retrieved October 23, 2020, from https://www.ncsbn.org/npa.htm

Paterick, T., Patel, N., Tajik, A., & Chandrasekaran, K. (2017). Improving health outcomes through patient education and partnerships with patients. *Proceedings (Baylor University. Medical Center)*, *30*(1), 112–113.

Becker, K., Biller, J., Brown, M., Demaerschalk, B. M., Hoh, B., Jauch, E. C., Kidwell, C. S., Leslie-Mazwi, T. M., Ovbiagele, B., Scott, P. A., Sheth, K. N., Southerland, A. M., Summers, D. V., Tirschwell, D. R. & American Heart Association Stroke Council.

Reif, K., deVries, U., Petermann, F., & Gorres, S. (2013). A patient education program is effective in reducing cancer-related fatigue: A multi-Centre randomised two-group waiting-list controlled intervention trial. *European Journal of Oncology Nursing*, *17*(2), 204–213.

Rymer, J., Kaltenbach, L., Anstrom, K., Fonarow, G., Erskine, N., Peterson, N., & Wang T. Y. (2018). Hospital evaluation of health literacy and associated outcomes in patients after acute myocardial infarction. American Heart Journal, 198, 97–107 10.1016/j.ahj.2017.08.02410.1016/j.ahj.2017.08.024 (2018). Hospital evaluation of health literacy and associated outcomes in patients after acute myocardial infarction. *American Heart Journal*, *198*, 97–107.

Ryoo, E. N., & Ha, E. (2015). The importance of debriefing in simulation-based learning. *CIN: Computers, Informatics, Nursing*, *33*(12), 538–545. doi:10.1097/cin.0000000000000194

Smith, P. C., & Hamilton, B. K. (2015). The effects of virtual reality simulation as a teaching strategy for skills preparation in nursing students. *Clinical Simulation in Nursing*, *11*(1), 52–58. doi:10.1016/j.ecns.2014.10.001

Smith, F., Carlsson, E., Kokkinakis, D., Forsberg, M., Kodeda, K., Sawatzky, R., Friberg, F., & Öhlén, J. (2014). Readability, suitability and comprehensibility in patient education materials for Swedish patients with colorectal cancer undergoing elective surgery: A mixed method design. *Patient Education and Counseling*, *94*(2), 202–209.

Spector, N. (2009). Approval: National council of state boards of nursing. In L. Caputi (Ed.), *Teaching nursing: The art and science* (2nd ed., Vol. 3). Glen Ellyn, IL: College of DuPage Press.

Spector, N., Blegen, M. A., Silvestre, J., Barnsteiner, J., Lynn, M. R., Ulrich, B., Fogg, L. & Alexander, M. (2015). Transition to practice study in hospital settings. *Journal of Nursing Regulation*, *5*(4), 24–38. doi:10.1016/s2155-8256(15)30031-4

Stellefson, M., Chaney, B., Ochipa, K., Chaney, D., Haider, Z., Hanik, B., Chavarria, E., & Bernhardt, J. M. (2014). YouTube as a source of chronic obstructive pulmonary disease patient education: A social media content analysis. *Chronic Respiratory Disease*, *11*(2), 61–71.

Straka, K., Ambrose, H., Burkett, M., Capan, M., Flook, D., Evangelista, T., Houck, P., Lukanski, Schenkel, K., & Thornton, M. (2014). The impact and perception of certification in pediatric nursing. *Journal of Pediatric Nursing*, *29*, 205–211.

The Joint Commission. (2018). 2018 Manual. (Retrieved October 23, 2020, from https://manual.jointcommission.org/

U.S. Department of Health and Human Services, Office of Disease Prevention and Health Promotion. (2010). National Action Plan to Improve Health Literacy [Brochure]. Washington, DC: Author. Retrieved October 22, 2020, from https://health.gov/sites/default/files/2019-09/Health_Literacy_Action_Plan.pdf

Wilson, A. B., Barger, J. B., Perez, P., & Brooks, W. S. (2017). Is the supply of continuing education in the anatomical sciences keeping up with the demand? Results of a national survey. *Anatomical Sciences Education, 11*(3), 225–235. doi:10.1002/ase.1726

Worral, P. S. (2019). Evaluation in healthcare education. In S. B. Bastable (Ed.), *Nurse as educator: Principles of teaching and learning for nursing practice* (5th ed.). Burlington, MA: Jones & Bartlett.

SUGGESTED READINGS

Dolansky, M. A., & Moore, S. M. (2013). Quality and safety education for nurses (QSEN): The key is systems thinking. *OJIN: The Online Journal of Issues in Nursing, 18*(3). doi:10.3912/OJIN.Vol18No03Man0

Easton, P., Entwistle, V. A., & Williams, B. (2013). How the stigma of low literacy can impair patient-professional spoken interactions and affect health: Insights from a qualitative investigation. *BMC Health Services Research, 13*, 1–12. doi:10.1186/1472-6963-13-319

Elder, L. (2017). A tool to assist nursing professional development practitioners to help nurses to better recognize early signs of clinical deterioration of patients. *Journal for Nurses in Professional Development, 33*(3), 127–130.

Peter, D., Robinson, P., Jordan, M., Lawrence, S., Casey, K., & Salas-Lopez, D. (2015). Reducing readmissions using teach back: Enhancing patient and family education. *The Journal of Nursing Administration, 45*(1), 35–42.

Pool, I., Poell, R., Berings, M., & Ten Cate, O. (2015). Strategies for continuing professional development among younger, middle-aged, and older nurses: A biographical approach. *International Journal of Nursing Studies, 25*, 939–950.

Smith, J., & Zsohar, H. (2013). Patient Education Tips for New Nurses. *Nursing*, online exclusive. doi:10.1097/01.NURSE.0000434224.51627.8a

Patient Outcomes and Evidence-Based Health Care

10

Parul Patel
Utilization Management Molina Healthare Healthcare, Oakbrook, IL, USA

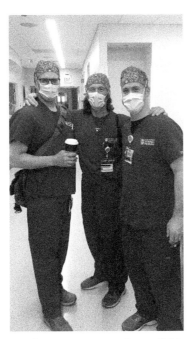

Working in today's complex environment, the nurse must use the available evidence to provide care and the best outcomes to all they care for, regardless of the practice setting.
Source: Photo used with permission.

A nurse's role in evidence-based practice includes asking important questions, realize that evidence is the foundation of practice, participate in EBP projects and disseminate findings, and collaborate with the health care team to provide quality care. Titler, (2008).

OBJECTIVES

Upon completion of this chapter, the reader should be able to:

1. Understand the nurse's role in evidence-based practice.

2. Explain importance of EBP.

3. Understand history and evolution of EBP.

4. Be familiar with evidence-based practice models and terminology.

5. Understand how to use evidence-based multidisciplinary practice models.

6. Identify and utilize resources for EBP.

7. Promote evidence-based best practices.

Kelly Vana's Nursing Leadership and Management, Fourth Edition. Edited by Patricia Kelly Vana and Janice Tazbir
© 2020 John Wiley & Sons Ltd. Published 2020 by John Wiley & Sons Ltd.
Companion Website: www.wiley.com/go/kelly-Nursing-Leadership

OPENING SCENARIO

Your nurse manager has shared with you that your unit has the highest number of surgical site infections. The nurse manager says that she is concerned because she has noticed variability in the management of patients pre and post operatively. The variability may be negatively affecting patient outcomes. She would like you to explore evidence-based practices (EBPs) and help determine what should be done in your organization. The nurse manager wants to appoint you to a task force to consider using EBP as a means of reducing variability and improving patient

outcomes. Where do you start? This type of scenario is becoming more and more common in health care institutions as nurse leaders explore new ways to improve the quality of care.

1. *What do you know about EBP and where do you begin?*

2. *What are some things you need to know before you can accept the appointment to the task force?*

3. *How will you prepare yourself for the task force and be able to make a positive impact?*

Nurse's Role in Evidence-Based Practice

Nursing plays a key role in the ability of a patient to heal, achieve optimal health, and transition back into the community. As nurses, there are many actions that we undertake to manage population health and help people attain optimal well-being. How do we really know that the actions we implement are the most effective for our patients? How do we ensure consistency and standardization but also incorporate patient individuality, preferences, social factors, etc.? Nursing knowledge is based on but not limited to tradition, authority, trial/error, personal experience, intuition/reasoning, and nursing research. How do we really know that what we are doing is at the top of our practice or the simply stated best practice? How many RNs challenge the status quo? How do we achieve excellence in care delivery? More than ever today it is imperative that tradition-based practice changes to scientific practice. This chapter will discuss the nurse's role related to EBP, the importance of EBP, and the history and evolution of EBP. Understanding the history of EBP and its evolution will allow the reader to really understand the criticality and significance of EBP. This chapter also focuses on how you can use EBP by reviewing various EBP models, terminology, and resources. The goal of this chapter is to provide you with the foundational elements required for you to promote and use EBP.

Demonstrating that outcomes of health care are effective, efficient, and safe is a major responsibility for nursing. This is where evidence-based care is integral to nursing practice. Using the term *evidence* in daily practice, as well as searching for and utilizing the best evidence when planning, implementing, and evaluating care goals and programs is essential. EBP is incorporating evidence-based research into practice to achieve desired outcomes.

The impact of evidence-based practice (EBP) has echoed across nursing practice, education, and science. The call for evidence-based quality improvement and health care

transformation underscores the need for redesigning care that is effective, safe, and efficient. In line with multiple direction-setting recommendations from national experts, nurses have responded to launch initiatives that maximize the valuable contributions that nurses have made, can make, and will make, to fully deliver on the promise of EBP.

(Stevens, 2013, p.1)

There is nothing more important to patients and professional nursing than evidence-based clinical interventions that can be linked to clinical outcomes and used as a basis for care within the institution. Makic & Rauen (2016) states "Practice interventions wedded in tradition need to be retired and evidence-based nursing interventions should be consistently implemented . . ." In 2010, the **Institute of Medicine** (IOM) provided a vision that all clinical decisions would be evidenced-based by 2020. EBP is a key component of nursing and removing barriers toward the utilization of EBP is imperative. One barrier of using EBP is the lack of a thorough understanding of what EBP is and how it is related to quality improvement and research.

Let's take a close look at quality improvement and EBP. Quality improvement usually consists of systematic and continuous actions that lead to measurable improvements in *processes*. For example, conducting chart audits to improve documentation is a quality improvement project. Nurse Moksha reviews the compliance of core measures bundles on patients in the ICU—this is a quality improvement activity. How does EBP differ? EBP is defined as the conscientious, explicit, and judicious use of current best evidence in making decisions about the *care* of individual patients (Sackett, Rosenberg, Gray, Haynes, & Richardson, 1996). EBP uses outcomes, research and other current research findings to guide the development of appropriate strategies to deliver quality, cost-effective care. Outcomes research provides evidence about benefits, risks, and results of treatments so that individuals can make informed decisions and choices to improve their quality of life. Research seeks to understand the end results of specific health care practices and interventions. End results may include changes in a person's ability to function and carry out routine activities of daily living (Mann & University of Florida, 2002). Outcomes research can also identify potentially effective strategies that can be implemented to improve the quality and value of care. Conducting research helps guide evidence. According to Hain (2017) "Conducting research to generate new evidence is extremely important, but so is translating the best available evidence into practice through quality improvement projects." Another barrier in using EBP relates to the presence of gaps in nursing literature. "Evidence-based practice is an approach to decision making in health care that brings together evidence from research, a clinician's expertise, and patient preferences and values to drive the best patient care and outcomes" (Melnyk, 2018, p. 1). However, this application of EBP is not the norm. For example, Melnyk (2018) found that children with asthma continue to be treated with nebulizers in many emergency rooms across the U.S., although numerous studies have indicated better outcomes and fewer hospitalizations when children are given a bronchodilator with a metered-dose inhaler and spacer. Nurses need to conduct research and share their findings via publications so others can gain important knowledge.

Conducting research can help reduce the gaps in EBP. When there is no EBP in the literature, research is the first step on how to acquire new knowledge. EBP bridges the gap between research and practice. It improves clinical practice. The 2011 report by the IOM recommends that all health care professionals possess certain skills and competencies in order to enhance patient care quality and safety. The competencies necessary for the continuous improvements of the quality and safety of the health care systems-patient centered care includes teamwork, and collaboration, EBP, quality improvement, safety, and informatics (Institute of Medicine (IOM), 2011). For nurses, these competencies are essential. The IOM Future of Nursing report (2011) focuses on knowledge in clinical decision making, quality, interpersonal team development, and EBP to transform health care. IOM also sponsored a landmark summit on education in the health professions and recommended five competencies for nurses: providing patient-centered care, applying quality improvement principles, working in interprofessional teams, using EBP, and using health information technologies (IOM, 2003, p. 49; John, 2016).

Nursing and EBP

Nurses are expected to manage the care of acutely ill patients. Beginning nurses should be encouraged to thoughtfully acknowledge their personal abilities and limitations. There must be a blend between knowing and doing. It is important that the beginning nurse realizes that gaining knowledge and skills is a gradual process. As the beginning nurse develops aspects of skilled know-how, the nurse will become aware of the ability to deliver safe patient care, minimize patient discomfort, decrease stress and anxiety, and assist in optimizing team performance. Guidelines based on EBP can help to direct care but cannot replace learning by hands-on delivery

of patient care. As beginning nurses gain clinical experience and learn new theoretical knowledge, they will be able to contribute to the development and revision of EBP guidelines. Remember, EBP guidelines outline practice parameters based on evidence or research, but they do not outline how to deliver individualized patient care.

A nurse's roles in EBP include asking important questions, realizing that evidence is the foundation of practice, participating in EBP projects and disseminating findings, and collaborating with the health care team to provide quality care. It was inevitable that nursing has moved to EBP. Established in 1996, one of the earlier proponents for EBP in nursing was the Joanna Briggs Institute for Evidence-based Nursing and Midwifery. Significant work has been done worldwide to implement EBP in Australian, Canadian, and UK institutions of care. The Joanna Briggs Institute recommends that many different types of evidence/combination can be utilized. Wyatt asserted that "By 2020 the goal is to ensure that 90% of all clinical decisions are individualized yet supported by the most current, relevant, and best available evidence and effective tools are in place to measure outcomes" (2017).

Role of the ANA

The **American Nurses Association** (ANA) has been an active advocate of outcomes evaluation as early as 1976. Outcomes were emphasized as a measure of quality care. The 1980 ANA Social Policy Statement said that one of the four defining characteristics of nursing is the evaluation of the effects of actions in relation to phenomena. In 1986, the ANA approved policies related to the development of a classification system, including outcomes. In 1995, the ANA developed a Nursing Report Card for Acute Care Settings, which lists indicators for patient-focused outcomes, structures of care, and care processes. In 2003, the ANA revised the Social Policy Statement and included:

> *Nurses use their theoretical and evidence-based knowledge of these phenomena in collaborating with patients to assess, plan, implement, and evaluate care. Nursing interventions are intended to produce beneficial effects and contribute to quality outcomes. Nurses evaluate the effectiveness of their care in relation to identified outcomes and use evidence to improve care (p. 7).*

EBP is also integral to accreditation and prestigious distinctions such as Magnet Recognition (designation by the American Nurse Credentialing Center). Nursing excellence is closely linked to EBP. The **American Nurses Credentialing Center** (ANCC) Magnet recognition program has been closely linked with environments in which nurses want and prefer to practice and where patients achieve the best outcomes. Nurses that are retained in a Magnet-accredited hospital are involved directly in making choices on patient care, and they are active in contributing to health care changes based on EBP (Nurse Leader Insider, 2017).

The Joint Commission (2019) National Patient Safety Goals and accreditation standards focus on implementing EBP.

Real World Interview

Evidence is critical to the work of The Joint Commission. We use the best evidence available in developing standards and elements of performance. We use evidence in the creation of Sentinel Event Alerts and our R3 (Requirement, Rationale, References) publications. And, when new evidence becomes available, we change.

One recent example is the work of our suicide risk expert panel. The panel reviewed existing literature to expand requirements around ligature resistance and updates to our National Patient Safety Goal 15.

Many of our standards require organizations to use evidence-based guidelines in determining their practice. Care based on evidence is safer and of higher quality than care practices that are

not. We are generally not prescriptive in which evidence-based guidelines to use—we want organizations to determine the best evidence for their particular patients and services. Examples of standard requirements that require the use of evidence-based guidelines or expert consensus is in the design of new services, including protocol development, and infection prevention and control strategies.

Lisa DiBlasi Moorehead, EdD, MSN, RN
RPI Certified Yellow Belt
Associate Nurse Executive
Accreditation and Certification Operations
Oakbrook Terrace, IL

With an understanding of the importance and evolution of EBP, how does one start? Hospital based nurses have the resource of: librarians to orientate them to key EBP Web sites for best evidence and clinical guidelines; using the PICO(T) search process to identify the best literature on a given topic; paying attention to the latest news, research, and standards; subscribing to one or more nursing and health care journals; starting a journal club for discussion of EBP articles; incorporating EBP guidelines into the revision of procedures and guidelines as they are reviewed; collaborating with researchers at their hospital or local university, as needed; and by partnering with faculty, other health care professionals, and students on EBP. With the support of nurse leaders, many teams have been formed and EBP has changed protocols and policies so patient care can be optimal.

Importance of EBP

EBP is a total process that begins with knowing what clinical questions to ask, how to find the best practice, and how to critically appraise the evidence for validity and applicability to the particular care situation. The best evidence is then applied by a clinician with expertise based on the patient's unique values and needs. A nurse needs to understand levels of evidence which will be discussed later in this chapter. The final aspect of EBP includes evaluation of the effectiveness of care and commitment to continuous improvement of the process of patient care. The use of EBP is crucial in nursing care delivery. Though written in 2000, a manual by Guyatt and colleagues remains a pivotal document that sets out the two fundamental principles of EBP:

- Evidence alone is never sufficient to make a clinical decision.

- EBP involves a hierarchy of evidence to guide decision making.

Historically, health care providers have relied primarily on biomedical parameters or measures such as laboratory and diagnostic tests to determine whether a health intervention is necessary and if it is successful. For example, outcome measures have included physical measures, such as blood pressure, to assess the effectiveness of antihypertensive medications. They have also sometimes included patient satisfaction measures to assess patient satisfaction with the care or services provided. However, these measures often do not fully reflect the multi-dimensional outcomes that matter most to patients such as quality of life, family, work, and overall level of functioning. There has been a lack of generally agreed-upon standards or processes that are based on evidence. This lack of standards has been addressed with the development of EBP.

There is a difference between EBP and evidence-based nursing practice. EBP has a medical focus, whereas evidence-based nursing practice considers the individual's needs and preferences based on nursing theory and research.

Although an older resource but worthy of highlighting, Ingersoll has defined **evidence-based nursing practice (EBNP)** as the conscientious, explicit, and judicious use of theory-derived, research-based information in making decisions about nursing care delivery to individuals or groups of individuals and in consideration of individual needs and preferences (Ingersoll, 2000). **Evidence-based nursing (EBN)** is an integration of the best evidence available, nursing expertise, and the values and preferences of the individuals, families, and communities who are served (Sigma Theta Tau International, 2005). This assumes that optimal nursing care is provided when nurses and health care decision makers have access to a synthesis of the latest research, a consensus of expert opinion, and are thus able to exercise their judgment as they plan and provide care that considers cultural and personal values and preferences. This approach to nursing care bridges the gap between the best evidence available and the most appropriate nursing care of individuals, groups, and populations with varied needs.

Scott and McSherry (2009) proposed that EBN could be defined as "an ongoing process by which evidence nursing

Real World Interview

"As a resident physician, EBP is an integral part of our training. We are encouraged and trained to identify and utilize appropriate scientific literature to make clinical decisions and deliver optimal patient care. Original papers, systematic reviews, meta-analyses, and other sources are ultimately used to develop patient care protocols that guide clinical decisions.

At Vanderbilt Medical Center, EBP is also critical for nurses and is used to make appropriate health care decisions for the patient at the bedside. Scientific literature is used to develop various nursing protocols which nurses are encouraged to implement into their everyday practice. Some of the areas where EBP is utilized in nursing care include proper means to verify enteric tube placement: auscultation vs. aspiration of fluid vs. radiographic imaging and proper methods for endotracheal tube suctioning. Nurses also take into account all the social, cultural, financial aspects when developing an appropriate plan of care. Important nursing care happens at the bedside and utilization of EBP in nursing is essential to deliver optimal patient care."

Dr. Yatrik J. Patel
Vanderbilt University Medical Center
Nashville, TN

theory and the practitioners' clinical expertise are critically evaluated and considered in conjunction with patient involvement, to provide delivery of optimum nursing care for the individual." This proposed definition of EBN indicates the use of evidence, theory, and expertise in making decisions about optimum care for and with the individual patient.

One must note that EBP is not a cookbook approach to patient care. The nurse and members of the health care team assess each patient and determine whether a guideline is appropriate. Many nursing theorists, such as Nightingale, Peplau, Benner, and others, have identified that the uniqueness of nursing is based upon the relational and integrative nature of healing, involving the person and environments. Nursing is the only discipline that views the whole person within the context of the person's environment. Nurses must not mimic medical practitioners, but must focus on the art and science of nursing that comforts, cares, nurtures, heals, and builds on nursing theory to guide practice. The role of the nurse is to participate in developing a comprehensive, interdisciplinary evidence-based plan of care in conjunction with the patient and members of the health care team. This plan of care integrates the art and science of caring, not merely the medical model of the absence or presence of disease. Nurses must use innovation, creativity, and technology to plan care. There is a need to define evidence in each agency, a need to use the term *evidence* in daily practice, and a need to look for the best evidence when evaluating new goals and programs.

A common misconception about EBP nursing is that it ignores patient values and preferences. This is not the case; rather, the nurse works with the patient in deciding treatment options based on which trade-offs the patient is willing to accept. EBP is crucial to successful patient care, and it is also a good tool for shaping policies, procedures, and safety regulations (Johnson, 2017). Nurses need to be on the alert for opportunities to improve practice. Some examples of EBP are implementing a nurse driven sepsis response algorithm based on the American Association of Critical Care Nurses EBP guidelines, and the creation of a nurse driven joint mobility program based on the National Association of Orthopedic Nurses practice. Marshall (2017, p.17) states:

As nurses practice in the current health care environment, they are integrating evidence-based nursing practice on a daily basis, even if they are not aware of where, when, and how much. Evidence surrounds nursing practice and begins with the collection of data, whether it is assessment or evaluation data on patients' condition. Nursing management and procedures are implemented based on policies that have been developed by an examination of the latest literature, which should be based on research and evidence.

According to the American Nurses Association Scope and Standards of Professional Nursing Practice (2015), the registered nurse integrates evidence and research findings into practice. The ANA Nursing Scope and Standards of Practice (2015, p. 77) states the competencies for the registered nurse:

- Uses current evidence-based knowledge, including research findings, to guide practice.

- Incorporates evidence when initiating change in nursing practice.

- Participates in the formulation of EBP through research.

- Articulates the value of research and its application relative to the health care setting and practice.

- Identifies questions in the health care setting and practice that can be answered by nursing research.

The use of EBP can significantly improve patient care. Some potential outcomes related to integrating EBP are a reduction in mortality, length of stay and readmission, and an improvement in patient experience. With advancement in EBP will come documented practice changes, practice guidelines, utilization patterns, advanced use of informatics, and workforce retention (Melnyk, Gallagher-Ford, Long, & Fineout-Overholt, 2014). Some of the effects of EBP in an organization include improved retention, recruitment, employee satisfaction, and an increase in pursuing/acquiring advanced nursing degrees. For significant impacts in the improvement of quality in health care, one needs to apply EBP. Without EBP "health care providers are at risk for variances in care that could seriously affect patient outcomes." (Becker's Hospital Review, 2016, p. 76). Patients deserve and expect that the care they receive is current and evidenced based (Makic & Rauen, 2016). Nursing care is advancing to the point where it is not enough to deliver treatment interventions. Rather, it is essential that it provides a significant role in ensuring quality care, and essential that it provides quality care using the best available evidence. EBP, therefore, is a widely accepted paradigm for professional nursing practice (John, 2016).

History and Evolution of EBP

It is worthwhile to look at the history and evolution of EBP to gain a thorough understanding of its importance and relevance in nursing care today. The term *evidence-based practice* (EBP) was coined at McMaster Medical School in Canada during the 1980s. D. L. Sackett, along with his Oxford colleagues, encouraged EBP as a way to integrate individual clinical medical experience with external clinical evidence, using a systematic research approach. The search for best evidence should be systematic. Then, practitioners use their clinical judgment to determine the relevance of evidence for changing practice. Subsequent to the alarming report, finding major deficits in health care caused significant preventable harm (IOM, 1999), a blueprint for health care redesign was advanced in the first Quality Chasm report (IOM, 2001; Stevens, 2013). The IOM released two landmark reports on health care safety and quality, *To Err is Human* (1999) and *Crossing the Quality Chasm* (2001). These studies provided a broad agenda for the nation in addressing quality improvement in health care. The IOM reported in *To Err is Human* (1999) that health care in the United States was in a poor state. The IOM began driving improvements in health care. "It accomplished this by supporting national projects focused on the six aims: safety, effectiveness, patient centeredness, timeliness, efficiency, and equity" (Pelletier & Beaudin, p. 138 & IOM). The report has since become a rallying call for evidence-based, knowledge-driven improvements in health care in order to improve more desirable outcomes (John, 2016). The Institute for Healthcare Improvement (IHI), in December 2004, decided to launch a national initiative, the 100,000 Lives Campaign, with a goal of saving 100,000 lives among patients in hospitals through improvements in safety and in the effectiveness of care (Berwick, Calkins, McCannon, & Hackbarth, 2006). Six areas for evidence-based interventions were identified:

1. Deploy rapid response teams.
2. Deliver reliable evidence-based care for acute myocardial infarction.
3. Prevent adverse drug events through medication reconciliation.
4. Prevent central line infections.
5. Prevent surgical site infections.
6. Prevent ventilator-associated pneumonia.

All of the nation's 5,759 hospitals were invited to join and share their progress in reducing mortality. Other organizations that joined the IHI to support the campaign interventions included the Agency for Healthcare Research and Quality (AHRQ), the Centers for Medicare & Medicaid Services (CMS), the Surgical Care Improvement Project, the Joint Commission (JC), and the Leapfrog Group. Approximately 3,100 hospitals participated in the initial IHI Initiative. Based on their work on the initiative's interventions, and combined with other national and local improvement efforts, the facilities saved an estimated 122,000 lives in 18 months.

The IHI then launched a second 2-year initiative in 2006, the 5 Million Lives Campaign for U.S. health care, focusing on protecting patients from 5 million incidents of medical harm over a 2-year period from December 2006 to December 2008. The 5 Million Lives Campaign challenged American hospitals to adopt 12 changes in care that would save lives and reduce patient injuries. In addition to the six interventions from the 100,000 Lives Campaign, six new interventions targeted at harm were identified:

1. **Prevent harm from high-alert medications**, starting with a focus on anticoagulants, sedatives, narcotics, and insulin.

2. **Reduce surgical complications** by reliably implementing all of the changes in care recommended by the Surgical Care Improvement Project (SCIP).

3. **Prevent pressure ulcers** by reliably using science-based guidelines for their prevention.

4. **Reduce methicillin-resistant *Staphylococcus aureus* (MRSA) infection** by reliably implementing scientifically proven infection control practices.

5. **Deliver reliable, evidence-based care for congestive heart failure** to avoid readmissions.

6. **Get boards on board** by defining and spreading the best-known leveraged processes for hospital boards of directors, so that they can become far more effective in accelerating organizational progress toward safe care.

The IHI 5 Million Lives Campaign engaged more than 4,000 U.S. hospitals to prevent 5 million incidents of medical harm over a 2-year period. The IHI campaign's how-to guides were developed to help organizations and providers implement EBPs that were available at no cost to institutions and health care providers—for example, the *How-to Guide: Improving Hand Hygiene*. New standards of care were developed at hospitals throughout the United States, with other countries also adopting the standards. The National Institute for Health also emphasize the importance of EBP. Stevens (2013) notes two additional federal initiatives that may be called the next big ideas in EBP, as each highlights evidence-based quality improvement. The initiatives call for wider use of the knowledge acquired from quality improvement efforts. Both initiatives are housed from the NIH and focus on amassing and appraising evidence needed to make systems improvements which will transform health care. The first program is on **Dissemination and Implementation** (D&I) science; the second is the development of the research network, the **Improvement Science Research Network** (ISRN) (Stevens, 2013)

The Patient Protection and Affordable Care Act was signed into law in 2010. The triple aim was introduced in health care. The Triple Aim, as defined by Slavitt (2018) as: (a) enhancing the experience of care for the patient, (b) improving the health of populations, and (c) reducing per capita costs of health care, has become the standard of American health policy in the last decade. Caregiver burnout has been added to the triple aim, now known as the quadruple aim. In 2013, the IOM released a report on Better Care at Lower Costs: The Path to Continuously Learning HealthCare in America calling for improving health and what is needed to achieve continuous improvement and better-quality care at lower cost. We will focus on EPB and how it can impact the outcomes of healthcare today.

Other organizations focusing on EBP and quality improvement have included the **Robert Wood Johnson Foundation** (RWJF), which has funded the **Quality and Safety Education for Nurses** (QSEN) (n.d.) project for three phases. The overall goal through all phases of QSEN is to address the challenge of preparing future nurses with the **knowledge, skills, and attitudes** (KSA) necessary to continuously improve the quality and safety of the health care systems in which they work. In the United States, the AHRQ has provided stimulus for the EBP movement through recognition of a need for evidence to guide practice throughout the health care system. In 1997, the AHRQ launched its initiative establishing 12 EBP centers (more information about the 12 centers is listed later in this chapter). This partnered AHRQ with other private and public organizations in an effort to improve the quality, effectiveness, and appropriateness of care. IHI is currently engaged in improvement initiatives in England, Scotland, Ghana, Malawi, and South Africa.

EBP evolved from a nice-to-know perspective to a need-to-know essential strategy in health care. This was a major paradigm shift. Nurses began to think about research and ways to transform health care. Patients, health care providers, and payors recognize the significance of collecting data and analyzing outcomes to achieve safe, quality, cost-effective care. Outcome strategies used in EBP by nurses and members of the health care team include the creation of clinical protocols, guidelines, pathways, algorithms, and so on, which become the tools for health care interventions. For example, the creation of a sepsis protocol is essential in the management of patients with sepsis. A **practice guideline** is a descriptive tool or a standardized specification for care of the typical patient in the typical situation. Guidelines are developed by a formal process that incorporates the best scientific evidence of effectiveness and expert opinions. Synonyms or near synonyms include *practice parameter, preferred practice pattern, algorithm, protocol,* and *clinical standard.* EBP is used to guide practice interventions and is most successful when the entire organization and interdisciplinary team buy into EBP and participate and support the process. By linking the care that people receive to the outcomes they experience, EBP or outcomes research has become key to identifying and developing better strategies to monitor and improve the quality of care. Decisions are based on information from clinical expertise, research evidence, and patient values and preferences. As Stevens states, "The intended effect of EBP is to standardize health care practices to science and best evidence and to reduce illogical variation in care, which is known to produce unpredictable health outcomes" (2013, p.1). The development of EBP is powered by increased public and professional demand for accountability, safety, and quality improvement in health care. (Stevens, 2013).

Evidence-Based Practice Models and Terminology

Many EBP models have been developed to help nurses move evidence into practice by providing an organized approach. Table 10.1 provides common EBP terms and their definitions. The models will assist in providing a framework to help maximize time and resources, and ease implementation.

Table 10.1 Important EBP Terms

Best practice	In application, best practice includes the use of rigorous scientific evidence to support the effectiveness of specific clinical interventions for explicit patients, groups, or populations; implementation monitoring to assure accurate application; and outcome measurement to validate effectiveness.
Case-control study	A case-control study compares certain characteristics of an individual, for example a child with asthma, with someone who does not have that characteristic, for instance a similar child without asthma. This type of study is conducted for the purpose of identifying variables that might predict the condition—e.g., exercise, environmental allergies.
Clinical practice guidelines (or practice guidelines)	Systematically developed statements or recommendations to assist practitioner and patient decisions about appropriate health care for specific clinical circumstances. Practice guidelines present indications for performing a test, procedure, or intervention, or the proper management for specific clinical problems. Guidelines may be developed by government agencies, institutions, organizations such as professional societies or governing boards, or by expert panels. Evidence-based clinical practice guidelines provide the strongest level of evidence to guide practice, as they are based on systematic reviews of RCTs of the best evidence on specific topic areas.

(Continued)

Table 10.1 (Continued)

Cohort study	A longitudinal study that begins by gathering two groups of individuals (the cohorts), one group that received exposure to a disease or condition—e.g., a developmental disability—and one that did not. The groups are then followed prospectively over time to measure the outcomes.
Control group	Subjects in an experiment who do not receive the experimental treatment and whose performance provides a baseline against which the effects of the treatment can be measured.
Dependent variable	The outcome variable of interest; the variable that is hypothesized or thought to depend on or be caused by another variable, called the independent variable.
Descriptive research	Research studies that have as their main objective the accurate portrayal of the characteristics of people, situations, or groups, and the frequency with which certain phenomena occur.
Independent variable	The variable that is believed to cause or influence the dependent variable; in experimental research, the independent variable is the variable that is manipulated.
Integrative review	A type of evidence summary; concludes with implications from research for practice.
Meta-analysis	A systematic review that uses quantitative measurement methods such as surveys and questionnaires to summarize the results of multiple studies. It often produces a summary statistic that represents the effects of an intervention across multiple studies and, therefore, is more precise than individual findings from any one study used in the review.
Nonexperimental research	A study in which the researcher collects data without introducing an intervention.
Outcomes research	Research designed to document the effectiveness of health care services and the end results of patient care.
Prospective study	A study that begins with an examination of presumed causes (e.g., cigarette smoking) and then goes forward in time to observe presumed effects (e.g., lung cancer).
Qualitative analysis	The organization and interpretation of non-numeric data for the purpose of discovering important underlying dimensions and patterns of relationships.
Quantitative analysis	The manipulation of numeric data through statistical procedures for the purpose of describing phenomena or assessing the magnitude and reliability of relationships among them.
Randomized clinical trial (RCT)	An experimental research study in which subjects are randomly assigned to experimental and control groups. The experimental group then receives an experimental preventive, therapeutic, or diagnostic intervention. This type of study is strong in internal validity, i.e., the ability to say that it was the experimental intervention that caused a change in the outcome variable of interest and not other extraneous variables.
Systematic review of the literature	Type of evidence summary that identifies all relevant research studies on a particular topic and uses a rigorous scientific process for retrieving, critically appraising, and synthesizing studies in order to answer a clinical question.
Variable	An attribute of a person or object that varies (i.e., takes on different values) within the population under study (e.g., body temperature, heart rate).

Source: Compiled by P. Patel.

Stevens (2013) states, "There are multiple EBP models used and the frameworks used guide the design and implementation of approaches intended to strengthen evidence-based decision making." The models all have various advantages and disadvantages. Regardless of the preferred model, the EBP process should tell the story of how a problem was recognized, addressed, and improved, and that story should be shared (Wyant, 2017). We will focus on several that are most commonly used in nursing. They were selected since they were most commonly found in the literature. The intent of this section is to provide you with an overview of selected models.

The Stevens STAR Model of Knowledge Transformation (a five-point star) is a frequently used model for EBP that provides a framework for nurses to transition through five stages (see Figure 10.1). The model helps transform knowledge into a form that is useful for clinical decision making. The stages are knowledge discovery, evidence summary, translation into practice, integration into practice, and evaluation (Stevens, 2013). The cycle starts at the discovery point and goes through each point systematically. During integration, individual and

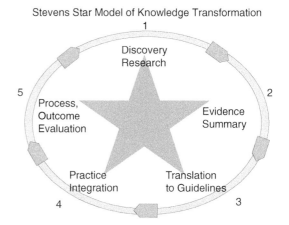

FIGURE 10.1 Stevens STAR Model of Knowledge Transformation. *Source:* Used with permission Stevens, K. R. (2015).

organizational practices are addressed. The final point of evaluation is when quality/performance improvement processes are initiated. The evaluation of the evidence based practice on the patient is conducted.

The Johns Hopkins Nursing EBP Model addresses nursing practice, research, and education. The model evaluates evidence within these domains as a core component of decision making. It uses at 3-step process known as PET: practice question, evidence, and translation. An important practice question is identified, and research is reviewed. The goal of this model is to allow the most current research findings to get quickly translated into clinical practice. The model uses clear criteria to rate the quality and level of evidence. A department protocol change or an institutional wide change may occur Figure 10.2.

The Iowa Model of Evidence-Based Practice to Promote Quality Care (Titler et al., 2001, Figure 10.3) starts by considering a trigger that focuses the nurse on new knowledge and research or one that focuses the nurse on a problem or opportunity for patient care improvement. The trigger concept is very unique to this model. Other triggers for seeking new evidence for practice may also occur. If the topic is a priority for the organization, the nurse can help form a team and assemble relevant research and related literature on the topic in order to critique and synthesize research for use in practice. If adequate evidence or a sufficient research base exists to propose a change in practice, the nurse can pilot the proposed change in practice. Within the Iowa Model, lack of sufficient evidence then prompts the nurse to seek evidence for best practices from other sources of information and/or to initiate the research process. Nurses in practice can seek answers to questions through collaboration with clinical nurse specialists and/or nurse scientists. Many times, these expert nurses can be found in the staff development department within a hospital. Nurse managers can also serve to provide direction and guidance for this purpose. Nurse manager support is particularly important, because the last element within the Iowa Model directs the nurse to ask if the change proposed is appropriate for adoption into practice. If it is, the nurse can institute the

change in practice and monitor and analyze structure, process, and outcome data and disseminate the results. If the change proposed is not appropriate for adoption in practice, the nurse will continue to evaluate the quality of care and review new knowledge until another trigger for seeking new evidence occurs. The original model from 1994 was revised in 2015 to focus on implementation of EBP.

When reviewing a study, the strength of the evidence is crucial, as levels of evidence help determine confidence about the study when making patient care decisions. There is a plethora of scales used. Professional organizations frequently use their own scales, (e.g., American Heart Association, American College of Chest Physicians,); publishing companies and EBP textbooks have developed their own scales too (Thompson, 2017). Table 10.2 is an example of a level of evidence scale (1 is the strongest level) that is frequently used.

Evidence-Based Multidisciplinary Practice Models

Over the past decade, nurses have been part of a movement that reflects perhaps more change than any two previous decades combined. The recommendation that nurses lead interprofessional teams in improving delivery systems and care brings to the fore the necessity for new competencies, beyond EBP, that are requisite as nurses transform health care (Stevens, 2013). The recently articulated vision for the future of nursing in the Future of Nursing report (IOM, 2011) focuses on the convergence of knowledge, quality, and new functions in nursing. The competencies focus on utilizing knowledge in clinical decision making and creating research evidence on interventions that promote use by individual and groups of providers (Stevens, 2013).

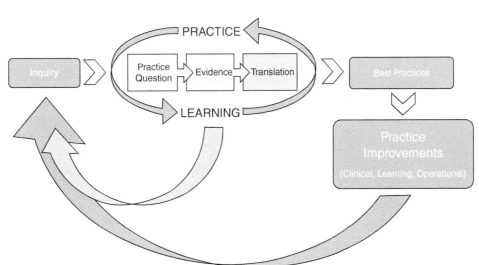

The Johns Hopkins Nursing Evidence-based Practice Model

FIGURE 10.2 Johns Hopkins EBP Model.
Source: Used with permission from: ©The Johns Hopkins Hospital/The Johns Hopkins University. Citation for tools: Dang, D., & Dearholt, S. (2017). Johns Hopkins nursing evidence-based practice: model and guidelines. 3rd ed. Indianapolis, IN: Sigma Theta Tau International

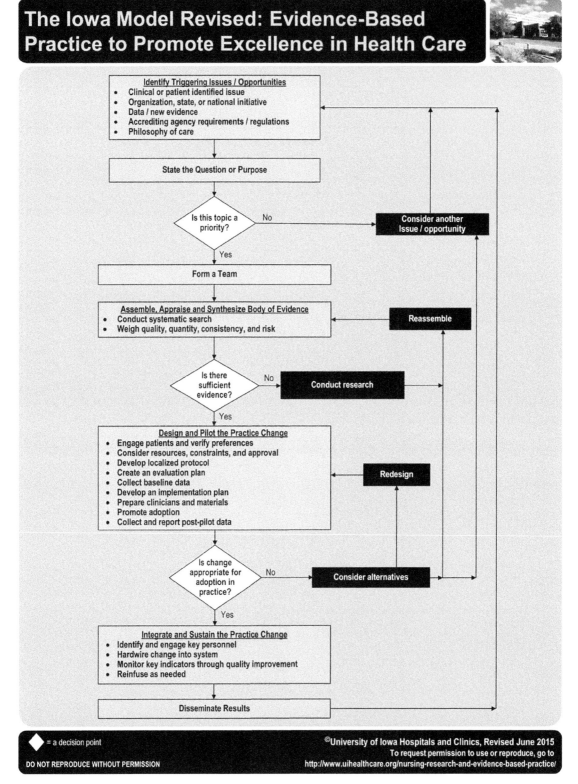

FIGURE 10.3   IOWA Model revised.
Source: Iowa Model Collaboration. (2017). Iowa Model of evidence-based practice: Revisions and validation. Worldviews on Evidence-Based Nursing, 14(3), 175-182. doi:10.1111/wvn.12223.

Table 10.2 **Levels of Evidence**

Level I:	Evidence from a systematic review or meta-analysis of all relevant randomized controlled trials (RCTs), or evidence-based clinical practice guidelines based on systematic reviews of RCTs
Level II:	Evidence obtained from at least one well-designed RCT
Level III:	Evidence obtained from well-designed controlled trials without randomization
Level IV:	Evidence from well-designed case-control and cohort studies
Level V:	Evidence from systematic reviews of descriptive and qualitative studies
Level VI:	Evidence from a single descriptive or qualitative study
Level VII:	Evidence from the opinions of authorities and/or reports of expert committees

Source: Table compiled by P. Patel.

Let's take a closer look at the University of Colorado Hospital model and the PDSA Cycle.

The University of Colorado Hospital Model

The University of Colorado Hospital model is an example of an evidence-based multidisciplinary practice model (Goode et al., 2000; Goode & Piedalue, 1999). This model presents a framework for thinking about how to use different sources of information to change or support practice. The health care team or team member uses valid and current research from sources such as journals, conferences, and clinical experts as the basis for clinical decision making. The model depicts nine sources of evidence that are linked to the research core. This model provides a way for the nurse to organize information and data needed not only to care for a patient, but also to evaluate the care provided. In other words, did this patient receive the best possible care, not only that this institution can offer, but that is available in this world?

The PDSA Cycle

Another model for using and implementing EBP is the PDSA Cycle (Langley, Nolan, Nolan, Norman, & Provost, 1996). The Cycle begins with these questions:

1. What are we trying to accomplish?

2. How will we know that a change is an improvement? What measures of success will we use?

3. What change can we make that will result in improvement? (What change concepts will be tested?)

The PDSA Cycle has 4 different stages: Plan, do, study, and act Figure 10.4.

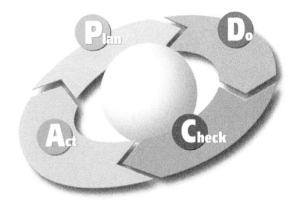

FIGURE 10.4   PDSA Cycle. Used with permission, Diagram by Karn G. Bulsuk (www.bulsuk.com).

How do you Formulate a Research Question? Let's PICOT. (the T is optional)

PICO(T)-Based Approach to Guiding an Evidence Search

The PICO(T) model is a technique that health care professionals can use to frame a clinical question and find an answer (Johnson, 2017). This mnemonic is used to help describe the elements of a good clinical question.

P—Population (Patient population, subject sample or group of interest)

I—Intervention (What is it that you want to consider—what treatment or intervention?)

C—Comparison (What alternative is this being compared to—what is your reference group?)

O—Outcome (What results will be measured?)

T—Time (How much time will be needed to evaluate/demonstrate the outcome? This element is not always included in formulating a question and is **optional**)

Resources for EBP

Currently, there are numerous excellent sites for finding information about evidence-based nursing and EBP. Since the early work of the McMaster's group, methods for review and summarization of evidence have undergone dramatic advances. A. Cochrane of the Cochrane Library group (www.cochrane.org) was a pioneer in the movement and preparation of high-quality reviews. In 1978, Cochrane suggested that only 15–20% of practitioner interventions were supported by objective evidence. This led to much variation in patient care delivery and patient care outcomes. Since then, with increasing technology, there have been major improvements in our ability to access information

Critical Thinking 10.1

When you start a PICO(T) question, it begins with a clinical question like: Do chlorhexidine products reduce CLABSI? Apply the question to the model:

An example of the PICO(T) model:

(P) IN THE ADULT POPULATION
(I) CHLORHEXIDINE (CHG) PRODUCTS
(C) COMPARED TO STANDARD PRECAUTIONS
(O) DECREASE THE INCIDENCE OF CENTRAL LINE ASSOCIATED BLOODSTREAM INFECTIONS (CLABSI)?
(T) NOT USED IN THE EXAMPLE AS THE T IS TIME FRAME AND NOT RELEVANT

PICO(T) Question: Does the use of CHG products decrease the incidence rate of CLABSI in adult patients?

Other examples of PICO(T) questions:

1. In the adult population, what is the effect of alternative pain management therapies on a patient's perceived pain level?
2. In post-operative patients, how does early ambulation and education impact the patient's hospital length of stay?
3. In children ages 6–10, what is the most effective antibiotic therapy for pneumonia?
4. In the adult population on an inpatient unit, what type of nursing interventions can decrease the number of falls?
5. In the adult population, does handwashing reduce the infection rate?
6. In women over 50, how does the use of Tylenol compare to Ibuprofen after the first hour post administration?
7. In men over 60 with total knee replacements, how effective is pain medication compared to aerobic stretching in controlling post-operative pain during the recovery period?

8. What is the impact on heart failure readmissions when a patient is seen by a provider within 7 days post discharge compared to a timeframe of 8–14 days post discharge?

Now that you have the idea, formulate your own PICO(T) question. Now that you have practiced PICO(T) questions, realize that is the first five fundamental steps of EBP:

Step 1: Formulating a well-built question
Step 2: Identifying articles and other evidence-based resources that answer the question
Step 3: Critically appraising the evidence to assess its validity
Step 4: Applying the evidence
Step 5: Reevaluating the application of evidence and areas for improvement

The PICO(T)-based approach can be applied to both clinical and organizational situations and can lead to improvement of care and/or function. Some common examples of types of evidence are listed in Table 10.3

Table 10.3   Common Examples of Types of Evidence

• Published research	• Policies, procedures, protocols
• Published quality improvement report	• Published guidelines
• Published meta-analysis	• Conference proceedings, abstracts, presentations
• Published systematic literature review	

Source: Compiled by P. Patel.

The first and most important tool in searching the literature for peer-reviewed, evidence-based journal articles are institution's librarians. Consult with them about the library's key journals and databases for nursing. While many databases exist for health care literature, MEDLINE (www.nlm.nih.gov/databases/databases_medline.html) and the **Cumulative Index to Nursing and Allied Health Literature** (CINAHL) (www.ebscohost.com/cinahl) are two of the most essential for nursing.

MEDLINE is the National Library of Medicine's electronic journal database, indexing thousands of journal publications in the fields of medicine, nursing, dentistry, veterinary medicine, the health care system, and the preclinical sciences. MEDLINE provides a complete citation for each article within those journals, with an abstract of the article provided in most cases. PubMed (www.pubmed.gov) is a free search engine for MEDLINE, provided by the National Library of Medicine. Ovid Medline and its electronic access to full-text journal articles is available if the institution's library subscribes to it.

CINAHL is an electronic database that indexes the contents of nursing and allied health publications, including journals, dissertations, and other materials. As with MEDLINE, the full text of an article found in CINAHL can be accessed electronically depends on if the institution's library subscribes to it.

Health policy makers and health care professionals recognize EBP as care based on state-of-the-art science reports. It is a process approach to collecting, reviewing, interpreting, critiquing, and evaluating research and other relevant literature for direct application to patient care. EBP uses evidence from research, performance data, quality improvement studies such as hospital or nursing report cards, program evaluations, and surveys, national and local consensus recommendations of experts and clinical experience.

The EBP process further involves the integrating of both clinician-observed evidence and research-directed evidence. This then leads to state-of-the-art integration of available knowledge and evidence in a particular area of clinical concern that can be evaluated and measured through outcomes of care. Refer to Table 10.4 for additional resources for EBP.

Table 10.4 **References for EBP**

Organization	Website
National guideline clearinghouse, Agency for Health Care Quality and Research	www.guideline.gov
The CINAHL Rehabilitation Guide, 7 Step Evidence-Based Methodology and Protocol	www.ebscohost.com/rrc_editorial
Evidence-Based Nursing	http://ebn.bmj.com
Sigma Theta Tau International	www.nursingsociety.org
Cochrane collaboration	www.cochrane.org
Joanna Briggs Institute for Evidence-based Nursing	www.joannabriggs.org
Sarah Cole Hirsh Institute for Best Nursing Practices Based on Evidence	http://case.edu/nursing/research/centers-of-excelllence/sarah-cole-hirsh-institute
Centre for Evidence-Based Medicine—Toronto	http://Ebm-tools.knowledgetranslation.net
Centre for Evidence-Based Medicine in Oxford, United Kingdom	www.cebm.net
The Canadian Medical Association	www.cma.ca
Royal College of Nursing	www.rcn.org.uk
Registered Nurses' Association of Ontario (guidelines available in English, French, and Italian)	www.rnao.org
Academic Center for Evidence-Based Nursing (ACE)	www.acestar.uthscsa.edu
Cumulative Index to Nursing and Allied Health (CINAHL)	https://guides.library.uab.edu
US National Library of Medicine	www.nlm.nih.gov
National Institute for Health and Clinical Excellence in the United Kingdom	www.nice.org.uk
Association of Women's Health Obstetrical and Neonatal Nurses	www.awhonn.org
Oncology Nursing Society	www.ons.org

Source: Table compiled by P. Patel.

EBP Centers in the United States

In response to this ongoing lack of evidence to make clinical decisions, in 1997 the AHRQ had undertaken the development and funding of 12 evidence-based centers to carry out development and dissemination of best practice models based on the available scientific information and data. Development of these special centers has been a driving force for state-of-the-art evaluations of current knowledge used in EBP in the United States. To visit the list of these centers, go to: www.ahrq.gov/research/findings/evidence-based-report/centers. Examples of evidence-based centers are Brown University, Duke University, ECRI Institute-Penn Medicine, Johns Hopkins University, and Kaiser Permanente Research Affiliates. The centers develop evidence reports on various topics to healthcare issues.

Case Study 10.1

Nurse Moksha has been working in the ICU for 5 years. In addition to working as a staff RN, her role is also to monitor compliance with important core measures. She had been noticing inconsistencies in the management of sepsis patients. Sepsis is a severe full body response to an infection. She was aware that there was a 20% turnover of staff RNs and there was variation in understanding the importance of making sure the hospitals 3-hr sepsis bundle is completed in a timely manner. The sepsis bundle includes a lactic acid level drawn, the completion of two blood cultures, fluid resuscitation (if systolic blood pressure is less than 90 or lactic acid is more than 4 mmol/L), and broad-spectrum antibiotics given within the 3 hr from time zero. The clock starts at time zero when the patient is in the emergency department or at the time that sepsis alert is triggered. She had noticed that the sepsis core measures had fall outs for various reasons. She brought this to the attention of her unit manager and they formed a sepsis committee to better understand the issue and how they can improve the current state. The interdisciplinary committee had members from the ICU, ED, and medical units. They brainstormed possible problems and solutions.

The team identified that there was a gap in the level of knowledge of the staff regarding sepsis education. The following PICO question was formed: In the adult medical surgical patient population, does education of new nurses and improved screening tools reduce the risk of patients developing severe sepsis compared to patients not receiving early interventions? They conducted a review of the literature.

Critical Thinking 10.2

1. What databases can be used to review the literature?
2. Can you identify the different levels of evidence?

The literature review identified that early intervention was key in reducing the possibility of severe sepsis. "The consensus is that sepsis needs to be recognized in the early stages to decrease the mortality rate. It is also agreed upon that education for health care staff is paramount in reducing mortality rates . . . the education of early signs and symptoms of sepsis and the importance of quickly implementing care bundles will improve mortality rates related to sepsis" (Bowman). The literature also identified the importance of screening tools. The sepsis committee

developed a sepsis alert algorithm and improved/streamlined the screening tool.

It was time for implementing interventions. The team refreshed sepsis education to all staff. A protocol for implementing this education was hard wired for all new staff as they completed nursing orientation. Superusers for sepsis were also formed to ensure ongoing education and refreshers to all staff. Screening tools were developed by working closely with physicians and key stakeholders. The screening tools were first trialed on paper and once finalized the team worked with information systems to modify the EMR. Policies and protocols were updated as appropriate.

Critical Thinking 10.3

How would you use the various EBP models with this sepsis scenario?

What would you measure prior to this EBP and post interventions to assess effectiveness?

What would you review monthly to ensure sustained compliance and effectiveness?

Evidence from the Literature

Source: Brown, R. G., Anderson, S., Brunt, B., Enos, T., Blough, K., & Kropp, D. (2018). Workplace Violence Training Using Simulation. *The American Journal of Nursing*, *118*(10), 56–68. https://doi.org/10.1097/01.NAJ.0000546382.12045.54

Discussion: Workplace violence in health care settings is increasing dramatically nationwide. In response, an interdisciplinary team at an Ohio health system developed and piloted a model of training to address workplace violence. The model included classroom learning, a code silver (person with a weapon or a hostage situation) simulation training, and hands-on self-defense techniques. Based on data collected in the pilot, the team revised the model to offer a more comprehensive approach; the new, revised training program is known as Violence: enABLE Yourself to Respond. The team designed four distinct five-minute simulation scenarios depicting a range of threats from "escalating behavior" to "active shooter" and enacted them with standardized participants (health care personnel trained to perform specific behaviors in educational scenarios). Immediately after each simulation, the instructors facilitated a debriefing of the participants.

Participants' pre- and post-training program self-evaluations of how prepared they felt to react to violent situations, as well as experts' evaluations of the participants' performance in simulations, provided evidence of the effectiveness of the model. Analysis of the data demonstrated a statistically significant positive difference in both participants' perception of their preparedness and experts' evaluation of their performance. The combination of classroom learning and simulation training is an effective, evidence-based method to prepare employees to respond when a situation escalates to violence, including the use of a weapon. This approach was designed for acute care but can be adapted to other settings. Skills learned can be used in both personal and professional life

Implications for Practice:

How can you use EBP to help employees respond to workplace violence?

Discuss how you can determine what strategies are effective?

Promoting Evidence-Based Best Practices

Chrisman, 2014, stated "Involving all disciplines, EBP is an approach to clinical practice that's been gaining ground since its formal introduction in 1992" and this holds true to date.

Starting in medicine, it then spread to other fields, such as nursing, psychology, and education. Currently, 55% of all nursing practices are based on research findings. The ANA predicts that: "By 2020, 90% of all nursing practice will be based on EBP research findings." As nurses, keeping abreast of EBP is integral in providing patient care supported through evidence.

Nurses are crucial members of the EBP team because of their clinical knowledge and expertise; thus, successful implementation of EBP, creative thinking, and advancement in technology can promote health care quality (John, 2016).

Below are some activities nurses can do to promote EBP:

1. Journal club to discuss EBP studies and how to implement them in your organization. Read and share findings for best practice and determine how to implement this into existing protocols—how do you translate research into practice?

2. Shared governance or EPB council to discuss relevant EBP findings

3. Conduct research on topics and share findings with others. Can you translate the research findings into practice?

Consider patient's unique preferences, concerns, goals, financial constraints, support systems, etc.

In summary, evidence-based practice is vital to nursing excellence. In this chapter you have discussed the nurse's role related to EBP, the importance of EBP, and the history and evolution of EBP. You have been provided tools including various EBP models, terminology, and resources.

Barriers to EBP practice need to be removed and nurses must integrate it into practice. Organizational support is critical to change and sustainment. The information learned in this chapter provides you with beginning tools and understanding of EBP that will contribute to improvements in population health and keeping the patient at optimal health.

KEY CONCEPTS

- Evidence-based practice (EBP) represents a multidisciplinary approach to the utilization of current research findings to guide the development of appropriate strategies to deliver quality, cost-effective care.

- Outcomes research provides evidence about benefits, risks, and results of treatment so that individuals can make informed decisions and choices to improve their quality of life.

- The ANA has been an active advocate of outcomes evaluation.

- EBP provides a "static" snapshot of a conclusion based on previous clinical trials about a condition or situation, but the clinician

must still make a clinical judgment about an individual, considering his or her unique characteristics (such as gender, age, clinical history, socioeconomic status, support system, ethical concerns, and the illness experience).

- The University of Colorado Hospital model is an example of a multidisciplinary EBP model for using different sources of information to change or support your practice.

- The Model for Improvement (PDSA) can be applied to a system or an individual.

KEY TERMS

Evidenced-based practice
Benchmarking

Evidenced-based practice models
Practice guidelines

PICO method

REVIEW QUESTIONS

1. What is the major purpose of evidence-based practice (EBP)?
   a. To increase variability of care
   b. To cause a link to be missing in clinical care
   c. To determine what medical models can be applied by nursing
   d. To provide evidence in support of clinical interventions

2. Which of the following is an accurate statement concerning EBP at this time?
   a. EBP takes the place of continuous quality improvement.
   b. Because we can already demonstrate effective and efficient care, EBP is redundant.
   c. Leaders and managers in nursing are not clinicians, generally speaking, and so do not have a part in EBP processes.
   d. EBP is recognized by nursing, medicine, and health policy makers as critical today in the management of patients and improving population health.

3. Which of the following organizations develops clinical practice guidelines on multiple clinical conditions?
   a. American Heart Association
   b. Agency for Healthcare Research and Quality (AHRQ)
   c. Pew Health Professions Commission
   d. Joint Commission (JC)

4. Which of the following is true about evidence for use in clinical practice?
   a. It is typically adopted quickly by clinicians.
   b. It always needs to be interpreted for appropriateness for a specific patient.
   c. It should never be challenged by nurses.
   d. It provides unarguable direction for patient care.

5. Which of the following is likely to provide the strongest evidence about diabetic patient care?

a. A study found in the literature about a patient with type 2 diabetes
b. An article about diabetes in a nursing research journal
c. An article about diabetes in a medical research journal
d. A systematic meta-analysis of the literature on diabetic nursing care.

6. Assessment of evidence from what source must be sought first when a patient complains of pain?
   a. The literature
   b. Your nursing textbook
   c. The patient
   d. Your unit's policy manual

7. Potential outcomes for organizations that adopt policies based on EBP include which of the following? Select all that apply.
   a. Improved quality of care
   b. Improved cost savings
   c. Decreased patient satisfaction
   d. Decreased lengths of stay
   e. Improved patient outcomes

8. Nurses must consider which of the following when working with patients?
   a. What the patient wants as well as what is medically best
   b. What science decides is best for the patient
   c. Only what the patient wants
   d. Only what the patient's family wants

9. The PICO strategy is used for
   a. Evidenced-based practice used to frame a research or clinical question
   b. A model used to implement EBP
   c. Formulating a plan of care
   d. Formulating a nursing diagnosis

10. Evidence-based practice should be
    a. Kept top secret as it is per each hospital
    b. Should only be practiced by Masters prepared nurses
    c. Shared with all as applicable
    d. Limited to physicians

REVIEW QUESTION ANSWERS

1. Answer: D is correct.
   Rational: The main purpose of evidence-based practice (EBP) is to provide evidence in support of clinical interventions (D). (A) To increase variability of care, (B) to cause a link to be missing in clinical care, and (C) to determine what medical models can be applied by nursing are incorrect.

2. Answer: D is correct.
   Rational: EBP is recognized by nursing, medicine, and health policy makers as critical today in the management of patients and improving population health (D). (A)
   EBP takes the place of continuous quality improvement, (B) because we can already demonstrate effective and efficient care, EBP is redundant, and (C) Leaders and managers in nursing are not clinicians and do not have a part in EBP processes are incorrect.

3. Answer: D is correct.
   Rational: The Joint Commission (JC) develops clinical practice guidelines on multiple clinical conditions (D). (A)
   The American Heart Association, (B) the Agency for Healthcare Research and Quality (AHRQ), and (C) the Pew Health Professions Commission are incorrect.

4. Answer: B is correct.
   Rational: Evidence for use in clinical practice always needs to be interpreted for appropriateness for a specific patient (B). (A)
   It is typically adopted quickly by clinicians, (C) it should never be challenged by nurses, and (D) it provides unarguable direction for patient care are incorrect.

5. Answer: D is correct.
   Rational: A systematic meta-analysis of the literature on diabetic nursing care provides the strongest evidence about diabetic patient care (D). (A)

A study found in the literature about a patient with type 2 diabetes, (B) an article about diabetes in a nursing research journal, and (C) an article about diabetes in a medical research journal are incorrect.

6. Answer: C is correct.
   Rational: When a patient complains of pain, assessment of the evidence must be sought first from the patient (C). Evidence cannot be found in the literature (A), your nursing textbook (B), or your unit's policy manual (D).

7. Answers A, B, D, and E are correct.
   Rational: Potential outcomes for organizations that adopt policies based on EBP include (A) improved quality of care, (B) improved cost savings, (D) decreased lengths of stay, and (E) improved pastient outcomes. (C) Decreased patient satisfaction is not relevent in this case.

8. Answer: A is correct.
   Rational: When working with patients, nurses must consider what the patient wants, as well as what is medically best (A). To consider (B) what science decides is best for the patient, (C) only what the patient wants, and (D) only what the patient's family wants are incorrect.

9. Answer: A is correct.
   Rational: The PICO strategy for evidence-based practice is used to frame a research or clinical question (A). A model used to implement EBP (B), formulating a plan of care (C), and formulating a nursing diagnosis are incorrect.

10. Answer: C is correct.
    Rational: Evidence-based practice should be shared with all applicable (C). To be kept secret as it is per each hospital (A), practiced by Masters prepared nurses (B), and limited to physicians (D) are incorrect.

REVIEW ACTIVITIES

1. Review Table 10.2, Levels of Evidence. Are the evidence levels clear to you? Look at a patient's condition that you encounter in your clinical lab experience. Which level of evidence supports the care delivery approaches for this patient? Are any clinical pathways or standards in use in caring for this patient?

2. Using the five-step process for EBP outlined in the Evidence from the Literature by Melnyk and Fineout-Overholt in this chapter, work to improve patient care on a health care condition of your choice. Use the PICO approach to focus your literature review.

DISCUSSION POINTS

- During your last clinical experience, how was quality nursing care visible?

- Were there any artifacts such as posters or graphs on the wall that explained quality initiatives on the unit?

- Consider the examples, models, or theories presented in this chapter.

- Which examples, models, or theories would you feel the most comfortable using in the hospital setting as a direct care clinical nurse?

- What appeals to you about the examples, models, or theories in this chapter?

- How can you improve quality as a direct care clinical nurse?

- How does the culture of a hospital affect nurse engagement with quality improvement (QI) projects?

- What kind of hospital culture would improve nurse participation in QI?

DISCUSSION OF OPENING SCENARIO

1. *What do you know about EBP and where do you begin?*

   It is critical to understand the role of EBP and its importance in practice. Before you begin to review evidence, familiarize yourself with EBP and your organization's resources.

2. *What are some things you need to know before you can accept the appointment to the task force?*

   What type of resources are available for you?
   Is there a research or nursing practice council in the organization?
   What is the baseline data related to surgical site infections?
   Engage physicians and key stakeholders on your team.

3. *How will you prepare yourself for the task and be able to make a positive impact?*

   Explore resources and research what strategies are effective in SSI reduction.
   Explore processes in other areas to better understand variation and its link to outcomes.
   Assemble a subcommittee or group to assist you as appropriate.
   Communicate findings with the key stakeholders and groups as per your organization.

EXPLORING THE WEB

Utilizing one of the Web sites listed, explore current evidence-based practice updates and/or specific clinical issues related to your area of practice (e.g., oncology, palliative care, wound care, etc.). Compare current practice guidelines utilized in your facility with current evidence-based practice guidelines and develop recommendations to share with your institution.

- American College of Physicians (ACP) ACP Journal Club. The ACP Journal Club's general purpose is to select from the biomedical literature those articles reporting original studies and systematic reviews that warrant immediate attention by clinicians attempting to keep pace with important advances in internal medicine. www.acpjc.org

- Agency for Healthcare Research and Quality (AHRQ): www.ahrq.gov

- Center for Evidence-Based Medicine, University of Toronto. Note the evidence-based nursing syllabi and resources. www.cebm.utoronto.ca

- Cumulative Index to Nursing and Allied Health (CINAHL). The CINAHL database covers nursing, allied health, biomedical and

consumer health journals, and publications of the American Nursing Association and the National League for Nursing. More than 350,000 records and 900 journals are included. www.cinahl.com

- Cochrane Library. The Cochrane Library contains four databases: the **Cochrane Database of Systematic Reviews (CDSR)**, the **Database of Abstracts of Reviews of Effectiveness (DARE)**, the **Cochrane Controlled Trials Register (CCTR)**, and the **Cochrane Review Methodology Database (CRMD)**. View introductory information for free: www.cochrane.org/index.htm

- Free access to Cochrane Reviewer's Handbook: www.cochrane.org/training/cochrane-handbook

- EBM Education Center of Excellence, North Carolina: http://library.ncahec.net

- Evaluating the Literature: Quality Filtering and Evidence-Based Medicine and Health. Available from the National Library of Medicine: www.nlm.nih.gov

- Evidence-Based Medicine: www.acponline.org

- Evidence-Based Medicine ToolKit: www.med.ualberta.ca

- Health Information Research Unit, McMaster University: http://hiru.mcmaster.ca
- Searching CINAHL Using the Ovid Web Gateway, Duke University Medical Center Library: www.mclibrary.duke.edu

- University of North Carolina Health Sciences Library: www.hsl.unc.edu

INFORMATICS

- Go to the QSEN site at: http://qsen.org/empowering-students-to-create-a-safer-clinical-environment-utilizing-evidence-based-practice

- Review the activity "Empowering students to create a safer clinical environment utilizing Evidence-Based Practice."
- How can you make your clinical environment safer utilizing EBP?

LEAN BACK

- How does this information impact you today?
- What is your role in EBP?
- What do you foresee as the role of the nurse leader and EBP?
- Review the levels of evidence. Are the levels of evidence clear to you? Look at a patient's condition that you encounter in your

experience. Which level of evidence supports the care delivery for this patient? Are there any clinical pathways or standards used in caring for this patient?

REFERENCES

American Nurses Association. (2015). *Nursing scope and standards of practice*. Washington, DC: American Nurses Association.

Becker, S. (2016). *Becker's hospital review*. Retrieved from www.beckershospitalreview.com

Berwick, D. M., Calkins, D. R., McCannon, B. A., & Hackbarth, A. D. (2006). The 100,000 lives campaign: Setting a goal and a deadline for improving health care quality. *Journal of the American Medical Association*, *295*(3), 324–327.

Brown, R., Anderson, S., Brunt, B., Enos, T., Blough, K., & Kropp, D. (2018). Workplace violence training using simulation. *The American Journal of Nursing*, *118*((10), 56–68.

Chrisman, J. (2014). *Exploring evidence based practice research, p. 8*. www.nursingmadeincredibleeasy.com

Dang, D., & Dearholt, S. (2017). *Johns Hopkins nursing evidence-based practice: model and guidelines* (3rd ed.). Indianapolis, IN: Sigma Theta Tau International.

Goode, C. J., & Piedalue, F. (1999). Evidence-based clinical practice. *Journal of Nursing Administration*, *29*, 15–21.

Goode, C. J., Tanaka, D. J., Krugman, M., O'Connor, P. A., Bailey, C., & Deutchman, M. (2000). Outcomes from use of an evidence-based practice guideline. *Nursing Economics*, *18*, 202–207.

Hain, D. J. (2017). Exploring the evidence. Focusing on the fundamentals: Comparing and contrasting nursing research and quality improvement. *Nephrology Nursing Journal*, *44*(6), 541–544.

Ingersoll, G. L. (2000). Evidence-based nursing: What it is, and what it isn't. *Nursing Outlook*, *48*, 151–152.

Institute of Medicine (IOM). (2003). *Health professions education : A bridge to quality*. Washington, DC: National Academies Press.

IOM. (1999). *To err is human*. Washington, DC: National Academies Press.

IOM. (2001). *Crossing the quality chasm: A new health system for the 21st century*. Washington, DC: National Academies Press.

IOM. (2011). *The future of nursing: Leading change, advancing health*. Washington, DC: The National Academies Press. doi.org/10.17226/12956

IOM. (2013). *Best care at lower costs: The path to continuous learning in healthcare in America*. Washington, DC: The National Academies Press.

Iowa Model Collaborative. (2017). Iowa model of evidence-based practice: Revisions and validation. *Worldviews on Evidence-Based Nursing*, *14*(3), 175–182. doi:10.1111/wvn.12223

John, S. (2016). *Assessing knowledge of evidence-based practice among nurses*. (Doctoral dissertation), (pp. 1-86). Minneapolis, MN: Walden University.

Johnson, S. (2017). Evidence-based practice. *Australian Nursing & Midwifery Journal*, *24*(10), 47.

Langley, G. J. Moen, R., Nolan, K. M., Nolan, T. W., Norman, C. L. & Provost, L. P. (2009). The improvement guide: A practical approach to enhancing organizational performance. San Francisco, CA: Jossey-Bass.

Makic, M. B. F., & Rauen, C. (2016). Guest editorial. Maintaining your momentum: Moving evidence into practice. *Critical Care Nurse*, *36*(2), 13–18. doi.org/10.4037/ccn2016568

Marshall, L. S. (2017). Is evidence-based practice in your nursing present and future? *Florida Nurse*, *65*(1), 13.

Melnyk, B. M. (2018). *Evidence-based health care: The care you want, but might not be getting.* . Retrieved from https://news.osu.edu/evidence-based-health-care-the-care-you-want-but-might-not-be-getting

Melnyk, B. M., Gallagher-Ford, L., Long, L. E., & Fineout-Overholt, E. (2014). The establishment of evidence-based practice competencies for practicing registered nurses and advanced practice nurses in real-world clinical settings: Proficiencies to improve healthcare quality, reliability, patient outcomes, and costs. *Worldviews on Evidence-Based Nursing*, *11*(1), 5–15.

Nurse Leader Insider. (2017). Relationship of Nursing Excellence to Evidenced Based Practice. Retrieved from www.hcpro.com

Quality and Safety Education for Nurses. : (n.d.). *Quality/Safety Competencies*. Retrieved from www.qsen.org/overview.php

Sackett, D. L., Rosenberg, W. M. C., Gray, J. A. M., Haynes, R. B., & Richardson, W. S. (1996). Evidence-based medicine: What it is and what it isn't. *British Medical Journal*, *312*(7023), 71–72.

Sigma Theta Tau International. (2005). *Evidence-based nursing position statement.* . Retrieved from www.nursingsociety.org/aboutus/PositionPapers/Pages/EBN_positionpaper.aspx.

Slavitt, A. (2018). *JAMA Forum. The Triple Aim Must Overcome the Triple Threat-news@JAMA.*Stevens, K. R. (2013). The impact of evidenced based practice in nursing and the next big ideas. *Online Journal of Issues in Nursing*, *18*(2), 1. Manuscript 4. Retrieved from 10.3912/OJIN.Vol18No02Man04

Stevens, K. R. (2015). *Stevens Star Model of Knowledge Transformation. Academic Center for Evidence-based Practice*. The University of Texas Health Science Center at San Antonio.

Thompson, C. J. (2017). *What Does "Levels of Evidence" Mean in Evidenced Based Practice?*

Titler, M. G. (2008). The Evidence for Evidence-Based Practice Implementation. In R. G. Hughes (Ed.), *Patient Safety and Quality: An Evidence-Based Handbook for Nurses*. Rockville, MD: Agency for Healthcare Research and Quality (U.S.), Chapter 7. Retrieved from www.ncbi.nlm.nih.gov/books/NBK2659

Titler, M. G., Kleiber, C., Steelman, V. J., Rakel, B. A., Budreau, G., Everett, L. Q., Buckwalter, K. C., Tripp-Reimer, T. & Goode, C. J. (2001). The Iowa model of evidence-based practice to promote quality care. *Critical Care Nursing Clinics of North America*, *13*(4), 497–509. Retrieved from www.mosescone.com/documents/public/Nursing%20Research/Iowa%20Model%201998.pdf

Wyant, T. (2017). Adopt an evidence-based practice model to facilitated practice change. *ONS Voice*, *32*(11), 50–51.

SUGGESTED READINGS

Boström, A.-M., Sommerfeld, D. K., Stenhols, A. W., & Kiessling, A. (2018). Capability beliefs on and use of evidence-based practice among four health professional and student groups in geriatric care: A cross sectional study. *PLoS One*, *13*(2), 1–15. doi.org/10.1371/journal.pone.0192017

Bourgault, A. M. (2018). Bridging evidence-based practice and research. *Critical Care Nurse*, *38*(6), 10–12.

Gradone, L. D. (2019). Integration of evidence-based practice at an Academic Medical Center. *Medsurg Nursing*, *28*(1), 53–58.

Graber ML, Johnston D, & Bailey R. (2016). *Report of the evidence on health IT safety and interventions*. Research Triangle Park, NC: RTI International.

Institute of Healthcare Improvement.(n.d.). *IHI Triple aim initiative.* www.ihi.org/engage/initiatives/tripleaim/pages/default.aspx

Jackson, D., & Kozlowska, O. (2018). Fundamental care—the quest for evidence. *Journal of Clinical Nursing*, *27*(11–12), 2177–2178.

Koffel, J., & Reidt, S. (2015). An interprofessional train-the-trainer evidence-based practice workshop: Design and evaluation. *Journal of Interprofessional Care*, *29*(4), 367–369.

Lavenberg, J. G., Cacchione, P. Z., Jayakumar, K. L., Leas, B. F., Mitchell, M. D. et al. (2019). *Sigma Theta Tau: Impact of a Hospital Evidence-Based Practice Center (EPC) on Nursing Policy and Practice.*

Porter, R. B., Cullen, L., Farrington, M., Matthews, G., & Tucker, S. (2018). Exploring Clinicians' perceptions about sustaining an evidence-based fall prevention program: A findings from this qualitative study may help improve sustainability. *AJN American Journal of Nursing*, *118*(5), 24–46.

McAllen, E. R., Stephens, K., Biearman, B. S., Kerr, K., & Whiteman, K. (2018). Moving shift report to the bedside: An evidence-based quality improvement project. *Online Journal of Issues in Nursing*, *23*(2), 1. doi:10.3912/OJIN.Vol23No02PPT22

Perry, L. (2018). The year of (evidence-based) nurse workforce planning? *International Journal of Nursing Practice*, *24*(1), 1.

Schaefer, J. D., & Welton, J. M. (2018). Evidence-based practice readiness: A concept analysis. *Journal of Nursing Management*, *26*(6), 621–629.

Scott, K., & McSherry, R. (2009). Evidence-based nursing: Clarifying the concepts for nursing in practice. *Journal of Clinical Nursing*, *18*(8), 1085–1095. doi:10.1111/j.1365-2702.2008.02588.x

Songur, C., Özer, Ö., Gün, Ç., & Top, M. (2018). Patient safety culture, evidence-based practice and performance in nursing. *Systemic Practice & Action Research*, *31*(4), 359–374.

Thorne, S. (2018). But is it "evidence"? *Nursing Inquiry*, *25*(1), 1.

Titler, M. G. (2018). Translation research in practice: An introduction. *Online Journal of Issues in Nursing*, *23*(2). Manuscript 1.

Warren, C., Medei, M. K., Wood, B., & Schutte, D. (2019). A nurse-driven Oral care protocol to reduce hospital-acquired pneumonia. *AJN American Journal of Nursing*, *119*(2), 44–51.

Wyant, T. (2018). A Spirit of inquiry leads to evidence-based answers to practice questions. *ONS Voice*, *33*(1), 43.

Xiang, X., Robinson-Lane, S. G., Rosenberg, W., & Alvarez, R. (2018). Implementing and sustaining evidence-based practice in health care: The bridge model experience. *Journal of Gerontological Social Work*, *61*(3), 280–294.

Zwakhalen, S. M. G., Hamers, J. P. H., Metzelthin, S. F., Ettema, R., Heinen, M., et al. (2018). Basic nursing care: The most provided, the least evidence-based – A discussion paper. *Journal of Clinical Nursing*, *27* (11–12), 2496–2505.

Zolot, J. (2016). Evidence-based care is highly valued but underused by many nurse executives. *AJN American Journal of Nursing*, *116*(6), 15.

11 Searching for the Evidence

Charlotte Beyer

Boxer Library, Rosalind Franklin University of Medicine and Science, North Chicago, IL, USA

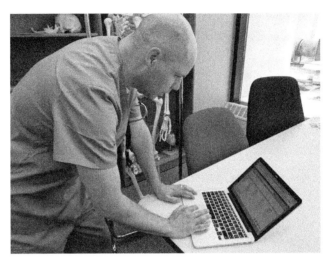

Source: John Scott Thomson

Although information is readily discoverable online, examination of the full set of evidence requires conducting a methodical literature search. An incomplete literature search, resulting in a partial selection of articles, could possibly mislead the one conducting the literature search to form biased conclusions in the literature review. To operate within an objective scientific framework, one must employ a strategic and systematic approach to formulating a literature search strategy; doing so will also make the most efficient use of time over the long term.

Gerberi & Marienau, 2017

OBJECTIVES

Upon completion of this chapter, the reader should be able to:

1. Use the Five A's (Assess, Ask, Acquire, Appraise, and Apply) to guide your literature search process.

2. Assess the patient or population and identify core literature search topics by using by using keywords or subject headings.

3. Ask answerable clinical questions using PICOT (**Patient/Population, Intervention, Comparison, Outcome, and Time**).

4. Acquire literature using Boolean Operators and Truncation in electronic databases.

5. Acquire literature using electronic databases.

6. Acquire literature and clinical practice guidelines by using mobile applications.

7. Appraise literature such as journals, mobile applications, and websites for relevancy and quality.

8. Discuss resources for lifelong learning.

9. Apply the literature to your patient or population.

OPENING SCENARIO

The head nurse on an orthopedic surgical unit audits her patient admissions monthly. She assesses the length of stay, discharge status, and notes if any patients were readmitted to the hospital within 30 days of discharge. She then reviews the patient records to determine the cause of any hospital readmissions. She noticed in the last month that there were three readmissions. When reviewing the charts, the head nurse recognized that all three patients were readmitted with an infection of the incision site, status post knee replacements.

She reviewed the literature on hospital readmissions for surgical patients post knee replacement and found that incisional wound infections are the major reason for re-admission for these surgical patients. She then further searched the literature for evidence-based practices (EBPs) to identify ways the health care system could be changed to reduce hospital readmissions from infection. In the end, she worked with other members of the interprofessional health care team such as physicians, pharmacists, physical therapist, wound care unit nurses, nurse educators, nurse practitioners, dietitians, and physician assistants.

Using the literature, this team developed recommendations including prescribing antibiotics prior to surgery and identifying other factors related to wound infection prior to hospitalization. They also developed new protocols for discharge to include patient education in areas such as recognizing signs/symptoms of wound infection, dietary recommendations, and medication adherence. In addition, the team developed a plan for the hospital's wound care nurse to call each patient 2 days after discharge to determine the patient's status and provide recommendations for further care if necessary, to promote wound healing and avoid readmission. To support a consistent level of patient care, a team of nursing educators and the wound care nurse held in-service staff education about best practices for wound care, sterile technique, medication administration, and basic hygiene.

Two months following the implementation of staff and patient education, the head nurse noted that here were no hospital readmissions for incisional wound infections.

1. What are the most effective ways for nurses to search the literature?

2. How does the literature support nursing practice? (Bridges, 2018)

In the scenario above, the members of the interprofessional team identified literature to guide their recommendations. Information such as research studies were identified using tools called electronic databases. **Electronic databases** are collections of information which can be searched and retrieved by a computer or mobile device such as a phone/tablet. Types of information in the electronic database include research studies, clinical trials, clinical practice guidelines, and more. As ease of access to these types of information has improved, so has the amount of published health sciences research. In 2019, there were 956,390 citations added to the citation database MEDLINE, which is the basis of the popular resource PubMed. This means in 1 year, almost a million citations were added to that one electronic database. It is also important to note that the 956,390 citations is almost double the number of citation than were added in 1998, where 411,921 citations were added. With the rapid rise in published literature due to new technological innovations like online resources, one major challenge health care professionals face is having the time and using their ability to sift through the large body of health research literature and identify the highest-quality information.

One overwhelming reality is that the knowledge nurses acquire in school may be altered just a few years after they graduate. The question then becomes not only, what do nurses need to know, but how do they locate the best information, as well as how do they keep up with changes in practice? (Sadoughi, Azadi, & Azadi, 2017)

The goal of this chapter is to provide nurses with effective information retrieval strategies designed to support nursing practice. This chapter opens with how to use five words which start with A (Assess, Ask, Acquire, Apprise, and Apply) to guide the literature searching process and locate evidence to support EBP. The literature searching process starts with Assessing the patient or population and identifying core keywords to use when searching for literature online in electronic databases, website, and mobile applications. To find the best resources, these core keywords can be used as natural language keywords or subject headings in electronic databases. Nurses will also learn how to Ask answerable clinical questions using those appropriate keywords and subject headings using PICOT. After the creation of an answerable clinical question, nurses will learn how to Acquire the evidence in online resources by using tools such as Boolean operators and truncation in resources such as electronic databases. Nurses will also learn how to Acquire literature evidence in electronic databases. Another method to Acquire evidence or literature is to use resources such as mobile applications. After literature such as research articles and clinical practice guidelines have been Acquired, the literature must be Appraised for relevance and quality. The chapter will close with how to Apply this information from the literature, as well as give a list of resources for lifelong learning.

Use the Five A's (Assess, Ask, Acquire, Appraise, and Apply) to Guide Your Literature Search Process

One component of the Patient-Centered Nursing Practice Model discussed in Chapter 5 is EBP. **Quality and Safety Education for Nurses** (QSEN) defines **evidence-based practice** as, "Integrate best current evidence with clinical expertise and patient/family preferences and values for delivery of optimal health care" (Cronwett et al., 2007). A core element of EBP is finding that best current evidence (Sackett, Rosenberg, Muir Gray, Haynes, & Richardson, 1996). Evidence is always changing and evidence in the field of health care comes in many forms including research articles, clinical practice guidelines, medical reference books, and more. In clinical practice, nurses need the ability to find the most appropriate evidence for a specific clinical situation. Nurses should think of EBP like a three-legged stool. If one leg of the stool is missing, the process will fall apart. The first leg is clinical expertise, which is what a nurse gains through clinical experiences with patients and other members of the interprofessional health care team. The second leg of the three-legged stool is that of patient values, which refers to a patient's values, preferences, and expectations. For example, a patient may have a religious objection to a specific treatment so an alternative must be identified to best help that patient. The third leg of the three-legged stool is the best available evidence for a clinical topic. One of the main objectives of this chapter is to help nurses identify strategies for gathering the best available evidence in EBP. One method for locating that best available evidence when practicing EBP is to think of five words which begin with A: Assess the patient or population, Ask an answerable clinical question, Acquire evidence to answer the clinical question, Appraise the evidence, and Apply the evidence to your patient or population (Table 11.1). Using the Five A's to frame the literature search process can provide a guide so the process of gathering literature feels less overwhelming.

Table 11.1 Information Retrieval Process Using the Five A's.

Assess the patient or population	You notice that multiple patients who go through renal dialysis often experience post-dialysis fatigue. You wonder if there are any specific treatments or interventions to help alleviate this problem. Before moving to the next step, identify a few keywords to describe the main topics in this clinical situation. Main ideas: <ul><li>Patients undergoing renal dialysis</li><li>Post-dialysis fatigue</li><li>Treatments or interventions</li></ul> To find the best terms, you use the MeSH database in PubMed to identify a few subject headings: <ul><li>Renal dialysis</li><li>Fatigue</li><li>Treatments</li></ul>
Ask an answerable clinical question	Next, weave together the main ideas identified during the Assess the patient or population part of the Five A's process into a question you can answer with information gathered in a literature search. In patients undergoing renal dialysis, what treatments can be used to alleviate post-dialysis fatigue?
Acquire evidence to answer the clinical question	Identify the types of evidence you want to find: <ul><li>Systematic reviews or review articles</li><li>Randomized controlled trials</li><li>Evidence-based clinical practice guidelines</li><li>Treatments or interventions</li></ul> Pick online resources to find articles and guidelines: <ul><li>PubMed, available at http://pubmed.gov (accessed on July 29, 2019)</li><li>CINAHL, The Cumulative Index to Nursing and Allied Health Literature, CINAHL, available via subscription at your hospital, accessed on 10/31/20 at https://www.ebscohost.com/nursing.</li></ul> Search the literature using the following keywords: <ul><li>Renal dialysis AND post dialysis fatigue AND treatments</li></ul> Limit your literature search results with the following criteria: <ul><li>Publication date within 5 years</li><li>Language—English</li><li>Article types—randomized controlled trials, review articles, systematic reviews, evidence-based clinical practice guidelines</li></ul>

Table 11.1 Continued

Appraise the evidence	Appraise the articles acquired and answer the following questions:
	• Who wrote the article? • What are the author's qualifications? • What journal is the article from? • How old is the article? • What is the article type? • Has the article gone through a review process by a professional group?
Apply the evidence to your patient or clinical problem.	While doing the literature search, one particular item stood out, which was a best practice implementation report from the Joanna Briggs Institute for use in helping to alleviate post-dialysis fatigue in patients undergoing renal dialysis. This report noted that one intervention which was successful was a nurse education program where the authors created a folder with resources of best practice recommendations in areas like sleep habits, exercise, fluid management, and other information the nurses could easily use to teach patients You mention this to your nurse manager and then develop a program at the hospital which greatly helps both nurses and patients manage this condition.

[a] CINAHL, The Cumulative Index to Nursing and Allied Health Literature available via subscription at your hospital, accessed on 10/31/20 at https://www.ebscohost.com/nursing.
Source: Charlotte Beyer

Expert Literature Searching with Librarians

One resource in a hospital that exists to guide members of the interprofessional health care team, including nurses, through the literature search process, are clinical librarians. **Clinical librarians** are librarians who specialize in supporting those in the health care environment, including all members of the interprofessional health care team as well as patients.

Some clinical librarians are stationed at patient care units from time to time, but one place they can always be found is in the hospital library. Some of the services found in the hospital library include interlibrary loan, a service where you can obtain a copy of an article not held in the hospital library; checking out library books; and literature search and reference assistance from the librarian.

In addition, the hospital library provides access to electronic databases and point-of-care tools such as Cochrane Reviews at www.cochrane.org (accessed August 15, 2019), UpToDate, at www.uptodate.com (accessed August 15, 2019); ClinicalKey, at www.elsevier.com/solutions/clinicalkey (accessed August 15, 2019), and more. As previously mentioned, clinical librarians can provide a literature search and reference assistance to guide you through the literature search with assistance on asking answerable clinical questions, including things such as identifying the best keywords or subject headings to use in a literature search, the best electronic databases to use to find literature, and more.

Assess the Patient or Population and Ask an Answerable Clinical Question by Using Keywords and Subject Headings

The first step in using the Five A's is to Assess the patient or population. During this step, nurses should identify a patient or population to be explored within a literature search. In Table 11.1, a nurse identified a problem of post-dialysis fatigue for patients undergoing hemodialysis. Once a problem is identified with a patient or a population, the next step is to identify keywords and subject headings which can be used in a literature search to Ask an answerable clinical question. **Keywords** are words or phrases used to describe a topic. Many

Real World Interview

Clinical librarians have many opportunities to teach, partner with, and mentor nurses, whether individually, on a unit-wide basis, through shared governance councils, or through other opportunities that arise. For example, at the University of North Carolina Medical Center, bedside nurses in two units learned about and conducted an evidence-based improvement project to reduce hospital noise and improve patients' ability to sleep. While some of the clinical team members measured the level of noise on their units, a librarian, nurses, and other team members undertook a literature review of interventions to improve sleep. Based on their literature review, the team then introduced interventions such as quiet time and a sleep menu to their patient care units. Follow-up assessments showed improvements in noise level and patient satisfaction. The team was able to publish their results and present their work at professional meetings.

Elizabeth Moreton, MLS
Nursing Liaison Librarian
University of North Carolina at Chapel Hill,
Chapel Hill, North Carolina

times, the reason a clinical question cannot be answered is that the best keywords to describe the topics are not identified in the literature search. These keywords are the foundation which the literature search process depends on. Many novice literature searchers may use the first keywords that come to mind. Often, these keywords are too specific, too broad, or not the most effective. Since keywords are in a person's natural language, the choice of keywords that those persons use will often reflect their life experiences. For example, some people use the keyword, soda, while others use the keyword, pop, to describe carbonated beverages. This is because choice of these keywords is often regional. For example, much of the northeastern United States (U.S.) use the keyword, soda; the northwestern U.S. uses the keyword, pop; and the southeastern U.S. uses the keyword, coke. A map of where individuals use the keywords, pop, soda, and coke, can be viewed at the Pop vs. Soda page (http://popvssoda.com), accessed July 26, 2019. With the multiple variations some keywords can possess, nurses need to be aware of not only what information they desire to find, but what keyword they need to use to search for that information.

What Is Keyword Literature Searching?

Keyword literature searching is the type of searching that occurs when individuals use keywords to do a literature search on a literature search topic. There are no defined rules or structure to keyword literature searching. The keywords used are usually in the literature searcher's own natural language. You perform a keyword search every time you search in Google. The good thing about a keyword search is that it is easy and you usually get plenty of Search results. The bad thing about a keyword search is that often too many search results appear, many of which are not what you are looking for. The keywords used are usually in the literature searcher's own natural language.

Literature searching with these keywords is how people often first search an electronic database. For example, if someone wants to find articles in the online resource, PubMed, about soda's effect on childhood obesity, keyword searching would entail entering any keywords they could think of, such as soda AND childhood obesity, or pop AND childhood obesity, in the literature search box. Another feature of keyword searching is that it searches anywhere in the bibliographic record for the keywords entered in the search box. **Bibliographic records** are records which include descriptive information such as article title, abstract, journal information, but not automatically the full text of the article or item. Electronic databases are collections of bibliographic records which can be searched and retrieved by a computer or mobile device such as a phone or tablet. Each bibliographic record has information describing that article broken into different sections which are called fields. These fields include article title, journal title, abstract, subjects, author names, etc. Think of a bibliographic record like a spreadsheet with the names of the authors in one row,

the name of the journal in another row, abstract of the article in another, etc. With keyword searching, the database will look for the keyword used in any of the spreadsheet rows, whether it is in the author name, journal title, etc.

Keyword literature searching is the most common type of computerized literature searching that people perform on a regular basis in resources such as Google, social media sites, and online databases. Keyword literature searching is the way most people search for information, and at a quick glance seems to be the simplest way to do a literature search. However, upon closer inspection, keyword literature searching presents challenges for members of the interprofessional team, including nurses. One challenge is having a variety of keywords with a similar meaning. In the earlier example, the nurse wanted to find articles about soda. However, one author from a northwestern state like Oregon may use the keyword, pop, while another author from northeastern Vermont will write a similar article and use the keyword, soda. Another author from southeastern Georgia may use the keyword coke, to identify the same idea. If the nurse searches an electronic database using a single version of a keyword, articles may be omitted from the search results list because the search will not retrieve articles with keywords which possess an identical or similar meaning. It will return just articles which mention the keywords entered. For example, if a nurse searches using only the keyword, soda, articles containing the keyword, pop, may be omitted because the database is only retrieving articles containing the keyword, soda. Another challenge of using keyword searching is having singular and plural forms of the same keyword, such as soda or sodas. A third challenge is having variations on spellings of the same word such as in British vs English spelling, such as pediatric or paediatric. Again, the database may not pick up both keywords in the literature search. Solutions to some of these challenges are presented in the next section with the use of subject headings.

Benefits of Using Subject Headings in a Controlled Vocabulary

Controlled vocabularies are standardized systems of words or phrases which provide a consistent framework for retrieving information. The reason it is called "controlled" is because there is a system of rules which define how the words or phrases are organized. **Subject headings** are words or phrases within a pre-defined controlled vocabulary, determined by a database, which can be used for locating information, and they often answer some of the challenges posed with keyword literature searching. Novice searchers often get frustrated in the literature search process when they must sift through articles which appear unrelated to their clinical question. This is because the electronic database looks for the keyword anywhere in the bibliographic record. The keyword could be in the title or abstract or even the author's name. For example, using the keyword, soda, may retrieve an article written by Hiroshi Soda and not retrieve an article about a soft drink.

Subject headings do some of the sifting work during the literature search process. When you do a literature search by subject headings, you will only retrieve articles that were assigned the subject heading you searched with and where the search topic is a main subject or topic of an article. When subject headings are used, the database only looks in the subject section of the record. The subject section of the bibliographic record is a listing of the main topics of the article. Reading the subject section can give you an idea of what topics are covered in the article. Even though the database only looks in one part of the record, this is a good thing. If the subject heading is found in the subject section of the bibliographic record, it means the retrieved article's content is related to your search topic. One example of a subject heading is, carbonated beverages, which is a subject heading used to describe drinkable liquids which utilize carbon dioxide. Using the subject heading, carbonated beverages, retrieves articles about soda, pop, or other soft drinks, which is what we were intending to find, instead of an article for a person with the last name, Soda, on an article that is unrelated to soft drinks.

Another benefit of using subject headings is that subject headings group words with similar meanings. Using carbonated beverages as a subject heading will tell an electronic database to not only include articles in the search results list with the subject heading of, carbonated beverages, but also include articles in the search results list with subject headings identified as soda, pop, soft drinks, or soda pop. This means that instead of doing a literature search for each individual keyword or doing five separate literature searches, a literature searcher can do one search, saving precious time. Remember the goal in literature searching for EBP is not to find simply a large quantity of articles, but to find high-quality articles which can help answer a clinical question. Therefore, the use of subject heading searching is an important tool in the literature search process. It is important to remember that to get all the benefits just mentioned, the database needs to know that the searcher wants to use a word as a subject heading term and not just as a keyword. To make sure it is formatted correctly, and to also provide a glossary or dictionary of subject heading terms used in an electronic database, many electronic databases have a database of subject headings within the larger database. Many databases also have tutorials on how to use these subject heading databases within their websites.

One electronic database which uses subject headings is PubMed. PubMed's medical-specific subject headings are produced and maintained by The National Library of Medicine and are called **Medical Subject Headings** (MeSH). These subject headings can be searched using the MeSH electronic database at www.ncbi.nlm.nih.gov/mesh (accessed May 20, 2019). These MeSH subject headings created by the librarians at the National Library of Medicine are used by literature searchers within areas of biomedical research such as medicine and within health care sciences like nursing, microbiology, immunology, neuroscience, and more. Using MeSH in the literature search process is a great method for retrieving search results closest to the desired topic. Note that MeSH

subject headings were created a with a set of rules and with a specific structure. Using MeSH can help guide nurses to using the best possible subject headings which will be used for the creation of a clinical question. If a nurse is struggling to find articles about childhood obesity, they could turn to the MeSH database www.ncbi.nlm.nih.gov/mesh (accessed May 20, 2019) and find out that the subject heading in the MeSH database is, pediatric obesity. Using that particular subject heading identifies a collection of more relevant articles.

To learn more about how to use MeSH within PubMed, go to the National Library of Medicine's MeSH tutorial at www.nlm.nih.gov/bsd/disted/meshtutorial/introduction (accessed August 8, 2019). This tutorial defines what MeSH is, as well as step-by-step instructions on how to use the MeSH electronic database (www.ncbi.nlm.nih.gov/mesh) (accessed May 20, 2019) .

Limitations of Using Subject Headings

Subject Headings are a great tool to use within your electronic literature search process, but they do have some limitations. One limitation is that not every keyword in the health care world has a corresponding subject heading. For example, MeSH terms are created by National Library of Medicine librarians who identify and define new subject headings which they see in the current body of scientific literature. A newer subject heading may not have been defined yet. For example, the phrase "social media" did not have a corresponding MeSH subject heading until 2012. Using the MeSH subject heading, social media, would retrieve articles published after 2012, but not necessarily before that date. One other problem is that a specific keyword may not match a subject heading well enough. For example, prior to 2019, the phrase "gun violence" was listed in the MeSH subject heading database under the subject heading, violence, which included any type of assertive behavior. Using the subject heading, violence, a literature searcher might have to sift through many articles about physical violence before finding articles specific to, gun violence. At times, limiting literature search results is not a good thing as relevant articles may be left off the literature search results list because the article does not meet your strict literature searching criteria for some of the reasons listed above. One best practice within literature searching is to use subject headings for the main topic of the search. For example, in the literature searching example above, a nurse may use the MeSH subject heading, carbonated beverages, and then use, pediatric obesity, as a keyword. The reason for using, carbonated beverages, as the MeSH subject heading is because there are a many variations for that particular topic. Using the MeSH subject heading for, carbonated beverages, will tell PubMed to retrieve articles with the keywords of pop, soda, soda pop, and soft drink. Instead of having to do four or five different literature searches, only one literature search needs to be done. Pediatric obesity is a newer subject heading created in 2014, so using it as a keyword instead of as a subject heading will help to not make the literature search too narrow. Starting broad

---

Critical Thinking 11.1

Review the National Library of Medicine's MeSH tutorial at www.nlm.nih.gov/bsd/disted/meshtutorial/introduction/ (accessed August 15, 2019) and then answer the questions below:

1. You want to find the best MeSH subject heading for the act and process of chewing and grinding food in the mouth. Using the MeSH database (www.ncbi.nlm.nih.gov/mesh) (accessed August 15, 2019). What is the best MeSH subject heading for the term, chewing?
2. Click on the checkbox next to the MeSH subject heading for chewing, then click on "Add to search builder," and then click on the Search PubMed button. How many results do you get?

---

with keywords at the beginning of your literature search and then refining the keywords while progressing through your literature search is a much easier process than broadening a narrow search topic.

Ask Answerable Clinical Questions Using PICOT (Patient/Population, Intervention, Comparison, Outcomes, and Time)

One popular model for asking answerable clinical questions is called PICOT. **PICOT** is a model used to assemble clinical questions within the EBP process. The core elements used to assemble PICOT questions include Patient/Population, Intervention, Comparison, Outcome, and Time. It is important to note that not all PICOT questions require the inclusion of Patient/Population, Intervention, Comparison, Outcome, and Time. The most basic form of a PICOT question requires only the Patient/Population, Intervention, and Outcome. PICOT gives the health care provider a model for easily creating answerable questions to be used in literature searching within the EBP process. One challenge many nurses face is how to ask a clinical question for the literature search process that is neither too specific nor too broad. Super-specific literature search questions may not generate enough literature search results to support a solid clinical decision, while literature search questions which are too broad might generate too many search results. These search results may not be relevant to a specific patient or clinical situation. Review Table 11.2 below to see a list of literature search questions which are too specific or too broad.

Using PICOT helps avoid literature search questions being too specific or too broad by requiring certain elements for an answerable clinical question. Remember the goal of finding literature is to support a clinical decision for a specific patient or population. Often these decisions must be made quickly, so the quicker you can find evidence to answer the clinical question, the better. One of the most frustrating situations for nurses or other members of the interprofessional team is to struggle finding the best evidence for a clinical decision. The P in Patient/Population ensures that you consider the patients or population this decision will impact. Is this for children, women, men, seniors, etc.? The I in Intervention ensures a search for an intervention or treatment. The C in Comparison ensures that if there is something to compare to, it is included. It is important to ask, is there something I want to compare the treatment to? For example, is there another medicine? Comparison is not always needed in the search question as sometimes the comparison is, no intervention. The O in Outcome ensures that the effect of the Intervention can be measured. Out of all the PICOT elements, the most critical is often the Outcome, as that is the element which usually focuses and grounds the PICOT question. In other

---

Table 11.2 Example of a Too Specific and a Too Broad Literature Search Question.

Question	Problem with question	Better question
Did the use of a Fitbit help 65-year-old men manage their Hemoglobin A1C in Lake Forest, Illinois in the past year?	This question has too many specific terms, i.e., Fitbit, 65-year-old man, Lake Forest, Illinois. It is unlikely that there will be enough literature search results to fully answer this question. If there are minimal results, it will be hard to make an effective clinical decision based on a trusted body of evidence.	Does the use of fitness trackers help seniors manage their hemoglobin A1C? Instead of using Fitbit, use the broader term, fitness tracker. Using the age group, seniors, will also broaden it as well.
What is the best exercise to manage diabetes?	This question is too broad. This literature search will result in thousands of results, which may not be relevant to the patient's or population's condition. Recommendations for exercises may vary based on age groups, other chronic health conditions, etc.	In the United States, do seniors who participate in yoga better manage their hemoglobin A1C? Picking a specific exercise such as yoga and hemoglobin A1C will focus the results better so a clinical decision can be made.

Source: Charlotte Beyer

words, what Outcome do you hope the evidence shows in relation to the Intervention? When applicable, T ensures that a time period is also included in the search question. In some situations, clinical decisions may vary based upon how long a period of time is indicated. For example, treatments for patients one-week post-surgery may be different than treatments for patients 2 months post-surgery. All these PICOT elements together assemble the most answerable clinical search question possible.

For example, an interprofessional team is caring for an elderly patient with mild dementia who has been recently diagnosed with diabetes. Before creating a customized treatment plan for the patient, the interprofessional team wants to identify how the patient's blood sugar fluctuates throughout the day. However, the dementia could cause the patient to forget to test their blood sugar multiple times a day, as needed. The nurse on the team has heard of the use of continuous blood sugar monitoring devices for patients who struggle with traditional home glucose monitoring systems with lancets (small needles) and test strips. These continuous blood sugar monitoring devices are implanted in the skin and monitor blood sugar levels around the clock. The patient does not need to remember to prick their finger at various times during the day and the team can track how the blood sugar fluctuates throughout the day. The interprofessional team wonders if this would be a good treatment to help monitor this patient's blood sugar so an effective treatment plan could be created.

The nurse could ask the clinical question, does continuous blood sugar monitoring track blood sugar levels effectively? However, this question does not take the whole clinical case into account. Using this clinical question, the interprofessional team might miss information specific to dementia, which could impact this patient's care. The interprofessional team may also miss information on patient compliance with diabetic treatment which is the reason for asking the question in the first place. The question also does not consider the time period of 3 months after diagnosis, since the goal of the use of this continuous blood sugar monitoring device is to monitor glucose levels to create a customized plan which helps this patient. The nurse instead could ask the question: In seniors with dementia (P), does the use of a continuous blood sugar monitoring device (I) effectively monitor blood glucose fluctuations (O) as compared to traditional glucose monitoring with lancets and test strips (C) 3 months post-diagnosis of diabetes?

After asking this clinical question using the PICOT format, the interprofessional team acquires a few articles which support the use of continuous blood sugar monitoring in patients with dementia. Using this continuous blood sugar monitoring device, the interprofessional team discovers that the patient's blood sugar spikes the worst overnight. This discovery leads to changing the patient's medication dosage to avoid blood sugar spikes while sleeping.

The example above demonstrates how important it is to Ask a focused literature search question in order to Acquire evidence which can be applied to specific Patients or Populations. With the first question, the team may have had to sift through literature search results which were not relevant to this clinical case. The second PICOT question better describes the clinical case and guides the interprofessional team to consider multiple aspects of the clinical case, so details are not missed. To see another example of asking a clinical question with the various PICOT elements, review Table 11.3.

The best situation to use this PICOT model is for searching the literature for focused questions about specific clinical situations which have multiple elements. Some examples of when PICOT is especially useful are when a nurse needs to locate literature to support a specific intervention with a specific patient/population or when a nurse wants to compare multiple interventions with a patient/population. This PICOT model guides nurses to Ask literature search questions which can be effectively answered through searching the literature. It is important to note that not all literature search questions fit into the PICOT model. Sometimes, to create a PICOT question, a nurse may need some additional background information. For example, before asking if the use of a continuous blood glucose monitoring device might be effective for the patient with dementia, the nurse may ask the question: What are some alternative methods for taking blood sugar? Why is compliance an issue for patients with dementia? When are the best times of day to take a blood sugar? These basic background questions can help inform the creation of a clear PICOT question. The most important part of asking any literature search question, whether you are using PICOT or you are using a simpler background information question, is to be flexible; your literature search questions can change throughout the literature search process. Creating effective clinical literature search questions is a skill which takes time and experience to master.

Table 11.3   How to Assemble a PICOT Question.

PICOT	In _____(P) is the use of _____(I) as effective as _____(C) at _____(O) within _____(T).
Example	In low risk post-surgical patients (P), is the use of aspirin (I) as effective as the use of anti-clotting drugs such as rivaroxaban (C) at preventing blood clots (O) within 1-week post-surgery (T)?

Source: Charlotte Beyer

Real World Interview

For the last 3 years, our health care system has organized a year-long fellowship opportunity for six nurses to increase their knowledge about investigating and implementing EBPs to improve the quality of patient care. The nurse fellows take a clinical idea, often framed as a PICOT question, through the process of finding, evaluating, and implementing a change in practice. Each nurse fellow works with a series of mentors to help guide them through their projects.

The library is invited to share expertise early in the process. Shortly after the fellows are selected, I provide an hour-long instruction session on literature searching using databases like CINAHL and PubMed and discuss citation management tools like Mendeley. At the end of the library session, I meet with the nurse fellows individually to develop a literature search strategy for their question. I continue to collaborate with these nurse fellows through the duration of their fellowship by providing individual consultations. The library is invited to the year-end celebration and presentation of the nurse fellows' projects. It's rewarding to see how the role of the library can directly impact and improve patient care.

Kate M. Saylor, MSI
Informationist, Taubman Health Sciences Library
University of Michigan, Ann Arbor, Michigan

Critical Thinking 11.2

You recently heard of alternating pressure mattresses which claim to reduce pressure ulcers and you want to know if they are more effective at preventing pressure ulcers than turning or rotating patients.

1. Identify the Patient/Population (P), Intervention (I), Comparison (C), and Outcome (O) and Time (T) for a literature search for this question.
2. Assemble the identified PICOT elements above to create a PICOT question.

Acquire Evidence in the Literature Using Boolean Operators and Truncation in Electronic Databases

Electronic databases acquire articles for a literature search through a specific process. The first step in this process is when a user enters a keyword or subject heading in a search box. The electronic database then reviews the records kept within the database and will retrieve only those articles which have the same keywords or subject headings which the user entered in the search box. This is why having the best keywords and subject headings is an important part of the literature search process. If there are multiple keywords or subject headings entered in the same search box, the electronic database will not automatically understand how to relate those keywords or subject headings to one another. To help the electronic database understand how to relate two or more keywords or subject headings to one another, Boolean opera-

tors can be used. **Boolean operators** are specific words that connect two keywords or subject headings with the goal of narrowing or broadening literature search results in electronic databases. Another strategy for helping the literature database know what to find in a literature search is to use something called truncation and wildcards. In the next few sections, these literature search strategies will be described. The best situations in which to use each of them will be identified.

Boolean Operators: AND, OR, NOT

Boolean operators are traditionally three words: AND, OR, NOT (Table 11.4). Each of these three words will help the electronic database be aware of how to connect multiple keywords or subject headings together when searching through article records for literature. These three Boolean operators communicate to the electronic database on how the user wants the two keywords or subject headings to be related to each

Table 11.4   **Boolean Operators.**

Boolean operators	Example of Boolean operator	What the database will retrieve.
AND	Childbirth AND Stress	Only information which includes both terms, Childbirth AND Stress is retrieved. Information that includes only one of the terms, e.g., Childbirth or Stress, will be left off the list. Use to narrow a literature search.
OR	PTSD OR Post Traumatic Stress Disorder	Information about either term will be retrieved. In other words, all information about PTSD as well as all information about post traumatic stress disorder will be retrieved. Use to broaden a literature search.
NOT	Dementia NOT Alzheimer's Disease	All information about Dementia except information about Alzheimer's Disease will be retrieved.

Source: Charlotte Beyer

Table 11.5   **Sample Truncation and Wildcards.**

Truncation or wildcard	When to use truncation or wildcard.	Example
*	Truncation used when you want to find records that match a root word.	Ther* will find therapy, therapeutic, and therapies.
#	Wildcard used if there are multiple spellings of a particular word.	P#ediatric will find pediatric or paediatric (British Spelling).
!	Wildcard used if you have a word where a character can change the words from singular to plural	Wom!n will find both woman or women.
+	Wildcard used if you have a word where an S will make it plural.	Drug+ will find drug or drugs.

Source: Charlotte Beyer

Critical Thinking 11.3

You are looking for studies about strategies for improving medication adherence with older patients. Go to the PubMed website, www. ncbi.nlm.nih.gov/pubmed, accessed April 4, 2019. Answer the following questions with Boolean Operators.

1. How many resources do you find if you type, medication adherence AND seniors, in the search box?
2. How many resources do you get if you type, seniors OR elderly, in the search box?

---

other when searching the literature. Table 11.4 outlines the various Boolean Operators and when to use each of them when searching electronic databases.

Using Truncation and Wildcards

Truncation and wildcards are used to format literature search terms, as described in Table 11.5. Truncation and wildcards are elements that are used to replace characters in words with the purpose of broadening literature searches without adding extra words. These elements should be available in any of the online databases, including free databases like Google. **Truncation** is a literature search technique where a character is used to replace the end of the word. Using this truncation literature search technique retrieves all words with the common root of the word. For example, searching for nurs* will retrieve articles about nurse, nurses, nursing, etc. **Wildcards** is a literature search technique used when only one character in a word needs to be replaced in a literature search. For example, searching for Nurse+ will retrieve articles about nurse in the singular or plural form.

Acquire Evidence in the Literature Using Electronic Databases

The next step in the literature search process is using resources like electronic or online databases to acquire search results. To learn about different electronic literature databases in the health sciences, review Table 11.6. Over the past 30 years, information retrieval has increasingly migrated to online databases, such as PubMed, Ovid Medline, and the **Cumulative Index of Nursing and Allied Health Literature** (Facchiano & Hoffman Snyder, 2012). Some of these databases, like PubMed, are available for free, while others, like CINAHL, are available by subscription through a hospital or university. Two main types of databases exist for retrieving information, bibliographic, or full text databases.

As mentioned earlier, **Bibliographical databases** are a collection of bibliographical records which include descriptive information such as article title, abstract, journal information, but not the full text of the article or item. PubMed, which is one of the most popular sources for biomedical articles, is a bibliographic database. This type of database is a great resource for finding information because you can identify if a piece of research exists, and then use resources like Interlibrary Loan at your hospital to access the full text of the article. Sometimes hospitals or universities will have software, called link resolvers, to facilitate access to online full text literature. The purpose of link resolvers is to connect or link full text subscriptions owned by the hospital or library to citations in a bibliographic database for easy access.

The other type of database is called a full text database. A **full text database** is an electronic database where the records are all full text. One example of a full text database is PsycARTICLES, a subscription database which has full text articles related to the field of the behavioral sciences or psychology. Those who use this literature database will enjoy immediate access to the articles, because all the articles are fully available.

Databases like CINAHL are a combination of the two types of databases with some of the citations having attached full text articles, but not all. If full text is not immediately available in your literature search, always remember to check with the medical librarian at your hospital or university to see if Interlibrary Loan is available for you to use.

In addition to literature searching databases, nurses should not forget to use the reference list of a relevant article to find other

Table 11.6 **Electronic Literature Databases.**

Electronic literature databases	What it covers.
PubMed https://pubmed.gov (accessed April 1, 2019)	PubMed comprises more than 28 million citations for biomedical literature from MEDLINE, life science journals, and online books. Citations may include links to full-text content from PubMed Central which is a free full text database of biomedical literature as well as links to publisher websites.
Cumulative Index of Nursing and Allied Health Literature (CINAHL) www.ebscohost.com/nursing/products/cinahl-databases/cinahl-complete (accessed August 19, 2019)	CINAHL stands for the Cumulative Index of Nursing and Allied Health Literature and is one of the main sources of literature in the field of nursing. Some of the tools included in this electronic database include literature search tools for limiting information as well as guidance on effectively using subject headings for literature searches specific to nursing and allied health. This electronic database may be available through a hospital subscription.
Ovid Medline www.ovid.com/product-details.901.html (accessed August 15, 2019)	This is an alternative subscription database for literature searching the MEDLINE content found in PubMed. Some of the features of this database include literature search tools for limiting information as well as guidance on effectively using subject headings for literature searches. This electronic database may be available through a hospital subscription.
Cochrane Library www.cochranelibrary.com (accessed April 4, 2019)	This database is a collection of systematic reviews in health care. This electronic database is produced by Cochrane, which is an independent network of literature searchers, professionals, patients, caregivers, and people interested in health. Some of the tools included in this electronic database include literature search tools for limiting information as well as guidance on effectively using subject headings for literature searches. This electronic database may be available through a hospital subscription.
EMBASE www.elsevier.com/solutions/embase-biomedical-research (accessed August 15, 2019)	This is a bibliographic database of biomedical and pharmacological citations. In addition to MEDLINE, EMBASE also includes drug information. Some of the tools included in this electronic database include literature search tools for limiting information as well as guidance on effectively using subject headings for literature searches. This electronic database may be available through a hospital subscription.
PsycINFO www.apa.org/pubs/databases/psycinfo (accessed August 15, 2019)	This is a database of peer-reviewed literature in behavioral science and mental health. Some of the tools included in this electronic database include literature search tools for limiting information as well as guidance on effectively using subject headings for literature searches specific to behavioral health. This electronic database may be available through a hospital subscription.
UpToDate www.uptodate.com (accessed August 1, 2019)	This is an evidence-based clinical resource. It includes a collection of medical and patient information, access to <u>Lexicomp</u> drug monographs and drug-to-drug, drug-to-herb and herb-to-herb interactions information, and a number of medical calculators. It is available both via the Internet and offline on personal computers or <u>mobile</u> devices. It requires a subscription for full access.
http://ClinicalKeyhttp://www.elsevier.com/solutions/clinicalkey (accessed August 1, 2019)	This site offers the latest evidence in a variety of formats, including full-text reference books and journals, point-of-care monographs, drug information, videos, practice guidelines, customized patient education handouts, and more. This site may be available through a hospital or personal subscription.
Essential Evidence Plus (accessed August 1, 2019)	This is a is a point of care tool that contains information on 9,000 common diagnoses and offers access to over 13,000 individual resource. This site may be available through a hospital or personal subscription.

Source: Charlotte Beyer

Real World Interview

Many nurses are taught in school how to perform a basic literature search in health and medical databases such as PubMed, OVID, or CINAHL. In clinical nursing practice, this skill in literature searching databases for current research becomes invaluable in finding ways to improve safety and quality of care. For example, to improve patient outcomes, an **Intensive Care Unit** (ICU) may want to implement a Progressive Mobility program. One step in this Progressive Mobility quality improvement program would be literature searching the health databases to find recent research, suggesting that a Progressive Mobility program actually *does*

improve patient outcomes. The results of this literature search would provide the most current evidence to determine the pros and cons of implementing the Progressive Mobility program. The ability to effectively search current literature allows clinical nurses to both understand the reasoning behind clinical practice guidelines and to be actively involved in the changes which affect their practice.

Kristi Cullor, RN, MSN.
Brodhead, Wisconsin

Critical Thinking 11.4

First review the PubMed for Nurses tutorial at, www.nlm.nih.gov/bsd/disted/nurses/cover.html, (accessed August 10, 2019) to learn how to apply filters. Next, answer the following questions.

1. Go to PubMed at, www.ncbi.nlm.nih.gov/pubmed. Do a literature search for hypertension. How many search results did you find?
2. With the search results list from the previous question, apply the 5-year publication date filter. How many results did you find?
3. How do you know a filter has been applied?

resources. This literature searching technique is called pearl growing because information grows from one core source. Using pearl growing or analyzing the references in a particular article helps nurses identify not only other good articles and core journals in a topic area, but it also helps identify what specific words are used to describe the topic. This is helpful because it provides additional keywords or subject headings options which may help you gather more literature for answering a clinical question.

Refining Literature Search Results in Electronic Databases with Filters

To guide an electronic database to information relevant to a literature search, nurses must ask the following question, "What are the characteristics of my perfect article for this topic?" Some possible answers might include things such as: being published within a certain date range, using a language like English, or coming from a particular article type, such as a randomized control trial or a systematic review. **Filters** are online tools used in electronic databases to restrict information retrieved to specific characteristics, such as publication date, article type, language, etc. Using these filters provides a database with clues to the types of evidence you hope to see in the literature search results list. Each database has a different set of filters, sometimes also called limits, so nurses should take some time to experiment with them to see what filters work the best with a literature search process. Remember, if there are too few items in the literature search results list, filters can always be taken off for a broader literature search. The only search filter which is recommended for most literature searches is language, since not all articles are published in English. Using a language filter ensures that nurses can read all of the articles in a search list. To learn how to use filters within PubMed, visit the Filters page within the PubMed Tutorial for Nurses: www.nlm.nih. gov/bsd/disted/nurses/cover.html (accessed August 10, 2019).

Acquire Evidence and Clinical Practice Guidelines by Using Mobile Applications

In addition to acquiring literature evidence though electronic databases, nurses may use other online resources to support patient care. With the rise in the use of personal devices such as tablets and smartphones, health care information has increasingly gone mobile. Nurses and other health professionals are now turning to mobile applications which can be used at the bedside point of care.

Mobile Applications in Clinical Practice

Mobile applications (apps) are software applications designed for gathering information through the use of a mobile device such as a smartphone or a tablet. One of the biggest areas of growth for gathering health information is in the form of mobile applications with health care content included. Health care mobile applications are often designed with an intended patient/population in mind. In other words, some mobile applications are designed for use by health care clinicians to deliver evidence-based clinical care, while other mobile applications are designed for use by patients to locate health care information or manage their personal health. For example, a nurse may use a mobile application to look up clinical practice guidelines on diabetes, while a patient may use a mobile application to track their blood glucose readings. The developers of the clinical practice guidelines on mobile applications would design it for the nurse's easy use within clinical cases. The developers of the blood glucose tracker mobile application would concentrate patient's easy use to encourage compliance. The language within the latter mobile application would be designed for use by patients who may have lower reading and technology literacy levels. The World Health Organization created a term for the use of mobile applications in the management of health care, called mHealth. With these new mobile health applications, it is easy for both clinicians and patients to be overwhelmed in finding the best app for their information needs (McNiel & McArthur, 2015). Every day, there seems to be a hot new app that everyone scrambles to download onto their tablet or smartphone. The sections below outline the various types of mobile applications nurses may encounter in their professional practice.

Mobile Applications for Point-of-Care Tools

One major group of mobile applications used by nurses is called point-of-care tools. **Point-of-care tools** are online clinical decision support resources that nurses can use to quickly look up information at the bedside. This information is often presented in summaries of clinical topics and clinical practice guideline

Table 11.7   Clinical Point of Care Tools

Point of care tool	Description
UpToDate www.uptodate.com (accessed May 20, 2019) (Paid Subscription)	Evidence-based clinical point of care tool that many clinicians use to find topic summaries, calculators, updates to practice, clinical guidelines, and more. This is the go-to resource for quick information for many in the clinical environment. A mobile application version of this tool is also available with the paid subscription.
DynaMedPlus www.dynamed.com (accessed May 20, 2019) (Paid Subscription)	Evidence-based clinical point of care tool which provides topic summaries, calculators, medical images, updates to practice, guidelines, and more.
Medscape: www.medscape.com (accessed May 20, 2019) (Free)	A free online point of care tool which provides topic summaries, calculators, drug information, and medical news. Free complementary app is also available.
Epocrates: www.epocrates.com (accessed May 20, 2019) (Free version or paid subscription for premium version)	Mobile Application which provides medical references on topics such as drug information, calculators, drug interaction checks, and clinical guidelines. There is a free mobile application with basic information. This tool also offers a paid subscription premium version which includes disease information, labs, and more.
Essential Evidence Plus www.essentialevidenceplus.com (accessed May 20, 2019) (Paid Subscription)	Evidence-based point of care tool which provides access to thousands of clinical topic summaries, abstracts, and guidelines.

Source: Compiled by C. Beyer.

recommendations. The point-of-care tools, such as UpToDate, DynaMed Plus, or Essential Evidence Plus, are normally in the form of a website. Many times, these point-of-care tools also offer a complementary mobile application for use at the point of care. To learn about these point of care tools, review Table 11.7. The comment, paid subscription, means there is a cost or fee required to access the point-of-care tool. Before using these mobile applications on mobile devices, nurses should always check with their institutions' policies on using mobile devices, especially in front of patients, as their use can vary based on those institutions' policies (Giles-Smith, Spencer, Shaw, Porter, & Lobchuck, 2017; McNally, Frey, & Crossan, 2017).

Mobile Applications for Journals

In addition to point of care tools, publishers are increasingly using mobile applications to advertise recently published articles in their journals. Nurses can use these apps to review citations and abstracts for new research studies and guidelines. Note that access to the application does not mean you will receive full access to the articles, but often only means you will just receive access to the abstract or summary of the article's content. If nurses personally subscribe to specific journals, they may have access to the full text of these articles but it is not guaranteed. To see if your desired journal has an app, review the journal's homepage.

Mobile Applications for Clinical Practice Guidelines

Another mobile application which may be useful in clinical practice is one focused on clinical practice guidelines. Many

different societies and organizations such as the World Health Organization will provide clinical practice guidelines on their individual websites. Two great sites for finding guidelines are Guideline Summaries in Guideline Central, available at, www.guidelinecentral.com/summaries (accessed March 1, 2019), and **Emergency Care Research Institute** (ECRI) Guidelines Trust, available at www.ecri.org/components/GuidelinesTrust/Pages/default.aspx (accessed March 1, 2019). Both sites provide clinical practice guidelines from multiple organizations at no cost.

Mobile Applications for Patient Use

Nurses can not only use mobile applications for locating information such as clinical practice guidelines or information at the point of care, they can also use mobile applications in patient education as well. Many patients use their smartphones and tablets on a regular basis. Patients are able to perform activities such as tracking glucose readings to manage diabetes, tracking the amount of exercise they do, learning about chronic health conditions through online games, and more. Since these patient activities are on a device familiar to them, little patient training is needed, so it is a low-cost intervention. However, how do health care professionals know if all of the popular apps are of high quality? One way to determine their quality is to appraise them using six words, i.e., who, what, when, where, why, and how (Table 11.8). Any information, whether it be a **Randomized Controlled Trial** (RCT), a website designed for patient education, or a mobile application, should be critically appraised using these six words at a minimum before including it as evidence or with patients.

Table 11.8 How to Appraise Information Using Who, What, When, Where, Why, and How.

Who • Who wrote it?	• What are a few specific hints that indicate the authors are qualified to write on the topic? ○ Are they literature searchers on this topic? ○ Are they faculty in an academic department? ○ Are they health care professionals? ○ Are they drug or equipment sellers, interested in selling their product?
What • What evidence is present that supports the author's statements?	• Are there references in the form of citations or surveys? • Is there research to support the author's statements?
When • When was information written, created, and/or updated?	• Was this material created more than 5 years ago? ○ If you are looking for the most current evidence, you may only want the most current information, unless it is a classic or gold standard article.
Where • Where did you find it? • Where (region) did it come from?	• Is this material from a journal, eBook, or professional website? ○ Is the region close to where you are located? ○ If you want to match the information to your population, you may only want to have evidence from the United States, United Kingdom, or Canada.
Why • Why was it created?	• Were the materials created to educate or convince? ○ Is there any evidence of bias in the item?
How • How does this piece of information help you answer your clinical question?	• What are the characteristics of the piece of information that make you want to include this in your body of evidence? For example: ○ Does it match your population? ○ Is the content of the material very relevant to your question?

Source: Charlotte Beyer

Case Study 11.1

You have been caring for patients with diabetes who struggle with getting the minimum recommended 150 min of exercise of moderate intensity per week (U.S. Department of Health and Human Services, 2018). Exercise is an integral part not only of glycemic control but also of overall health. You are wondering if small bursts of exercise throughout the day are as effective as a single exercise session per day. Conduct a literature search to help answer this question.

1. What did you find?
2. How will you share these results?

Appraise Evidence Such as Journals, Mobile Applications, and Websites for Relevancy and Quality

After nurses have Assessed the patient or population, Asked an answerable clinical question, and Acquired evidence to answer the clinical question, the next step in the literature search process is Appraising the evidence. This is one of the most vital pieces of the literature search process, as the quality of the evidence can directly impact the effectiveness of clinical decision making. Examples of evidence used in clinical practice can include journal articles, websites, clinical topic summaries, and mobile apps. Just because a piece of evidence is available, however, does not mean it is of high quality, which is why health care professionals must appraise evidence before including it in clinical decision making (Friesen-Storms, Beurskens, & Bours, 2017). As mentioned above, six words which can be used in appraising the evidence for relevancy and quality within the literature search process are, who, what, when, where, why, and how. **Critical appraisal** is the act of evaluating evidence for its quality and relevance to a specific topic. The rest of this section is devoted to strategies for practicing critical appraisal throughout the literature search process.

Appraising the Evidence: Journals

The main form of evidence needed to answer clinical questions within EBP is in the form of articles published in academic/research journals. Not all research is created equal. Just because something was published does not mean the study/data is of high quality. One of the core elements of EBP is using the evidence from scientific literature in clinical decision making. This means a nurse needs to use evidence which could be replicated and applied to clinical situations. If the data was gathered poorly or the process for collecting the data was flawed or influenced by the researcher, the use of that evidence could negatively impact a clinical decision.

In the past few decades, open access publishing has grown in many fields including nursing (Oermann et al., 2016). In the traditional model of publishing, the publisher will offset the costs of publishing by charging subscription fees to individual or group subscribers, such as libraries or hospitals. In open access publishing, reader access to articles is free of charge and often has less restrictive copyright restrictions. The benefits of open access publishing are that more people can readily access research in an easier way. However, the downside to this is that some publishers can take advantage of the system.

In open access publishing, readers do not have to pay to access the published content, as full text content is available for free. However, the costs to produce the journal and articles still exist. Therefore, many open access publishers charge the authors a fee to publish their articles instead of charging readers to access the article. One of the challenges with the open access publishing model is that certain publishers become less concerned with providing access to high-quality journals at little cost to the reader, and more concerned about publishing as many articles as possible to make the largest profit.

Some of the problems associated with predatory journals or publishing include a fast review process with little attention paid to the quality of the research, or no review process at all, and/or no digital preservation, so the articles disappear when the journal stops publishing. When some of these journals stop publishing, not only is there no new content, the website where the journal lived is shut down so there is no record that older articles existed. As open access publishing continues to be more prevalent in scientific research, the problem of predatory publishers will only continue to grow. Jeffery Beall, an academic librarian, defined predatory publishing or predatory journals as publishers or journals who, "unprofessionally abuse the author-pays publishing model for their own profit" (Beall, 2013). He compiled a list of journals and publishers which exhibited signs of being predatory. In 2011, there were 18 open access publishers, while in 2016 that number had grown to 923 open access publishers. With the pressure to publish, predatory publishing will not stop anytime soon. Strategies and guidelines for clearly identifying predatory journals are still emerging (McCann, & Polacsek, 2018). Until these strategies and guidelines are established, nurses can appraise journal content by evaluating the methods sections of research articles. Ideally, the data should be able to stand on its own without the influence of external factors, either with the research participants or with the researchers who review the data. Note that, if the participants in a study know what the researchers are hoping to find, study participants may tailor their responses to state what they think the researchers want to hear, instead of giving their true responses. Also, if researchers can identify individual participants, they may begin to hypothesize and make false connections based on the participants' characteristics, such as race, gender, socioeconomic status, etc., rather than solely on the participants' responses. Not all research studies are of high quality, so it becomes very important to do an evaluation before including an article in the literature search and EBP process.

Use the Methods Section to Appraise and Evaluate the Quality of the Research Articles

One method for evaluating articles is to review the methods section of the research articles. The methods section is where the author(s) outline in a step-by-step process how the study was conducted. Think of the methods section like the foundation of a house. If the foundation has cracks in it, the rest of the house may crumble. A research study with a solid foundation

Evidence from the Literature

Source: Oermann, M. H, Conklin, J. L., Nicoll, L. H., Chinn, P. L. et al. (2016). Study of Predatory Open Access Nursing Journals. *Journal of Nursing Scholarship,* **48**, 624–632.

Discussion: In recent years, open access journals have become a popular part of the EBP process, due to their ease of access and low cost to the reader, such as a member of an interprofessional team. However, with the rise of this new type of publishing comes another challenge in health care publishing called predatory journals. Often the purpose of these journals is to make money from **Article Processing Charges** (APC) instead of sharing high-quality knowledge in the areas of research. The authors of this study sought to identify predatory journals in the field of nursing, as well as distinguishing their predatory characteristics and editorial practices. To find journals that appeared predatory, the authors reviewed Beall's List of Predatory Publishers and Beall's list of Standalone Journals. Using these Lists, the authors located 140 journals from 75 publishers which met the criteria for predatory journals outlined by Jeffery Beall and included the word "nursing" in the title. One troubling characteristic the authors identified was that 104 of these journals published a first volume, and out of those 104 journals, only 51 journals published a second volume, and only 26 journals produced a third volume. In fact, the median number of volumes per journal was only two before ceasing publishing. Journal content was also unfocused with pediatric, midwifery, and critical care nursing all publishing articles within the same volume. Also, the peer review process was rushed, with some journals having less than a 3-day peer review process. The APC also ranged from $75.00 to $1,500.00 dollars per article. One challenge is that there is no one defining characteristic for these journals, so the authors noted that nurses must practice due diligence if they wish to publish quality scholarship.

Implications for Practice: As nurses search for evidence in the literature search process, they must be aware that predatory journals exist and put an extra effort into appraising the evidence they find for quality. With some of these predatory journals accepting articles regardless of quality, nurses in clinical care must be aware that not all the evidence they find in the literature search process will be of merit. Evaluating the study designs in the methods section will become even more important, as more predatory journals are published online. For nurses who wish to publish clinical research of their own, being able to identify the characteristics of potential predatory journals is an important skill in the publishing process.

usually has solid results, which can be used as evidence in clinical care. One great feature about evaluating the methods section of a research article is that it can be done quickly, as time in the clinical environment is precious. Evaluating the methods section can tell a clinician a wide variety of information in a small period of time. The one thing to keep in mind when appraising the methods section is evidence of bias. **Bias** is defined as factors outside the research study that could affect the results. One example of bias could be in a drug trial for weight loss. Instead of randomly selecting patients in one group to receive a drug and then selecting patients in another group who receive a placebo, researchers select patients with healthy lifestyles to receive the weight loss drug. These patients may do better not simply because of the drug, but because of their healthier lifestyles. At its most basic level, the purpose of research in health care is to identify interventions or treatments' cause and effect. Did an intervention or treatment alone cause some effect on a patient that impacted them in a positive, negative, or neutral way? Bias complicates the interpretation of the research results because it adds factors outside of a treatment. Was it the impact of the drug alone or the impact of the healthier lifestyles which contributed to the patients' weight loss success? Bias is especially problematic in health care research because this type of research is used in clinical decision making. Bias in research leads to clinicians not being aware of the full picture of why the research results happened. This can lead to clinical decisions being ineffective or dangerous to a patient's health and well-being. To help you identify examples of bias in the methods sections of research studies in the literature search process, review Table 11.9 for five questions to ask about the research study. Then read below

to view examples of why each of these questions is an important part of the appraisal process.

Question 1: How Many Participants Began the Study?

The reason that the number of participants who began a study is important is because if there are not many participants, study generalizations/recommendations are harder to verify. Researchers may try to make big generalizations based on a small number of participants, and bias may appear. For example, say there is a study about how free weekly massages impacted anxiety in a senior center in an affluent area. In reviewing this study, you note it only reviewed 15 participants at one senior center, and it found that anxiety levels decreased after the free weekly massages. The participants all were ladies who had been doing monthly spa treatments elsewhere for a few decades before the study. Could the participants' receptivity to free weekly massages be possibly impacted by their prior spa treatments and possibly, by their economic level? If this study was repeated at a few different sites with females with different experiences and economic levels, the evidence for free weekly massages as a treatment for anxiety might be different. Remember, evidence in clinical decision making should be applicable to as many types of patients as possible.

Question 2: How Many Participants Completed the Study?

Another important point to evaluate is how many participants completed the study. If there are not many participants who completed the study, generalizations/recommendations are harder to verify, as the study data only reflects a portion of the

Table 11.9   Five Questions to Ask When Reviewing a Methods Section of a Research Article.

Questions to ask	
How many participants began the study?	If there are not many participants, study generalizations/recommendations are harder to verify.
How many participants finished the study?	If there are not many participants who finished the study, generalizations/recommendations are harder to verify as data only reflects a portion of the participants and not all participants. Researchers may not know how the intervention impacted the majority of participants, or researchers may omit negative data to make their treatment or intervention look more effective than it was, either accidentally or on purpose.
Were the participants blind to the treatment or intervention?	A way to minimize bias is to not let the participants know what the researchers are hoping to find and what treatment or intervention the participants received. The participants may act in a way which reflects what they think the researchers want to capture instead of demonstrating the impact of the treatment or intervention alone.
Were the researchers blind to the treatment or intervention?	Another way to minimize bias is for the researchers to be blind to the treatment or intervention as well as the participants. First it prevents the researchers from hinting to the participants the treatment or intervention they are getting. Secondly, it prevents the researchers from having expectations of what the results will be, as these expectations could be tainted with the researchers' own bias.
Were the participant assignments randomized?	Another way to minimize bias is to randomize the participants assignments in both the treatment and intervention group and the control group. This means distributing participants with particular characteristics among all groups instead of placing participants more likely to get a positive result in the treatment or intervention group and placing the participants more likely to have negative results in the control group.

Source: Created by Charlotte Beyer

participants and not all the participants. For example, if there is a study about the effects of a ketogenic diet on weight loss for patients with **Polycystic Ovarian Syndrome** (PCOS), and only 250 out of 750 patients complete the study, it would be difficult to use the study as evidence for use of the ketogenic diet. It may have been successful for 250 patients, but what about the other 500? Were they not successful, so they dropped out of the study on their own? Was the data omitted by the researchers because it indicated negative results, which did not support the researchers' hypothesis? When negative data is not listed at all, it cannot be evaluated. This is an example of how author bias can have a negative effect in research.

Question 3: Were the Participants Blind to Treatment?

As you search for evidence in literature searching, you may see the phrase, "double blind study." A double-blind study is a study where neither the research participants nor the researchers know what treatment the research participants are receiving until the study is over. The next section will discuss why it may be important for the researchers to be blinded. However, a single blind study is a study where only the research participants are unaware of what the researchers are looking to find. This is important because if research participants know what the researchers want to find, the research participants may change their answers. For example, say a researcher is doing a study to see if the nausea medicine, Zofran, makes research participants sleepy. If the research participants know the goal of the study, some research participants may trick themselves into feeling sleepy to meet that goal, either accidentally or on purpose. The study results data would be tainted. Therefore, the study results could not be used as evidence in answering a clinical question.

Question 4: Were the Researchers Blind to the Treatment?

In the last section, the idea of a double-blind study was discussed, where not only the subjects but also the researchers were blind to what treatment the subjects were getting. The reason this is a desirable type of study is that it prevents a few things from happening. First, it prevents the researchers from hinting to the subjects what treatment they are getting. Second, it prevents the researchers from having expectations of what the results will be, as those expectations could be tainted with the researchers' own bias. For example, a group of researchers are doing a study to see if the antidiabetic medication, metformin, should be given to patients with insulin resistance for weight loss. The study consists of researchers giving some subjects a placebo and giving other subjects, metformin. In a single blind study, the subjects would not know which medication they were being given. What could happen in this single blind study is that the researchers could choose subjects who had a better chance at weight loss while using the drug, such as patients with healthier lifestyles. This finding would inflate the positive results of the study and not be a truthful example of

evidence that metformin is a good intervention used in weight loss for these patients. If a clinician used this study as evidence in the EBP process, then they may not have the full picture, and their patients could suffer from this lack of knowledge.

In a double-blind study, neither the researchers nor the participants would be aware of which medication was given to which participant. Therefore, the study results would only reflect the effect of the drug regardless of what participant it was given to. The evidence from this study would give the clinicians a better picture of whether or not participants would benefit from this treatment.

Question 5: Were the Participants Assignments Randomized?

Another way to minimize bias in research is to randomize the assignment of participants into various groups, such as participants in the group with an intervention and participants in the group without an intervention. The participant group without an intervention is called the control group. Participant assignment is often done electronically, and the researchers have no say in this assignment process. A type of study which uses this method of randomized participant assignment is called a randomized control study and it is a very common type of evidence used in the EBP process. A randomized control study minimizes bias because it takes away the possibility that another factor could make an intervention or treatment more or less effective. For example, a study is done to see if the breast cancer drug, letrozole, is effective at treating breast cancer post-surgery. If the researchers assign the subjects to the various groups, they may assign the healthier patients to a treatment group that has a better chance of a positive outcome. Instead of evaluating if the cancer drug, letrozole, was successful in preventing new breast cancer tumors by itself, the initial health of the subject may be a factor in who has positive or negative results. Clinicians would not have a full picture of the effect of the drug, letrozole. This could result in future ineffective care of the patient with breast cancer.

The five questions listed above are just a few questions to ask when reviewing a methods section of a research article to identify if the researchers took steps to minimize bias. The great thing about reviewing the methods section for these questions is that it can be done quickly and efficiently. Not all studies will meet all of these criteria, but these are the questions that should be asked before including evidence into your EBP Process.

Appraising Evidence: Websites and Mobile Applications

Other than academic research journal articles, another vital type of evidence nurses might use is in the form of websites or mobile applications. However, with so many choices, how do nurses ensure resources recommended to patients are high quality? The first main question you want to concentrate on as you do your appraisal/evaluation process of websites or mobile

Table 11.10   Questions to Ask When Appraising Websites or Mobile Applications.

For health care professionals	For patients/consumers
• What organization or group sponsored the website or mobile application? • What are the references used to support their claims? • Do the authors go into enough detail for a professional audience? • Are the authors trying to sell something which may impact the objectivity of the information presented?	• How user-friendly is the resource? • Do the authors use plain language when designing the materials for those with limited literacy levels? • Does the content match the user's level of health literacy? • Are there privacy concerns (HIPAA)* with patients sharing information?

ª The Health Insurance Portability and Accountability Act (HIPAA).
Source: Created by Charlotte Beyer

applications is, "Was this material designed for a consumer/patient use or was it designed for use by health professionals?" This answer is important because there are different questions you need to ask based on the type of audience. For example, a nurse needs to be concerned with things such as the possibility of distribution of patients' personal health information via a website or mobile application. Also, does the patients' level of literacy or reading levels match the language on the site? One site which is a great resource for health professionals is iMedicalApps, www.imedicalapps.com (accessed April 1, 2019), which is a site created and maintained by physicians dedicated to reviewing new apps and mobile health care resources. Review Table 11.10 to discover questions to ask when reviewing websites or mobile apps.

Resources for Lifelong Learning

A major challenge nurses face is keeping up with all of the new changes in health care practice. One tool nurses can use to stay current with these changes is something called personal accounts. **Personal accounts** are online tools in electronic databases or websites that provide a customized space for the user to store things such as saved searches, set up database alerts, and more. **Personal accounts** are present in many different electronic databases and electronic resources such as PubMed, CINAHL, Ovid Medline, etc.

Two common features of personal accounts which all members of the interprofessional team can use to stay current are database alerts and saved literature searches. A **database alert** is an online tool where a database will notify the user when a research citation has been released. In other words, instead of having to initiate a literature search to find citations, the citations come to the user. One nice feature of database alerts is that nurses can dictate how often they receive the database alerts, such as daily, weekly, or monthly.

Saved literature searches are where nurses can save literature search topics, such as hyperglycemia and surgery, in their personal accounts. Every time a nurse logs into their personal account, instead of having to type in their topic, they can re-run the literature search of the saved topic via a link, thus saving time. These are just a few features available in personal accounts in the various electronic databases and resources. To learn how to set up personal accounts in the various resources, visit the home page for the database or ask your clinical librarian for assistance.

Final Step: Apply the Evidence to Your Patient or Clinical Problem

Now that you have assessed the patient or population, asked an answerable clinical question, acquired the evidence to answer the clinical question, and appraised the evidence, the final step is to apply the evidence to your patient or clinical problem. This entails taking what you have learned and making a treatment plan for the patient or population. In the opening scenario, the evidence found within a literature search turned into a few new protocols to prevent hospital readmissions due to post-surgical incision site infections. The first part of applying the evidence is simply digesting the evidence and making clinical decisions to support future interventions or treatments. After clinical decisions have been made, the next step is to evaluate if the result of the interventions or treatments improved the patient's health or solved a clinical problem. If it did, then that experience will add to your body of knowledge as a clinician for future patient care. If it did not produce a desired result, try to identify why it did not. Then, use the Five A's again to start another literature search process. Most importantly, do not get discouraged. Effective literature searching is a skill which you will develop and improve over your career as a nurse.

KEY CONCEPTS

• A nurse must have the ability to locate and analyze high-quality health information and use EBP.

• One resource nurses can use to become more familiar with information retrieval processes needed for EBP are clinical librarians.

• One process nurses can use to direct their literature search for health care research literature is to use the words Assess, Ask, Acquire, Appraise, and Apply during their literature search process.

• Finding the best keywords and subject headings to create answerable clinical questions is vital to successful literature searching.

- The main system for searching subject headings in the health sciences is called MeSH.

- PICOT is a format for creating questions in the clinical setting. PICOT stands for Patient/Population (P), Intervention (I), Comparison (C), Outcome (O), and Time (T).

- Boolean operators can be used in literature searches to inform online resources such as electronic databases on how to relate one term to another.

- Another tool nurses can use to identify important information on a topic is to analyze the reference list of an important article. This analysis of the reference list is called pearl growing.

- Online point of care tools such as UpToDate or Essential Evidence Plus can be used to answer questions emerging in clinical practice.

- Mobile applications (apps) on devices such as smartphones and tablets are helpful to find research or answer patients' questions at the bedside. Before using, nurses should check their institution's policies for using apps in front of patients.

- Before including information as evidence in the EBP process, nurses should appraise or evaluate information resources for quality and relevance. Six words nurses can use to appraise or evaluate information include: who, what, when, where, why, and how.

- To appraise or evaluate research studies as potential evidence, nurses should first review the methods section of the research to see the quality of the researchers' methodology.

- When evaluating websites and mobile apps, nurses should first identify if the intended audience for the website is a professional or a patient audience. The audience for the website will direct the types of appraisal and evaluation questions needed.

- To stay current on upcoming research and practice changes, nurses can take continuing education courses or set up topic alerts in various electronic databases.

KEY TERMS

Bibliographic Databases	Critical Appraisal	PICOT
Bibliographic records	Electronic Databases	Subject Headings
Bias	Filters	Truncation
Boolean Operators	Mobile Applications	Wildcards
Clinical Librarians	Full Text Databases	Personal Accounts
Controlled Vocabularies	Keyword Literature Searching	Database alerts

REVIEW QUESTIONS

1. An Obstetrics and Gynecology nurse heard of an intervention where feeding test weights (weighing the babies before and after feeding) are used to encourage breastfeeding in infants with congenital heart disease. What is the first thing the nurse should do?
   a. Start using feeding test weights to encourage breastfeeding.
   b. Perform a literature search to find the evidence on this topic.
   c. Meet with the physician to discuss the intervention.
   d. Brainstorm a pilot study.

2. When you begin a literature search, what five words should you keep in mind?
   a. Activate, Acquire, Asses, Appraise, Apply.
   b. Assess, Ask, Acquire, Appraise, and Apply.
   c. Ask, Acquire, Absorb, Appraise, Apply.
   d. Ask, Acquire, Assess, Advance, Apply.

3. You are an ICU nurse and want to find articles about the best techniques for administering drugs via a feeding tube. What is the best literature search strategy you could use?
   a. Feeding Tube AND Drug Administration.
   b. Feeding Tube OR Drug Administration.
   c. Feeding Tube NOT Drug Administration.
   d. Do not combine the two topics, and instead search one topic at a time.

4. You are doing a literature search on the effect of cinnamon supplements on glycemic control. How should you approach finding the information?
   a. Literature search free websites like Google to see if anything exists.
   b. Use a few different scholarly databases such as PubMed and CINAHL to find multiple articles on this topic.
   c. Find one good article and base your recommendations on that one piece of evidence.
   d. Use a single piece of evidence, such as an entry in a nursing textbook.

5. One of your diabetic patients is struggling to track their carbohydrate intake while managing their blood sugar. You notice this is a common problem with many of your patients and want to periodically search electronic databases for literature to identify new interventions for tracking glucose levels. What is one online tool you could use to help you identify evidence like articles on an ongoing basis?
   a. Do a Google search once a month.
   b. Search the American Diabetes Association website for ideas
   c. Create a personal account in an electronic database like CINAHL or PubMed to save searches, set up database alerts, and preserve search histories.
   d. Email a colleague to ask for ideas new interventions

6. After doing some research on mobile applications, there are a few different mobile applications which might help the patient manage their food intake and track nutrients such as carbohydrates. Within your literature search, you notice the mobile application, MyFitnessPal, keeps coming up. What should be your next step?

   a. Evaluate the mobile application, MyFitnessPal, by using the words who, what, when, where, why, and how.
   b. Recommend the mobile application, MyFitnessPal, to the patient.
   c. Recommend the mobile application, MyFitnessPal, to your nurse manager for use with all of your patients.
   d. Do not recommend mobile applications for patient use.

7. You are a nurse working in a long-term care facility. One of your major concerns is your patients' stability and their danger of falling. You want to identify interventions which are effective at prevention of falls in senior residents. You have heard that yoga can be an effective exercise for improving balance and preventing falls. What is the best question you could ask in the PICOT format?

   a. Does yoga prevent falls in seniors?
   b. What is the best treatment to prevent falls in seniors?
   c. In seniors, is the use of yoga an effective treatment for preventing falls in long-term care facilities?
   d. Does exercise help improve balance in long-term care facilities?

8. Many of your patients have COPD. You wonder, what are the various interventions which could be used to minimize airway infections? You find one literature search article which mentions oral hygiene as a possible intervention for preventing these infections. What should you do next?

   a. Use the article as evidence in your recommendations to a patient.
   b. Evaluate the study's quality by reviewing the methods section.
   c. Share the article with your nurse manager.
   d. Make recommendation to the physician.

9. You are a surgical nurse and notice that patients are being readmitted with infections in their incision sites. You are struggling to find helpful literature resources and suspect the search terms you are using are not helpful. You find one really good article. What is one strategy you could use to find better terms for literature searching the literature?

   a. Brainstorm more terms.
   b. Look in the reference list of the article to identify common key phrases and terms.
   c. Use a term that is marginally related to the topic.
   d. End the literature search and use the evidence you found, even if lower quality.

10. You are a perioperative nurse and want to identify the recommended practices for preventing infections via transfusion in the perioperative practice setting. What is the best resource to find the most current practices/recommendations?

    a. Nursing Textbook.
    b. Practice Guideline websites such as Guideline Central or ECRI Guideline Trust.
    c. Journal article from 2010.
    d. Website geared toward patients about preparing for a procedure.

REVIEW QUESTION ANSWERS

1. Answer: B is correct.

   Rationale: Part of the EBP process is incorporating literature into making clinical decisions (B). Prior to incorporating this intervention into clinical care (A), speaking to a physician (C), or brainstorming a pilot study (D), the nurse should have a clear understanding of the topic which comes from the literature.

2. Answer: B is correct.

   Rationale: The five words which describe the literature search process in EBP are assess, ask, acquire, appraise, and apply (B). (A) does not include the word ask, which is an integral part of the process for finding information. (C) does include the word assess. Nurses need to assess the patient or situation before asking the clinical question. (D) does include the word appraise. Appraising literature for quality is another vital part of the literature search process.

3. Answer: A is correct.

   Rationale: The best situation is to being able to locate articles about feeding tubes as well as drug administration in one results list (A). Searching feeding tube OR drug administration will bring back all articles about feeding tubes and all articles about drug administration. However, the articles will not be about both concepts, so the nurse would have to sift through the results to see if any articles have the two concepts in common which could be

time consuming (B). Feeding tube, not drug administration, will exclude articles about drug administration, which is the opposite of what is desired (C). Finally, searching one concept at a time and then trying to sift through articles to find which ones have both concepts in common would be inefficient (D).

4. Answer: D is correct

   Rationale: The best strategy would be to use multiple electronic databases such as PubMed and CINAHL to locate quality articles (D). Google includes a lot of information including advertisements for supplements which may have false or misleading information. There is so much information that it can be hard to sift through the results to get the highest-quality information (A). Finding one good article is good; however, clinical recommendations should not be based on a single piece of evidence in the EBP process (B) or (C).

5. Answer: C is correct

   Rationale: The best online tool for helping nurses keep up with a particular topic is to create a personal account in an electronic database (C). Using this tool, nurses can set up database alerts, where the database will send an email informing when a new citation has been published. The nurse can also save searches for later use while also viewing what was searched in the past. Doing a Google search is not as efficient, as it may not identify relevant information (A). The American Diabetes Association website may not have all of the newest interventions listed on their website (B). Likewise, a colleague may not be aware of all of the newest interventions (D).

6. Answer: A is Correct

Rationale: Before recommending any app to a patient, the app should just be evaluated with at least the words who, what, when, where, why, and how (A). Answering these questions informs you the desired audience, the purpose and more. If an app is recommended which is not designed for patients, the patient could get frustrated and not get the maximum benefit from using this tool (B). Likewise, it should be evaluated before recommending to the nurse manager (C). Also, this app has the potential to help the patient manage their condition, so it would be a shame to not recommend it if it is of higher quality (D).

7. Answer: C is Correct

Rationale: PICOT questions need to have multiple elements such as population, intervention, comparison, and outcome (C). (A) does not include long-term care facilities, which are an integral to the clinical situation. (B) looks at exercise in general for seniors which is really broad and may not be relevant to this particular clinical situation. (D) does not include seniors or yoga as the exercise. Using this question might not retrieve evidence which helps this clinical situation.

8. Answer: B is correct

Rationale: After you find an article which is relevant to your clinical question or need, the next step should be to evaluate the

article's quality. One way you can do this is by reviewing the methods section of an article to identify things such as sample size, how the information was gathered, etc. (B). An article should not be used as evidence until an evaluation or appraisal is conducted (A). Before sharing with a nurse manager, nurses need to take the time to evaluate the quality of the article (C). One piece of evidence such as an article should not be the basis of any clinical recommendation (D).

9. Answer: C is correct.

Rationale: The best strategy listed in the options above is looking in the reference list to identify common phrases and terms (C). Additionally, nurses might be able to identify key authors and journals in a particular field. If not familiar with a topic, brainstorming terms may be problematic (A). Using a term that is marginally related to the topic may not generate relevant results (B). Ending the search using only the available evidence may miss critical pieces of information (D).

10. Answer: A is correct.

Rationale: Two resources nurses can use to find current practice guidelines are Guideline Central or ECRI Guideline Trust, which are free websites designed to list practice guidelines (A). A nursing textbook may not have the all the guidelines needed (B). A journal article from 2010 may not have the most current guidelines (C). If a website is geared toward patients, it probably will not be specific enough for health professionals such as nurses (D).

REVIEW ACTIVITIES

1. Pick a patient's condition that you want to learn more about and apply the Five A's process to find evidence and literature on the condition. What types of resources did you find in your literature search? How will you communicate what you find?

2. Locate a website, app, or article of your choice that relates to the patient's condition you chose for the last question and evaluate it using Table 11.10 Was there anything surprising or unexpected you found as you appraised the website, app, or article for its quality?

DISCUSSION POINTS

• With the changing nature of information, what are some strategies you can use to stay up to date in your clinical practice?

• What are some strategies you can use to find the best terms for your literature search process?

• What are some evaluation criteria you can use to evaluate quality of articles you find in a literature search?

DISCUSSION OF OPENING SCENARIO

1. The most effective way to search the literature is to have a literature search process in place which you can draw from when you need to. The nurse in this example might first ask a possible background question such as: "What are some specific interventions for preventing hospital readmissions due to incision site infection after knee replacement surgery?" Once the nurse gathers a list of interventions, the nurse will

next create a PICOT question to research specific interventions with the patient population. For example, in this situation, the nurse may ask the PICOT question, In post-surgical knee replacement patients (P), is the prescription of antibiotics prior to surgery (I) as compared to no antibiotics prior to surgery (C) effective at preventing post-surgical infection (O) 2 days post discharge (T)? Once the nurse has that question answered, the next step is using keywords, such as post-surgical knee replacement patients, antibiotics, 2 days post discharge, and preventing post-surgical infection, to find the evidence. Once the evidence is located, the nurse would review the evidence for quality and then apply it to the clinical situation. In this case, it could include suggesting changing protocols such as requiring nurses to call patients 2 days past discharge to assess if they are developing any signs of infection.

2. The literature supports nursing practice by providing the best available evidence which is a core element of EBP. New research and new discoveries are being made every day. In order for patient care to continuously improve, this evidence needs to be integrated with clinical practice. Information retrieval of this evidence is a critical skill all nurses must possess.

EXPLORING THE WEB

- Nursing CEU Directory: www.nurseceu.com (accessed April 1, 2019)

- Institute for John Hopkins Nursing www.ijhn-education.org (accessed April 1, 2019)

- CEConnection: www.nursingcenter.com/continuing-education (accessed April 1, 2019)

- American Association of Critical care Nurses, Continuing Education (CE) Courses: www.aacn.org/education/free-continuing-education-nurse-courses (accessed April 1, 2019)

- Essential Evidence Plus: www.essentialevidenceplus.com (accessed August 15, 2019)

INFORMATICS

Go to the QSEN website (http://qsen.org) Accessed March 1, 2019 and click on Education>Competencies>QSEN Competencies. Next click on Informatics.

1. What is the first checkpoint mentioned in the Attitudes section?

2. How does this relate to the research or literature searching process?

LEAN BACK

- Now that you have learned about searching for literature, what is one change you will make in your literature search process?

- What is one database or mobile application you might try to use with your literature search process?

REFERENCES

Beall, J. (2013). Medical publishing triage—chronicling predatory open access publishers. *Annals of Medicine and Surgery, 22*, 49.

Bridges, D. (2018). *Opening Scenario on prevention of hospital readmission due to incision site infection*. Unpublished manuscript.

Cronenwett, L., Sherwood, G., Barnsteiner, J., Disch, J., Johnson, J., Mitchell, P., Sullivan, D. T., & Warren, J. (2007). Quality and Safety Education for Nurses. *Nursing outlook, 55*(3), 122–131 https://doi.org/10.1016/j.outlook.2007.02.006.

Facchiano, L., & Hoffman Snyder, C. (2012). Evidence-based practice for the busy nurse practitioner: Part two: Literature searching for the best evidence to clinical inquiries. *Journal of the American Academy of Nurse Practitioners, 24*, 640–648.

Friesen-Storms, J., Beurskens, A., & Bours, G. (2017). Teaching and implementing evidence-based practice in a hospital unit with secondary vocational trained nurses: Lessons learned. *Journal of Continuing Education in Nursing, 48*, 407–412.

Gerberi, D., & Marienau, M. S. (2017). Literature searching for practice research. *AANA Journal, 85*, 195–204.

Giles-Smith, L., Spencer, A., Shaw, C., Porter, C., & Lobchuck, M. (2017). A study of the impact of an educational intervention on nurse attitudes and behaviours toward mobile device and application use in hospital settings. *Journal of the Canadian Health Libraries Association/Journal de l'Association des bibliothèques de la santé du Canada, 38*, 12–29.

McCann, T. V., & Polacsek, M. (2018). False gold: Safely navigating open access publishing to avoid predatory publishers and journals. *Journal of Advanced Nursing, 74*(4), 809–817.

McNally, G., Frey, R., & Crossan, M. (2017). Nurse manager and student nurse perceptions of the use of personal smartphones or tablets and the adjunct applications, as an educational tool in clinical settings. *Nurse Education in Practice, 23*, 1–7.

McNiel, P., & McArthur, E. C. (2015). What's app-ropriate for your clinical practice? *Clinical Advisor, 18*, 80–88.

National Library of Medicine. (2020). Citations Added to MEDLINE by Fiscal Year. Retrieved May 23, 2020, from https://www.nlm.nih.gov/bsd/stats/cit_added.html

Oermann, M. H., Conklin, J. L., Nicoll, L. H., Chinn, P. L., Ashton, K. S., et al. (2016). Study of predatory open access nursing journals. *Journal of Nursing Scholarship, 48*, 624–632.

Sackett, D. L., Rosenberg, W., Muir Gray, J. A., Haynes, R. B., & Richardson, W. S. (1996). Evidence based medicine: What it is and what it isn't. *Britiah Medical Journal, 312*, 71.

Sadoughi, F., Azadi, T., & Azadi, T. (2017). Barriers to using electronic evidence based literature in nursing practice: A systematized review. *Health Information and Libraries Journal, 34*, 187–199.

U.S. Department of Health and Human Services. (2018). *Physical activity guidelines for Americans* (2nd ed.). Washington, DC: U.S. Department of Health and Human Services.

SUGGESTED READING

Baumann, N. (2016). How to use the medical subject headings (MeSH). *International Journal of Clinical Practice, 70*(2), 171–174.

Bramer, W. M., de Jonge, G. B., Rethlefsen, M. L., Mast, F., & Kleijnen, J. (2018). A systematic approach to literature searching: An efficient and complete method to develop literature searches. *Journal of the Medical Library Association, 106*, 531–541.

Brandt Eriksen, M., & Faber Frandsen, T. (2018). The impact of patient, intervention, comparison, outcome (PICO) as a literature search strategy tool on literature search quality: A systematic review. *Journal of the Medical Library Association, 106*, 420–431.

Buccheri, R. K., & Sharifi, C. (2017). Critical appraisal tools and reporting guidelines for evidence-based practice. *Worldviews on Evidence-Based Nursing, 14*, 463–472.

Dang, D., & Dearholt, S. L. (2018). *John Hopkins nursing evidence based practice: Model and guidelines* (3rd ed.). Indianapolis, IN: Sigma Theta Tau International.

Fink, A., & Beck, J. C. (2015). Developing and evaluating a website to guide older adults in their health information literature searches: A mixed-methods approach. *Journal of Applied Gerontology, 34*, 633–651.

LoBiondo-Wood, G., & Haber, J. (2018). *Nursing literature search: Methods and critical appraisal for evidence-based practice* (9th ed.). St. Louis, MO: Mosby.

Martín-Martín, A., Orduna-Malea, E., & Delgado López-Cózar, E. (2018). Coverage of highly-cited documents in Google Scholar, Web of Science, and Scopus: A multidisciplinary comparison. *Scientometrics, 116*, 2175–2188.

Pilcher, J. (2016). Mobile apps for educational purposes. *Journal for Nurses in Professional Development, 32*, 306–308.

Wernersson, I., & Orwehag, M. H. (2016). Scholarly skills as everyday practice—implications for education. *Higher Education, Skills and Work-based Learning, 6*, 224–236.

Yucha, C. (2015). Predatory publishing: What authors, reviewers, and editors need to know. *Biological Research for Nursing, 17*, 5–7.

Quality Improvement of Patient Care

Christine Rovinski Wagner[1], Catherine C. Alexander[2]

[1] Office of Veterans Access to Care, Veterans' Health Administration, Washington, D.C. USA

[2] Quality Management, San Francisco VA Medical Center, CA, USA

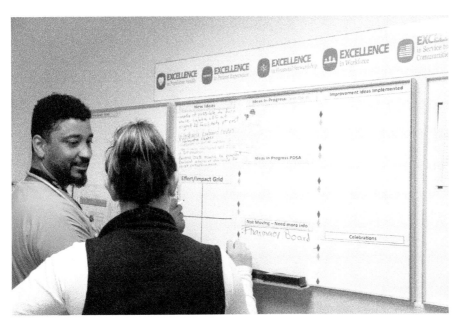

Health care team members reviewing a huddle board.
Source: Used with permission from Tessa Corilss

Everyone in health care really has two jobs when they come to work every day: to do their work and to improve it.

Paul Batalden & Frank Davidoff, 2007

OBJECTIVES

Upon completion of this chapter, the reader should be able to:

1. Discuss the importance of **Quality Improvement** (QI) in Health Care.

2. Explain why quality improvement is important for the patient, the nurse, and the organization.

3. Discuss the major principles of QI, including customer identification; the need for participation at all levels; and a focus on improving the structures, processes, and outcomes of patient care.

4. Explain how QI decisions are made based on data (Pareto charts, Pie charts, time series data).

5. Identify benchmarking resources.

6. Review a Balanced Scorecard and a Clinical Value Compass.

7. Identify that QI is a continuous process.

Kelly Vana's Nursing Leadership and Management, Fourth Edition. Edited by Patricia Kelly Vana and Janice Tazbir
© 2021 John Wiley & Sons Ltd. Published 2021 by John Wiley & Sons Ltd.
Companion Website: www.wiley.com/go/kelly-Nursing-Leadership

8. Discuss the QI focus on simplification and standardization of work processes.

9. Review the FOCUS Methodology for QI and the **Plan Do Study Act** (PDSA) Cycle.

10. Discuss STEEEP and Evaluation of a Health Care Organization's QI Program.

OPENING SCENARIO

A hospital that participated in a benchmark study on patients with total hip arthroplasty noted that compared to other organizations, its average length of stay (LOS) was longer than the benchmark average LOS by 1.29 days. The hospital also noticed that the percentage of their patients that used a pneumatic compression device to decrease the postoperative rate of deep vein thrombosis was 32% lower than the benchmark average. The percentage use of indwelling catheters in post-operative patients with total hip arthroplasty at the hospital was 53%. Although this indwelling catheter use was lower than the benchmark average, the team believed it was important to decrease the rate further, since indwelling catheters are associated with an increase in postoperative urinary tract infections (UTIs). The hospital also noted an average of three physical therapy (PT) visits postoperatively per patient, whereas the benchmark average was five postoperative visits per patient. Finally, the cost of total care for patients with total hip arthroplasty was higher at the hospital versus the average hospital cost in the benchmark study.

The hospital assigned an interprofessional team the responsibility of identifying opportunities for improvement. The team began by developing a clinical pathway based on the most recent research in this area. Using data and evidence-based research, the team looked for ways to improve the patient care process. The team incorporated the best practices that they found. This meant designing into the clinical pathway increased use of the pneumatic compression device, more physical therapy, earlier indwelling catheter removal, and an earlier postoperative discharge date. To prepare the patient properly for the earlier discharge,

the team added a preoperative home visit to the clinical pathway. The home care agency would make the home visit and then make a recommendation for discharge planning prior to the patient's admission. This process expedited initiation of referrals to a postoperative rehabilitation facility or home care following hospital discharge, if needed. If the family home had to be rearranged to accommodate limited ambulation or stair use, these recommendations were made early in an effort to allow the family to prepare ahead of time and assure the patient's safety.

When the cost of health care for patients with total hip arthroplasty was examined, the higher costs at the hospital seemed to be related to the number of prosthetic vendors. Different surgeons preferred using different prosthetic devices from different vendors. When more vendors are used, there is little to no incentive for the vendor to decrease their costs. When fewer vendors are used, the volume of prosthetic devices used in total hip arthroplasty with each vendor is higher, allowing more competitive price negotiation among vendors. The hospital worked with the surgeons on the team to decrease the number of vendors to a ratio of 0.25 vendors to surgeons.

1. *If you were a staff nurse on the QI team, how would you encourage the decreased use of postoperative indwelling catheters?*

2. *How could you bring your ideas to other staff members without making them feel that the quality of their care was being criticized?*

3. *If you were a staff nurse not on the QI team, how could you support the efforts of the team?*

Quality improvement (QI) is the use of data to monitor the outcomes of care processes and improvement methods to design and test changes to continuously improve the quality and safety of health care systems (QSEN Institute, 2019). The science of QI is the development of new ideas, the testing of those ideas, and the implementation of change, as needed. QI approaches are used to refocus health care delivery systems from provider- centered to patient-centered where health care services are reliable, coordinated, and respond to the needs of the patient. QI is not research. The intent of QI is not to generate new knowledge, but rather to use existing evidence and tools to change practices to prevent potential or actual harm (Stausmire & Ulrich, 2015). Patient safety comes first. QI is about systematically testing evidence-based practices at all levels of health care to improve patient care. It is a proactive approach that emphasizes doing the right thing, at the right time, for the right reason, in the right way, in the right place, and obtaining the best possible results for the patient. QI is an overall management approach rather than a single program. Integrating concepts of QI into daily organizational operations is key to successful outcomes.

Table 12.1 Patient Experience Data

Patient experience quality topic	Your hospital (%)	State average (%)	National average (%)
Patients who reported that their nurses "Always" communicated well	84	83	80
Patients who reported that they "Always" received help as soon as they wanted	72	74	70
Patients who reported that their room and bathroom were "Always" clean	76	80	75
Patients who reported that the area around their room was "Always" quiet at night	63	66	62
Patients who "Strongly Agree" they understood their care when they left the hospital	59	57	53

Source: Adapted from Centers for Medicare and Medicaid Services (2019c).

This chapter will discuss the importance of QI in health care and explain the importance of it for the patient, the nurse, and the organization. It will discuss the major principles of QI, including customer identification; the need for participation at all levels, and a focus on improving the structures, process, and outcomes of patient care. QI decision-making based on data (Pareto charts, Pie charts, time series data) and benchmarking resources are reviewed. The chapter identifies Balanced Scorecards and a Clinical Value Compass and identifies that QI is a continuous process.

It discusses the QI focus on simplification and standardization of work processes and reviews the FOCUS Methodology for QI and the PDSA Cycle. The STEEEP principles of health care, that is, Safe, Timely, Effective, Efficient, Equitable, and Patient-Centered Care and evaluation of a Health Care Organization's QI Program are reviewed.

The Importance of Quality Improvement in Health Care

The Importance of QI to the Patient

A health care delivery system, or health care organization, is a set of people, institutions, and resources that deliver health care services to meet the health needs of target populations. Individual patients are the core of target populations. Patients value what they experience during health care service delivery. They also value the end results of the health care services they receive. It is important for nurses to know what the patient values from his or her health care experience as this is the basis of patient-centered care. **Patient-centered care** is recognizing the patient or designee as the source of control and full partner in providing compassionate and coordinated care based on respect for patient's preferences, values, and needs (QSEN Institute, 2019).

To more fully understand the patient's perception of their health care experience, organizations obtain patient experience and satisfaction data utilizing several methods, such as,

mail-in surveys, telephone surveys, focus groups and "real time" surveys, such as patient interviews, that take place immediately prior to discharge. These surveys require that organizations use the same data collection tools in the same way to assure accuracy of results. Patient experience and satisfaction data are most helpful when compared with data from other organizations (Table 12.1). All patient experience and satisfaction data are put into a database so the results can be statistically analyzed. The process of comparing this data is discussed later in the chapter.

The **Hospital Consumer Assessment of Healthcare Providers and Systems** (HCAHPS) Survey, also known as the CAHPS® Hospital Survey or Hospital CAHPS, is a standardized survey instrument and data collection methodology that has been in use since 2006 to measure patients' perspectives of hospital care (Press Ganey, 2019). The HCAHPS results posted on Hospital Compare www.medicare.gov/hospitalcompare/search.html (accessed February 18, 2019) helps patients make fair and objective comparisons between hospitals and with state and national averages on important measures of patients' perspectives of care. Hospitals also use private companies, such as Press Ganey (2019) (www.pressganey.com/solutions/service-a-to-z/hcahps-regulatory-survey accessed February 18, 2019) to further understand the quality of their patients' experiences. For example, how well was information about medication provided in addition to how often.

The terms patient experience and patient satisfaction are often used interchangeably, but they are not the same thing. Patient experience encompasses all the interactions that patients have with the health care system. It includes several aspects of health care delivery that patients value when they seek and receive care, such as receiving patient care in the timeliest manner possible, easy access to information, and good communication with health care providers. Data on patient experience shows whether patients are receiving care that is respectful of and responsive to their needs. The question in Table 12.2 about how often did nurses treat the patient with courtesy and respect is a measure of patient experience.

Table 12.2   Patient Experience and Satisfaction Survey Questions

Survey topic	Survey question
How often did nurses communicate well with patients?	• How often did nurses treat you with courtesy and respect? • How often did nurses listen carefully to you? • How often did nurses explain things in a way you could understand?
How often did patients receive help quickly from hospital staff?	• How often did you get help as soon as you wanted after you pressed the call button? • How often did you get help in getting to the bathroom or in using a bedpan as soon as you wanted?
How often did staff explain about medicines before giving them to patients?	• How often did hospital staff tell you what the medicine was for? • How often did hospital staff describe possible side effects in a way you could understand?
Were patients given information about what to do during their recovery at home?	• Did hospital staff talk with you about whether you would have the help you needed when you left the hospital? • Did you get information in writing about what symptoms or health problems to look out for after you left the hospital?
Would patients recommend the hospital to friends and family?	• Would you recommend this hospital to your friends and family?

Source: Centers for Medicare and Medicaid Services (CMS). (2019b). Hospital Consumer Assessment of Healthcare Providers and Systems. Retrieved at https://www. medicare.gov/hospitalcompare/search.html, Centers for Medicare and Medicaid Services (CMS). (2019b). Equity Initiative. Retrieved at https://www.cms.gov/About-CMS/Agency-Information/OMH/equity-initiatives/index.html

Patient satisfaction encompasses how patients feel about the health care they receive. Patient satisfaction is about whether a patient's expectations about a health encounter were met. For example, two people who receive the exact same care can give different satisfaction ratings because of their different expectations for how that care was supposed to be delivered (AHRQ, 2017a). The question in Table 12.2 about whether the patient would recommend a hospital to family and friends is a measure of patient satisfaction.

The Importance of QI to the Nurse

The fact that the health care organization is a complex system challenges all health care providers to function as part of an interprofessional team. Interprofessional team models are designed to provide better care coordination and improved patient experiences and outcomes at a lower overall cost of care (International Council of Nurses, 2015; IOM, 2010; Sullivan, Kiovsky, Mason, Hill, & Dukes, 2015). Nurses today are providing care in a constantly changing health care environment that requires increased awareness and attention to the performance of all health care staff. QI is an essential part of the entire health care team's daily work.

Daily team huddles are one way to ensure that the health care team incorporates QI into daily practice (AHRQ, 2017). A **team huddle** is a brief, in-person, scheduled meeting with relevant team members to anticipate and prepare to meet patient needs so the work day runs more smoothly. Huddles provide an opportunity for staff to raise safety concerns in real time. Many health care teams use huddles to identify problems, discuss QI activities, and review outcomes. Some organizations have standard huddle board templates to document, track, and celebrate QI work. The opening photo shows two health care team members working on a huddle board.

Huddles enable the nurse to work collaboratively with the other health care team members. A daily team huddle is an opportunity for the nurse to demonstrate the nurse's four key roles in the health care delivery system: professional, advocate, innovator, and collaborative leader (Baker & Williams, 2016) (Table 12.3). QI is sustained over time when nurses collaborate with interprofessional teams and use data to support their decisions. The nurse who fully engages with the health care team in daily improvement, and works to full scope of nursing practice, provides the greatest value to the health care system (Lucatorto, Thomas, & Siek, 2016).

Leadership is a critical element for the provision of quality health care (Sfantou et al., 2017). Without it, successful QI is jeopardized. Leadership is inherent in all nursing positions, from the bedside to the executive suite. The nurse who demonstrates professional accountability in the delivery of safe high-quality care on a daily basis demonstrates personal leadership.

The Importance of QI to the Organization

Health care organizations today are structured to maximize QI efforts by encouraging accountability, communication, and the focus of all staff on the mission, vision, values, and priorities of the organization. Accountability, communication, and staff who are focused on the mission, vision, values, and priorities of the organization are elements of a **high reliability organization** (HRO). The goal of an HRO is to increase patient safety and quality outcomes through standardization of care delivery structures and processes. Health care organizations value a combination of quality outcomes, patient satisfaction outcomes, and cost outcomes. Quality outcomes include a patient's clinical or functional outcomes. For example, did the patient survive? Can the patient go back to work? Patient sat-

Table 12.3   The Nurse's Key Roles in the Health Care Delivery System

Nurse's key role	Examples during a daily huddle
Professional	Making attendance at team huddle a personal priority. Being prepared and participating in team huddles.
Advocate	Identifying patient care issues that need improvement. Sharing concerns that focus on the health care process, not people.
Innovator	Countering resistance to change with professional candor. Brainstorming with team members
Collaborative leader	Helping the team separate the issues and solutions that are under the control of the staff and those that need support from those further up the organizational chain of command. Volunteering to lead a quality improvement team.

Note. Created by C. Wagner & C. Alexander.

Table 12.4   Structure, Process, and Outcome in an Operating Room

Structure	+	Process	=	Outcome
Sterile operating Room	+	Interprofessional team follows sterile protocol	=	Low infection rate

Note. Created by Patricia Kelly Vana.

isfaction outcomes include, would the patient recommend this health care facility to someone else? Cost outcomes include the cost of both direct and indirect patient care delivery. Direct cost is the cost of the care of the patient, for example, cost of medications, operating room equipment, and direct patient caregiver salaries. Indirect costs are the costs of indirect care activities, including, for example, electricity and salaries of indirect patient caregivers such as secretaries or human resource staff. See Table 12.4 for an example of how quality structures and quality processes lead to quality outcomes in an Operating Room.

Quality care delivery directs the use of evidence-based care and ensures that finite health resources are used wisely to improve patient outcomes. Patient care that is based upon the best science available will be effective care. Effective care is achieved by proactively seizing opportunities to continuously improve care before a problem or error occurs. In most, but not all QI efforts, as quality is improved by standardizing care delivery work processes and applying evidence-based

principles, the cost of care decreases (New Jersey Hospital Association, 2017).

Within an organizational structure, it is vital that nursing leadership be represented at all levels. The Nurse Executive should participate in board councils, executive management councils, and quality councils. The Nurse Executive and all nurses are champions for QI. Communicating QI priorities at all levels in the organization is essential. One method to do this is through shared governance councils so there is broad representation of QI activities. The day-to-day work of all nurses, in collaboration with the interprofessional team and staff from other departments, helps achieve the strategic goals of the organization.

Nurses are entering a profession that has a wide-reaching impact by providing and affecting safe, high-quality, patient-centered, accessible, and affordable health care. The expectation of nurses' colleagues is that you will look for opportunities to lead and share collaborative improvement efforts (National Academies of Sciences, Engineering, and Medicine, 2016).

Real World Interview

There are many ways for a nurse leader to engage nursing staff in Quality Improvement. I believe that it is first important to find out what is meaningful to each nurse. This requires relationship building. I make myself visible to the staff by conducting listening sessions for all shifts on a monthly basis. The nurses are invited to tell me their concerns and share their ideas for how to make our medical center better. I make myself transparent in helping the nurses understand the necessary steps for evaluating their suggestions for implementation. Sometimes it is as simple

as a "just do it." Sometimes a suggestion must go up to the rest of the medical center's leadership for approval. I have found that nurses who believe they can be a voice for change demonstrate a more robust understanding of how to integrate QI into the work they do every day.

Bernadette Y. Jao, DNP, MSN, RN-BC
Associate Director Patient and Nursing Services/CNE
VA Medical Center, Manchester, New Hampshire

Major Principles of Quaity Improvement (QI)

QI principles include the following:

1. The priority of QI is to identify and benefit patients and all other internal and external customers.

2. Quality is achieved through the participation of everyone at all levels of the organization.

3. Improvement opportunities are developed by focusing on the work structures, processes, and outcomes, not criticizing individual performance.

4. Decisions to change or improve a system or process are made based on data.

5. Improvement in the quality of service is a continuous process.

QI Benefits Patients and All Health Care Customers

Early quality-focused literature focused on fixing problems, "doing it right," and having zero defects. Over time, a gap was found between theory and practice. It was determined that quality is not about being perfect. Quality is about being better, doing the right thing the first time, and being better than the competition. Being better than the competition brings financial stability as more people want the service the quality organization provides.

Quality is about health care professionals seeing themselves as having customers. This notion requires a shift in the mindset of health care professionals. A customer is anyone who receives the output of health care team efforts. There are internal and external health care customers. An internal health care customer is anyone who works within the organization and receives the output of another employee. Internal customers include health care staff such as medical and nursing practitioners, nurses, pharmacists, physical therapists, respiratory therapists, occupational therapists, and pastoral caregivers. An external customer is anyone who receives the output of the organization. External customers include patients, private medical and nursing practitioners, insurance payers, and regulators such as the state Department of Health, the Joint Commission (TJC), and the community served.

Designing health care processes from the customer's point of view versus the professional's point of view requires a change in thinking about how health care is delivered. Health care involves work processes in which one step leads to the next step. Improving these steps in the work process is an important part of quality care, customer satisfaction, and a patient's experience. Patient satisfaction and experience are rooted in the way health care professionals treat their patients/customers and in the quality of patient outcomes.

QI looks at every problem as an opportunity for improvement. Empowering staff to identify problems and implement improvement strategies improves staff satisfaction, staff engagement in their work, and patient outcomes. Other QI concepts include designing health care work processes to meet the patient's needs, rather than the health care provider's needs, and reducing waste and rework (Table 12.5). Patient care should be efficient and avoid waste of time, money, and resources. QI concepts should be emphasized until they become part of an organization's daily operations and the organizational culture.

Table 12.5 Examples of Waste in Health Care

Waste	Definition	Example
Defect	Time spent doing something incorrectly or fixing errors	Incomplete instrument kits in the Operating Room.
Overproduction	Doing more than is needed by the customer.	Filling out assessment forms that ask for the same information in different places on the form.
Waiting	Waiting for the next event to occur or the next step in a process.	Low risk patients spending hours in the emergency department.
Non-utilized talent	Not using staff experiences, skills, knowledge, or creativity.	Employees who are not heard, engaged, or supported.
Transportation	Unnecessary movement of materials, information, or equipment.	Poor hospital design so that radiology services are located a long distance from the emergency department.
Inventory	Excessive cost through accumulation of supply beyond that which is needed, and storage and spoilage of supplies.	Letting supplies expire and then disposing of them.
Motion	Unnecessary movement by employees in the system.	Equipment room shared by two or more units that is conveniently located for only one of the units.
Extra processing	Doing work that is not valued by the customer.	Medical record forms that require information that is never used.

Note. Created by C. Wagner & C. Alexander.

QI Requires the Participation of Staff at All Levels of the Organization

QI is achieved through the participation of staff at all levels of the health care organization. A new staff member can participate in the design and improvement of daily work practices and processes on an individual, unit, or organizational level. For example, as an individual, a nurse could change the organization of his/her day to spend more time on patient education. On a unit level, a nurse could work with colleagues on the unit to redesign how patient report is given in order to improve efficiency (McAllen, Stephens, Swanson-Biearman, Kerr, & Whiteman, 2018). On an organizational level, a nurse could suggest a QI project that improves the process for notifying pharmacy about a missing medication and then join a QI team to find a solution.

Membership on a QI team is defined by the specific goals of the QI project. For example, if you were trying to decrease the time a patient waits outside the radiology suite for a test, you would need to include the patient transportation staff, unit clerks, unit RNs, and radiology staff in your QI efforts. If you wanted patients with congestive **heart failure** (HF) to understand the importance of weighing themselves daily after discharge, you would include the patient and patient's family, the cardiac unit's RNs, the clinical dietician, the primary care practitioner, the cardiologist, the pharmacist, and the home care agency staff. A key feature of successful QI teams is including the point-of-service staff who are directly involved in the work process you are trying to change. Point of service staff has the most knowledge of the work process and can quickly identify potential areas of improvement. Organizations should provide all staff with the opportunity to suggest improvements in their day-to-day work. For example, an X-ray technologist identifies that the current process for scheduling and transporting patients is creating a long wait time for X-ray testing. If the organization has a built-in mechanism for QI process improvement, the X-ray technologist could begin small tests of change to improve efficiency, decrease the waiting time, and increase patient satisfaction.

QI Focuses on Structure, Process, and Outcomes

Quality improvement opportunities are focused on the structures, processes, and outcomes of patient care. When an interprofessional team performs well in terms of structure,

it also tends to perform well in terms of clinical processes, which in turn have a favorable influence on patient outcomes (Moore, Lavoie, Bourgeois, & Lapointe, 2015). The model of structure, process, and outcomes in health care was pioneered by Avedis Donabedian and has direct consequences on how emerging global health issues are tackled (Abrampah et al., 2018).

Structure refers to the physical and organizational characteristics of a hospital such as its buildings, human resources, financing, and equipment. An example of structure is a hospital policy that requires a nurse to check the code cart each shift to verify that the cart contains the necessary equipment and medications.

A **process** is a series of steps and decisions that interact to produce a result. The people involved in these steps and decisions include all types of health care workers, such as nursing and medical practitioners, technicians, housekeeping, and so on. An example of a health care work process is illustrated by a patient who presents in the emergency department with chest pain. When it is determined that the patient has had a myocardial infarction (MI), several work processes must occur to achieve a quality outcome for the patient. These work processes include an appropriate set of interventions for the patient with an MI, such as taking an electrocardiogram; starting an intravenous line; drawing pertinent blood work; choosing the right medications in the right time frame; and doing patient assessments on a regular interval to identify complications early or before they happen. All these steps and decisions of a work process can be measured. These measurements are then reviewed, applying evidence-based principles as appropriate to improve patient care. Steps of the work process may be eliminated or changed and then standardized so that all staff use the improved work process. For instance, in the example of the patient with an MI, health care evidence shows that all patients with an MI should receive aspirin within a specific time frame. In an organization with a focus on quality improvement, the steps of aspirin administration to the patient are reviewed and changed, as needed, until the measurement data shows that all patients with an MI receive aspirin in the specific time frame. This would mean a review of when the health care practitioner ordered the drug, when the order was transcribed, when the pharmacy got the aspirin to the staff, when the staff gave it to the patient, and so on. In addition, if this patient care is standardized with a protocol to decrease variability in the work process, this leads to the best end result or outcome for the patient.

Case Study 12.1

You have developed a good working relationship with the other nursing and medical staff on your unit as you have been caring for many patients with a **myocardial infarction** (MI). You believe that the care delivery on your unit could improve, thus improving patient satisfaction and clinical outcomes and decreasing the LOS.

1. How would you proceed to improve care delivery?
2. Whose support would you enlist first?
3. Who else should be involved?
4. What quality indicators could be measured?

Outcomes are the end results of all the work processes as well as the relationships among the work processes. You can improve outcomes by examining both the work processes and the relationships. In a system, every step of a work process affects the next step. For example, if the X-ray technician places the patient in the hall and calls the transport service to take the patient back to his room, but does not monitor the transportation process, this may decrease the total time a patient is in radiology but increase the patient's time in the hall waiting for transportation. Note that improvement in the structure and process of health care leads to improved outcomes. You cannot improve care outcomes unless you review all the structures and work processes leading to an outcome.

Of all the efforts to achieve QI, monitoring patient outcomes is the most significant criteria for the delivery of safe, competent care. Patient outcomes measure actual clinical achievement. Outcomes can be short-term outcomes, such as the average LOS for a patient population, or long-term outcomes, such as a measure of patients' progress over time, for example survival rate for a transplant patient, 1, 2, and 3 years after treatment. Outcomes are studied to identify potential areas for QI. A negative outcome may lead to an investigation of structure and process to determine any root causes of the outcome. Outcomes influence ongoing decision making in the provision of health care services by each health care discipline. Ongoing monitoring of health care outcomes is captured through data collection and interpretation.

QI Decisions Are Based on Data

Improvements in the quality of health care services is a continuous process in which decisions to change or improve a work system or work process are made based on data. When someone says, "The patients are waiting too long to return from radiology," it is time to look at the data. Collecting data helps nurses and the interprofessional team understand the work process and clarify current issues. Using data correctly is important. Data should be used for learning, not for judging. It is critical to focus on improving work processes rather than criticizing people. In the radiology example above, if we jumped to conclusions, we might criticize the transportation staff person who returned the patient from radiology. This would not stimulate QI ideas. By not analyzing the work process (patient has chest X-ray, is put in hall, clerk at desk calls transportation, transportation clerk pages transportation aide, and so on) and the relationships among the work processes (waiting times between calls, transportation phone process, page system, and so on), we could miss where the real opportunity for QI lies. Reviewing the wait time data is an example of examining the work process, not the people carrying out the work process. If the people in the work process are slowing it down, this will be demonstrated in the outcome data. QI will only happen if the health care team works together to improve the entire work process.

Pareto Charts, Pie Charts, and Time Series Data

Several different types of charts and graphs are used to examine data in QI efforts. Each type of chart and graph shows data with a different perspective. For example, a Pareto, or bar, chart compares differences between groups of data. For example, in the opening scenario data is grouped as reasons for extended LOS (Figure 12.1). The Pareto chart compares the reasons for extended LOS from the most frequent reason, that is, limited PT visits, to the least frequent reason, that is indwelling urinary catheters. Pareto charts can also be used to show changes in data over time when the data changes are large. Pie charts are circular statistical charts that show data as part of a whole (Figure 12.2). The pie chart provides a proportional view and makes it easier to compare parts of the whole. For example, in Figure 12.2 the pie chart is comprised of all the reasons for extended LOS lengths and provides the team with a simple visual comparison of the data. Pie charts do not measure change over time. Time series graphs show data over a period of time (Figure 12.3). The time series graph shows the effect of the improvement solutions. A decrease in all of the percentages of all the reasons for extended LOS shows that the care provided to these patients is improving because the clinical pathway is now being followed. Standardized formatting in the charts and graphs in conjunction with statistical methods enables reliable interpretation of the data.

The **Agency for Healthcare Research and Quality** (AHRQ) (www.ahrq.gov/professionals/systems/hospital/qitoolkit/index.html accessed November 12, 2018) provides a set of readily available QI programs to track and improve hospital care and patient safety. These can be downloaded from their website without charge. The AHRQ site also includes a tool on how to use Excel worksheets to produce charts based on your hospital's data and a PowerPoint presentation template. Most health care organizations are also members of larger associations that make available QI software and data for benchmarking of outcome measures. Off-the-shelf computer software can also be used to create tables and figures with graphs, charts, flowcharts, and tables. Figures 12.1–12.3 and 12.9 in this chapter were made using Microsoft Excel. All of the tables and Figures 12.4–12.7

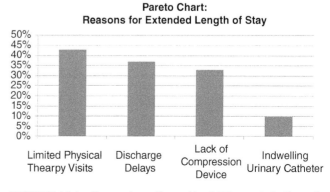

FIGURE 12.1 Pareto chart. Created by C. Wagner & C. Alexander.

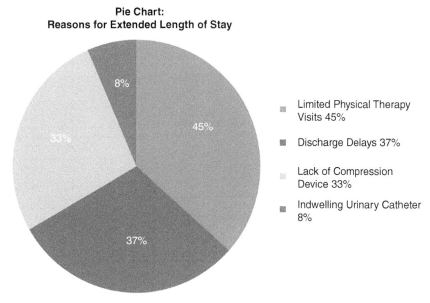

FIGURE 12.2   Pie chart. Created by C. Wagner & C. Alexander.

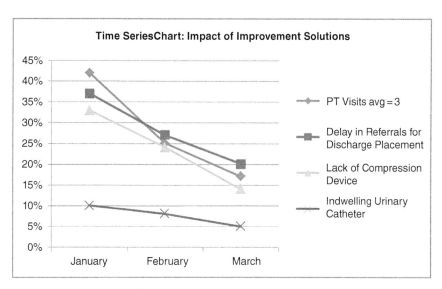

FIGURE 12.3   Time series graph. Created by C. Wagner & C. Alexander.

and 12.10 in this chapter were created with Microsoft Word (Use, Insert Table, with its Columns and Rows to show alignment; Use Insert, Smart Art to select a Diagram). Diagrams, such as Figure 12.8 and Figure 13.4 were made using Microsoft Visio.

Benchmarking

Benchmarking is the public reporting of data that helps patients make more informed choices about where to obtain their health care based on their individual needs and preferences. It is the continual and collaborative practice that measures and compares the outcomes of key work processes with those of the best performers on a national scale. A key

characteristic of all benchmarking is that it is part of an organization's comprehensive and participative policy of continuous quality improvement. A benchmark study will identify gaps in performance and provide organizations with the information necessary to redesign health care delivery or develop strategies to enhance customer expectations. There are various types of benchmarking studies, such as clinical, financial, and operational benchmarking (Table 12.6).

A clinical benchmark study will review grouped outcomes of patient care, for example patients who have had a stroke. Financial benchmarking studies examine cost/case charges and LOS. Operational benchmarking studies review the health care systems that support care, for example, the case management system in an organization. The outcomes of clinical, financial, and operational

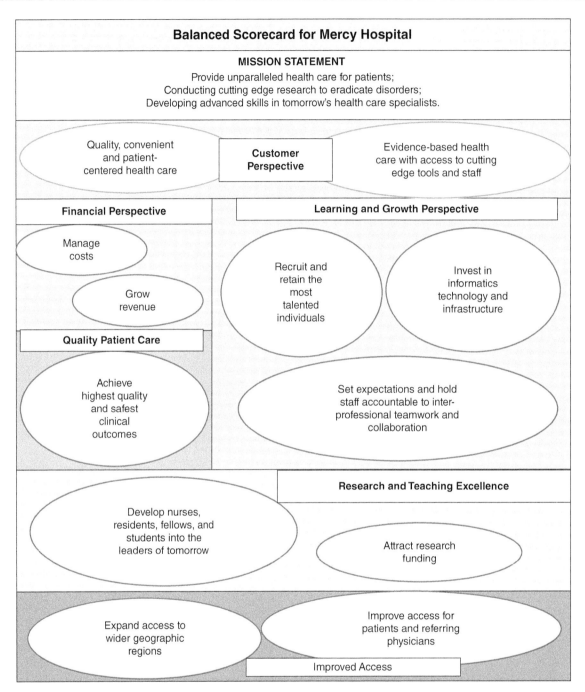

FIGURE 12.4   Example of a hospital's balanced scorecard.
Source: Adapted from ClearPoint Strategy (2018).

studies are compared or benchmarked with the outcomes of high-quality services or organizations. Looking at high-quality performing services or organizations and finding out what they do to achieve their high quality helps to spread improvements in the quality and effectiveness of care. Effective care means the patient's care will be based on the best science available. Using benchmarks gives nursing teams a relatively easy way to identify practices where performance can be improved, or where new initiatives can be introduced to help raise standards of care.

Health care organizations collect and report measures at various levels in the organization to assess and monitor outcomes.

Two examples of data collection and measuring performance at both the strategic and operational levels in the organization are a Balanced Scorecard and a Clinical Value Compass.

A **Balanced Scorecard** (Figure 12.4) is a tool used by hospital executive leadership to identify, track, and manage their strategy for achieving desired quality outcomes. The Balanced Scorecard reflects the hospital's mission, vision, and values. It usually has four perspectives: patient, financial, internal processes, and staff development and organizational culture. Health care quality improvement work should always be linked to the organization's mission, vision, and values.

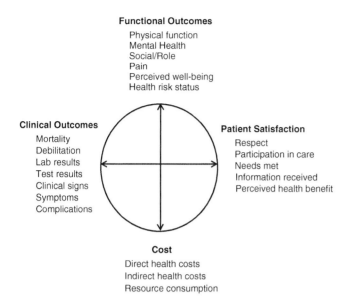

Functional Outcomes
Physical function
Mental Health
Social/Role
Pain
Perceived well-being
Health risk status

Clinical Outcomes
Mortality
Debilitation
Lab results
Test results
Clinical signs
Symptoms
Complications

Patient Satisfaction
Respect
Participation in care
Needs met
Information received
Perceived health benefit

Cost
Direct health costs
Indirect health costs
Resource consumption

FIGURE 12.5 Clinical value compass. Created by C. Wagner & C. Alexander with material from ClearPoint Strategy, 2018. https://www.clearpointstrategy.com/full-exhaustive-balanced-scorecard-example/

Data can be arranged to create a Balanced Scorecard in an approach that uses the organization's priorities as categories for quality indicators. For example, three priorities might be customer service, cost-effectiveness, and positive clinical outcomes. These priorities help sort out what should be measured to give a balanced view of whether a QI strategy is working. Quality indicators are selected based on what they have in common, so that if a change occurs in the cost-effectiveness category, it will affect the data in another category. For example, if we decrease cost for orthopedic surgery, does that affect the customer's satisfaction positively or negatively? If we decrease the LOS for these patients, does it increase or decrease complication rates? After quality indicators are selected, data are tracked over time at regular intervals, for example every month or every quarter. These quality indicators are utilized to monitor organizations' priorities. The goal is to assess that changing a strategy in one area does not negatively impact another quality indicator. For example, as an organization increases patient volume and reduces LOS, is there any change noted in the patient hospital readmission rate or patient satisfaction?

The implications of quality improvement for patient care can be measured by the overall value of care. **The Clinical Value Compass** is a visual tool for evaluating the balance or imbalance between patient clinical status, functional status, cost, and patient satisfaction outcomes. The Clinical Value Compass measures the overall value of care. The Clinical Value

Compass can efficiently communicate clinical, patient satisfaction, and economic endpoints of interest to patients, providers, and policy makers (Weinstein et al., 2014). For example, in the clinical setting, a plan of care may be medically appropriate, but may be inconvenient, unpleasant, unfeasible, and very costly to the patient. The Clinical Value Compass allows those reviewing data to examine all aspects of the plan of care and can help providers determine a course of treatment that is balanced, medically sound, and satisfying to the patient.

QI Is a Continuous Process

Improvement in quality of service is a continuous process. Walter Shewhart, the Director of Bell Laboratories in the mid-1920s, is credited with the concept of the cycle of continuous improvement. This concept suggests that products or services are designed and made based on knowledge about customer needs. The product or service is then marketed to and judged by the customer. Data is collected and evaluated about the product or service which leads to continued improvement. Hence, the process of QI is continuous, because it is linked to changing customer needs and judgments.

Simplification and Standardization

In addition to QI being a continuous process, QI focuses on simplification and standardization of work processes. Variation in a work process increases complexity, that is, too many steps in a work process increase variation opportunities and the risk of error. **Simplification** of work processes is the act of reducing a work process to its basic components. For example, the six rights of medication administration, that is, right patient, right medication, right dose, right route, right time, and right documentation, is a simplification of the work process needed to safely administer medications to patients. **Standardization** of a work process is the use of a single set of terms, definitions, practices and/or clinical tools in a work process. For example, the use of a Clinical Practice Guideline for the care of the patient with Type 2 diabetes mellitus is a standardized work process (Figure 12.6). Together, simplification and standardization improve health care quality and reduce risk.

See the complete list of U.S. Department of Veterans Affairs, VA/DoD Evidence-Based Clinical Practice Guidelines (2017) including Guidelines for Chronic Disease, Mental Health, Pain, Rehabilitation, Women's Health, etc. at, www.healthquality.va.gov/index.asp, accessed July 5, 2019.

Technology increasingly offers tools for standardization of work processes. For example, some electronic medical records use standard templates or forms for nursing assessment that

Case Study 12.2

Reread the opening scenario. Identify one patient outcome to measure in each of the four areas of the Clinical Value Compass, patient clinical status, functional status, cost, and patient satisfaction outcomes.

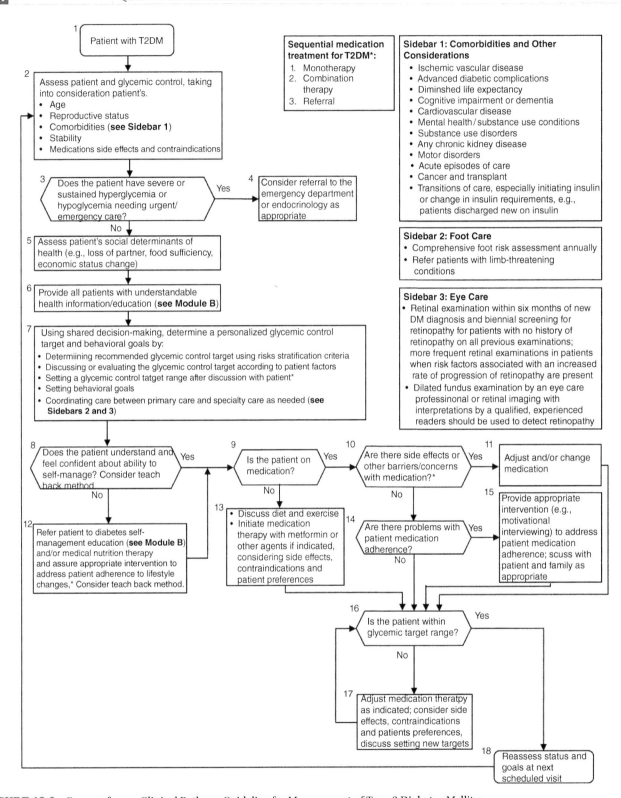

FIGURE 12.6 Excerpt from a Clinical Pathway Guideline for Management of Type 2 Diabetes Mellitus.
Source: Clinical Practice Guideline for the Management of Type 2 Diabetes Mellitus in Primary Care (2017). U.S. Department of Veterans Affairs and Department of Defense. Public Domain.

require certain fields be filled in before more information can be entered. As we increase the use of technology to further standardize work processes, we need to bear in mind the need to standardize the technology itself. For example, the Veterans Health Administration and the Department of Defense have collaborated for many years to improve the sharing of Veteran's patient information. One of the most challenging aspects of the work has been standardization of two very different

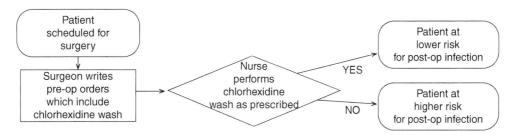

FIGURE 12.7   Example of a macro or high level flowchart. Created by C. Wagner & C. Alexander.

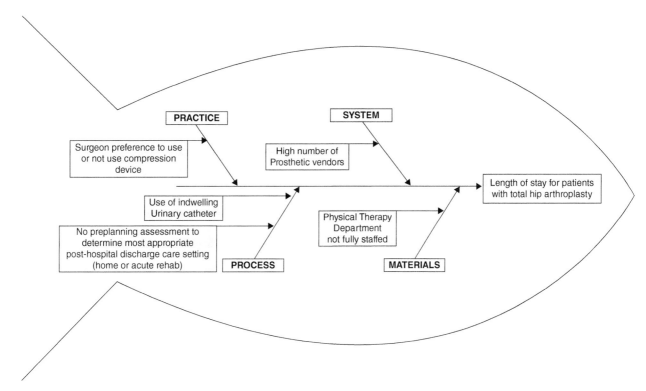

FIGURE 12.8   Fishbone diagram: length of stay for patients with total hip arthroplasty. Created by C. Wagner & C. Alexander.

Table 12.6   **Benchmark Sources**

Benchmark type and source	Data
Clinical: Agency for Healthcare Research and Quality https://nhqrnet.ahrq.gov/inhqrdr/National/benchmark/summary/Setting_of_Care/Hospital Accessed March 14, 2019	The National Healthcare Quality Report's quality measures specific to hospitals are compared to achievable benchmarks, which are derived from the top-performing States
Financial: Becker's Hospital Chief Financial Officer (CFO) Report www.beckershospitalreview.com/finance/65-financial-benchmarks-for-hospital-executives-022117.html accessed March 14, 2019	Financial benchmarks from a variety of sources are provided so hospital executives can compare their health care organization against local and regional competitors as well as national leaders.
Operational: ProPublica https://projects.propublica.org/emergency/state/DC Accessed March 14, 2019	Emergency Department average wait times are benchmarked with data from the Centers for Medicare and Medicaid Services.
Clinical, Financial, and Operational: Centers for Medicare and Medicaid Services (CMS) www.medicare.gov/hospitalcompare/search.html Accessed March 14, 2019	Information from over 4,000 Medicare-certified hospitals, including over 130 Veterans Administration (VA) medical centers, across the country, is compared in the following categories: patient experience, timely and effective care, complications and death, unplanned hospital visits, medical imaging, and payment and value of care.

Note. Compiled by C. Wagner & C. Alexander.

Critical Thinking 12.1

A group that was developing a simplified and standardized clinical pathway for the care of patients with acute myocardial infarction noted evidence showing that these patients should receive acetylsalicylic acid (ASA) before transferring from the Emergency Department if the patient did not receive it within 24 hr of arrival. The research in this area was very clear, and most providers believed this was being done. When a chart audit was performed to determine whether this was the practice on the Emergency Department, it was discovered that only 48% of the patients were receiving ASA within 24 hr of arrival or before transferring from the Emergency Department. The team added that patients with acute myocardial infarction should receive ASA before transfer from the ED to the inpatient unit if the patient did not receive it within 24 hr of arrival to the clinical pathway. After this was implemented, 85% of the patients received ASA before transfer from the ED to the unit if the patient did not receive it within 24 hr of arrival to the ED.

1. What clinical practices do you see on your clinical units that are based on an evidence-based clinical pathway?
2. How can you participate in improving the care of more patients using clinical pathways?

---

electronic medical records into one record that achieves seamless and accurate care coordination.

Standardization and evidence-based clinical guidelines are meant to communicate the latest evidence as to the best practice for a given patient problem. The use of large amounts of data with standardization can result in algorithms which can improve decision-making. Algorithms, such as Figure 12.6, are increasingly used by health care organizations to guide safe treatment decisions, improve diagnostic and treatment timeliness, efficiency and effectiveness, increase health care equity, and lower costs (Rajkomar, 2018). In the absence of evidence-based practices, consensus of the team should be used to develop algorithms and clinical guidelines. Simplified and standardized algorithms and guidelines must always be used with clinical judgment and individualized to individual patients.

The FOCUS Methodology and the Plan Do Study Act (PDSA) Cycle

Implementing methods for QI requires consideration of the environment of care, the data collection methodologies, and the response to the interpretation of the evidence. There are many ways to do QI. The FOCUS Methodology and the PDSA Cycle are two examples of methods for QI. Sometimes the PDSA Cycle is done within the FOCUS Methodology. Sometimes the PDSA Cycle is done alone. The decision to use the FOCUS Methodology and a PDSA Cycle or a PDSA Cycle alone is usually based on the size and scope of the process being improved.

FOCUS Methodology

The **FOCUS Methodology** is a standardized approach to problem-solving and QI that helps the health care team look at an entire process which has many dimensions. It describes in a stepwise way how to move through the QI process.

F: Find a work process to improve. This step asks, "What is the problem?" "What is the opportunity?" During this step, an improvement opportunity is articulated and data are obtained to support the hypothesis that an opportunity for improvement exists.

O: Organize a team that knows the work process. This step identifies a group of team members who are direct participants in the work process to be examined—the point-of-service staff. These team members are appointed to roles on the team, such as leader, coach/facilitator, timekeeper, and scribe.

C: Clarify what is happening in the current work process. A **flowchart**, which is a visual representation of the sequential steps of a work process, is very helpful for this (Figure 12.7). A detailed flowchart can be analyzed in two ways to uncover possible problems—at a macro or high level and at the micro or detailed level.

At the macro level, this flowchart usually has a few steps showing the major parts of a work process. It is commonly used at the beginning of a project to get an overview of the process. The macro flowchart is scanned for any indication that the work process is broken.

Red flags used to indicate problem areas on the macro flowchart include the following:

- Many steps that represent quality checks or inspections for errors. When you notice too many boxes in your flow diagram describing similar steps, this could indicate rework or lack of clarity in roles.

- Areas in the work process that are not well understood or cannot be defined. If the work process defies definition, you can be certain it is not being performed efficiently, with maximized outcomes. For example, in the macro flowchart in Figure 12.7, "The nurse performs chlorhexidine wash as prescribed," the diamond is a decision point. Either the action is completed or it is not. Why would a nurse not follow the order for the chlorhexidine wash? Does the nurse consider it low priority during a busy evening shift? Does the nurse understand the evidence-based rationale underlying this particular wash and its importance in preventing post-operative infections?

- Many wait times between work processes. Wait times should always be minimized to improve efficiency of the process.

- Multiple paths that show lots of people involved in the activity or delivering the service to the customer. Too many staff involved is wasteful and confusing to the patient.

If the existing work process seems reasonable on the macro flowchart, with only one or two areas needing improvement, then a micro or detailed level analysis of your work process in a micro flowchart is needed. For example, Figure 13.4 shows a micro flowchart of the process for transferring a patient from the Primary Care clinic to the inpatient unit. Refer to Figure 13.4 as you read about micro flowcharts.

The micro flowchart has many steps. As a result, the team is able to pinpoint specific problem areas. The team:

- Examines decision symbols (diamonds) that represent quality inspection activities. Examination of each of decision points by creating micro flowcharts will ensure maximum clarity in understanding the work process.

- Examines each step in the work process in the flowchart for redundancy and value. If a step in the work process is repeated or does not have any value for the patient, it should be eliminated.

- Examines all work processes for areas of wait time. The work process should be changed to eliminate these wait times.

- Examines all work processes for rework loops. A step in the work process should not be repeated. Resources are always limited, especially in hospitals today.

- Checks that all hand-offs are smooth and necessary. Hand-offs are times when a work process is handed from one staff person or department to another. Problems with hand-offs are a longstanding, common problem in health care.

U: Understand the degree of change needed. In this step, the team reviews what it knows. It looks at the variability and the capabilities of the work process. A fishbone or Ishikawa diagram can be helpful (Figure 12.8). A fishbone diagram is also called a cause-and-effect diagram. The team identifies the potential causes of a problem in order to understand its root causes. This is important when team members have different ideas about what is causing the problem in a work process. A fishbone diagram visually shows the team where change is needed and where they need to consolidate their improvement efforts.

The team then enhances its knowledge by reviewing the literature, available data, and competitive benchmarks. The health care organization's librarian is a valuable resource and can be helpful with the literature search. The team seeks to answer the question, "How can we improve and how are other health care organizations implementing the work process."

S: Select a solution for improvement. The team brainstorms and then choose the best solution. It can use the PDSA Cycle to test this solution (Table 12.7). A solution implementation plan should be used to track progress and the steps required. This implementation plan can be in the form of an action plan or Gantt chart, as shown in Figure 12.9. This action plan or Gantt chart is in the form of a table that identifies what activity is to be completed, who is responsible for it, and when is it going to be done. It outlines the steps needed to implement the change.

Plan Do Study Act (PDSA) Cycle The **PDSA Cycle** is a test of change on a small scale that examines the effect of one change on one aspect of a work process. The PDSA Cycle involves Planning a change, Doing the change, Studying the results of the change, and Acting on what is learned from the results of the change. In the Plan step, the team creates the structure for the test of change. They ask themselves what are we trying to improve, how will we know that a change is an improvement or what are we going to measure, and what

Table 12.7 PDSA Cycle

Plan	Plan a change that might result in improvement. Ask: • What are we trying to improve? • How will we know that a change is an improvement or what are we going to measure? • What changes can we make that might result in improvement? Identify: • Who will do what? • When they will do it? • Where they will do it? • How will data be collected?
Do	Do (Implement) the selected change.
Study	Study and analyze data and observations about the effect of the change. Determine if the change resulted in an improvement.
Act	Act to • Adopt the change, or • Adapt the change, or • Abandon the change.

Note. Created by C. Wagner & C. Alexander.

ACTION PLAN		STATUS	Green = On Schedule	Last Review Date: 1-Jun-19			
Unit: 3 West Medical			Yellow = Possible Delay	Coach: Susie Smith, Improvement Advisor			
			Red = Not on Schedule/Delayed	Ted Jones, RN, Infection Prevention			
Focus Area: Hand Hygiene			Blue = Completed	Team Lead: Advisor			
			Black = Canceled				
Opportunity/ Issue	Status	Actions Taken		Active Date	Estimated Completion Date	Actual Completion Date	Lead Responsible Point of Contact for Action Item
Less than 85% of the observed opportunities resulted in appropriate hand hygiene.		Education is being provided to all staff assigned to the unit, including per diem staff.		15-May-19	31-Jul-19		Jenny Smith, RN, Clinical Nurse Leader

FIGURE 12.9   Action plan for hand hygiene compliance improvement. Created by C. Wagner & C. Alexander.

changes can we make that might result in improvement? They then select a change that might result in improvement. The team identifies who will do what, when they will do it, where they will do it, and how data will be collected. In the Do step, the team implements the selected change following the who, what, when, where, and how structure identified in the Planning step. In the Study step, the team collects the data and observations about the effect of the change. They analyze the data and observations to determine if the change resulted in an improvement. In the Act step, several questions are asked and answered to guide further action. For example, will the proposed change be adopted for use without further change because the desired improvement occurred? Will the proposed change be adapted, meaning will there be another PDSA cycle to further refine the change and study the effect on improvement? Will the proposed change be abandoned since it did not lead to the improvement that was anticipated? The goal of repeated PDSA Cycles is to increase the amount of actual improvement.

For example, a cardiology team identifies a problem with readmissions within 30 days of hospital discharge for patients with heart failure at a rate higher than the benchmark rate. The team is concerned because the patients are being admitted through the ED with acute symptoms of fluid overload. The team also expresses concern because the cost of care for these patients is higher than the benchmark cost at similar sized hospitals. The team progresses through the FOCUS Methodology (Table 12.8) and then uses a PDSA Cycle (Figure 12.10) to improve the health care provided to patients with heart failure, which may also decrease the cost of care for the hospital.

STEEEP and Evaluation of a Health Care Organization's QI Program

Evaluation of a Health Care Organization's QI Program can be guided by measurement of the six domains of health care quality: **Safe, Timely, Effective, Efficient, Equitable, and Patient-Centered** (STEEEP) (Table 12.9).

Health care organizations pay for outside monitoring of their QI programs. For example, the cost of participation in The Joint Commission (TJC) monitoring program can range from

Table 12.8   FOCUS Methodology Used by a Cardiology Team

Find a process to improve.	Rates of hospital readmission within 30 days of discharge for patients with heart failure are higher than rates at benchmarked facilities. The team believes that by addressing a potential cause of acute fluid overload in patients with heart failure, ED visits and costs will decrease. Further analysis of the data, including medical record reviews, reveals inconsistent patient education about self-management of weight.
Organize a team that knows the work process.	Cardiology nurse practitioner, cardiologist, nurse from the unit that receives most of the heart failure patients, clinical dietician, clinical pharmacist, and the hospitalist will be on team.
Clarify what is happening in the work process.	The team creates a flowchart of the current patient discharge process.
Understand the degree of change needed.	The team collects data including what type of discharge education patients with heart failure are receiving, such as, education in an individual versus group setting, the date when education starts, the use of written and verbal methods of instruction, and so forth. The team discovers that patients are not being taught how to use their home scales for weight monitoring in a consistent manner.
Select what to improve.	The team decides to do a PDSA Cycle to see the effect on hospital readmissions within 30 days of discharge if patients with heart failure are taught how to monitor their weights in a standard way using an evidence-based check list.

Note. Created by C. Wagner & C. Alexander.

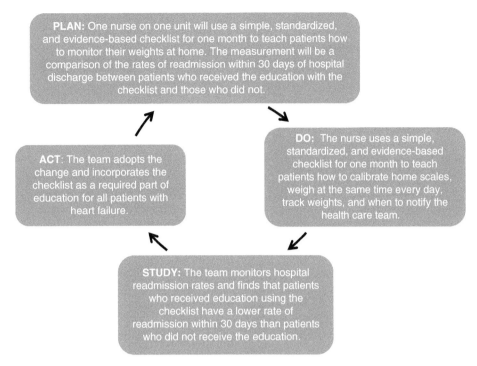

FIGURE 12.10   PDSA Cycle used by a cardiology team. Created by C. Wagner & C. Alexander.

Table 12.9   Six Domains of Health Care Quality (STEEEP) and Examples of QI Measures

Domain	Definition	Example of QI Measure
Safe	Avoid harm to patients from care that is intended to help them. The patient's safety comes first.	The hospital monitors medication errors for trends.
Timely	Reduce wait times and harmful delays for those who give care and those who receive care. Patient care will be delivered in the timeliest manner possible.	The organization monitors wait times for health care appointments.
Effective	Provide evidence-based services. Patient care will be based upon the best science available.	The organization regularly reviews and updates its procedures to assure they are effective.
Efficient	Avoid waste of equipment, supplies, ideas, and energy. Patient care will avoid waste of time, money, and resources.	The organization has a system to ensure that the right supply in the right quantities is delivered at the right time for a reasonable cost.
Equitable	Provide care that does not vary in quality because of personal characteristics such as gender, ethnicity, geographical location, and socioeconomic status. Access to care will be provided to all in an equitable manner.	The organization educates the staff about diversity so health care is provided to all patients in the same way.
Patient-centered	Provide care that is respectful and ensure that patient values guide all clinical decisions. Patients will participate fully in care decisions.	The organization teaches the staff how to include patients as a member of the health care team.

Source: Adapted from Agency for Healthcare Research and Quality (AHRQ), The Six Domains of Health Care Quality (2016), and Institute of Medicine (IOM) (2001).

about $8,500.00 to over $50,000, depending on the number of locations a health care organization has and the volume of individuals it serves (TJC, 2015). Some monitoring is required by state law, for example, monitoring of licensure. Some monitoring, for example by TJC or the **Commission on Accreditation of Rehabilitation Facilities** (CARF), is required by insurance companies before reimbursement contracts are signed. Other monitoring, for example, by Magnet or Baldrige programs, is

desired by health care organizations that wish to be recognized for their exemplary status as a professional work environment and provider of high-quality patient care. A health care organization's QI program is monitored at the local, state, and national levels. For example, local monitoring is done when the QI Department staff reviews the Department's structures, processes, and outcomes against the hospital's policies and procedures related to QI to determine the degree of compliance and identify any areas that need improvement. Balanced scorecards are also a form of local monitoring of the QI program and the effectiveness of its structures and processes. State level monitoring occurs during licensure surveys and site visits.

TJC has developed standards for patient safety and quality of care that guide the critical activities performed by health care organizations. TJC surveys occur about every 38 months and grant accreditation if the organization achieves the target levels of standards compliance. TJC does more frequent surveys if they learn of significant complaints or issues about health care delivery. Therefore, the cycle of readiness for survey is continuous when an organization commits to providing safe and effective health care of the highest quality and value. TJC makes data that health care organizations self-report about specific monitors available to the public (www.quality-check.org/ Accessed November 21, 2018).

Nurses participate in interprofessional hospital committees like Infection Control or Patient Safety. These committees continually monitor hospital performance to maintain adherence to TJC standards of practice. Nurses also participate with the interprofessional team in TJC site visit surveys, for example, when TJC surveyors ask nurses and the interprofessional team questions about how they implement hospital procedures that reflect TJC standards. If deficits are identified during the survey, such as lack of compliance with hand hygiene protocols, nurses and the interprofessional team participate in the development, implementation, and monitoring of action plans for improvement (Figure 12.8). If no deficits are identified during the survey, nurses and the interprofessional team can volunteer to participate in ongoing quality improvement activities that enhance patient outcomes.

United States federal regulations and national standards set by organizations such as the **Centers for Medicare and Medicaid Services** (CMS), the Joint Commission (TJC), and the **National Quality Forum** (NQF) require the development of clinical indicators of safe and competent care within the health care organization. Clinical indicators are sometimes called quality indicators. **Clinical indicators** are outcome data measured over time to assess the quality and safety of health care at a system level. Clinical indicators are publicly reported (Table 12.10). Due to the standardization of measurements and volume of data collected by the monitoring organizations,

Table 12.10   Monitoring Organizations, Clinical Indicators, and the Nurse

Monitoring organization	Clinical indicator	Example of how a nurse affects the clinical indicator
Centers for Medicare and Medicaid Services Public access to data. www.medicare.gov/HospitalCompare/Data/patient-and-caregiver-centered-experience-of-care-care-coordination-domain.html Accessed November 23, 2018	Patient- and caregiver-centered experience of care/care coordination.	The nurse explains things clearly, listens carefully, and treats the patient with courtesy and respect.
The Joint Commission Public access to data. www.qualitycheck.org/data-download accessed November 23, 2018	Hours of physical restraint use on older adults, age 65 or older.	The nurse follows the health care organization's restraint policy, including documentation requirements.
National Quality Forum Public access to data. www.qualityforum.org Accessed 11/23/2018	Documented patient falls with an injury level of minor or greater.	The nurse assesses each patient for fall risk and implements the organization's policy for fall-reduction.
Baldrige Public access www.nist.gov/sites/default/files/documents/2017/02/09/2017-2018-baldrige-excellence-builder.pdf Accessed November 23, 2018	The way an organization improves the quality of care provision through reduction of variability.	The nurse assures that all colleagues provide care using the organization's approved evidence-based standardized clinical practice guidelines
Magnet Member-only access www.nursingworld.org/organizational-programs/magnet Accessed November 23, 2018	Benchmarking structure and process of nurse-sensitive quality indicators at the unit level against a database at the highest/broadest level possible (i.e., national, state, specialty organization, regional, or system) to support quality improvement initiatives.	The nurse volunteers for a Hand Hygiene Improvement Team as the unit's Hand Hygiene Champion and ensures that graphs with benchmarked results are posted on the unit.
US News and World Reports Public access https://health.usnews.com/best-hospitals/area/mn/mayo-clinic-6610451/gastroenterology-and-gi-surgery accessed November 23, 2018	Fewer patient complications post-surgery.	The nurse initiates an improvement project to increase the number of patients who receive education on how to properly use chlorhexidine prior to surgery.

Note. Created by C. Wagner & C. Alexander.

Table 12.11   Monetary Impact of a Reduction in DRG Payment

DRG payment per inpatient care of a patient with heart failure (HF)	=	$14,631.00
Number of patients admitted with heart failure per year	=	× 96
Annual DRG payment for inpatient admissions of patients with HF	=	$1,404,576.00
1% reduction of DRG payment	=	−$14,045.76
Reduce annual DRG payment for inpatient care of 96 patients with HF	=	$1,348,392.96

Note. Created by C. Wagner & C. Alexander.

Evidence from the Literature

Source: Adapted from Salmond, S., & Eschevarria, M (2017). Healthcare Transformation and Changing Roles for Nursing. Orthopedic Nursing. January. 36(1): 12–25.

Discussion: This article discusses the role of the nurse in leading and being a fully contributing member of the interprofessional team as health care changes from episodic, provider-based, fee-for-service care to team-based, patient-centered care. Cost and quality concerns, the driving forces behind health care reform, are reviewed within an historical context, noting health care reimbursement is swiftly changing to value or outcome-based models where payment is linked to specified quality outcomes. Nursing practice must be dramatically different to deliver the expected level of quality care, including enhanced competencies in wellness and population care with a stronger focus on patient-centered care, care coordination, data analytics, and quality improvement.

Implications for Practice: It is critical for nurses to understand how health care reform impacts future nursing practice, and which skill sets are essential for nurses to be viable members and leaders of the health care team.

clinical indicators can also be benchmarked, or compared, between similar services in different health care systems or against national averages. Nurses who understand how clinical indicators reflect patient outcomes can more easily see the importance of QI in their daily work.

CMS requires eligible providers, eligible hospitals, and critical access hospitals organizations to report clinical indicators. CMS payment for services is based on achieving specific quality and cost outcomes. This is called **value-based payment** for health care services. For example, CMS will reduce the payments by 1% to a hospital with a total **hospital-acquired condition** (HAC) score greater than the 75th percentile of all total HAC scores (i.e., the worst-performing quartile) (Table 12.11). By tying the measuring and reporting of QI data to payment, CMS helps to ensure that our health care system is delivering Safe, Timely, Efficient, Equitable, and Patient-centered (STEEEP) care. CMS is the nation's largest health care insurer, and leads the way in innovative QI programs. For example, CMS has designed several initiatives to eliminate disparities in health care quality and access so that access to quality care is provided to all patients in an equitable manner (CMS, 2019b). Another CMS initiative is a patient-centered chronic care management program where the patient participates fully in care decisions by creating a personalized health care plan with help from their interprofessional health care team (CMS, 2019a). Expert assistance with setting and meeting health goals is part of patient-centered care. As a result, nurses can anticipate a future of increased interprofessional partnerships in planning and implementing continuous QI methods to understand, and at least meet, if not exceed, customer needs and expectations, and improve patient outcomes.

KEY CONCEPTS

- Quality improvement (QI) is important in health care for the patient, the nurse, and the organization.

- QI is a continuous process focused on maintaining regulatory compliance and improving patient care structures, processes, and outcomes.

- Patient preferences, values, and care needs should drive QI opportunities.

- The major principles of QI that are implemented in an organization include customer identification; the need for participation at all levels; and a focus on improving the process, not criticizing individual performance.

- The nurse who fully engages in QI and works to their full scope of practice is of greatest value to patients and the health care organization.

- An organization's mission, vision, and values should be communicated up and down the organizational hierarchy.

- Health care organizations use quality structures and quality processes to achieve quality outcomes.

- Customers of health care are patients, nurses, doctors, the community, and so on.

- Everyone in a health care organization is part of QI efforts.

- QI decisions should be driven by data.

- Different types of charts and graphs, e.g., Pareto charts, Pie charts, and time series data, are used to analyze QI data.

- Benchmarking resources are reviewed to monitor quality.

- QI work should be linked to the organization's mission, vision, and values.

- There should be a balance in QI goals focused on patient clinical status, functional status, cost, and patient satisfaction outcomes.

- QI focuses on improving work processes rather than criticizing individual performance.

- The FOCUS Methodology and the PDSA Cycle are used to improve quality in an organization.

- A Balanced Scorecard and a Clinical Value Compass are used to review quality in an organization.

- Systems for QI improve care in an organization continuously.

- QI focuses on simplification and standardization of work processes

- Patient care should meet the STEEEP principles, namely, Safe, Timely, Effective, Efficient, Equitable, and Patient-centered.

- Monitors of a health care organization's quality may include some or all of the following: The Joint Commission, state law, Commission on Accreditation of Rehabilitation Facilities, Magnet, and Baldrige.

KEY TERMS

Quality Improvement (QI)	Outcomes	Plan Do Study Act (PDSA) Cycle
Patient Satisfaction	Simplification	Flowchart
Patient Experience	Standardization	FOCUS Methodology
Team Huddle	Benchmarking	Clinical Value Compass
Structure	Balanced scorecard	Value-Based Payment
Process	Clinical indicator	

REVIEW QUESTIONS

1. Hospital QI programs are monitored at the local, state, and national levels using measurements. These measurements include which of the following? Select all that apply.
   a. The health care organization's proposed budget
   b. The balance of employee education with hospital values
   c. The comparison of actual work processes to hospital policies
   d. The collection of clinical outcomes
   e. The patient's satisfaction or dissatisfaction with health care

2. The nurse is orienting a new employee to the unit's QI program. Which one of the following best describes the primary goal of quality improvement?
   a. Continuous improving the quality and safety of health care systems
   b. Continuously reviewing past violations of clinical practices
   c. Involving the consumer in the decision-making process
   d. Continuously improving response time to health care requirements

3. The nurse is assigned to lead the benchmarking process for the QI team. Which of the following best describes the benchmarking process?
   a. Reviewing your own unit's data for opportunities to improve

   b. Collecting data on an individual patient to deploy small tests of change
   c. Reviewing data in the literature for evidence-based comparisons
   d. Comparing your data to that of other organizations to identify improvement opportunities

4. The nurse continues to teach new employees about QI. Who of the following are responsible for identifying QI opportunities in the health care area? Select all that apply.
   a. Hospital leadership
   b. Nurses and licensed clinicians
   c. Patients and their families
   d. All health care personnel
   e. Only designated staff

5. Standardizing a work process has which one of the following effects?
   a. It removes unwanted variation and all chance of error from a work process.
   b. It removes unwanted variation from a work process, decreasing risk for error.
   c. It increases complexity, because it is hard to communicate the standard to everyone.

d. It advocates for the same care for everyone regardless of individual differences.

6. The nurse is part of a QI team that has changed the way referrals are made for home care oxygen. What tool could be used to track the effect of changes in the referral process?
   a. Flowchart
   b. Pareto chart
   c. Time series chart
   d. Pie chart

7. A nurse has been assigned as leader for a team charged with decreasing the LOS for patients with **Chronic Obstructive Pulmonary Disease** (COPD). What actions by this nurse leader will help create a well-functioning team? Select all that apply.
   a. Designating a role for each member
   b. Ensuring that everyone understands the team purpose
   c. Using effective communication practices
   d. Preparing for each team meeting
   e. Including staff who are involved in the process on the team

8. Cost of care decreases with QI initiatives such as which of the following? Select all that apply.
   a. Standardizing care delivery work processes
   b. Applying evidence-based principles

c. Improving patient care outcomes
d. Maintaining continuous quality improvement surveillance
e. Benchmarking with other health care organizations

9. The patient says, "The nurses are very nice here, but I don't like it when they wake me up to give me medication." The patient is expressing which of the following?
   a. Patient satisfaction
   b. Patient experience
   c. Patient-centered care
   d. Clinical value of care

10. The nurse volunteers to participate on a team whose purpose is to improve transfers of patients from the ED to the inpatient units. Three aspects of the transfer process are being measured: the cost of keeping a patient in the emergency room, the effect on the patient's care when transfer to the unit is delayed, and the length of time to coordinate and complete transfers. What type of benchmarking will be done to provide the team with desirable target outcomes?
   a. Financial, Internal, Clinical
   b. Operational, Financial, Geographical
   c. Clinical, Financial, Operational
   d. Operational, Geographical, Financial

REVIEW QUESTION ANSWERS

1. Answers A, B, C, D, and E are correct.
   Rationale: The hospital's proposed budget (A) and the balance of employee educations with hospital values (B) are used locally in monitoring the QI program through the use of a balanced scorecard which uses four perspectives: patient, financial, internal processes, and staff development and organizational culture to identify, track, and manage their strategy for achieving desired quality outcomes. The hospital assesses if there is enough money in a proposed budget for achieving the desired level of quality patient health care. The hospital also evaluates if employee education, such as new-hire orientation, is aligned with hospital values, such as every employee participates in quality improvement. The comparison of actual processes to hospital policies (C) including those related to the hospital's QI program is monitoring done during the state survey for licensure. The collection of clinical outcomes (D), or clinical indicators, to monitor a hospital's QI program and its ability to provide safe and competent care within the health care organization is mandated for payment national organizations such as CMS. Patient satisfaction or dissatisfaction with health care (E) encompasses whether a patient's expectations about a health encounter were met and is measured nationally by such organizations as Press Ganey. Patient satisfaction or dissatisfaction is a monitor of a QI program, because it reflects the participation of staff at all levels of the health care organization in QI.

2. Answer: A is correct.
   Rationale: The goal of quality improvement is to use data to monitor outcomes and to test changes to improve the delivery of health care practices (A). QI's focus is on current outcomes of clinical care and does not review past violations of clinical

practices. Review of past violations of clinical practice (B) is done by risk management. Consumers can be involved in making decisions (C) related to care processes in order to get their input and points of view but their involvement is not the primary goal of QI. Improving response time to health care requirements (D) does not necessarily improve the delivery of health care practices.

3. Answer: D is correct.
   Rationale: Benchmarking is the continual and collaborative practice that measures and compares the results of key work processes with those of the best performers on a national scale to help improve patient and organizational outcomes, so you can compare your data to that of other organizations to identify improvement opportunities (D). Reviewing your own unit's data for opportunities to improve (A) is the PLAN step of the PDSA Cycle and the first step of the FOCUS methodology which is "Find a process to improve." Clinical benchmarking reviews grouped outcomes of patient care (i.e. patients who have had a stroke), not the data of an individual patient (B). Benchmarking helps organizations identify gaps in their performance and provide organizations with the data necessary to guide redesign of health care delivery. Benchmarking data is mathematically produced so that the data comparisons between health care organizations are equal. Data from the literature (C), even if it is evidence-based, does not guarantee mathematical accuracy when data is compared.

4. Answer: A, B, and D are correct.
   Rationale: Hospital leadership (A) is responsible for identifying QI opportunities through use of clinical, financial, and operational benchmarking, and the use of the hospital's balanced scorecard. The nurse and other licensed clinicians (B) are responsible for

identifying QI opportunities through observations made in their daily work and through comparisons with evidence-based literature. All health care personnel (D), not designated staff (E), are responsible for identifying QI opportunities in their daily work, since every one touches at least one work process in the health care organization. Patients and their families (C) can provide information about their satisfaction with the health care experience, but they are not responsible for identifying opportunities for QI.

5. Answer: B is correct.

Rationale: Standardization of a work process is use of a single set of terms, definitions, practices, and/or clinical tools in a work process. When work is standardized it decreases variation in the process and reduces the potential risk of error (B). Standardization does not guarantee the removal of all chance of error (A). Standardization reduces the complexity of a process by reducing the steps in the process (C). When care processes are standardized, patient care is still individualized based on the unique needs of the patient (D).

6. Answer: C is correct.

Rationale: The Time series chart (C) show data over a period of time. It allows QI team members to track the effects of changes in the referral process to study if a new process is more efficient. A flowchart (A) is a visual representation of the sequential steps of a work process. Pareto charts (B) group data in descending order to compare the most common problem to the least common problem. Pie charts (D) illustrate each segment of data as part of a whole to more easily view a proportional comparison of the data.

7. Answers A, B, C, D, and E are correct.

Rationale: The leader designates a role for each team member (A) to create the team's structure for QI work. The leader ensures everyone understands the team purpose (B) by discussing the problem and what the targeted improvement is so that the team is focused on a shared goal. The leader uses effective communication practices (C) to facilitate the team's collaboration. The leader prepares, that is, creates an agenda or process for each team meeting (D) so that meetings are productive and time is not wasted. When the team leader is prepared for the team meetings, the team knows the leader values them and their time. The leader includes staff who are involved in the process on the team (E), because these are the people who have the most knowledge of the work process and can quickly identify potential areas of improvement.

8. Answers A and C are correct.

Rationale: Standardizing care delivery work processes (A) reduces cost of care through the reduction of variation in a work process, for example, the hospital can stock one type of procedure kit rather than several different kinds. Improving patient outcomes (C) leads to decreased cost of care through reduced length of stay in inpatient units or reduced readmissions within 30 days of discharge for the same diagnosis, and reduced utilization of ambulatory care clinics. Evidence-based principles (B) reduce cost in most but not all QI efforts. Maintaining continuous quality improvement surveillance (D) helps the health care facility find where gains made in improvement work have or have not been sustained, and can increase cost of care due to the additional time needed for surveillance and follow-up activity. Benchmarking (E) helps a health care organization understand where there may be gaps in care and areas for improvement but does not alone reduce cost of care.

9. Answer: A is correct.

Rationale: Patient satisfaction (A) encompasses how patients feel about the health care they receive and whether a patient's expectations about a health encounter were met. Patient experience encompasses all the interactions that patients have with the health care system and shows whether patients are receiving care that is respectful of and responsive to their needs (B). Patient-centered care (C) is recognizing the patient or designee as the source of control. The clinical value of care (D) is visualized by a Clinical Value Compass, which is a visual tool for evaluating the balance or imbalance between patient clinical and functional status, cost, and patient satisfaction outcomes.

10. Answer: C is correct.

Rationale: Clinical, financial, and operational benchmarks will provide the team with desirable target outcomes. Clinical benchmarking reviews group outcomes of patient care (i.e. patients who have had a stroke). Financial benchmarking examines cost/case charges and length of stay. Operational benchmarking reviews the health care systems that support care, for example, the case management system in an organization. Internal benchmarking (A) will not provide comparisons with outside high-quality health care organizations. Geographical benchmarking (B and D) refers to selecting health care organizations in physical proximity for comparison to your hospital, not to the specific target outcomes.

REVIEW ACTIVITIES

1. Risk management, infection control practitioners, and a benchmark study have revealed that your unit's utilization of indwelling urinary catheters is above average. Brainstorm reasons and categorize why this may be occurring. Create a fishbone diagram to help with this.

2. After you have identified possible causes for the overuse of indwelling urinary catheters, use the PDSA Cycle to identify improvement strategies.

3. Think about your last clinical rotation experience. Identify one work process that you believe could be improved, and describe how you would begin improving the process. Use the FOCUS Methodology.

DISCUSSION POINTS

1. During your last clinical experience, were there any posters or graphs on the wall of the unit that explained their quality initiatives?

2. Which of the four key roles of nursing, that is professional, advocate, innovator, collaborative leader, would you feel most comfortable demonstrating in an interprofessional meeting as a staff nurse?

3. What appeals to you about any of the QI methods in this chapter?

4. During your last clinical experience, did the organization support nursing engagement in QI activities?

DISCUSSION OF OPENING SCENARIO

1. If you were a staff nurse on the QI team, how would you encourage the decreased use of postoperative indwelling catheters?

   Discussion: As a staff nurse, you will want to collect data about the patients who had a catheter inserted after surgery. Specifically, you would want to gather information about the patient population, age, gender, and overall health status of the patients. For example, the team may find after investigating that there is a higher incidence of catheter insertion in patients over 65 years old. You may also want to suggest that the QI team collect data regarding the time of day the catheter is placed (night shift vs day shift), who placed the catheter, and what health care provider wrote the order.

2. How could you bring your ideas to other staff members without making them feel that the quality of their care was being criticized?

   Discussion: Interprofessional staff engagement is a key component of quality improvement work. Collaborate with a member of the medical staff, as the physicians write the orders for urinary catheter insertion. Start the process by sharing comparison data (benchmark vs hospital data) with all the team to identify where the gaps in care are. Find opportunities to share best practices found in the literature and explain why and how use of catheters may contribute to infections, longer hospitalizations, and potentially poorer outcomes for patients. Use opportunities to share information at staff meetings or daily huddles. Use social media such as twitter to post articles of interest for staff. Be sure to support the interprofessional team and recall that change can be difficult.

3. If you were a staff nurse not on the improvement team, how could you support the efforts of the QI team?

   Discussion: The nurse can ask improvement team members to communicate relevant information about the improvement project. This communication could happen during staff meetings, lunch-and-learn sessions, or by posting PDSAs and data graphs on the unit. The nurse can use team huddles, patient care rounds, or shift report to discuss this improvement strategy being used in patient care. Ongoing collaboration with members of the improvement team is an important way to ensure best practices are implemented.

EXPLORING THE WEB

- Institute for Healthcare Improvement (IHI), www.ihi.org (accessed November 4, 2018)

- HealthGrades, www.healthgrades.com/quality/hospital-ratings-awards (accessed November 4, 2018)

- National Guideline Clearinghouse: www.guideline.gov (accessed November 4, 2018)

- American Nurses Credentialing Center (ANCC) Magnet Recognition Program, www.nursingworld.org/organizational-programs/magnet (accessed December 10, 2018)

- Substance Abuse and Mental Health Services Administration-Health Resources and Services Administration (SAMHSA-HRSA) Center for Integrated Health Solutions, www.integration.samhsa.gov/search?q=quality+process+toolkit (accessed December 12, 2018)

- The Joint Commission: www.jointcommission.org (accessed November 4, 2018)

- Commission on Accreditation of Rehabilitation Facilities (CARF), www.carf.org/home (accessed November 4, 2018)

INFORMATICS

1. Go to the Commission on Accreditation of Rehabilitation Facilities (CARF) site, www.carf.org/home (accessed November 4, 2018). Search the "Promising Practices" section for ways that technology can be used to enhance health care service delivery.

2. Review the Constructive Feedback Power Point at qsen.org/giving-and-receiving-constructive-feedback (accessed November 4, 2018)

Identify a difference between what you observed in nursing care on your assigned unit and what you have been taught as a nursing student. Select a QI strategy from Slide 19 "Strategies" that you could use to lead any need for change improvement. Why do you think this strategy will work?

LEAN BACK

- How does this information about QI impact you today as a student nurse?

- How do you see it impacting you as a graduate nurse?

REFERENCES

Abrampah, N. A., Syed, S. B., Hirschhorn, L. R., Nambiar, B., Iqbal, U., Garcia-Elorrio, E., Chattu, V. K., Devnani, M., & Kelley, E. (2018). Quality improvement and emerging global health priorities. *International Journal for Quality in Health Care, 30*(1), 5–9. doi:10.1093/intqhc/mzy007

Agency for Healthcare Research and Quality (AHRQ). (2017.-a). *Daily huddle component kit.* Content last reviewed June 2017. Rockville, MD: Agency for Healthcare Research and Quality. Retrieved from www.ahrq.gov/professionals/quality-patient-safety/hais/tools/ambulatory-surgery/sections/sustainability/management/huddles-compkit.html

AHRQ. (2016). *The six domains of health care quality.* Rockville, MD: Agency for Healthcare Research and Quality. Retrieved from www.ahrq.gov/professionals/quality-patient-, afety/talkingquality/create/sixdomains.html

AHRQ. (2017-b). *Toolkit for using the AHRQ quality indicators.* Content last reviewed March 2017. Rockville, MD: Agency for Healthcare Research and Quality. Retrieved from www.ahrq.gov/professionals/systems/hospital/qitoolkit/index.html

Baker, K., & Williams, T. E. (2016). Overview and summary: Elimination of barriers to RN scope of practice: Opportunities and challenges. *The Online Journal of Issues in Nursing, 21*(3). Retrieved from http://ojin.nursingworld.org/MainMenuCategories/ANAMarketplace/ANAPeriodicals/OJIN/TableofContents/Vol-21-2016/No3-Sept-2016.aspx

Batalden, P. B., & Davidoff, F. (2007). What is "quality improvement" and how can it transform healthcare? *BMJ Quality & Safety, 16,* 2–3. doi:10.1136/qshc.2006.022046

Centers for Medicare and Medicaid Services (CMS). (2019a). *Connected care: The chronic care management resource.* Retrieved from www.cms.gov/About-CMS/Agency-Information/OMH/equity-initiatives/chronic-care-management.html

Centers for Medicare and Medicaid Services (CMS). (2019b). *Equity initiative.* Retrieved from www.cms.gov/About-CMS/Agency-Information/OMH/equity-initiatives/index.html

Centers for Medicare and Medicaid Services (CMS). (2019c). *Hospital consumer assessment of healthcare providers and systems.* Retrieved from www.medicare.gov/hospitalcompare/search.html

Department of Veterans Affairs and Department of Defense. (2017). *VA/DoD clinical practice guideline for the management of type 2 diabetes mellitus in primary care.* Retrieved from www.healthquality.va.gov/guidelines/CD/diabetes/VADoDDMCPGFinal508.pdf

Institute of Medicine (IOM). (2001). *Crossing the quality chasm: A new health system for the 21st century.* Washington, DC: National Academy Press. Retrieved from www.ncbi.nlm.nih.gov/books/NBK222274

Institute of Medicine (IOM). (2010). *Report: The future of nursing; leading change, advancing health.* Retrieved from www.iom.edu/Reports/2010/The-Future-of-Nursing-Leading-Change

International Council of Nurses. (2015). *Nurses: A force for change.* Geneva, Switzerland: International Council of Nurses.

Lucatorto, M. A., Thomas, T. W., & Siek, T. (2016). Registered nurses as caregivers: Influencing the system as patient advocates. *The Online Journal of Issues in Nursing, 21*(3). Retrieved from http://ojin.nursingworld.org/MainMenuCategories/ANAMarketplace/ANAPeriodicals/OJIN/TableofContents/Vol-21-2016/No3-Sept-2016

Lucco, J. (2018). A Full & Exhaustive Balanced Scorecard Example. retrieved from https://www.clearpointstrategy.com/full-exhaustive-balanced-scorecard-example/

McAllen, E. R., Stephens, K., Swanson-Biearman, B., Kerr, K., & Whiteman, K. (2018). Moving shift report to the bedside: An evidence-based quality improvement project. *The Online Journal of Issues in Nursing, 23*(2). Retrieved from http://ojin.nursingworld.org/MainMenuCategories/ANAMarketplace/ANAPeriodicals/OJIN/TableofContents/Vol-23-2018/No2-May-2018.aspx

Moore, L., Lavoie, A., Bourgeois, G., & Lapointe, J. (2015). Donabedian's structure-process-outcome quality of care model: Validation in an integrated trauma system. *Journal of Trauma and Acute Care Surgery, 78*(6), 1168–1175. Retrieved from www.ncbi.nlm.nih.gov/pubmed/26151519

National Academies of Sciences, Engineering, and Medicine. (2016). *Assessing progress on the Institute of Medicine report: The future of nursing.* Washington, DC: The National Academies Press.

New Jersey Hospital Association. (2017). *Partnership for patients-NJ 2012-2016 progress report.* Retrieved from www.njha.com/media/405402/P4P-Report-2017.pdf

Press Ganey. (2019). *HCAHPS regulatory survey.* Retrieved from www.pressganey.com/solutions/service-a-to-z/hcahps-regulatory-survey

QSEN Institute. (2019). *Pres-licensure KSAs: Quality improvement.* Retrieved from http://qsen.org/competencies/pre-licensure-ksas

Rajkomar, A., Oren, E., Chen, K., Dai, A. M., Hajaj, N., Hardt, M., Lui, P., Xiaobing, L., Marcus, J., Sun, M., Sunberg, P., Yee, H., Zhang, K., Zhang, Y., Flores, G., Duggan, G., Irvine, J., Le, Q., Litsch, K., Mossin, A., Tansuwan, J., Wang, Wexler, J., Wilson, J. Lidwig, D., Volchenboum, S., Chou, K., Pearson, M., Madabushi, S., Shah, N., Butte, A., Howell, M., Cui, C., Corrado, J. & Dean, J. (2018). Scalable and accurate deep learning with electronic health records. *Npj Digital Medicine, 1*(1). doi:10.1038/s41746-018-0029-1.

Salmond, S., & Eschevarria, M. (2017). Healthcare transformation and changing roles for nursing. *Orthopedic Nursing, 36*(1), 12–25.

Sfantou, D., Laliotis, A., Patelarou, A., Sifaki-Pistolla, D., Matalliotakis, M., & Patelarou, E. (2017). Importance of leadership style towards quality of care measures in healthcare settings: A systematic review. *Healthcare, 5*(4). doi:10.3390/healthcare5040073

Stausmire, J. M., & Ulrich, C. (2015). Making it meaningful: Finding quality improvement projects worthy of your time, effort, and expertise. *Critical Care Nurse, 35*(6), 57–62.

Sullivan, M., Kiovsky, R. D., Mason, D. J., Hill, C. D., & Dukes, C. (2015). Interprofessional collaboration and education: Working together to ensure excellence in health care. *American Journal of Nursing*, *115*(3), 47–53.

The Joint Commission. (2015). *Fee examples*. Retrieved from www.jointcommission.org/assets/1/6/Fee_examples.pdf

Weinstein, J. N., Tosteson, A. N., Tosteson, T. D., Lurie, J. D., Abdu, W. A., Mirza, S. K., Zhao, W., Morgan, T. S., & Nelson, E. C. (2014). The SPORT value compass: Do the extra costs of undergoing spine surgery produce better health benefits? *Medical Care*, 52(12), 1055–1063.

SUGGESTED READINGS

Bender, M. (2017). Clinical nurse leader–integrated care delivery: An approach to organizing nursing knowledge into practice models that promote interprofessional, team-based care. *Journal of Nursing Care Quality*, *32*(3), 189–195.

Braithwaite, J., Hibbert, P., Blakely, B., Plumb, J., Hannaford, N., Hannaford, N., Long, J. C., & Marks, D. (2017). Health system frameworks and performance indicators in eight countries: A comparative international analysis. *SAGE Open Medicine*. doi:10.1177/2050312116686516

Cleary, P. D. (2016). Evolving concepts of patient-centered care and the assessment of patient care experiences: Optimism and opposition. *Journal of Health, Politics and Policy Law*, *41*(4), 675–696.

Donabedian, A. R. (2003). *An introduction to quality assurance in health care.* New York: Oxford University Press.

Hirschhorn, L. R., Ramaswamy, R., Devnani, M., Wandersman, A., Simpson, L. A., & Garcia-Elorrio, E. (2018). Research versus practice in quality improvement? Understanding how we can bridge the gap. *International Journal for Quality in Health Care*, *30*(1), 24–28. doi:10.1093/intqhc/mzy018 2018

Magalhães, A. L. P., Erdmann, A. L., da Silva, E. L., & dos Santos, J. L. G. (2016). Lean thinking in health and nursing: An integrative literature review. *Revista Latino-Americana de Enfermagem*, *24*, e2734. doi:10.1590/1518-8345.0979.2734

Moore, J., Everly, M., & Bauer, R. (2016). Multigenerational challenges: Team-building for positive clinical workforce outcomes. *The Online Journal of Issues in Nursing*, *21*(2). Retrieved from http://ojin.nursingworld.org/MainMenuCategories/ANAMarketplace/ANAPeriodicals/OJIN/TableofContents/Vol-21-2016.aspx

Ogrinc, G., Davies, L., Goodman, D., Batalden, P., Davidoff, F., & Stevens, D. (2016). SQUIRE 2.0 (Standards for QUality Improvement Reporting Excellence): Revised publication guidelines from a detailed consensus process. *Journal of Nursing Care Quality*, *31*(1), 1–8.

Ryan, R. W., Harris, K. K., Mattox, L., Singh, O., Camp, M., & Shirey, M. R. (2015). Nursing leader collaboration to drive quality improvement and implementation science. *Nursing Administration Quarterly*, *39*(3), 229–238.

13 Improving Quality at the Bedside

Christine Rovinski Wagner[1], Catherine C. Alexander[2]

[1]Office of Veterans Access to Care, Veterans Health Administration, Washington, DC, USA
[2]Department of Community & Family Medicine, Dartmouth-Hitchcock, Lebanon, NH, USA

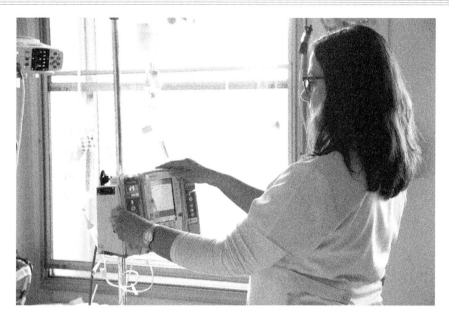

Nursing practice decisions culminate in quality health care.
Source: Regina Summermatter

Good, better, best. Never let it rest, until your good is better and your better is best.

Source: Childhood saying from C. Wagner & C. Alexander.

OBJECTIVES

Upon completion of this chapter, the reader should be able to:

1. Discuss how the daily work of the nurse uses **Quality Improvement** (QI) competencies at the bedside, on the unit, and in the organization to fulfill the nurse's professional role.

2. Explain the skills needed by the nurse to do QI including self-awareness, ability to work as a collaborative team member, ability to work as a nurse leader, and the ability to manage crucial conversations with the interprofessional team.

3. Choose behaviors that support interprofessional collaboration in QI work.

4. Explain the process and rationale for deciding who should be included on QI teams.

5. Identify structure and process resources needed to generate outcomes and meet or surpass benchmarks in clinical practice.

6. Apply the QI processes of the **Plan Do Study Act** (PDSA) Cycle and the **Find-Organize-Clarify-Understand-Select** (FOCUS) methodology to implement **Evidence-Based Practice** (EBP) in specific patient situations.

7. Discuss how to use QI tools such as the fishbone diagram, the affinity diagram, and **Specific, Measurable, Achievable, Realistic, and Timely** (SMART) goals.

Kelly Vana's Nursing Leadership and Management, Fourth Edition. Edited by Patricia Kelly Vana and Janice Tazbir
© 2021 John Wiley & Sons Ltd. Published 2021 by John Wiley & Sons Ltd.
Companion Website: www.wiley.com/go/kelly-Nursing-Leadership

OPENING SCENARIO

It's a busy morning on the medical surgical unit. All of the beds are occupied. You are participating in patient rounds with the interprofessional team. You learn that one of your patients, Mr. Sullivan, is going to be discharged in the afternoon. He is a newly diagnosed diabetic and will need education about his insulin, as well as coordination of home health services. You contact the continuity of care nurse to help with the discharge. While you are on the phone with the continuity of care nurse, the charge nurse interrupts to say there is an unexpected admission coming in from the primary care clinic. The Primary Care Clinic reports the patient had chest pain while doing yard work, is denying any pain now, and has stable vital signs. The patient is being admitted for observation. The nurse manager tells you the only open bed will be Mr. Sullivan's and you will be admitting the patient once Mr. Sullivan leaves. You acknowledge the assignment but know there is a lot to do before the Mr. Sullivan is ready to go home. Despite your best efforts, his discharge has been delayed until mid-afternoon.

As the day goes on the charge nurse keeps asking when the bed will be available. The nurse from the Primary Care Clinic is calling repeatedly. The new patient is in the Primary Care Clinic waiting room and getting increasingly anxious. At 2 p.m., you let the charge nurse know that Mr. Sullivan has been discharged and the room is being cleaned. The charge nurse tells you that the patient had a cardiac arrest while waiting to be admitted. Despite the Code Team's interventions, the patient died.

You are bothered by the patient's death and feel the need to do something. You decide to meet with the nurse manager to discuss the case and how the situation could have been handled differently. The nurse manager appreciates your concern and tells you that the hospital's risk manager has talked to the primary care staff, started to review the existing medical record documentation, and the facility's transfer and handoff protocols. Hospital leadership has also sent a notice effective immediately that all patients who complain of chest pain or have a possible heart attack who are waiting for admission to an inpatient unit from the Primary Care Clinic will be sent to the Emergency Department until there is an open bed on the inpatient unit. The nurse manager also asks if you would be willing to participate in a root cause analysis. The nurse manager reminds you that a root cause analysis examines adverse patient outcomes or near misses that could negatively affect patient safety. The nurse manager also tells you that root cause analyses do not blame people but look for ways to improve health care work processes to avoid harm to patients.

Several days later, you are invited to be part of the root cause analysis team. The team creates a flow chart from the patient coming in for his primary care appointment to when he died in the waiting room. Examination of the completed flow chart reveals that the patient handoff from the clinic to the patient care unit could be improved. You learned in school that patient handoff is an important link in making sure patients are safe. You volunteer to lead a quality improvement project focused on patient handoffs.

1. Who would you ask to participate on the QI team?

2. How will you know what changes can be made in the process of patient handoff that will result in an improvement in care?

3. How will you know that the process of handoff from the primary care clinic to the inpatient unit has been improved?

Quality improvement (QI) is the use of data to monitor the outcomes of care processes and use improvement methods to design and test changes to continuously improve the quality and safety of health care systems (QSEN Institute, 2018). It is easy to think about QI as something apart from the work a nurse does every day in a health care organization. There is a QI department with staff that is dedicated to making sure the health care organization demonstrates quality improvement in all services including nursing. While the ultimate responsibility for QI in nursing is delegated to the Nurse Executive, you have a duty to make nursing practice decisions that culminate in safe, quality, and evidence-based health care (Bickford, Marion, & Gazaway, 2015).

This chapter will discuss how the nurse uses QI at the bedside, on the unit and in the organization to fulfill the nurse's professional role. The skills needed by the nurse to improve quality at the bedside, including self-awareness, ability to work as a collaborative team member and as a nurse leader, and the ability to manage crucial conversations with the interprofessional team will be illustrated. Behaviors that support interprofessional collaboration in QI work will be reviewed. The process and rationale for deciding who to include on a QI team will be discussed. Structure and process resources that are needed to generate outcomes and surpass benchmarks in clinical practice will be identified. The QI processes of the PDSA Cycle and the FOCUS methodology will be demonstrated. QI tools such as the fishbone diagram and the affinity diagram, and SMART goals will be reviewed and illustrated.

QI is Part of the Nurse's Work at the Bedside

QI is fundamental to the nurse's daily work. The nurse reports to work knowing that the goal or outcome that is desired for each patient is to get the right care at the right time in the right way in the right place. For this to happen, the right patient care structures and processes must be in place. Quality patient care structures that must be in place include a unit layout that is safe for patients, food service and medication delivery that is timely, good staffing, good computers, etc. Once on duty, the nurse receives and reviews assignments. Planning has begun. Patient information is received from nurses going off duty. Personnel resources, such as nursing assistants, are allocated for the work process. The work process is organized and delegated. The day's schedule is modified for attendance at staff huddles, committee meetings, and staff development programs. Nursing care, in collaboration with other health care staff, is provided to patients. Nurses are the primary providers of clinical care. They are a constant bedside presence and have stewardship as well as legal and ethical responsibility for the patient's safety and high-quality care outcomes. Throughout the shift, the nurse assesses the outcomes of care for each patient. The nurse provides this information to interprofessional team members so that decisions can be made to continue the same care, improve the care, or change the care totally. When necessary, the nurse consults with the interprofessional team members and the nursing supervisor and uses the chain of command to assure quality care for patients and avoid hospital acquired negative outcomes. The daily work of a competent and respected nurse, which includes QI, patient-centered care, interprofessional teamwork and collaboration, EBP, and safety, and informatics, is a series of PDSA Cycles (Figure 13.1).

QI is Part of the Nurse's Work as a Team Member on the Unit

The structure of professional development combined with the processes in professional socialization leads to an outcome where the nurse's work is animated by quality improvement. (Table 13.1). A nurse has a professional responsibility to continually monitor patient outcomes, assess the unit's climate and needs, structures, and processes, and identify areas for outcome improvement personally and in concert with co-workers. For example, if infections increase on the unit, a nurse can highlight the need for a QI project. The nurse will contribute to planning and implementing unit changes. Perhaps the communication flow on the unit is erratic. The nurse could partner with others on the unit to create a standardized method of communicating new or changed policies, available continuing education, and training opportunities. Nurses also provide input into front-line decision making and QI by joining unit-based QI councils (Needleman et al., 2016).

The National Database of Nursing Quality Indicators (NDNQI®)

The **National Database of Nursing Quality Indicators** (NDNQI) is a voluntary database of unit-specific quality indicators that are directly related to nursing care, including nursing satisfaction with job and work environment (Table 13.2) (National Database of Nursing Quality Indicators, 2011). If your health care organization participates in NDNQI's RN Survey, you and your colleagues can use the data to assess your unit's quality outcomes to identify areas for improvement.

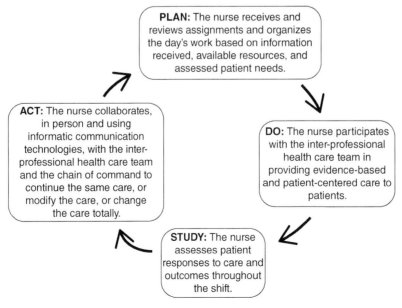

FIGURE 13.1   Daily work of a nurse as a PDSA Cycle. Created by C. Wagner & C. Alexander.

Table 13.1   Structures, Processes, and Outcomes that Develop Nursing Engagement in QI

	Definition	Example of a how a Nurse Engages in QI
Structure	The physical and organizational characteristics of a hospital such as its buildings, patient care units, human resources, financing, and equipment that support the process of nursing care.	Have professional library available. Offer continuing education courses. Utilize structures on unit that support quality patient outcomes, e.g., informatics, sterile equipment, etc. Offer funding of courses for advanced degree or specialized certification. Have guideline for your unit's specific QI plan. Have clear chain of command guideline for staff use.
Process	The series of actions, steps, and decisions that interact to produce a professional nursing outcome.	Use Evidence-based Practice (EBP) guidelines in daily work. Have clear policies and procedures. Be a role model in discussion and application of EBP. Attend interprofessional clinical rounds. Ask questions when patient care processes appear incomplete or need clarification. Speak up about discrepancies in patient care. Be aware of your unit's issues and priorities.
Outcome	The end result of work structures and processes.	Monitor patient outcomes and identify need for QI. . Identify and champion potential QI projects such as monitoring nurse-sensitive patient outcomes such as pain management or hospital-acquired pressure ulcers. Deliver a presentation to nursing students about the unit's QI activities, incorporating use of the national "Partnering to Heal" program to prevent hospital-acquired infections (https://health.gov/hcq/training-partnering-to-heal.asp accessed February 18, 2019).

Source: Created by C. Wagner & C. Alexander.

Table 13.2   Examples of Data on the NDNQI RN Survey:

- Patient falls with injury
- Unit-acquired Pressure Ulcers
- Restraints prevalence
- Healthcare-associated infections:
  - Ventilator-Associated Pneumonia (VAP)
  - Central Line-Associated Blood Stream Infection (CLABSI)
  - Catheter-Associated Urinary Tract Infections (CAUTI)

Source: Adapted from NDNQI: Transforming.
Data into Quality Care. Retrieved at http://public.qualityforum.org/action-registry/Lists/List%20of%20Actions/Attachments/141/NDNQIBrochure.pdf?Mobile=1 Accessed April 27, 2019.

The NDNQI RN Survey measures nursing's contribution to quality care and positive patient outcomes. Your unit can be compared to similar health care organizations and benchmarked against all participating health care organizations nationally. The benchmark data is only available to organization's that are members of NDNQI. You and your colleagues can develop and implement a targeted intervention based on the initial assessment, evaluate the effectiveness of the intervention using subsequent reports, and retain or adapt the intervention to improve your work environment (Lockhart, 2018). Selected NDNQI indicators are monitored on the Press Ganey patient satisfaction and experience surveys (Table 13.3) also. Press Ganey is a well-regarded consulting firm that uses integrated data, advanced analytics, and strategic advisory services to help health care organizations improve the quality, safety, and experience of their patients.

The Centers for Medicare and Medicaid (CMS) Hospital Value-Based Purchasing Program

The **Centers for Medicare and Medicaid (CMS)** adjusts payments to hospitals based on the quality of care that the

Table 13.3   Press Ganey Patient Experience Survey Questions

Degree to which your provider talked to you in words you could understand.

Concern your provider showed for your worries and concerns.

Care provider's efforts to include you in decisions about your treatment.

Amount of time your care provider spent with you.

Source: Adapted from material from University of Utah (2018).
Retrieved from https://healthcare.utah.edu/fad/pressganey.php Accessed April 27. 2019.

Real World Interview

I became involved with quality improvement following my sophomore year in nursing school. We learned about **Quality and Safety Education in Nursing** (QSEN) in one of my sophomore level nursing classes and I became interested. I wanted to make a difference and have a voice in the world of health care as a nursing student. I contacted Dr. Mary Dolansky, a national nurse leader in QI education and practice. She was supportive and together we created QStudent (http://qsen.org/category/qs accessed December 16, 2018), a portion of QSEN that is directed toward nursing students. The goal of QStudent is to get students involved earlier in QI and create more competent quality-focused nurses.

Rachel Jalowiec, BSN, RN-BC
Ridgeville, Ohio

hospitals deliver to patients. Under their Hospital Value-Based Purchasing Program, CMS holds back 2% of a hospital's diagnostic related group payment. The hospital can earn back none, some, all, or more than the 2% based on their performance in quality measures, which include patient experience, in such areas as communication with nurses and responsiveness of staff. Communication with nurses is measured as the percentage of patients who reported that their nurses "Always" communicated well. This means nurses explained things clearly, listened carefully, and treated the patient with courtesy and respect. Responsiveness of staff is measured as the percentage of patients who reported that hospital staff were "Always" responsive to their needs. This means the patient was helped quickly when he or she used the call button or needed help in getting to the bathroom or using a bedpan. All of the quality measures can be accessed at www.medicare.gov/HospitalCompare/Data/patient-and-caregiver-centered-experience-of-care-care-coordination-domain.html, accessed July 16, 2019.

QI is Part of the Nurse's Work as an Employee of a Health Care Organization

A nurse must be aware of the health care organization's efforts to deliver quality health care to patients. The health care organization's mission, vision, goals, and strategies play a pivotal role in whether or not structures, processes, and outcomes of QI projects will be successful. Leadership must be open to admitting that its health care structures and processes can be improved, and willing to take steps to improve and allocate the necessary resources. Without support from leadership, staff nurses and hospital employees are less likely to be dedicated to the improvement of patient care. Organizational support and the availability of hospital resources and dedicated staff together are the most important contributions to a successful QI culture. A nurse can influence QI culture through participation in a health care organization's shared governance council. The nurse can advocate for the necessary elements to support quality patient outcomes, including the health care organization's involvement in national improvement campaigns such as the **Hospital Engagement Network** (HEN) (Foster, Kenward, Hines, & Maulik, 2017). The HEN is part of the CMS Partnership for Patients campaign that intends to help improve the quality, safety, and affordability of health care for all Americans. There are 10 areas of quality improvement focus (Table 13.4).

The Skills Needed by the Nurse to do QI

The nurse who wants to do QI needs four essential skills: self-awareness, the ability to work as a collaborative team member, the ability to manage crucial conversations with the interprofessional team, and the ability to work as a nurse leader.

Self-Awareness

First, the nurse needs to be self-aware. **Self-awareness** means to be able to look at yourself critically and identify your strengths and your weaknesses. A mentor can guide and support you through the self-awareness process. A **mentor** is someone who helps you with your career and with specific work projects. If you have a particularly hard time with changing a weakness, a good mentor can help you understand what is standing in your way. A mentor motivates you to do more than you think you can. A mentor will help you see the big picture and can put health care and QI practices in context for you. For example, in the opening scenario, the nurse manager understood the nurse's need to participate in a constructive activity. A mentor can draw from a wide range of strategies that could

Table 13.4   Quality Improvement Focus

- Adverse Drug Events (ADE)
- Catheter-Associated Urinary Tract Infections (CAUTI)
- Central Line-Associated Blood Stream Infections (CLABSI)
- Injuries from falls and immobility
- Obstetrical adverse events
- Pressure ulcers
- Surgical site infections
- Venous ThromboEmbolism (VTE)
- Ventilator-Associated Pneumonia (VAP)
- Preventable readmissions

Source: Adapted from Centers for Medicare & Medicaid Services. U.S. Government. Public Domain. https://innovation.cms.gov/initiatives/partnership-for-patients.

help you reach your goals. A mentor tells you things you need to hear, not necessarily things you want to hear. Being able to take constructive criticism is a necessary skill in QI. For example, if you have a difficult time with one person on a QI team, your mentor will work with you on how to collaborate more effectively with that individual. You might find through discussions with your mentor that it is your behavior not the other person's behavior that is causing the difficulty.

Some health care organizations have formal mentoring programs, and match mentors and mentees. Sometimes the organization will expect that supervisors will be mentors to their staff. If an organization doesn't have a formal program for mentoring, the nurse can take the initiative. Find out which nurses are involved in QI, and who are regarded as QI experts by the nursing members of the interprofessional team. Look for a nurse who is more experienced than you, and is well-respected by team members. Ask other staff who they would recommend as a mentor. Once you have identified a nurse that you admire and believe shares your values, reach out and ask this nurse to be your mentor. The worst that will happen is the nurse will say no. If you have selected carefully, the nurse you ask will be happy to help and provide recommendations to you.

Collaborative Team Member

Second, the nurse needs to work in **collaboration** with others, in other words to work as a member of a team. Nurses are like the hub of a wheel with all of the other health professionals branching out from it (Lampert, 2015). The nurse can be deliberate in using behaviors that ensure that collaboration with the interprofessional team is one of trust and mutual respect (Table 13.5).

Interprofessional collaboration results in the best health care experiences and outcomes for patients. Think about the opening scenario. Did the nurse ask anyone for help in discharging Mr. Sullivan? Perhaps the nurse could have used more help than she requested. Nurses interact with many other health professionals every day as part of the health care team. Communication behaviors can help or hinder conversations and patient outcomes (Table 13.6).

Crucial Conversations

The third skill needed by a nurse who does QI is the ability to manage crucial conversations with the interprofessional team. Crucial conversations occur when the stakes are high,

---

Real World Interview

When I began my master's degree program, I was required to have a mentor to support my capstone graduation project. This individual provided many experiences for me to learn and grow in QI. Mainly, she empowered me to lead a QI project on my unit related to postpartum hemorrhage. This was accomplished by implementing a system for measuring blood loss instead of visual estimation. The project contributed to a reduction in maternal morbidity at the hospital. Moving from peer to leader-among-peers was very difficult and my mentor's weekly guidance and support was a key to my success. Nursing and its culture can sometimes be described like a bucket of crabs (Nance, 2008).

When one tries to rise up and lead, the others grab hold and pull them back down to assimilate. My director's mentorship enabled me to grow, persevere, and avoid being pulled down. That gave me the courage to follow my QI passion to help lead patient safety and QI initiatives.

Amber Weiseth, MSN, RNC-OB
Associate Director, Delivery Decisions Initiative,
Ariadne Labs, Brigham and Women's Hospital,
Harvard T.H. Chan School of Public Health Collaboration
Boston, Massachusetts

Table 13.5   Behaviors that Enhance Interprofessional Collaboration

The nurse uses positive and healthy communication techniques.	The nurse is assertive and kind in interactions with others.
The nurse offers help and jumps in to help co-workers.	The nurse understands how the work of others impacts the patient's health care.
The nurse asks for help.	The nurse smiles and says, thank you, to others.
The nurse is organized and plans the day's work with co-workers.	The nurse appreciates that others have work to do and doesn't waste their time.
The nurse shares power and information.	The nurse energizes others by staying focused on them during interactions.
The nurse acknowledges the contribution of others in the delivery of patient care.	

Note. Created by C. Wagner & C. Alexander.

Table 13.6   Helping versus Hindering Communication Behaviors

Helping Behaviors	Hindering Behaviors
The nurse listening completely to what team members are saying, even when not in agreement.	The nurse interrupts team members in mid-sentence.
The nurse paraphrases a team member's points before contradicting the team member.	The nurse ignores and does not acknowledge a team member's ideas.
The nurse gives appropriate praise to the ideas of team members.	The nurse criticizes the ideas of team members without offering useful feedback.
The nurse builds on ideas of team members and gives them credit for the ideas.	The nurse pushes her own ideas while ignoring how they could be made better by using the ideas of all team members.
The nurse is open and receptive to feedback and critique.	The nurse responds defensively to feedback.
The nurse is open to alternative ideas and actions.	The nurse is closed to ideas from anyone else.
The nurse is focused on facts.	The nurse lets feelings guide arguments with others.

Source: Adapted from Ingrid Bens, Facilitating with Ease!: Core Skills for Facilitators, Team Leaders and Members, Managers, Consultants, and Trainers, 2017.

opinions vary, and emotions run strong, for example when the interprofessional team has differing opinions about whether handwashing has to be done when members of the interprofessional team visit the patient but don't touch the patient or anything in the room. The nurse must be able to talk with others during crucial conversations in a manner that gets the job done and doesn't destroy a healthy team environment or the individual feelings of team members. Strong communication skills are essential for the nurse in order to thrive during all the interactions and activities of a busy day. The outcome of a crucial conversation can be the difference between a high performing and a low performing team. The nurse can respond in various ways.

The nurse can avoid a crucial conversation by being silent. Silence undermines the nurse's ability to demonstrate any of the key roles of nursing discussed in Chapter 12. The nurse can also choose to participate in a crucial conversation but handle it poorly, for example by giving a sharp response. This behavior undermines the nurse's ability to be well-regarded as a professional team member.

The best option in crucial conversations is for the nurse to participate in the conversation and handle it well. Strategies for productively handling a crucial conversation are staying impartial, actively listening, asking questions, paraphrasing, and summarizing periodically throughout the conversation and at the end of the conversation. It is important to note that staying impartial does not mean not having your own opinions or values. It means being able to converse with another person in a manner that is respectful and calm, no matter how sharp the differences are between your perspectives. The process of health care delivery requires that nurses have productive crucial conversations with the interprofessional team and the chain of command as needed to assure quality patient outcomes.

For example, in the opening scenario, team members working on improvement of the patient handoff have different ideas about what is causing the problem. The nurse in primary care believes that the nurses on the inpatient unit don't appreciate the urgent need for action when primary care calls for a transfer. The primary care provider thinks the hospitalist should read the progress notes as soon as the decision to admit is shared over the phone. The nurse on the unit thinks there isn't enough staff on the inpatient units which negatively impacts discharges from the inpatient unit. The housekeeper believes that nursing does not understand the time it takes to clean a room between patients. Productive crucial conversations and helping behaviors can help lead the team through the work of quality improvement.

The team must make a decision about where to start in the quality improvement issues. There are three techniques that are useful for categorizing and prioritizing these issues: brainstorming, affinity diagrams, and multi-voting. **Brainstorming** is a way to gather a lot of ideas very quickly. You encourage the team to freely discuss their ideas to fix the patient handoff issue. You ask them to write their ideas on sticky notes. You collect the sticky notes and begin, with input from the team, to group them into categories. This is called making an affinity diagram.

An **affinity diagram** places items that are similar together so that the team can see where their individual ideas from brainstorming are similar. This facilitates the team having a shared understanding about what idea each member is bringing forward. Each of the team members is then given three sticky notes and votes for the top three issues they believe are most critical to a safe patient handoff. Since each team member has three votes, this is referred to as multi-voting.

Multi-voting is a way to achieve team consensus about which problem from the affinity diagram should be improved first (Figure 13.2). Multi-voting may reveal to the team that the priority issue needing improvement is the variation in the communication practices, that is the patient handoff, between the primary care staff and the inpatient staff when a patient is being transferred for admission.

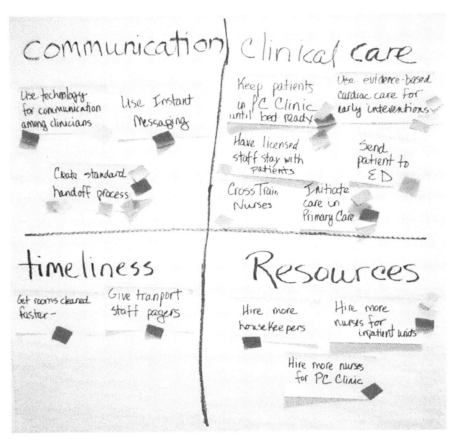

FIGURE 13.2   Affinity diagram with multivoting.
Source: Created by C. Wagner & C. Alexander.

You could then remind that team that it is important to know how other health care organizations implement patient handoffs, since that knowledge can provide a benchmark for best practice changes in the patient handoff process. If one of the nurses on the team volunteers to work with the health care organization's medical librarian to get that information, the resultant literature search for resources about evidence-based outcomes related to the patient handoff process can be shared with the team (Table 13.7).

Nurse Leader in QI

The ability to work as a nurse leader is the fourth skill needed by the nurse who does QI. Interprofessional collaboration requires the nurse to use leadership skills, even if the nurse is not in a stated leadership position, such as charge nurse or nurse manager (Table 13.8). The nurse leader at the bedside has a strong sense of direction and facilitates agreement among others about what needs to be done to achieve certain goals. The nurse leader at the bedside is at the center of the work but may allow others to direct the path forward toward goal achievement. For example, a patient insists that only one nursing assistant can do his care. The nurse gains consensus from the team during a case conference that other staff has to participate in the patient's care to provide particular aspects of care. As a leader, the nurse then facilitates a discussion with the team that encourages all staff to contribute ideas and create a plan for how to motivate and monitor patient acceptance of care from others. The nurse would also talk to the patient so that his input is considered as well (Green et al., 2016). The nurse leader's behavior is guided by self-awareness and self-reflection. It reflects honesty and integrity. The nurse builds trustworthy relationships and makes sure everyone has a voice on the team, including the patient.

A nursing student can build leadership skills by participating in the NSNA Leadership University. This is an online educational offering that allows students to build their leadership skills by learning how to work in shared governance and cooperative relationships with peers, faculty, students in other disciplines, community service organizations, and the public (NSNA, 2018 Leadership U FAQs.pdf www.nsna.org/leadership-university.html, accessed December 12, 2018).

Applying QI Methodologies at the Bedside

Part of the role for the nurse leader in QI is review of patient outcomes. The reviews can be done individually or as a group. The outcomes needing review are usually negative patient outcomes such as a psychological or physical injury. In the open-

Table 13.7   Resources to Generate Outcome Benchmarks in Clinical Practice

Resource	Example of use by the nurse doing QI
Joanna Briggs Institute http://joannabriggs.org accessed December 14, 2018. Identifies evidence-based healthcare practices to assist in the improvement of health care outcomes.	The nurse shares an evidence summary from the Johanna Briggs Institute that states effective standardized practices in patient handoffs include face-to-face communication, standardized documentation, identification of patients, care plan handover and transfer of responsibility (Yu et al., 2017).
The Cochrane Library www.cochranelibrary.com accessed December 14, 2018. Provides databases tha, contain different types of high-quality, independent evidence to inform healthcare decision-making	The nurse shares the results of a systematic literature review that concludes face-to-face communication, structured documentation, patient involvement and the use of Information Technology (IT) supports the handoff process (Smeulers et al., 2014).
Agency for Healthcare Research and Quality (AHRQ) (2020) https://innovations.ahrq.gov/ accessed 1 May 27, 2020. Shares evidence-based innovations and tools suitable for a range of health care settings and populations.	The nurse reports on a standardized transport tool that can be used when transferring a patient from one area of the hospital and which provides critical patient information and a checklist of steps to ensure patient safety during the transport and accurate care at each destination (Scholle et al., 2014).
Centers for Medicare and Medicaid Services (CMS) www.cms.gov/Medicare/Quality-Initiatives-Patient-Assessment-Instruments/HospitalQualityInits/HospitalCompare.html Provides information on how well hospitals provide recommended care to their patients.	The nurse shares that this site benchmarks timely and effective health care, that is, how often and how quickly hospitals provide care that research shows gets the best results for patients with chest pain or a possible heart attack.

Note. Created by C. Wagner & C. Alexander.

Table 13.8   Leadership Skills Shown by Nurses Working in QI

Leadership skills	Example of how a nurse demonstrates leadership in QI
The nurse sees self as a leader	The bedside nurse prepares to work on a patient care unit by identifying common patient diagnoses and medications for patients cared for on that unit.
	The bedside nurse develops a plan for quality patient care structures and processes needed to assure quality patient outcomes.
	The bedside nurse recognizes their primary responsibility is to the patient and uses the chain of command, when necessary, to assure safe, high-quality patient care.
The nurse is a professional.	The nurse uses critical thinking skills to identify a patient care issue and then takes action by using knowledge and skills to develop an intervention.
The nurse has a plan.	The nurse volunteers to lead a QI project when opportunities to improve care occur at the bedside.
The nurse invests in self.	The nurse continually looks for opportunities to expand knowledge in quality improvement and evidence-based practice by taking classes or attending conferences and then applying these skills at the frontline of care.
The nurse gets involved.	The nurse leads QI initiatives by: 1. Joining a unit-based council or a hospital-wide quality improvement committee; 2. Joining a national nursing organization like The Institute for Quality and Safety Education for Nurses (QSEN) and volunteering to be on a task force.

Source: Adapted from Keast, 2016 and Northouse, 2016.

ing scenario, the patient's death related to a long wait time and poor patient handoffs was reviewed by a root cause analysis team. You volunteered to lead a quality improvement project focused on patient handoffs. Part of that work was to gather a team of people who touched the process of patient handoff and determine team roles and responsibilities (Table 13.9).

The **FOCUS** QI methodology describes, in a stepwise process, how to move through the quality improvement process in patient handoffs (Table 13.10).

The team also wants to test that patients who are being admitted to the inpatient unit from the Primary Care Clinic received the most appropriate care based on their acuity and health care needs. In the opening scenario, the patient had a cardiac arrest while in the Primary Care Clinic waiting room. The team creates and implements a Flow Chart that incorporates evidence-based interventions for patients who complain of chest pain or who have a possible heart attack while they are in the Primary Care Clinic (Figure 13.3). The team continues to review other parts

Table 13.9   Roles and Responsibilities on a Quality Improvement Team

Team Role	Responsibilities
Leader	Oversees and guides all aspects of the quality improvement project. Keeps the team focused and manages team discussions to achieve meeting objectives. Communicates meeting decisions and distributes any needed updates or materials to the team, Executive Sponsor, and stakeholders.
QI coach	Collaborates with the Leader to accomplish the above activities. Assists the Leader in planning meetings and developing agendas. Ensures the participation of all team members. Guides and mentors the team, building their capacity for QI work, as they go through the steps of the organization's QI methodology, using the appropriate QI tools.
Members	Contribute their knowledge and insights to the QI project. Support suggested improvements in their areas of the organization to facilitate buy-in for changes that result in improvement. Work with others to achieve or exceed project goals. Represent the interprofessional team, as appropriate.
Timekeeper	Monitors the agenda and keeps track of time so that meetings start and end on time and discussions are kept to the time limits noted on agenda.
Scribe	Takes notes during team meetings and coordinates them with the Leader.
Executive sponsor	Holds the QI project team accountable for results. Helps team overcome organizational barriers. Approves and/or allocates resources, such as staff, space, access to data, etc. Provides visible organizational leadership in support of the QI project.
Data analyst	Accesses, compiles, analyzes, and reports clinical and operational data to the team.

Note. Created by C. Wagner & C. Alexander.

Critical Thinking 13.1

You have attended a national conference to learn about preventing pressure ulcers. After returning from the conference, the Nurse Executive designates you as the Leader for a QI project to reduce the organization's rate of hospital-acquired pressure ulcers. The Nurse Executive asks you to decide who should be on the team.

1. Who do you ask to be on the team and why?
2. What do you do if someone declines your invitation to be on the team?
3. What action do you take if someone has agreed to be part of the team but does not attend any of the team meetings?

---

of the flow map that show opportunities for improvement. The team creates a fishbone diagram of the improved patient handoff process (Figure 13.4). The team creates and implements a PDSA Cycle that incorporates evidence-based interventions for patients who complain of chest pain or who have a possible heart attack while they are in the Primary Care Clinic (Figure 13.5).

The team continues to do PDSA cycles on other parts of the flow map that show opportunities for improvement. The team creates a flow chart of the improved patient handoff process (Figure 13.6.).

Finishing and Sustaining the Quality Improvement Changes

Decisions for change are made on data. The QI team conducts interviews with the inpatient unit and Primary Care Clinic teams to assess their satisfaction with the improved patient handoff process. Interview results indicate a higher level of satisfaction with the new process than with the old. The number

of steps in the process of patient handoffs during the admission process from the Primary Care Clinic to the inpatient unit has been reduced by 50%. Additionally, there have been no adverse patient outcomes associated with admissions from the Primary Care Clinic to the inpatient unit during the 3 months of the QI project's implementation.

You and several of the team members present the results of the QI project to the hospital's leadership. Leadership compliments you on your work and asks what contributed to the success of the team. You share the lessons you learned from the experience as a QI team leader (Table 13.12).

One of the leadership team states that sustainment of changes that result from a QI project can be challenging for health care organizations (Scoville, Little, Rakover, Luther, & Mate, 2016). The leader asks for recommendations to help sustain the change in the patient handoff process. You reply that holding the interprofessional teams in the Primary Care Clinic and the inpatient unit accountable for maintaining the improved patient handoff process will be critical to long-term

Table 13.10   FOCUS Methodology Used by the Patient Handoff Quality Improvement Team

FOCUS	Actions of the patient handoff quality improvement team
Find a process to improve.	Based on a review of a patient's unexpected death, a root cause analysis concludes that the process of patient handoffs for admission from the Primary Care Clinic and the inpatient unit did not communicate appropriate information to meet the patient health care needs. The team decided that the process of patient handoff needed improvement.
Organize a team that knows the work process.	You find interprofessional colleagues in your organization who are involved and "touch the process" of patient hand-off from the patient's point of entry into the health care system, that is, the Primary Care Clinic, through to admission to the inpatient unit. Included on the interprofessional team are you, a charge nurse, a nurse from the Primary Care Clinic, a primary care provider, a hospitalist, a nurse from the Emergency Department (because Emergency Department staff are the Code Team staff), the Continuity of Care nurse, a housekeeper, and a coach/facilitator. The team decides to not include a patient or lay person on the team due to legal issues. Through consensus, the interprofessional team agrees to team roles and responsibilities (Table 13.9). The Executive Sponsor of the quality improvement team is the Nurse Executive.
Clarify what is happening in the work process.	The interprofessional team creates a Flow Chart (Figure 13.3) of the patient's admission transfer from the Primary Care Clinic to the inpatient unit. The team does not know some details of the transfer process, so a team member is assigned to talk to staff responsible for those sections of the transfer process. The Flow Chart identifies many communication and handoff issues in the patient handoff process and a lack of timeliness in the patient transfer process. The team also realizes that there is variation between what they think happens in each step of the process and what actually happens.
Understand the degree of change needed.	The interprofessional team creates a Fishbone Diagram (Figure 13.4) using the categories of Practice, Process, Materials, and System to achieve the outcome of safe patient transfer from the Primary Care Clinic to the inpatient unit. Major organizational categories in a Fishbone Diagram often include: Equipment or Supply factors, Environmental factors, Rules/Policy/Procedure factors, and People/Staff factors. You ask the team what are the Practice, Process, Materials, and System factors that led to the outcome of the patient death. The team reviews the Fishbone Diagram and the Flow Chart to identify the opportunities for improvement in the handoff process.
Select what to improve.	The interprofessional team prioritizes opportunities for improving the handoff process using brainstorming, an affinity diagram, and multi-voting. The team realizes they need a way to know how to the measure the improvement. You ask the coach for input on the best way to do this. The coach suggests that the team use the SMART format to create the goal. SMART goals are Specific, Measureable, Actionable, Realistic, and Time-bound. You lead the team's discussion and create a SMART goal (Table 13.11).

Note. Created by C. Wagner & C. Alexander.

Case Study 13.1

You are the nurse member of an interprofessional team working on decreasing inpatient days of stay for patients awaiting home oxygen assessment and needs. One of the PDSA Cycles suggests the addition of an oxygen-weaning evaluation to daily nurse assessments. However, the Nurse Executive is concerned about assigning additional duties to the bedside nurses. One nurse leader says that respiratory therapists should be doing the oxygen-weaning evaluation.

1. How could you work with the Nurse Executive to measure the added burden on bedside nurses if an oxygen-weaning evaluation was included in the daily RN assessments?

2. What actions could you take to determine whether oxygen-weaning evaluations should be done by nurses or by respiratory therapists?

3. How could you approach the Nurse Executive about your findings if they indicate nurses have the time to do oxygen-weaning evaluations?

---

success. You suggest that this can be facilitated by a senior leader such as the Executive Sponsor visiting the Primary Care Clinic and the inpatient unit and asking staff about the patient handoff process for admission (Silver et al., 2016). You share evidence from the literature that when QI outcome data is monitored by a leadership team, staff perceives that the improvement has a higher value and sustainment is more likely (Hayes & Goldmann, 2018).

The leaders thank you and your team for the hard work. They express hope that the experience has been a good one and that you will continue to participate in QI. You leave the meeting knowing you have made accountable and responsible nursing practice decisions in collaboration with colleagues on your unit and in the health care organization. You have improved the high risk, high volume, and problem prone process of patient handoffs. You are ready to lead change!

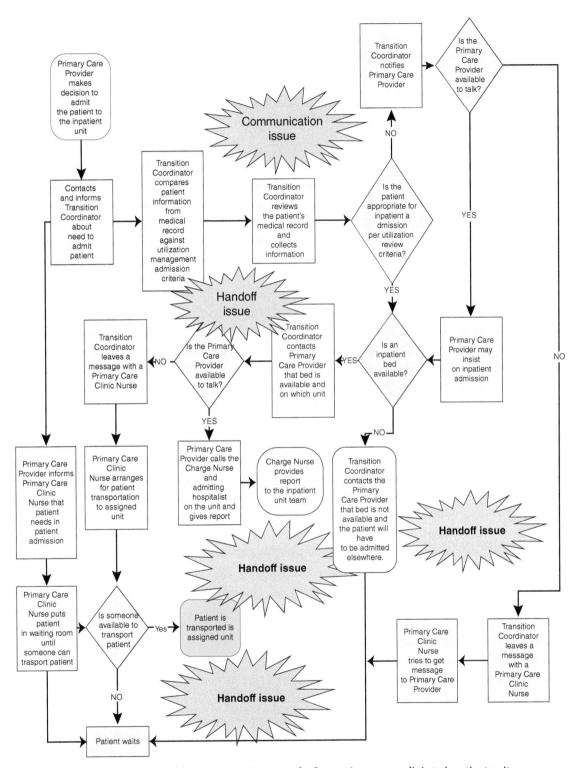

FIGURE 13.3   Flow chart: problem-prone patient transfer from primary care clinic to inpatient unit.

Table 13.11   Creating SMART Goals for an Improvement Project

Specific	The handoff process for patients admitted from the Primary Care Clinic to the inpatient unit will be standardized, timely, and safe.
Measureable	The number of process steps in the handoff process will be reduced by 50% from 19 process steps as of August 1 to 10 process steps by October 31, with no resulting adverse patient outcomes.
Actionable	The health care organization's leadership supports the improvement and it is within the purview of the team to implement.
Realistic	The specific goal can be achieved.
Time-bound	The QI project can be completed within 3 months.

Note. Created by C. Wagner & C. Alexander.

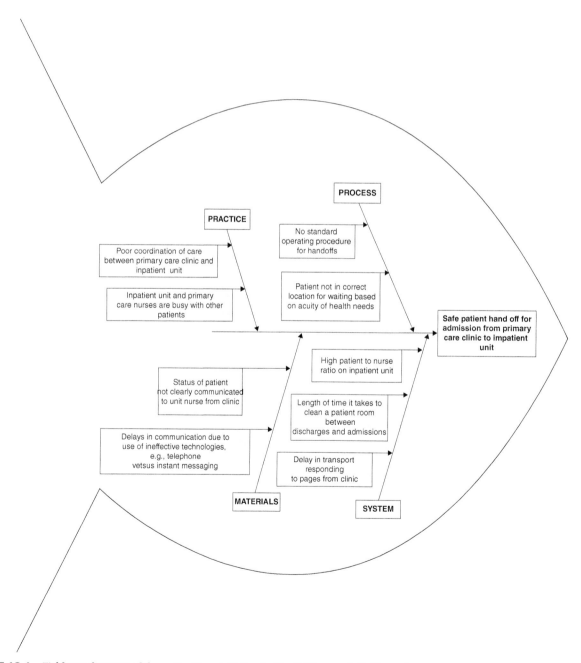

FIGURE 13.4   Fishbone diagram of the patient handoff. Created by C. Wagner & C. Alexander.

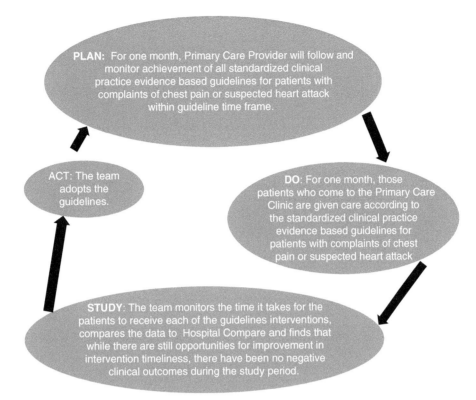

FIGURE 13.5   PDSA Cycle use by the Patient Handoff Improvement Team.
Source: Created by C. Wagner & C. Alexander.

Table 13.12   Lessons Learned as a Leader of a QI Project

Patience: It takes time to see improvement in a new process.
Good communication: The team leader must schedule ongoing meetings to discuss the project, review the data, and help the team use PDSA cycles to test changes to the process as indicated by the data.
Consistency in data collection: The team leader needs to monitor data collection to assure consistency.
Measurable improvement: Data must demonstrate outcome improvement from the process.
Administrative support: The team and team leader need the support of administration to do QI projects, including selection and implementation of changes.
Team recognition: The team leader needs to take the time to recognize the efforts of team members throughout the project to maintain team engagement and enthusiasm.

Note. Created by C. Wagner & C. Alexander.

Critical Thinking 13.2

Makary and Daniels noted that death certificates in the U.S., used to compile national statistics, have no way to identify medical error and that the death reporting system should be revised to facilitate better understanding of deaths due to medical error, the third leading cause of death in the U.S. (Makary & Daniels, 2016). What can nurses and other health care providers do to improve the identification and reporting system?

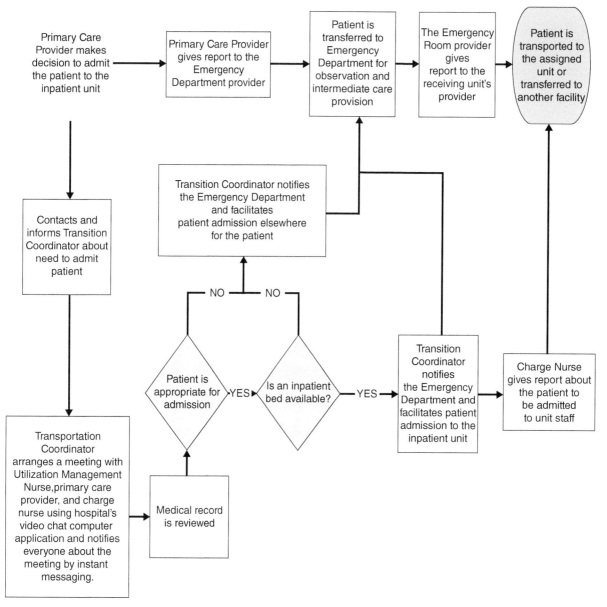

FIGURE 13.6. Flow Chart: Improved Patient Handoff Process.
Source: Created by C. Wagner & C. Alexander.

Evidence from the Literature

Source: Meehan, A., Loose, C., Bell, J., Partridge, J., Nelson, J., & Goates, S. (2016) Health System Quality Improvement: Impact of Prompt Nutrition Care on Patient Outcomes and Health Care Costs. Journal of Nursing Care Quality. 31(3):217–223.

Discussion: Disease-associated malnutrition is a common and widespread problem. Nurses are ideally positioned to identify patients at risk for malnutrition and facilitate their treatment. An interdisciplinary nurse-led team implemented a quality improvement project that positioned early nutritional care into the nursing workflow. The team's objectives were to (a) identify specific work process reforms to improve the efficiency and rate of providing nutritional support for patients admitted to the hospital, and (b) determine whether such reforms would lead to positive outcomes, both clinical and economic.

The outcomes measured included a reduction in delay time of 1 day for patients needing **oral nutritional supplements** (ONSs) by having nurses order ONS based on nursing assessments, even though there was a significant increase in the proportion of patients receiving ONS. The average hospital length of stay decreased for all patients, with greater reduction achieved for patients typically treated with nutritional supplementation. This was attributed to the patients receiving the nutritional supplements earlier in their hospital stay. The rate of readmission to the hospital within 30 days of discharge decreased. The QI project was associated with a 50% reduction in incidence of hospital-acquired pressure ulcers. Patients whose diagnoses are commonly treated with nutrition support and patients with diagnoses not commonly treated with nutrition support both experienced a reduction in their hospital bills.

Implications for Practice: Nurse-led quality improvements can result in better health outcomes and lower costs of care.

KEY CONCEPTS

1. QI uses data to monitor the outcomes of care processes.

2. QI uses improvement methods to design and test changes to continuously improve the quality and safety of health care systems.

3. Nurses' engagement and leadership in QI occurs at the bedside, the unit level, and the organizational level.

4. Nurses make QI a fundamental responsibility of their daily work by providing the right care, at the right time, in the right way, and in the right place.

5. The daily work of a competent and respected nurse includes QI, safety, patient-centered care, teamwork and collaboration, EBP, and informatics.

6. Leadership skills of frontline bedside nurses who are engaged in QI include self-awareness, ability to work as a collaborative team member and nurse leader, and the ability to manage crucial conversations.

7. At the unit level, a nurse has a professional responsibility to continually assess the unit's climate and needs and to identify areas for improvement personally and in concert with co-workers.

8. Self-awareness means to be able to look at yourself critically and identify your strengths and your weaknesses.

9. Crucial conversations are productively handled by staying impartial, actively listening, asking questions, paraphrasing, and summarizing periodically throughout the conversation and at the end of the conversation.

10. Improvement teams should be made up of people who are involved in the work process, in other words, they "touch the process."

11. There are many useful tools, such as brainstorming, affinity diagrams, and SMART goals, to help a QI team do its work.

KEY TERMS

Self-awareness	SMART goal	Multi-voting
Collaboration	Brainstorming	Mentor
Crucial conversation	Affinity diagram	

REVIEW QUESTIONS

1. The nurse is having a discussion with colleagues during their break. There is some disagreement about what QI is and how the QI process should be completed. The nurse listens respectfully to what is being said and then states "Quality improvement is" which of the following? Select all that apply.
   a. Critical to the delivery of safe patient care
   b. Delegated to the clinical nurse by the nurse manager
   c. Identified as the right care, at the right time, in the right place
   d. Work that is led by the physician
   e. Fundamental to nurses' daily work

2. You have accepted the role of leader for a hand hygiene improvement team. You want to be effective as a team leader, and consider purchasing a book about techniques to practice self-awareness. Which of the following is true about self-awareness? Select all that apply.
   a. It is an essential behavior of being an authentic leader
   b. It is only about knowing your strengths and weaknesses
   c. It does not make you a better leader in QI work
   d. It is a way of being self-reflective about your leadership abilities
   e. It is a behavior that only expert leaders use due to its difficulty

3. You are a recent graduate and have been paired with a nurse mentor. Your mentor will help you by doing which one of the following?
   a. Pointing out your mistakes in front of the team
   b. Taking credit for your hard work
   c. Guiding you through leading an improvement team
   d. Giving you advice on who to avoid

4. The bedside nurse is a clinical leader. Which of the following nursing behaviors indicate that the nurse has accepted responsibility for safe quality patient care? Select all that apply.
   a. Reviewing and delegating work assignments
   b. Assessing the outcomes of care for each patient
   c. Collaborating with others to provide patient care
   d. Covering for another nurse who has is going to lunch

5. The patient asks you why nurses are meeting at his bed when one nurse is starting their shift and another nurse is going home. You tell the patient the nurses are doing bedside rounding to improve patient handoff between shifts. Which of the following describes a patient handoff? Select all that apply.
   a. An infrequent occurrence in health care that occurs when critical patient information is needed
   b. A handshake about patient care between members of the health care team
   c. A good way to check on the status of a patient's condition when accepting responsibility for the care of a patient
   d. A high risk occurrence because they are used to convey critical information about the patient from one person to another
   e. A standardized communication tool used to keep the patient safe

6. The five steps in the FOCUS methodology of QI include all or which of the following?
   a. Find a process to improve
   b. Organize a team that can make things happen
   c. Clarify what is happening in the work process
   d. Understand the degree of change needed
   e. Select what to improve

7. You are the lead on a QI project and you want to build a flow chart illustrating the usual activities that occur during the overnight shift with a goal of reducing noise and patient complaints about noise at night. The QI team says noise is not related to a process and the members don't understand why you want to build a flow chart for this project. You explain to the team that the purpose of a flow chart is which of the following? Select all that apply.
   a. Help the team understand the steps in the overnight work process
   b. Justify more staff for the overnight shift
   c. Identify who is to blame for making all the noise during the overnight shift

   d. Help identify which steps of the overnight work process need improvement
   e. Fix all of the staff's complaints about the overnight work process

8. A brainstorming session will help an improvement team do which of the following? Select all that apply.
   a. Find a quick solution to the QI problem
   b. Gather a lot of ideas quickly
   c. Allow the team to develop friendships
   d. Save a lot of time in the QI process
   e. Build trust among the team members

9. You have been asked to participate in a discharge planning improvement team. You work in the operating room. When their surgeries are completed, patients are transferred to the recovery room. From there, patients are either transferred as an inpatient or discharged home. You should decline the invitation to participate in the discharge planning improvement team because of which of the following?
   a. You are not friends with the team leader
   b. You do not "touch the process" of discharge
   c. You are not a member of the QI department
   d. You know there are already two other nurses on the team

10. You have worked hard on an improvement team on your unit to decrease interruptions during the medication administration process. You want to make sure that the changes which dramatically decreased interruptions and medication errors are sustained. Which of the following support sustainment of QI changes? Select all that apply.
   a. Regular and ongoing collection and sharing of the data measurements
   b. Recognition from the hospital's leadership about the value of the improvement
   c. Bonuses for the improvement team members
   d. Holding the interprofessional staff accountable for the new process
   e. Review and re-education of the new medication process during staff meetings

REVIEW QUESTION ANSWERS

1. Answers A, C, and E are correct.
   Rationale: Quality improvement (QI) is to use of data to monitor the outcomes of care processes and use improvement methods to design and test changes to continuously improve the quality and safety of health care systems (QSEN Institute, 2018). QI is critical to the delivery of safe patient care (A). The nurse's goal in the provision of nursing care is to ensure the patient receives the right care at the right time in the right way in the right place (C). QI is a fundamental part of the work the nurse does every day (E) as an employee of a health care organization. QI is a responsibility of every clinical nurse, not simply a delegation to the clinical nurse by the nurse manager (B). QI is led by different members of the health care team, including but not limited to the physician (D).

2. Answers A and D are correct.
   Rationale: Self-awareness is an essential behavior for the nurse who wants to be a leader (A) and do QI. Self-awareness is a way

of being self-reflective about your leadership abilities (D). Self-awareness includes both the ability to look at yourself critically and identify your strengths and your weaknesses (B). Self-awareness guides the nurse leader's behavior and makes the nurse a better leader (C). Self-awareness is a learned behavior can be used by all leaders (E).

3. Answer: C is correct.
   Rationale: A mentor provides support for the nurse to grow and develop as a professional in a positive atmosphere, for example, by guiding you when you are leading an improvement team (C). A mentor provides feedback, but never in a critical, a judgmental, or a cruel manner (A). A mentor does not take credit for your work (B). A mentor does not gossip about you or others. A mentor treats you as an adult capable of making your own decisions about colleagues and does not tell you who to avoid (D).

4. Answerw A, B, C, and D are correct.

   Rationale: The nurse reports to work knowing that the goal is for each patient to get the right care at the right time in the right way in the right place. Reviewing and delegating work assignments (A) enables the most appropriate use of staff resources. Assessing the outcomes of care for each patient (B) and collaborating with others to provide patient care (C) assures that decisions can be made to continue the same care, or improve the care, or change the care totally. Covering for another nurse who is going to lunch (D) communicates teamwork and its importance of rested and healthy staff in the provision of quality and safe patient care. Disciplining colleagues is a supervisory function and not part of the bedside nurse's role (E).

5. Answers C, D, and E are correct.

   Rationale: A patient handoff is a good way to check on the status of a patient's condition when accepting responsibility for the care of a patient (C). Patient handoffs are high risk because they are used to convey critical information about the patient from one person to another (D). Patient handoff improves communication between providers and nurses by reducing the chance of miscommunication and errors. It is a standardized way to communicate with all members of the health care team when patients are transferred between departments, at shift report or at discharge (E). Patient handoffs are frequent or high-volume occurrences because they occur every time responsibility for a patient's care is transferred from one inter-disciplinary team member to another or from one hospital department to another (A). Patient handoffs are more than a handshake about patient care between members of the health care team (B), because if a patient handoff is not done correctly the patient is harmed or has the potential to be harmed by the health care system.

6. Answer: B is correct.

   Rationale: The team is organized from colleagues in the health care organization who are involved in the work process that will be improved. In other words, the team is organized with members of the inter-disciplinary staff and other staff members who "touch the process." They are the experts of their respective steps in the process. They are not necessarily the people who can "make things happen," (B) such as an executive leader. Finding a process to improve (A), clarifying what is happening in the work process (C), understanding the degree of change needed (D), and selecting what to improve (E) are steps in the FOCUS methodology.

7. Answers A and D are correct.

   Rationale: A flow chart is a QI tool that helps the team understand how a process is functioning in its current state, for example, the steps in the overnight work process (A). A flow chart identifies which steps in the process are problematic and need to be improved (D). A flow chart identifies opportunities to improve a process but is not used to justify solutions such as increasing staff (B). A flow chart does not assign blame (C). A flow chart helps the team identify variation between what they think happens in each step of the process and what actually happens but does not fix all of the staff's complaints about the overnight work process (E).

8. Answers B and D are correct.

   Rationale: Brainstorming is a way to gather a lot of ideas very quickly from the group (B). Brainstorming saves time (D) by increasing the efficiency of the QI process. Brainstorming does not produce quick solutions to a QI problem (A). Brainstorming can help the team collaborate on the task of gathering ideas but it does not include interpersonal exercises to help the team develop friendships (C). Brainstorming does not include exercises to build interpersonal relationships so it does not build trust among team members (E).

9. Answer: B is correct.

   Rationale: Improvement teams should be made up of people who are involved in the work process, in other words, they "touch the process" (B). Members of the QI team should be chosen because they touch the process, not because they are friends of the team leader (A). Members of the QI should be chosen because they touch the process, not because they are members of the QI department (C). There is no limit on the number of nurses or other disciplines that can be on a QI team, although the team should have representation from all the people who touch the process (D).

10. Answers A, B, D, and E are correct.

   Rationale: Regular and ongoing collection and sharing of data measurements (A) ensures that the improvement is maintained and monitored. Recognition from the hospital's leadership (B) will reinforce for the inter-disciplinary team and others that QI is valued as part of the essential operations of the health care system. Holding the interprofessional staff accountable to the new process (D) is critical to long-term success. Review and re-education of a new process during staff meetings (E) reinforces knowledge about the improvement and gives staff the opportunity to ask questions about the improvement as they are using it. Bonuses for staff who participate on the QI team (C) provide recognition but do not contribute to sustaining use of the improvement.

REVIEW ACTIVITIES

1. Find graphs or displays related to QI posted in your clinical area. Ask the staff what QI interventions were implemented and how work was affected in the clinical area.

2. Ask several nurses in your clinical area about their involvement in QI. If the nurse indicates much involvement, ask how the nurse got interested in QI. If the nurse states little or no involvement, ask the nurse if there are any barriers to QI involvement.

3. Collaborate with your classmates to combine your findings about barriers to involvement in QI. Identify categories and sort the findings to create a fishbone diagram. Identify possible changes that could be tested in a PDSA.

4. Review the health care organization's priorities for improvement during your clinical rotation. The Nurse Manager or the organization's QI department can help you locate these. Ask how nursing is involved in each of the improvement efforts. If nursing does not have a direct role in an improvement effort, ask how nursing supports the improvement.

5. Make a list of what quality structures and processes are available and that you can incorporate into your daily practice as a nurse to assure quality patient outcomes.

DISCUSSION POINTS

1. What are some examples of teamwork and collaboration you have seen during your clinical rotations? What are some examples of when teamwork could have been demonstrated but was not?

2. Discuss a time when you witnessed a bedside nurse or other member of the health care team do something that improved a patient's health care experience.

3. What are the characteristics of a good bedside nurse leader? How can you be a good nurse leader at the bedside and in other QI activities now and once you graduate?

4. What do you think is the role of technology in nursing QI? Discuss what generational differences there might be in a patient's willingness to use computer technology, for example, as a means of answering patient survey questions about satisfaction with health care.

DISCUSSION OF THE OPENING SCENARIO

1. Who would you ask to participate on the QI team?

   Answer: You would invite people in the organization who touch the process you are trying to improve. You may also want to invite a leader, manager, or supervisor in the department where you are conducting the process improvement project. It would be important to keep this leader in the "loop of communication" especially at the beginning and throughout the project. A leader's support is an essential component of a successful QI project.

2. How will you know what changes can be made in the process of patient handoff that will result in an improvement in care?

   Answer: You will use QI tools such as a process flow map to identify the source of the problem. Brainstorming, affinity diagrams and multi-voting are also QI tools that can help you "drill down" to find the source of the problem and help the team define the problem and improve care.

3. How will you know that the process of handoff from the primary care clinic to the inpatient unit has been improved?

   Answer: You will use the power of data analysis to identify if the handoff process was improved after the intervention.

EXPLORING THE WEB

1. Agency for Healthcare Research and Quality (AHRQ), www.ahrq.gov accessed December 10, 2018.

2. Quality and Safety Education in Nursing (QSEN) Institute, http://qsen.org accessed December 9, 2018.

3. National Committee for Quality Assurance, www.ncqa.org accessed December 10, 2018.

4. The Leapfrog Group, www.leapfroggroup.org accessed December 10, 2018.

5. National Association for Healthcare Quality, https://nahq.org accessed December 10, 2018.

6. Emergency Care Research Institute (ECRI) Institute, www.ecri.org accessed December 10, 2018.

INFORMATICS

1. Go to the National Association for Healthcare Quality website, https://nahq.org accessed October 12, 2018. Click on the box "HEDIS Measures." Then click on "Effectiveness of Care." Open each of the categories and review the variety of health care measures reported by health care organizations.

2. Go to http://qsen.org accessed September 12, 2018 Click on, Resources, and then scroll down. Click on "Culture Cues-University of Washington Medical Center." Review one or two of the tip sheets. How could you use this material to improve the patient experience?

LEAN BACK

- Think about the nurses you observed and worked with during your clinical rotations. Did the nurses have dedicated time in their schedules for QI?

- How could you structure your work day as a new nurse to assure quality structures and processes are in place to achieve quality outcomes for your patients?

- How will you as a new nurse leader at the bedside step up to assure quality patient care outcomes? How will you incorporate QI activities?

REFERENCES

Agency for Healthcare Research and Quality. (2020). *SHARE approach curriculum tools*. Content last reviewed September 2016. Rockville, MD: Agency for Healthcare Research and Quality. Retrieved from https://innovations.ahrq.gov/

Bens, I. (2018). *Facilitating with ease* (4th ed.). Hoboken, NJ: John Wiley & Sons, Inc.

Bickford, C. J., Marion, L., & Gazaway, S. (2015). *Nursing: Scope and standards of practice* (3rd ed.). American Nurses Association. Retrieved from www.augusta.edu/nursing/cnr/documents/seminar-files/pp8.28.pdf

Foster, G. L., Kenward, K., Hines, S., & Maulik, S. J. (2017). The relationship of engagement in improvement practices to outcome measures in large-scale quality improvement initiatives. *American Journal of Medical Quality*, *32*(4), 361–368.

Green, S. A., Evans, L., Matthews, R., Jayacodi, S., Evered, R., Parker, C., Polledri, L., Tabb, E., Green, J., Manickam, A., Williams, J., Deere, R. & Tiplady, B. (2016). Service user engagement in quality improvement: Applying the national involvement standards. The Journal of Mental Health Training, Education and Practice, 1(5), 279–285.

Hayes, C. W., & Goldmann, D. (2018). Highly adoptable improvement: A practical model and toolkit to address adoptability and sustainability of quality improvement initiatives. *The Joint Commission Journal on Quality and Patient Safety*, *44*(3), 155–163.

Keast, K. (2016). How to become a nurse leader. *Health Times*. Retrieved from https://healthtimes.com.au/hub/leadership/35/guidance/kk1/how-to-become-a-nurse-leader/1460

Lampert, L. (2015). *Collaborating with your healthcare colleagues*. Retrieved from www.ausmed.com/articles/collaboration-in-healthcare

Lockhart, L. (2018). Measuring nursing's impact. *Nursing Made Incredibly Easy*, *16*(2), 55.

Markary, M. A., & Daniel, M. (2016). *British Medical Journal*, *353*, i2139. doi:10.1136/bmj.i.2139

Nance, J. (2008). *Why hospitals should fly: The ultimate flight plan to patient safety and quality care*. Boseman, MT: Second River Healthcare.

National Database of Nursing Quality Indicators. (2011). NDNQI:Transforming Data into Quality Care [Brochure]. South Bend, IN: Author. Retrieved from http://public.qualityforum.org/actionregistry/Lists/List%20of%20Actions/Attachments/141/NDNQIBrochure.pdf?Mobile=1

National Student Nurses Association. (2018). *Leadership U FAQs.pdf*. Retrieved from www.dropbox.com/s/2mww968ga0lci6u/Leadership%20U%20FAQs.docx?dl=0

Needleman, J., Pearson, M. L., Upenieks, V. V., Yee, T., Wolstein, J., & Parkerton, M. (2016). Engaging frontline staff in performance improvement: The American Organization of Nurse Executives implementation of transforming care at the bedside collaborative. *The Joint Commission Journal on Quality and Patient Safety*, *42*(2), 61–69.

Northouse, P. G. (2016). *Leadership: Theory and practice*. Los Angeles, CA: Sage Publications.

Quality and Safety Education in Nursing (QSEN) Institute. (2018). Retrieved from http://qsen.org

Scholle, C., Rack, L. & Pesanka, D. (2014). Transition "Tickets" Reduce Adverse Events During Patient Transports. Retrieved from https://innovations.ahrq.gov/profiles/transition-tickets-reduce-adverse-events-during-patient-transports accessed 10/31/2020

Scoville, R., Little, K., Rakover, J., Luther, K., & Mate, K. (2016). *Sustaining improvement*. IHI white paper. Cambridge, MA: Institute for Healthcare Improvement.

Silver, S. A., McQuillan, R., Harel, Z., Weizman, A. V., Thomas, A., et al. (2016). How to sustain change and support continuous quality improvement. *Clinical Journal of the American Society of Nephrology*, *11*(5), 916–924.

Smeulers, M., Lucas, C., & Vermeulen, H. (2014). Effectiveness of different nursing handover styles for ensuring continuity of information in hospitalised patients. *Cochrane Database System Review*, (6), CD009979. doi:10.1002/14651858.CD009979.pub2

University of Utah. (2018). *About the Press Ganey survey*. Retrieved from https://healthcare.utah.edu/fad/pressganey.php

Yu, Z., Zhang, Y., Gu, Y., Xu, X., & Mcarthur, A. (2017). Pediatric clinical handover: A best practice implementation project. *JBI Database of Systematic Reviews and Implementation Reports*, *15*, 2585–2596. doi:10.11124/JBISRIR-2016-003296

SUGGESTED READINGS

Affairs Blog. (2017). *Empowering nurses to innovate at the bedside, then spread their innovations*. Health Affairs Blog. Retrieved from www.healthaffairs.org/do/10.1377/hblog20171121.831571/full

Barnhorst, A., Martinez, M., & Gershengorn, H. B. (2015). Quality improvement strategies for critical care nursing. *American Journal of Critical Care*, *24*(1), 87–92.

Dilts Skaggs, M. K., Daniels, J. F., Hodge, M. J., & DeCamp, V. L. (2018). Using the evidence-based practice service nursing bundle to increase patient satisfaction. *Journal of Emergency Nursing*, *44*(1), 37–45.

Goodyear-Bruch, C., Altman, M, & Cox, K. (2017). Empowering nurses to innovate at the bedside, then spread their innovations. Health Affairs. Retrieved from https://www.healthaffairs.org/do/10.1377/hblog20171121.831571/full/

Hargwood, P., & Duffy, C. (2016). Out of the library and on to the floors: Librarian participation in nursing rounds. *Journal of Hospital Librarianship*, *16*((3)), 209–214.

Izumi, S. (2012). Quality improvement in nursing: Administrative mandate or professional responsibility? *Nursing Forum*, *47*(4), 260–267.

Jimenez, R. A., Swartz, M., & Mccorkle, R. (2018). Improving quality through nursing participation at bedside rounds in a pediatric acute care unit: A Pilot Project. *Journal of Pediatric Nursing*, *43*, 45–55.

Mette Bach, A., Forman, A., & Seibaek, L. (2018). Postoperative pain management: A bedside perspective. *Pain Management Nursing*, *19*(6), 608–618.

Moore, L., Lavoie, A., Bourgeois, G., & Lapointe, J. (2015). Donabedian's structure-process-outcome quality of care model: Validation in an integrated trauma system. *Journal of Trauma and Acute Care Surgery*, *78*(6), 1168–1175.

Patterson, K., Grenny, J., McMillan, R., & Switzler, A. (2012). *Crucial conversations tools for talking when stakes are high* (Vol. 2). New York: McGraw Hill.

Start, R., Matlock, A. M., Brown, D., Aronow, H., & Soban, L. (2018). Realizing momentum and synergy: Benchmarking meaningful ambulatory care nurse-sensitive indicators. *Nursing Economics*, *36*(5), 246–251. Retrieved from www.nursingeconomics.net/necfiles/2018/SO18/246.pdf

Tobiano, G., Bucknall, T., Sladdin, I., Whitty, J. A., & Chabover, W. (2017). Patient participation in nursing bedside handover: A systematic mixed methods review. *International Journal of Nursing Studies*, *77*, 243–258.

14

Safety: Patient and Health Care Team

Christine Rovinski-Wagner[1], Peter Mills[2,3]

[1] Office of Veterans Access to Care, Veterans' Health Administration, Washington, DC, USA

[2] VA National Center for Patient Safety Field Office, Veterans Affairs Medical Center, White River Junction, VT, USA

[3] The Geisel School of Medicine at Dartmouth, Hanover, New Hampshire, USA

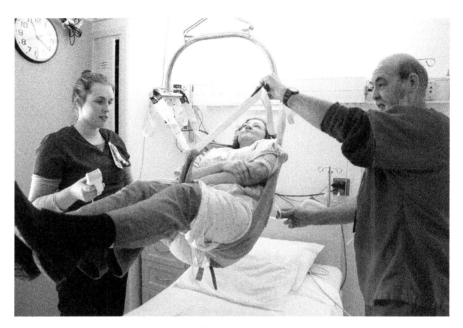

Nurses practice how to use safe patient handling equipment.
Source: Katherine Tang.

First do no harm.

Hippocrates.

OBJECTIVES

Upon completion of this chapter, the reader should be able to:

1. Define safety.

2. Illustrate how the nurse and the inter-professional team create a culture of safety using leadership, measurement, team work, and risk identification and reduction.

3. Differentiate between a person approach and a system approach to patient safety.

4. Identify the five safety behaviors that are seen in a **high reliability organization (HRO)**, i.e., preoccupation with failure, reluctance to simplify, sensitivity to operations, commitment to resilience, and deference to expertise.

5. Relate simplification and standardization of work processes to patient and health care staff safety.

6. Identify organizations that spread and sustain health care safety.

7. Discuss current safety initiatives for patients such as suicide prevention, safe patient handoff, reduction and avoidance of patient suffering, medication management, hand hygiene, and **Rapid Response Teams (RRTs)**.

Kelly Vana's Nursing Leadership and Management, Fourth Edition. Edited by Patricia Kelly Vana and Janice Tazbir
© 2021 John Wiley & Sons Ltd. Published 2021 by John Wiley & Sons Ltd.
Companion Website: www.wiley.com/go/kelly-Nursing-Leadership

8. Discuss current safety initiatives for nurses and other health care staff, such as **safe patient handling and mobility (SPHM)**, avoidance of falls, slips and trips, environmental safety and biological hazards, and management of violence in the workplace.

OPENING SCENARIO

Mr. Jones is a 62-year-old male brought into the Emergency Department (ED) by local police after he was found standing on the top of a parking garage. The police report that Mr. Jones had been drinking and said he "just wants to end it all." He was brought to the ED for evaluation and possible admission to the mental health unit. You are the triage nurse in the ED and accept the patient from the police. Mr. Jones is relatively calm and does not want to talk about his suicidal ideation at this time. You place him in a mental health safe room and initiate one-to-one observation. You assist Mr. Jones to change into hospital pajamas. You ask Mr. Jones about any family or friends in the area. He reports that his wife of 35 years recently died of cancer and he has been devastated ever since. His responses are short and he doesn't initiate conversation. You orient Mr. Jones to the safe room as a specially designed place where you and the other health care staff can help him be free from harm. In addition, you instruct the sitter who will be providing one-to-one observation for Mr. Jones that he is on observation for suicidal ideation and should be kept under observation at all times, including when using the bathroom. You tell the sitter and Mr. Jones that he is under continuous observation until he can be moved to the safer environment of the mental health unit. You page the mental health team for a STAT evaluation of the patient. Next, you give Mr. Jones a breathalyzer test to determine his blood alcohol level, and find that the level is under the legal limit. The mental health team arrives and continues to evaluate Mr. Jones. The team determines that he is appropriate for admission to the hospital's mental health unit. There is an available bed so, once he is medically cleared by the ED physician, Mr. Jones is escorted to the mental health unit for further treatment.

1. *Why is it important to keep Mr. Jones under continuous one-to-one observation, even while using the bathroom?*

2. *Why does the nurse have Mr. Jones change out of his street clothes?*

3. *What techniques can you use to assess Mr. Jones while he is in the ED?*

Safety minimizes the risk of harm to patients and providers through both system effectiveness and individual performance (QSEN, 2018). Safety is a process. Nurses work with inter-professional teams to create health care systems that provide safe care for patients and reduce preventable harm to patients and health care staff. They use safe, reliable activities and processes such as standardized methods for handoffs to achieve positive health care outcomes. Safety improvement teams are composed of people who are involved in or "touch" the process being improved. In a safe health care system, nurses, doctors, and the inter-professional team identify and remove safety problems before anyone in the system is harmed or subject to an adverse event. An **adverse event** is an occurrence caused during health care delivery in which the patient suffers injury resulting in prolonged hospitalization, disability, or death (Rafter et al., 2015). For example, if a nurse gives a patient the wrong dose of a medication and the patient is harmed, it is an adverse event. This adverse event is preventable if the health care organization has a number of systems in place to prevent giving a wrong dose, for example, a bar code medication administration system or prefilled syringes. Many negative outcomes in health care that were once considered normal complications, such as **Catheter-Associated Urinary Tract Infections (CAUTI)** and hospital-acquired pressure ulcers, are now considered preventable adverse events (Cullen Gill, 2015; Feinmann, 2018).

This chapter will define safety. The behaviors of the nurse and inter-professional team will be illustrated as components of a culture of safety, for example leadership, measurement, teamwork, and risk identification and reduction. The safety behaviors that are visible in an HRO will be reviewed. A person approach to safety and a system approach to safety in a health care organization will be discussed in relation to the nurse's daily work. The chapter will review the Swiss Cheese Model of Safety. A selection of organizations that sustain and spread health care safety will be identified. It will review the quality improvement strategies of simplification and standardization of work processes. Safety initiatives for patients and health care staff will be discussed.

Safety

The problem of preventable medical harm has been estimated to be the third leading causes of death in the United States, after heart disease and cancer (Makary & Daniel, 2016). The estimate is more startling as it does not include harm in which the patient survives but is left with lasting disability or in need of additional medical care (Gandhi, 2017). Every year there are almost 3 million **Hospital-Acquired Conditions** (HACs) among all hospital inpatients of 18 years and older. Many HACs are preventable adverse events (Table 14.1).

Nurses are in a unique position to directly influence the use and spread of best practices to reduce harm to patients. Nurses are with patients around the clock in hospitals. They are typically left in charge of entire hospitals during evening and over-night hours, weekends, and holidays. Nurses understand the organization's processes for delivering health care. Nurses are intimately involved with patient care more than any other health care provider. This results in countless opportunities to support patient safety on a daily basis. Nurses monitor patients for clinical deterioration and respond to ensure patients receive high-quality care in response. As a result, nurses can be the first to detect weaknesses in health care systems that have the potential to harm patients, staff, and visitors (Patient Safety Network (PSNET), 2018). Nurses play a critically important role in ensuring patient safety.

However, there are obstacles in health care organizations that challenge safety. Communication breakdowns, inadequate staffing, poor judgment, lack of skill, and inconsistent adherence to standardized and evidence-based practices can directly result in patient harm and death. Nurses who use the health care organization's quality and safety structures and processes counteract these possibilities and support the outcome of safe quality care for patients.

For example, in the opening scenario, you are assigned the mental health safe room as part of your duties as the triage nurse. You check all the health care system's safety structures, that is, you make sure the mental health safe room does not have any objects that could be used for patient self-harm, such as medications, sharps, or anchor points for hanging. You verify that safe health care processes are in place by checking your assignment and duties with the ED physician, other nurses, and nursing support personnel. You are ready for the arrival of a patient needing emergency mental health care because you have ensured the safety structures and safety processes necessary to ensure patient safety and quality patient care are in place.

Table 14.1 Hospital-Acquired Conditions

Adverse drug events
Catheter-Associated Urinary Tract Infections (CAUTI)
Central-Line Associated Blood Stream Infections (*CLABSI*)
Pressure ulcers
Surgical Site Infections
Ventilator-Associated Pneumonias

Source: Adapted from Declines in Hospital-Acquired .Agency for Healthcare Research and Quality (AHRQ). U.S. Department of Health & Human Services (2018).

A Culture of Safety

Culture is the sum of all the characteristics, values, thinking, and behaviors of people in organizations (Braithwaite, Herkes, Ludlow, Testa, & Lamprell, 2017). Culture refers to the consistent practices, beliefs, and attitudes of a whole organization such as a hospital. It also refers to more specific workplace characteristics within the larger organization. For example, hospital departments such as inpatient units and laboratories, or employee groups such as doctors and nurses, have their own identifiable subcultures, each with their own characteristics, values, thinking, and behaviors. Culture is a product of what is done on a consistent daily basis.

A **culture of safety** is one where everyone feels responsible for safety, pursues it on a daily basis, and is comfortable reporting unsafe conditions and behaviors. The health care organization values safety designs, safety structures, and safety processes, so the safety outcome of greatest reduction in accidental harm to patients and staff is achieved. The nurse and the inter-professional team become personally involved in making safety a priority by identifying gaps in the organization's safety operations and committing to finding ways to provide a culture of safety for patients and staff (Table 14.2).

A culture of safety is critical in keeping preventable harm from reaching patients and health care staff. The four components of a culture of safety are: leadership, measurement, teamwork, and risk identification and reduction.

Leadership

Leadership establishes and nourishes the health care organization's safety culture. Health care staff, patients, and the community measure an organization's commitment to culture by what leaders do, rather than what they say should be done (Joint Commission, 2017b). For a culture of safety to flourish, the leaders must constantly reinforce a just environment where staff are not punished for making unintentional mistakes or errors. Instead, health care staff receive positive reinforcement for bringing errors or problems in the system to leadership so that problems can be studied and resolved. Good leaders understand that when unintentional mistakes or errors are punished, it can lead to staff keeping errors hidden. Hiding errors increases the chance of harm to patients, staff, or visitors.

Incident Report

An **incident report** is a mechanism used by health care organizations for staff reporting any adverse event such as a fall, medication error, or close call. For example, if a nurse is about to give a patient a wrong dose but at the last minute double-checks and sees that it is a wrong dose, then no harm comes to the patient and it is considered a close call. In a health care organization where the leadership is committed to safety, and the staff are educated to report close calls, the nurse has no fear of punishment, and reports the close call on an incident report. The study of close calls provides good

Table 14.2 **Nursing Commitment to a Culture of Safety**

Quality measure	Gap in health care organization's safety operations	Nursing commitment to a culture of safety
Structure, i.e., the physical and organizational characteristics of a hospital, such as its buildings, patient care units, unit design, staffing, equipment and supplies, policies and procedures, computers, human resources, financing, etc.	Participation of bedside nurses on the Environment of Care Committee and Infection Committee is low due to chronic short-staffing on the units.	The nurse reads committee minutes and shares the summary with colleagues during unit staff meeting. The nurse asks the nurse manager what can be done to obtain more staffing.
Process, i.e., a series of steps, actions, and decisions, e.g., diagnosis, treatment, preventive care, and patient education, that interact to produce an outcome.	New-hire health care staff receive minimal orientation to the health care organization's Safe Patient Handling and Movement (SPHM) program.	The nurse teaches new employees on the unit how to use patient-lifting equipment. All staff regularly assess what health care processes are needed to improve patient care.
Outcome, i.e., the end result of all the structures and work processes as well as the relationships among them.	The health care organization's rates for nurse injury are higher than benchmarked rates from other organizations.	The nurse collaborates with colleagues to implement a Comprehensive Unit-based Safety Program (CUSP), a method that can help clinical teams make care safer by combining improved teamwork, clinical best practices, and the science of safety.

Nursing care that develops quality patient care structures also tends to perform well in terms of developing quality clinical processes, which in turn tends to lead to quality patient outcomes.

Note. Created by C. Rovinski-Wagner & P. Mills.

information about how a patient or staff member could have been harmed in a process. This knowledge guides quality improvements to reduce the chance of these incidents happening in the future.

An incident reporting system strengthens patient and staff safety within the health care organization. It helps staff identify the factors that lead up to a situation and what to look out for in similar situations in the future. Health care leadership cultivates a culture of safety by managing the incident report process with a system, rather than a person, approach.

Person Approach to Safety

The **person approach to safety** is the perspective that each health care staff member is responsible for keeping patients safe and in order to do that, no one can make mistakes while doing their jobs. While all staff must take personal responsibility for doing the best job possible, everyone can eventually make a mistake or error. Leadership relying on health care staff perfection as a strategy to keep patients safe is a formula for patient harm. A person approach to safety blames the person who makes the error regardless of any other factors that may have contributed to the error. For example, a nurse who is floated to a different unit administers the wrong dose of an intravenous medication because the pump is similar but not the same as the one the nurse uses on the nurse's regularly assigned unit. The nurse is blamed for the error despite the similarity of the pumps. A person approach to safety is a barrier to nurses and other health care staff reporting errors (Peyrovi, Nasrabadi, & Valiee, 2016).

System Approach to Safety

On the other hand, the **system approach to safety** is a system of patient care that takes into account human error and strives to keep the harm potentially caused by an error from reaching patients. A system approach to safety takes a broad view of an adverse event.

For example, a nurse realizes that she has drawn up and administered the wrong dose of a medication to a patient and the patient experiences no demonstrable ill effect. No one but the nurse is aware of the error, creating a situation where the nurse has to choose whether or not to submit an incident report. The nurse may decide to not report the occurrence if the organization has a person approach to safety. The nurse in a health care organization that uses a system approach to safety is more likely to submit an incident report. This nurse understands that all components of a system of medication administration will be reviewed after a medication error, in order to determine how to prevent the error from happening again in the future. Many questions will be asked. For example, was the staffing on the unit sufficient, how many interruptions did the nurse have during the medication administration process, how was the medication preparation area configured, etc. The nurse also understands that a culture of safety is not a punitive culture.

In a culture of safety, however, the nurse is not absolved of personal accountability. The nurse's characteristics are also considered. For example, individual mentoring might be recommended if the nurse is a new graduate and needs further training on time management and patient care accuracy. If analysis reveals that the nurse is well-experienced and has a pattern of similar errors despite re-education and counseling, escalated discipline, such as a written warning, suspension, or termination, might be implemented.

Measurement

A health care organization, with a culture of safety, measures and monitors its patient care delivery processes and outcomes to ensure that the organization is consistently utilizing best practices for patient and staff safety. Measurement of safety measures provides feedback to leadership and health care staff about the outcomes of its culture of safety.

For example, a hospital has implemented a plan of action that all inpatients assessed to be at high risk for falling will be monitored using a specific set of interventions to reduce the chance of falls. The hospital measures and monitors the rate of falls for each unit. Measuring a fall rate as opposed to just counting the number of falls provides a more accurate picture of the occurrence of patient falls (Table 14.3). When only the number of falls is tracked, the census, meaning how full or empty the unit is at any given time, is not considered. Patient falls are lower when the census is lower, regardless of the care that is provided (**Agency for Healthcare Research and Quality (AHRQ)**, 2013).

There are no national benchmarks available to the public for fall rates since there is no way to guarantee a reliable and valid measurement of falls, since some patients are more likely to fall than others and hospitals care for different types of patients. In assessing fall rates, it is more important to focus on improvement over time within your units and your hospital overall, rather than focusing strictly on your hospital's performance compared with an external benchmark. However, there are two ongoing initiatives to determine fall rates using a standardized method across a large number of hospitals, the National Database of Nursing Quality Indicators (www.pressganey.com/resources/white-papers/the-role-of-workplace-safety-and-surveillance-capacity-in-driving-outcomes accessed May 4, 2019) and the Collaborative Alliance for Nursing Outcomes (https://calnoc.org/page/8 accessed May 4, 2019) (AHRQ, 2013).

The fall rate data from one unit looks variable on the time series graph but the linear line shows a slight downward trend (Figure 14.1). The nurse executive is concerned with the higher rate of falls over the summer months, and measures the process, that is, how often the fall prevention interventions are provided by staff to high-risk patients. The fall prevention intervention data offers a picture of the frequency of the interventions to prevent falls in patients at high risk. It shows the interventions were used less frequently in the summer months. The nurse executive and the nurse managers begin looking at staffing on various units during the times of higher falls rates and lower use of the fall prevention interventions. Their concern is with both patient and staff safety and safe patient handling and mobility. They develop safety improvement strategies based on their findings from data analysis. On-going measurement and monitoring will guide further improvement actions toward the goal of not only increased patient safety but also health care staff safety.

Teamwork

Health care is complex and is not provided by a single clinician. Organizations with a culture of safety demonstrate integrated and inter-professional teamwork in the provision of health care. Teamwork involves communication with colleagues. For example, the plan of care for patients at high risk for falls, mentioned above, includes input and treatment from nursing, pharmacy, physical therapy, as well as the physicians. Monitoring of the plan of care can be done during the inter-professional daily team huddle.

Table 14.3   How to Calculate the Fall Rate on a 30-Bed Unit

Step 1: Count the number of falls that occurred during the month of October from the incident reporting system	There were four falls in the month.
Step 2: Determine for each day of the month at the same point in time, how many beds were occupied on the unit. (A data source for this is the daily hospital census since the calculation is done at the same time every day.)	On the first day of the month, there were 26 beds occupied; on the second day of the month, there were 28 beds occupied, and so on.
Step 3: Add up the total occupied beds each day of the month. The month has 30 days. (If the hospital can calculate the total number of occupied bed days on the unit during the month, use that number and skip Step 2 and 3.)	The total adds to 846 (out of a maximum of 900, since if all 30 beds were occupied on all 30 days, 30×30 would equal 900).
Step 4: Divide the number of falls by the number of occupied bed days for the month.	$4/846 = 0.0047$
Step 5: Multiply the result in Step 4 by 1,000.	$0.0047 \times 1,000 = 4.7$
Step 6: State the fall rate or how many falls occurred per 1,000 occupied bed days of care. (This creates a standardized benchmark to compare fall rates between units.)	Fall rate for the month = 4.7

Source: Adapted from Agency for Healthcare Research and Quality (AHRQ). (2013). How do you measure fall rates and fall prevention practices. Agency for Healthcare Research and Quality, Rockville, MD. U.S. Department of Health & Human Services.

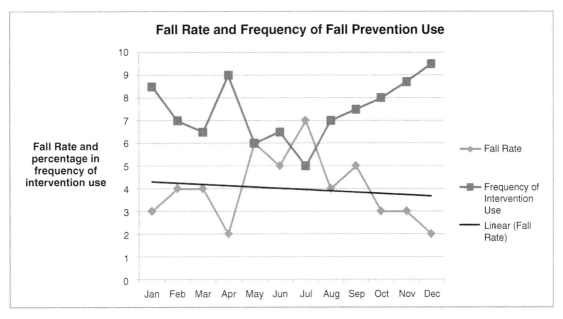

FIGURE 14.1 Fall rate and frequency of fall prevention intervention use. Created by C. Rovinski-Wagner & P. Mills, made with Excel.

Teamwork relies on team members knowing and trusting that others on the inter-professional team will function fully in their respective roles. Building relationships with other team members supports team cohesion. For example, socializing with inter-professional colleagues at breaks facilitates interactions on a personal level and supports the development of rapport among team members. Effective teamwork creates a safe environment for patients and health care staff.

Risk Identification and Reduction

Risk identification and reduction is the identification, mitigation, monitoring, and prevention of potential threats or actual harm to an organization, patients, and staff. Risk identification and reduction is also called risk management. A health care organization with a culture of safety identifies and manages risks to safety, through processes such as the incident reporting system mentioned earlier, the **Healthcare Failure Modes and Effects Analysis (HFMEA)**, a **Root Cause Analysis (RCA)**, and aggregate reviews.

High Failure Mode and Effect Analysis (HFMEA)

The **HFMEA** is a step-by-step standardized method that examines activities having a high possibility for a negative outcome, identifies possible ways that the system can fail in those activities, and recommends actions to improve patient and staff safety when doing activities with a high possibility of a negative outcome (Figure 14.2). It is proactive and occurs before a negative event happens. The purpose of an HFMEA is to prevent tragedy. It doesn't require a previous bad experience or a close call. For example, what will happen on the **Intensive Care Unit (ICU)** when the power goes out? An HFMEA examines possible failures in care or the reasons health care could not be pro-

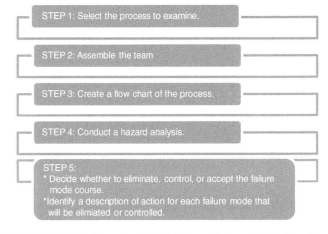

FIGURE 14.2 Steps in a Health Failure Mode and Effect Analysis (HFMEA),
Source: Adapted from VA National Center for Patient Safety, Healthcare Failure Mode and Effect Analysis (HFMEA), 2019.

vided to critically ill patients. Measures to eliminate or control the potential failures are identified. If the electricity goes out in the ICU, the staff cannot use intravenous pumps, computers, ventilators, etc. The HFMEA identifies an action plan for each failure in care that needs to be addressed. For example, battery backup needs to be provided for every intravenous infusion pump, a standard operating procedure to ensure complete written documentation in the event of a power failure needs to be established, and a generator specifically dedicated to the ICU needs to be obtained. This is all addressed in an HFMEA.

Root Cause Analysis (RCA)

An **RCA** is a process that investigates the underlying main cause of an adverse event or near miss. An RCA seeks to discover what happened, why it happened, and how to prevent it from happening again. In an RCA, the inter-professional team interviews clinicians involved in an adverse event or near miss to get an accurate picture of what happened. For example, a patient receives a double dose of anticoagulant medication. The RCA team gathers information from the clinician interviews and builds a fishbone diagram to view the double dose medication error from a system perspective and identify the root cause. A fishbone diagram, also called a cause and effect diagram or Ishikawa diagram, is a visual tool for categorizing the potential causes of a problem in order to view it from a system perspective and identify its root cause. The fishbone diagram guides the RCA team as it asks questions about the double dose medication error, such as, did the nurse accidentally double the dose at the bedside, did the pharmacy double the dose and send it to the floor, or did the doctor order a double dose? And if one or all of these errors happened, why didn't the system, including the electronic medical record and the barcoding system, catch the error? Once the root causes are determined, then an action plan to address each root cause is developed. The RCA helps the health care organization understand what caused an adverse event or near miss after the occurrence and make plans to prevent its reoccurrence.

Aggregate reviews are when a series of similar adverse events or near misses are examined by an inter-professional team to determine if a pattern of breakdowns exists in the health care system that has caused these adverse events. For example, the inter-professional team looks at falls that have occurred on a medical unit. All the falls are listed and the important elements of each case (such as patient's age, illness, and risk for falling) are recorded. Then the team attempts to understand if there are any common threads or patterns in the series of falls. The team may find that all of the falls occurred on the night shift when the nurse to patient ratio is lower and the patients are getting up to go to the bathroom by themselves because their call bells are not answered quickly. Once common threads or patterns are determined, an action plan, such as toileting all patients after dinner and every 2 hr, is implemented. A measurement and monitoring system is established to see if this action plan reduces the falls on the unit.

A health care organization with a culture of safety has high-quality structures and processes of leadership, measurement, teamwork, and risk identification and reduction that result in patient and staff safety. The health care staff in this organization share similar high-quality attitudes, beliefs, perceptions, and values in relation to safety. The staff is committed to creating, strengthening, improving, and sustaining safety constantly throughout the system. The health care staff consistently deliver the right care to the right patient at the right time in the right setting. The same safe outcomes are achieved regardless of patient transfers, patient background, the day of the week, or the area of patient care. The health care organization with a culture of safety demonstrates reliability. This reliability, with its high-quality safety structures, processes, and outcomes, is reproducible in other health care organizations.

Safety Behaviors in a High Reliability Organization

HROs are organizations that achieve a culture of safety in dangerous environments, such as aviation, nuclear energy, and health care. Health care is included as a dangerous environment due to the complex and interwoven components involved in providing safe quality care to patients (Institute for Healthcare Improvement (IHI), 2018). A health care organization that wants to strengthen its culture of safety incorporates the five behaviors of HROs: preoccupation with failure, reluctance to simplify, sensitivity to operations, commitment to resilience, and deference to expertise (Robertson & Kirsh, 2018). HRO behaviors are discussed briefly below, as they apply to safety. They are discussed more extensively in Chapter 4.

Preoccupation with Failure

Leaders in a health care organization with a culture of safety have a preoccupation with failure. **Preoccupation with failure** occurs when leaders want to study errors and undesirable outcomes to improve care. They are willing to hear bad news. They want staff to feel comfortable reporting errors that led to or nearly missed having an undesirable outcome.

Leaders who are preoccupied with failure remove barriers and hierarchies that may impede the flow of bad news because they understand the flow of bad news is an opportunity to prevent or reduce potential harms. For example, leaders preoccupied with failure are visible throughout the organization as they seek both to understand the risks of daily work to patients and staff, and to obtain feedback about what needs to change to improve patient and staff safety.

These leaders also create a health care organization that embraces a just culture as a backbone for patient and health care staff safety. A just culture promotes an atmosphere of trust in which staff are encouraged, even rewarded, for providing essential safety-related information. Health care staff and others can report errors or close calls without fear of reprimand or reprisal. Individuals trust that they will not be held accountable for system failures. However, a just culture is still an environment in which accountability exists.

Accountability is often seen as a response to a wrong act, but it is more complex than that. In a just culture, the health care staff is clear about the difference between acceptable and unacceptable behavior. If reckless behavior is left unpunished, staff will see this as unjust. However, if an honest mistake is punished, staff will also see this as unjust. What matters is that staff in a just health care organization feel assured that they will receive fair treatment when they are involved in adverse events, or when they report them. Leaders who are preoccupied with failure promote accountability but also foster a non-punitive environment in order to keep open lines of communication in support of patient and health care staff safety.

Reluctance to Simplify

Reluctance to simplify is a disinclination to apply a one-size-fits-all solution to a problem. For example, a patient may develop a CAUTI for a variety of reasons, including catheter kits that are not sterile, staff that have not properly washed their hands, insertion kits that are awkward to use, catheters left in too long, and catheters used when they are not called for. Consequently, the process of reducing CAUTIs is not simply replacing catheter kits. The process is multi-faceted and must address all the possible causes of the infection.

In a safe and highly reliable health care organization, human factor engineering might be used when deciding which urinary catheter insertion kits to purchase. Human factor engineering is an applied science that focuses on how systems work in actual practice, with real human beings at the controls. It attempts to design systems that optimize safety and minimize the risk of error in complex environments such as hospitals (PSNET, 2019). For example, a nurse might be asked to use different types of catheter insertion kits in a simulation lab to test which kit is easier to use and less likely to contribute to CAUTI through breaks in sterility. Once the decision is made regarding the preferred kit, a standardized and simple evidence-based procedure for urinary catheter insertion is written.

A reluctance to simplify recognizes all the complexities in a problem situation in order to evaluate and choose the best solution. A reluctance to simplify prevents the health care organization from jumping to conclusions about what will work to keep patients and health care staff safe.

Sensitivity to Operations

Sensitively to operations is when leadership is aware of the day-to-day operations of the health care organization. Leadership wants to hear if problems are occurring more often in a particular area as soon as possible, so that the necessary adjustments can be made before there is an adverse event. For example, if there are usually four staff members that are able to help move bariatric patients and one staff member is injured, the work and strain for the remaining three staff members increases and can lead to further injuries. Nurse leaders, who are sensitive to operations, will anticipate this problem and make adjustments in staffing before other staff members are injured. A nurse who is committed to safety demonstrates leadership by notifying the nursing office and asking for assistance in providing or strategizing how to provide safe care to patients while also protecting all staff from harm.

Commitment to Resilience

Commitment to resilience is when leaders in the health care organization think about what could go wrong in a complex system and attempt to create backup systems to catch errors before any harm comes to the patient. Humans make many errors every day.

There two broad types of errors, execution failure and planning failure. Execution failure occurs when the correct action is taken but, because of problems with attention or memory, the desired goal is not achieved. For example, there is an execution failure when a nurse takes a patient's vital signs but forgets to document them in the medical record. Planning failures occur when the wrong action is applied to the situation. For example, it is a planning failure when a nurse does not bring all necessary supplies into a patient room and has to interrupt patient care in order to retrieve the supplies.

Swiss Cheese Model

Attempts to make humans perfect are futile. The best way to prevent harm to patients is to anticipate human error and build systems that will keep harm from coming to the patient (PSNET, 2019). The **Swiss Cheese Model** is a tool that helps visualize checks and barriers in a system of health care so there is no harm caused to patients or staff due to failures in execution or planning (Reason, 1990) (Figure 14.3). In the Model, the checks and barriers to patient harm in a complex health care system are represented by slices of Swiss Cheese with holes. When by chance, all the holes are aligned, random harm can reach the patient. This Model draws attention to randomness in a health care system as opposed to deliberate action by individuals in the occurrence of health care errors.

For example, a nurse is running late and rushes through administering medications. The nurse does a workaround and overrides the barcode medication system so that late medication can be delivered. The barcode system appears to be running effectively. But there are two patients with the same name on the unit. The nurse's workaround causes the barcode system to not catch the error. As a result, medication is given to the wrong patient. The cheese slices, that is checks and barriers of the five rights of medication administration, the bar code system, and the hospital policy for medication administration, were not enough to prevent the error.

The Swiss Cheese Model does not blame front line clinicians when errors are made. It looks at the holes in the checks and barriers that could cause harm to patients and asks what can be done to close a hole and increase patient safety. For example, what caused the nurse to be late with medication administration? Are there ways to make overrides to the barcode system harder to do? Does the procedure used when two patients with the same name are on the unit have sufficient checks and balances to ensure the safety of each patient during medication administration? Subsequent actions are determined based on the answers to the questions asked.

Another example of a health care organization's commitment to resilience is contingency planning. Contingency planning helps avoid or minimize harm to patients and health care staff by proactively providing a process to follow in the event of an unexpected event such as when a staff shortage occurs during the flu season.

One day, during the flu season, there are many call-outs. The charge nurse follows the hospital's flu season contingency plan. The plan instructs the charge nurse to coordinate assignments

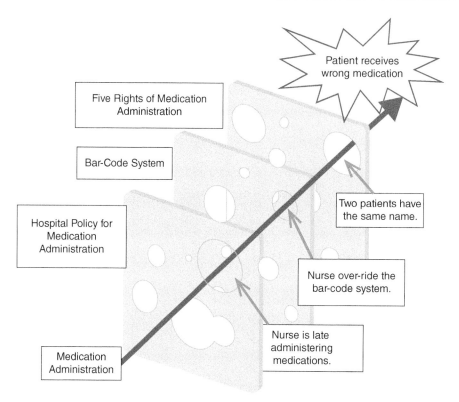

FIGURE 14.3   Swiss Cheese Model and medication administration safety. Concept adapted from Reason (1990), figure created by C. Rovinski-Wagner.

and tasks with the inter-professional team and the nursing office. Nursing leaders come to the unit and accept assignments for the tasks for which they have current competencies. The participation of nursing leaders helps prevent the fatigue that the staff might feel if they did not have the extra nurses. The visible presence of the nursing leaders helps to improve the mental health of the staff as they see leadership that is truly committed to working together with them to deliver the best care possible to patients in the safest way available. Various members of the inter-professional team, such as physical therapists, take on extra tasks such as helping turn patients to ensure that patient needs are safely met and the nursing staff is not injured by doing more than is physically safe. A commitment to resilience by the leadership and the inter-professional team contributes to positive organizational cultures and workplace subcultures. Positive cultures and subcultures in health care are consistently associated with improved patient outcomes such as reduction in mortality, falls, and hospital-acquired infections, and increased patient satisfaction (Braithwaite et al., 2017).

Deference to Expertise

Deference to expertise is the practice of seeking advice from the person with the most experience or expertise in a specific situation, regardless of their position in the organizational hierarchy. For example, there is a new nurse on the ICU who worked at another hospital for 10 years on the mental health unit. When the ICU receives a medically ill patient with a bipolar disorder, the nurse manager asks the new nurse during care

plan construction with the inter-professional team for suggestions on how to manage mental health issues that may arise. In this way, the nurse manager is showing deference to expertise. The nurse manager is using the new nurse's knowledge to get the best input possible to care for the patient, even though she is senior to the new nurse in the organizational hierarchy. Deference to expertise also demonstrates to the new nurse and other health care staff that the nurse manager values teamwork.

Organizations that Spread and Sustain Health Care Safety

Many organizations help spread and sustain patient and health care staff safety. Their materials are accessible through the internet (Table 14.4). These organizations value partnerships with a wide variety of health care organizations including but not limited to specialized international health care organizations and large national health care organizations. This provides nurses with opportunities to work with national and international colleagues in the development of standardized clinical tools usable by many hospitals. Organizations that spread and sustain health care safety collect, analyze, validate, and distribute evidence-based best practices.

Best practices for safe health care provision reflect simplification of work practices and standardization of work processes. Simplification and standardization of work processes reduces variation which is associated with increased harm to patients and health care staff.

Table 14.4 Organizations that Spread and Sustain Patient and Health Care Staff Safety

Organization	Safety focus
Agency for Healthcare Research and Quality www.ahrq.gov/professionals/education/curriculum-tools/ cusptoolkit/index.html accessed December 30, 2018	The Comprehensive Unit-based Safety Program (CUSP), a method that can help clinical teams make care safer by combining improved teamwork, clinical best practices, and the science of safety.
Occupational Safety and Health Administration www.osha.gov/dts/oom/clinicians accessed December 30/, 2018	Work-related health and safety information for health care staff.
Veterans Health Administration www.patientsafety.va.gov accessed December 20, 2018	Reduction and prevention of inadvertent harm to patients and the health care team as a result of patient care.
Children's Hospitals' Solutions for Patient Safety www.solutionsforpatientsafety.org accessed December 30, 2018	Improvements in safe pediatric care for patients and the health care team.

Note. Created by C. Rovinski-Wagner & P. Mills.

Simplification of Work Processes

Simplification of work processes is the reduction of a work process to its essential steps, making it easier to understand and complete. For example, assigning staff to patient care in rooms in close proximity to each other may simplify the work process and improve efficiency.

Standardization of Work Processes

Standardization of work processes is the use of a single set of terms, definitions, practices and/or clinical tools, such as bundles, checklists, or protocols. Standardization makes it easier to do the right step every time to improve health care safety. For example, a nurse wants to reduce the occurrence of CAUTI on the surgical unit. The nurse uses the Catheter Out clinician and researcher resources, at www.catheterout.org/resources.html, accessed January 4, 2019, for guidance to increase nurse and physician engagement in the reduction of CAUTI. This helps to ensure that the resulting structures and processes for urinary catheter management at the health care

organization will be evidence-based and reliable and will support the outcome of reduction of the occurrence of CAUTI on the surgical unit.

Health care organizations incorporate evidence-based best practices into safety initiatives to reduce potential and actual harm to their patients, their nurses, and their other health care staff (Table 14.5).

Safety Initiatives for Patients

Suicide Prevention

Suicide is a leading cause of death in the United States, and suicide rates are increasing. The Centers for Disease Control and Prevention (**CDC**) estimates that over half the people who died by suicide did not have a known mental health condition (Centers for Disease Control (CDC), 2018). Risk factors for suicide include personal characteristics such as age, gender, and race, as well as previous suicide attempts and suicidal thoughts, mood disorders (such as depression), and access to lethal weapons. Suicide is the second leading cause of death

Table 14.5 Safety Initiatives to Protect Patients, Nurses, and Other Health Care Staff

Disaster planning and disaster drills	Double checks on blood for transfusions
Patient identification bands	Annual tuberculosis testing of staff
Incident reports	Fit-testing for N95 respirator masks for staff
Air control rooms for isolation patients	Patient lift equipment
Disinfectant cleaning of patient and procedure rooms	Hourly rounding for patient status and needs, such as toileting
Visitor sign-in	Training for staff on how to prevent and manage disruptive behavior by patients, staff, and visitors
Fire prevention education and fire drills	ID badges for hospital personnel to access to hospital
Locked hospital units	Suicide prevention protocol

Note. Created by C. Rovinski-Wagner & P. Mills.

for adolescents 15–19 years old (Shain & AAP Committee on Adolescence, 2016). White males over 50 are at higher risk. Additionally, individuals who are members of the Armed Forces or in the Lesbian, Gay, Bisexual, and Transgender populations are at higher risk for suicide than the general population (U.S. Department of Health and Human Services (HHS) Office of the Surgeon General and National Action Alliance for Suicide Prevention, 2012).

Suicide prevention involves evaluating individual patients for their intention to harm themselves. It is important to understand that if a patient is reporting an intention to harm themselves, it must be taken seriously and acted upon. The suicidal patient should be kept under observation and mental health professionals should be immediately called to the scene. Nurses can encounter suicidal patients in all areas of the hospital (Joint Commission, 2017). Nurses need to understand how to care for these patients and how to avoid an inpatient suicide.

When working with a patient whom you think is suicidal, ask if the patient is thinking about hurting himself or herself or committing suicide. This does not push a patient toward suicide. Rather, it informs the patient that you are actively concerned with the patient's safety. This contributes to eliciting the patient's trust in you and the provision of high-quality comprehensive care. The structure for quality care provision to a patient with suicidal ideation or intent is important in the prevention of self-harm. For example, hanging accounts for more than 70% of suicides in hospital inpatient suicides (Williams et al, 2017). Almost 54% of the time the fixture point for the hanging device was a door, door handle, or door hinge. Psychiatric units should not have clothes hooks and unnecessary doors since these could be used for a suicide by hanging. If the suicidal patient is getting care on a medical unit, all objects that could be used for self-harm should be removed except when they are needed for patient care.

The process of safe care for a patient with suicidal ideation includes notification of the patient's primary care provider and the psychiatry department per your facility's protocol. This facilitates a more thorough patient assessment and determination of the appropriate level of care. For example, in the opening scenario, Mr. Jones' blood alcohol level did not indicate a need for detoxification on a medical unit. With these findings of the ED physician and mental health team, the most appropriate level of care was determined to be admission to the mental health unit. Typically, suicidal patients are only feeling suicidal for a short period of time. Nurses are responsible for getting these patients through this time without allowing the patients to hurt or kill themselves.

Safe Patient Handoff

A **patient hand-off** involves passing patient specific information from one caregiver to another or from one team of caregivers to another, for the purpose of ensuring the continuity and safety of the patient's care (Joint Commission, 2017a). It is a transfer and acceptance of patient care responsibility. For example, in

the opening scenario, handoffs occur when you transfer responsibility for constant observation to the patient's bedside sitter, when you give intake information to the ED physician, when information is shared with the mental health team, and when Mr. Jones is admitted to the mental health unit. Patients are at risk if handoffs are not communicated thoroughly and carefully. For example, one study of malpractice cases found that over half of the cases involving nurse communication failures resulted in either a high-severity injury or death in health care organizations (CRICO Strategies, 2015) (Figure 14.4).

Patient safety can be improved and miscommunication avoided when the process of patient handoff is standardized. Two common techniques to standardize patient handoff communication are **I-PASS** (Illness severity, Patient summary, Action lists, Situational awareness and contingency planning, and Synthesis by receiver) and **SBARR** (Situation, Background, Assessment, Recommendation, and Response) (Table 14.6).

Patient handoffs must be interactive to be safe. Nurses can interact and contribute to safe patient handoffs during shift report by using standardized processes such as I-PASS or SBARR, by giving, asking and verifying information, and by using relational behaviors. Relational behaviors are deliberate behaviors. They include being approachable, using clear and concrete language, taking steps to make the other person feel comfortable, and being respectful. Patients can be included in handoffs when they are able, for example, during shift reports at the bedside. These relational behaviors and standardized processes, such as I-PASS and SBARR, strengthen interprofessional and patient-centered collaboration. They protect patient safety (Eggins & Slade, 2015).

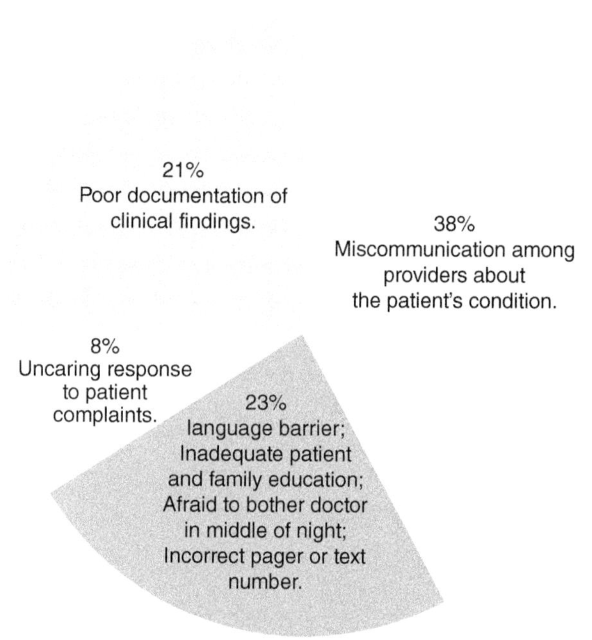

21%
Poor documentation of clinical findings.

38%
Miscommunication among providers about the patient's condition.

8%
Uncaring response to patient complaints.

23%
language barrier; Inadequate patient and family education; Afraid to bother doctor in middle of night; Incorrect pager or text number.

FIGURE 14.4   Communication breakdowns involving nurses resulting in patient harm.
Source: Data from CRICO Strategies (2015). Figure created by C. Rovinski-Wagner & P. Mills.

Table 14.6   Opening Scenario Handoff Using I-PASS and SBARR for Patient Safety

I-PASS	SBARR	Example from opening scenario
Illness severity	Situation	Mr. Jones is on 1 : 1 observation in the mental health safe room with a sitter. He is answering questions but not questions about his suicidal ideation. He says he is devastated by the death of his wife and "just wants to end it all."
Patient summary	Background	Mr. Jones was brought in by the police earlier this evening. They found him on a garage roof. He had been drinking. He was verbalizing suicidal ideation.
Action lists	Assessment	Mr. Jones hasn't made any attempts to self-harm since being in the ED. The breathalyzer was within legal limits. The medical team and the mental health team have cleared Mr. Jones for admission to the mental health unit.
Situational awareness and contingency planning	Recommendation	Please continue 1 : 1 observation during the transfer and admission to the mental health unit. The sitter will go with you. Mr. Jones' clothes are in this bag, including a belt and a very stretchy t-shirt. Please don't let Mr. Jones have access to the bag or any other item than can be used for self harm right now.
Synthesis by receiver	Response	I will have the sitter accompany me and Mr. Jones during the transfer and admission. I will make sure that Mr. Jones does not have access to the bag containing his personal belongings until any items that can be used for self-harm have been removed.

Note. Created by C. Rovinski-Wagner & P. Mills.

Evidence from the Literature

Source: White-Trevino, K., & Dearmon, V. (2018). Transitioning Nurse Handoff to the Bedside: Engaging Staff and Patients. Nursing Administration Quarterly. 42(3): 261–268.

Discussion: A standardized patient-centric bedside handoff report process was implemented in an emergency department. 46 hospital-based nurses participated. Outcomes were measured through observations of the bedside report process and nurse and patient surveys. Off-going nurses used most elements of the handoff process more often than the nurses coming on-shift. All the nurses believed that the new handoff report process positively influenced their ability to respond to patient needs. More than half of the patients observed during the bedside handoff report actively participated in the handoff report process. Overall, patients were more satisfied with their nursing care.

Implications for Practice: A standardized, patient-centered bedside handoff report process ensures reliable communication between the patient and nurses that increases patient safety and promotes patient satisfaction with care.

Reduction and Avoidance of Patient Suffering

Suffering is often part of the patient experience and has the potential to cause harm to the patient (Card & Klein, 2016). Some suffering is avoidable and some is not. Unavoidable patient suffering is associated with their diseases or treatments. For example, pain is an unavoidable suffering when caused by disease, such as cancer, or by a treatment, such as surgery. The patient's suffering can be reduced by treating the underlying illness and managing side effects and symptoms.

Avoidable patient suffering is the result of dysfunction in the health care delivery system. Examples of avoidable patient suffering are delaying response to a patient's call bell and speaking too quickly for the patient to understand what is being said. Poor care coordination such as in non-informative patient hand-offs, ignorance about the individual details of a patient's treatment plan, or less than collegial behavior among the patient's inter-professional health care team also contribute to a patient's experience of suffering. A nurse reduces avoidable patient suffering by: giving information to patients, such as introducing the team members at the start of shift and letting patients know the basics of the shift routine; orienting patients to unfamiliar health care environments, such as where the nurse's station is in relation to the patient's room; and showing courtesy, such as not talking from the patient's doorway and using the patient's preferred form of address when conversing with the patient.

Health care staff in a culture of safety know that avoidable and unavoidable patient suffering erodes patient trust in the health care system and elevates the patient's existing anxiety, fear and frustration. This suffering becomes a barrier to the patient's ability to achieve safe, high-quality health care outcomes.

The hospitalized patient is in a situation that is often life-changing. In a culture of safety, a nurse recognizes that what the nurse considers normal may not be what the patient considers normal. The nurse makes a conscious effort to eliminate avoidable suffering. One way to do this is to anticipate the patient's pain and consider the impact the nurse's words and approach may have on the patient. For example, the nurse coaches the patient with bilateral knee replacements through

Critical Thinking 14.1

You are the charge nurse on an overnight shift. One of the patients, Mr. Smith, is well-known to you and the other nurses. He has been hospitalized many times since a serious car accident to treat the initial injuries and the subsequent related health issues. Mr. Smith has been characterized as a "difficult" patient because of his many questions about the health care being provided to him. Toward the end of the shift, Mr. Smith calls you to his room. He says that a new nurse brought his medication 2 hr early. He told the nurse he normally took his medications at a different time and that the pills looked different. The nurse replied that his illness was making him forgetful. When Mr. Smith continued to refuse the medication, the nurse became more and more irritated. Mr. Smith insisted that the nurse check his medical record. The nurse returned and confirmed that she had, indeed, made an error, and had been trying to give him the wrong patient's medication. The nurse told Mr. Smith that now everything was fine and left the room without further discussion.

1. What would you say to Mr. Smith about the incident?
2. What behaviors of the medication nurse constitute patient harm?
3. What would you say to the nurse?
4. What would your follow-up actions be?

---

the patient's first walk to the bathroom. When the nurse has the forethought to coordinate the patient's walk and toileting with the timing of analgesic administration, the nurse has made an effort to reduce the patient's unavoidable suffering due to pain. The nurse's encouragement and assurances of stand-by assistance reduces the patient's avoidable suffering.

However, if the nurse does not assess or ask about pain prior to the walk and toileting, the pain is avoidable suffering due to pain, plus the patient is not able to focus on safe ambulation techniques without distraction. The nurse decreases the patient's avoidable suffering from pain and increases the patient's trust in the health care system by being attentive to pain signals such as facial cringing, anticipating and asking about levels of pain, and then responding with empathy and urgency in medication administration.

Medication Management

A nurse is likely to be involved in a medication management error through individual mistakes or lapses in concentration. An individual mistake is a lack of problem solving, such as not contacting the physician when a prescribed medication dosage seems too large. Lapses in concentration are associated with competing sensory or emotional distractions, fatigue, and stress, such as when the nurse doesn't follow the five rights (right patient, right medication, right time, right dose, and right route) because of multiple interruptions during the medication management process. Medication management errors also result from health care organization failures such as understaffing or purchasing equipment such as a medication cart that is poorly designed.

The nurse protects patient safety by adhering to the organization's procedure for medication administration (van der Veen et al., 2018). For example, when the health care organization uses a **BarCode Medication Administration (BCMA)** scanner, the nurse does not use a workaround when the patient's armband is smudged and the bar code is unreadable. Instead the nurse replaces the patient's arm band with one that is clear and readable by the BCMA scanner.

The nurse can also use quality improvement to improve patient safety. For example, the nurse can form a team that uses **Plan-Do-Study-Act (PDSA)** Cycles to evaluate the effectiveness of different strategies and ideas in reducing the number of interruptions during medication administration. The PDSA Cycle is not used to evaluate near misses or adverse events. Refer to Chapter 12 for an example of how a cardiology team used a PDSA Cycle to reduce the occurrence of fluid overload in patients with heart failure.

Hand Hygiene

Nosocomial, or hospital-acquired, infections are a major threat to patient safety. Every year, an estimated 2 million patients get a hospital-related infection and 90,000 die from their infection (CDC, 2018). Frequent handwashing, using the proper procedure, is associated with decreased morbidity and mortality rates (Rodziewicz & Hipskind, 2018).

Health care providers might need to wash their hands as many as 100 times per 12 hr shift, depending on the number of patients and intensity of care. On average, health care staff wash their hands less than half as often as they should (CDC, 2018). This puts patients and staff at risk for infection transmission.

A nurse contributes to patient and health care staff safety by role modeling hand hygiene, offering feedback to peers who do not follow hand hygiene practices, volunteering to be the unit's hand hygiene champion, and participating in infection control improvement projects that require real time performance monitoring. A nurse also increases the effectiveness and frequency of hand hygiene compliance by identifying structures, processes, and outcomes related to hand hygiene and by educating patients about handwashing (Table 14.7).

Rapid Response Team

An RRT is a team of expert clinicians who provide additional care for patients on acute care units who are experiencing unexpected acute changes in their conditions. Its use provides

Table 14.7 Hand Hygiene Structure, Process, and Outcome

Structure	Sinks, soap, paper towels, and antibacterial hand wash are easily accessible in and around patient rooms. Signage about hand-washing procedures is posted near sinks.
Process	The nurse explains how and why the health care team members clean their hands before, after, and sometimes during patient care. The nurse encourages patients to ask health care team members about hand hygiene. The nurse discusses how and why patients should keep their hands clean.
Outcome	Patients are involved in their care. Health care team members wash their hands per standard. Patients and health care team members experience fewer infections.

Note. Created by C. Rovinski-Wagner & P. Mills.

the greatest potential for reduced risk of harm to the patient who is experiencing unexpected acute changes in their condition. The goal of the RRT is to prevent avoidable patient progression to cardiopulmonary arrest or unexpected death. The RRT is different than a code blue team. The goal of a code blue team is to resuscitate a person who has stopped breathing, or who does not have a heartbeat.

The composition of RRTs is variable. Some are physician led, some are nurse led, and all are dependent on the health care organization's resources in personnel and funding. Typically, an RRT consists of critical care nurses, physicians, and respiratory therapists. The nurse on the acute care unit has a pivotal role in relation to the RRT. The nurse is responsible for early recognition of clinical deterioration of the patient, early calls to the RRT for assistance, and timely interventions to counteract patient clinical deterioration. When a nurse does not recognize signs of clinical deterioration in a patient, it is called Failure to Rescue.

The nurse is responsible for improving the patient's safety through proactive assessments of patients at risk for clinical deterioration. Responsible actions include educating other staff, patients, and families about how to recognize warning

signs that need to be brought to the nurse's attention. In some health care organizations, anyone, including family, hospital staff, nursing staff, physicians, and visitors are allowed to call the RRT. Patient safety is supported when the nurse in a health care organization identifies early warning signs in a patient and calls an RRT.

Safety for Nurses and Other Health Care Staff

Health care has one of the highest occurrences of nonfatal occupational injury and illness than any other industry sector (U.S. Bureau of Labor Statistics (BLS), 2017). Historically, nurses have experienced some of the highest injury and illness rates in the health care sector (Dressner, 2017). Nurses working in health care organizations are subject to musculoskeletal conditions related to patient handling, falls, slips, and trips, blood-borne pathogens and tuberculosis (TB), and workplace violence (Occupational Safety and Health Administration (OSHA), 2015). The distribution of injuries and illnesses differs between nurse age groups (Figure 14.5).

Safe Patient Handling and Mobility (SPHM)

It is easy in the heat of the moment to attempt to lift a patient by one's self. However, the nurse who is injured will not be available to work and help other patients for weeks or months. Additionally, the remaining staff will be at risk for injury if the open position is not covered or filled due to less people to do the same work.

The most common event in hospitals leading to injuries in 2015 was injury sustained during physical interactions such as lifting and moving patients (Dressner, 2017). Nurses accounted for a substantial portion of these injuries. Nurses had almost as many reported days away from work as construction laborers in 2016 due to workplace injuries (BLS, 2017). Excessive physical effort, bending, twisting, lifting, and repetitive motion in the daily workday of nurses lead to musculoskeletal disorders such as sprains, strains, and tears of muscles. More than a quarter of these disorders are back injuries

---

Critical Thinking 14.2

The number of employed nurses who are 55 or older has increased from 13% in 2000 to 24% in 2017. However, during the same time frame, the median age of employed nurses has only increased by about 1 year due to a major increase in RNs under the age of 35. This data indicates that employers are gaining younger nurses who are lacking experience, but losing older nurses who have necessary experience (Karp, 2018). Refer to Figure 14.5 as you answer these questions.

1. What might account for the variation in overexertion and bodily reaction between the younger and older age ranges?
2. What might account for the reduction in exposure to harmful substances and environments from younger nurses to older nurses?
3. How can novice nurses and experienced nurses collaborate to reduce the work-related injuries and illnesses?
4. What is the hospital's responsibility to nurses to reduce these work-related injuries and illnesses?

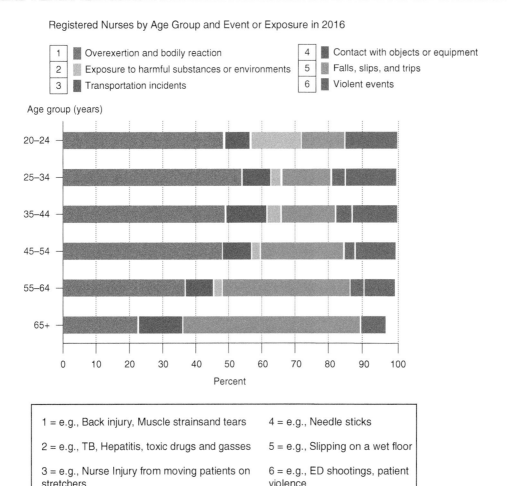

Registered Nurses by Age Group and Event or Exposure in 2016

1	Overexertion and bodily reaction	4	Contact with objects or equipment
2	Exposure to harmful substances or environments	5	Falls, slips, and trips
3	Transportation incidents	6	Violent events

Age group (years)

Percent

1 = e.g., Back injury, Muscle strainsand tears	4 = e.g., Needle sticks
2 = e.g., TB, Hepatitis, toxic drugs and gasses	5 = e.g., Slipping on a wet floor
3 = e.g., Nurse Injury from moving patients on stretchers	6 = e.g., ED shootings, patient violence

FIGURE 14.5   Percent of distribution of non-fatal occupational injuries and illnesses to registered nurses by age group and event or exposure in 2016.
Source: Dressner, M. A. and Kissinger, S. P. (2018). Occupational Injuries and Illnesses Among Registered Nurses. Monthly Labor Review, U.S. Bureau of Labor Statistics. Public Domain.

(Dressner & Kissinger, 2018). In 2016, registered nurses had a higher rate of musculoskeletal disorders than all other occupations combined in the private sector (Figure 14.6). A study in China, which examined low back pain in orthopedic nurses, revealed that almost 67% of the 797 nurses studied suffered low back pain during the 1-year study period and over half planned to quit due to low back pain (Li et al., 2019). The

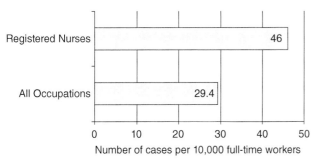

FIGURE 14.6   Incidence rates of sprains, strains, and tears of muscles.
Source: Adapted from Bureau of Labor Statistics (2016).

study also found that nurses in this region of China experienced an incidence of low back pain similar to those in other regions in the world. Nurses can work collaboratively with the physical and occupational therapy staff during construction of patient care plans to ensure that instructions are included about the minimum number of staff and type of equipment needed to move or ambulate a patient. This team collaboration should also include any assessments of the patient that might influence the patient's ability to participate in safe handling and mobility. For example, the patient with bilateral knee replacements says the incisions feel like they are going to rip open when his legs are bent and the patient is resistant to repositioning and ambulation. The care plan includes this information so staff can re-educate the patient that the feeling is normal and related to the post-operative swelling and healing. The care plan also includes interventions for analgesic administration as prescribed and 1 hr before ambulation, having two or more staff, as needed, when repositioning and ambulating the patient, and using a walker for ambulation that has been adjusted for the patient's height. Patient education

Table 14.8   Ergonomics Components and Examples in Health Care Needed to Eliminate All Manual Lifting to Avoid Patient and Staff Injury

Ergonomic component	Examples in health care
Work being performed	Nursing care of patients
Physical environment where the work is performed	Intensive care unit
The tools used to help perform the work	Ceiling mounted patient lifts and other Safe Patient Handling and Mobility (SPHM) Technology
Methods	Establish a Culture of Safety
	Establish a System for Staff Education, Training, and
	Maintaining Competence
	Develop a "zero-lift" program or policy to minimize direct patient lifting by using specialized lifting equipment, transfer tools, and lift teams. Include SPHM in Reasonable Accommodation and Post-Injury
	Return to Work Standards
	Emphasize to all team: Manual lifting, such as lifting, repositioning and transferring, is **NOT** safe for patients and staff members (Zwerdling, 2015).
Organization of work	Use specialized lift teams and equipment to move patients out of bed.

Note. Created by C. Rovinski-Wagner & P. Mills.

about post-operative swelling and healing and its effects on the lower extremities is also to be provided.

It is critical for nurses to learn and follow the procedures for SPHM. The basis for SPHM is ergonomics. **Ergonomics** is the scientific study of the relationship between the work being performed, the physical environment where the work is performed, the tools used to help perform the work, the methods used to perform the work, and the way the work is organized (Table 14.8). There is a positive significant correlation between the prevalence of low back pain and the use of body mechanics (Hossein, Elham, & Mohammed, 2019).

SPHM strategies protect patients and health care staff against injury by ensuring that the biomechanical, physiological, and psychosocial limits of people are not exceeded. 75% of nurses working have access to SPHM technology, but only half use it consistently (Francis & Dawson, 2016). Nurses can only ensure their patients' and their own safety through consistent use of SPHM practices. The American Nurses Association has developed Interprofessional Standards of Safe Patient Handling and Mobility (American Nurses Association (ANA), 2014). They are:

- Establish a culture of safety.

- Implement and sustain a SPHM program.

- Incorporate ergonomic design principles to provide a safe environment of care.

- Select, install, and maintain SPHM technology.

- Establish a system for education, training, and maintaining competence.

- Integrate patient-centered SPHM assessment, plan of care, and use of SPHM technology.

- Include SPHM in reasonable accommodation and post-injury return to work.

- Establish a comprehensive evaluation system.

Adherence to these standards should reduce staff injuries, improve quality of care, and improve patient and staff satisfaction.

Critical Thinking 14.3

Note that the American Nurses Association recommends policies and practices that lead to the elimination of all manual lifting. The National Institute for Occupational Safety and Health (**NIOSH**) recommends lifting no more than 35 lb under the best ergonomic conditions. Go to, www.nursingworld.org/~498de8/globalassets/practiceandpolicy/work-environment/health--safety/ ana-sphmcover__finalapproved.pdf, accessed July 12, 2019. Review the Myths and Realities of Patient Handling, identified by the ANA at the site (ANA, 2015).

1. Were you surprised by any of the information?

2. How will you incorporate this information into your patient care?

Avoidance of Falls, Slips, and Trips

Falls, slips, and trips are common occurrences in health care for both patients and staff. In 2015, 7 out of 24 fatal work-related injuries in hospitals were the results of falls, slips, and trips (Dressner, 2017). Improvements in the workplace such as decentralization to reduce walking distances, adequate lighting, and non-slip floor surfaces can reduce falls, slips, and trips. Nurses reduce the risk of falls, slips, and trips by being proactive. For example, the nurse cleans up coffee spills to dry the floor of the break room, or moves equipment to a storage closet to reduce the obstructions in a hallway. The nurse also collaborates with nonclinical staff in preventing falls, slips, and trips. For example, the nurse notices that people walking down the corridor are stumbling because their footwear is catching on a broken floor tile. The nurse places a warning sign over the tile, and contacts the facilities management department and requests a repair. The nurse also submits an incident report about the observed near misses of falls, slips, and trips to ensure that the health care organization repairs the tile and has an opportunity to determine a system-wide improvement, such as regularly scheduled environment of care rounding to identify where similar repair is needed.

Environmental Safety and Biological Hazards

Nurses and other health care staff are potentially exposed to a great number of biological hazards. Laboratory personnel might be exposed when collecting or processing biological materials from patients. Nurses and doctors can be exposed during surgical or invasive procedures, when they treat wounds, when they take body fluid samples, or even when doing clinical examinations. Health care staff face potential exposure to biological hazards when personal care is provided to patients who are incapable of looking after themselves. Potential exposure to biological hazards can also happen when health care staff are disinfecting, cleaning, transporting contaminated equipment, or working in contaminated areas (Sacadura-Leite et al., 2018). The blood borne pathogens that are most commonly involved in occupational exposures in health care workers are hepatitis B, hepatitis C, and human immunodeficiency virus (**HIV**) (OSHA, 2018). The risk of becoming infected with a blood-borne virus is highest for hepatitis B, followed by hepatitis C, and then HIV (Cooke & Stephens, 2017).

Occupational health departments in hospitals have protocols to manage the potential occupational risks of biological hazard exposure. For example, there are protocols to manage exposures to blood-borne pathogens through accidental needle sticks and other protocols to manage *Mycobacterium tuberculosis* exposure. Special challenges arise when health care staff are exposed to bacteria that are resistant to antibiotics. The exposed person can become colonized with the resistant bacteria and be a vehicle for hospital-acquired, or nosocomial, spread of infection. Patient and health care staff safety in the face of potential biological hazards relies upon consistent adherence to all protective procedures, such as not recapping needles and using personal protective equipment.

It has been estimated that more than 50% of nurses will experience at least one needle stick injury in their careers (Rohde, Dupler, Postma, & Sanders, 2013). A study of 158 hospitals in 2016 revealed that nurses experienced over 36% of all the sharps injuries (Good & Grimmond, 2017). A nurse should not take short-cuts when feeling pressured for time. Consistent adherence to evidence-based procedures by the nurse reduces the chance of the nurse being exposed to a blood-borne pathogen. If the nurse does experience a needle-stick, the nurse must report the occurrence immediately to the nurse manager, and complete an incident report. This starts the health care organization's protocol to ensure the nurse receives the proper treatment. The organization's Occupational Health Department guides the nurse through the protocol which may include long-term follow up. Similarly, the Occupational Health Department will coordinate immediate and continued care if the nurse has an exposure due to a needle stick in order to reduce harm to the nurse.

In a similar fashion, tuberculosis (TB) may be avoided by making sure that all procedures for isolating and caring for patients with tuberculosis are followed. This includes using the appropriate personal protective equipment such as gowns, gloves, and specially fitted N95 disposable particulate-filtering respirator masks every time the nurse comes in contact with the patient with TB. This can seem cumbersome but it is critical to safety. Annual TB testing of staff by health care organizations is done to screen for TB infection so that treatment can be initiated. Exposure to tuberculosis has the potential to spread and cause severe physical harm to nurse, family, co-workers, other patients, visitors, and the general community.

Case Study 14.1

Mrs. Smith is an 84-year-old woman who was just returned to your medical-surgical unit after having surgery to repair a broken hip. She is no longer under anesthesia and she is beginning to complain of pain in her hip. Mrs. Smith also has high blood pressure, osteoporosis and type-2 diabetes, for which she takes medications. When she first returned from the operating room, she had a catheter in place and was not allowed to get out of bed.

The catheter was removed on the second day to avoid a CAUTI. Mrs. Smith is instructed to call the nurse if she needs to get up or use the bathroom. Mrs. Smith also has a bedpan available for use.

1. What safety precautions should you take with Mrs. Smith?

2. What other actions by the inter-professional team will help keep Mrs. Smith safe?

Evidence from the Literature

Source: Katz, A. (2013). Exposed to patient's body fluids? Now what? American Nurse Today. December 2013, Vol. 8, No. 12. Retrieved from www.americannursetoday.com/exposed-to-patients-body-fluids-now-what, July 11, 2019.

Discussion: Occupational exposure to a patient's body fluids may occur through needle stick, splash of body fluids to eye, nose, or mouth mucous membrane, and contact with a patient's blood, body fluids, secretions, and excretions, with nonintact skin. Most exposures are caused by a failure to follow standard precautions. Note that it only takes a small paper cut on a finger to expose one to a mucocutaneous infection with a potentially deadly virus. The estimated annual number of needle stick and sharps injuries in the United States is around 385,000. These injuries may expose health care workers to more than 20 different blood-borne pathogens, for example, hepatitis B, hepatitis C, and HIV.

The risk of developing HIV after a needle stick injury is about 0.3% (after a splash 0.09%), the risk for hepatitis B is 6–30%, and the risk for hepatitis C after a needle stick is about 1.8% (much lower after a splash).

Implications for Practice: If you experience a needle stick or are exposed to a patient's body fluids during the course of your work, remember these key points: clean the injured site immediately, notify your supervisor, and seek health care evaluation.

Critical Thinking 14.3

Makary (2016) found that more than 250,000 people in the United States die every year because of medical mistakes, making medical mistakes the third leading cause of death after heart disease and cancer. Makary (2016) defines a death due to medical error as a death that is caused by inadequately skilled staff, an error in judgment or care, a system defect, or a preventable adverse effect. What does the health care system need to do in order to stop these deaths from medical mistakes?

Management of Violence in the Workplace

Workplace violence is any act or threat of physical violence that occurs at the work site. Workplace violence includes patient attacks on nurses, harassment, intimidation, and threatening or disruptive behavior (OSHA, 2017). Bullying and active shooter events are also two types of violence seen in health care settings.

Bullying manifests in humiliating behaviors such as teasing or name-calling, withholding information that is needed to get work done, being the target of gossip, and not being told when meetings are scheduled. Bullying undermines a culture of safety by inhibiting teamwork, obstructing communication, and impeding implementation of new practices. It is estimated that 46–100% of nurses' experience bullying and incivility (Roberts, 2015). For nurses, bullying by other nurses has a stronger negative effect on job satisfaction, emotional exhaustion, and mental and physical health outcomes than supervisor and co-worker incivility (Read & Laschinger, 2015). Bullying is also associated with negative patient outcomes and staff turnover (Wallace & Gipson, 2017).

New nurses are particularly susceptible to bullying in the work place. If you are subjected to bullying in the workplace, there are steps to take. First, be assertive with the person who is bullying you. Practice what you will say. For example, practice a phrase such as "Please stop and let me do my work." The practice will give you confidence to respond in a respectful and productive way. If this does not stop the bullying, talk with your nurse manager, and continue up the hierarchy as necessary. You might consider submitting an incident report. Keep a dated and timed log of the occurrence or occurrences.

Include what you did to improve the situation. You may need the information when leadership of the organization investigates. Build support among your colleagues for a no bullying culture. Speak up when you see others being bullied. If your situation doesn't improve, consider looking for another job. Taking care of yourself is one of the strongest ways you can take care of your patient's safety. The American Psychiatric Nurses Association Task Force on Workplace Violence (www.apna.org accessed January 4, 2019) provides strategies for helping nurses deal with workforce bullying, and creating a safe and healthy work environment.

Another type of work place violence seen in health care organizations is an active shooter event. Active shooter events had been relatively rare in the past but this is changing. Four of the 50 active shooter incidents that occurred in 2016 and 2017 happened in a health care setting (Federal Bureau of Investigations, 2018). Studies reveal active shooter events in health care occurred primarily inside hospitals, with the majority in emergency departments, and resulted in 5% of the shooting victims being nursing staff (Rege, 2017). Health care organizations are considered soft targets because they have a high concentration of people, a low degree of security against assault, and lack the capacity to fight back against an attack (Kalvach et al., 2016). However, due to the increase of attacks against or within health care organizations, many health care organizations have revised their emergency preparedness plans to include drills for events that involve weapons or explosives.

The nurse who is committed to the safety of self, patients, and others acknowledges that these types of events can happen in the workplace and is proactive in preparing for such an event. Situational awareness, with staff awareness and adherence to

Table 14.9   Actions to Take in an Active Shooter Event

Run	If there is an accessible escape path, attempt to evacuate the premises.
Hide	If evacuation is not possible, find a place to hide where the active shooter is less likely to find you.
Fight	As a last resort, and if your life is in imminent danger, attempt to disrupt and/or incapacitate the active shooter.

Source: Adapted from Federal Emergency Management Agency (FEMA). (2018). Be Prepared for an Active Shooter. FEMA V-1000 Catalog No. 17233-1.

the health care organization's current security measures, emergency preparedness plan, and code system may be the difference between life and death. The nurse also participates in the health care organization's emergency drills so that decisions in a real situation are made rapidly and have a higher probability for the safest course of action. In the event of an active shooter, all involved persons should quickly determine the most reasonable way to protect their own lives (Table 14.9).

The Healthcare and Public Health Sector Coordinating Council (2017) offers more specific guidance for each of the Federal Emergency Management Agency's (**FEMA**s) active shooter recommendations, including ethical decisions that the nurse and other health care staff may face during an active shooter incident. These are available at, www.calhospitalprepare.org/sites/main/files/file-attachments/as_active-shooter-planning-and-response-in-a-healthcare-setting_1.pdf accessed February 16, 2019.

Active shooter events are also classified as disasters. Disasters cause widespread destruction of the environment, of the economic, social and health care infrastructures, as well as loss of life. Disasters overwhelm the ability of individuals and the community to respond using their own resources (ICN, 2009). Disasters can be natural, such a hurricanes or floods, or man-made such as acts of terrorism or active shooter incidents. A major goal of disaster preparedness is to maintain an efficient health care system.

Nurses are the largest group in the health care workforce. They are often found on the frontline in disaster preparedness and management, because their wide range of skills is applicable in a variety of disaster settings and situations. These include care giving skills, creativity and adaptability, and leadership (Achora et al., 2017). The skills of the nurse are integrated throughout the disaster continuum (Table 14.10).

Table 14.10   Examples of the Nurse's Skills in the Disaster Continuum

Phase of a disaster	Objective of the phase	Example of the Nurse's Caregiving, Creativity, Adaptability, and Leadership Skills.
Pre-Incident		
Prevention	Identify risks at community and individual level.	The nurse helps plan for the evacuation and relocation of patients in a disaster.
Preparedness	Achieve a satisfactory level of health care system readiness to respond.	The nurse participates in the creation of policies related to use of licensed and unlicensed personnel during a disaster.
Incident		
Response	Save as many lives as possible.	The nurse manages scarce resources and provides care in a variety of settings under challenging conditions.
	Provide for the immediate needs of the survivors.	The nurse works with a health care team and other responders to provide assistance to as many survivors as possible.
	Reduce the long-term health impact of the disaster.	The nurse identifies patterns of illness to detect any threat of communicable disease.
Post-Incident		
Recovery	Meet the needs of the population while assisting them to recover and restore their lives to normal.	The nurse provides care, support, and monitoring to the injured, ill, and those with chronic disease, mental health illness, or disability to reduce the risk of complications and facilitate recovery.
Reconstruction	Restore vital services.	The nurse makes referrals to appropriate health care providers, government or relief agencies for housing, food, medications, etc., to connect survivors to vital services for help in reconstructing their lives.
Rehabilitation	Rebuild infrastructure and meet the needs of the population while assisting them to restore their lives	The nurse collaborates with appropriate agencies to re-establish health care services within the community, and participates in reconstruction and rehabilitation activities to assure that patient needs can be met.

Source: Adapted from material from International Council of Nurses (2009).

Evidence from the Literature

Source: Adapted from Inaba, K., Eastman, A., & Jacobs, L. M. (2018). Active-Shooter Response at a Health Care Facility. New England Journal of Medicine, 379(6), 583–586.

Discussion: The FEMA recommendation, to run, hide, and fight in an active shooter event, faces implementation barriers in hospital settings. These barriers include vertical building construction, patients with limited mobility, and the moral responsibility of health care professionals to not abandon their patients. Other barriers include large common areas such as lobbies and nursing units designed for maximum visibility of patients and patients who cannot run, hide, or fight due to physical or mental disabilities or being on continuous life sustaining therapy. An alternative strategy suggested by the authors is to Secure the location immediately, Preserve the life of the patient and self, and Fight only if necessary. Strategies to strengthen a Secure-Preserve-Fight response are discussed within the context of the principles of emergency management: mitigation, preparation, response, and recovery. These principles include proactively securing hospital areas by using enhanced security measures such as use of an identification card or buzzer-only entrances, preserving lives of patients and staff by widespread availability of emergency kits containing essential supplies for hemorrhage control with ongoing training for staff about use, ensuring that emergency notification systems are easily accessed and heard, and doing advanced coordination with law enforcement agencies to maximize the response by trained resources to an active shooter event, and prevent harm. The authors believe a Secure-Preserve-Fight strategy allows health care providers to fulfill their ethical obligations to their patients while responding in a way that maximizes the odds of survival for both their patients and themselves.

Implications for care: A hospital that wants to provide the highest degree of patient and health care staff safety in the event of an active shooter should include clinical staff as members of the emergency preparedness and management team. These staff must be taught the Secure-Preserve-Fight strategy.

Real World Interview

Opioid use can impact the patient's ability to engage in meaningful conversations related to treatment plans and patient education. When patients present to the Emergency Department or outpatient clinic, they often are displeased with the reluctance of their health care providers to refill opioid prescriptions. Differing cultural expectations about pain management can complicate the situation. Aberrant behavior that threatens patient and health care staff safety may ensue. Close management of patients is needed to support safety. Excellent communication, including verbal and nonverbal de-escalation techniques, displays of empathy, and being versed in alternative modalities to treat chronic pain will aid in effective patient discussions and reduce the risk of harm to patients and health care staff when opioid prescriptions are not refilled.

Debra Lee, RN, MS, BSBM, CRC, CCM, CDMS
Ambulatory Care Operations Director/Group
Practice Manager
Boise VA Medical Center, Idaho

Safety for patients and health care staff ranges from a seemingly non-injurious event such as catching oneself from tripping over a misplaced piece of equipment to extraordinarily courageous responses such as actions to save survivors in a natural disaster or active shooter. Nurses are exposed to all types of physical, mental, and emotional harm that can negatively affect patient safety. They are responsible for the lives and safety of their patients and their colleagues, and not least of all, their own. Nurses who understand how to use the tools and strategies of a culture of safety will be able to meet the challenges of supporting patient and health care staff safety throughout their careers.

KEY CONCEPTS

- Safety activities minimize the risk of harm to patients and providers through both system effectiveness and individual performance.

- Nurses work with inter-professional teams to create health care systems that provide safe care for patients and reduce preventable harm to patients and health care staff.

- The four components of a culture of safety are leadership, measurement, teamwork, and risk identification and reduction.

- A culture with a person approach to safety blames the individual person for error, while a culture with a system approach to safety reviews the total system to seek out all possible causes of error, not just individual error.

- Safety behaviors in an HRO demonstrates a preoccupation with failure, sensitivity to operations, a reluctance to simplify, a commitment to resilience, and deference to expertise.

- Organizations that spread and sustain health care safety collect, analyze, validate, and distribute evidence-based best practices.

- Safety initiatives for patients include suicide prevention, safe patient handoffs, reduction and avoidance of patient suffering, medication management, hand hygiene, and RRTs.

- Current safety initiatives for nurses include SPHM, avoidance of falls, slips, and trips, environmental safety and biological hazards, and management of violence in the workplace.

KEY TERMS

Safety	Reluctance to simplify	Root Cause Analysis (RCA)
Culture	Sensitivity to operations	Patient handoff
Culture of safety	Commitment to resilience	Rapid Response Team (RRT)
Incident report	Deference to expertise	Ergonomics
High reliability organization	Adverse event	Simplification of the work process
Person approach to safety	Aggregate reviews	Standardization of the work process
System approach to safety	Healthcare Failure Mode and Effect	Swiss cheese Model
Preoccupation with failure	Analysis (HFMEA)	

REVIEW QUESTIONS

1. Tonight is the first time you have been designated as charge nurse on a medical unit. According to the recommended nurse to patient ratio for the unit, there is sufficient staffing. How could you organize your activities so that you know you are prepared for the shift? Select all that apply.
   a. Check the schedule to see who else is assigned to the unit
   b. Contact the nursing office to request more help, just to be safe
   c. Huddle with the on-coming staff to discuss anticipated problems
   d. Verify that on-coming staff has received reports from off-going staff
   e. Find out if any of the physicians left new orders on the previous shift

2. The nurse is concerned about the increased number of falls on a medical unit. Which of the following best demonstrates teamwork supporting a culture of safety? Select all that apply.
   a. Calculating the fall rate for the unit and posting it in the break room
   b. Requesting that the nurse manager arrange an in-service on fall prevention
   c. Submitting an incident report about the increase in the number of falls
   d. Collaborating with colleagues to identify patients at high risk of falls
   e. Identifying patients who should be transferred to the ICU

3. The nurse thinks her assigned 30-bed medical unit is experiencing a lot of patient falls. The number of falls for this month is 5. The occupied bed days for this month equal 615. The fall rate for the unit during this month is which of the following?
   a. 3.10
   b. 0.31
   c. 8.10
   d. 0.81
   e. 3.80

4. An overhead announcement is made using a code for "active shooter in the hospital." According to FEMA what do you do?
   a. Run, Hide, Escape
   b. Secure, Preserve, Defend
   c. Run, Hide, Fight
   d. Hide, Secure, Defend
   e. Secure, Preserve, Fight

5. You are working with your nurse manager to examine a recent increase in days with unexpected staff shortages. No adverse events occurred during those days, but there were several near misses. Which one of the following tools is not appropriate for this examination?
   a. Swiss Cheese Model
   b. PDSA cycle
   c. Root Cause Analysis
   d. Aggregate Review

6. The patient suffers an acute episode of fluid retention which extends the patient's hospitalization. The RCA reveals that several nurses did not document the patient's fluid intake and output. Which of the following will appropriately hold the nurses accountable? Select all that apply.
   a. Person approach to safety
   b. Preoccupation with failure
   c. Commitment to resilience
   d. System approach to safety
   e. Deference to expertise

7. The definition of safety includes which one of the following?
   a. Standardizing policies and procedures about how health care staff complete and submit incident reports
   b. Reducing risk of harm to patients and providers through system effectiveness and individual performance
   c. Simplifying the steps used by health care organizations to measure and analyze data related to adverse events
   d. Ensuring safety improvement teams are composed of people who supervise the care delivery systems

8. You work in the ED of a large metropolitan hospital. You have been asked to participate in an HFMEA that is going to address active shooter scenarios. Your role on the HFMEA team is to provide information about which of the following? Select all that apply.
   a. What happens in the ED on a typical day
   b. The ethical perspectives and responsibilities of clinicians
   c. Level of staff knowledge about current security measures
   d. How overhead paging is poorly heard in the ED
   e. How often staff tape the breakroom door lock open for ease of entry

9. A post-operative patient has been transferred from the recovery room to the inpatient unit. You are receiving reports from the recovery room nurse. Which part of the SBARR handoff process is your responsibility?

   a. Situation
   b. Background
   c. Assessment
   d. Recommendations
   e. Response

10. You are making rounds and a patient who you know has been oriented to person, place, and time isn't responding appropriately to your questions. Which one of the following actions provides the greatest potential for reduced risk of harm to the patient?
    a. Call a Code Blue
    b. Call the Rapid Response Team
    c. Call the nursing supervisor
    d. Call for a bedside sitter

REVIEW QUESTION ANSWERS

1. Answers A, B, C, D, and E are correct.
   Rationale: Checking the schedule to see who else is assigned to the unit (A) lets you know what your staffing resources are for the shift and helps you to identify who will be responsible for what work during the shift. Contacting the nursing office to request more help is a safe action (B) based on the comparison of the recommended nurse to patient ratio and the actual staffing provided for the shift. A huddle with the rest of the on-coming staff to discuss anticipated problems (C) is contingency planning so that if a problem does occur, the team will know what is supposed to be done by each team member. Verifying that the on-coming staff has received reports from the off-going staff (D) ensures that the team members are aware of the status of each patient for whose care they are responsible. Finding out if new physician orders were written on the previous shift (E) can help you identify whether they need follow-up during your shift.

2. Answers A, B, and D are correct.
   Rationale: Calculating the fall rate for the unit and posting it in the breakroom (A) provides a blame-free way to bring attention to the unit's fall rate. Requesting the nurse manager to arrange an in-service about falls for the staff (B) is collaborative and demonstrates teamwork by thinking about the potential educational needs of the rest of the staff. Collaborating with colleagues to identify patients at high risk for falls (D) demonstrates teamwork, because the expertise of inter-professional team members is sought and used to provide safe health care for patients. Submitting an incident report about the fall rate (C) is a misuse of the incident report system, since an incident report is used to report a single adverse event or a close call. Identifying patients for transfer to the intensive care unit (E) does not address the issue of why the individual patients are falling and does not support team work in a culture of safety.

3. Answer: C is correct.
   Rationale: Divide the number of falls in the month (i.e., 5) by the number of occupied bed days for the month (i.e., 615). 5/615 = 0.00813. Multiply the result in by 1,000. $0.00813 \times 1,000 = 8.13$. The fall rate or how many falls occurred per 1,000 occupied bed days of care, is 8.13.

4. Answer: C is correct.
   Rationale: FEMA recommends that you Run, Hide, and Fight (C). Run if there is an accessible escape path, and attempt to evacuate the premises. If evacuation is not possible, find a place to hide where the active shooter is less likely to find you. Fight as a last resort, and if your life is in imminent danger. You would not Run, Hide, Escape (A) as you might be seen by the active shooter. Secure, Preserve, and Defend (B) and Hide, Secure, and Defend (D) combine recommendations from FEMA and the Evidence from the Literature. Defend is a term used by security companies and while it means to fight, it can be confusing since people often associate the word with use of firearms which may not be available. Secure, Preserve, and Fight (E) is the recommendation in Evidence from the Literature and incorporates strategies for protecting vulnerable populations in health care organizations.

5. Answer: B is correct.
   Rationale: The PDSA Cycle evaluates the effectiveness of different improvement strategies and ideas (B). The PDSA Cycle is not used to evaluate near misses or adverse events. The Swiss Cheese Model (A) is a tool that helps visualize checks and barriers in a system of health care, so there is no harm caused to patients or staff due to execution or planning failure. Failures in the system, whether they are adverse events or near misses, are represented by holes in the slices of Swiss cheese where harm might occur. An RCA (C) is a process that investigates the underlying main cause of an adverse event or near miss. Aggregate reviews (D) are when a series of similar adverse events or near misses are examined by an inter-professional team to determine if a pattern of breakdowns exists in the health care system that has caused these adverse events.

6. Answers B and D are correct.
   Rationale: Leaders who have a preoccupation with failure (B) create a just culture where staff are held accountable for their own behaviors but not for system failures. A system approach to safety (D) does not absolve the individual of personal accountability but considers the individual's characteristics as part of a broader view of an adverse event. A person approach to safety (A) blames the person who makes the error, regardless of any other factors that may have contributed to the error. Commitment to resilience

(C) is when leaders in the health care organization think about what could go wrong in a complex system and attempt to create backup systems to catch errors before any harm comes to the patient. Deference to expertise (E) is the practice of seeking advice from the person with the most experience or expertise in a specific situation regardless of their position in the organizational hierarchy.

7. Answer: B is correct.

Rationale: Safety minimizes the risk of harm to patients and providers through both system effectiveness and individual performance (QSEN, 2018) (B). Standardizing policies and procedures about how health care staff complete and submit incident reports (A) focuses on the documentation and process for incident reports, and is needed for system effectiveness. But alone, it does not minimize risk of harm to patients and providers. Promoting techniques that nurses and physicians can use to protect themselves in a variety of patient care situations can be part of both system effectiveness and individual performance. However, safety encompasses reduction of risk to patients and other health care staff as well. Simplifying the steps used by health care organizations to measure and analyze data related to adverse events (C) is only one part of system effectiveness to reduce safety and does not include individual performance. Safety improvement teams are composed of people who touch the process being improved (D), but that is not part of the definition of safety. Nurses work with inter-professional teams to create health care systems that provide safe care for patients and reduce preventable harm to patients and health care staff.

8. Answers A, B, C, D, and E are correct.

Rationale: You are the HFMEA team's expert on daily operations in the ED. Your information about what happens during a typical day in the ED (A) helps the team understand the daily work flow of the ED and when it would be easiest for an active shooter to attack. As a licensed health care professional, you can discuss the ethical perspectives and responsibilities held by clinicians. (B)

Situational awareness, such as the level of staff knowledge about the facility's current security measures, (C) may be the difference between life and death. Poorly heard overhead paging in the ED identifies a communication problem (D) in the event of an active shooter. How often the staff tape the breakroom door lock open for ease of entry (E) identifies an avenue for unobstructed access to staff that may hide in the breakroom during an active shooter event.

9. Answer: E is correct..

Rationale: You are responsible for the response (E) to the recovery room nurse. Your response demonstrates that you correctly understand the information being given by the recovery room nurse. A correct understanding of the information enables you to provide safe care to the post-operative patient. The recovery room nurse is responsible for telling you the patient's situation (A), which is the post-operative patient's status and the background (B) of the surgical procedure. The recovery room nurse is also responsible for giving you an assessment (C) of care provided to the post-operative patient in the recovery room and the recommendations (D) or orders for further post-operative.

10. Answer: B is correct.

Rationale: Inappropriate responses by a patient who was previously oriented to person, place, and time may signal a declining physical status. A Rapid Response Team is a team of expert clinicians who provide additional care for patients on acute care units who are experiencing unexpected acute changes in their conditions. (B) The goal of a code blue (A) team is to resuscitate a person who has stopped breathing, or who does not have a heartbeat. Calling the nursing supervisor (C) or calling for a bedside sitter (D) first will not provide the greatest potential for reduced risk of harm to the patient. Notify the supervisor as soon as possible after the Rapid Response Team has been called, so the supervisor is aware of the situation and can provide further assistance if needed. A bedside sitter is not used in situations when the patient's condition has acutely deteriorated.

REVIEW ACTIVITIES

1. Collaborate with your classmates in a clinical rotation and ask members of the inter-professional team during your rotation which of the health care organization's safety initiatives is most important. If you can, ask the same question of staff who work the evening or night shift. Do the answers vary based on the health care discipline questioned or the shift worked?

2. Think about your clinical rotations. What topics do you recall staff discussing? Did their discussions reflect problem solving or did they focus on concerns without taking action? As a new nurse, how would you participate productively in these conversations?

3. Look for posters or data graph about safety initiatives in your clinical area. Select one and ask staff to review the poster or data graph with you.

DISCUSSION POINTS

1. Think about your clinical experiences and whether you have ever been assigned a patient described as "difficult." How did it influence the way you interacted with that patient? How could that have affected the patient's safety?

2. Consider the safety behaviors associated with preventing errors in medication administration. How would you respond to a nurse colleague who clearly resents being questioned about her actions?

3. How would you evaluate a health care organization's safety culture during your job hunt, when you are applying and when you are being interviewed for a nursing position?

4. How can you contribute to safety as a direct care clinical nurse?

DISCUSSION OF OPENING SCENARIO

1. Why is it important to keep Mr. Jones under continuous one-to-one observation, even while using the bathroom?

   Answer: Suicidal behavior usually happens in private areas when the patient is alone, such as the bathroom and private rooms. The presence of another person provides a protection structure visible to the patient and a person to intervene in the event the patient attempts self-harm.

2. Why does the nurse have Mr. Jones change out of his street clothes?

   Answer: Suicidal patients in the ED are at risk of using any material for self-harm. Hospital pajamas for patients are designed for safety. Drugs or sharps in a patient's clothing can be used for self-harm and need to be removed immediately. The separation of Mr. Jones from his personal belongings is part of the process of reducing the potential for harm. This process also reinforces for Mr. Jones that the nurse and other health care staff value his safety. When done respectfully, the process shows compassion and helps reduce patient suffering.

3. What techniques can you use to assess Mr. Jones while he is in the ED?

   Answer: When working with a patient whom you think is suicidal, ask if the patient is thinking about hurting himself or herself or committing suicide. Mr. Jones did not want to talk about his suicidal ideation but he says that he is devastated since his wife's death. You ask Mr. Jones about how his life has changed since his wife died. Your goal is to establish a relationship with Mr. Jones. During your conversation with Mr. Jones, you observe his nonverbal behaviors. For example, Mr. Jones avoids eye contact but keeps looking around the mental health safe room. By paying attention to what Mr. Jones is focusing on, you will have clues as to how to further provide a secure environment for Mr. Jones.

EXPLORING THE WEB

1. Children's Hospitals' Solutions for Patient Safety National Children's Network: www.solutionsforpatientsafety.org accessed December 19, 2018

2. The American Association of Occupational Health Nurses: American Association of Occupational Health Nurses (AAOHN) accessed December 19, 2019

3. Migrant Clinicians Network: www.migrantclinician.org accessed December 19, 2018

4. AHRQ Patient Safety Net: psnet.ahrq.gov accessed 12December /19, /2018

5. Joint Commission International: www.jointcommission international.org/ accessed December 19, 2018

6. U.S. Food and Drug Administration: www.fda.gov/ accessed December 19, 2018

7. QSEN Institute:; http://qsen.org accessed December 12/29, 2018

8. World Health Organization: www.who.int/features/factfiles/patient_safety/en accessed December 28, 2018

9. Centers for Disease Control and Prevention (CDC). The National Institute for Occupational Safety and Health (NIOSH). Intervention Tools. Available at, www.cdc.gov/niosh/topics/ohsn/link.html, accessed June 11, 2019.

INFORMATICS

1. Go to the Joint Commission International website at www.jointcommissioninternational.org accessed December 19, 2018. Scroll down and select "JCI Publishes White Paper on Communicating Clearly and Effectively to Patients." Scroll down and open the complimentary link to the white paper. Review the Executive Summary to learn that the effect of poor communication on patient safety is the same world-wide.

2. Go to http://qsen.org/publications/related-links accessed December 19, 2018. Scroll down and select "Tubing Misconnections—A Systems Failure with Human Factors: Lessons for Nursing Practice." The link into Medscape will ask you to sign in. This is free—please sign-in. Read the article and note the publication date. Then go to the Food and Drug Administration site, www.fda.gov/MedicalDevices/ProductsandMedicalProcedures/GeneralHospitalDevicesandSupplies/TubingandLuerMisconnections/default.htm (accessed December 19, 2018), and read the article "Medical Device Connectors" and note the publication date. What is your reaction to the length of time between the two articles and the fact that medical device connectors continue to be a risk to patient safety?

LEAN BACK

You plan to apply at a hospital that has many open nursing positions and is aggressively recruiting new graduates. A fellow student tells you she heard the hospital is always short-staffed because nurses are quickly promoted. Consider the impact this information might have on patient and health care staff safety.

REFERENCES

Achora, S., & Kamanyire, J. K. (2016). Disaster Preparedness: Need for inclusion in undergraduate nursing education. *Sultan Qaboos University medical journal*, 16(1), e15–e19. https://doi.org/10.18295/squmj.2016.16.01.004

AHRQ. (2013). *How do you measure fall rates and fall prevention practices*. Rockville, MD: Agency for Healthcare Research and Quality. Retrieved from www.ahrq.gov/professionals/systems/hospital/fallpxtoolkit/fallpxtk5.html.

Agency for Healthcare Research and Quality. (AHRQ). (2018). *Declines in hospital-acquired conditions save 8,000 lives and $2.9 billion in costs*. Retrieved from www.ahrq.gov/news/newsroom/press-releases/declines-in-hacs.html

American Nurses Association (ANA). (2014). *Safe patient handling and mobility: Interprofessional national standards. Across the care continuum*. Silver Spring, MD: Nursesbooks.org.

ANA. (2015). *Safe patient handling & mobility*. Retrieved from www.nursingworld.org/~498de8/globalassets/practiceandpolicy/work-environment/health--safety/ana-sphmcover__finalapproved.pdf

Braithwaite, J., Herkes, J., Ludlow, K., Testa, L., & Lamprell, G. (2017). Association between organizational and workplace cultures, and patient outcomes: Systematic review. *British Medical Journal Open*, 7(11). doi:10.1136/bmjopen-2017-017708

Card, A. J., & Klein, V. R. (2016). A new frontier in healthcare risk management: Working to reduce avoidable patient suffering. *Journal of Healthcare Risk Management*, 35(3), 31–37.

Centers for Disease Control (CDC). (2018). *Vital Signs*. Retrieved from www.cdc.gov/vitalsigns/pdf/vs-0618-suicide-H.pdf

Cooke, C. E., & Stephens, J. M. (2017). *Clinical, economic, and humanistic burden of needlestick injuries in healthcare workers. Medical Devices (Auckland, N.Z.)*, 10, 225–235. doi:10.2147/MDER.S140846. Retrieved from www.ncbi.nlm.nih.gov/pmc/articles/PMC5628664

CRICO Strategies. (2015). *Malpractice risk in communication failures; 2015 annual benchmarking report*. Boston, MA: The Risk Management Foundation of the Harvard Medical Institutions, Inc.

Cullen Gill, E. (2015). Reducing hospital acquired pressure ulcers in intensive care. *British Medical Journal Quality Improvement Reports*, 4(1). doi:10.1136/bmjquality.u205599.w3015

Dressner, M. A. (2017). *Hospital workers: An assessment of occupational injuries and illnesses*. Monthly Labor Review, U.S. Bureau of Labor Statistics. doi: 10.21916/mlr.2017.17

Dressner, M. A. Kissinger, S. P. (2018). *Occupational injuries and illnesses among registered nurses*. Monthly Labor Review, U.S. Bureau of Labor Statistics. doi:10.21916/mlr.2018.27

Eggins, S., & Slade, D. (2015). Communication in clinical handover: Improving the safety and quality of the patient experience. *Journal of Public Health Research*, 4(3), 666. doi:10.4081/jphr.2015.666

Federal Bureau of Investigation. (2018). *Active shooter incidents in the United States in 2016 and 2017*. Retrieved from www.fbi.gov/file-repository/active-shooter-incidents-us-2016-2017.pdf

Federal Emergency Management Agency (FEMA). (2018). *Be prepared for an active shooter*. FEMA V-1000 Catalog No. 17233-1. Retrieved from www.fema.gov/media-library-data/1523561958719-f1eff6bc841d-56b7873e018f73a4e024/ActiveShooter_508.pdf

Feinmann, J. (2018). *Nobody wants to talk about catheters. Our silence could prove fatal*. Mosaic. Retrieved at https://mosaicscience.com/story/catheters-foley-uti-cauti-amr-dri-hospital-acquired-bacterial-infection-sepsis

Francis, R., & Dawson, J. M. (2016). Safe patient handling and mobility: The journey continues. *American Nurse Today*, 11(5), 38.

Gandhi, T. K. (2017). Can we get a national action plan for patient safety? HFM Magazine. Retrieved from www.hfma.org/Content.aspx?id=54280

Good L. & Grimmond T. (2017). Proven Strategies to Prevent Blood-borne Pathogen Exposures in EXPO-S.T.O.P. Hospitals. *AOHP Jrl* 38(4):10-13.

Healthcare & Public Health Sector Coordinating Council. (2017). *Active shooter planning and response: Learn how to survive a shooting event in a health care setting*. Retrieved from www.calhospitalprepare.org/sites/main/files/file-attachments/as_active-shooter-planning-and-response-in-a-healthcare-setting_1.pdf

Hossein, Y., Elham, H., & Mohammed, A. (2019). Relation between body mechanics performance and nurses' exposure of work place risk factors on the low back pain prevalence. *Journal of Nursing Education and Practice*, 9(3), 25–32. doi:10.5430/jnep.v9n3p25

IHI Multimedia Team. (2018). *How to conduct safety huddles that stick. Daily huddles can improve patient safety, hospital flow, and joy in work*. Retrieved from www.ihi.org/communities/blogs/how-to-conduct-safety-huddles-that-stick?utm_campaign=tw&utm_source=hs_email&utm_medium=email&utm_content=67694841

Institute for Healthcare Improvement (IHI). (2018). *Patient safety 100: Introduction to patient safety*. Retrieved from www.ihi.org/education/ihiopenschool/Courses/Documents/SummaryDocuments/PS%20100%20SummaryFINAL.pdf

International Council of Nurses. (2009). ICN framework of disaster nursing competencies. Retrieved from www.apednn.org/doc/resourcespublications/ICN%20Framework%20of%20Disaster%20Nursing%20Competencies%20ICN%202009.pdf

Joint Commission. (2017). Perspectives preview: Special report: Suicide prevention in health care settings. Retrieved from www.jointcommission.org/issues/article.aspx?Article=GtNpk0ErgGF%2B7J9WOTTkXANZSEPXa1%2BKH0%2F4kGHCiio%3D

Joint Commission. (2017a). *Inadequate hand off communication*. Sentinel Event Alert 58:1–6. Retrieved from www.jointcommission.org/assets/1/18/SEA_58_Hand_off_Comms_9_6_17_FINAL_(1).pdf

Joint Commission. (2017b). *The essential role of leadership in developing a safety culture*. Sentinel Event Alert, 57, 1–8. Retrieved from www.jointcommission.org/assets/1/18/SEA_57_Safety_Culture_Leadership_0317.pdf

Kalvach, I. Z. (2016). *Basics of soft targets protection—guidelines (2nd version)*. Prague: Soft Targets Protection Institute. Retrieved from www.mvcr.cz/cthh/soubor/basics-of-soft-target-protection-guidelines.aspx

Karp, M. (2018). *Health care staffing report*. Retrieved from www2.staffingindustry.com/site/Editorial/Healthcare-Staffing-Report/March-8-2018/Median-age-of-employed-registered-nurses-declines-from-2011-to-2017

Li, L., Deng, X., Zhang, H., Yang, H., Chen, J., Chen, J., Hou, X., Ning, N. & Li, J (2019). A cross-sectional survey of low back pain in nurses working in orthopedic departments. *Workplace Health Safety*, 67(5), 218–230. doi:10.1177/2165079918807231

Makary, M. A., & Daniel, M. (2016). Medical error—The third leading cause of death in the US. *British Medical Journal*, 353. doi:10.1136/bmj.i2139

Occupational Safety and Health Administration (OSHA). (2018). Bloodborne Pathogens and Needlestick Prevention. https://www.osha.gov/bloodborne-pathogens/hazards accessed 10/21/2020

Occupational Safety and Health Administration (OSHA). (2015). *Inspection guidance for inpatient healthcare settings*. Retrieved from www.osha.gov/dep/enforcement/inpatient_insp_06252015.html

Patient Safety Network (PSNET). (2018). *Patient safety primer: Nursing and patient safety.* Retrieved from https://psnet.ahrq.gov/primers/primer/22/Nursing-and-Patient-Safety

Peyrovi, H., Nasrabadi, A. N., & Valiee, S. (2016). Exploration of the barriers of reporting nursing errors in intensive care units: A qualitative study. *Journal of the Intensive Care Society, 17*(3), 215–221.

PSNET. (2019). Systems approach. Retrieved from https://psnet.ahrq.gov/primers/primer/21

Quality and Safety Education in Nursing (QSEN). (2018). *QSEN Institute Competencies.* https://qsen.org/competencies/pre-licensure-ksas/ accessed 10/20/2020

Rafter, N., Hickey, A., Condell, S., Conroy, R., O'Connor, P., O'Connor, P., Vaughn, D. & Williams, D. (2015). Adverse events in healthcare: Learning from mistakes. *Quality Journal of Medicine, 108*(4), 273–277.

Read, E., & Laschinger, H. K. (2015). Correlates to new graduate nurses' experiences of workplace mistreatment. *Journal of Nursing Administration, 45*(Suppl 10), S28–S35.

Reason, J. (1990). *Human error.* New York: Cambridge University Press.

Rege, A. (2017). Hospital shootings: How common are they? Becker's Hospital Review. Retrieved from www.beckershospitalreview.com/population-health/hospital-shootings-how-common-are-they-8-things-to-know.html

Roberts, S. J. (2015). Lateral violence in nursing: A review of the past three decades. *Nurse Science Quarterly, 28*(1), 36–41.

Robertson, D. W., & Kirsh, E. R. (2018). Systems science: A primer on high reliability. *Otolaryngologic, 52*(1), 1–9. doi:10.1016/j.otc.2018.08.001 Epub September 20, 2018.

Rodziewicz, T. L., & Hipskind, J. E. (2018). *Medical error prevention.* Treasure Island, FL: StatPearls Publishing. Retrieved from www.ncbi.nlm.nih.gov/books/NBK499956

Rohde, K. A., Dupler, A. E., Postma, J., & Sanders, A. (2013). Minimizing nurses' risks for needlestick injuries in the hospital setting. *Workplace Health & Safety, 61*(5), 197–202. doi:10.1177/216507991306100503

Sacadura-Leite, E., Mendonça-Galaio, L., Shapovalova, O., Pereira, I., Rocha, R., & Sousa-Grape, A. (2018). Biological hazards for healthcare workers: Occupational exposure to vancomycin-resistant *Staphylococcus aureus* as an example of a new challenge. *Portugese Journal of Public Health, 36*(1). doi:10.1159/000487746

Shain, B., & AAP Committee on Adolescence. (2016). Suicide and suicide attempts in adolescents. *Pediatrics, 138*(1), e20161420.

U.S. Bureau of Labor Statistics (BLS). (2017). 2016 Survey of occupational injuries and illnesses charts package. Retrieved from www.bls.gov/iif/osch0060.pdf

U.S. Department of Health and Human Services (HHS) Office of the Surgeon General and National Action Alliance for Suicide Prevention. (2012). *National strategy for suicide prevention: goals and objectives for action.* Washington, DC: HHS. Retrieved from www.surgeongeneral.gov/library/reports/national-strategy-suicide-prevention/full-report.pdf

VA National Center for Patient Safety. (2019). *Healthcare failure mode and effect analysis (HFMEA)* Retrieved from www.patientsafety.va.gov/professionals/onthejob/hfmea.asp

van der Veen, W., van den Bemt, P. M. L. A., Wouters, H., Bates, D., Twisk, J. W. R., de Gier, J. J., Taxis, K., BCMA Study Group, Duyvendak, M., Oude Luttikhuis, K., Ros, J. J. W., Vasbinder, V. C., Atrafi, M., Brasse, B. & Mangelaars, I. (2018). BCMA Study Group. (2018). Association between workarounds and medication administration errors in bar-code assisted medication administration in hospitals. *Journal of American Medical Informatics Association, 25*, 385–392.

Wallace, S. C., & Gipson, K. (2017). Bullying in healthcare: A disruptive force linked to compromised patient safety. *Pennsylvania Patient Safety Authority, 14*(2), 64–70.

White-Trevino, K., & Dearmon, V. (2018). Transitioning nurse handoff to the bedside: Engaging staff and patients. *Nursing Administration Quarterly, 42*(3), 261–268.

Williams, S. C., Schmaltz, S. P., Castro, G. M., & Baker, D. W. (2018). Incidence and method of suicide in hospitals in the United States. *Joint Commission Journal on Quality and Patient Safety, 44*(11), 643–650.

Zwerdling, D. (2015). *Even 'Proper' technique exposes nurses' spines to dangerous forces.* Retrieved from www.npr.org/2015/02/11/383564180/even-proper-technique-exposes-nurses-spines-to-dangerous-forces

SUGGESTED READINGS

Bauer, A. (2018). First, do no harm: The patient's experience of avoidable suffering as harm. *Patient Experience Journal, 5*(3). Retrieved from https://pxjournal.org/journal/vol5/iss3/3

Gandhi, T. K., Berwick, D. M., & Shojania, K. G. (2016). Patient safety at the crossroads. *Journal of the American Medical Association, 315*(17), 1829–1830.

Joint Commission Resources Alliance. (2017). OSHA and worker safety: Handling with care practicing: Safe patient handling. Retrieved from www.jcrinc.com/assets/1/7/Pages_from_ECN_20_2017_08-2.pdf

Seshia, S. S., Young, G. B., Makhinson, M., Smith, P. A., Stobart, K., & Croskerry, P. (2017). Gating the holes in the Swiss Cheese (part I): Expanding professor reason's model for patient safety. *Journal of Evaluation in Clinical Practice, 24*, 187–197. doi:10.1111/jep.12847

da Silva, B. A., & Krishnamurthy, M. (2016). The alarming reality of medication error: A patient case and review of Pennsylvania and National data. *Journal of Community Hospital Internal Medicine Perspectives, 6*(4), 31758. doi:10.3402/jchimp.v6.31758

Starmer, A. J., Schnock, K. O., Lyons, A., Hehn, R. S., Graham, D. A., Keohan, C. & Landrigan, C. P. (2017). Effects of the I-PASS nursing handoff bundle on communication quality and workflow. *British Medical Journal of Quality and Safety, 26*(12), 949–957.

Stolldorf, D. P., & Jones, C. B. (2015). Deployment of rapid response teams by 31 hospitals in a statewide collaborative. *Joint Commission Journal on Quality and Patient Safety, 41*(4), 186–191.

The National Patient Safety Foundation. (2015). *Free from harm: Accelerating patient safety improvement fifteen years after to err is human.* Boston, MA. Retrieved from www.aig.com/content/dam/aig/america-canada/us/documents/brochure/free-from-harm-final-report.pdf

Uthaman, T., Chua, T. L., & Ang, S. Y. (2016). Older nurses: A literature review on challenges, factors in early retirement and workforce retention. *Proceedings of Singapore Healthcare, 25*(1), 50–55. doi:10.1177/2010105815610138

15 Nursing Informatics

Rebecca J. Rankin
Nursing Informatics, UW Health, Madison, WI, USA

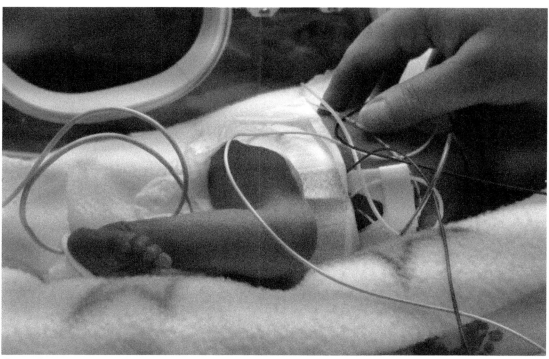

Photo of neonate with technology in incubator.
Source: Used with permission.

> Why it's simply impassible! Alice: Why, don't you mean impossible? Door: No, I do mean impassible. (chuckles) Nothing's impossible! (Lewis Carroll, 1865).

We are continually faced by great opportunities brilliantly disguised as insoluble problems.
Source: Lee Iacocca, GM of Ford

Don't limit your thinking to what is possible technically. Figure out what you want and then bend and stretch the technology to meet your needs.

(Rebecca Rankin, 2011)

OBJECTIVES

Upon completion of this chapter, the reader should be able to:

1. Understand the need for **nursing informatics** (NIs).

2. Describe nursing informatics history, definition, and tenets.

3. Introduce a collaborative model of Nursing Informatics.

4. Explain decision support, error prevention, high reliable organizations, and a just culture.

5. Discuss critical thinking, security risk and compliance, big data, social determinants of health, and population wellness.

6. Describe how to become certified or specialized in nursing informatics.

OPENING SCENARIO

Weston Miller is a 37-year-old construction worker who was struck by a vehicle and thrown 20 ft from the site of impact while working on Highway 104. Weston was stabilized in the field for transport via medical air lift to Northview Central, a trauma certified facility fully equipped with the latest technologies used to treat complex trauma cases. He sustained multiple injuries including a mandibular fracture, open fracture of the right humerus, broken ribs with a perforated lung, a liver contusion, bowel injury, and right renal laceration. A CT of his head was cleared for any subdural bleeding or additional head trauma beyond the mandibular fracture. Weston is moderately overweight, is taking Lovastatin for high cholesterol and started Zyban (bupropion) 1 week ago to help him quit smoking. He was otherwise healthy prior to the accident. He and his fiancé have a 3-month-old daughter and are engaged to be married in 4 months.

You are fortunate to work in a facility that has invested in life saving technologies to ensure optimal patient care and outcomes. In the brief time you care for Weston in the Emergency Department before he is transferred for emergent surgery, you use multiple technologies including an electronic health record (EHR) accessed from a fixed computer in the trauma bay, infusion pumps that automatically send and receive information from the EHR, and a wireless scanning device that integrates with the EHR for checking and documenting the administration of medications and blood products as well as the collection of laboratory specimens. You have a communication device that acts as a backup scanning device when a fixed or other mobile computer isn't available. Your name badge has tracking system technology that is integrated with the hospital's real-time locating system (RTLS), which shows where equipment and staff are located within seconds in time and meters in space. Your name badge has a button that you can discreetly press to alert staff that you are in an unsafe situation or need immediate assistance. You also have a button on your communication device configured to connect you to the charge nurse for voice-to-voice communication. There is a program on your computer and communication device that integrates with RTLS to show you where to find additional staff and equipment. You use this to find the closest mobile physiologic monitoring device to continuously monitor and automatically record Weston's heart rate, blood pressure, and pulse oximetry in the EHR while he is being transported to the operating suite.

1. *What is your role in using technology to care for patients?*

2. *How can you be confident that the technologies you use are safe, efficient, and appropriate for your patient?*

3. *How can you be confident you are using technologies appropriately?*

Computers, the internet, and other technological advances have changed the way we communicate, obtain information, work, entertain, and make important health decisions.

Nurses are immersed in the changes that computers and technologies are bringing to both everyday life and nursing practice. As professionals, information technology and computer science can help achieve the goals of quality patient and family-centered care and increased patient safety. The use of health information technologies has evolved over the past 50 years. Technologies are rapidly moving from the automation of data and data processing to fully integrated software, devices, and networks that make up the complex health care ecosystem and underpin all aspects of care delivery in modern medicine. To ensure optimal patient experiences and health outcomes, it is imperative that health care professionals are competent in interacting with and using health care technologies (Skiba, 2017).

The Human Resources chapter of the Joint Commission accreditation manual describes the relationship between "education" and "training" and how they provide the foundation for competency.

> *Education is the process of receiving systematic instruction resulting in the acquisition of theoretical knowledge. Training differs from education in that "training" focuses on gaining specific—often manually performed—technical skills. Competency requires a third attribute—ability. Ability is simply described as being*

able to "do something." The ability to do something "competently" is based on an individual's capability to synthesize and correctly apply the knowledge and technical skills to a task. Competency differs from education and training in that competency incorporates all three attributes: Knowledge, technical skills, and ability— all are required to deliver safe care, correctly perform technical tasks, etc. (Joint Commission Standards, 2018, HR.01.05.03, HRM.01.05.01).

Whether you are a nursing student learning a clinical procedure using a computer-based instruction program; a nurse on the floor using electronic devices such as ventilators, intravenous pumps, telemetry, and **the EHR (or digital version of a patient's chart)**; a nursing administrator using a spreadsheet and database to plan a budget; or a nursing researcher or clinician keeping updated with the latest evidence-based nursing care, it is evident that information technology and computers are essential parts of professional nursing practice, both at the individual and institutional level. The competent use of technologies is central to achieving desired outcomes.

Some nurses have chosen to fully immerse themselves in information management and technology-related work. These nurses specialize in Nursing Informatics (NI). NI supports nurses, consumers, patients, the interprofessional health care team, and other stakeholders in their decision making in all roles and settings to achieve desired outcomes. This support goes beyond the competent use of technologies and is accomplished through the use of information structures, information processes, and information technology.

As the proliferation of information and technology continues to grow at an exponential rate, nursing informatics will remain an essential element of health care delivery. The professional nurse of the twenty-first century will not be effective in the nursing role without a solid base of knowledge related to the impact of nursing informatics, computers, and information technology on nursing practice, patient and family-centered care, and patient outcomes. This chapter will introduce you to the world of nursing informatics and outline informatics competencies that nurses in all roles should possess. In this chapter we will understand the need for nursing informatics, and describe nursing informatics history, definition, and tenets. We will introduce a collaborative model of Nursing Informatics, explain decision support, error prevention, high reliable organizations, and a just culture. We will also discuss critical thinking, security risk and compliance, big data, social determinant of health, and emerging technologies outside traditional health care. Finally, we will describe how to certify or specialize in nursing informatics.

The Need for Nursing Informatics

The idea that all health care professionals needed knowledge and skills in computer science and information management began as far back as the 1970s (Skiba, 2017). Nursing informatics as a specialty grew in earnest in the 1980–1990s, but it wasn't until the turn of the century that the urgency for health care professionals to have knowledge and skills in informatics fully emerged. In Nursing Informatics Education: From Automation to Connected Care (2017), Diane Skiba describes the driving forces for this urgency as:

- *Institute of Medicine (*IOM*) Reports stressed the importance of health information tools to provide safe and quality care. These reports had impacts on patient safety measure around the globe.*

- *Health Profession Education: A Bridge to Quality recommended the following goal: "All health professional[s] should be educated to deliver patient centered care as members of an interdisciplinary team, emphasizing evidence-based practice, quality improvement approaches and informatics." Informatics tools are considered essential for communication, management of information and knowledge, mitigation of error, support for decision making and health care interventions.*

- *Creation of the Office of the National Coordinator of Health Information Technology and its federal mandates served as a catalyst for the adoption of EHRs.*

- *The Technology Informatics Guiding Educational Reform (Tiger) Initiative, which many countries have engaged in.*

- *Robert Wood Johnson Foundation funded Quality and Safety Education for Nurses (QSEN) initiative. The QSEN project emphasizes the integration of knowledge, skills, and attributes related to the IOM six core competencies in their nursing programs and are sharing their work on the QSEN web site (www.qsen.org).*

- *Web-based applications, mobile devices, and EHRs were part of the global technology landscape (Skiba, 2017, pp. 13–14).*

- In 2009, the **Health Information Technology for Economic and Clinical Health** Act (HITECH), which was part of the American Recovery and Reinvestment Act, was passed with the goals of addressing computer interoperability issues. Interoperability is the ability of a computer to connect with other computers in various settings in a secure, accurate, and efficient way without special effort on the part of the user and without any restricted access or implementation. HITECH also established a **National Health Information Network** (NHIN) (HITECH Act Summary, 2018).

It was the convergence of these varied publications, mandates, economic incentives, and technologic advances that created the perfect storm to increase and accelerate **the demand for health professionals that** could navigate and apply the necessary expertise to meet the needs of the rapidly changing health care landscape, particularly in the case of nurses.

Nursing Informatics: Evolution of a Definition

Florence Nightingale (1820–1910) is credited with being the founder of modern nursing. In addition, she is recognized as a statistician and public health pioneer of her time. Betts and Wright (2003) even propose that Florence Nightingale was the first nursing informaticist as evidenced by her collection and analysis of data, and her organization and subsequent report writing using data to convey important information regarding the health of the British nation at home and abroad, as well as how to improve that health (Betts & Wright, 2003).

The **American Nurses Association** (ANA, 2015) defines **Nursing informatics** (NI) as the specialty that integrates nursing science with multiple information and analytical sciences[1] to identify, define, manage and communicate data, information, knowledge, and wisdom in nursing practice. NI supports nurses, consumers, patients, the interprofessional health care team, and other stakeholders in their decision making in all roles and settings to achieve desired outcomes. This support is accomplished through the use of information structures, information processes, and information technology.

The nursing informatics specialty and its constituent members contribute to achieving the goal of improving the health of populations, communities, groups, families, and individuals. Supporting activities include, but are not limited to, the identification of issues and the design, development, and implementation of effective informatics solutions and technologies within the clinical, administrative, educational, and research domains of practice (ANA, 2015, pp. 1–2).

In 1985, Hannah defined nursing informatics as the use of information technology by nurses carrying out their duties in relation to any function in the purview of nursing (as cited in Ball, Hannah, Newbold, & Douglass, 2000). Graves and Corcoran (1989) state that nursing informatics is a combination of computer science, information science, and nursing that is designed to assist in the management and processing of nursing data, information, and knowledge to support the practice of nursing and the delivery of nursing care. Grobe, cited in Ball et al. (2000), adds a further dimension to the definition by asserting that nursing informatics is the application of the principles of information science and theory to the study, scientific analysis, and management of nursing information for the purposes of establishing a body of nursing knowledge. This added dimension suggests that the contribution of nursing informatics is not limited to clinical and administrative nursing practice, but it also contributes to the development of nursing knowledge.

Romano, as cited in Ball et al. (2000), departs from the view that nursing informatics is the integration of information science, computer science, and nursing by maintaining that the focus of nursing informatics is the nature of nursing and how nursing information is acquired, manipulated, and used. Goossen (1996) adds that nursing informatics is the multidisciplinary scientific endeavor of analyzing, formalizing, and modeling how nurses collect and manage data, process data into information and knowledge, make knowledge-based decisions and inferences for patient care, and use this empirical and experiential knowledge to broaden the scope and enhance the quality of their professional practice.

The definitions can be categorized as technology-focused, conceptually focused, or role-oriented. In sum, several definitions of nursing informatics have been proposed and the definition continues to evolve as the nursing informatics specialty moves quickly from its infancy through adolescence on its way to full maturity. Further research is needed to define what is uniquely nursing informatics and develop models to understand and promote its practice (Staggers, 2002).

Tenets of Nursing Informatics

A tenet is a principle, belief, or doctrine generally held to be true, especially one held in common by members of an organization, movement, or professions. As with the definitions of nursing informatics, nursing informatics tenets have also evolved through the years. The ANA published *Nursing informatics: scope and standards of practice (2nd Edition)* in 2015 and outlines the most recent tenets. Nursing informatics:

- Has a unique body of knowledge, preparation, and experience that aligns with the nursing profession. NI incorporates informatics concepts in specific application to the role of nursing and nurses in the health care continuum.

- Involves the synthesis of data and information into knowledge and wisdom.

- Supports the decision making of health care consumers, nurses, and other professionals in all roles and settings to achieve health care consumer safety and advocacy.

- Supports data analytics, including quality-of-care measures, to improve population health outcomes and global health. The IN [**informatics nurse**] and INS [**informatics nurse specialist**] understand that the teal-time [sic] application of accurate information by nurses and other clinicians is a mechanism to change health care delivery and affect patient outcomes.

- Promotes data integrity and the access and exchange of health data for all consumers of health information.

- Supports national and international agendas on interoperability and the efficient and effective transfer and delivery of data, information, and knowledge.

- Ensures that collaboration is an integral characteristic of practice.

---

[1]A listing of sciences that integrate with nursing informatics includes, but is not limited to: computer science, cognitive science, the science of terminologies and taxonomies (including naming and coding conventions), information management, library science, heuristics, archival science, and mathematics.

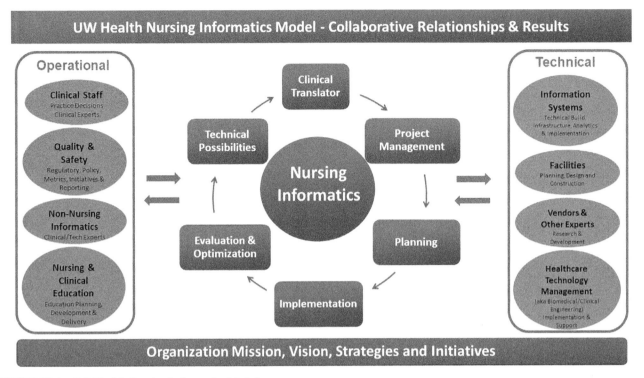

FIGURE 15.1　UW Health Nursing Informatics Model.
Source: Rebecca Rankin, 2016. © 2020 University of Wisconsin Hospitals and Clinics Authority.

- Interweaves user experience and computer-human interaction concepts throughout practice.

- Incorporates key ethical concerns of NI such at advocacy, privacy, and assurance of the confidentiality and security of data and information.

- Considers the impact of technological changes on patient safety, health care delivery, quality reporting, and the nursing process.

- Leads in the design and promotion of useful, innovative information technologies that advance practice and achieve desired outcomes.

These tenets form a framework that characterizes the thinking and actions of informatics nurses in all aspects of practice and in every setting (ANA, 2015, pp. 8–9).

A Collaborative Model of Nursing Informatics

It is certain that, as nursing science, information management, computer science, and other technologies continue to evolve, so will the practice and definition of nursing informatics. Regardless, nursing informatics will continue to ensure that collaboration is an integral characteristic of the practice. Just as there is a interprofessional team with unique knowledge, skills, and roles to provide direct patient care, so too, a nursing informaticist relies on a interprofessional team to meet the needs of staff and ultimately the patients and families everyone serves.

The Nursing Informatics Model at UW Health

The Nursing Informatics Model at UW Health illustrates these various interprofessional team members and their roles (Figure 15.1):

Operational

- Clinical Staff—Practice Decisions, Clinical Experts

- Quality & Safety—Regulatory, Policy, Metrics, Initiatives, & Reporting

- Non-Nursing Informatics—Clinical/Technical Experts within their field

- Nursing & Clinical Education—Education Planning, Development, & Delivery

Technical

- Information Systems (IS)—Technical Build, Infrastructure, Analytics, & Implementation

- Facilities—Planning, Design, & Construction

- Vendors & Other Experts—Research & Development

- **Healthcare Technology Management** (HTM)—(sometimes known as Biomedical or Clinical Engineering) Implementation & Support

Nursing informatics is the bridge between the operational and technical team members. Nursing informatics' key

Real World Interview

"In my experience with Nursing Informatics, what they bring to the table is a wealth of knowledge and a broad perspective when it comes to how we use the clinical record and what makes sense from a documentation standpoint. As a risk manager, I appreciate the collaboration with us to say where are the risks when it comes to using the EHR. Where do we need to use flowsheets versus progress notes? I think that finding that balance is really important because otherwise you can't tell the patient story. You need to know what is happening in that patient's care and what we are doing for that patient clinically so that we can actually tell the patient's story. Nursing Informatics makes clinicians critically think about how they are currently using or how they want to use the EHR versus just having someone else put it together and say here it is.

They're a crucial part of providing leadership. They understand how nurses work and even if nursing informatics isn't actively doing clinical work, they know the questions to asks because they've been there. Nursing informatics can help facilitate discussions because they have the clinical experience and they can work with individual groups but still have a broad perspective to think about the need or application across the organization too. It's so important to know how technology fits into your tasks and what you have to accomplish when taking care of a patient. The technology needs to enhance and support the patient's care and nursing informatics knows how to make that happen."

Jan Haedt, BS, RN, CPHRM,
Risk Management, UW Health, Madison, Wisconsin

---

functions on the interprofessional team include but are not limited to:

- Clinical Translator
- Project Management
- Planning
- Implementation
- Evaluation and Optimization
- Identifying Technical Possibilities

This model is a visual representation of the various partnerships and roles commonly leveraged to meet the technology, data, and information needs of the front-line clinician. The model outlines the unique skills that each discipline contributes to satisfying the needs of the patient and family and can be applied in a variety of settings. Underpinning and directing all the work are the organization's mission, vision, strategies, and initiatives. The remainder of the chapter will illustrate how the model works in practice.

Decision Support and Error Prevention

Weston is out of surgery being cared for in an intermediate care trauma unit. He is doing very well considering the extent of his injuries and may be able to move to general care status soon. He is completing a course of antibiotics for his open humerus fracture and other injuries, and his jaw is wired shut due to the mandibular fracture. He has a **nasogastric** (NG) tube for decompression for his bowel injury and is currently NPO except for medications via his NG tube. His medical team is monitoring bowel activity so they can begin tube feedings. Weston was taking Lovastatin for high cholesterol and Zyban once a day for smoking cessation prior to his hospitali-

zation. Lovastatin was discontinued due to Weston's renal and liver injuries as well as the orthopedic trauma with increased risk of bleeding should he continue taking it. Zyban was also discontinued. Weston types on the bedside tablet he was issued on admission to your unit that he is feeling anxious and jittery and wants to smoke again. He was taking Zyban for a week prior to the hospitalization and reports his last cigarette was 2 days before the accident. He wonders about taking Zyban again as he felt that was making a difference in his withdrawal symptoms and desire to use tobacco. During interdisciplinary rounds, you talk with Weston, his doctor, and the pharmacist about the possibility of restarting Zyban. A decision is made to restart his once daily Zyban and to apply nicotine patches for a short period of time for additional symptom relief. Since Weston last smoked a cigarette 2 days before his hospitalization, the physician will order a lower dose of the nicotine patch than what you would see in a patient that is actively smoking.

Three hours after seeing Weston, the physician has entered the orders discussed during interdisciplinary rounds, the pharmacist has processed the orders, and the medications have been delivered to the unit for you to administer them. This is the first time Weston is receiving transdermal nicotine patches, so you educate him on the possible side effects which include vivid dreams and difficulty sleeping among other things. You direct him to additional educational materials about nicotine patches and smoking cessation that he can access on his tablet. You show him what the patch looks like and use the wireless barcode scanner on the computer at the bedside to confirm that the dose on the nicotine patch packaging matches the physician's orders. Weston has a lot of body hair, so you have a hard time finding an area to place the patch, but soon find a promising site that you clean and dry before applying the patch. Weston's once daily extended release Zyban was ordered by mouth. He is not able to swallow medication due to his mandibular fracture but is cleared to receive medications via his NG tube. Like the nicotine patch, you scan the packaging for the extended release Zyban to confirm it matches the order. You show Weston the tablet and he nods indicating it looks like what he was taking before he was hospitalized. You crush the medication to administer via the NG tube. It takes a little longer to prepare his medication because the coating is so hard, but you are able to crush the Zyban into small enough pieces so that it will go down the NG tube. You wonder if there is a liquid version of the medication and make a mental note to ask the pharmacist and physician to change the order for future doses. Standard practice on your unit when administering medication via an NG tube is to flush the tube with 30 mL of room temperature tap water and clamp the tube for 20 min for medication absorption before putting patients back on suction. Weston no longer has suction to his NG tube, so you don't need to clamp it, but you decide to add another 30 mL to be sure all the Zyban cleared the tube before capping it.

Fifteen minutes later while caring for another patient, you receive a high alert notice on your communication device that Weston is having a tachycardic event. At the same time, you get a message that he may be in early stages of sepsis based on significant changes in his heart rate and blood pressure (hypotension). This makes no sense to you since he has been doing so well after his surgeries. All his surgical sites look great and his vitals and laboratory results have been stable with no trending that might suggest sepsis. Sepsis just doesn't feel right. Shortly after you arrive in Weston's room to assess him, he reports some difficulty breathing and begins to have a seizure. You press a button on your phone to notify the charge nurse that you need immediate assistance in the room and to alert the rapid response team.

The rapid response team is able to stabilize Weston and stay with him until he can be transferred to intensive care. There is an immediate debriefing after the event to try to identify why Weston's condition changed so dramatically and so quickly. You share with the interdisciplinary team that the only changes since earlier rounds were application of the nicotine patch and restarting Zyban. The clinical nurse specialist for your unit asked how Weston was able to swallow the Zyban since his jaw was wired and he has an NG tube. After you shared that you crushed the tablet, the team realized Weston's symptoms were related to an overdose of Zyban since the extended release medication no longer had its protective coating to regulate administration of the drug over 24 hr.

High Reliability Organizations and a Just Culture

Northview Central recently adopted the concepts of high reliability and just culture to help reduce defects in care processes, increase the consistency of care delivery, and improve patient outcomes. High reliability concepts emerged from learning how dangerous industries like aviation, air traffic control, and nuclear power plants could have such excellent safety records. **High Reliability Organizations** (HRO) have a number of characteristics in common. These include:

- They operate in unforgiving social and political environments;
- Their technologies are risk prone and present a high potential for error;
- The scale of possible consequences from things going wrong precludes learning through experimentation;
- The organizations use complex processes to manage complex technologies and complex work to avoid failures (Gallis & Zwetsloot, 2014).

The concept of high reliability is attractive for health care, due to the complexity of operations and the risk of significant and even potentially catastrophic consequences when failures occur in health care (Zwetsloot et al., 2013).

System Failures

Systemic failures in the delivery of health care have more of an impact on patient safety than poor performance by individual health care providers. Focusing on creating a just culture where individuals are not penalized for error disclosure, helps create an environment that welcomes and encourages open reporting of errors and near misses. This allows an organization to learn from and develop systems to reduce or prevent future errors. A just culture shifts the focus from errors and outcomes to system design and the facilitation of good behavioral choices. This in turn creates better and safer patient outcomes (Marx, 2019).

Research shows that highly reliable organizations are able to correct errors and adapt to unexpected events through identifying and discussing potential sources of system failure, questioning assumptions, learning from errors and near misses, and deferring to others' expertise when needed (McFarland & Doucette, 2018). Nurses play an important role in the surveillance and identification of potential adverse events that could negatively impact patient outcomes. As the frontline providers of patient care, nurses use their professional skill, critical thinking, and judgment to make decisions that are in the best interest of their patients and conversely identify potential areas of risk. Through this critical role, nurses are in a perfect position to contribute their knowledge, skills, and expertise to the strategies that ensure high reliability in the practice environment (McFarland & Doucette, 2018).

One of the strategies Northview Central has adopted as part of their high reliability work is to debrief all care team members involved in a serious patient safety event. Because they have a just culture, staff are able to disclose information about errors or near miss events without fear of reprisal. Rather than focusing on the failure of a single individual, the group identifies system flaws that may have led to the error. After discussing and identifying potential sources of system failure, the hospital review group decides to focus on the actual error and how it occurred.

In this particular case, the review group decides to focus on how a medication that was not appropriate for the patient could have been ordered and administered. In the course of the debriefing, the pharmacist shared that her medication verification queue does not include information about the patient's PO status or the presence of any tubes. The physician ordering the Zyban mentioned all the pop-up messages that are built into the system alerting him about what to order and what not to order for any given patient. He reported that based on his previous experience with these types of alerts, he thought the system would stop him from ordering something the patient shouldn't receive. Similar to the physician, the nurse shared that she did not receive a warning that the medication was not appropriate for the patient when she scanned the packaging. Based on these findings, the review group recommended mistake proofing the EHR system with a particular focus on eliminating the possibility of error, improving clinical decision support, and addressing alert fatigue.

> *Mistake proofing uses changes in the physical design of processes to reduce human error. It can be used to change designs in ways that prevent errors from occurring, to detect errors after they occur but before harm occurs, to allow processes to fail safely, or to alter the work environment to reduce the chance of errors (Grout, 2006, p. 44).*

> *Good mistake proofing designs would be very effective in preventing errors or harm. They would be inexpensive, easy to implement, make life easier for staff, and speed up the process. Ideally and when appropriate, they should involve patients and families. They should be mistake proofed themselves and should be informed by other good design practices (Grout, 2006, p. 46)*

It is the role of the nursing informaticist to help design, test, and in some cases, build the EHR or other clinician or patient-facing technology to reduce the likelihood of human error or the opportunity for workarounds that could result in unintended consequences of the technology. The likelihood and severity of downstream errors can be reduced by mistake proofing the system upfront. Unfortunately, mistake proofing does not always eliminate the possibility of error, especially in processes that rely on an individual's attention, skill, or experience (ASQ, 2020).

The most effective principle or method in mistake proofing a process is to eliminate the possibility of the error even occurring by redesigning the product or process so that the task or part is no longer necessary, or in this case is no longer a possibility. In essence, the error is eliminated or designed out of the system so it could never happen (Grout, 2006). For this system failure, this might mean configuring the EHR to eliminate the possibility that the clinician could order any medication that should not be crushed for a patient that has a tube of any sort that goes to or through the stomach, such as NG tube, Dobhoff, gastric tube, jejunostomy tube, etc.

Unfortunately, in this instance, the design recommendation to not allow medications that should not be crushed to be ordered for patients with tubes has limitations, as there are many times when patients with tubes are able to take medications orally or are transitioning away from the tube altogether. The system would also need to be configured to recognize when a new tube has been placed, identify any existing medications that should not be crushed for administration while the tube is in place, and then alert the health care team to evaluate these medications. The EHR technology used at Northview Central isn't advanced enough at this point to support the complex logic and decision points needed to eliminate the possibility of error by designing it out of how the EHR is built. On the other hand, it is easy to include additional print groups to the Pharmacist's medication verification screen that will display the patient's PO status and any tubes or lines the patient may have in place. This additional information supports the clinical decision making of the pharmacist and could add a layer of safety to catch the error before it reaches the patient but still depends on the evaluation and critical thinking of the pharmacist.

Clinical Decision Support

The physician ordering the Zyban mentioned all the pop-up messages that are built into the system alerting him about what to order and what not to order for any given patient. The physician made an erroneous assumption that the system would stop him from ordering something for the patient that could cause harm. Trusting and becoming overly dependent on technology can lead to errors and patient harm. On the other hand, overriding or ignoring technology can also lead to errors and patient harm.

Electronic systems are well suited to collect and compare data and present information to clinicians based on logic applied to those data including complex algorithms. **Clinical decision support systems** (CDSS), which provide alerts at the point of ordering, can reduce medication errors and adverse drug events. CDSS can be used throughout the care delivery process to prevent errors, not just at the point of order entry. CDSS is promoted by several agencies, including the **American Health Information Management Association** (AHIMA), the **Agency for Healthcare Research and Quality** (AHRQ), and the **Office of the National Coordinator** for Health Information Technology (ONC). CDSS are spearheaded by the Clinical Decision Support Collaborative for Performance Improvement.

Clinical Decision Support Rights

A good CDSS considers five key "rights" to improve the likelihood that an alert will aid in timely, effective decision making (AHRQ, 2020) (Table 15.1).

Adding key information to the pharmacist verification work queue is an effective use of DCSS. Alerting a nurse manager via hospital email that a nurse crushed and administered an extended release medication to a patient is not an effective use of DCSS. In this case, the alert has gone to the wrong person, at the wrong point in the workflow, i.e., after the error

Table 15.1   The Clinical Decision Support Rights

1. Getting the *right information*: evidence-based, actionable, relevant
2. To the *right person*: considering all members of the care team, including clinicians, patients, and their caretakers
3. In the *right CDS intervention format*: such as an alert, order, or reference information to answer a clinical question
4. Through the *right channel*: for example, through the EMR (Electronic Medical Record) on a mobile device
5. At the *right time in workflow*: such as when a decision/action/need arises

Source: Retrieved 9/16/19 from https://healthit.ahrq.gov/ahrq-funded-projects/current-health-it-priorities/clinical-decision-support-cds/Chapter-1-approaching-clinical-decision/section-2-overview-cds-five-right.

occurred, and via an unsecure message channel that is outside the clinical record. (Table 15.1)

In Weston's case, Weston and the nurse would have benefitted from the nurse critically thinking about the five rights of medication administration: the right patient, the right drug, the right dose, the right route, and the right time. Errors can happen at a variety of junctures that are not caught by the system or by individual clinicians collaborating in care delivery, so critically thinking about every action you personally take, particularly when performing high risk, high volume, problem prone procedures like medication administration, are essential for patient safety.

CDSS have been shown to provide clinically relevant and accurate information; however, in practice, 49–96% of alerts are overridden (Ancker et al., 2017). This raises questions about the effectiveness of decision support. Although overrides are frequently justified, they can be associated with errors and serious adverse events (including death) if clinically important information is inadvertently ignored. It is widely accepted that "alert fatigue" explains high override rates for clinical decision support alerts (Ancker et al., 2017).

Alert Fatigue

The term **alert fatigue** describes how busy workers, such as health care clinicians, become desensitized to safety alerts, and as a result ignore or fail to respond appropriately to such warnings. Alert fatigue in health care is a symptom of improperly configured technology systems that present excessive, false,

or irrelevant warnings, leading users to mentally tune them out over time. The danger is that a clinically relevant warning will eventually appear but be ignored (Newman, 2019). This phenomenon occurs because of the sheer number of alerts, and it is compounded by the fact that the vast majority of alerts generated by EHR systems (and other health care technologies) are clinically inconsequential—meaning that in most cases, clinicians can and should ignore them without negative clinical consequences. The problem is that clinicians then ignore both the bothersome, clinically meaningless alerts and the critical alerts that warn of impending serious patient harm. In essence, a proliferation of alerts that are intended to improve safety actually results in a paradoxical increase in the chance patients will be harmed. Although little discussed prior to the widespread use of electronic medical records, alert fatigue is now recognized as a major unintended consequence of the computerization of health care and a significant patient safety hazard (Jacques & Williams, 2016).

Alarm Fatigue

Excessive noise is disruptive. There is a large body of literature reporting the benefits of a quiet environment as a healing environment. While it may be quieter and more calming to mute an alarm, silencing or muting a critical alarm to the point you can't hear it can increase the possibility of error which can lead to patient harm, and in this case, even death. In 2013, The Joint Commission issued a Sentinel Event Alert regarding medical device alarm safety in hospitals. This alert highlighted that alarm signals per patient can be a hundred/per day, so the noise level is high within units and hospitals. This Sentinel Event Alert highlighted that injuries and deaths occurred from ignoring alarms, turning alarms down, or off, with the majority of cases occurring in the **intensive care units** (ICUs), telemetry, general medicine, and emergency room (Ross, 2015). Despite the Sentinel Event Alert in 2013, issues with alarms continued and by 2016, The Joint Commission required hospitals to establish policies and procedures for managing alarms and to educate staff about the purpose and proper operation of alarm systems for which they are responsible (Short & Chung, 2016).

Case Study 15.1

Monica, a 17-year-old girl, was monitored following a routine tonsillectomy at Southtowne Heights surgery center. She was given fentanyl for pain and a call button to alert staff if there was anything she needed. The nurse turned down the pulse oximeter alarm attached to Monica's finger to let her rest in a quieter environment and pulled her curtain for privacy. Twenty-five minutes later when the nurse checked on Monica, the nurse realized that the pulse oximeter alarm had been alerting of low oxygenation for an unknown period of time. Monica had severe respiratory depres-

sion and a code was called. Unfortunately, Monica had already suffered profound and irreversible brain damage before the code team even arrived (Ross, 2015).

1. How could this event have been prevented?
2. Have you ever ignored an alarm?
3. Have you ever thought of the consequences of alarm fatigue?

Hospital noise levels have been increasing steadily since 1960s, as the hospital environment has become more complex and interactive. Health care providers are more distracted by the noise as well. The noise levels lead to alarm fatigue, defined as when clinicians become immune or desensitized to the noise or overwhelmed by the information. Alarm fatigue results in the health care provider either not responding to the alarm or being slow to respond to the alarm. This delay or failure to respond leads to error (Ross, 2015).

> *Hospital units have so much equipment with alarms that nurses and other health care providers can become overwhelmed. In reality, many of the alarms are false positives and do not require a clinical intervention from a nurse. The alarm is likely set too high or the threshold is too tight. Other common causes include electrocardiogram (EKG) electrodes that have dried out and become disconnected from the patient or sensors that are not positioned well. Another system process issue is that the default settings are not adjusted for the individual patient or to various patient populations (Ross, 2015, p. 351).*

ECRI Institute (formerly the "**Emergency Care Research Institute**") is an independent nonprofit organization authority on the medical practices and products that provide the safest, most cost-effective care. ECRI published their first Top 10 Technology Hazards list in 2007 for 2008. The list is updated each year based on information found in ECRI Institute's medical device problem reporting databases, ECRI Institute Patient Safety Organization, and the judgment, analysis, and expertise of the organization's multidisciplinary patient safety staff (ECRI Institute, 2012). Some hazards remain on the list for several years if still deemed critical, and others are removed to make room for new more pressing safety concerns. Each of the hazards on the report meet one or more criteria:

- It has resulted in injury or death

- It has occurred frequently

- It can affect a large number of individuals

- It has had a high profile or wide-spread news coverage

- There are clear steps an organization can take to minimize the risk from the hazards.

What is significant about the list is that alarm hazards have been the top one or two highest hazards from 2007, when the list was first published for 2008, until 2016 when three of the top five hazards all related to monitors and alarms (Figure 15.2, Carr, 2011; ECRI, 2007, 2008, 2009, 2013, 2014, 2015, 2016, 2017, 2018, 2019; Schmidt, 2010; Zabel, 2016). Monitor-related alerts and alarms fell out of the top five list for the first time in the 2020 list when Alarm, Alert, and Notification Overload moved to sixth place.

Given the combinations and challenges of technologies and alerts and alarms, it's easy to see how a clinician can become quickly overwhelmed. What is the role of the direct care nurse when facing these challenges? What is the role of NI? The direct care nurse needs to be competent in using the technologies to safely and appropriately care for the patient. This means the nurse is able to synthesize and correctly apply the knowledge and technical skills needed for using any particular technology in completing the task at hand. First and foremost, the nurse needs to recognize the importance and value of using the technology and keeping it in good working order. The nurse needs to know how to set alerts and adjust parameters within the technology based on individual patient needs using established policies and procedures for the organization. The nurse needs to recognize when technology doesn't appear to be working and know how to escalate issues. If the nurse works in an HRO with a just culture, it will be easy to collaborate with other care team members to effect change in optimizing the use of the technology.

Roles of the Nurse Informaticist

Nursing informatics has a unique body of knowledge, preparation, and experience that incorporates informatics concepts in the role of nursing and nurses in the health care continuum. Nursing informatics' role is to collaborate with the various team members to ensure the technologies are optimally configured and working for nurses when caring for the patient and family. This means working with the quality and safety experts and the clinical nurse specialists to define alert and alarm parameters for various patient populations, for example, pediatric and adult, and general care versus ICU, then working with Healthcare Technology Management (HTM) and physiologic monitoring vendors to build and test default parameters in the monitors specific to those populations. This cuts down on the number of false positive alarms for staff and decreases staff time needed to configure devices for specific patients and patient populations.

The nurse informaticist promotes data integrity and the access and exchange of health data for all consumers of health information. The nurse informaticist partners with HTM, the Information Systems (IS) interface team, the IS network team, and the IS EHR application builders to configure the physiologic monitors to automatically send information to the patient's EHR. This reduces staff documentation time and transcription errors as well as supporting **real-time** documentation, which makes information immediately available for all team members to view and use. This also aids in timely system generated data analytics that can inform Clinical decision support systems (CDSS) and support the decision-making of nurses and other health care professionals to promote patient safety.

The nurse informaticist collaborates with the clinical experts and the IS application builders to develop CDSS that gets the right information, to the right person, in the right place in the workflow, in the right format, through the right channel. In addition, the nurse informaticist can inventory and coordinate

ECRI Top 5 Health Technology Hazards 2008-2020

Top 5	1	2	3	4	5
2020	Misuse of Surgical Staplers	Adoption of Point-of-Care Ultrasound Is Outpacing Safeguards	Infection Risks from Sterile Processing Errors in Medical and Dental Offices	Hemodialysis Risks with Central Venous Catheters	Unproven Surgical Robotic Procedures May Put Patients at Risk
2019	Hackers Can Exploit Remote Access to Systems, Disrupting Healthcare Operations	"Clean" Mattresses Can Ooze Body Fluids onto Patients	Retained Sponges Persist as a Surgical Complication Despite Manual Counts	Improperly Set Ventilator Alarms Put Patients at Risk for Hypoxic Brain Injury or Death	Mishandling Flexible Endoscopes after Disinfection Can Lead to Patient Infections
2018	Ransomware and Other Cybersecurity Threats to Healthcare Delivery Can Endanger Patients	Endoscope Reprocessing Failures Continue to Expose Patients to Infection Risk	Mattresses and Covers May Be Infected by Body Fluids and Microbiological Contaminants	Missed Alarms May Result from Inappropriately Configured Secondary Notification Devices and Systems	Improper Cleaning May Cause Device Malfunctions, Equipment Failures, and Potential for Patient Injury
2017	Infusion Errors Can Be Deadly If Simple Safety Steps Are Overlooked	Inadequate Cleaning of Complex Reusable Instruments Can Lead to Infections	Missed Ventilator Alarms Can Lead to Patient Harm	Undetected Opioid- Induced Respiratory Depression	Infection Risks with Heater-Cooler Devices Used in Cardiothoracic Surgery
2016	Inadequate Cleaning of Flexible Endoscopes before Disinfection Can Spread Deadly Pathogens	Missed Alarms Can Have Fatal Consequences	Failure to Effectively Monitor Postoperative Patients for Opioid- Induced Respiratory Depression Can Lead to Brain Injury or Death	Inadequate Surveillance of Monitored Patients in a Telemetry Setting May Put Patients at Risk	Insufficient Training of Clinicians on Operating Room Technologies Puts Patients at Increased Risk of Harm
2015	Alarm Hazards: Inadequate Alarm Configuration Policies and Practices	Data Integrity: Incorrect or Missing Data in EHRs and Other Health IT Systems	Mix-Up of IV Lines Leading to Misadministration of Drugs and Solutions	Inadequate Reprocessing of Endoscopes and Surgical Instruments	Ventilator Disconnections Not Caught because of Mis- set or Missed Alarms
2014	Alarm hazards	Infusion Pump Medication Errors	CT Radiation Exposure in Pediatric Patients	Data Integrity Failures in EHRs and other Health IT Systems	Occupational Radiation Hazards in Hybrid ORs
2013	Alarm hazards	Medication administration errors using infusion pumps	Unnecessary exposures and radiation burns from diagnostic radiology procedures	Patient/data mismatches in EHRs and other health IT systems	Interoperability failures with medical devices and health IT systems
2012	Alarm hazards	Exposure hazards from radiation therapy and CT	Medication administration errors using infusion pumps	Cross-contamination from flexible endoscopes	Inattention to change management for medical device connectivity
2011	Radiation overdose and other dose errors during radiation therapy	Alarm hazards	Cross-contamination from flexible endoscopes	The high radiation dose of CT scans	Data loss, system incompatibilities, and other health IT complications
2010	Cross contamination from flexible endoscopes	Alarm hazards	Surgical fires	CT radiation dose	Retained devices and unretrieved fragments
2009	Alarm hazards	Needlesticks and other sharps injuries	Air embolism from contrast media injection	Retained devices and unretrieved fragments	Surgical fires
2008*	Alarm hazards	Burns during electrosurgery	Burns during magnetic resonance imaging	Caster failures	Infusion pump programming errors

Alarm/Monitor Hazards (16)
Infection Control/Cleaning (12)
Radiation Hazard (7)
Infusion Pump Errors (5)
Data Integrity (4)
Retrained Device (3)
Cybersecurity Hazards (2)

*Top 5 Health Technology Hazards for 2008 are listed alphabetically. In subsequent years, hazards are listed by level of risk with the number 1 hazard being the highest risk.

ECRI Institute (formerly the "Emergency Care Research Institute") is an independent nonprofit organization authority on the medical practices and products that provide the safest, most cost-effective care. Since 2007, the ECRI Institute produces a Top 10 Health Technology Hazards list each year that identifies the potential sources of danger ECRI believes warrant the greatest attention for the coming year. The list does not enumerate the most frequently reported problems or the ones associated with the most severe consequences—although they do consider such information in their analysis. Rather, the list reflects their judgment about which risks should receive priority now. All the items on their list represent problems that can be avoided or risks that can be minimized through the careful management of technologies.

FIGURE 15.2   ECRI top five health technology hazards 2008–2020.
Source: ECRI Institute. Reproduced with permission from ECRI Institute.

regular review of CDSS alerts evaluating how frequently they are triggered, their clinical effectiveness, and any **evidence-based practice** (EBP) updates needed. The nurse informaticist will consider and facilitate discussion concerning the likelihood and burden for alert fatigue versus the timely provision of data and information to support key decision making.

The nurse informaticist collaborates with nursing and other clinical education experts to develop training tools and strategies for educating current and future staff on new technologies, or changes to existing technologies, always considering and reflecting the impact of those changes on patient safety, health care delivery and the nursing process.

Finally, the nurse informaticist leads in the design and promotion of useful, innovative information technologies that advance practice and achieve desired outcomes. The nurse informaticist collaborates with pharmacy informaticists, IS clinical application teams, IS user support resources, and EHR and mobile device vendors to configure scanning technologies for medication administration. The nurse informaticist collaborates with HTM, IS network, IS security, IS application experts; and communication, nurse call, and real-time location system (RTLS) vendors to configure mobile devices that can support voice, text, and alert/alarm communication; as well as track equipment and staff, and discreetly alert staff of an unsafe situation.

Unfortunately, despite all the collaboration and innovation, and using all the technologies and tools at hand, in this case the long and short of it is that Weston was the victim of a health care error. This illustrates how technology has its limitations and puts the focus back on the importance of mistake proofing the broader care delivery system, including the support and development of the clinicians that work within the system.

Critical Thinking

Rapid changes in the health care environment have expanded the decision-making role of the nurse. Patient care is becoming more and more complex, and patient acuity both within and outside traditional health care environments is rising. Decision making and critical thinking are necessary for safe patient care. Nurses deal with the lives of patients on a daily basis where crucial clinical judgments have to be made. Committing themselves to the development of critical thinking is essential in ensuring optimal patient outcomes (Chabeli, 2007).

Decision Making

Critical thinking often has been used interchangeably with other terms, for example decision making, problem-solving, clinical reasoning, and nursing process. In practice, critical thinking refers to clinicians' awareness of complexity, their willingness to work at analyzing situations, and the skills in processing information (Chen, Chang, & Pai, 2018, p. 197).

Reflective Thinking

One of the strategies to becoming a good critical thinker, is to practice reflective thinking. Critical thinking is reflective in that one does not jump to conclusions or make hurried decisions but takes the time to collect evidential information, think the matter through in a disciplined manner, weigh facts, make conclusions, and consider alternatives (Chabeli, 2007). When preparing Weston's Zyban, the nurse was reflecting on how hard it was to crush the tablet and thinking that another form of the medication might be better for future doses. Unfortunately, while insightful, this reflective thinking did not translate into a pause to consider the consequences of crushing a medication with a hard coating and administering it via an NG tube. Reflection upon a situation or problem after a decision is made allows the individual to evaluate and learn from the decision. The debriefing exercise is an excellent way of reflecting on what happened in the situation with Weston and learning from that experience. Ideally, during reflection one can think beyond the immediate event and apply the lessons learned to similar situations. In this case, the nurse might consider what other extended release or sustained release medications should not be crushed regardless of how hard or soft the coating is. We all make mistakes; the important point is reflecting on and learning from those mistakes to help prevent future errors.

Intuitive Thinking

Intuition and **intuitive thinking** are described as an innate feeling that nurses develop that helps them to act in certain situations. It has also been described as a "gut" feeling that something is wrong. Intuitive thinking may result from unconscious assessment and analysis of data based on an individual's past experience. Nurses may make decisions about patient care based, in part, on intuitive thinking. This may seem contrary to using the logical, evidenced-based practice with reasoning that is so prevalent in nursing literature. Intuition guides expert nurses to use a small amount of clinical information and arrive at a conclusion drawing from the ability to recognize patterns and themes from past experiences in a very short time period (Root-Bernstein & Root-Bernstein, 2003).

Pretz and Folse (2011) studied intuition in nursing and found more experienced nurses reported using intuition than those with little experience. Brenner, Tanner, and Chesla (2009) support this by saying, "intuition constitutes a significant part of everyday practice of expert nurses" (p. 210). Weston's nurse received a message on the communication device indicating Weston was showing signs of early sepsis. The nurse had a "gut" feeling this message was not accurate. It made no sense since Weston had *"been doing so well after his surgeries. All his surgical sites look great and his vitals and laboratory results have been stable with no trending that might suggest sepsis. Sepsis just doesn't feel right."* This is an example of intuitive thinking. Perhaps the nurse was recognizing a pattern of how septic patient's present and Weston's did not appear to fit this pattern. Reflectively thinking on this intuitive thinking could help strengthen the nurse's critical thinking skills.

Evidence from the Literature

Source: Adapted from Henneman, E. A., Cunningham, H., Roche, J. P., & Curnin, M. E. (2007). Human patient simulation: Teaching students to provide safe care. *Nurse Educator, 32*(5), 212–217.

Discussion: The use of human patient simulation as a teaching methodology for nursing students has become popular. It effectively demands paying careful attention to the details of the simulation, debriefing staff after use, and employing good evaluation processes. When used properly, human patient simulation offers a unique opportunity to teach nursing students important patient safety principles and strengthen teamwork. For example, one simulator model allows the insertion of a chest tube or the application of a trauma or wound care kit. Such features support educators' abilities to create learning situations that address a variety of specific clinical problems or needs. Human patient simulation can also provide clinicians with an opportunity to care for a simulated patient with other acute clinical problems, such as airway obstruction, cardiac arrest, hemorrhage, or shock.

Implications for Practice: Working with patient simulators allows students to solve problems, utilize teamwork, and communicate effectively with the inter-professional team. Role-playing provides an opportunity to practice teamwork and collaboration, improve communication, and enhance patient safety. By integrating concepts related to patient safety—such as human factors engineering, staff management, and situational awareness—participants learn approaches and concepts related to patient safety and develop clinical skills that reduce the potential for errors. Patient safety and avoidable medical errors are a concern in any institution. The IOM report *To Err Is Human: Building a Safer Health System* recommends simulation training as one strategy to prevent errors in the clinical setting.

Simulation

Simulation is a safe, nonthreatening way to hone critical thinking and clinical decision-making skills. Simulation is widely used in the academic setting and is being used more frequently in the hospital setting. In the IOM report *To Err is Human: Building a Safer Health Care System* (Kohn, Corrigan, & Donaldson, 2000), simulation training is recommended as one strategy that can be used to prevent errors in the clinical setting. The report states that "health care organizations and teaching institutions should participate in the development and use of simulation for training novice practitioners, problem solving, and crisis management, especially when new and potentially hazardous procedures and equipment are introduced" (p. 179). The use of simulation as a teaching strategy can contribute to patient safety and optimize outcomes of care, providing learners with opportunities to experience scenarios and intervene in clinical situations within a safe, supervised setting without posing a risk to a patient (Durham & Alden, 2008).

Simulation promotes teamwork, fosters effective communication, and develops critical thinking and clinical decision-making skills. Simulation is utilized for staff development while introducing new equipment or protocols to give nurses a safe way to practice skills until proficient (Durham & Alden, 2008). Reflection is used as part of simulation and is an effective tool to objectively review situations, actions, communication, and outcomes. It is a nonthreatening way to further critical-thinking skills without the potential for patient harm.

Facilities Planning, Design, and Construction

Simulation has long been used for health care education and training. Simulation is also good for planning, design, and construction decisions, especially when investing in new facilities or remodeling existing spaces. It's one thing to conceptualize how a space will be used and configure it accordingly. It's another thing to actually practice in a space and evaluate its suitability for supporting optimal care delivery, particularly when considering expensive technologies and equipment that

Case Study 15.2

Manny Kin is a 28-week gestational male being cared for in the brand-new neonatal unit at Northview Central. Manny was inadvertently extubated while being transported for a radiologic procedure when his incubator hit the transition in the threshold between the linoleum in the patient room and the carpet in the hall. Manny is taken back into his room to reintubate and stabilize him. The nurse is not able to activate the STAT Assist/Code button in the room for additional help as the button is centrally located in the head wall behind the incubator. The incubator is moved aside so the nurse can activate an internal unit code. The code team is quickly assembled except for the neonatal resident who is napping in the resident call room after a busy night shift. After the patient is stabilized, the nurse documents the event in the EHR and discovers that key documentation elements and prompts are missing from the record.

- How can simulation help in facility design?
- What are some of the key findings in this simulation exercise?
- Does an organization need a simulation lab to benefit from simulation?

might be planned for that space. Simulation offers several advantages in health care delivery:

1. Predictions are possible for situations that do not necessarily exist. An example of this would be disaster planning for a given unit.

2. Solutions that would be very difficult, disruptive, or risky to test under real life conditions can be easily tested in simulation. An example of this is having new nurses practice "code" situations with simulation instead of waiting for the opportunity to arise in the clinical setting; or as in the case above, urgently transferring a vulnerable patient with multiple technologies to another location.

3. Interactions can be identified and considered when making process improvement. This might include testing out what a new workflow might look like when adding a second person to assist with weighing a neonate.

4. Different configurations can be tested in a short period of time. Once the initial process flow model is created, scenarios are relatively straightforward to set up and test. Answers that normally would take many days or weeks to obtain can be acquired in a matter of seconds (McGinley & Stockhoff, 2009).

In the case study above, key findings from the simulation event include problems with the threshold transition, the location of the STAT Assist/Code button above and behind the incubator, lack of nurse call enunciation equipment in the resident sleep room, and missing documentation elements and prompts in the EHR. These are significant findings from a patient safety standpoint. Identifying these opportunities to configure and build the patient care area and technologies so that they support and promote safe patient care ensures optimal outcomes and decreases work and stress for staff. Additionally, it saves time and money by eliminating rework to address these issues after the unit is occupied.

In this exercise, the interprofessional team role-played standard day-to-day work in the simulated environment. Imagine if the team collected around a table in a conference room with bagels and just talked through how they would transport a neonate in an incubator to a radiologic procedure. They might even go so far as to put post-it notes on a board outlining each step in the process. Using this approach, the probability of recognizing the physical barriers and limitations of the space, as it was currently configured, are far less likely than what could be quickly identified when actually interacting in the space, or in this case, a mockup of the unit and patient room. To get the most out of a simulation exercise, it is important to mock up the space to resemble the actual environment as much as possible and have the interprofessional team interact in the space as they would in the actual environment.

The interprofessional team were instrumental in testing standard workflows and interacting with the equipment and in the simulation space as they would in their day-to-day work. Their full immersion in the exercise provided rich feedback

that could be used to optimally configure the work environment and ensure the best care possible when the unit opened. The nurse informaticist had a key role in coordinating the simulation event and considering the user experience and computer-human and other technology-human interactions throughout the exercise. The nurse informaticist developed the test scenarios and scripts with the clinical team and other informatics experts. He added patient details in the EHR test environment to be used during the simulation event and coordinated with the IS security team for the direct care staff to have temporary access to the test environment during the simulation event. He developed the data collection tool, observed and noted anytime there was a barrier, delay in care, or risk of patient harm during the simulation event, and used those data to inform workflow and design changes needed to the physical space and technology configuration and set-up. Those design decisions could then be catalogued and used to standardize specifications for building new units and remodeling existing spaces going forward.

Standardizing building configurations provides predictability and potential for huge time and cost savings for subsequent construction projects. That said, lessons learned and standardization from a construction project in one unit may not apply to or be all inclusive for another care setting. For example, an Emergency Department received a generous donation that would allow them to double their space. Rather than assembling a team to determine the build considerations for the treatment bays in the ED, they decided to use the latest construction specifications developed by a multidisciplinary team, including nursing informatics, for remodeling inpatient ICUs (see Figure 15.3). Their thinking was that if the building and technology specifications met the ICU needs, they would meet the ED needs.

While standardizing build specifications can save time and money, regulatory, patient population, space, staffing models, and myriad other factors need to be considered when remodeling or building a new space. In the ICU design, the computer is located at the head of the patient bed along the same wall as the door. This allows for optimal nurse-patient-computer interaction and a clear path for the nurse to come and go from the patient's bedside. Planners for the ED maintained the nurse-patient-computer configuration at the head of the bed but pivoted the computer/bed design used in the inpatient room layout by 90° to allow for easier transport of carts in and out of the smaller treatment bays. This resulted in a safety/trapping hazard for staff as the computer was now on the furthest wall diagonal to the door and the nurse had to navigate a small opening between a counter and the cart to exit the treatment bay. There was an additional cost to remove and replace nurse call equipment for the newly built behavioral health rooms in the ED. The nurse call equipment specifications were suitable for an ICU setting but posed a safety risk for patients in the ED related to strangulation or other harm from some components in the nurse call equipment not being flush with the wall. Finally, there was a significant technology investment for a bed exit alarm system built into the headwall of each bay in the ED to match the build specifications in the ICU; however, the ED uses carts instead

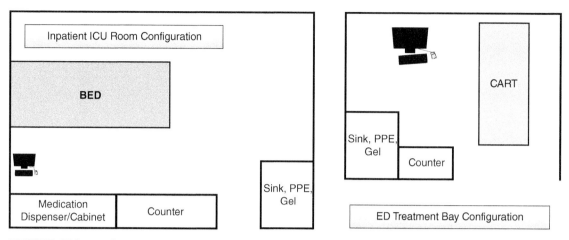

FIGURE 15.3   Applying a nurse-computer-patient technology configuration for an ICU to an ED treatment bay.
Source: Rebecca Rankin, 2011. Reproduced with permission from Rebecca Rankin.

of beds, and carts do not have the technology to interface with the bed exit system. Here is another instance where mocking up the space and simulating care would have saved significant time and expense). It also showcases the importance of considering regulatory requirements for various care settings, unique patient population needs, and the impact of those requirements and needs on building a safe, healing space. This is a classic example where one size does not fit all.

Nurse informaticists bring a unique body of knowledge, preparation, and experience that aligns with the nursing profession and assimilates information from diverse disciplines. In this case, the nurse informaticist could have consulted on the best room design to keep patients and staff safe, while still allowing for easy transport of carts in and out of the treatment bays. Knowing the nurse call technologies needed and available, the nurse informaticist could have envisioned the technical possibilities to meet the particular needs of behavioral health patients and comply with regulatory requirements rather than requiring rework to make the rooms safe after they were built. These are two examples of how the nurse informaticist's understanding of computer-human interactions in combination with other technologies, and collaborative relationships with operational and technical experts alike, makes nurse informaticists a valuable partner in any facility planning, design and construction project.

Security, Risk, and Compliance

You are the nurse that cared for Weston in the Emergency Department at Northview Central. You heard a rumor that he had a significant event that was "being investigated" and that he was transferred to intensive care. You got close with his fiancé and remember how fragile she seemed in the Emergency Department. You have some time after your shift and you think you'd like to visit Weston if he is able to receive visitors. You look in his EHR to see what room he is in and whether he is conscious and alert enough to receive visitors. Unfortunately, he is not doing well and visitors are restricted to family only. Two days later you are called into your man-

ager's office to meet with your manager and the compliance officer to discuss why you accessed Weston's chart when you were no longer providing care to him.

Privacy

Viewing a patient's record without authorization or a valid clinical reason is a serious employee offense. In 2019, a Chicago-based hospital fired approximately 50 staff members who inappropriately accessed the record of a local actor thought to be a victim of racially motivated violence (Drees, 2019b). A Charleston-based hospital reported firing 13 employees in 2017 for viewing patient records without clinical justification (Drees, 2019b). Some employees have even been incarcerated for breaches as in the case of a Pennsylvania woman who illegally accessed and disclosed the medical records of 111 patients (Drees, 2019b).

Another type of privacy breach is emerging with social media. A Charleston-based hospital employee posted a photo on social media without parental consent of a baby being cared for at the facility (Drees, 2019b). This was not an isolated event. The hospital reported six social media-related privacy breaches in the past 3 years by other staff posting content without consent on social media (Drees, 2019b).

There are important issues regarding privacy—who controls sharing and accessing of the information in the health record, how to optimally design an EHR in order to allow patients to maximize the security of their information, and how to develop authentication methods that ensure both privacy and security, yet do not present a major barrier to access (Kaelber, Jha, Johnston, Middleton, & Bates, 2008).

The HITECH Act addresses computer interoperability, privacy, and security concerns associated with the electronic transmission of health information over the internet through funding assistance, incentives, disincentives, and education. In 2009, it widened the scope of privacy and security protections available under The **Health Insurance Portability and Accountability Act** (HIPAA) of 1996 in anticipation of

Table 15.2   Ten Common HIPAA Privacy Violations

1. Employees disclosing information
2. Medical records mishandling
3. Lost or stolen devices
4. Texting patient information
5. Social media
6. Employees illegally accessing patient files
7. Social breaches
8. Authorization requirements
9. Accessing patient information on home computers
10. Lack of training

Source: Retrieved 10/15/19 from https://www.beckershospitalreview.com/healthcare-information-technology/10-common-hipaa-violations-and-preventative-measures-to-keep-your-practice-in-compliance.html

a massive expansion in the exchange of electronic protected health information. The HIPAA Privacy Rule was put in place to provide right to access and amend protected health information, appropriate disclosures and help reduce fraud, waste, and abuse. In addition to widening the scope of privacy and security protections, HITECH increased the potential legal liability for HIPAA non-compliance and provided for more enforcement. For the ten most common HIPAA privacy violations, see Table 15.2.

When appropriately secured, EHR systems may provide better protection of confidential health information than do paper-based systems, because they support controls that ensure that only authorized users with legitimate uses have access to health information. Security functions address the confidentiality of private health information and the integrity of the data. Security functions must be designed to ensure compliance with applicable laws, regulations, and standards. Security systems must ensure that access to data is provided only to those who are authorized and have a legitimate purpose for using the data and provide a means to audit for inappropriate access.

It is the role of every nurse to diligently guard the confidentiality and privacy of patients and families. This includes protecting health information that should only be accessed, used, or disclosed to satisfy a legitimate purpose or carry out a function; and when accessing a record, to only access the minimum necessary information needed to satisfy that legitimate purpose or carry out a function (HHS Office of the Secretary, Office for Civil Rights (OCR), 2013). Nursing informatics has a role in

supporting confidentiality and privacy by working with clinical experts, regulatory experts, compliance resources, and IS analytics and application builders to create reports and chart views that allow clinicians appropriate access to clinical information in a HIPAA-compliant manner.

Access to the EHR and associated communication about care has become more mobile with the advent of smartphones and tablet technologies. Nursing informatics incorporates key ethical concerns such as advocacy, privacy, and assurance of the confidentiality and security of data and information by ensuring staff have the technologies they need, such as facility-issued phones and messaging software, to communicate securely with other health care team members about patient and family needs. Nursing informatics' role when considering phones or other mobile technologies includes imagining the technical possibilities based on current clinical communication needs and technologies available; collaborating with IS and organizational leaders to plan the scope and budget for providing the necessary technologies to ensure HIPAA-compliant communication; coordinating and participating in the selection, configuration, and testing of a device with IS teams and clinical experts; planning and developing educational resources and strategies with education and clinical experts; implementing the technologies; then evaluating and optimizing the use of the technologies.

Providing the technologies necessary to ensure a HIPAA-compliant, secure means for communication to health care team members protects both the patient and the clinician. Three important terms are used when discussing protection of patient information: privacy, confidentiality, and security. It is important to understand the differences among these concepts.

- ***Privacy*** refers to the right of individuals to keep information about themselves from being disclosed to anyone. If a patient had an abortion and chose not to tell a healthcare provider this fact, the patient would be keeping that information private.

- ***Confidentiality*** refers to the act of limiting disclosure of private matters. After a patient has disclosed private information to a health care provider, the provider has a responsibility to maintain the confidentiality of that information.

- ***Security*** refers to the means of controlling access and protecting information from accidental or intentional

Evidence from the Literature

Source: Levine, C. (2006). HIPAA and talking with family caregivers. *American Journal of Nursing, 106*(8), 51–53.

Discussion: HIPAA has alarmed and confused many conscientious health care providers. Providers can share needed information with family and friends or with anyone a patient identifies as involved in his care as long as the patient does not object and/or the provider believes that doing so is in the best interests

of the patient. The article shares the U.S. Department of Health & Human Services Web site for a list of frequently asked questions about HIPAA (available at www.hhs.gov/hipaafaq).

Implications for Practice: Health care providers concerned with quality patient care will want to review HIPAA and ensure that they do not use HIPAA to avoid difficult conversations.

disclosure to unauthorized persons and from alteration, destruction, or loss. When private information is placed in a confidential EHR, the system must have controls in place to maintain the security of the system and not allow unauthorized persons access to the data (Hebda, Czar, & Mascara, 2008).

Medical identify theft is the fastest growing crime in America, followed closely by Medicare fraud. With this in mind, the heightened awareness about data security on the part of the public is not surprising, particularly where the individual consumer or patient has little control and can only take remedial action once a breach has occurred (Andrews, 2016).

An Insider Data Breach survey completed in 2019 asked more than 4,000 employees based in the United States and United Kingdom their thoughts on data breaches and acceptable behaviors when sharing data (Drees, 2019a). Ninety-two percent of employees said they have not accidentally broken company data sharing policy in the last 12 months; however, 35% of employees said they are unaware that certain information should not be shared. Of the employees who reported they had accidentally shared data, 48% listed rushing and making mistakes, 30% listed high-pressure work environment, and 29% listed being tired/not as careful as reasons for the breach data (Drees, 2019a).

In terms of protecting patient privacy, Kendall (2009) notes that the loss of privacy seems to be a foregone conclusion in the information age. Polls show that most Americans believe they have lost all control over the use of personal information by companies. Americans are also concerned about the threats posed by identity theft and fraudulent internet deceptions like phishing. People are learning the hard way to withhold personal information unless it is absolutely necessary to disclose it. A reluctance to provide personal health and financial information is not difficult to understand, given the many high-profile reports of data security breaches from top companies and organizations.

Cybersecurity and Phishing

Cybersecurity is an increasingly important threat to health care delivery. The ECRI Institute identified cybersecurity as the number one technology hazard for 2018 and 2019 (Figure 15.2, Carr 2011; ECRI, 2007, 2008, 2009, 2013, 2014, 2015, 2016, 2017, 2018, 2019; Schmidt, 2010; Zabel, 2016). A cyberattack is a malicious and deliberate attempt by an individual or organization to breach the information system of another individual or organization (CISCO, 2019a). In 2019, more than 33 million people were affected by data breaches across the United States alone. Many of the top 10 data breaches came about due to a security incident with a single vendor partner (Garrity, 2019). Some of the breaches were the result of phishing attempts. Phishing is a cyberattack where the malicious hacker sends a fake email with a link or attachment in order to trick the receiving user into clicking them. In most cases, either the link launches a malware infection, or the attachment itself is a malware file. There are clues to spotting a phishing email (Table 15.3).

Phishing is one type of cybersecurity threat but there are other threats. Smaller hospitals and freestanding facilities are particularly at risk for cyberattack and breaches. They are vulnerable because they are more likely to lack resources to staff cybersecurity roles and are more likely to have outdated equipment that is easy to hack. Regardless of the size of a health care organization or facility, cyber threats and attacks can affect care providers in three ways (Drees, 2014):

1. Threats that jeopardize patient safety and result in harm or death. Attacks against connected medical devices, including insulin pumps, defibrillators, and cardiac monitors, present a large risk for hospitals, because they require constant updating and patching.

2. EHR disruption. Ransomware and cyberattacks that compromise the EHR will impact a hospital's ability to provide patient care. Prolonged disruption from ransomware attacks will affect scheduling of appointments and procedures They also impact revenue cycle and disrupt cash flow, which ultimately impacts hospital margins.

3. Increased sharing of health data. As more patient and health systems share health data with vendors and third parties, data will become more vulnerable because it opens more avenues for hackers to access.

Case Study 15.3

You are the nurse manager for a complex surgical unit at Southtowne Heights. You and your staff order a lot of specialty supplies for your patient population. Southtowne Heights recently completed a yearlong project to move all their procurement and inventory processes to the cloud. Southtowne Heights is the first organization making this transition with the external vendor **Everything and Then Some Solutions** (EaTSS). You have been receiving daily reports listing individual staff that haven't completed the mandatory training required to order supplies and are getting pressure from your director to have all staff complete the training before the deadline. Now you just received a message from EaTSS that you need to provide key information on the EaTSS portal to ensure there are no interruptions in your ability to order supplies. You click on the link embedded in the email and provide the necessary information before racing to your next meeting. Forty minutes into the meeting your phone vibrates, as do the phones of all the leaders in the room. You have just been notified that Southtowne Heights is the victim of a cyberattack by way of a phishing event.

- How would you know to avoid potential phishing emails?

- Who would you contact if you were concerned about the authenticity of an email?

Table 15.3 Phishing Tips

Detecting a Phishing Email

LogRhythm Labs

10 Things to Watch

With the uptick in ransomware infections that are often instigated through phishing emails, **it's crucial to take proactive measures to help protect yourself and your organization's security.**

Having a computer that is up to date and patched makes a big difference in reducing an organization's overall risk of infection.

But being vigilant in detecting phishing emails and educating employees in your organization to also be proactive is a critical step in protection.

Here is a quick top ten list for how to spot and handle a phishing email.

1 Don't trust the display name of who the email is from.

Just because it says it's coming from a name of a person you know or trust doesn't mean that it truly is. Be sure to look at the email address to confirm the true sender.

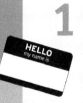

2 Look but don't click.

Hover or mouse over parts of the email without clicking on anything. If the alt text looks strange or doesn't match what the link description says, don't click on it—report it.

3 Check for spelling errors.

Attackers are often less concerned about spelling or being grammatically correct than a normal sender would be.

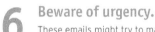

4 Consider the salutation.

Is the address general or vague? Is the salutation to "valued customer" or "Dear [insert title here]?

5 Is the email asking for personal information?

Legitimate companies are unlikely to ask for personal information in an email.

6 Beware of urgency.

These emails might try to make it sound as if there is some sort of emergency (e.g., the CFO needs a $1M wire transfer, a Nigerian prince is in trouble, or someone only needs $100 so they can claim their million-dollar reward).

7 Check the email signature.

Most legitimate senders will include a full signature block at the bottom of their emails.

8 Be careful with attachments.

Attackers like to trick you with a really juicy attachment. It might have a really long name. It might be a fake icon of Microsoft Excel that isn't actually the spreadsheet you think it is.

9 Don't believe everything you see.

If something seems slightly out of the norm, it's better to be safe than sorry. If you see something off, then it's best to report it to your security operations center (SOC).

10 When in doubt, contact your SOC.

No matter the time of day, no matter the concern, most SOCs would rather have you send something that turns out to be legit than to put the organization at risk.

Source: Carden, J. (2016, March 28). 10 Things to Watch: Detecting a Phishing Email. Retrieved October 27, 2020, from https://logrhythm.com/blog/detecting-a-phishing-email/ Used with permission from LogRhythm.

Real World Interview: Downtime Interview

Interviewer: "What is the one technology that you think you would have the hardest time doing without in trying to do your day-to-day work?"

Answer: "You mean like including the charting?"

Interviewer: "Yeah, and then we can include what your second one is."

Answer: "Honestly, the communication, so important. The fact that if I don't know where my preceptor is, the fact that I can send her a quick message, 'hey, I'll be in room 80 if you need me.' The next step is for her being able to send me a message back and say, 'sounds good, can you bring the meds or do a quick assessment while you're in there?' Just being able to communicate while on the floor is a great ability."

Question: "Yeah, I can see that. But the chart would be your first? Or would you make it the communication?"

Answer: "I think I would make the communication first because the chart is important for other people. It's important for the doctor, it's important for JCAHO [The Joint Commission], it's important for everyone else, but for me in the moment, I would say communication is the most important thing."

Leah Alexander, BS, RN,
nurse resident, practicing as a nurse for 4 months
Madison, Wi.

It is estimated the total volume of cyberattack events increased almost four-fold between January 2016 and October 2017. Usually, the attacker seeks some type of benefit from disrupting the victim's network, often seeking ransom and in essence holding the individual or organization hostage by interrupting access to the EHR until the ransom is paid (CISCO, 2019b).

Downtime

A cyberattack, with or without phishing, is one circumstance that can impact computer availability, and by extension, EHR access. Human error, software and hardware failures, severed power cables, software viruses, and disruptions caused by climate or natural disasters can all result in unplanned system outages or downtime. "The immediate effect of any unexpected downtime of a clinical system is the risk to patient safety. Information may be lost or compromised, and care providers must revert to a system of manually reporting patient data. For example, during system downtime, orders are handwritten and transcribed into a manual system, and test results are called to the floor or delivered by a messenger. Without the electronic guidance provided by an order form, critical information such as a patient's allergies or medication lists can often be overlooked. Therefore, side effects of system downtime include disruption to clinical workflow, limited access to patient data, increases in patient wait time, staff overtime hours related to reentry of data, and frustration of staff and patients (Coffey, Postal, Houston, & McKeeby, 2016). Because downtimes are inevitable and lengthy ones can be catastrophic, it is important to have policies, processes, and procedures in place, both for the information services staff to recover from the downtime and for the clinical staff to continue to provide appropriate care during the downtime" (Brazelton & Lyons, 2018).

System downtimes can impact more than just the EHR. There may also be disruptions in the transmission of physiologic alarm notifications and nurse call requests and alerts; paging and phones may not work, depending on how an organization configures their communication systems; medication, blood, and specimen scanning technologies may be down; staff and equipment location systems may not work; and staff duress or STAT assist technologies may also be impacted. Isolated systems may be compromised, depending on the type and extent of a disruption. A fire in an IS network closet can incapacitate the pharmacy or lab systems for the whole organization for several hours. A flood in a facility maintenance closet can compromise positive and negative pressure airflow in isolation rooms and temperature control throughout an organization.

Nursing informatics has a key role in preparing staff for unexpected as well as planned EHR and broader system outages. Nursing informatics' unique body of knowledge, preparation, and experience, along with their collaborative relationships, provides insights and direction when considering the impact of technological changes on patient safety, health care delivery, quality reporting, and the nursing process during a system outage. Nurse informaticists work with IS, HTM, clinical and education experts, and other non-nursing informatics specialists to develop downtime policies and procedures, downtime resources, non-electronic documentation tools, and testing plans to prepare staff for both planned and unplanned downtimes. Nurse informaticists work with clinical experts and IS application teams to ensure appropriate electronic reports and resources are available in a suitably maintained back-up system or downtime environment. This ensures staff have the tools to provide safe, high-quality care in the event of an EHR or broader system downtime. Nurse informaticists consider the individual downtime preparation and recovery for each type of patient care-related technology that may be impacted by a system outage. They then develop resources for the clinician to continue to provide care without the technology and identify steps to recover information from that technology if possible once the downtime has passed.

Disaster Planning

An aspect of security that many people fail to consider is disaster planning. Natural disasters, such as fires, tornadoes, hurricanes, earthquakes, landslides, and floods, may impact an organization's ability to safely care for patients. Even if there is no compromise to the EHR or other technologies, patients, families, and staff may need to be rapidly evacuated from a facility for their own safety. Nursing informatics supports the decision making of nurses, and other professionals in all roles and settings to achieve patient safety and advocacy by assisting in the timely placement of patients in alternate care facilities that can meet their clinical needs. The case above illustrates the importance of having data readily available for critical decision making at a moment's notice. Knowing which patients are close to discharge versus those that need continued care makes a difference in placement considerations. Identifying which patients are in isolation, and what type of isolation, informs transportation and placement considerations along with personal protective equipment needs for patients, staff, and others. Patients with specialized medications, treatments, and care needs may be more difficult to place. Bariatric patients may need special transfer equipment and transport vehicles to be safely evacuated. The same goes for patients that are ventilated or have traction. The list of placement considers based on unique patient needs goes on and on. Figuring out the considerations and options in the midst of a crisis is not the best time for making these decisions, which in some cases have life and death implications.

Nursing informatics can work with the nursing coordinators or supervisors, non-nursing informatics experts, and other clinical experts to identify conditions, orders and equipment that can make a patient more challenging to transfer or place. Using this information, the nurse informaticist can collaborate with the IS application experts to build a dynamic report that continually updates and displays all patients being cared for and highlights those with special transfer or placement needs. The nurse informaticist can partner with the organization's disaster planning or emergency management and safety staff to develop processes and infrastructure for ensuring key patient information is available whenever needed. The nurse informaticist may even collaborate with the regional safety coalition to develop databases that can help match patients with facilities best suited to care for them. The key in these cases is to be able to quickly process data and to present the data in such a way that decision makers can easily make informed decisions about the fastest and safest way to evacuate patients, families, and staff.

Big Data

Developing ways to quickly process data and present it in such a fashion that staff can easily make informed decisions resonates with nursing informatics. One benefit of EHRs already discussed is the promise of using data within the EHR to assist in decision support. You may recall earlier in the chapter that the nurse caring for Weston received a message on the communication device that Weston was showing signs of sepsis. This alert was generated as part of a predictive analytics pilot that the intermediate trauma care team was testing. Predictive analytics encompasses a variety of statistical techniques using data mining, machine learning, and predictive modeling that analyze current and historical facts to make predictions about future or otherwise unknown events (Nyce, 2007).

Data mining is a component of predictive analytics whereby data are analyzed to identify trends, patterns, or relationships among the data. Information from this analysis can then be used to develop a predictive model (Nyce, 2007). Machine learning is a kind of artificial intelligence that provides

Case Study 15.4

You are a nursing leader that covers weekend and off-hour call for urgent and emergent issues. You are invited to participate in a statewide tabletop simulation exercise scheduled to take place on Tuesday morning beginning at 10:00 a.m. The previous year your facility participated in the exercise as a receiving hospital and did quite well, accepting 28 patients in transfer from a hospital with a simulated flooding event 20 miles north of your facility. This year, your facility will act as the evacuating hospital. The event involves a hazardous gas leak that requires full evacuation and safe patient placement for your 580-bed facility within 90 min of initial knowledge of the event. Your facility cares for both adult and pediatric patients. It is the regional burn and trauma center, has an active transplant program, and provides complex orthopedic care. Your facility is nationally recognized for your cancer, neurology, cardiac, and pulmonary programs as well. Patient acuity is particularly high at this time, including two adult and two pediatric patients receiving ECMO (**extracorporeal membrane**

oxygenation), a treatment that uses a pump to circulate blood through an artificial lung back into the patient's bloodstream. You receive a page at 10:07 a.m. to report to the Incident Command Center to begin the evacuation exercise. At 11:37 a.m. the event clock is stopped. Only 39 of your 558 patients were successfully placed in the 90 min allocated to evacuate the facility. While debriefing after the event, the group identified trying to find placement for the two adult and two pediatric patients on ECMO as consuming the majority of the group's time.

1. What are considerations for emergently evacuating unique patient populations?

2. How could you quickly find the information needed to safely transfer patients?

3. Is it a HIPAA violation to access patient records when trying to coordinate patient placement during an emergency?

computers with the ability to learn about newer data sets, as in identifying trends, patterns, or inferring relationships among the data, without being explicitly programmed to do so (Bishop, 2006). "Machine learning algorithms are designed to identify the hidden patterns of the data and generate output predictions based on what they have seen in the past" (Yu & Kohane, 2018). With machine learning, computers can predict the likelihood of certain outcomes based on the data analyzed. But what if the data are incomplete or inaccurate, or worse yet, biased to reflect underlying human biases used to collect the data or set the parameters for machine learning?

The accuracy of the outcome from machine learning is dependent on the accuracy of the data evaluated and how representative the data are of the population(s) being considered. For example, using population health data from residents in rural Alabama to predict the likelihood or probability of certain health outcomes for an Asian-Pacific American woman in Hawaii is not likely to be especially accurate or useful. To make meaningful health-related predictions for either a gentleman in Alabama or a woman in Hawaii would take analysis of enormous amounts of data. This is where the power of big data is realized. Data bias aside, data mining and machine learning can garner information from huge databases that were previously incomprehensible and unknown and use that information to suggest relevant health care decisions (Koti & Alamma, 2018).

Along with their clinical judgment, clinicians can use predictive analytics to assist in assessing the likelihood that a patient's condition warrants hospitalization or other interventions. For instance, if a patient presents to the Emergency Department with new onset chest pain, it is often hard to predict whether the patient needs to be hospitalized or not. Predictive analytics can assist the clinician in making that clinical decision. Similarly, predictive analytics can assist in preventive medicine and public health decisions and recommendations. Many diseases can be prevented or reversed in early stages. Using predictive analytics, a clinician can recognize patients who are at-risk for, or have a higher probability of, developing certain conditions or diseases. The clinician can then share the information with the patient and engage the patient in making lifestyle choices to reverse or avoid further risk of the likely condition or disease in the future (Koti & Alamma, 2018). In Weston's case, predictive analytics were used to alert the nurse that Weston might be septic based on changes in his physiologic data, for example, heart rate and blood pressure. These changes were consistent with changes in heart rate and blood pressure of other patients who were actually septic and whose data were included in the data mining and machine learning used to develop the predictive analytics that triggered the alert. Based on the correlation between Weston's physiological changes and those in the predictive analytic model, a sepsis alert was presented to the nurse. In this case, however, the nurse thought "*sepsis just doesn't feel right*." The nurse based this assessment on a gut feeling as well as clinical observation and assessment, specifically: *All his surgical sites look great and his vitals*

and laboratory results have been stable with no trending that might suggest sepsis.

Frontline nurses providing direct patient care have a role in improving the use of data for predictive analytics and how alerts are triggered and presented to support clinical care. The trauma team, which included the nurses from the trauma unit, were participating in a pilot to test a clinical alert to the nurse of possible sepsis. While Weston presented with life threatening physiological changes that needed immediate attention, the changes were not due to sepsis. The nurse's role in this case might be to provide feedback to the pilot group to include other indicators such as wound documentation, lab results, and trended vital signs over time to increase the specificity of the predictive analytic to alert for sepsis. This example also highlights the importance of accurate, complete, and timely clinical documentation, which is the building block for any data analytics. Waiting to document at the end of a shift renders real-time decision capabilities useless in an EHR. Data mining, machine learning and subsequent predictive analytic alerts are dependent on and only as good as the underlying data used to develop predictions about future or otherwise unknown events. With this in mind, nurses' attention to scrupulously document a patient's clinical care is paramount for building reliable data sets and realizing the full potential of big data.

The nurse informaticist role in the use of big data in this pilot study included partnering with quality and safety specialists to facilitate project management for the pilot. Other collaborative partners included IS analytics and EHR application builders, physician champions, clinical nurse specialists, pharmacists, representatives from infection control, the EHR vendor, and even representatives from the school of medicine and the school of engineering associated with the healthcare facility.

As the pilot continued, the nurse informaticist identified a gap in nursing staffs' understanding of predictive analytics and its role in patient care. Information generated from predictive analytics appears as messages on the nurse's communication device similar to alert and alarm messages. This type of messaging potentially contributes to alert/alarm fatigue and risks staff ignoring the message. To help staff synthesis the information generated from predictive analytics to better support decision making for patient safety and advocacy, the nurse informaticist partnered with the nurse education specialist to develop computer-based learning curriculum to increase staff knowledge and improve attitudes about predictive analytics.

Health care organizations generate huge amounts of data from a variety of sources. Further investigation of big data and its application has the potential to identify and better understand trends in improving health care outcomes, extend life expectancy, and reduce health care costs by providing early and effective treatment across the health care continuum (Koti & Alamma, 2018). With their focus on content and representation of data and information, nursing informatics is well suited to collaborate with the health care team on the synthesis of those data and information into knowledge and wisdom that in turn can be used to optimize patient care and health outcomes.

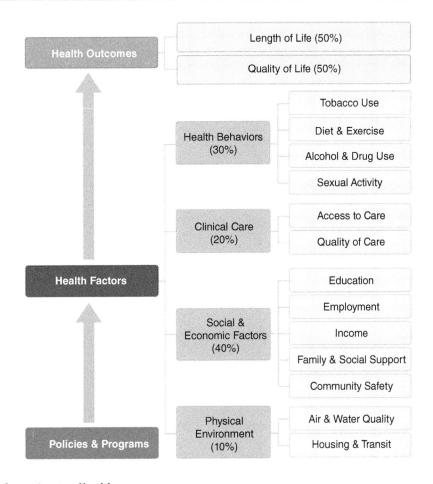

FIGURE 15.4   Social determinants of health.
Source: County Health Rankings model. University of Wisconsin Population Health Institute. www.countyhealthrankings.org/county-health-rankings-model. Copyright 2014 UWPHI.

Population Health and Social Determinants of Health

Whether a data set is big or small, the power of data analysis can have a huge impact on population health. This is particularly evident in the case of the Flint, Michigan water crisis. The Flint water crisis began in 2014, after the drinking water source for the city of Flint, Michigan was changed from Lake Huron and the Detroit River to a less costly source of the Flint River. Due to insufficient water treatment, lead (a known neurotoxin) leached from aging water pipes into the drinking water, exposing an estimated 140,000 residents to lead and other contaminants in their drinking water. Dr. Mona Hanna-Attisha, a pediatrician in Flint Michigan, used lab data readily available in the EHR, to compare lead levels in the blood of children ages 1 and 2 years old before and after the change in the source of the city's drinking water. She found the percentage of children in Flint with lead poisoning had doubled with the change in the drinking water source. In some neighborhoods the rate actually tripled, going from about 5% to almost 16% of children with detectable levels of lead in their blood. At the same time, findings across the country showed lead levels dropping every year (Hanna-Attisha, 2018).

Flint city officials recommended the drinking water be boiled for bacteria and denied it was otherwise harmful to health. It wasn't until Dr. Hanna-Attisha and other data scientists were able to consistently show the level and types of contaminants contained in the water and their impact on the health of local residents that the city became accountable for the crisis. The consequences of lead poisoning are far reaching and a significant cost to individuals, families, and society. This is one example of how where a person lives and what a person consumes impacts their overall health.

Health is promoted or inhibited by many factors beyond access and use of traditional health care. The University of Wisconsin Population Health Institute developed a model in collaboration with the Robert Wood Johnson Foundation using County Health Rankings from 2015 to describe a holistic view of population health. Data were analyzed for 45 states using 35 measures of factors that impact health. Findings were compiled into composite scores for four groups of health factors and one composite score for health outcomes (Figure 15.4). Although understood to be an important predictor of health, genetics was excluded from the model because it is primarily non-modifiable—so far (Hood et al., 2016).

The model performed better in some states than others; however, the results provided broad support for the model and its relative weightings, which empirically estimated the strength of association between the health factors and health outcomes. Factors that influence quality of health and life expectancy (with associated weights) include: social and economic factors (40%), including indicators for community safety, education, employment, family and social support, and income; healthy behaviors (30%), which includes indicators for alcohol use, diet and exercise, sexual activity, and tobacco use; clinical care (20%), including access to and quality of care; and physical environment (10%), consisting of air and water quality, housing, and transit. The results of the model provide a framework by which to prioritize health-related investments (Hood et al., 2016). Based on the findings, it is interesting to note that the greatest improvements in population health can be gained by addressing social and economic factors, and promoting behaviors that positively impact health.

A better understanding of what factors contribute to overall population health can help focus resources and efforts to ultimately improve the health of individuals and communities alike. Now more than ever, organizations have an opportunity to innovate and partner with communities to think collaboratively about how healthy living occurs outside the walls of their own organization. Forward-thinking organizations are considering how investments in services and resources outside of hospitals and conventional clinics can positively impact the health and quality of life for an entire community. Organizations focusing on transportation, social services, and data directories are helping to improve a community's overall health through creating additional avenues for people to get to appointments, maintain their health regime, make social connections, build a more diverse and accurate data set to inform health-related decision making, etc.

> *New reimbursement codes specifically for mental health and efforts around digital health entrepreneurs [are] coming together to support Medicaid populations. And more and more health systems are exploring how they can take accountability for the social determinants of health, ranging from mental health to culturally appropriate engagement (HIMSS, 2019). Source: HIMSS, 2019, Is the Digital Health Bubble Bursting? Retrieved October 17, 2019 from https://www.himss.org/news/digital-health-bubble-bursting-health-20-weighs-in.*

An explosion of technology, shifts in where and how care can be provided, and what services will be reimbursed, create an environment of endless possibilities for improving the health and quality of life for all.

The nurse informaticist is uniquely suited to see the technical possibilities of new models for care delivery and to lead in the design and promotion of useful, innovative information technologies that advance practice and achieve desired outcomes.

E-Health and Telehealth

One such innovative technology that has the potentially to advance the health and wellbeing of a population is the internet. The internet created new opportunities and challenges to the traditional health care information technology industry. These "new" challenges were mainly: (a) the capability of healthcare consumers to interact with healthcare systems online, (b) improved possibilities for institution-to-institution transmissions of data, and (c) new possibilities for consumer to consumer communication (Eysenbach, 2001). E-health emerged from this happy collision of health care and the internet. E-health is "the intersection of medical informatics, public health, and business, referring to health services and information delivered or enhanced through the internet and related technologies. In a broader sense, the term characterizes not only a technical development but also a state of mind, a way of thinking, an attitude, and a commitment for networked, global thinking to improve health care locally, regionally, and worldwide by using information and communication technology" (Eysenbach, 2001).

Telehealth is the delivery of health-related services and information for health promotion, disease prevention, diagnosis, consultation, education, and therapy, via telecommunications technologies and computers to patients and providers at another location. It may be as simple as two health professionals discussing a case over the telephone or as sophisticated as using satellite technology to broadcast a consultation between providers at facilities in two countries, using videoconferencing equipment or robotic technology. It may include transmission of patient images or data, such as pulse oximetry, heart rate, blood pressure, etc., for diagnosis or disease management; groups or individuals exchanging health services, education, health care advice, or research via live videoconference; or home monitoring of dialysis or cardiac patients. Telehealth can improve health care access in vulnerable patient populations through the use of electronic devices in patients' homes that monitor and assess for early complications (Prinz, Cramer, & Englund, 2008).

By 2018, an estimated 22 million households were using virtual care solutions such as telehealth and e-health, up from less than a million in 2013. Average health care visits among these adopter households were expected to increase from 2 per year in 2013 to 6 per year in 2018, which includes both acute care and preventive follow-up services in a variety of care settings such as at home, at retail kiosks, or at work (Wang, 2014).

Ubiquitous Computing

Computers are no longer distinct objects but are integrated into the environment, thus enabling people to interact with information-processing devices more naturally and casually. Computers have become so fundamental to our human experience that they have "disappeared," and we have ceased to be aware of them. The result is "calm technology," in which computers do not cause stress and anxiety for the user but, rather, recede into the background of life. Our information and news are accessed through computers or mobile devices; many books are read through wireless reading devices (Kindle, iPad); mobile phones are part of daily life; and **global positioning systems** (GPSs) are in many phones, watches, etc. There are even self-driving cars.

One only has to look around a typical house to see how ubiquitous computing is becoming part of our lives. Microprocessors exist in every room: appliances in the kitchen, remote controls throughout a home, advanced gaming and **virtual reality** (VR) systems. Many homes even have voice activated technologies that can turn on lights, turn off appliances, make a shopping list, tell you a joke, and let you know how long it will take you to get to work and whether you should bring an umbrella.

Technologies are not limited to the home or place of work. A lot of wearable devices have emerged in the past decade with a good portion of them attempting to bridge the data gap by sharing medical information with health care providers. A survey from the research firm Accenture reported that 9 out of 10 people are willing to share wearable health data with their physician. Consumer adoption of wearable health technology is increasing exponentially, with over a 50% increase from 21% in 2016 to 33% in 2018. These medical technologies are aiming to get a better sense of people's health outside of the 0.1% of the patient's life spent in a provider's office. The majority of patients surveyed in the Accenture study felt that wearable health devices improved the understanding of their condition, their quality of care, and it helped them communicate with their physician (Berry, 2018).

Computers and health care are becoming so ingrained in all aspects of life that even toilet manufacturers are finding a niche. Toto and Matsushita, two toilet manufacturing giants in Japan, released WiFi-connected toilets that measure body mass index, biochemical makeup (sugar, protein), urine flow rate, and temperature of urine. Inui Health (formerly known as Scanadu) announced FDA approval for its smartphone-connected urine analysis that can detect bladder infections, pre- and gestational diabetes, and kidney disease, all in the comfort of one's home (Berry, 2018).

Mobile Applications and Digital Health

The rapid uptake of smartphones, tablets, and other technologies by both consumers and providers for health care purposes is astounding. Mobile applications (commonly called apps) are software programs for smartphones and other handheld computing devices. The creation of health care apps for these mobile devices is also moving quickly. What is it that makes these mobile devices so attractive? Unlike any other **health information technology** (HIT) platform, they are basically inexpensive, attractive, and easy to use anytime they are needed. They are so intuitive and user-friendly that most people can download and use the many computer applications available for them quickly without much training or basic computer literacy. In 2017, iTunes offered 95,851 Health and

Fitness apps. Not to be outdone, Google offered 105,912 (Bol, Helberger, & Weert, 2018).

According to Accenture research posted in March 2018, health care consumers continue to show strong use of digital technology, with numbers rising each year. In fact, 75% of consumers surveyed said technology is important to managing their health. This research also showed increases across the board in the use of mobile devices, EHRs, social media, wearables, and use of online communities. More specifically, nearly half (48%) of health care consumers are using mHealth apps, compared to just 16% in 2014 (Liquid State, 2019).

Networking and connecting data from various devices and applications can assist in improving individual patient health outcomes, such as reminding patients to take their medications at home, tracking blood glucose responses to changes in medication, providing just-in-time support for smoking cessation coaching, and contributing to big data for research. The emerging field of "digital health," which includes mobile apps, e-Health, telemedicine, EHR, and consumer data, shows promise in reducing the cost of health care due in part to remote processes and the ability to treat a higher number of patients. In addition, digital tools allow for more "consumer-centric" health care by engaging consumers in managing their own health care and that of their families (Iakovleva, Oftedal, & Bessant, 2019, pp. 1–2). It also provides a platform for impacting social determinants of health that may not otherwise be addressed during the brief face-to-face encounters between patients and health care professionals.

There are some challenges with digital health. While digital health "ecosystems promise a future for universally accessible and more intelligent healthcare, the privacy of patients, doctors, nurses, and health care providers is of greater concern today than ever" (Iyengar, Kundu, & Pallis, 2018). In addition to privacy concerns, Bol et al. (2018) explored factors associated with mobile app use and considered whether health app use may contribute to new digital inequalities. They found "a person's age, education level, and e-health literacy skills were predictors of mobile health app use in general. Importantly, the findings also suggest that different populations select different types of mobile health apps such that gender, age, education levels, and privacy concerns are differently associated with use of specific types of mobile health apps."

Their findings suggest there are "different gradations of mobile health app users, differentiated either by their demographic background and/or their level of privacy concern for mobile health apps use" (Bol et al., 2018).

Differences in individuals and individual use of mobile health app make data challenging, but consider how a researcher accounts for health-related data for the population who do not use mobile apps at all or is not reflected in data sets in other ways? Health care is one of the most challenging industries when it comes to data, primarily due to the fact that health care operational systems were not designed for modern analytics and are often not fully integrated with internal or external data systems (Nelson, 2019). Outputs resulting from artificial intelligence and machine learning, used for health-related decision making, need to be guarded and regarded with caution understanding the potential impact of privacy, incomplete data sets, and data bias.

Social Network Sites

Social network sites are also exerting a prevalent presence in health care. They have been growing in popularity across broad segments of internet users and are a convenient means to exchange information and support. For example, Facebook groups (www.facebook.com) have become a popular tool for awareness-raising, fundraising, and support-seeking related to breast cancer, attracting over 1 million users (Bender, Jimenez-Marroquin, & Jadad, 2011). Patient communities, such as PatientsLikeMe (www.patientslikeme.com) are flourishing. PatientsLikeMe is committed to providing patients with access to the tools, information, and experiences that they need to take control of their disease.

A Pew Research Center study completed in 2012 measured how many people use online resources to find information or connect with others about health conditions. The study found that 72% of adult internet users say they have searched online for information about a range of health issues, the most popular being specific diseases and treatments. One-in-four (26%) adult internet users say they have read or watched someone else's health experience about health or medical issues in the past 12 months. And 16% of adult internet users in the U.S. have gone online in the past 12 months to find others who share the same health concerns (Fox, 2014).

Given the popularity of social media and online marketing, health care organizations are developing an online presence using conventional web sites and social media. This work is proceeding with caution keeping in mind potential confidentiality, privacy, and security risks associated with the technologies. The **Association for Healthcare Social Media** (AHSM), which opened for public membership in May 2019, knows that many people look to the internet for their daily health care information. AHSM was founded by doctors and nurses who recognize the potential gains and risks for using the internet for health care information. One of AHSM's goals is to show hospitals and institutions how they can advance their own goals of spreading good information via social media (Uitti, 2019).

Virtual Reality

Another computer-driven technology expanding its footprint in health care is virtual reality (VR). VR puts people inside a computer-generated world. VR has enormous potential in health care applications, such as health games like Ruckus Nation: An Online Idea Competition to Get Kids Moving! (Delicious.com, 2019). With VR, a person can see, move through, and react to computer-simulated items or environments. Using certain tools such as a head-mounted computer display and a handheld input device, the user feels immersed in and can interact with this world. The virtual world can represent the current world or a world that is difficult or impossible to experience firsthand—

for example, the world of molecules, the interior of the human body, or the surface of Pluto. By putting the sensors on the person (head-mounted computer display, sensors in gloves, shoes, and glasses), the person can move and experience the world in a typical way—by walking, moving, and using the senses of touch, sight, smell, and hearing.

Applications in health care education also exist. VR allows information visualization through the display of enormous amounts of information contained in large databases. Through 3-D visualization, students can understand important physiological principles or basic anatomy. Students can go "inside" the body to visualize structures and see how they work. It is also possible to observe changes in physiological functioning. For example, a student can visualize the vascular system of a patient going into shock (Kilmon, Brown, Ghosh, & Mikitiuk, 2010).

VR has allowed practitioners to develop minimally invasive surgical techniques. This allows direct viewing of internal body cavities through natural orifices or small incisions. The manipulation of instruments by the surgeon or assistants can be direct or via virtual environments. In the latter case, a robot reproduces the movements of humans, using virtual instruments. The precision of the operation may be augmented by data or images superimposed on the virtual patient (Nunes, 2008).

For students learning clinical procedures, VR gives them the opportunity to practice invasive and less commonly occurring procedures in the lab, so that they have both the skill and the confidence necessary when encountering a patient requiring the procedure for the first time. Likewise, VR enhances patient education materials. Diabetic patients needing to understand the physiological processes of the pancreas may visualize the organ to more fully understand their disease and treatment. Patients requiring painful or unusual procedures may experience a VR simulation as a means of preparation. By providing an alternate environment, VR also has the potential to mitigate or minimize the side effects of certain procedures such as chemotherapy in patients with cancer.

A popular use of VR in psychology has been in exposure therapy for patients with specific phobias. VR simulation has been used to treat patients with a fear of flying, agoraphobia, fear of spiders, fear of falling, fear of the dentist, and other phobias (Brinkman et al., 2010). Some researchers have also found improvements using VR in patients with **post-traumatic stress disorder** (PTSD) and some anxiety disorders (Carl et al., 2019); however, a meta-analysis of VR interventions for anxiety and depression outcomes shows mixed efficacy in the use of VR suggesting more research is needed (Fodor et al., 2018).

Trends in Computing

The explosion of technologies and the increased availability of electronic information requires nurses to be computer literate in order to provide optimal care to patients and families. Computer literacy is defined as the knowledge and understanding of computers, combined with the ability to use them effectively (McDowell & Ma, 2007). For health care professionals, computer literacy requires having an understanding of systems used in clinical practice, education, and research settings. In clinical practice, for example, electronic patient records and clinical information systems have become the norm. A clinical information system draws information from multiple systems into an electronic patient record. The computer literate nurse must be able to use these systems effectively and address issues discussed earlier, such as confidentiality, security, and privacy. At the same time, the more advanced nurse must be able to effectively use applications typically found on PCs, such as word-processing software, spreadsheets, and PowerPoint. The nurse will want to develop the ability to use statistics for research. Finally, the computer literate nurse must know how to access information from a variety of electronic sources and how to evaluate the appropriateness of the information at both the professional and patient level. The computer literate nurse has information literacy. Information literacy is the ability to identify when and what information is needed, understand how the information is organized, identify the best sources of information for a given need, locate those information sources, evaluate the information sources critically, and share that information as appropriate (ANA, 2015).

Internet and Searching for Evidence

Information literacy is a necessary skill for extracting evidence from research and practice resulting in EBP. EBP is the process of systematically finding, appraising, and using contemporaneous research findings as the basis for clinical decisions. Evidence-based health care asks questions, finds and appraises the relevance based on accurate analysis of current nursing knowledge and practice, and harnesses that information for everyday clinical practice. The primary sources for this type of information are web-based resources such as online databases (e.g., Medline, CINAHL) and also electronic practice documents, such as EHRs.

Evidence-based health care follows four steps:

1. Formulate a clear clinical question from a patient's problem;

2. Search for clinical research articles or prior practice applications relevant to the intervention at hand;

3. Evaluate and critically appraise the evidence for its validity and usefulness;

4. Implement useful findings in clinical practice (Magrabi, Westbrook, & Coiera, 2007).

The skills that underpin evidence-based clinical practice and nursing are:

• Forming a good clinical question.

• Finding evidence using effective search techniques.

• Using resources for EBP including databases, e-journals, e-textbooks and other internet sites (Cushing/Yale Medical Library, 2019).

For nurses, sources of evidence are studied and the wealth of information that exists is confronted. The challenging question is how to integrate a more evidence-based approach into the every-day practice of nurses. Although the nursing profession recognizes that research is the basis for knowledge development, lack of organizational support for providing nursing time to access, use, and conduct research on clinical units can limit the ability of nurses to practice EBP.

Using the Internet for Clinical Practice

Information literacy is critically important for EBP; especially since the amount and complexity of information is expanding daily (Barnard et al., 2010). Not all information is created equal: some is authoritative, current, reliable, but some is biased, out of date, misleading, and false. Also, to find the "right" information, keep in mind that the clinician must be persistent. No one search strategy is going to work all the time, nor is any one search engine more effective than any other. Here are some strategies and tactics to render internet searches more efficient and to reduce search time (Anderson & Klemm, 2008):

• Use Web sites published by trusted governmental or professional organizations for the information they specialize in.

  ○ American Heart Association (http://heart.org) or the National Heart, Lung & Blood Institute (http://nhlbi.nih.gov), cardiovascular diseases.

  ○ NIH National Cancer Institute (http://cancer.gov), cancer.

  ○ National Institute of Diabetes and Digestive and Kidney Diseases (http://niddk.nih.gov), diabetes and digestive disorders.

  ○ Center for Disease Control and Prevention (http://cdc.gov), a primary resource for developing and applying disease prevention and control, environmental health, and health promotion activities.

  ○ National Institute on Aging (http://nia.nih.gov), well-being and health of older adults.

  ○ American Dietetic Association (http://eatright.org), offering information related to food and diet.

  ○ American Medical Association's consumer health information site (http://ama-assn.org), resource for general health information.

• Use Consumer health sites organized by health care librarians. These offer a wealth of organized information on disease management and include MEDLINE*plus* (http://medlineplus.gov), maintained by the National Library of Medicine.

• Use precise terms, such as "diabetes type 1" instead of just "diabetes," to reduce the number of hits when searching for very specific information.

- Draw on search engines such as Mayo Clinic (www.mayoclinic.com), WebMD (www.webmd.com), and others that collect information from reliable online health resources rather than relying on the "bots," or robots, typically used by search engines to "crawl" the Web, as with Google.

- Refine your internet searches with filters. Filtering is mechanically blocking internet content from being retrieved through the identification of key words and phrases. For example, you can narrow your search by the type of medical viewpoint (traditional or alternative), reading level (easy, moderate, or complex), and type of site (commercial, noncommercial, government, or nonprofit) that you use in your key words to filter your search.

The result of the searches after using these strategies will probably be a more focused and helpful list of links matching the clinician's specific request. The clinician will then want to evaluate the search data.

Internet Resources for Patients

The internet can be used by patients to manage their health or diseases. A major problem with using the internet for this purpose is that information on the internet lacks the conventional standards by which traditional published resources are evaluated. Though many general instruments can be used in evaluating health-related Web sites, most of them are incomplete, and many do not measure what they claim to measure (Anderson & Klemm, 2008). In addition, they are geared toward professional and regulatory organizations, and some patients may lack the knowledge to understand the information provided.

Yet, it is critical that non-clinicians be able to evaluate health information on the internet. Helping patients determine this quality and relevance of information available via the internet becomes a key responsibility for clinicians. Criteria to evaluate internet health information have developed over the years; however, these criteria often assume knowledge of healthcare content and some familiarity with traditional standards for evaluating such resources.

One creditable resource for helping patients find reliable internet sites is **Health On the Net** (HON). HON is a not-for-profit organization associated with the World Health Organization. HON promotes transparent and reliable health information online and accredits web sites that adhere to eight HON principles, i.e., authority, complementarity, confidentiality, validity, justifiability, and objectivity, user's practice, financial disclosure, and advertising policy. Patients and families can feel confident in the information they get from web sites that have the HON certification; however, many web sites do not pursue HON certification. In these cases, based on published criteria and taking into account patient context and needs, the nurse can provide the patient with a simple set of criteria, subjective and objective, to evaluate website content, design, navigation, and credibility (Alpay, Overberg, & Zwetsloot-Schonk, 2007).

Here is an instance where the clinic nurse could collaborate with NI to ensure consumer safety and support informed decision making. Partners in the work might include education experts and patient and family advisory representatives. Developing resources to help patients and families find information on the internet safely and with confidence can help address questions about the new diet as well as other health information patients and families might search for on the internet.

Case Study 15.5

You are a nurse in a busy internal medicine clinic. You are seeing a new patient, Weston Miller, a 37-year-old construction worker who was struck by a car 3 months ago while working on Highway 104. He has made a full recovery from his injuries, despite one rocky event early in his hospitalization, and is here to establish a relationship with a new primary care provider. Weston is looking forward to marrying his fiancé in a month and would really like to lose some weight before the wedding. He asks you about a new diet he saw online. The diet helps reduce inflammation, decreases risk for 17 different diseases, and if followed exactly, guarantees significant weight loss in just weeks. Several other patients have also asked you about this diet, which has been recommended by friends and friends of friends via social media and on the internet.

1. How do you advise Weston and other patients concerning this popular life-changing diet?

Case Study 15.6

You have been working as a nurse for 3 years and really love what a difference you've been able to make in the lives of your patients and their families. As part of your work, you've had the opportunity to participate in a pilot project to evaluate patient use of tablets to review their medications and labs, watch and read educational materials, order meals, and complete other useful tasks. After deploying the tablets, patient satisfaction scores for your work area have significantly increased compared to other areas that aren't using the tablets. You also proposed affixing Quick Response (QR) codes on infrequently used equipment and technology, so that staff can scan the code and access educational materials for just-in-time training when they have questions about using the equipment/technology. Your colleagues naturally gravitate to you when they have a technology question, because you just seem to "get technology" and you don't make them feel stupid when they ask questions. You've been thinking about exploring some advanced studies in nursing informatics but aren't sure where to begin.

1. What resources can you use to explore your options related to nursing informatics?

Nursing Informatics Specialist

Formal Programs in Informatics

As the health care industry relies more on information technology for the delivery of care, it is imperative that basic computer skills and nursing informatics competencies are incorporated in all levels of professional nursing education programs.

The first Master's program in Nursing Informatics was established at the University of Maryland in 1989, followed by a doctoral program in 1992. Now, there are numerous universities nationwide offering master's degrees, doctoral degrees, and postgraduate certifications in Nursing Informatics easily searchable on the internet.

Informal Education

There are numerous venues for all nurses to stay abreast of emerging health information technologies and trends. Groups such as the **American Medical Informatics Association** (AMIA) and the **Healthcare Information and Management Systems Society** (HIMSS) have annual conferences that attract thousands of Health Information Technology (HIT) professionals and vendors, offering educational and networking opportunities for all informatics appetites. Many regions have formed nursing informatics groups that function at the local, national, and even international levels. These groups offer vital networking and educational services to their members. In 2004, many regional nursing informatics groups, representing 2,000 nurses, formed the **Alliance for Nursing Informatics** (ANI) in collaboration with HIMSS and the ANA (www.allianceni.org/about. asp). There are several nursing and health informatics scholarly journals, such as *Computers, Informatics, and Nursing* (https:// journals.lww.com/cinjournal/pages/default.aspx), *Journal of Medical Informatics Association* (https://journals.lww.com/ cinjournal/pages/default.aspx), and *Applied Clinical Informatics* (www.amia.org/aci-applied-clinical-informatics-journal-0), that provide essential elements of continuing industry trends and nursing informatics education.

Certification

Certification in a specialty is a formal, systematic mechanism whereby nurses can voluntarily seek a credential that recognizes their quality and excellence in professional practice and continuing education (Jones & Nicoll, 2011). For many nurses, becoming certified is a professional milestone and validation of their qualifications, knowledge, and skills in a defined area of nursing practice. The **American Nurses Credentialing Center** (ANCC) offers certification examinations for a variety of specialties in nursing, including informatics. The ANCC Website (www.nursingworld.org/ancc) details the nursing candidate's requirements for the Informatics Nurse Certification Exam.

Conclusion

The nursing informatics specialty and its constituent members contribute to improving the health of populations, communities, groups, families, and individuals. This chapter covered key concepts in using technology to provide safe, high-quality care to patients and families. It introduced a model illustrating the role of the nurse informaticist in working with a multidisciplinary team to meet the needs of staff and ultimately the patients and families everyone serves. We also stressed the importance of diligently guarding patient confidentiality and the changing landscape of where and how care is provided, including social determinants of health and the emerging field of digital health.

Career opportunities in the fields of computer science and information technology are growing at an exponential rate, and nursing is no exception. Nurses working in informatics can look forward to multiple job opportunities, with new roles continuously being developed as technology changes and matures.

> *The unfolding of new health care paradigms will bring greater connectivity between care providers and patients, include a wider array of emerging technologies and an increasing emphasis on data analytics will make the integration of informatics competencies into every area of nursing imperative. (Nagle, Sermeus, & Junger, 2017).*

KEY CONCEPTS

- **Nursing informatics** (NI) is the specialty that integrates nursing science with multiple information and analytical sciences to identify, define, manage, and communicate data, information, knowledge, and wisdom in nursing practice. NI supports nurses, consumers, patients, the interprofessional health care team, and other stakeholders in their decision making in all roles and settings to achieve desired outcomes.

- Nursing informatics ensures that collaboration is an integral characteristic of practice.

- High Reliability Organizations (HRO) are able to correct errors and adapt to unexpected events through identifying and discussing potential sources of system failure, questioning assumptions,

learning from errors and near misses, and deferring to others' expertise when needed.

- Organizations with a Just Culture identify system flaws that may have led to an error rather than focusing on the failure of a single individual.

- Alert, alarm, and notification fatigue describes how busy workers, such as health care clinicians, become desensitized to safety alerts/alarms/notifications, and as a result ignore or fail to respond appropriately to such warnings.

- E-Health, telehealth, and mobile applications are developing rapidly in healthcare.

- As more patient and health systems share health data with vendors and third parties, data will become more vulnerable because it opens more avenues for hackers to access.

- It is important to evaluate information found on the internet and to educate your patients about the importance of evaluating the information found on the internet.

- Nurses can pursue formal education in nursing informatics at both the graduate and undergraduate levels. Informal education in informatics can be pursued through self-study, attendance at conferences, and reading the informatics literature.

- Certification in nursing informatics is voluntary and recognizes superior achievement and excellence in the specialty.

KEY TERMS

Nursing informatics	Critical thinking	Social Determinants of Health
Electronic health record systems (EHR)	HIPAA	Digital health
Clinical decision support systems	Cyberattack	Computer literacy
Alert fatigue	Downtime	Information literacy
Alarm fatigue	Predictive analytics	

REVIEW QUESTIONS

1. A person who is HIV positive and chooses not to reveal this information to a nurse during an admission assessment is keeping this information
   a. anonymous.
   b. secure.
   c. private.
   d. confidential.

2. You are interested in learning more about **amyotrophic lateral sclerosis (ALS)**. You find a Web site where the author states that he is a worldwide leading researcher into causes for this disease. As part of your evaluation of the author's credentials, you will do which of the following?
   a. Take him at his word.
   b. E-mail him and ask for a list of references.
   c. Ask several colleagues whether they are familiar with his research.
   d. Do an author search on MEDLINE.

3. Informatics nursing is distinguished from other nursing specialties by its focus on which of the following?
   a. Electronic health records.
   b. Data coding and the use of abbreviations.
   c. Content and representation of data and information.
   d. Training and education.

4. You are caring for 5-month-old baby boy Armaan who is being treated for a respiratory syncytial virus infection and is receiving formula during his hospitalization. Armaan's family are practicing Muslims and maintain strict dietary practices by only consuming halal certified food (foods permissible according to Islamic law). You notice that the formula Armaan is receiving is not halal certified. You talk to the nutritionist and provider to get an order to substitute a halal certified formula. What is the most effective strategy for preventing a future error of this sort?
   a. Develop a flyer to educate other staff on your unit about recognizing and honoring patient's and family's cultural needs.
   b. Request nutrition services clearly label key attributes on formula such as halal-certified, kosher, vegan, etc.
   c. Work with someone to see if there is a way to trigger warnings to staff of religious and cultural counterindications for certain foods similar to how allergy alerts work.
   d. Complete the five rights of medication administration, i.e., right patient, right drug, right dose, right route, and right time.

5. You are working on a low acuity unit dedicated to providing palliative care. Your patient Mary is a 58-year-old woman receiving end of life comfort care after a 4-year battle with ovarian cancer. Mary is receiving intravenous morphine for pain control. The hospital has a policy that requires blood pressure, pulse, and respiratory documentation every 2 hr for patients receiving opioids. Your unit is one of the poorer performing units in meeting these documentation requirements. Worse than that, you feel bad every time you need to interrupt Mary and her family to take vital signs, especially since the blood pressure cuff seems to cause Mary extra discomfort. What should you do?
   a. Work with someone to evaluate possible changes to the existing policy to exclude palliative care patients from requiring frequent vital signs and update the documentation report parameters accordingly.
   b. Leave the blood pressure cuff continuously in place to minimize movement when you take Mary's blood pressure.
   c. Ask the provider if Mary can have an arterial line placed to automatically monitor blood pressure and pulse.
   d. Ask the provider to order no further vital signs for Mary.

6. You are working on a complex cardiac unit and have just returned from a 2-week vacation backpacking in the Alps. You noticed you don't seem to be getting as many alerts to your communication device about abnormal cardiac rhythms for your patients that you used to receive. You remember there was a recent update to the physiological monitoring equipment while you were gone. What should you do?

a. Don't worry about it. The change has been in place long enough that someone would have already noticed it and reported it if it was a problem.

b. Check if your colleagues have seen a similar decrease in the number of alerts coming to their communication devices.

c. Assume the updates to the system removed nuisance alarms that your unit council has been working to address as part of an alert fatigue improvement project.

d. Report your concerns to someone who can investigate the issue further.

7. Your manager shares a report with you that shows you are not documenting the patient's primary support contact, a key regulatory requirement. You are confused because you know you always document this information. Upon further review, you and your manager discover there are two different places for documenting the data in the EHR but only one data field is considered in the compliance report. What should you and your manager do? Check all that apply.

a. Document the primary support contact data in the EHR field that is used for the report; then you will be 100% compliant in your documentation and no further follow-up is needed.

b. Request that someone evaluate how staff are documenting the patient's primary support contact data on your unit and across the organization.

c. Request that the primary support contact field that is not used for the report be removed from the EHR.

d. Request both primary support contact data fields be added to the report parameters to satisfy the regulatory requirement.

8. Which of the following is a characteristic of an HRO?

a. Their technologies are risk prone and present a high potential for error.

b. They shift the focus from errors and outcomes to system design and the facilitation of good behavioral choices.

c. They use the five key elements of the Clinical Decision Support Rights.

d. They have clearly defined policies and procedures for ensuring confidentiality of patient data.

9. Which of the following introduces a risk to an organization for a cyberattack?

a. Alert fatigue.

b. Social media.

c. Phishing.

d. Data mining.

10. Which of the following is an example of simulation?

a. Evaluating two scanning technologies by using them throughout a shift.

b. Practicing sterile technique when inserting an IV into a colleague.

c. Showing a nursing assistant how to use a new glucometer.

d. Putting post-it notes on a board to outline a new process.

REVIEW QUESTION ANSWERS

1. Answer: C is correct.
   Rationale: The person is withholding their HIV status from the nurse, not their name, so the information is not anonymous. Because the person chose not to share the information, there is not an opportunity to keep the disclosure confidential. Similarly, there is no information to secure from accidental or intentional disclosure to unauthorized persons. The person has chosen to keep the information private.

2. Answer: D is correct.
   Rationale: As Ronald Reagan said after signing a treaty with Mikhail Gorbachev in 1987, "Trust but verify"—as in don't take the author at his word. Emailing the author for a list of references is not reliable for two reasons: (a) the author may be too busy doing research and other work that he won't get back to you in a timely manner, or at all, and (b) the author could fabricate a body of work. Asking your colleagues about the author is also not helpful unless your colleagues are especially interested in or experts themselves in ALS. On the other hand, a worldwide leading researcher should have a body of work and peer-reviewed publications easily searched on MEDLINE.

3. Answer: C is correct.
   Rationale: A great deal of informatics nursing work involves the EHR; however, the scope and breadth of NI goes beyond the EHR; nor is the nurse informaticist the only specialty focused on and expert in the EHR. Data coding and the use of abbreviations is not a primary focus of informatics nursing; and while nurse informaticists have unique knowledge and expertise to aid in training and education, it does not distinguish from other education experts. Nursing informatics is distinguished from other nursing specialties by its focus on content and representation of data and information.

4. Answer: C is correct.
   Rationale: Developing a flyer is a great educational resource for the unit where you work, but it is not the most effective in preventing this problem from happening in the future for your patient population or other patients that could be similarly impacted. Visual labeling of nutritional products may help in alerting staff to key information, but there is still opportunities for labeling errors and the actual labels risk becoming overlooked or ignored over time. Making sure you are giving the right patient, the right drug (tube feeding), in the right dose, via the right route, and at right time is never a bad idea but it is not as foolproof or as effective as working with someone to eliminate the possibility of even ordering the wrong tube feeding to begin with, which will ensure that you and no one else can make this error again.

5. Answer: A is correct.
   Rationale: Leaving the blood pressure cuff in place could result in skin breakdown and further discomfort. It also poses a ligature risk and could make repositioning challenging. Generally, advanced monitoring technologies, such as arterial lines, require the patient receive care in an ICU or other higher acuity location. Asking the provider to write an order for no vital signs could be contraindicated by hospital policy. Asking someone to evaluate possible policy changes within the parameters of existing regulatory requirements, then updating the EHR and reports accordingly is the best approach.

6. Answer: D is correct.
   Rationale: Always worry about it and celebrate your intuitive thinking! Trust your gut and check it out. Don't assume someone else has noticed a change or taken the time to question it. Asking your council members and colleagues if they've noticed any change, and if so, whether they confirmed it was due to the alert fatigue project and system changes is a good start, but never assume this is the reason for the change. Report your concerns and any feedback from your colleagues to someone who can investigate the change further with IS or a HTM expert to verify the monitors and alerts are working as intended.

7. Answer: B is correct.
   Rationale: Changing where you document this information does not correct the underlying issue. If you are confused about where to document primary support contact data, chances are other people are confused as well. Continuing to include both fields for data entry can result in reporting errors and confusion in future data analysis. Removing a data field without investigating who is using it for what purpose can also cause confusion and error. The best approach is to request that someone evaluate how staff are documenting the patient's primary support contact data on your unit and across the organization, then have them take steps to retire a data field if appropriate and develop a single shared data field that can be used in various parts of the records as needed.

8. Answer: A is correct.
   Rationale: Shifting the focus from errors and outcomes to system design and the facilitation of good behavioral choices is a characteristic of a just culture. Using the Clinical Decision Support Rights helps ensure clinically useful messages are presented to support clinician decision making. By law, every health care organization needs to have policies and procedures in place for ensuring confidentiality of patient data. HROs are characterized by having risk prone technologies that present a high potential for error.

9. Answer: C is correct.
   Rationale: Alert fatigue describes how health care clinicians become desensitized to safety alerts, and as a result ignore or fail to respond to their warnings. Data mining is a component of predictive analytics whereby data are analyzed to identify trends, patterns, or relationships among the data. Social media can pose a confidentiality breach but is not an example of a cyberattack. Phishing occurs when a malicious party sends a fake email with a link or attachment in order to trick the receiving user into giving the malicious party access to the organization's data. Fun fact: phishing can occur through attachments in social media.

10. Answer: B is correct.
    Rationale: Simulation is the imitation of a situation or a process. Evaluating scanning technology to determine which device might be better used in practice is part of device selection and not simulation in this case. Educating someone on how to use a piece of equipment is not simulation. Putting post-it notes on a board is an intellectual exercise, not the physical imitation of a situation or a process. Practicing sterile techniques when inserting an IV into a colleague is imitating what it would be like to insert an IV into a patient.

DISCUSSION POINTS

- During your last clinical experience, how did nursing informatics shape your day?

- How can you use technology to improve patient care?

- Reflecting on the case study with Wesley, did you realize how nursing informatics affects the delivery of care?

DISCUSSION OF OPENING SCENARIO

1. What is your role in using technology to care for patients?
   The nurse's first role in using technology to care for patients is to use the technology in a competent fashion. This means synthesizing and correctly applying the knowledge and technical skills required to use a technology to perform the intended task. This could be as simple as knowing how to turn on or change the battery of a device to the complex set-up and integration of a technology that interfaces with the EHR. It means adjusting the technology to meet the unique needs of the patient, as in adjusting physiological alarm parameters; and using the technology to know more about what the patient wants personally and needs medically, such as using a nurse call system or tablet for patient requests and not turning off pulse-ox alarms to allow patients to sleep more easily. It also means interacting with technology in a timely fashion, especially in the case of infusion pumps or documenting in the EHR.

   Informatics competencies needed by every nurse go beyond safely interacting with and managing the technologies at the elbow or bedside of the patient. Integral to the basic skills of interacting with technology is an attitude of openness to innovation and continual learning, as information systems and patient care technologies are constantly changing. In 2008, the American Association of Colleges of Nursing developed a publication entitled The Essentials of Baccalaureate Education for Professional Nursing Practice. Informatics competencies identified in this publication, many of which are still relevant, include:

   1. Demonstrate skills in using patient care technologies, information systems, and communication devices that support safe nursing practice.

   2. Use telecommunication technologies to assist in effective communication in a variety of healthcare settings.

   3. Apply safeguards and decision-making support tools embedded in patient care technologies and information systems to support a safe practice environment for both patients and health care workers.

4. Understand the use of **Computer Information Systems** CIS systems to document interventions related to achieving nurse sensitive outcomes.

   5. Use standardized terminology in a care environment that reflects nursing's unique contribution to patient outcomes.

   6. Evaluate data from all relevant sources, including technology, to inform the delivery of care.

   7. Recognize the role of information technology in improving patient care outcomes and creating a safe care environment.

   8. Uphold ethical standards related to data security, regulatory requirements, confidentiality, and clients' right to privacy.

   9. Apply patientcare technologies as appropriate to address the needs of a diverse patient population.

   10. Advocate for the use of new patient care technologies for safe, quality care.

   11. Recognize that redesign of workflow and care processes should precede implementation of care technology to facilitate nursing practice.

   12. Participate in evaluation of information systems in practice settings through policy and procedure development.

2. How can you be confident that the technologies you use are safe, efficient, and appropriate for your patient?

The nurse is the first and best line of defense to know if a technology is safe, efficient, and appropriate for a patient. If a technology is broken or does not appear to be working as intended, the nurse should follow organization processes to alert the appropriate support staff to evaluate the technology. This might be IS end-user support staff, HTM staff, NI, or others. If the technology does not enhance the care delivery process, nurses can work with NI and other technology experts to evaluate any unanticipated safety concerns or inefficiencies introduced by using the technology. In some cases, it could be that additional education or training is needed to ensure competency, or a workflow incorporating the technology needs to be reconsidered and tweaked. In other cases, the technology may not be suited to the task at hand as expected. Technology should enhance and support practice; it should not drive practice nor be used just for the sake of using technology. By leveraging the partnership with NI and other support staff, the nurse can be confident the technology is safe, efficient, and appropriate for patient care.

3. How can you be confident you are using technologies appropriately?

   You can be confident you are using technologies appropriately if you are able to synthesize and correctly apply the knowledge and technical skills required to use the technology to perform the intended task in a safe, efficient, and appropriate manner.

EXPLORING THE WEB

Check these sites for more informatics information (All sites accessed September 9, 2019): Agency for Healthcare Research and Quality: https://psmet.ahrq.gov

Alliance for Nursing informatics (ANI): www.allianceni.org

American Health Information Management Association (AHIMA): www.ahima.org

American Medical Informatics Association (AMIA): www.amia.org

American Nursing Informatics Association (ANIA): www.ania.org

Becker's Hospital Review: www.beckershospitalreview.com

Canadian Nursing Informatics Association (CNIA): cnia.ca

Clinical Decision Support Collaborative for Performance Improvement: https://sites.google.com/site/cdsforpiimperativespublic

Health Canada: www.canada.ca/en/health-canada.html

Healthcare Information and Management Systems Society (HIMSS): www.himss.org

Healthforce Center at UCSF: http://healthforce.ucsf.edu

Institute for Healthcare Improvement (IHI): www.ifi.org

International Medical Informatics Association (IMIA): www.imia.rog

Online Journal of Nursing Informatics (OJNI): www.ojni.org

INFORMATICS

• Search for the American Nurses Credentialing Center at www.nursingworld.org Click on Certification and choose another specialty in which a nurse can be certified, comparing it to the certification in informatics.

• How are they similar? How are they different?

LEAN BACK

• How has Weston's story enriched your understanding of informatics and the impact it has on nursing?

• How will this new understanding impact or change your care?

REFERENCES

Agency for Healthcare Research and Quality (AHRQ). (2019). *Digital healthcare research: clinical decision support clinical decision section 1: Introduction.* Retrieved from https://digital.ahrq.gov/ahrq-funded-projects/current-health-it-priorities/clinical-decision-support-cds/chapter-1-approaching-clinical-decision/section-1-introduction

Alpay, L. L., Overberg, R. I., & Zwetsloot-Schonk, B. (2007). Empowering citizens in assessing health related websites: A driving factor for healthcare governance. *International Journal of Healthcare Technology and Management, 8*(1–2), 141–160.

American Association of Colleges of Nursing. (2008). *The essentials of baccalaureate education for professional nursing practice* (pp. 18–19). Washington, DC: American Association of Colleges of Nursing. Retrieved from https://nursing.lsuhsc.edu/Docs/Quality/AACN%20Essentials%20of%20Baccalaureate%20Education%20for%20Professional%20Nsg%20Practice%20(2008).pdf

American Nurses Association (ANA). (2015). *Nursing informatics: Scope and standards of practice* (2nd ed.). Silver Spring, MD: American Nurses Association.

Ancker, J. S., Edwards, A., Nosal, S., Hauser, D., Mauer, E., & Kaushal, R. (2017). *Effects of workload, work complexity, and repeated alerts on alert fatigue in a clinical decision support system.* Retrieved from https://bmcmedinformdecismak.biomedcentral.com/articles/10.1186/s12911-017-0430-8.

Anderson, A., & Klemm, P. (2008). The Internet: Friend or foe when providing patient education? *Clinical Journal of Oncology Nursing, 12*(1), 55–63. doi:10.1188/08.CJON.55-63. Retrieved from https://search.proquest.com/openview/02e008cad4f17371ee58ae1b1a9dba5d/1/advanced

Andrews, M. (2016). *The rise of medical identify theft.* Consumer Reports. Retrieved from www.consumerreports.org/medical-identity-theft/medical-identity-theft

ASQ. (2020). *What is mistake proofing?* Retrieved from https://asq.org/quality-resources/mistake-proofing

Ball, M. J., Hannah, K. J., Newbold, S. K., & Douglass, J. V. (2000). *Nursing informatics: Where caring and technology meet* (3rd ed.). New York: Springer Verlag.

Barnard, A. G., Nash, R. E., & O'Brien, M. (2010). Information literacy: Developing lifelong skills through nursing education. *Journal of Nursing Education, 44*(11), 505–510.

Bender, J. L., Jimenez-Marroquin, M., & Jadad, A. R. (2011). Seeking support on Facebook: A content analysis of breast cancer groups. *Journal of Medical Internet Research, 13*(1), e16.

Berry, S. K. (2018). *A 'smart' toilet could stop us from flushing away our most valuable health information, argues this doctor.* CNBC. Retrieved from www.cnbc.com/2018/11/21/smart-toilets-would-be-a-huge-boon-to-public-health-commentary.html

Betts, H., & Wright, G. (2003). *Was florence nightingale the first nursing informatician?* International Congress in Nursing Informatics. Retrieved from www.researchgate.net/file.PostFileLoader.html?id=59ca5fc6eeae3922d8345715&assetKey=AS%3A542841950932992%40150643 5014110

Bishop, C. M. (2006). *Pattern recognition and machine learning.* New York: Springer. ISBN: 978-0-387-31073-2

Bol, N., Helberger, N., & Weert, J. C. M. (2018). Differences in mobile health app use: A source of new digital inequalities? *The Information Society, 34*(3), 183–193. doi:10.1080/01972243.2018.1438550

Brazelton, N. C., & Lyons, A. M. (2018). Downtime and disaster recovery for health information systems. In R. Nelson & N. Staggers (Eds.), *Health informatics: An interprofessional approach* (2nd ed., pp. 560). St. Louis, MO: Elsevier. ISBN: 978-0-323-40231-6

Brenner, P., Tanner, C. T., & Chesla, C. A. (2009). *Expertise in nursing practice: Caring, clinical judgment & ethics* (2nd ed.). New York: Springer Publishing Company, LLC.

Brinkman, W. P., Mast, C. V. D., Sandino, G., Gunawan, L. T., & Emmelkamp, P. M. G. (2010). The therapist user interface of a virtual reality exposure therapy system in the treatment of fear of flying. *Interacting with Computers, 22*(4), 299–310.

Carl, E., Stein, A. T., Levihn-Coon, A., Rogue, J. R., Rothbaum, B., Emmelkamp, P., Asmundson, G. J., Carlbring, P. & Powers, M. B. (2019). Virtual reality exposure therapy for anxiety and related disorders: A meta-analysis of randomized controlled trials. *Journal of Anxiety Disorders, 61,* 27–36. doi:10.1016/j.janxdis.2018.08.003

Carr, S. (2011). ECRI Institute announces its top 10 health technology hazards for 2012. *Patient Safety & Quality Healthcare.*

Carroll, L. (1865). *"Why it's simply impassible! . . .".* Retrieved from www.brainyquote.com/search_results?q="Why+it's+simply+impassible!+Alice:+Why,+don't+you+mean+impossible?+Door:+No,+I+

Chabeli, M. M. (2007). Facilitating critical thinking within the nursing process framework: A literature review. *Health SA Gesondheid, 12*(4), 69–89.

Chen, S. Y., Chang, H. C., & Pai, H. C. (2018). Caring behaviors directly and indirectly affect nursing students' critical thinking. *Scandinavian Journal of Caring Sciences, 32,* 197–203. doi:10.1111/scs.12447

CISCO. (2019a). *Cyber attack—what are common cyberthreats?* Retrieved from www.cisco.com/c/en/us/products/security/common-cyberattacks.html?dtid=osscdc000283.

CISCO. (2019b). *Cisco cybersecurity report series—download PDFs.* Retrieved from www.cisco.com/c/en/us/products/security/security-reports.html?CCID=cc000160&DTID=esootr000515&OID=ebksc018563#~new-report.

Coffey, P. S., Postal, S., Houston, S., & McKeeby, J. (2016). Lessons learned from an electronic health record downtime. *Perspectives in Health Information Management,* 1–7. Retrieved from www.delicious.com/gamesforhealth

Drees, J. (2014). *Moody's: Healthcare cyberattacks on the rise, small hospitals most vulnerable.* The interconnected nature of hospital operations and information technology presents a significant and growing cyberattack risk for hospitals, particularly smaller organizations that lack enough resources to absorb any financial impact, according to a September 12 Moody's Investors Service report. Retrieved from www.beckershospitalreview.com/cybersecurity/moody-s-healthcare-cyberattacks-on-the-rise-small-hospitals-most-vulnerable.html

Drees, J. (2019a). *61% of CIOs think employees leak data maliciously, survey finds.* More than half of company CIOs believe their employees have purposefully put their organizations' data at risk in the last year, according to an Egress software company survey. Retrieved from www.beckershospitalreview.com/cybersecurity/61-of-cios-think-employees-leak-data-maliciously-survey-finds.html

Drees, J. (2019b). *EHR snooping: Best efforts to bust, punish and prevent it.* Whether it's the result of sheer curiosity or motivated by an act of malice, EHR snooping is a serious employee offense that can occur at any hospital. Retrieved from www.beckershospitalreview.com/ehrs/ehr-snooping-best-efforts-to-bust-punish-and-prevent-it.html

Durham, C. F., & Alden, K. R. (2008). Enhancing patient safety in nursing education through patient simulation. In R. G. Hughes (Ed.), *Patient safety and quality: An evidence-based handbook for nurses* (pp. 1403). Rockville, MD: Agency for Healthcare Research and Quality (US).

Emergency Care Research Institute (ECRI). (2007). Top 10 health technology hazards: are you protecting your patients from these high-priority risks? *Health Devices, 36*(11), 345–351.

ECRI Institute. (2008). Top 10 health technology hazards. *Health Devices, 37*(11), 343–350.

ECRI Institute. (2009). Top 10 health technology hazards: high-priority risks and what to do about them. *Health Devices, 38*(11), 364–373.

ECRI Institute. (2012). *Top 10 health technology hazards for 2013*. Retrieved from www.ecri.org/Resources/Whitepapers_and_reports/2013_Health_Devices_Top_10_Hazards.pdf

ECRI Institute. (2013). *Top 10 health technology hazards for 2014*. Retrieved from www.ecri.org/Resources/Whitepapers_and_reports/2014_Top_10_Hazards_Executive_Brief.pdf

ECRI Institute. (2014). *Top 10 health technology hazards for 2015*. Retrieved from www.ecri.org/Resources/Whitepapers_and_reports/Top_Ten_Technology_Hazards_2015.pdf

ECRI Institute. (2015). *Executive brief: Top 10 health technology hazards for 2016*. Retrieved from www.ecri.org/Resources/Whitepapers_and_reports/Haz16.pdf

ECRI Institute. (2016). *Executive brief: Top 10 health technology hazards for 2017*. Retrieved from www.ecri.org/Resources/Whitepapers_and_reports/Haz17.pdf

ECRI Institute. (2017). *Executive brief: Top 10 health technology hazards for 2018*. Retrieved from www.ecri.org/Resources/Whitepapers_and_reports/Haz_18.pdf

ECRI Institute. (2018). Retrieved from www.ecri.org/Resources/Whitepapers_and_reports/Haz_19.pdf

ECRI Institute. (2019). *Special report: Top 10 health technology hazards for 2020*. Retrieved from assets.ecri.org/PDF/White-Papers-and-Reports/ECRI-Top-10-Technology-Hazards-2020.pdf?utm_campaign=2020%20Top%2010%20Tech%20Hazards&utm_source=hs_automation&utm_medium=email&utm_content=77690309&_hsenc=p2ANqtz-8L1g2Up4t-56sgY3uKYGMcgL8yJspKx1gH72tEY-9__34FMUjxPevDU56bw0h_el-dP4FtwEk6uQIS4Wu37TEK0BfJYag&_hsmi=77690309

Eysenbach, G. (2001). What is e-health? *Journal of Medical Internet Research, 3*(2), e20. doi:10.2196/jmir.3.2.e20

Fodor, L. A., Cotet, C. D., Cuijpers, P., Szamoskozi, S., David, D., & Cristea, I. A. (2018). The effectiveness of virtual reality based interventions for symptoms of anxiety and depression: A meta-analysis. *Scientific Reports, 8*, 1–13. Retrieved from www.nature.com/articles/s41598-018-28113-6

Fox, S. (January 2014). The social life of health information. *Pew Research Center*. Retrieved from www.pewresearch.org/fact-tank/2014/01/15/the-social-life-of-health-information/

Gallis, R., & Zwetsloot, G. I. J. M. (2014). High reliability organizations. *NARCIS*. Retrieved from www.narcis.nl/publication/RecordID/oai:tudelft.nl:uuid%3Abeebe965-3ab9-4c3f-9577-77aba6a99805

Garrity, M. (2019). *10 largest data breaches in 2019*. Since the start of the year, nearly 33 million people have been affected by data breaches across the country as of August 5, according to HHS data and cited by Gov Info Security. Retrieved from www.beckershospitalreview.com/cybersecurity/10-largest-data-breaches-in-2019.html?oly_enc_id=2782C1212156H0G.

Goossen, W. T. F. (1996). Nursing information management and processing: A framework and definition for systems analysis, design and evaluation. *International Journal of Bio-Medical Computing, 40*(3), 187–195. doi:10.1016/0020-7101(95)01144-7

Graves, J. R., & Corcoran, S. (1989). The study of nursing informatics. *Image: The Journal of Nursing Scholarship, 21*(4), 227–231. doi:10.1111/j.1547-5069.1989.tb00148.x

Grout, J. R. (2006). Mistake proofing: Changing designs to reduce error. *Quality & Safety in Health Care, 15*(Suppl I), i44–i49. doi:10.1136/qshc.2005.016030

Hanna-Attisha, M. (2018). *What the eyes don't see: A story of crisis, resistance, and hope in an American city*. New York: Random House Large Print.

Hebda, T. L., Czar, P., & Mascara, C. M. (2008). *Handbook of informatics for nurses and healthcare professionals* (4th ed.). Upper Saddle River, NJ: Prentice Hall.

Henneman, E. A., Cunningham, H., Roche, J. P., & Curnin, M. E. (2007). Human patient simulation: Teaching students to provide safe care. *Nurse Educator, 32*(5), 212–217. 210.1097/1001.NNE.0000289379.0000283512.fc

HHS Office of the Secretary, Office for Civil Rights (OCR). (2013). *Minimum necessary requirement*. Retrieved from www.hhs.gov/hipaa/for-professionals/privacy/guidance/minimum-necessary-requirement/index.html.

HIMSS. (2019). *Is the digital health bubble bursting?* Retrieved from www.himss.org/news/digital-health-bubble-bursting-health-20-weighs-in.

HITECH Act Summary. (2018). Retrieved from www.hipaasurvivalguide.com/hitech-act-summary.php

Hood, C. M., Gennuso, K. P., Swain, G. R., & Catlin, B. B. (2016). County health rankings: Relationships between determinant factors and health outcomes. *American Journal of Preventive Medicine, 50*(2), 129–135. doi:10.1016/j.amepre.2015.08.024

Iakovleva, T., Oftedal, E. M., & Bessant, J. (2019). Responsible innovation in digital health. In T. Iakovleva, E. M. Oftedal, & J. Bessant (Eds.), *Responsible innovation in digital health: Empowering the patient* (pp. 259). Northampton, MA: Edward Elgar Publishing, Inc. doi:10.4337/9781788975063

Iyengar, A., Kundu, A., & Pallis, G. (2018). Healthcare informatics and privacy. *IEEE Internet Computing, 22*(2), 29–31. Retrieved from https://ieeexplore.ieee.org/abstract/document/8345561

Jacques, S., & Williams, E. (2016). Retrieved from https://psnet.ahrq.gov/perspective/reducing-safety-hazards-monitor-alert-and-alarm-fatigue?q=/perspective/reducing-safety-hazards-monitor-alert-and-alarm-fatigue

Jones, J., & Nicoll, L. H. (2011). Nursing and health care informatics. In P. V. Kelly (Ed.), *Nursing leadership and management* (3rd ed.). Clifton Park, NY: Delmar, Cengage Learning.

Joint Commission Standards. (2018). Retrieved from, www.jointcommission.org/facts_about_joint_commission_accreditation_standards/

Kaelber, D. C., Jha, A. K., Johnston, D., Middleton, B., & Bates, D. W. (2008). A research agenda for personal health records (PHRs). *Journal of the American Medical Informatics Association, 15*(6), 729–736. doi:10.1197/jamia.M2547

Kendall, D. B. (2009). Protecting patient privacy through health record trusts. *Health Affairs, 28*(2). doi:10.1377/HLTHAFF.28.2.444

Kilmon, C., Brown, L., Ghosh, S., & Mikitiuk, A. (2010). Immersive virtual reality simulations in nursing education. *Nursing Education Perspectives, 31*(5), 314–317.

Kohn, L. T., Corrigan, J. M., & Donaldson, M. S.. (Eds.). (2000). *To err is human: Building a safer health system*. Washington, DC: National

Academies Press (US). Institute of Medicine (US) Committee on Quality of Health Care in America. doi:10.17226/9728

Koti, M. S., & Alamma, B. H. (2018). Predictive analytics techniques using big data for healthcare databases. In S. Satapathy, V. Bhateja, & S. Das (Eds.), *Smart intelligent computing and applications* (pp. 689).

Levine, C. (2006). HIPAA and talking with family caregivers. *American Journal of Nursing, 106*(8), 51–53.

Liquid State. (2019). *The rise of mHealth apps: A market snapshot.* Retrieved from https://liquid-state.com/mhealth-apps-market-snapshot/

Magrabi, F., Westbrook, J. I., & Coiera, E. W. (2007). What factors are associated with the integration of evidence retrieval technology into routine general practice settings? *International Journal of Medical Informatics, 76*(10), 701–709.

Marx, D. (2019). Patient safety and the just culture. *Obstetrics and Gynecology Clinics of North America, 46*(2), 239–245. doi:10.1016/j.ogc.2019.01.003

McDowell, D. E., & Ma, X. (2007). Computer literacy in baccalaureate nursing students during the last 8 years. *Computers, Informatics, Nursing: CIN, 25*(1), 30–36.

McFarland, D. M., & Doucette, J. N. (2018). Impact of high-reliability education on adverse event reporting by registered nurses. *Journal of Nursing Care Quality, 33*(3), 285–290. doi:10.1097/NCQ.0000000000000291

McGinley, P., & Stockhoff, B. A. (2009). *Tests of change: simulated design of experiments in healthcare delivery.* Retrieved from www.psqh.com/analysis/tests-of-change/

Nagle, L. M., Sermeus, W., & Junger, A. (2017). Evolving role of the nursing informatics specialist. In J. Murphy, W. Goossen, & P. Eeberen (Eds.), Proceedings of the Nursing Informatics Post Conference 2016*Forecasting informatics competencies for nurses in the future of connected health* (pp. 212). Amsterdam, Netherlands: IOS Press. doi:10.3233/978-1-61499-738-2-212

Nelson, G. (2019). Bias in artificial intelligence. *North Carolina Medical Journal, 80*(4), 220–222. doi:10.18043/ncm.80.4.220. Retrieved from www.ncmedicaljournal.com/content/80/4/220.short

Newman, D. (2019). *Alert fatigue.* Retrieved from https://healthcareitskills.com/alert-fatigue/

Nunes, F. L. S. (2008). *The virtual reality challenges in the health care area: A panoramic view.* Paper presented at the Proceedings of the 2008 ACM symposium on Applied computing. SAC '08.

Nyce, C. (2007). *Predictive modeling white paper.* Retrieved from www.the-digital-insurer.com/wp-content/uploads/2013/12/78-Predictive-Modeling-White-Paper.pdf

Pretz, J. E., & Folse, V. N. (2011). Nursing experience and preference for intuition in decision making. *Journal of Clinical Nursing, 20*(19–20), 2878–2889. doi:10.1111/j.1365-2702.2011.03705.x

Prinz, L., Cramer, M., & Englund, A. (2008). Telehealth: A policy analysis for quality, impact on patient outcomes, and political feasibility. *Nursing Outlook, 56*(4), 152–158. doi:10.1016/j.outlook.2008.02.005

Rankin, R. (2011). Unpublished quote. [Interview by R. Rankin].

Root-Bernstein, R., & Root-Bernstein, M. (2003). Intuitive tools for innovative thinking. In L. Shavinina (Ed.), *The international handbook on innovation* (pp. 1171). Oxford, UK: Elsevier Science Ltd.

Ross, J. (2015). Alarm fatigue: Are you tuning out? *Journal of PeriAnesthesia Nursing, 30*(4), 351–353. doi:10.1016/j.jopan.2015.05.007

Schmidt, B. (2010). ECRI Institute Releases Top 10 Health Technology Hazards for 2011. *Patient Safety & Quality Healthcare.* Retrieved from www.psqh.com/news/ecri-institute-releases-top-10-health-technology-hazards-for-2011/

Short, K., & Chung, Y. (2016). Solving alarm fatigue with smartphone technology. *Nursing Critical Care, 13,* 43–47. doi:10.1097/01.CCN.0000532370.33226.77

Skiba, D. J. (2017). Nursing informatics education: From automation to connected care. In J. Murphey, W. Goossen, & P. Weber (Eds.), *Forecasting informatics competencies for nurses in the future of connected health.* Proceeding of the nursing informatics post conference 2016 (pp. 255). Amsterdam, Netherlands: IOS Press BV. doi:10.3233/978-1-61499-738-2-9

Skiba, D. J. (2017). *Nursing informatics education: from automation to connected care.* Retrieved from www.researchgate.net/publication/325950378_Nursing_Informatics_Education_From_Automation_to_Connected_Care

Staggers, N. (2002). The evolution of definitions for nursing informatics: A critical analysis and revised definition. *Journal of the American Medical Informatics Association, 9*(3), 255–261. doi:10.1197/jamia.m0946

Uitti, J. (2019). *Doctors and nurses team up to launch the association for healthcare social media.* Retrieved from https://nurse.org/articles/association-for-healthcare-social-media-guidelines/

Wang, H. (2014). *Virtual health care will revolutionize the industry, if we let it.* Forbes. Retrieved from www.forbes.com/sites/ciocentral/2014/04/03/virtual-health-care-visits-will-revolutionize-the-industry-if-we-let-it/

Yu, K. H., & Kohane, I. S. (2018). Framing the challenges of artificial intelligence in medicine. *BMJ Quality & Safety, 28*(3), 238–241. doi:10.1136/bmjqs-2018-008551. Retrieved from https://qualitysafety.bmj.com/content/qhc/28/3/238.full.pdf

Zabel, L. (2016). *10 common HIPAA violations and preventative measures to keep your practice in compliance.* Retrieved from www.beckershospitalreview.com/healthcare-information-technology/10-common-hipaa-violations-and-preventative-measures-to-keep-your-practice-in-compliance.html

Zwetsloot, G. I. J. M., Aaltonen, M., Wybo, J. L., Saari, J., Kines, P., & Op De Beeck, R. (2013). The case for research into the zero accident vision. *Safety Science, 58,* 41–48.

SUGGESTED READING

Amith, M., Manion, F., Liang, C., Harris, M., Wang, D., et al. (2019). Architecture and usability of OntoKeeper, an ontology evaluation tool. *BMC Medical Informatics and Decision Making, 19*(Suppl 4), 152. doi:10.1186/s12911-019-0859-z

Ammenwerth, E., Hoerbst, A., Lannig, S., Mueller, G., Siebert, U., & Schnell-Inderst, P. (2019). Effects of adult patient portals on patient empowerment and health-related outcomes: A systematic review. *Studies in Health Technology and Informatics, 264,* 1106–1110. doi:10.3233/SHTI190397

Arcia, A., Suero-Tejeda, N., & Bakken, S. (2019). Development of pictograms for an interactive web application to help Hispanic caregivers learn about the functional stages of dementia. *Studies in Health Technology and Informatics, 264,* 1116–1120. doi:10.3233/SHTI190399

Bakken, S., Arcia, A., Koleck, T., Merrill, J. A., & Hickey, K. T. (2019). Informatics and data science for the precision in symptom self-management center. *Studies in Health Technology and Informatics, 264,* 1827–1828. doi:10.3233/SHTI190668

Beleigoli, A. M., Maeder, A., Button, D., Lange, B., & Tiemann, J. (2019). The care informatics and technologies project—enhancing capability, motivation and opportunities in digital health among health professionals and students. *Studies in Health Technology and Informatics, 266*, 25–29. doi:10.3233/SHTI190768

Borycki, E. M., & Kushniruk, A. W. (2019). Educational electronic health records at the University of Victoria: Challenges, recommendations and lessons learned. *Studies in Health Technology and Informatics, 265*, 74–79. doi:10.3233/SHTI190141

Chang, X., Lober, W. B., Evans, H. L., Wang, Z., Qian, X., & Huang, S. (2019). Artificial intelligence methods for surgical site infection: Impacts on detection, monitoring, and decision making. *Surgical Infections*. doi:10.1089/sur.2019.150

Chung, I. Y., Jung, M., Lee, S. B., Lee, J. W., Park, Y. R., et al. (2019). An assessment of physical activity data collected via a smartphone app and a smart band in breast cancer survivors: Observational study. *Journal of Medical Internet Research, 21*(9), 13463. doi:10.2196/13463

Downey, C., Ng, S., Jayne, D., & Wong, D. (2019). Reliability of a wearable wireless patch for continuous remote monitoring of vital signs in patients recovering from major surgery: A clinical validation study from the TRaCINg trial. *BMJ Open, 9*(8), e031150. doi:10.1136/bmjopen-2019-031150

Giannini, H. M., Ginestra, J. C., Chivers, C., Draugelis, M., Hanish, A., et al. (2019). A machine learning algorithm to predict severe sepsis and septic shock: Development, implementation, and impact on clinical practice. *Critical Care Medicine*. doi:10.1097/CCM.0000000000003891

Gordon, J. S., McNew, R. E., Weiner, E. E., & Trangenstein, P. (2019). Using contemporary e-learning tools to teach staff how to use new online documentation systems. *Studies in Health Technology and Informatics, 264*, 1672–1673. doi:10.3233/SHTI190590

Hubner, U., Thye, J., Shaw, T., Elias, B., Egbert, N., et al. (2019). Towards the TIGER international framework for recommendations of core competencies in health informatics 2.0: Extending the scope and the roles. *Studies in Health Technology and Informatics, 264*, 1218–1222. doi:10.3233/SHTI190420

Jaen, S. H., Batalla, M. F., Aguna, A. G., Duque, A. C., Garcia, J. M. S., et al. (2019). Technology in the determination of people health level: Design of a computational tool. *Studies in Health Technology and Informatics, 264*, 1478–1479. doi:10.3233/SHTI190493

Jahne-Raden, N., Gutschleg, H., Wolf, M. C., Kulau, U., & Wolf, K.-H. (2019). Wireless sensor network for fall prevention on geriatric wards: A report. *Studies in Health Technology and Informatics, 264*, 620–624. doi:10.3233/SHTI190297

Jefferson, U. T., Zachary, I., & Majee, W. (2019). Employing a user-centered design to engage mothers in the development of a mHealth breastfeeding application. *Computers, Informatics, Nursing: CIN*. doi:10.1097/CIN.0000000000000549

Jenkins, M. L., & Davis, A. (2019). Transforming nursing documentation. *Studies in Health Technology and Informatics, 264*, 625–628. doi:10.3233/SHTI190298

Kim, J., Kim, H., Bell, E., Bath, T., Paul, P., et al. (2019). Patient perspectives about decisions to share medical data and biospecimens for research. *JAMA Network Open, 2*(8), e199550. doi:10.1001/jamanetworkopen.2019.9550

Liang, C., Miao, Q., Kang, H., Vogelsmeier, A., Hilmas, T., et al. (2019). Leveraging patient safety research: Efforts made fifteen years since to err is human. *Studies in Health Technology and Informatics, 264*, 983–987. doi:10.3233/SHTI190371

Liu, Y., Chen, J., Lamb, K. V., Wu, P., Chang, P., et al. (2019). Smartphone-based self-empowerment app on secondary prevention of patients with cardiovascular disease. *Studies in Health Technology and Informatics, 264*, 1712–1713. doi:10.3233/SHTI190610

Lo, Y., Lynch, S. F., Urbanowicz, R. J., Olson, R. S., Ritter, A. Z., et al. (2019). Using machine learning on home health care assessments to predict fall risk. *Studies in Health Technology and Informatics, 264*, 684–688. doi:10.3233/SHTI190310

Lober, W. B., & Evans, H. L. (2019). Patient-generated health data in surgical site infection: changing clinical workflow and care delivery. *Surgical Infections*. doi:10.1089/sur.2019.195

Luo, S. (2019). Special focus issue on nursing informatics: Challenges of utilizing electronic health records. *International Journal of Nursing Sciences, 6*(1), 125. doi:10.1016/j.ijnss.2018.11.001

Magdalinou, A., Mantas, J., Sendelj, R., Ognjanovic, I., Knaup, P., et al. (2019). A framework for enhancing and updating study programs in public health and medical informatics fields in Montenegro. *Studies in Health Technology and Informatics, 264*, 1964–1965. doi:10.3233/SHTI190736

Mansoori, M. H., Benjamin, K., Ngwakongnwi, E., & Al Abdulla, S. (2019). Nurses' perceptions of the clinical information system in primary healthcare centres in Qatar: A cross-sectional survey. *BMJ Health & Care Informatics, 26*(1). doi:10.1136/bmjhci-2019-100030

Martin, C., & Janeway, L. (2019). The intersection of mobile health and nursing knowledge: Big data science. *Computers, Informatics, Nursing: CIN, 37*(8), 394–395. doi:10.1097/CIN.0000000000000571

McCall, T., Schwartz, T., & Khairat, S. (2019). Acceptability of telemedicine to help African American women manage anxiety and depression. *Studies in Health Technology and Informatics, 264*, 699–703. doi:10.3233/SHTI190313

McNew, R., Weiner, E., & Gordon, J. (2019). Designing new buildings to accommodate current technologies. *Studies in Health Technology and Informatics, 264*, 1283–1287. doi:10.3233/SHTI190433

Meher, S. K., Gupta, S., Sharma, S., Ibrahim, M., & Ajmera, K. (2019). Nursing informatics as a specialization in India: Present and future. *Studies in Health Technology and Informatics, 264*, 1955–1956. doi:10.3233/SHTI190731

Nantschev, R., Hackl, W. O., & Ammenwerth, E. (2019). Developing a model for using clinical routine data to analyze nursing sensitive patient outcome indicators. *Studies in Health Technology and Informatics, 264*, 1863–1864. doi:10.3233/SHTI190686

Nelson, R., & Staggers, N. (2014). *Health Informatics - E-Book: an Interprofessional Approach*.

Schaller, M., Hackl, W. O., Ianosi, B., & Ammenwerth, E. (2019). Towards a systematic construction of a minimum data set for delirium to support secondary use of clinical routine data. *Studies in Health Technology and Informatics, 264*, 1026–1030. doi:10.3233/SHTI190380

Schnall, R., Liu, J., Mohr, D. C., Bakken, S., Hirshfield, S., et al. (2019). Multimodal methodology for adapting digital health tools to new populations: Adaptation of the video information provider (VIP) for persons living with HIV with HIV-associated non-AIDS (HANA) conditions. *Studies in Health Technology and Informatics, 264*, 1347–1351. doi:10.3233/SHTI190446

Schweitzer, M., Huber, L., Gorfer, T., & Hoerbst, A. (2019). Real-time & autonomous data transmission for vital-sign telemonitoring: requirements & conceptualization. *Studies in Health Technology and Informatics, 267*, 28–36. doi:10.3233/SHTI190801

Senathirajah, Y., Borycki, E. M., Kushniruk, A., Cato, K., & Wang, J. (2019). Use of eye-tracking in studies of EHR usability—The current state: A scoping review. *Studies in Health Technology and Informatics, 264*, 1976–1977. doi:10.3233/SHTI190742

Sockolow, P. S., Bass, E. J., Yang, Y., Le, N. B., Potashnik, S., & Bowles, K. H. (2019). Availability and quality of information used by nurses while admitting patients to a rural home health care agency. *Studies in Health Technology and Informatics, 264*, 798–802. doi:10.3233/SHTI190333

Sockolow, P. S., Le, N. B., Yang, Y., Potashnik, S., Bass, E. J., & Bowles, K. H. (2019). Incongruence of patient problem information across three phases of home care admission: There's a problem with the problem list. *Studies in Health Technology and Informatics, 264*, 803–807. doi:10.3233/SHTI190334

Soni, H., Grando, A., Aliste, M. P., Murcko, A., & Todd, M. (2019). Perceptions and preferences about granular data sharing and privacy of behavioral health patients. *Studies in Health Technology and Informatics, 264*, 1361–1365. doi:10.3233/SHTI190449

Stonbraker, S., Halpern, M., Bakken, S., & Schnall, R. (2019). Developing infographics to facilitate HIV-related patient-provider communication in a limited-resource setting. *Applied Clinical Informatics, 10*(4), 597–609. doi:10.1055/s-0039-1694001

Syed-Abdul, S., Malwade, S., Nursetyo, A. A., Sood, M., Bhatia, M., et al. (2019). Virtual reality among the elderly: A usefulness and acceptance study from Taiwan. *BMC Geriatrics, 19*(1), 223. doi:10.1186/s12877-019-1218-8

Tiase, V. L., Sward, K. A., & Cummins, M. R. (2019). Navigating the search for patient generated health data. *Studies in Health Technology and Informatics, 264*, 1992. doi:10.3233/SHTI190750

Veinot, T. C., Ancker, J. S., & Bakken, S. (2019). Health informatics and health equity: Improving our reach and impact. *Journal of the American Medical Informatics Association: JAMIA, 26*(8–9), 689–695. doi:10.1093/jamia/ocz132

Weiner, E., Gordon, J., Rudy, S., & McNew, R. (2019). Expanding virtual reality to teach ultrasound skills to nurse practitioner students. *Studies in Health Technology and Informatics, 264*, 893–897. doi:10.3233/SHTI190352

Weiner, E., McNew, R., Gordon, J., Trangenstein, P., & Wood, K. (2019). Twenty plus years of distance learning: Lessons learned. *Studies in Health Technology and Informatics, 264*, 1807–1808. doi:10.3233/SHTI190658

Xiao, Q., Wang, J., Wang, Y., & Wu, Y. (2019). Data mining in nursing: A bibliometric analysis (1990-2017). *Studies in Health Technology and Informatics, 264*, 1616–1617. doi:10.3233/SHTI190562

Xing, Z., Yu, F., Qanir, Y. A. M., Guan, T., Walker, J., & Song, L. (2019). Intelligent conversational agents in patient self-management: A systematic survey using multi data sources. *Studies in Health Technology and Informatics, 264*, 1813–1814. doi:10.3233/SHTI190661

Zaidi, H., Bader-El-Den, M., & McNicholas, J. (2019). Using the National Early Warning Score (NEWS/NEWS 2) in different intensive care units (ICUs) to predict the discharge location of patients. *BMC Public Health, 19*(1), 1231. doi:10.1186/s12889-019-7541-3

Zangerle, C. (2019). Risk, resilience, and creating balance: An interview with Gail Latimer. *The Journal of Nursing Administration, 49*(7–8), 345–346. doi:10.1097/NNA.0000000000000763

Interprofessional Teamwork and Collaboration

16

Dianne Hoekstra and Janet Chaney
College of Nursing, Purdue University Northwest, Hammond, IN, USA

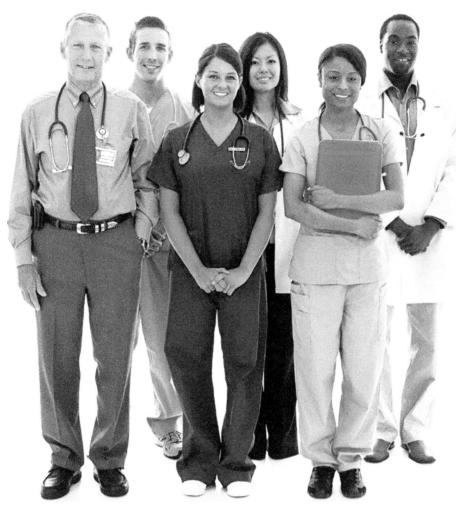

Interprofessional team.
Source: Sean Locke/Alamy Stock

Coming together is a beginning. Keeping together is progress. Working together is success.

Source: Henry Ford. (1863–1947)

OBJECTIVES

Upon completion of this chapter, the reader should be able to:

1. Define team, interprofessional teamwork, and collaboration.

2. Stages of team process.

Kelly Vana's Nursing Leadership and Management, Fourth Edition. Edited by Patricia Kelly Vana and Janice Tazbir
© 2021 John Wiley & Sons Ltd. Published 2021 by John Wiley & Sons Ltd.
Companion Website: www.wiley.com/go/kelly-Nursing-Leadership

3. Identify advantages and disadvantages of teamwork.

4. Description of formal and informal teams.

5. Review key concepts of creating an effective team.

6. Focus on the elements of the communication process within a team.

7. Describe organizational communication and communication skills in the workplace.

8. Identify barriers to communication and strategies to overcome them.

9. Define conflict, the sources and types of conflict.

10. Explain the steps in the conflict management process within a team.

OPENING SCENARIO

You are a nurse with six months of experience working on a hospital inpatient oncology unit. Your nurse manager has observed your skill and compassion for terminally ill patients and your warm interaction and interpersonal relationship with the other staff on the unit. Complimenting you on your skills and professional work ethic, the nurse manager has asked if you would be interested in joining an Interprofessional Cancer Support Committee to help address pain management and other issues to improve

patient care. If you accept this responsibility, this will be your first committee membership.

1. *Would you be ready at this point to accept the responsibility?*

2. *How would you prepare yourself for this unfamiliar role?*

3. *What qualities or skills do you need to possess to become a productive member of the team?*

In today's health care environment, great demands are placed on each health care professional to optimize patient care outcomes by providing the best quality of care efficiently, safely, and cost-effectively. Teamwork, with effective communication and collaboration, is needed to accomplish this monumental task. In the interest of creating a safe patient care environment, health care professionals recognize that each discipline cannot work alone. Collaboration among health care professionals with varying specialties is a complex process. It requires careful planning, time, and effort to achieve the common goal of positive patient care outcomes.

This chapter focuses on collaboration and effective team building within and between professions. The process of team development and the stages are considered. The advantages and disadvantages of teamwork are shared. The chapter also dissects components of a successful team, including workplace communication skills and conflict management. Tools for improving communication, strategies for teams, and tools to enhance performance and patient safety are introduced via the TeamSTEPPS® model. As the leader and manager of assigned patients, the nurse is not only responsible for managing patient care but functioning as a member of a health care team and collaborating for high quality patient care.

Team, Collaboration, and Interprofessional Teamwork

According to the Agency for Healthcare Research and Quality (AHRQ, 2013), the definition of **team** in health care is two or more people who interact dynamically, interdependently, and adaptively toward a common and valued goal, have specific roles or functions, and have a time-limited membership. That common and valued goal is the best possible outcome for the patient.

Collaborate has been described as the ability to co-labor (AACN, 2017). In nursing, the definition of **collaboration** is a process of sharing involving both professionals within nursing (intra-professional) and other members of the health care team (**interprofessional**). Together the health care team members collaborate and work together to solve patient care or system problems by respectfully sharing knowledge and resources. An example of this is interprofessional team members coordinate care to create seamless transitions for patients and families when discharged home from a hospital setting. While each discipline has its own focus, the scope of health care mandates that health professionals work collaboratively with other related disciplines. Collaboration stems

Critical Thinking 16.1

Teamwork on a patient care unit—day shift routine:

Throughout the day shift, nursing and the interdisciplinary team communicate and work together to deliver quality patient care.

0700   Charge nurse reviews patient care assignments with all nurses and unit staff; goals and priorities are set.

0705   Day shift RN takes hand-off patient shift report from night shift RN.

0725   RN gives report to the UAP and discusses plan of care for their shared patients. Results reviewed of previous diagnostic testing. Night shift and Day shift RN complete bedside rounds, involving the patient in plan of care.

0730   Day shift RN completes Patient assessment with vital sign assessment, IV assessment, etc.

0730   Breakfast served by the UAP.

0745   UAP begins morning care and hygiene.

0800   Medications given, practitioners make rounds, patient sent for diagnostic tests, documentation completed, hourly regular patient rounds.

0830   RN calls physician or HCP regarding critical lab results and/or changes in assessment findings.

1000   RN discusses plan of care with Charge nurse and Case Manager. Needs for home recuperation discussed with Social Worker. Progress discussed with Physical Therapist and Occupational Therapist.

1130   Vital sign assessment. RN discusses patient care needs and staffing for following shift.

1200   Lunch served by UAP

1300   Medications given by RN.

1400   Intake and output reports completed with assistance of UAP; documentation completed.

1500   Hand-off patient shift report from day shift to evening shift.

How does teamwork get patient care completed?

Does patient care on your clinical unit follow a time sequence similar to the routine above?

---

from an understanding and appreciation of the roles and contributions that each discipline brings to the care delivery experience.

Most health care professionals today were educated in isolation with only those from their own profession. Few were trained to work as part of interprofessional teams. During patient care, however, health care professionals must interact with providers from other professions to share information, execute quality and safety checks and help patients understand and comply with treatment plans. Interdisciplinary health-care teams can help each of the disciplines better understand and relate to other team members to enhance quality care (Brunt, 2015). "Working as a member of an interprofessional team is like learning a dance in which you learn not to step on each other's toes, but rather demonstrate fluid movements." (Witt Sherman et al., 2017, p. 229).

Before health care team members are able to collaborate there must be a willingness to participate in the team, good communication skills, a common vocabulary, strong interpersonal skills, opportunity to meet and collaborate, understanding of one's own roles as well as each other's roles, and finally a willingness to accept the final decisions of the group (Emich, 2018). The ability to resolve conflict is also key to successful collaboration in healthcare (Darlow et al., 2015).

Consider, for example, the case of a 67-year-old female patient just diagnosed with terminal cancer. All health care providers are concerned about this major life changing event

and the impact for the patient and her family. Yet each of the health care providers have differing roles and goals. The physician also has a plan for her oncological care, including surgery during this admission followed by chemotherapy and radiation after discharge. Her bedside nurses want to control her pain, prevent complications and injury, provide emotional support to the patient and her family, and ensure a safe transition back to her home. The physical therapists are focused on resuming independent mobility with tolerable pain levels. The occupational therapists are assessing and intervening to maintain independence in activities of daily living like eating and dressing. The social worker is identifying needs for home care after discharge. Length of stay is a concern for the case managers. The registered dietitian has suggestions for dietary modifications to meet the patient's caloric and protein needs. As active members of the health care team, the patient and her family will seek guidance and participate with the interdisciplinary group of professionals who are providing care. All of these varying professionals need to share information, agree upon the priorities of care, develop a plan with input from all team members, and monitor and evaluate the execution of that plan. At the heart of the team is the patient and their needs and desires.

Stages of a Team Process

Teams do not evolve by happenstance, nor is the path to effective teamwork easy. Developing an effective team requires

Case Study 16.1   Improving Patient Satisfaction

You are a nurse in a busy 42-bed telemetry unit. Both the staff nurses and unlicensed assistive personnel (**UAP**) work 12-hour shifts. Change of shift hand-off report occurs at 0700 and 1900 daily. During the staff meeting, the nurse manager charges everyone to think of ways to improve patient satisfaction. You note that patients are dissatisfied during the change of shift hand-off report times when the unit hallways become crowded and noisy. Most nurses and UAP are not available to answer call lights and attend to patient needs during this time.

What are some suggestions you can make to improve patient care during the change of shift hand-off report?

If you are asked to lead a team to problem-solve and identify solutions to these issues, what qualities do you possess that will be essential in this team leadership role?

What roles should some of the team members hold?

What qualities would you look for in selecting your team members?

How can you use the five stages of team development in Table 16.1—forming, storming, norming, performing, and adjourning—to develop your team?

Table 16.1   Tuckman and Jensen's Stages of Team Process

Stages	Description
Forming	*Relationship development:* Team orientation, identification of role expectations, beginning team interactions, explorations, and boundary setting occurs. Purpose is identified. Members of the team will ask, "What can I contribute?"
Storming	*Interpersonal interaction and reaction:* Dealing with tension, conflict, and confrontation occurs. Differences need to be openly confronted and addressed.
Norming	*Effective cooperation and collaboration:* Personal opinions are expressed and resolution of conflict with formation of solidified goals and increased group cohesiveness occurs. Learn to respect differences of opinion.
Performing	*Group maturity and stable relationships:* Team roles become more functional and flexible and structural issues are resolved, leading to supportive task performance through group-directed collaboration and resource sharing.
Adjourning	*Termination and consolidation:* Team goals and activities are met, leading to closure, evaluation, and outcomes review. This may also lead to reforming when the need for improvement or further goal development is identified. A sense of accomplishment.

Source: Adapted from Polifko-Harris and Anunciado (2012).

ample planning, with conscious and deliberate intentions focused on building its foundation through an organized system. Teams will develop at various paces, depending on the team's composition, experiences, relationships, and type of tasks, yet the development process for teams is predictable. A widely used theory of the team development was introduced by Tuckman (1965) and then modified by Tuckman and Jensen (1977). They identified five stages of team development: forming, storming, norming, performing, and adjourning. Understanding the phases of the team development process may help improve team development and participation.

Forming Stage

The first phase of the team process is the forming stage. This stage occurs when the group is created and they meet as a team for the first time. The team members come to the meeting with zest and a sense of curiosity, adventure, and even apprehension as they orient themselves to each other and get to know each other through personal interaction and perhaps team-building activities. With the help of the team leader or facilitator, they will explore the purpose of the team, why they are called to be a part of the team, and what contribution they can bring to the table. When the purpose of the team is clearly identified, they may proceed to establishing their team goals and expectations and setting boundaries for the teamwork.

Storming Stage

The second phase of the team process is the storming stage. As the group relaxes into a more comfortable team setting, interpersonal issues or opposing opinions may arise that may cause conflict between members of the team and with the team leader. This may cause feelings of uneasiness in the group. It is important at this stage to understand that conflict is a healthy and natural process of team development. When members of the team come from various disciplines and specialties, there is always a tendency to approach an issue from several completely

Evidence from the Literature

Citation: Witt Sherman, D., Maitra, K., Gordon, Y., Simon, S., Olenick, M. et al., (2017). Illustrating and analyzing the processes of interprofessional collaboration: A lesson learned from palliative care in deconstructing the concept. *Journal of Palliative Medicine, 20*(3). doi: 10.1089/jpm.2016.0332 .

Discussion: An **Interprofessional educational** (**IPE**) team was organized by faculty from a Florida college of nursing and representatives from **physical therapy** (**PT**), **occupational therapy** (**OT**), communication sciences and disorders, athletic training, and health services administration. The team developed a simulated case study for the palliative care of a veteran with

a traumatic brain injury. Through the process of developing the case study and follow-up interviews with the team members, seven steps for the interprofessional process were developed as well as the identification of key attitudes and behaviors critical to teamwork. The team identifies Palliative Care as a specialty which requires interprofessional collaboration and thus leads by example.

Implications for Practice: Specialty care, such as palliative care, requires an interprofessional approach where members must identify attitudes and behaviors as well as skills to ensure the best possible care.

---

different standpoints. These differences need to be openly confronted and addressed so that effective resolution of the issue may occur in a timely manner. Real teams don't emerge unless individuals on them take risks involving conflict, trust, interdependence, and hard work (Katzenbach & Smith, 2003).

Norming Stage

The third stage is called norming. After resistance is overcome in the storming stage, a feeling of group cohesion develops. Team members master the ability to resolve conflict. Although complete resolution and agreement may not be attained at all times, team members learn to respect differences of opinion and may work together through these obstacles to achieve team goals. Communication of ideas, opinions, and information occurs through effective cooperation among the team members. Overcoming barriers to performance is how groups become teams (Katzenbach & Smith, 2003).

Performing Stage

The fourth phase of the team development process is the performing stage. In this stage, group cohesion, collaboration, and solidarity are evident. Personal opinions are set aside to achieve group goals. Team members are openly communicating, know each other's roles and responsibilities, are taking risks, and are trusting or relying on each other to complete assigned tasks. The group reaches maturity at this stage. One of the biggest strengths of this stage is the emphasis on maintaining and improving interpersonal relationships within the team as members function as a whole.

Adjourning Stage

The fifth and final stage of team process development is the adjourning stage. Termination and consolidation occur in this stage. When the team has achieved their goals and assigned tasks, the team closure process begins. The team reviews their

activities and evaluates their progress and outcomes by answering the questions: Were the team goals sufficiently met? Was there anything that could have been done differently? The team leader summarizes the group's accomplishments and the role played by each member in achieving the goals. It is important to provide closure or feedback regarding the team process to leave each team member with a sense of accomplishment.

Advantages of Teamwork

Teamwork and collaboration among health care professionals from multiple disciplines optimizes patient care outcomes. Outcomes, such as improved patient and employee safety, reduction in errors, improved patient mortality statistics, and decreased length of hospitalization, are benefits of teamwork (Emich, 2018).

In addition to improved patient care outcomes, benefits for health care worker includes personal and professional growth, an increase in morale, and a decrease in staff turnover rates (Emich, 2018). Teamwork equalizes power through shared governance and facilitates interprofessional collaboration by working toward common goals. Teamwork increases respect from colleagues, develops trust and role clarity, addresses negative stereotypes, and enhances well-being (Darlow et al., 2015). When nursing staff are valued as team members and included in the decision-making process, there is a boost in professional autonomy, which in turn improves the standard of care. Joining forces with members of other professional disciplines allows other perspectives in the decision-making processes. Interprofessional teamwork deconstructs the silos created by professional education that occurs in isolation from other health care specialties.

Disadvantages of Teamwork

Although it is often true that "two heads are better than one," there are some disadvantages of teamwork. Teams may take longer to achieve a goal than would one individual. On a team composed of varied disciplines, or even on a team with all members from the same discipline but with various levels of experiences and backgrounds, a single patient care situation may produce varied and diverse solutions. The team members may have disagreements on the best course of action to take for a specific situation.

The time, effort, and resources the team process requires is a disadvantage. Selecting the right members for the team, organizing the team goals and roles, and the actual time spent brainstorming and collaborating as a team can be lengthy. Providing time away from direct patient care may consume precious financial resources. Creating physical space that is conducive for teamwork may not be feasible at all institutions.

Another negative of teamwork involves using it when the situation may best be handled by an individual or single profession. (Emich, 2018). Which situations require a team to collaborate and which are best handled by an individual team member or professional? Should the resources required for teamwork be a consideration in this decision? What is best for the patient is the question that should be pondered.

Some team members may lack interest, motivation, ability, time, or skill to participate in the team process. These members may have been appointed or self-appointed for whatever reason, but they may not do the work as expected. Factors such as personality differences, variation in personal work ethics, and disparities of perception of the team goals may impede effective team collaboration.

Team size may be a disadvantage. Team size affects performance in that too few or too many members will reduce performance and too many members may slow down or complicate the task. Smaller groups are less cumbersome, easier to create and manage, and have lower incidences of social down time. Individuals in large teams are able to maintain a sense of anonymity and gain from the work of the group without making a suitable contribution and may be difficult to create and manage (Table 16.2).

Formal and Informal Teams

In a hospital setting, there are a variety of formal teams involved in patient care. The **Core Team** includes those who are providing direct and continuous patient care and is located on the unit to which the patient is assigned. In a hospital setting, the staff nurse and the unlicensed assistive personnel are part of the core team. The **Coordinating Team** involve those are who are responsible for the day-to-day management and direction of care provided by the core team, such as the unit manager. **Ancillary services teams** complete specific tasks for the patient for a limited period of time, such as a Radiology Tech who completes a chest X-ray. **Contingency Teams** are formed for emergencies, such as the code blue team or the rapid response team. Members of these contingency teams may include one or two nurses from critical care, a respiratory therapist, an EKG technician, a phlebotomist, a pharmacist, and a physician from the ER. **Support Services Team** create a comfortable, safe, and clean health care environment for all patients and staff. Dietary personnel, maintenance, and housekeeping staff are part of the support services team (AHRQ, 2013).

Anyone working in an organization needs to be aware of the informal teams that influence the organization. Informal groups or teams are not directly established or sanctioned by the administrators or top leadership of the organization but are often formed naturally by individuals in the organization to fill a personal or social interest need. Informal teams can have a negative impact on an organization and can become so powerful that they undermine the formal authority structure. Informal teams can assume a change agent role. They are often responsible for facilitating improvements in working conditions and sometimes evolve into formal groups. Informal groups or teams may also emerge to deal with a particular organizational problem or to work toward changes in organizational policies and procedures. In sum, informal teams play a unique role in organizations. These roles may be positive or negative.

Table 16.2 Barriers to Team Performance

Barriers to team performance	
Inconsistency in team membership	Lack of time
Hierarchy (i.e., nurses may not be identified as full and equal partners of the team)	Conventional thinking (i.e., the way things have always been done)
Defensiveness	Lack of information sharing
Varying communication styles	Conflict
Lack of coordination and follow-up	Distractions
Fatigue	Workload
Misinterpretation of clues	Lack of role clarity

Source: Adapted from Team STEPPS 2.0 pocket guide. Agency for Healthcare Research and Quality. 2013.

Creating an Effective Team

Effective teamwork is essential in any setting, whether it be in a large business corporation, in a complex health care system, in social assemblies, and even within the close network of a family unit. In today's health care setting, effective teamwork is not considered an option, it is a necessity. Patient welfare and safety depends on health care professionals, with varying specialties and training, collaborating together. According to Polifko-Harris and Anunciado (2012), effectiveness of a team can be anticipated when six key requirements are incorporated:

1. Common Purpose
2. Assessment of team's composition
3. Clear communication
4. Active participation
5. Agreed upon action plan
6. Ongoing assessment and evaluation

Common Purpose

In order to succeed as a team, first and foremost the team must have a *clearly stated purpose*: What are the goals? What are the objectives? What is the timeline? What does the leader see the team accomplishing? An effective team keeps the larger organization's goals in mind as it progresses; otherwise, its goals will be inconsistent with those of the parent organization. Are any budget requirements, decision-making ability, and lines of authority for the team spelled out? Is the role of the team clear from the beginning of the team's work as to who has the final power to make a decision? Administrative support means leadership support for team efforts. Does administration empower staff by encouraging decision making at the team level? Does administration allow for individual creativity and self-governance? Developing a supportive and conducive environment for teamwork to succeed requires ongoing time and effort. Physical facility design can impact teamwork by influencing productivity, work attitudes, confidentiality, and the professional image of the health care personnel. Factors to consider in facility design include noise control, privacy, seating space, and convenience. Are there enough resources available to the team—that is, financial, support staff, time allotted, and so on? Examine and adjust the team's physical work space to optimize communication and coordination (AHRQ, 2013).

Assessment of Team's Composition

Second, an *assessment of the team's composition* is needed. What are the team members' personal strengths and weaknesses? Each team member has unique talents that can be maximized to benefit the team's goals. How do the team members see themselves as individuals? Do they see themselves as part of a cohesive team? Are the contributions of all team members valued? Are all team members' opinions respected? Does the team have a plan to avoid **groupthink**? Groupthink occurs when the desire for harmony and consensus within the group or team overrides the member's efforts to appraise the situation. Are any additional members with special expertise needed? The team members need clear roles and responsibilities. What is the role of each team member?

In well-managed interprofessional teams, all individuals are encouraged to contribute to the team goals. Each team member of an interprofessional team brings the skills and expertise of their specialty to share with the group. It is important to develop a team where all members are highly regarded and respected if the team's goals are to be fully achieved. Psychological safety describes individuals' perceptions about the consequences of interpersonal risks in their work environment—that is, beliefs, largely taken for granted about how others will respond when one puts oneself on the line. In psychologically safe teams, people believe that if they make a mistake, other team members will not penalize them or think less of them for it. This belief fosters the confidence to experiment, discuss mistakes and problems, and ask others for help. Psychological safety is created by mutual respect and trust among team members. Each team member has confidence in the good intentions of fellow team members.

It is important to note that psychological safety is distinct from team cohesiveness, which can lead to groupthink. There is a reduced willingness to disagree and challenge others' views and a lack of interpersonal risk-taking in groupthink (Janis, 1972).

Clear Communication

Third, *clear communication* is required for effective teams: Are successful communication patterns in place? Are closed loop communication methods being used? Is there a need to improve communication, either in written or verbal format? Does the team work well together, and is communication open with minimal hidden agendas of the members? Can the truth be told in a compassionate and sympathetic manner in order to reach a difficult decision? Communication needs to be timely to ensure that all members of the team have the information needed to contribute and share. Communication within the interprofessional team and workplace communication are covered in more detail later in this chapter.

Active Participation

Active participation by all team members is the critical fourth item needed for a team to succeed: Does everyone have a designated responsibility? Do people listen to one another? Is "we versus they" thinking discouraged? Are all team members involved in shaping plans and decisions? Are they all carrying their weight on the team, or are some members not doing their part? What are the relationships of the team members? Is there mutual trust and respect for members and their decisions, however unpopular? Are there political institutional issues that must be resolved before proceeding? The climate of the team should be relaxed but supportive. Use open, honest communication and discussion on tough issues to foster the team's goals. Team members should focus on the positive and not the negative. Being part of a team is an opportunity to learn and grow. Believe strongly in the team's collective ability to succeed (AHRQ, 2013). If conflict occurs, the ability to address and manage conflict is an essential part of teamwork. Conflict is covered in more detail later in this chapter.

Agreed upon Active Plan

The fifth element of a successful team is an *agreed upon action plan,* determined early in the process and revisited at designated times. Ask if is there a clear plan as to how to proceed? Each team member collaborates to create a vision or goal that helps facilitate professional and personal growth. The vision is shared with all team members and a plan is mutually developed. This inspires a more desirable team spirit and team environment. Responsibility for keeping the vision alive belongs to each member of the team. Plans to differentiate between higher and lower priorities is also a necessary part of the plan, as well as regular feedback to one another and the team. Feedback by team members and others affected by the team's decisions is necessary to monitor progress and to see if any changes are necessary as part of the action plan.

A target of the action plan that may not be considered is to allow appropriate work life balance for the team members. It is imperative that team members allow themselves personal downtime. There should be a good balance of work and personal life to allow team members to regroup, renew, and revitalize.

Ongoing Assessment and Evaluation

Linked to the action plan is the sixth guideline for a successful team: *ongoing assessment and evaluation*. Team effectiveness needs to be analyzed, including its results, processes, morale, energy, and retention of members. Team goals and plans need to be revised based on feedback of team members, feedback from those in authority and feedback from those benefitting from the team's efforts. Outcomes have to be consistent and related to the expectations of the organization. The pros and cons of all reasonable ideas should be freely discussed within the team. Creativity is encouraged; perhaps a member has an idea to solve a problem that no one has ever tried. In this supportive environment, creativity keeps the vision of the team alive and drives positive achievements. With each goal achieved, the team should celebrate. Celebration is a central part of a successful team.

When integrating new team members, make a conscious effort to welcome and include the new members of the health care team. Share the purpose, composition, and preferred communication methods with the new recruits. Encourage their active participation, reminding the new team member that they bring a fresh perspective to the group's activities. Ensure the new team member is aware of the action plan and the methods for ongoing assessment and evaluation (Table 16.3).

Qualities of Effective Team Members

To be an effective team member, you need to possess certain characteristics conducive to team collaboration. You must be proactive, motivated, have a certain personal sense of purpose or mission, and possess personal and time management skills (Covey, 1989).

Being proactive and motivated means taking charge of your life and the circumstances around you. Proactive, motivated people are not easily affected by situations in their

Table 16.3   Team Evaluation Checklist

	Yes	No
1. Is the environment/climate conducive to team building?	_____	_____
2. Do the team members have mutual respect and trust for one another?	_____	_____
3. Are the team members honest with one another?	_____	_____
4. Does everyone actively participate in the decision making and problem solving of the team?	_____	_____
5. Are the purpose, goals, and objectives of the team obvious to all participants?	_____	_____
6. Are the goals met?	_____	_____
7. Are creativity and mutual support of new ideas encouraged by all team members?	_____	_____
8. Does the team work to avoid groupthink?	_____	_____
9. Is the team productive, and does it see actual progress toward goal attainment?	_____	_____
10. Does the team begin and end its meetings on time?	_____	_____
11. Does the team leader provide vision and energy to the team?	_____	_____
12. Do any persons on the team serve as ambassador, task coordinator, or scout?	_____	_____

Source: Adapted from Polifko-Harris and Anunciado (2012).

Real World Interview

A good team leader is an objective outlier to all situations. They are able to provide feedback and criticism using language which encourages improvement and development within the career. The team leader builds the team's confidence by gathering examples of positive interactions between the nurse and patient. On the other hand, a good team is comprised of individuals who work toward the same goals. Every member is aware of what is expected of them during their shift, while understanding that there will be times when not every task can be completed on their shift. The nurses, their charge, and the patient care techs work together in order to provide safe care in a professional and courteous manner. When another nurse is occupied and one of their patients are in need of something, other members of the team step forward to care for the patient. Recently, we have had a situation where a more senior patient care technician was encouraging the junior PCT to use down time to ensure the floor was organized and well stocked. The junior PCT took this as an unnecessary criticism of her job. The two shared an unpleasant exchange and the manager was notified. The manager resolved the issue by gathering all patient care techs to ensure that they were clear about the expectations of their job. She encouraged the group to divert criticisms to the charge nurse on duty in order to avoid any future conflicts between techs.

Lauren Mikolajczyk
Wheat Ridge, CO

surroundings, because they avoid being reactive. Being proactive and motivated is to take full responsibility for your own actions, decisions, and behavior. Proactive and motivated people end up with the jobs because they are problem solvers. They seize the initiative to do whatever is necessary, consistent with correct principles, to get the job done (Covey, 1989).

To succeed in nursing as a new graduate and as a member of a team, you need to develop a personal sense of purpose, mission, and professional goals early on and work toward meeting them. Covey (1989) calls this "working toward goals and beginning with the end in mind." When joining a team, nurses need to examine their own skills, assess what contributions they can provide, and be confident in their role as team members. Knowing your priorities and managing personal and professional time wisely and efficiently will go a long way toward teamwork.

Qualities of Effective Team Leaders

A team leader will organize, facilitate, and manage the entire team. Nurse leaders need to examine their own leadership styles, strengths, and weaknesses, and learn to capitalize on their strengths. Effective team leaders must understand how various learning styles, cultural diversity, and personality differences play into the dynamics of teamwork. Qualities of a good team leader should include good communication skills, conflict resolution skills, and leadership skills.

Open and honest communication is an essential skill to develop as a team leader. Respectful negotiations, clear and tactful expression of ideas and messages, and empathetic listening must occur. The team leader must work to develop these skills. Empathetic listening allows a leader to seek first to understand the other person, become truly interested in and attentive to what the other person has to say, and then place himself or herself in the other person's shoes (Covey, 1989). See Table 16.4 for guidelines for meetings.

Communication Within the Interprofessional Team

Communication errors are a frequent cause of adverse health care events and suboptimal patient care. Safe and effective patient care requires effective communication within the members of the health care team and the patient and families. Communication is central in effective interprofessional collaboration (Darlow et al., 2015).

Table 16.4 Guidelines for Meetings

In managing meetings, leaders should be aware of the following principles:

- Set a time frame for meetings and stick to it.
- Send out an agenda prior to the meeting
- At the beginning of the meeting, review the agenda, progress made to date and clarify the task facing the group.
- Help group members feel comfortable with one another.
- Establish ground rules governing group discussions.
- As early in a meeting as possible, get a report from each member who has been preassigned a task.
- Sustain the flow of the meeting by using informational displays.
- Manage the discussion to achieve equitable participation.
- Work to avoid groupthink by using critical appraisal of all ideas.
- Close the meeting by summarizing what has been accomplished and reviewing assignments.
- Identify a time frame for future meetings.

Source: Adapted from Schwarz, R. (2016, September 24). 8 Ground Rules for Great Meetings. Retrieved October 30, 2020, from https://hbr.org/2016/06/8-ground-rules-for-great-meetings

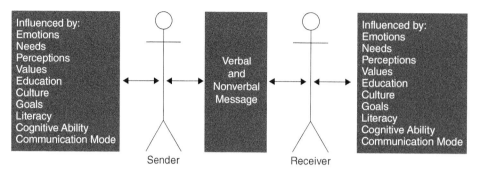

FIGURE 16.1   Communication process.
Source: Dianne Hoekstra.

Elements of the Communication Process

Communication is an interactive process that occurs when a person (the sender) sends a verbal or nonverbal message to another person (the receiver) and receives feedback citation (Wikipedia, 2020). The communication process is influenced by emotions, needs, perceptions, values, education, culture, goals, literacy, cognitive ability, and the communication mode. The input comes from visual, auditory, and kinesthetic stimuli.

Effective communication in care delivery is essential to ensure positive patient outcomes. Effective communication is a critical component to meeting patient needs, providing safe, high-quality, patient-centered care, as wells as how health care delivery is managed (Merlino, 2017). Good communication skills within the health care team has been shown to have positive effects on patient outcomes, decrease adverse events, increase positive work environments, decrease patient transfers, and lengths of stay (Merlino, 2017). The ability of the sender and receiver to accurately interpret messages is required and takes training (Figure 16.1).

Because no system can catch all errors, all hospital staff must take seriously their role in stopping the error cascade.

Modes of Communication

Face to Face

Face-to-face encounters usually allow for verbal and nonverbal exchange and have been regarded as the most effective modes of communication and hence have been preferred. Verbal communication is a conscious process, so the sender has the ability to control what is said. While it is generally accepted that tone of voice is more important than the words spoken, it has long been suggested that nonverbal facial expression is even more important than either tone of voice or the words used. Nonverbal communication tends to be unconscious and more difficult to control.

Electronic Communication

When face-to-face encounters are not possible or practical, other approaches are used. Historically, the next most effective approach is the telephone, followed by voice messages, electronic pages, e-mail messages, and written documents. These electronic methods comprise the third mode of communication, and they will grow in importance as nurses increasingly rely on technology, particularly computers, to communicate interpersonally.

Patients are being monitored long distance and connecting to their health care providers using a variety of technologies. These methods, where caregiver and care receiver interact using technology rather than the traditional face-to-face or voice-to-voice encounter, require careful communication to maintain patient safety. For example, e-mail now allows almost instantaneous communication around the world, but it also accommodates individual preferences with respect to the timing of the response. This allows a patient to provide an update on a condition early in the day and affords the caregivers the opportunity to respond as their schedules permit. Therefore, the first tip when communicating using technology is that it is important that both parties have an understanding about the circumstances under which different modes of communication will be used. Although one practitioner who is "connected" may be comfortable receiving an electronic message with urgent patient information such as an elevated potassium level, other practitioners expect a telephone call if the data being shared is potentially life threatening. Often, organizations have policies that guide under what circumstances a particular mode of communication is used, so be sure to understand your institution's policy for communicating urgent information.

Another tip is to respond in a timely manner. Timeliness is defined by what information is being shared and the route being used. E-mail, in general, provides greater immediacy, but the telephone remains the primary tool for communicating urgent information. Other tips for communicating on e-mail include the following:

- Be brief and reply sparingly, as appropriate.

- Use clear subject lines.

- Cool off before responding to an angry message. Answer tomorrow if not urgent.

- Spell out your message clearly; avoid abbreviations, as patients and others may not understand them.

- Forward e-mail messages from others only with their permission.

- Use good judgment; e-mail may not be private.

Always proofread correspondences prior to sending them. Imagine yourself the recipient of the document.

Electronic health records (EHRs) have been adopted by health care systems. The American Recovery and Reinvestment Act, requires that all public and private health care providers and other eligible professionals (EPs) to adopt and demonstrate "meaningful use" of electronic medical records (EMRs) by January 1, 2014, to maintain their existing Medicaid and Medicare reimbursement levels and avoid penalties of a 1% decrease in Medicare reimbursements (Office for Civil Rights, 2017). Orientation to each institution likely includes an introduction to the system(s) in use. In general, as with all patient records, issues of confidentiality are of utmost importance, so nurses must be mindful of their important role in maintaining privacy and appropriately accessing and granting access to the system.

Levels of Communication

The level of communication involves who the audience is at the time of communication. Communication can be thought of as having three levels: public, intrapersonal, and interpersonal. Examples of each are provided below:

Public Communication

The nurse educator presenting a workshop on signs and symptoms of menopause to a room full of middle-aged women engages in **public communication**. **Public communication** happens when individuals and groups engage in dialogue in the **public** sphere in order to deliver a message to a specific audience. Their audience is a group of people with a common interest. As presenter, he or she acts primarily as a sender of information. By design, feedback is typically limited in public speaking, though it does occur.

Intrapersonal Communication

Another level is **intrapersonal communication**, which can be thought of as self-talk. As the name suggests, it is what individuals do within themselves, and it can present as doubts or affirmations. A new nurse may engage in intrapersonal communication as he simultaneously doubts and affirms his ability to complete a procedure. For example, the first time the newly licensed RN has to catheterize a patient, he may simultaneously doubt his ability to insert a Foley catheter, with one message, "I have only done this on a mannequin," while affirming his ability to insert a Foley catheter with an "I can do this" message to himself. He is engaging in intrapersonal communication. The so-called competing voices within himself act as sender and receiver in this intrapersonal conversation whose outcome will be influenced by the feedback that follows.

From self-awareness and understanding of oneself, a nurse can move confidently into one-to-one interactions with others, and then into interactions with smaller and larger groups.

Interpersonal Communication

The last level, **interpersonal communication**, involves communication between individuals, person-to-person or in small groups. Not surprisingly, nurses engage in this level regularly. Interpersonal communication allows for a very effective level of communication to occur and incorporates all of the elements, channels, and modes previously discussed. The nurse, who observes a patient grimace when he moves, interprets the nonverbal cue as indicating that the patient is experiencing pain. Using verbal communication, the nurse clarifies her perception by asking the patient to describe and rate his pain. He describes it as tolerable and states that he is expecting a visitor and he does not want to be drowsy. The communication goes back and forth until, ideally, both parties' understanding of the message match. This is the goal of communication.

Organizational Communication

Networks of communication are often defined by an organization's formal structure. The formal structure establishes who is in charge and identifies how different levels of personnel and various departments relate within the organization. Some of these relationships are typically depicted by an organizational chart. When the chief executive officer of an organization announces that the company will adopt a new policy that all employees will follow, that is downward communication. The message starts at the top and is usually disseminated by levels through the chain of communication. Upward communication is the opposite of downward communication. The idea originates at some level below the top of the structure and moves upward. For example, when a nurse recommends a more efficient approach to organizing care to his nurse manager, who takes the recommendation to her superior, who uses the recommendation to develop a new policy, that is upward communication. Besides the upward and downward chain network of communication, other common networks of communication have been identified, for example, a Y network, a wheel network, a circle network, and an all-channel network of communication (Maharjan, 2018). In a Y pattern of communication, all communication is funneled through one individual. An example is two staff nurses who report to the nursing unit director, who reports to the vice president for nursing, who reports to the president. A wheel network of communication looks like an *X in a wheel* and could be a situation in which four nurses report to one nurse manager. There is no interaction among the four nurses, and all communications are channeled through the nurse manager at the center of the wheel. This network is rare in health care organizations. Even though this type of network communication is not used routinely, it may be used in circumstances in which urgency or secrecy is required. For example, the president of an organization who has an emergency might communicate with the vice presidents in a wheel network because time does not permit using other modes.

A circle network of communication allows communicators in the network to communicate directly only with two others, next to them in the circle. Because each communicates with another communicator in the circle network, the effect is that everyone communicates with someone, and there is no central authority or leader.

Communication networks vary along several dimensions. The most appropriate network depends upon the situation in which it is used. The wheel and all-channel networks tend to be fast and accurate compared with the chain and Y-pattern networks. The chain and Y-pattern networks promote clear-cut lines of authority and responsibility but may slow communications. The circle and all-channel networks enhance morale among those in the networks better than other patterns. Nurses must construct communication networks to fit the various communication situations they face.

Grapevine

A final avenue worth mentioning, which is not a formal avenue, is the grapevine. The **grapevine** is an informal avenue in which rumors circulate. It ignores the formal chain of command. The major benefit of the grapevine is the speed with which information is spread, but its major drawback is that it often lacks accuracy. For example, nurses who inform an oncoming shift about a rumor that layoffs or mandatory overtime is imminent, in the absence of any information from the hospital's administration, are participating in grapevine communication.

Communication Skills

Because nurses are often placed in positions of leadership and are responsible for representing nursing's concerns to others, including the patient, it is important that they have the requisite skills to be effective communicators. There is no one correct way to ensure effective communication. Rather, effective communication requires that both parties engaged in communicating use skills that enhance that particular interaction. In general, the most important considerations for facilitating communication are to be open, assertive, and willing to give and receive feedback. Some of the most important communication skills upon which nurses rely to do this are listed in Table 16.5.

Barriers to Communication

Barriers are obstacles to effective communication. The nurse who can identify potential barriers to communication will be better equipped to avoid them or to compensate for them. Some barriers can be physical, such as trying to communicate with someone on a poor phone connection. Some of the other most common barriers are language, gender, culture, anger, generational differences, illiteracy, and conflict.

Use of Language

Language is the primary means that we use to communicate with each other. Humans have developed written, sign, and oral languages to share messages. In a health care setting, oral language is used to verbally communicate with patients and other health care professionals. As you work with patients, you will encounter a great diversity in spoken languages. For instance, more than 6,900 languages and dialects are spoken today, with Mandarin Chinese topping the list, with 1.28 billion speakers (Eberhard, Simons, & Fennig, 2019). The other top five languages spoken are Spanish, numbering 437 million speakers; English, 372 million; Arabic, 295 million; Hindi, 260 million; and Bengal, 242 million (McCarthy, 2018).

Table 16.5 Communication Skills

Skill	Description
Attending	Active listening for what is said and how it is said as well as noting nonverbal cues that support or negate congruence, for example, making eye contact and posturing.
Responding	Verbal and nonverbal acknowledgement of the sender's message, such as "I hear you."
Clarifying	Restating, questioning, and rephrasing to help the message become clear, for example, "Can you restate that? I lost you there."
Confronting	Identifying the conflict, for example, "We have a problem and it is X" and then clearly delineating the problem. Confronting uses knowledge and reason to resolve the problem.
Supporting	Siding with another person or backing up another person: "I can see why you would feel that way."
Focusing	Centers on the main point: "So your main concern is . . ."
Open-ended questioning	Allows for patient-directed responses: "How did that make you feel?"
Providing information	Supplies one with knowledge they did not previously have: "It's common for people to experience frustration when doing this for the first time."
Using silence	Allows for intrapersonal communication.
Reassuring	Restores confidence or removes fear: "I can assure you that tomorrow . . ."
Expressing appreciation	Shows gratitude: "Thank you" or "You are so thoughtful."
Using humor	Provides relief and gains perspective; may also cause harm, so use carefully.
Conveying acceptance	Makes known that one is capable or worthy: "It's okay to cry."
Asking related questions	Expands listener's understanding: "How painful was it?"

Source: Dianne Hoekstra.

Individuals also communicate nonverbally using body language. It is important to remember that there are many cross-cultural similarities in body language, but there are also key differences. The meaning of different gestures varies from culture to culture. Never assume that a gesture holds the same meaning for you and your patient, especially if your patient is from another culture.

Generational Differences

Generational differences can create tensions among workers because of the divergent outlooks on life. Different generations can have different values about work, motivation, lifestyle, and communication. It is important to be aware that even though generalizations can be misleading and unfair, four generations make up the current workforce. This is discussed more in Chapter 24.

Health Literacy

Nurses need to be mindful that many patients and their families lack the health literacy skills to understand the health care system and function successfully as health care consumers. Health literacy is an individual's ability to read, understand, and use health care information to make decisions and follow instructions for treatment. Health Literacy is defined as an individual's ability to obtain, communicate, process, and understand basic health information and services to make appropriate health decisions (Centers for Disease Control and Prevention, 2019).

This definition encompasses the elements of personal empowerment and action and views health literacy as an outcome of health promotion and health education efforts that have both personal and social benefits. Patients, families, and even subordinates simply do not always understand what nurses and other health care providers are trying to communicate. Almost a quarter of the adult population in the United States is functionally illiterate, and nearly half have limited literacy skills. There is a correlation between illiteracy and higher health care costs and poor patient outcomes. According to Proliteracy.org (2019), 43% of adults with low literacy levels live in poverty

and 70% receive welfare; of those adults, their children have a 72% chance of having low literacy levels themselves. It is estimated that low literacy levels result in over $230 billion per year in health care costs. Literacy challenges are increased for patients whose primary language is not English.

Anger

Anger is a universal, strong feeling of displeasure that is often precipitated by a situation that frustrates or prevents a person from attaining a goal or getting what is wanted from life. Anger is influenced by one's beliefs. According to Kassinove (2019), anger is a negative feeling state that is typically associated with hostile thoughts, physiological arousal, and maladaptive behaviors. Anger is a result of the perception of an individual who feels another is being disrespectful, demeaning, threatening, or neglectful. Rational and appropriate responses are feelings of disappointment. Anger, on the other hand, can be unmanageable and self-defeating. Physical manifestations of anger include muscle tension, headaches, and heart rate elevation. Some signs of anger include raising a fist, yelling, and throwing or breaking things.

Anger can be dealt with in one of several ways. Three methods that may work from time to time but that may have serious and potentially destructive drawbacks are denying and repressing anger, which may lead to resentment; expressing anger, which may lead to defensiveness on the part of the respondent; and turning the other cheek, which may lead to continued mistreatment and lack of trust. Anger can stem from deep-seated feelings of unassertiveness. Assertiveness involves taking a stand, whereas aggression involves putting another down. If unassertiveness is the source of anger, then a solution is to learn to act assertively.

Overcoming Communication Barriers

Additional barriers to communication are seen in Table 16.6. Ways to overcome these communication barriers are seen in Table 16.7

Table 16.6 Additional Barriers to Communication.

Barrier	Description
Offering false reassurance	Promising something that cannot be delivered.
Being defensive	Acting as though one has been attacked.
Stereotyping	Unfairly categorizing someone based on his or her traits.
Interrupting	Speaking before another has completed her message.
Inattention	Not paying attention.
Stress	A state of tension that gets in the way of reasoning.
Unclear expectations	Ill-defined direction to perform tasks or duties that make successful completion unlikely.
Incongruent responses	When words and actions in a communication don't match the inner experience of self and/or are inappropriate to the context. This response commonly presents itself as blaming, placating, being super-reasonable, or using irrelevant information when communicating with another person.
Giving advice	Assumes that the other person is unable to solve his or her own problems. It is better to share problem solving options when communicating. This allows the other person to choose one of the options for solving a problem.

Source: Dianne Hoekstra.

Table 16.7   Overcoming Communication Barriers. Note: Table created by chapter authors.

Method	Actions
Understand the receiver	Ask yourself what's in it for the other person. Work to develop understanding of the other person's needs.
Communicate Assertiveness	Be direct. Explain ideas clearly and with feeling. Repeat important messages. Use various communication channels, for example, written, e-mail, verbal, and so on.
Use two-way communication	Ask questions. Communicate face to face.
Unite with a common vocabulary	Define the meaning of important terms, such as *high quality*, so that everyone understands their meaning.
Elicit verbal and nonverbal feedback	Request and offer verbal feedback often. Document important agreements. Observe nonverbal feedback.
Enhance listening skills	Pay attention to what is said, what is not said, and to the nonverbal signals. Continue listening carefully even when you don't like the message. Give summary reflections to assure understanding; for example, "You say you are late giving medications because the pharmacy did not deliver meds on time." Engage in concluding discussions, such as, "Has your unit been late with medications due to problems with pharmacy deliveries before?" Ask questions to explore problems. Paraphrase a speaker's words to decrease miscommunication rather than blurting out questions as soon as the other person finishes speaking.
Be sensitive to cultural differences	Know what cultural communication barriers exist. Show respect for all workers. Minimize use of jargon specific to your culture. Be sensitive to cultural etiquette such as use of first names, eye contact, hand gestures, personal appearance.
Be sensitive to gender differences	Be aware that men and women may have some differences in communication style; for instance, men may call attention to their accomplishments, and women may tend to be more conciliatory when facing differences. Know that male-female stereotypes often don't fit the person you are working with. Avoid barriers by knowing that differences exist, and don't take things personally. Males can improve communication by showing more empathy and females by becoming more direct.
Engage in metacommunication	Communicate about your communication to resolve a problem; e.g., "I'm trying to get through to you, but either you don't react to me or you get angry. What can I do to improve our communication?"

Source: Adapted from DuBrin (2000).

Trends in Society that Affect Communication

Good communication will grow in importance because of trends in our culture. Among the trends affecting nursing practice is the increasing diversity in society. The United States is made up of people with different ethnic, racial, cultural, and socioeconomic backgrounds. Increased diversity causes once-dominant values and beliefs to be replaced or diluted with diverse values and beliefs. These differences become a source of possible misunderstanding that can be bridged by effective communication.

Another trend is our aging population. It is estimated that one in five persons in the United States will be of retirement age and by 2035 individuals over 65 will be the majority to those under 18 at a rate of 78 million to 76.7 million respectively (United States Census Bureau, 2018). Our aging society will challenge nurses to maintain effective communication to compensate for the diminished sensory abilities that typically accompany aging. Multiple sensory deficits can occur simultaneously so that patients may experience losses in a variety of combinations that include hearing, seeing, smelling, tasting, and touching. The potential diminished input challenges nurse and patient alike to creatively compensate for these deficits.

At the same time as the population is aging, it is also shifting to an electronic mode, with computer technology playing an increasingly dominant role. As electronic communication assumes this role, the nurse's ability to effectively communicate in writing will grow in importance. Reliance on written communication using electronic input shifts the source of input away from traditional visual, auditory, and kinesthetic modes to the written word. To use electronic tools effectively, tomorrow's nurses will require keen writing skills. These trends have influenced nursing today.

Workplace Communication

It is probably clear by now that how individuals communicate depends, in part, on where communication occurs and in what relationship. Patterns of communication in the workplace are sensitive to organizational factors that define relationships. Nurses have diverse roles and relationships in the workplace that call for different communication patterns with supervisors, coworkers, subordinates, practitioners, and other health care professionals, patients, families, and mentors. Nurses need to keep in mind what the educational levels are of the people with whom they are communicating. Using medical terminology is appropriate with another practitioner who shares a common understanding. Discussions with others such as licensed practical nurses (LPNs), nursing assistive personnel (NAP), patients, and family members will more likely result in understanding when language is adjusted to their level of understanding. Always remember that the goal is to communicate effectively. We more clearly share information between practitioners with progress notes. Each part of the team documents care and progress based on their part in the health care team. Progress notes should be read to get a fuller picture of the patients' status. Interdisciplinary rounds on patients is another way that the interprofessional teams share information and communicate to provide the best possible care to patients and their families.

Supervisors

Communicating with a supervisor can be intimidating, especially for a new nurse. Observing professional courtesies is an important first step. For instance, begin by requesting an appointment to discuss a problem when it arises. This demonstrates respect and allows for the conversation to occur at an appropriate time and place. Dress professionally. Arrive for the appointment on time and be prepared to state the concern clearly and accurately. Provide supporting evidence and anticipate resistance to any requests. Separate out your needs from your desires. State a willingness to cooperate in finding a solution and then match behaviors to words. Persist in the pursuit of a solution

Co-workers

Nurses depend on their coworkers in many ways to collectively provide quality patient care. Nowhere is this more important than in the acute care setting where nursing services are non-stop around the clock. Transfer of patient care from nurse to nurse is one of the most important and frequent communications between coworkers. Fluid communication in end of shift hand-off reports are crucial for achieving quality nursing care. However, time constraints demand that the change of shift handoff report be accurate, informative, and succinct. How the nursing care is organized influences who gets the report. Tips for communicating with coworkers include remembering professional courtesies and being mindful of an appropriate time and place to share your concerns. Stay focused on what is needed to get the job done, and seek a win-win solution to conflicts, where all parties are satisfied with the outcome (Table 16.8).

An excellent guide for directing communication with coworkers is the golden rule: "Do unto others as you would have them do unto you." As a nurse who will be responsible for overseeing others' work, a valuable perspective for you to maintain is that all members of the team are important to successfully realize quality patient care. Communication between nurses and co-workers will most likely involve delegating. In addition to delegating, a few other communications skills are worth mentioning. Offering positive feedback such as "I appreciate the way you interacted with Mr. T to get him to ambulate twice this shift" goes a long way toward team building, and it improves coworkers' sense of worth. Nurses also have an opportunity to act as teachers to coworkers. Often in a hospital setting, nurses teach by example. Demonstrating the desired behavior allows the coworker the opportunity to copy the behavior. It is important to allow time for return demonstrations to evaluate that the coworker has learned the intended skill. Offer constructive feedback. Be patient. Remember your own learning curves when mastering new skills and behaviors and allow those you supervise the opportunity to grow. Be open to the possibility that coworkers, particularly those with experience, may have a few pearls of wisdom to share with you as well.

Table 16.8   How to Improve Your Ability to Work with Your Boss

Know your boss's:	• Strengths and weaknesses
	• Working style
• Goals and objectives	• Predisposition toward dependence on authority figures
• Pressures	
• Strengths, weaknesses, and blind spots	*Develop a relationship that:*
• Working style	
	• Meets both your objectives and styles
Understand your own:	• Keeps your boss informed
	• Is based on dependability and honesty
• Objectives	• Selectively uses your boss's time and resources
• Pressures	

Note. Adapted from Gabarro and Kotter (1993).

Table 16.9   Signs of Horizontal/Lateral Violence

Aggressive or mocking behavior
Verbal retorts, abrupt responses, vulgar language
Belittling gestures such as deliberate rolling of eyes, folding arms, staring into space
Undermining behavior such as constantly ignoring questions, devaluing comments
Criticizing or excluding an individual from discussion
Withholding needed information or advice
Sabotage, such as setting up a new-hire nurse for failure
Constant confrontation, demonstrating negativity
Infighting and bickering
Scapegoating
Blaming and gossiping behind a colleague's back
Humiliation and confrontations in public
Failure to respect privacy, broken confidences
Shouting, yelling, or other intimidating behaviors
Judging others based on age, gender, sexual orientation, etc.
Punishing activities by management, e.g., bad schedules, chronic understaffing
Physical violence

Source: Adapted from Incivility, Bullying, and Workplace Violence - ANA Position Statement. (2015, July 15). Retrieved January 30, 2020, from https://www.nursingworld.org/practice-policy/nursing-excellence/official-position-statements/id/incivility-bullying-and-workplace-violence/

Horizontal/Lateral Violence

New nurses need to be aware that not all working environments are hospitable. **Horizontal violence** are behaviors exhibited by a single nurse or group of nurses such as hostile, aggressive, or harmful actions toward another nurse or group of nurses (Taylor, 2016). This may also be called bullying. Manifestations of horizontal violence include overt or covert hostile behaviors that are a symptom of a hostile "system" or work group culture rather than individual pathology. See Table 16.9 for signs of horizontal/lateral violence.

There are several explanations for horizontal/lateral violence in nursing, including role, gender, self-esteem, anger as an unacceptable emotion, and nursing as an oppressed group. Whatever its origins, violence in the nursing workplace is demoralizing for nurses and also negatively patient and nursing safety. Several organizations have developed no-tolerance policies (Figure 16.2).

Personal strategies to avoid horizontal violence and create a safe and happy workplace include: (a) name the problem using the term, horizontal violence, to label the situation; (b) break the silence about horizontal violence by raising the issue at staff meetings; (c) ask about the process for dealing with horizontal violence; (d) engage in reflective practices such as journaling to raise your self-awareness about your own behaviors, beliefs, values, and attitudes; (e) engage in self-care activities to maintain your own health and happiness; (f) be willing to speak up when you observe horizontal violence behaviors; and (g) discuss strategic options with your union representative or nursing or hospital administrators (American Nurses Association, 2015).

Physicians, Nurse Practitioners, and Other Health Care Professionals

One of the most intimidating experiences for new nurses may be communicating with physicians, **nurse practitioners** (**NP**), or **physician assistants** (**PA**s). Despite gender and role challenges that have already been discussed, this need not be a stressful event. The nurse's goal is to strive for collaboration, keeping the patient goal central to the discussion. It involves seeking creative, integrative solutions while also working through emotions. To communicate effectively with the practitioner, the nurse presents information in a straightforward manner, clearly

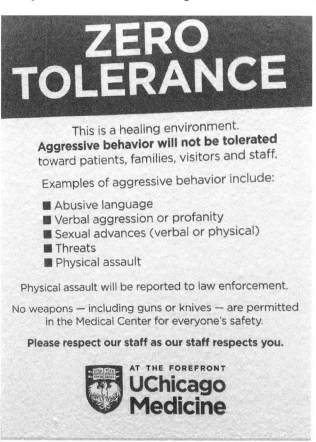

FIGURE 16.2   Zero tolerance.
Source: Used with permission from P. Zemansky (2019).

delineating the problem, supported by pertinent evidence. This is especially important when reporting changes in patient conditions. Nurses are responsible for knowing classic symptoms of conditions, apprising the practitioner of changes, and recording all observations in the chart. It is important that the nurse remains calm and objective, even if the practitioner does not cooperate. For example, if a practitioner hangs up, document that the call was terminated and fill out an incident report. If the practitioner gives an inappropriate answer or gives no orders, for example for a patient complaint of pain, document the call, the information relayed, and the fact that no orders were given. In addition, document any other steps that were taken to resolve the problem, for example notifying the nursing supervisor. If a practitioner cannot be reached, first follow the institution's procedure for getting the patient treated and then document the actions taken. The SBAR tool can be very useful for all communication with other nursing or medical practitioners and is discussed later in this chapter.

According to the Institute for Health Improvement (2019),

> *Medication reconciliation is the process of creating the most accurate list possible of all medications a patient is taking— including drug name, dosage, frequency, and route—and comparing that list against the physician's admission, transfer, and/or discharge orders, with the goal of providing correct medications to the patient at all transition points within the hospital.*

The reconciliation process involves communication between members of an interdisciplinary team that includes nurses, physicians, and pharmacists. While the process may vary from one institution to another, members of the interdisciplinary team engage in checks and balances to prevent medication errors. Communication between members of the interdisciplinary team is important to resolve any medication discrepancies and prevent medication errors.

From the time a medication order is placed in the system to the time that the medication is administered to the patient, there are numerous opportunities for medication errors to occur in health care settings today. Nurses must be aware that medication administration is the most interrupted nursing activity. Sources of interruptions include people (health care professionals, patients, and family members) and technical interruptions (missing equipment, IV infusion pump failure, etc.). Nurses and NAP are the primary source of interruptions, with discussions related to patient care issues or personal issues. While little research has been done to test interventions to help nurses create a culture of safety and cope with interruptions, some hospitals have attempted to reduce errors by creating interruption-free medication preparation zones.

Patients and Families

Communication with patients and families is optimized by the many skills previously described in this chapter. There are a few additional skills that have not yet been mentioned. The first is touch. Nurses routinely use touch as a way to communicate caring and concern. Occasionally, language barriers will limit communication to the nonverbal mode. For instance, a stroke patient who cannot process words can still interpret a gentle hand on their shoulder.

Communication requires an openness and honesty with concurrent respect for patients and families. In addition, it is important to honor and protect patients' privacy with the nurse's actions and words. Information that patients share with nurses and other health care providers is to be held in confidence. Verbal exchanges regarding patient conditions are private matters that should not occur in the hallway or just outside a patient's room where others will hear them. Nurses are obligated to not discuss patient conditions with others, even family members, without patient permission.

Mentor and Prodigy

The final pattern of communication that occurs in the workplace that will be discussed is between mentor and prodigy. Mentoring may be an informal process that occurs between an expert nurse and a novice nurse, but it may also be an assigned role. This one-on-one relationship focuses on professional aspects and is mutually beneficial. The optimal novice is hardworking, willing to learn, and anxious to succeed. Communication entails using the skills previously described in this chapter to help the novice develop expert status and career direction. The novice accomplishes this by gleaning the mentor's wisdom. This wisdom is typically shared through listening, affirming, counseling, encouraging, and seeking input from the novice. A strategy that facilitates mentoring is to share the same work schedule so that the novice is exposed to the mentor. This allows for sharing and shadowing opportunities. The mentor can also anticipate added challenges that will likely occur with increasing responsibility. Role-playing, in which the expert preceptor nurse describes a theoretical situation and allows the novice to practice his response to new and sometimes challenging situations, is another strategy that can be used.

Conflict

An important part of the change process is the ability to resolve **conflict**. Conflict management skills are leadership and management tools that all registered nurses should have in their repertoire. Conflict itself is not bad. Conflict is healthy. It, like change, allows for creativity, innovation, new ideas, and new ways of doing things. It allows for the healthy discussion of different views and values and adds an important dimension to the provision of quality patient care. Without some conflict, groups or work teams tend to become stagnant and routinized. Nothing new is allowed to penetrate the "way we have always done it" mentality. Conflict can be stimulated by such things as scarce resources, invasion of personal space, safety or security issues, cultural differences, scarce nursing resources, increased workload, group competition, and various nursing demands and responsibilities.

Definition of Conflict

Conflict can be generally defined as two or more parties experiencing a breakdown in relations. Effective management of a conflict results in minimized negativity and positive outcomes (SHRM, 2018). Not all disagreements become conflicts, but all disagreements have the potential for becoming conflicts, and all conflicts involve some level of disagreement. It is the astute manager who can determine which disagreements might become conflicts and which ones will not.

Sources of Conflict

Whenever there is the opportunity for disagreement, there is a potential source of conflict. The common sources of conflict in the professional setting include disputes over resource allocation or availability, personality differences, differences in values, threats from inside or outside an organization, cultural differences, and competition. Organizational, professional, and unit goals serve as a major source of conflict. Nurses frequently see financial goals and patient care goals as being in direct conflict with one another.

Sources of conflict in personal arenas include differences in values, threats to security or well-being, financial problems, and cultural differences. Living conditions and social contacts can increase or decrease sources of conflict in someone's personal life. When people believe they have control over their living conditions and their social contacts, they can work to minimize conflict. Family relationships may present sources of conflict because of the complexity of these relationships.

Types of Conflict

There are three broad types of conflict: intrapersonal, interpersonal, and organizational. Intrapersonal conflict occurs within the individual. When opposing values or differences in priority arise within an individual, they may suffer intrapersonal conflict. For example, if Marilyn is not granted her requested day off, she may have internal conflict about whether or not to call in sick or to take the day off without pay or to go to work. Or Marilyn may have a conflict about priorities. Should she attend her daughter's softball game or write her paper for school? Individuals often have internal conflict about values. For example, in Marilyn's case, the requested day off may have been to attend the softball game, so the values in conflict would be the values of family versus the values of the work ethic.

In interpersonal conflict, the source of disagreement may be between two people or groups or work teams. There may be disagreement in philosophy or values, or policy or procedure. It may be a personality conflict; for example, two people just openly dislike each other. This type of conflict is not unusual in the work situation. People new to a team may bring ideas with them that are not totally acceptable to the members in place. Individuals who transfer from one unit to another often stir up a certain amount of conflict over processes and procedures. For example, the nurse transferring from the intensive care unit (ICU) to the coronary care unit (CCU) may be comfortable with one way of making assignments and then try to encourage his new peers to adopt that methodology without sharing the rationale for why his way is better.

On occasion, there may be some interpersonal conflict between ICU nurses and medical-surgical nurses when they are required to work in one another's areas. Little regard is sometimes offered to each other about differences among patients, equipment, or required organizational skills. This lack of regard may sometimes lead to conflict based on preconceived notions rather than fact.

Organizational conflict is often referred to as intergroup conflict. It is at times a healthy way of introducing new ideas and encouraging creativity. Competition for resources, organizational cultural differences, and other sources of conflict help organizations identify areas for improvement. Conflict helps organizations identify legitimate differences among departments or work teams based on corporate need or responsibility. When organizational conflict is highlighted, corporate values and differences are aired and resolved.

In today's health care environment, conflict between the organizational goals of quality patient care and the need for a healthy financial bottom line can occur. These are both important values to the organization. Organizational conflict may help individual work groups or teams clarify goals and become more cohesive, hopefully with few interpersonal disagreements. This process may also work for organizations in direct competition with one another as they unite internally against an outside threat to their well-being.

The Conflict Process

In 1975, Filley suggested a process for conflict management that is widely accepted. In this process, there are five stages of conflict:

1. antecedent conditions,

2. perceived and/or felt conflict,

3. manifest behavior,

4. conflict resolution or suppression, and

5. resolution aftermath.

In Filley's model, conflict and conflict management proceed along a specific process that begins with specific preexisting conditions called antecedent conditions. The situation develops so that there is perceived or felt conflict by the involved parties that initiates a behavioral response or manifest behavior. The conflict is either resolved or suppressed, leading to the development of new feelings and attitudes, which may create new conflicts. Conflict management is vital in change. The antecedent conditions that Filley suggests may or may not be the cause of the conflict, but they certainly move the disagreement to the conflict level. The sources of these conditions include those discussed earlier: disagreement in goals, values, or resource utilization. Other issues may also serve as antecedent conditions, such as the dependency of one group on another. For instance, the nursing department is dependent on the pharmacy department to provide drugs for the nursing unit in a timely fashion. The goals and priorities of pharmacy and nursing may be different at the time the nurse requests the drugs, so a source of disagreement arises. If the circumstances for disagreement continue, a conflict will develop. Differing beliefs regarding steps to achieve goals and quality of relationships are the most frequent predisposing factors of conflict (McKibben, 2017).

An example of this is the incompatibility of quality nursing care and financial goal setting. There is often suspicion on the part of nurses that cutting costs in any area of nursing will lead to poor-quality nursing care, and the antecedent condition of goal disagreement is established. If the cost cutting occurs too often, patient care may or may not be negatively affected. There is no way of actually knowing the exact impact of financial cuts on quality, but there is some predictability that at some point continual financial cuts will negatively affect the quality of care provided for the patient. The antecedent condition or preexisting condition for conflict are present with apparently incompatible goals, such as, financial goals and quality-care goals are not always compatible.

The antecedent conditions lead to frustration, and a conflict is born. The frustration is often described as a felt conflict—that is, when one party feels in conflict with another and perceives conflict and when each party believes he or she knows what the other party's position is in the conflict. Of course, in the case of groups, one group or person may not be aware of another person's or group's feelings of conflict. This adds to the frustration. In the case of intrapersonal conflict, the frustration surrounds the internal conflict and how to resolve it. Once frustration has been felt, then resolution of some kind is necessary. The emotional components of frustration are anger and resignation. Both of these are powerful emotions that require some kind of action. For example, if Julio is not aware of the conflict between him and Tamika, Tamika may feel frustrated and upset. She is then obligated to let Julio know of her feelings so the conflict can be managed. If Tamika does not let Julio know of her feelings, then the frustration builds to anger, and Tamika will not be able to resolve the issues with Julio until that frustration is alleviated. This often results when frustration erupts into anger over some little thing rather than over the actual conflict.

Meaning of the Conflict

Conceptualization of the meaning of a conflict develops when individuals form an idea or concept of what the conflict is about, such as a conflict over control, professional standards, values, goals, and so on. Each party may or may not be aware of the other's conceptualization of the meaning of the conflict, but the parties do have what they believe is a clear concept of the conflict in their own minds. To determine the accuracy of the beliefs about the conflict, both parties need to sit down and determine the existence and nature of the conflict and the reasons it exists. The four most common themes that lead to conflict include facts, goals, methods of goal achievement, and the values or standards used to select the goals or methods (McKibben, 2017). This means that the actual facts of the dispute may be in question, the goals each side wishes to achieve may not be the same, how to achieve the agreed-upon goal is not acceptable to one side or the other, or values are in dispute. After the nature of the conflict or the points of disagreement are known, then conflict management can begin.

The actions taken to resolve the conflict can take many forms:

- Discussion of the conflict may move it toward resolution.

- Someone in power may take steps to end the conflict or at least suppress it.

- One or both parties may decide to do nothing to resolve the conflict.

Successful conflict management will be discussed later. It is important to point out that failure to successfully manage the conflict leads to more frustration and a further heightening of the conflict. Communication breaks down and fighting spreads to the pettiest of issues. After it is apparent that a conflict is occurring, conflict management of some type must occur. People simply do not get over it and move on. The conflict is a source of friction and pain that must be resolved.

Outcomes are, of course, the result of any action taken. Positive resolution of conflict leads to positive outcomes; negative resolution or no resolution of conflict leads to negative or angry consequences. The hope is that each side has gained some measure of trust and respect, but if they are at least still talking, progress has been made. The best outcome is one in which both sides feel that something is won and their self-respect is intact.

Conflict Management

There are essentially seven methods of conflict management. These methods dictate the outcomes of the conflict process. Although some methods are more desirable or produce more successful outcomes than do others, there may be a place in conflict management for all the methods, depending on the nature of the conflict and the desired outcomes. Table 16.10 is a summary of these methods, highlighting some of their advantages and disadvantages. The five techniques most commonly acknowledged are avoiding, accommodating, competing, compromising, and collaborating. Other techniques are negotiating and confronting.

Strategies to Facilitate Conflict Management

Open, honest, clear communication is the key to successful conflict management. The nurse and all parties to the conflict must agree to communicate with one another openly and honestly.

Table 16.10   Summary of Conflict Management Techniques

Conflict management technique	Advantages	Disadvantages
Avoiding—ignoring the conflict	Does not make a big deal out of nothing; conflict may be minor in comparison to other priorities	Conflict can become bigger than anticipated; source of conflict might be more important to one person or group than to others
Accommodating—smoothing or cooperating; one side gives in to the other side	One side is more concerned with an issue than is the other side; stakes not high enough for one group, and that side is willing to give in	One side holds more power and can force the other side to give in; the importance of the stakes is not as apparent to one side as to the other
Competing—forcing; the two or three sides are forced to compete for the goal	Produces a winner; good when time is short and stakes are high	Produces a loser; leaves anger and resentment on losing side
Compromising—each side gives up something and gains something	No one should win or lose, but both should gain something; good for disagreements between individuals	May cause a return to the conflict if what is given up becomes more important than the original goal
Negotiating—high-level discussion that seeks agreement but not necessarily consensus	Stakes are very high, and solution is rather permanent; often involves powerful groups	Agreements are permanent, even though each side has gains and losses
Collaborating—both sides work together to develop the optimal outcome	Best solution for the conflict and encompasses all important goals of each side	Takes a lot of time; requires commitment to success
Confronting—immediate and obvious movement to stop conflict at the very start	Does not allow conflict to take root; very powerful	May leave impression that conflict is not tolerated; may make something big out of nothing

Source: Table created by Dianne Hoekstra.

Courtesy in communicating is to be encouraged. This includes listening actively to the other side. This does not include interrupting, being aggressive, or being overbearing in demeanor. Most importantly, use of derogatory language or gestures is not acceptable or tolerable. Voice level should be calm and at a normal tone. This sounds easy, but it may not always be easy to do in practice.

The setting for the discussions for conflict management should be private, relaxed, and comfortable. If possible, external interruptions from phones, pagers, overhead speakers, and personnel should be avoided or kept to a minimum. The setting should be on neutral territory so that no one feels overpowered. The ground rules, such as not interrupting, who should go first, time limits, and so on, should be agreed upon at the beginning. Adherence to ground rules should be expected.

The management of conflict should be entered into by both sides in the spirit of expectation of compliance to the results. Threats on either side of the conflict should not be tolerated. Conflict management cannot be achieved if either party is threatening one another. If one party cannot agree to comply with the decisions or outcomes, there is no point to the conflict management process.

Leadership and Management Roles in Conflict Management

Leadership role model and implement conflict management methods as soon as the conflict is evident. This strategy demonstrates awareness of the intrapersonal or interpersonal conflict and works to resolve it and set the goal of conflict management so that both parties win. The leader also works to lessen the perceptual differences of the conflicting parties

about the conflict and tries to encourage each side to see the other's view. The nurse assists conflicting parties to identify techniques that may resolve the conflict and accepts differences between the parties without judgment or accusation. The leader fosters open and honest communication.

The nursing manager role includes the creation of an environment conducive to conflict management. The manager uses their authority to solve conflicts, including the use of competition for immediate or unpopular decisions. The manager facilitates conflict resolution in a formal manner when necessary. The manager negotiates consensus or compliance to conflict resolution outcomes or goals. Although the roles of leader and manager often appear in the same person, the leadership roles in conflict management are often more important to resolution and compliance. The manager has formal power that can be used when necessary, but it should be reserved for truly unmanageable or important issues.

Conflict Management and Change

Conflict management is an important part of the change process. Change can often threaten individuals and groups, so conflict is an inevitable part of the process. It is important to keep in mind that some conflicts resolve themselves, so the change agent should not be too quick to jump into an intervention mode. Figure 16.3 provides a guide for assessment of the level of conflict. A low conflict level supports change and encourages the healthy exchange of thoughts and ideas. This level of conflict is often resolved between individuals or between groups in an organization. Note that a conflict level that is too low may lead to complacency or a sense of dread regarding change. On the other hand, conflict that is too high

Real World Interview

Good manager and leader skills are essential for the workflow of a nursing department. As a nurse with 28 years' experience, a good manager must have consistent and equally fair follow through with all decisions that are made. This consistency is important from balancing the budget of the department, to the schedule, to reprimanding or praising staff. The team must respect the decisions of the manager. When the leader is consistent and equally fair, the team can thrive even if certain nurses think things are unfair. A great leader and team must be balanced, like our bodies, with acid/base and normal ph.

There was a situation where a charge nurse gave too many patients to a nurse. This situation was not resolved until days later when a significant group of nurses complained to the manager regarding the decision-making process of this charge nurse. That specific day, I believe the charge RN should have rearranged the staff to assist the triage nurse. The charge nurse should have consulted the doctor on duty in the emergency department to help decide what patients could be moved or discharged to elevate the unclogging of the triage area. The assistance of the house supervisor should have been utilized. The other nurses were busy, but instead of talking behind the charge nurse back, direct communication should have been established.

On this particular day, things were not consistent and equally fair—the way I feel leadership should be.

Kristi Holmes
Hammond, IN

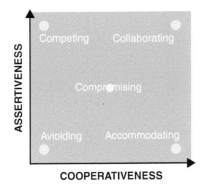

FIGURE 16.3 Guide for the assessment of level of conflict.
Source: Kilmann, T. & Thomas, K. (2009).

is not healthy, as it promotes anxiety and anger. It may dissolve into conflict that cannot be managed without drastic steps by the manager or change agent. These drastic steps may include a change in group composition or assignment of some members of the group to another type of project. Successful change may be difficult to achieve when groups or individuals have either too little or too high levels of conflict. It is the nurse manager's responsibility to assure that the conflict level is neither too low nor too high. Both of these levels of conflict can interfere with achievement of the objectives of the change project. Both change and conflict are positive processes that promote creativity, idea exchange, and innovation. Leaders, managers, and staff should be encouraged to embrace them and explore them as opportunities for positive growth development and professional expansion.

Crew Resource Management and TeamSTEPPS

Patient care, like other technically complex and high-risk fields, is a codependent process carried out by teams of individuals with advanced technical training who have varying roles and decision-making responsibilities. While technical training assures proficiency in specific tasks, it does not address the potential for errors created by poor communication and decision making in rapidly changing environments. Experts in the aviation industry have developed safety training focused on effective team management, known as **Crew Resource Management (CRM)**. Improvements in the safety record of commercial aviation may be due, in part, to this training. CRM training encompasses a wide range of knowledge, skills, and attitudes, including communication, assertiveness, situational awareness, problem solving, decision making, and teamwork.

TeamSTEPPS (AHRQ, 2013) is an evidence-based framework to optimize team performance across the health care delivery system. Building on more than 30 years of research, evidence has been accumulated on teams and team performance in aviation, the military, nuclear power, health care, business, and industry. TeamSTEPPS has evolved from research in these high stakes fields and CRM. TeamSTEPPS provides team strategies and tools to enhance performance and patient safety.

Four Teachable Skills

Built upon an evidenced-based framework, there are four teachable skills at the core of the model:

1. Communication
2. Leadership
3. Situation Monitoring
4. Mutual Support

From the TeamSTEPPS framework, several communication techniques are provided to enhance performance and promote safety. Sharing critical information that requires immediate attention and action can be presented to another health care provider in the SBAR format. Situation reflects what is going on with the patient. Background is the clinical background or context. Assessment refers to my assessment of the problem, what I think the problem is. Recommendation and Request includes what I think should be done to correct the problem. For example, Mr. Plum, who is in room 372, has extreme pain in the left leg (Situation). Mr. Plum is a 57-year-old male patient who underwent surgery earlier today to repair a crushing injury and fractures of the left fibula and tibia. Medical history for Mr. Plum is hypertension and current smoking 1 ppd (Background). Despite receiving his maximum allowed dose of IV push hydromorphone (Dilaudid) and IV acetaminophen (Ofirmev), Mr. Plum is still rating his pain as 9 or 10 on a scale of 0–10 (Assessment). I feel strongly that this patient should be assessed and evaluated for possible compartment syndrome; can you come to room 372 now please? (Recommendation and Request).

Communication

During emergency situations, a communication technique known as "**Call-Out**" is encouraged to communicate critical or important information. This technique informs all team members of the patient status simultaneously and allows the team to anticipate the next steps. For example, during the evaluation of a patient who is deteriorating during a Rapid Response situation, the team leader may call out "Airway?" and a team member will respond "Airway clear, oxygen saturation 88%." The team leader asks, "Breath sounds?" A nurse responds, "Clear to all lung fields." "Blood pressure?" the team leader calls out. A team member will respond loudly "92/56 left arm and dropping."

"**Check-Back**" is a closed loop communication technique which ensures that the message the sender intended was received by the intended recipient. The recipient acknowledges the communication by repeating back the information. During the above situation, the team leader may order "Start a liter 0.9 Normal Saline at 125 ml hr⁻¹ and get oxygen nasal cannula to bring oxygen saturation up to 90%." Team member replies "0.9 normal saline at 125 and oxygen nasal cannula to bring saturation to 90% or greater." Team leader confirms "That is correct!"

A final communication tool recommended by TeamSTEPPS is called "I PASS THE BATON." (Agency for Healthcare Research and Quality, 2019). See Table 16.11. This tool is intended for any handoff situation, for example at change of shift or transfer of a patient from one level of care to another.

Leadership

Leading teams in the second teachable skill in the TeamSTEPPS model. The **Brief** provides a list of responsibilities of effective team leaders as well as checklists for sharing the plan. Prior to the start, the team meets to share the plan, assign roles, establish expectations, and anticipate outcomes and issues. **Huddles** are encouraged throughout the process to monitor and modify the plan as needed (Figure 16.4). During the **Debrief** the team exchanges information about what went well, reinforcing these positive behaviors, and the team makes plans for improvement.

Situation Monitoring

Situation Monitoring is the third teachable skill involving continuous scanning and evaluation of what is going on around you. Four components of situation monitoring involve the patient, the team members, the environment, and the progress toward meeting the established goal. These four components of situation monitoring are summarized in the acronym STEP:

1. Status of the patient
2. Team members
3. Environment
4. Progress toward the goal

Involved in situation monitoring is a strategy called cross-monitoring, also known as "watching each other's back." By monitoring the actions of the team, mistakes can be prevented or can be caught quickly and remedied. Each team member has the responsibility to assess their own safety status using the I'M SAFE checklist:

- I = Illness
- M = Medications
- S = Stress
- A = Alcohol and drugs
- F = Fatigue
- E = Eating and Elimination

Evidence from the Literature

Source: Adapted from Bittle, M., O'Rourke, K., & Srinivas, S. K. (2018). Interdisciplinary skills review program to improve team responses during postpartum hemorrhage. *Journal of Obstetric, Gynecologic & Neonatal Nursing (JOGNN), 47*, 254–263. https://doi.org/10.1016/j.jogn.2017.09.002

Discussion: Clinical practice leaders and nursing faculty in a university-based hospital system in Pennsylvania undertook a quality improvement project to develop a standard hemorrhage protocol for a multidisciplinary comprehensive team. RNs, physicians, residents, advanced practice nurses, and ancillary staff completed the educational program consisting of online didactic modules, interactive skills stations, and simulation. After completing the training, team members reported an increased confidence and preparation for post-partum hemorrhage.

Implications for Practice:

Using simulation and an interprofessional approach, team members can become more confident and prepared for life saving situations.

Table 16.11 **I PASS THE BATON**

I	Introduction	"My name is Shenay and I am the nurse who has been for Jenny Brown for the past 8 hr."
P	Patient	"Jenny Brown is a 57-year-old female on the Ortho inpatient unit."
A	Assessment	"Earlier today, Jenny had an Open Reduction and Internal Fixation of her right leg following a crushing right leg injury in a car accident. Despite giving her Morphine 4 mg IVP and Toradol 30 mg IVP within the past hour, her pain is still a 10/10 in her right leg. Her BP is elevated 158/92, Heart rate is 102 BPM. She states the pain is 'worse than ever'. Her right full leg cast in intact. Her right toes are pale, cool, with capillary refill of 3 s."
S	Situation	"Her pain is increasing; her BP and Heart rate are rising. Her capillary refill, color and warmth to her right toes are worsening. I am worried she is developing compartment syndrome."
S	Safety concern	"She is a fall risk and is maintaining bed rest at this time. She is also at risk for Venous Thrombo Embolism (VTE)."
The		
B	Background	"Jenny has no previous hospital admissions other than three surgeries for c-sections 24, 26, and 30 years ago. She has hypertension and takes a low dose Beta blocker daily."
A	Actions	"I have removed the pillow from under her right leg. I have attempted to call the surgeon's cell phone, and also had the surgeon's answering service try to contact him. The Nursing House Supervisor is on her way to our Ortho unit."
T	Timing	"If the surgeon does not return my call within the next couple of minutes, I am going to call one of the Hospitalists to assess her state."
O	Ownership	"If the surgeon is not available, the Hospitalist can assume care for now."
N	Next	"Charge nurse Ron, could you please help me locate the cast saw so it is immediately available. UAP Sue, let's keep her NPO for now, just in case she needs to go to the OR for a fasciotomy."

Source: Adapted from: Agency for Healthcare Research and Quality. (2019, March). TeamSTEPPS Fundamentals Course: Module 3. Communication. Agency for Healthcare Research and Quality, Rockville, MD.

The final of the four teachable skills from TeamSTEPPS is Mutual Support. Helping others with their tasks builds a strong team. Team members must protect each other from situations where they are overloaded with work. Asking for help and offering help is part of patient safety and does not reflect the quality or capability of the team member who needs help. Team members expect that assistance will be sought and offered.

Ashley is a new RN and is halfway through her orientation on an inpatient oncology unit. Ashley, together with her preceptor, have just switched to working the midnight shift. After several midnight shifts, Ashley excitedly calls her former classmate and brags about the teamwork she has observed. The nurses working the midnight shift on this unit frequently ask each other how they are doing and if they need help. The unit generally becomes really busy 2 hr before their shift ends and everyone pitches in and helps each other. Needing help is not interpreted as something negative. Not one of the midnight nurses will leave until they have confirmed that everyone has finished their work. They all walk out to their cars together. Ashley is impressed with the mutual support and is thankful to be part of this team.

Mutual Support

Mutual support involves encouraging and re-directing through feedback. Providing information to the team members for the purpose of improving team performance is the definition of feedback. Feedback should be prompt, specific, respectful, directed toward improvement, and considerate of the feelings of the team member.

Evan works 12-hr rotating day and night shifts in the ICU, while Vanessa often works the shift opposite. Every time Evan receives report from Vanessa, she whines about how busy she was and how difficult the patients and their families were that shift. Regularly she left tasks for Evan to complete, tasks that she should have completed on her shift. For weeks, Evan has quietly listened to Vanessa complain and picked up after her. One day, in the nurses' station during shift change, Evan finally loses his temper and starts yelling at Vanessa, "What is your problem? You are always leaving things for me to finish! All I hear are your excuses. What do you do all day? Other than complain!"

Unfortunately, not all feedback is respectful, considerate, constructive, and timely. Evan should have addressed his concerns with Vanessa weeks ago. He should have brought his concerns to her privately and stated the observed facts without losing his temper. Evan might have softened his negative comments by sharing one or two positive instances while sharing the specific examples of Vanessa's negative behaviors. Feedback can motivate Vanessa to improve and provide excellent nursing care while strengthening the team of ICU nurses.

During patient care, there may be situations when a member of the team, such as a nurse, disagrees with recommendations or actions of a team member. Mutual support requires nurses to advocate for the patient and perhaps use assertive behavior. The Two-Challenge Rule empowers all members of the team to halt all activity if they sense or discover a breach of

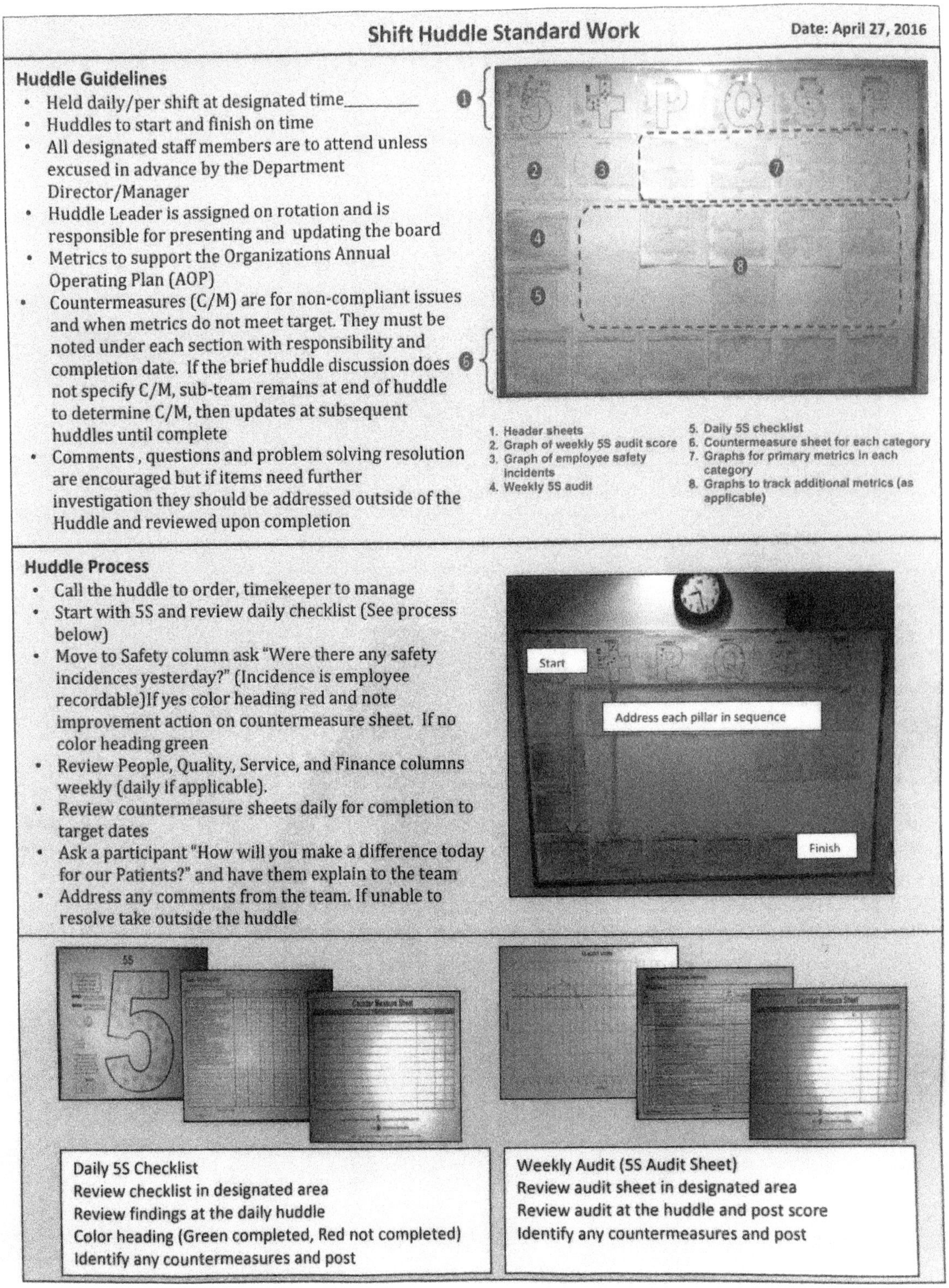

Shift Huddle Standard Work Date: April 27, 2016

Huddle Guidelines

- Held daily/per shift at designated time_____
- Huddles to start and finish on time
- All designated staff members are to attend unless excused in advance by the Department Director/Manager
- Huddle Leader is assigned on rotation and is responsible for presenting and updating the board
- Metrics to support the Organizations Annual Operating Plan (AOP)
- Countermeasures (C/M) are for non-compliant issues and when metrics do not meet target. They must be noted under each section with responsibility and completion date. If the brief huddle discussion does not specify C/M, sub-team remains at end of huddle to determine C/M, then updates at subsequent huddles until complete
- Comments, questions and problem solving resolution are encouraged but if items need further investigation they should be addressed outside of the Huddle and reviewed upon completion

1. Header sheets
2. Graph of weekly 5S audit score
3. Graph of employee safety incidents
4. Weekly 5S audit
5. Daily 5S checklist
6. Countermeasure sheet for each category
7. Graphs for primary metrics in each category
8. Graphs to track additional metrics (as applicable)

Huddle Process

- Call the huddle to order, timekeeper to manage
- Start with 5S and review daily checklist (See process below)
- Move to Safety column ask "Were there any safety incidences yesterday?" (Incidence is employee recordable)If yes color heading red and note improvement action on countermeasure sheet. If no color heading green
- Review People, Quality, Service, and Finance columns weekly (daily if applicable).
- Review countermeasure sheets daily for completion to target dates
- Ask a participant "How will you make a difference today for our Patients?" and have them explain to the team
- Address any comments from the team. If unable to resolve take outside the huddle

Daily 5S Checklist
Review checklist in designated area
Review findings at the daily huddle
Color heading (Green completed, Red not completed)
Identify any countermeasures and post

Weekly Audit (5S Audit Sheet)
Review audit sheet in designated area
Review audit at the huddle and post score
Identify any countermeasures and post

FIGURE 16.4 The huddle.
Source: Used with permission from P. Zemansky (2019).

safety. It is the responsibility of the team member to respectfully and assertively voice their concerns at least two times to ensure they have been heard. Assertive statements follow the CUS acronym.

- I am <u>C</u>oncerned.
- I am <u>U</u>ncomfortable.
- This is a <u>S</u>afety issue. Stop the line!

Managing and resolving conflict, a portion of the final teachable skill in the TeamSTEPPS model was covered earlier in this chapter.

TeamSTEPPS is not intended to replace clinical expertise. The knowledge, skills, and attitudes of teamwork will complement clinical expertise and improve patient outcomes . . . the foundation of teamwork builds on technical proficiency and protocol compliance.

In this chapter we focused on collaboration and effective team building within and between professions. The process of team development and the stages were considered and the advantages and disadvantages of teamwork are shared. The chapter also dissected formal and informal teams, components of a successful team, including workplace communication skills and conflict management. Tools for improving communication, strategies for teams, and tools to enhance performance and patient safety were introduced via the TeamSTEPPS model. As the leader and manager of assigned patients, the nurse is not only responsible for managing patient care but functioning as a member of a health care team and collaborating for high-quality patient care. As a registered nurse, you will always be part of a team. Learning how to be an effective part of a team is essential to you and your success, as well as optimal patient outcomes.

KEY CONCEPTS

- Effective teamwork and collaboration are essential to improving patient care outcomes.

- Teams and committees are formed for a variety of reasons, depending on the level of collaboration required or the specific purpose desired.

- Each team goes through the stages of a team process.

- Successful teamwork requires a conducive physical, social, and political environment for it to succeed.

- An effective team member must be proactive, be motivated, have a certain personal sense of purpose or mission, and possess personal and time management skills.

- Teams are affected by team size, status differences, and psychological safety.

- Guidelines for conducting meetings are useful when managing meetings.

- Successful teams work to avoid groupthink, which can cause the group to fail to analyze a problem.

- The team leader must possess effective communication skills, conflict resolution skills, and leadership skills.

- Great teams have clear goals, well-defined role delineation, organized processes that are outcomes oriented, and open and honest interpersonal relationships.

- Crew Resource Management training encompasses a wide range of knowledge, skills, and attitudes including communication, assertiveness, situational awareness, problem solving, decision making, and teamwork.

- Groupthink occurs when the desire for harmony and consensus overrides members' rational efforts to appraise a situation.

- Nurses rely on basic principles of communication.

- Trends, such as increasing diversity, an aging population, generational differences, illiteracy, and changing technology affect nursing practices.

- At the most basic level, communication involves a sender, a message, a receiver, and feedback. The input comes from visual, auditory, and kinesthetic stimuli.

- There are three levels of communication: intrapersonal, interpersonal, and public.

- Nurses may participate in chain, Y, wheel, circle, and all-channel communication networks and/or communicate through the grapevine.

- Nurses use linguistically appropriate services.

- Barriers to effective communication exist.

- Communication happens with patients, families, supervisors, coworkers, physicians, nurses, other health care workers, and mentors.

- Nurses must work to eliminate horizontal violence from the workplace.

- A clear medication reconciliation process helps to avoid errors and maintain patient safety.

- Conflict is a normal part of any change project and is often healthy and positive.

- Conflict comes from many sources, including value differences, fear, goal disagreement, and cultural differences.

- The four steps in the conflict management process are frustration, conceptualization, action, and outcomes.

- There are several strategies for conflict management. Clear, open communication is key. There must be commitment to conflict management.

- Useful tools for conflict management include a guide for the assessment of conflict and a guide for the assessment of the level of conflict.

- The techniques for conflict management include avoiding, accommodating, compromising, competing, negotiating, confronting, and collaborating.

- Conflict can move the change process along if it is handled well. Conflict can stop the change process if it is handled poorly or allowed to get out of control.

- TeamSTEPPS is an evidence-based framework to optimize team performance across the health care delivery system. TeamSTEPPS provides team strategies and tools to enhance performance and patient safety.

KEY TERMS

Ancillary services team
Brief
Call-out
Check-back
Collaboration
Communication
Conflict
Contingency teams
Coordinating team

Core team
Crew Resource Management (CRM)
Debrief
Grapevine
Groupthink
Horizontal violence
Huddles
Interpersonal communication
Interprofessional

Intrapersonal communication
Public Communication
SBAR
Situation monitoring
Support Services team
Team
TeamSTEPPS

REVIEW QUESTIONS

1. Based on the Tuckman and Jensen team process, what stage of team development is it when team members work harmoniously together, have open communication, take risks, and trust each other to complete assigned tasks?
   a. Forming
   b. Storming
   c. Norming
   d. Performing

2. A good leader does all except which of the following?
   a. Encourages open communication and interpersonal relationship
   b. Uses only an authoritative leadership style
   c. Actively listens to team members' concerns and opinions
   d. Clearly identifies goals, roles, and the team process

3. Which of the following are characteristics of a successful team? Select all that apply.
   a. They socialize outside of the work environment.
   b. They understand the role of each team member.
   c. They communicate effectively.
   d. They possess identical expertise.
   e. They have an explicit purpose.

4. A new RN has received a medication order from the physician that is higher than the maximum recommended dose. How should the nurse proceed?
   a. Refuse to give the medication since it is greater than the maximum dose.
   b. Inform the physician via text and then choose a lower, safe dose of the medication.
   c. Give the medication as ordered since the doctor probably intended to give a high dose.
   d. Call the physician and ask for confirmation of the ordered dose explaining that your reference materials state this is higher than the maximum recommended dose.

5. All but which of the following are steps to improve communication using the SBARR technique?
   a. Share the situation.
   b. Provide background information.
   c. Assure patient safety.
   d. Ask for a recommendation from the practitioner.

6. Nurses can proactively create a safe and happy workplace by using which techniques? Select all that apply.
   a. Engage in self-care activities.
   b. Exclude an individual from discussion.
   c. Name the problem, labeling horizontal violence, as appropriate.
   d. Use reflection to raise self-awareness.
   e. Withhold needed information.

7. Identify the least reliable form of communication on a nursing unit.
   a. The grapevine
   b. Minutes from a staff meeting
   c. A memo from the unit director
   d. A medical center newsletter

8. Select the best reason why change is necessary.
   a. To maintain the status quo
   b. To enhance the quality of health care
   c. To encourage staff turnover
   d. To increase the cost of patient care

9. What is often the most desirable conflict resolution technique?
   a. Avoiding
   b. Competing
   c. Negotiating
   d. Collaborating

10. Jose has just completed his first assessment of a critically ill patient in the ICU. He approached the physician about the patient and states that he is concerned about the patient's frequent coughing, night sweats, bloody sputum, and history of being homeless. Jose is concerned and shares with the physician that he thinks this is a safety issue and requests the patient be placed in isolation, tested, and treated for Tuberculosis. This is an example of which of the following TeamSTEPPS® techniques?
    a. SBARR
    b. Brief, Huddle, and Debrief
    c. Call-out
    d. CUS

REVIEW QUESTION ANSWERS

1. Answer: D is correct.
    (D) The performing stage occurs as the group shows cohesiveness and collaboration, when the group reaches maturity while maintaining interpersonal relationships. Forming is the first stage and involved are still exploring their purpose establishing team goals (A). Storming occurs as the group relaxes into more comfortable team settings and opposing opinions may arise (B). Norming occurs when the resistance of storming is overcome and the team overcomes (C).

2. Answer: B is correct.
    Rational: Good leaders will have open communication (A), be a good listener (C), and clearly identify goals, roles and team process (D) Good leaders will not have an authoritative style exclusively (B).

3. Answers B, C, and E are correct.
    Rational: A successful team will have a common purpose, assessment of the team's composition (B), clear communication (C), active participation, and an agreed upon action plan and ongoing assessment and evaluation (E). Socializing outside of the work environment (A) and possessing identical expertise (D) are not characteristics of a successful team.

4. Answer: D is correct.
    Rational: If a nurse has a concern, it should be shared with the provider at least 2 times (D). Therefore, (A), (B), and (C) are incorrect. The CUS acronym is a potential guideline. CUS: "I am concerned," "I am uncomfortable," and "This is a safety issue."

5. Answer: C is correct.
    Rational: Situation (A), Background (B), Assessment and Recommendation (D) is SBAR. Patient safety is not part of SBAR (C).

6. Answers A, B, and C are corect.
    Rational: Personal strategies to avoid horizontal violence and create a safe and happy workplace include engaging in self-care activities (A), engaging in reflective practices to raise your self-awareness about your own behaviors, beliefs, values, and attitudes (B), and naming the problem using the term, horizontal violence, as appropriate (C). Excluding an individual from discussion (D) and withholding needed information (E) will not create a safe and happy workplace.

7. Answer: A is correct.
    Rational: The **grapevine** is an informal avenue of communication in which rumors circulate. It ignores the formal chain of command and it often lacks accuracy (A). Therefore, minutes from a staff meeting, (B), a memo from the unit director (C), and a medical center newsletter are more effective forms of communication.

8. Answer: D is correct.
    Rational: The core team consists of nurses and unlicensed assistive personnel who provide direct and continuous care on the same unit to which the patient is assigned (D).
    The Ancillary Services team includes radiology technicians and phlebotomists who provide care for a limited time period (A). The Coordinating team involves nurse/unit managers who manage the care provided by the Core team (B). The Contingency team includes interprofessional health care providers who respond in emergency situations only (C).

9. Answer: A is correct.
    Rational: Open and honest communication is key to successful conflict management (A). Competing, avoiding, and confronting are commonly acknowledged techniques in conflict management (B, C, and D), but not key to successful management of conflict.

10. Answer: C is correct.
    Rational: CUS
    Call-Out is a method of communication used to share critical information with all team members simultaneously (A). Therefore, SBAR (A), a Brief, Huddle, and Debrief (B), and CUS (D) are incorrect.

REVIEW ACTIVITIES

1. Note a team of which you are a member. Have you ever seen groupthink operate in the team? What did you do?

2. Your nursing care manager has asked you to serve on a committee to explore how your unit might communicate more effectively. What elements of communication might affect the group's plan?

3. The charge nurse apologizes as she informs you that your assignment includes the "problem patient" on the unit. What communication skills will you use to enhance communication with this patient? How will you avoid barriers to communication?

4. Recall a conflict with which you have been involved in the clinical situation. Discuss each of the methods of conflict management identified in the chapter. Identify which ones would have worked. Did the conflict ever get resolved? How?

DISCUSSION POINTS

• During your last clinical experience, how was team work visible?

• Did you observe interprofessional teamwork during your last clinical experience? What were specialties of the health care team members involved?

• Imagine you are the nurse caring for a nonverbal elderly patient. The patient's daughter is very critical of the nursing care her mother is receiving and has confronted you. Review the conflict management techniques in Figure 16.3 and decide which technique may be appropriate for you at this time. Which technique would not be appropriate?

• During a clinical experience, a nursing student observes a health care provider yelling at one of the staff nurses. Which of the tips or strategies suggested by TeamSTEPPS would be appropriate to use in this situation?

DISCUSSION OF OPENING SCENARIO

1. Would you be ready at this point to accept the responsibility?
   Yes absolutely! Stretch yourself. This would be a great learning experience and will help to advance your career in the future. As an RN, you are expected to be a part of interprofessional teams.

2. How would you prepare yourself for this unfamiliar role?
   Pull out your Leadership and Management textbook from nursing school and review the chapters on teamwork and communication. Ask for a copy of the agenda for the next meeting. If the committee has met previously, ask for minutes from the previous meetings.

3. What qualities of skills do you need to possess to become a productive member of the team?
   Review the qualities of effective team members recommended by Covey (1989), including a personal sense of purpose or mission, being proactive and motivated, and possessing personal and time management skills.

EXPLORING THE WEB

- Visit the **Quality and Safety Education for Nurses (QSEN)** web site at qsen.org and search for the 6 QSEN competencies. Review the definition and **KSA's (Knowledge, Skills and Attitudes)** for teamwork and collaboration. Download the pdf version of the table containing the 6 QSEN competencies with KSAs. Accessed August 9, 2019.

- **National Council of State Boards of Nursing (NCSBN)** can be accessed at www.ncsbn.org/index.htm. Download the most current version of the NCLEX-RN Examination test plan. Review the content related to collaboration with interdisciplinary teams. Accessed August 9, 2019.

- Healthy People 2020 identifies health communication strategies and health information technology as goals. Go to www.healthypeople.gov/2020/topics-objectives/topic/health-communication-and-health-information-technology?_ga=2.27446204.1005427468.1565403010-33808072.1565403010 and review the objectives. How can you provide nursing care that meets these objectives? Objectives include providing easy to understand instructions and asking how a patient will follow instructions. Accessed August 9, 2019.

- Visit the following website www.franklincovey.com/Events/webcast-series.html, click on the picture of the 7 Habits of Highly Effective People webcast and watch the video (5:09 min). Now imagine your 80th Birthday party. Write your personal mission statement. Accessed August 9, 2019.

- **American Organization for Nursing Leadership (AONL)** has educational programs available for nurses who hope to advance their career in nursing leadership. Visit www.aonl.org/aonl-education and identify a course or webinar that interests you. Accessed August 9, 2019.

INFORMATICS

- Go to the Joint Commission website at www.jointcommission.org. Search for the National Patient Safety Goals and download the latest simplest version of the Hospital National Patient Safety Goals. Or if you hope to work in another type of facility, download the appropriate goals for that facility, such as Behavioral health, Home care, etc. Is communication or team work included in the goals? Think of a recent clinical experience. How are the RNs on the unit meeting the NPSG for communication on that unit? Is there room for improvement? Accessed August 9, 2019.

LEAN BACK

- What have you learned about yourself and your role as a team member?

- What can you do to become a better part of the interprofessional team at your facility? When you first went into nursing, did you ever realize how many other professions you would be working with in patient care settings?

REFERENCES

Agency for Healthcare Research and Quality. (2013). *TeamSTEPPS®2.0 pocket guide*. Retrieved from www.ahrq.gov/sites/default/files/wysiwyg/professionals/education/curriculum-tools/teamstepps/instructor/essentials/pocketguide.pdf

Agency for Healthcare Research and Quality. (2019, March). TeamSTEPPS Fundamentals Course: Module 3. Communication. Agency for Healthcare Research and Quality, Rockville, MD. Retrieved October 30, 2020, from https://www.ahrq.gov/teamstepps/instructor/fundamentals/module3/ig-communication.html

American Association of Colleges of Nursing (AACN). (2017). *Interdisciplinary education and practice*. Retrieved from www.aacnnursing.org/News-Information/Position-Statements-White-Papers/Interdisciplinary-Education-Practice

American Nurses Association. (2015). *Incivility, bullying, and workplace violence—ANA position statement*. Retrieved from www.nursingworld.org/practice-policy/nursing-excellence/official-position-statements/id/incivility-bullying-and-workplace-violence/

ANA Position Statement. (2015). Retrieved from www.nursingworld.org/practice-policy/nursing-excellence/official-position-statements/id/incivility-bullying-and-workplace-violence

Andersen, E. (2014). *21 quotes from Henry Ford on business, leadership and life.* Retrieved from www.forbes.com/sites/erikaandersen/2013/0/31/21-quotes-from-henry-ford-on-business-leadership-and-life/

Bittle, M., O'Rourke, K., & Srinivas, S. K. (2018). Interdisciplinary skills review program to improve team responses during postpartum hemorrhage. *Journal of Obstetric, Gynecologic & Neonatal Nursing (JOGNN)*, *47*, 254–263. doi:10.1016/j.jogn.2017.09.002

Brunt, B. (2015). Interprofessional education to promote collaboration. *Ohio Nurses Review*, *90*(4), 20–21.

Centers for Disease Control and Prevention. (2019). *What is health literacy?* Retrieved from www.cdc.gov/healthliteracy/learn/

Covey, S. (1989). *The 7 habits of highly effective people.* New York, NY: Fireside.

Darlow, B., Coleman, K., McKinlay, E., Donovan, S., Beckingsale, L., et al. (2015). The positive impact of interprofessional education: A controlled trial to evaluate a program for health professional students. *BMC Medical Education*, *15*, 98. doi:10.1186/s12909-015-0385-3

DuBrin, A. J. (2000). *The active manager.* United Kingdom: South-Western Publishing.

Eberhard, D. M., Simons, G. F., & Fennig, C. D.. (Eds.). (2019). *Ethnologue: Languages of the world* (22nd ed.). Dallas, TX: SIL International. Online version: www.ethnologue.com

Emich, C. (2018). Conceptualizing collaboration in nursing. *Nursing Forum*, *53*, 567–573. doi:10.1111/nuf.12287

Ford, Henry (1863–1947). Retrieved from www.goalcast.com/2017/12/24/henry-ford-quotes

Gabarro, J., & Kotter, J. P. (1993). Managing your boss. *Harvard Business Review*, 71, no. 3 (May–June) 150–157.

Institute for Healthcare Improvement. (2019). *Medication reconciliation to prevent adverse drug events.*

Janis, L. (1972). *Victims of groupthink.* Boston, MA: Houghton-Mifflin.

Kassinove, H. (2019). *How to recognize and deal with anger.* American Psychological Association. Retrieved from www.apa.org/helpcenter/recognize-anger

Katzenbach, J. R., & Smith, D. K. (2003). *The wisdom of teams: Creating the high-performance organization.* New York, NY: HarperCollins Publishers Inc.

Kilmann, T. & Thomas, K. (2009). *An Overview of the Thomas-Kilmann Conflict Mode Instrument (TKI).* Retrieved from: http://www.kilmanndiagnostics.com/overview-thomas-kilmann-conflict-mode-instrument-tki

Maharjan, P. (2018). *Communication patterns.* Businesstopia. Retrieved from www.businesstopia.net/communication/communication-patterns

McCarthy, N. (2018). *The world's most spoken languages.* Statista. Retrieved from www.statista.com/chart/12868/the-worlds-most-spoken-languages

McKibben, L. (2017). Conflict management: Importance and implications. *British Journal of Nursing*, *26*(2), 100–103. https://doi-org.pnw.idm.oclc.org/10.12968/bjon.2017.26.2.100

Merlino, J. (2017). *Communication: A critical healthcare competency.* Patient Safety and Quality Healthcare. Retrieved from www.psqh.com/analysis/communication-critical-healthcare-competency

Office for Civil Rights. (2017). *HITECH Act enforcement interim final rule.* U.S. Department of Health and Human Services. Retrieved from www.hhs.gov/hipaa/for-professionals/special-topics/hitech-act-enforcement-interim-final-rule/index.html

Polifko-Harris, K., & Anunciado, C. J. (2012). Effective team building. In P. Kelly & J. Tazbir (Eds.), *Nursing leadership and management* (pp. 267–282). Clifton Park, NY: Delmar.

Proliteracy. (2019). *Adult literacy facts.* Proliteracy. Retrieved from www.proliteracy.org/Adult-Literacy-Facts/gclid/EAIaIQobChMI-bPY0NrQ4QI-VjP7jBx2-oQkWEAAYASAAEgK_cfD_BwE

Society for Human Resource Management (SHRM). (2018). *Managing workplace conflict.* Retrieved from www.shrm.org/resourcesandtools/tools-and-samples/toolkits/pages/managingworkplaceconflict.aspx.

Taylor, R. (2016). Nurses' perceptions of horizontal violence. *Global Qualitative Nursing Research*, *3*. doi:10.1177/2333393616641002 Retrieved from www.ncbi.nlm.nih.gov/pmc/articles/PMC5342647

Tuckman, B. W. (1965). Developmental sequences in small groups. *Psychological Bulletin*, *63*, 384–399.

Tuckman, B. W., & Jensen, M. A. C. (1977). Stages of small group development revisited. *Group and Organizational Studies*, *2*, 419–427.

United States Census Bureau. (2018). *Older people projected to outnumber children for first time in U.S. history.* United States Census Bureau. Retrieved from www.census.gov/newsroom/press-releases/2018/cb18-41-population-projections.html

Wikipedia. (2020, October 28). Communication. Retrieved October 30, 2020, from https://en.wikipedia.org/wiki/Communication

Witt Sherman, D., Maitra, K., Gordon, Y., Simon, S., Olenick, M., et al. (2017). Illustrating and analyzing the processes of interprofessional collaboration: A lesson learned from palliative care in deconstructing the concept. *Journal of Palliative Medicine*, *20*(3). doi:10.1089/jpm.2016.0332

SUGGESTED READING

Agreli, H. F., Peduzzi, M., & Bailey, C. (2017). The relationship between team climate and interprofessional collaboration: Preliminary results of a mixed methods study. *Journal of Interprofessional Care*, *31*(2), 184–186. doi:10.1080/13561820.2016.1261098

Bedoya, P., Neuhausen, K., Dow, A. W., Brooks, E. M., Mautner, D., & Etz, R. S. (2018). Student hotspotting: Teaching the interprofessional care of complex patients. *Academic Medicine: Journal of the Association of American Medical Colleges*, *93*(1), 56–59. doi:10.1097/ACM.0000000000001822

Bentley, M., Freeman, T., Baum, F., & Javanparast, S. (2018). Interprofessional teamwork in comprehensive primary healthcare services: Findings from a mixed methods study. *Journal of Interprofessional Care*, *32*(3), 274–283. doi:10.1080/13561820.2017.1401986

Dahlke, S., Meherali, S., Chambers, T., Freund-Heritage, R., Steil, K., & Wagg, A. (2017). The care of older adults experiencing cognitive challenges: How interprofessional teams collaborate. *Canadian Journal on Aging = La Revue Canadienne Du Vieillissement*, *36*(4), 485–500. doi:10.1017/S0714980817000368

Dahlke, S., Steil, K., Freund-Heritage, R., Colborne, M., Labonte, S., & Wagg, A. (2018). Older people and their families' perceptions about their experiences with interprofessional teams. *Nursing Open*, *5*(2), 158–166. doi:10.1002/nop2.123

Darlow, B., McKinlay, E., Gallagher, P., Beckingsale, L., Coleman, K., et al. (2017). Building and expanding interprofessional teaching teams. *Journal of Primary Health Care*, 9(1), 29–33. doi:10.1071/HC16053

Duffy, P. A., Ronnebaum, J. A., Stumbo, T. A., Smith, K. N., & Reimer, R. A. (2017). Does including public health students on interprofessional teams increase attainment of interprofessional practice competencies? *The Journal of the American Osteopathic Association*, 117(4), 244–252. doi:10.7556/jaoa.2017.042

Feather, R. A., Carr, D. E., Garletts, D. M., & Reising, D. L. (2017). Nursing and medical students teaming up: Results of an interprofessional project. *Journal of Interprofessional Care*, 31(5), 661–663. doi:10.1080/1356182 0.2017.1322563

Fox, L., Onders, R., Hermansen-Kobulnicky, C. J., Nguyen, T.-N., Myran, L., Linn, B., & Hornecker, J. (2018). Teaching interprofessional teamwork skills to health professional students: A scoping review. *Journal of Interprofessional Care*, 32(2), 127–135. doi:10.1080/13561820.2017.1399868

Golom, F. D., & Schreck, J. S. (2018). The journey to interprofessional collaborative practice: Are we there yet? *Pediatric Clinics of North America*, 65(1), 1–12. doi:10.1016/j.pcl.2017.08.017

Gould, K., Day, K. H., & Barton, A. T. (2017). Changing student attitudes through interaction: Findings from an interprofessional workshop. *Journal of Interprofessional Care*, 31(4), 540–542. doi:10.1080/13561820.2017.1287165

Grohmann, B., Espin, S., & Gucciardi, E. (2017). Patients' experiences of diabetes education teams integrated into primary care. *Canadian Family Physician Medecin de Famille Canadien*, 63(2), e128–e136.

Haque, F., Daniel, M., Clay, M., Vredeveld, J., Santen, S., & House, J. B. (2017). The interprofessional clinical experience: Introduction to interprofessional education through early immersion in health care teams. *MedEdPORTAL: The Journal of Teaching and Learning Resources*, 13, 10564. doi:10.15766/mep_2374-8265.10564

Housley, C. L., Neill, K. K., White, L. S., Tedder, A. T., & Castleberry, A. N. (2018). An evaluation of an interprofessional practice-based learning environment using student reflections. *Journal of Interprofessional Care*, 32(1), 108–110. doi:10.1080/13561820.2017.1356808

Hudak, N. M., Melcher, B., & Strand de Oliveira, J. (2017). Preceptors' perceptions of interprofessional practice, student interactions, and strategies for interprofessional education in clinical settings. *The Journal of Physician Assistant Education: The Official Journal of the Physician Assistant Education Association*, 28(4), 214–217. doi:10.1097/JPA.0000000000000168

Hustoft, M., Biringer, E., Gjesdal, S., Abetamus, J., & Hetlevik, O. (2018). Relational coordination in interprofessional teams and its effect on patient-reported benefit and continuity of care: A prospective cohort study from rehabilitation centres in Western Norway. *BMC Health Services Research*, 18(1), 719. doi:10.1186/s12913-018-3536-5

Leclair, L. W., Dawson, M., Howe, A., Hale, S., Zelman, E., et al. (2018). A longitudinal interprofessional simulation curriculum for critical care teams: Exploring successes and challenges. *Journal of Interprofessional Care*, 32(3), 386–390. doi:10.1080/13561820.2017.1405920

Lockeman, K. S., Appelbaum, N. P., Dow, A. W., Orr, S., Huff, T. A., et al. (2017). The effect of an interprofessional simulation-based education program on perceptions and stereotypes of nursing and medical students: A quasi-experimental study. *Nurse Education Today*, 58, 32–37. doi:10.1016/j.nedt.2017.07.013

MacKenzie, D., Creaser, G., Sponagle, K., Gubitz, G., & MacDougall, P. (2017). Best practice interprofessional stroke care collaboration and simulation: The student perspective. *Journal of Interprofessional Care*, 31(6), 793–796. doi:10.1080/13561820.2017.1356272

McKibben, L. (2017). Conflict management: Importance and implications. *British Journal of Nursing (Mark Allen Publishing)*, 26(2), 100–103. doi:10.12968/bjon.2017.26.2.100

Meyer, B. A., Seefeldt, T. M., Ngorsuraches, S., Hendrickx, L. D., Lubeck, P. M., et al. (2017). Interprofessional education in pharmacology using high-fidelity simulation. *Currents in Pharmacy Teaching & Learning*, 9(6), 1055–1062. doi:10.1016/j.cptl.2017.07.015

Patel, S., O'Brien, B. C., Dulay, M., Earnest, G., & Shunk, R. L. (2018). Team retreats for interprofessional trainees and clinic staff: Accelerating the development of high-functioning teams. *MedEdPORTAL: The Journal of Teaching and Learning Resources*, 14, 10786. doi:10.15766/mep_2374-8265.10786

Peeters, M. J., Sexton, M., Metz, A. E., & Hasbrouck, C. S. (2017). A team-based interprofessional education course for first-year health professions students. *Currents in Pharmacy Teaching & Learning*, 9(6), 1099–1110. doi:10.1016/j.cptl.2017.07.006

Rousseau, C., Pontbriand, A., Nadeau, L., & Johnson-Lafleur, J. (2017). Perception of interprofessional collaboration and co-location of specialists and primary care teams in youth mental health. *Journal of the Canadian Academy of Child and Adolescent Psychiatry = Journal de l'Academie Canadienne de Psychiatrie de l'enfant et de l'adolescent*, 26(3), 198–204.

Schug, V., Finch-Guthrie, P., & Benz, J. (2018). Interprofessional education and team-based learning in a research methods course. *Nursing Education Perspectives*, 39(6), 380–382. doi:10.1097/01.NEP.0000000000000264

Smith, T., Fowler-Davis, S., Nancarrow, S., Ariss, S. M. B., & Enderby, P. (2018). Leadership in interprofessional health and social care teams: A literature review. *Leadership in Health Services (Bradford, England)*, 31(4), 452–467. doi:10.1108/LHS-06-2016-0026

Sonke, J., Pesata, V., Lee, J. B., & Graham-Pole, J. (2017). Nurse perceptions of artists as collaborators in Interprofessional care teams. *Healthcare (Basel, Switzerland)*, 5(3). doi:10.3390/healthcare5030050

Stone, R. (2017). Interprofessional learning: Benefits for healthcare teams and patients. *British Journal of Nursing (Mark Allen Publishing)*, 26(10), 571. doi:10.12968/bjon.2017.26.10.571

Ulrich, B., & Crider, N. M. (2017). Using teams to improve outcomes and performance. *Nephrology Nursing Journal: Journal of the American Nephrology Nurses' Association*, 44(2), 141–151.

Vogel, M. T., Abu-Rish Blakeney, E., Willgerodt, M. A., Odegard, P. S., Johnson, E. L., et al. (2018). Interprofessional education and practice guide: Interprofessional team writing to promote dissemination of interprofessional education scholarship and products. *Journal of Interprofessional Care*, 1–8. doi:10.1080/13561820.2018.1538111

Wellmon, R., Lefebvre, K. M., & Ferry, D. (2017). Effects of high-Fidelity simulation on physical therapy and nursing Students' attitudes toward interprofessional learning and collaboration. *The Journal of Nursing Education*, 56(8), 456–465. doi:10.3928/01484834-20170712-03

Young, G. J., Cohen, M. J., Blanchfield, B. B., Jones, M. M., Reidy, P. A., & Weinstein, A. R. (2017). Assessing Interprofessional education in a student-faculty collaborative practice network. *Education for Primary Care: An Official Publication of the Association of Course Organisers, National Association of GP Tutors, World Organisation of Family Doctors*, 28(4), 223–231. doi:10.1080/14739879.2017.1298406

Members of the Interprofessional Team

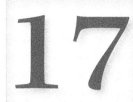

17

Patrick D. Reed[1], Bryan J. Camus[2]
[1] College of Nursing, Purdue University Northwest, Hammond, IN, USA
[2] Charity/Delgado School of Nursing, New Orleans, LA, USA

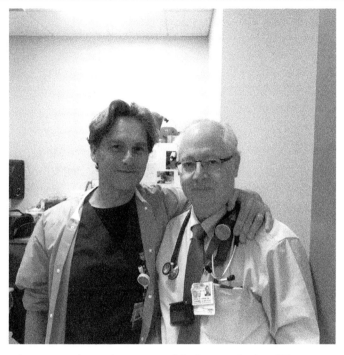

Physicians and nurses work together as part of the Interprofessional Team.
Source: Photo used with permission from Dr. Michael O'Connor and Johnny Tazbir

"Alone we can do so little; together we can do so much." Helen Keller (1888) in Lash, J. P. (1981) p. 489.

OBJECTIVES

Upon completion of this chapter, the reader should be able to:

1. Define the concept of a team.

2. Identify QSEN competency of team work and collaboration.

3. Identify members of a team.

4. Discuss advantages and disadvantages of teamwork.

5. Define key concepts of creating an effective team.

6. Define the stages of a team process.

7. Identify the qualities of an effective team leader.

8. Discuss the concept of teamwork environment.

9. Discuss crew resource management.

Kelly Vana's Nursing Leadership and Management, Fourth Edition. Edited by Patricia Kelly Vana and Janice Tazbir
© 2021 John Wiley & Sons Ltd. Published 2021 by John Wiley & Sons Ltd.
Companion Website: www.wiley.com/go/kelly-Nursing-Leadership

OPENING SCENARIO

You are a new graduate nurse who has six months of clinical experience working on an oncology unit. Your nurse manager has observed your skill and compassion for terminally ill patients and your warm interaction and interpersonal relationship with the other staff nurses on the unit. Complimenting you on your skills and personal work ethic, the nurse manager has also asked if you would be interested in joining the Interdisciplinary Cancer Support Committee to help address pain management and other issues to improve patient care. If you accept this responsibility, this will be your first committee membership.

1. How would you respond to this request?

2. Would you be ready at this point to accept the responsibility?

3. How would you prepare yourself for this unfamiliar role?

4. What qualities or skills do you need to possess to become a productive member of the team?

We begin this chapter by considering the question, what is a team? A **team** is:

A group of people with a full set of complementary skills required to complete a task, job, or project. Team members (a) operate with a high degree of interdependence, (b) share authority and responsibility for self-management, (c) are accountable for the collective performance, and (d) work toward a common goal and shared reward(s). A team becomes more than just a collection of people when a strong sense of mutual commitment creates synergy, thus generating performance greater than the sum of the performance of its individual members (team).

Source: Wikapedia. (2020, October 23). Team. Retrieved November 10, 2020, from https://en.wikipedia.org/wiki/Team.

Quality and Safety in Nursing Education (QSEN) (2019) defines the importance of teamwork in nursing as intricately woven into the function of nurses within nursing and in interprofessional relations to achieve a common goal of excellence in patient care. Contrasting the concept of a group versus a team, Oalkey, Felder, Brent, and Elhhaij (2004) state "With a group, the whole is often equal to or less than the sum of its parts; with a team, the whole is always greater" (p. 13). While the article is a little dated, the concept is relevant today. In health care, teams exist at all levels to provide care for patients. There are roles for each member and differing levels of expertise. Each role is critical to the mission and goal of the team, thus the whole is greater than the sum of its parts. Consider a hospital code team, a group of people with expertise in providing advanced life support for a patient experiencing cardiopulmonary arrest. The team consist of a **licensed independent practitioner** (LIP), registered nurses, and a respiratory technician. An **LIP** is a person that may independently practice and prescribe under their license in a given state. Other members may include a **certified registered nurse anesthetist** (CRNA), phlebotomy, r-ray technical, clerical support, and the house supervisor. Other examples of teams are Stroke Teams, Trauma Teams, and Rapid Response Teams, and each may comprise different members to best facilitate the team's purpose. In this chapter we will explore many aspects of teams and creating an effective team. We will also explore the stages of the team process, crew resources management, and the qualities of an effective leader.

Roles

Each role in a team is decided based on the skill of the team members and the specific task required to achieve the mission and goal of the team. In a code team, an expert in **advanced cardiac life support** (ACLS) would most likely be the team leader. Depending on the situation of the event, this person might be a physician, a nurse practitioner, a registered nurse, or any other individual who is ACLS certified. The defined roles in ACLS are specific to the function of the team. The functional roles/positions in an ACLS team are: (a) team leader, (b) compressor (the person(s) providing chest compressions), (c) monitor/defibrillator, (d) airway management, (e) medications (IV/IO), and (f) recorder (**American Hospital Association,** (AHA), 2014). In team building, priority is always given to the person with the highest level of training in the field. Usually, the LIP (a physician, nurse practitioner, or physician assistant), trained in ACLS, would be the leader but this is not always the case. Expertise and experience are the critical components of any team.

QSEN

According to QSEN, nurses must acquire and maintain competencies to engage interprofessional teams for better patient outcomes (QSEN, 2019). QSEN identifies three competencies required by nurses: (a) knowledge, (b) skills, and (c) attitudes (see Table 17.1). Understanding these competencies entails a bit of self-reflection. Knowledge refers to one's knowledge of self, values, expectations, strength, and limitations (QSEN, 2019). Individuals must be skilled at using their strengths and limitations to leverage the goal of the team in favor of the patient and support of members of the team. Team members' attitude must be conducive to the mission. Honesty

Table 17.1   Quality and Safety in Education for Nurses: Teamwork and Collaboration

Definition: Function effectively within nursing and interprofessional teams, fostering open communication, mutual respect, and shared decision making to achieve quality patient care.

Knowledge	Skills	Attitudes
Describe own strengths, limitations, and values in functioning as a member of a team	Demonstrate awareness of own strengths and limitations as a team member Initiate plan for self-development as a team member Act with integrity, consistency and respect for differing views	Acknowledge own potential to contribute to effective team functioning Appreciate importance of intra- and interprofessional collaboration
Describe scopes of practice and roles of health care team members Describe strategies for identifying and managing overlaps in team member roles and accountabilities Recognize contributions of other individuals and groups in helping patient/family achieve health goals	Function competently within own scope of practice as a member of the health care team Assume role of team member or leader based on the situation Initiate requests for help when appropriate to situation Clarify roles and accountabilities under conditions of potential overlap in team member functioning Integrate the contributions of others who play a role in helping patient/family achieve health goals	Value the perspectives and expertise of all health team members Respect the centrality of the patient/family as core members of any health care team Respect the unique attributes that members bring to a team, including variations in professional orientations and accountabilities
Analyze differences in communication style preferences among patients and families, nurses, and other members of the health team Describe impact of own communication style on others Discuss effective strategies for communicating and resolving conflict	Communicate with team members, adapting own style of communicating to needs of the team and situation Demonstrate commitment to team goals Solicit input from other team members to improve individual, as well as team, performance Initiate actions to resolve conflict	Value teamwork and the relationships upon which it is based Value different styles of communication used by patients, families and health care providers Contribute to resolution of conflict and disagreement
Describe examples of the impact of team functioning on safety and quality of care Explain how authority gradients influence teamwork and patient safety	Follow communication practices that minimize risks associated with handoffs among providers and across transitions in care Assert own position/perspective in discussions about patient care Choose communication styles that diminish the risks associated with authority gradients among team members	Appreciate the risks associated with handoffs among providers and across transitions in care
Identify system barriers and facilitators of effective team functioning Examine strategies for improving systems to support team functioning	Participate in designing systems that support effective teamwork	Value the influence of system solutions in achieving effective team functioning

Source: Cronenwett, L., Sherwood, G., Barnsteiner J., Disch, J., Johnson, J., Mitchell, P., Sullivan, D., Warren, J. (2007). Cronenwett, L., Sherwood, G., Barnsteiner J., Disch, J., Johnson, J., Mitchell, P., Sullivan, D., Warren, J. (2007). Quality and safety education for nurses. Nursing Outlook, 55(3)122–131. Quality and Safety Education for Nurses. (2019). *Team work and collaboration.* Retrieved from http://qsen.org/competencies/pre-licensureksas/#teamwork_collaboration.

and integrity are critical to positive contributions and success of the team. According to QSEN, team members must "Appreciate [the] importance of intra-and interprofessional collaboration" (QSEN, 2019, Cronenwett, L., et al. (2007) Table 17.1).

Leadership Competencies

Understanding leadership competencies is necessary when working in a team, as it relates to the various roles and skills required. Team members must have knowledge of their scope of practice as well as the scopes of their team mates (QSEN, 2019).

QSEN continues to stress that team members must show respect for one another and the scope of practice for each member. This must be demonstrated in attitude toward one another. In any health care team, the "respect [for] the centrality of the patient/family as core members of the team" must be evident (QSEN, 2019, Cronenwett, L., et al. (2007) see Table 17.1).

Leadership on the Nursing Unit

Another example of a team is the organization of the patient care team on a nursing unit. Managers/directors are deemed

Case Study 17.1

Amanda is in orientation and is asked to review (Table 17.1) Quality and Safety in Education for Nurses: Teamwork and Collaboration and review the knowledge, skills, and attitudes. She reads, "Explain how authority gradients influence teamwork and patient safety" and states, "I don't know what that means?"

- How do you define the "authority gradients influence" at your institution?
- Are the roles and their authorities clearly understood?
- How would you explain this to Amanda?

Critical Thinking 17.1

1. What teams have you been a part of in the past?
2. What are the similarities and differences in becoming a part of an interprofessional team versus the other teams you have been on?

---

to be those individuals with effective critical thinking skills in patient care, organizational management, and team leadership (Sullivan, 2013). A leader is one who inspires, supports, and empowers other individuals with supportive roles on the team. The leader develops and promotes the vision and mission for the team/unit. Their ability to transmit their enthusiasm, energy, and passion for the task at hand is derived from their ability to harness the strength of **emotional intelligence** (EI). EI refers to the ability to harness and focus the strengths of human emotions (Goleman, 2005). For leaders, EI enhances the skill to lead effectively by encouraging, inspiring, and empowering others. Key components of EI are: (a) self-awareness, (b) self-regulation, (c) social skills (recognition of other's emotion), (d) empathy, and (e) motivation (Cherry, 2018).

Roles and Expectations

If the focus of nursing is patient-centered care then, in order to achieve that patient–centered focus, nurses must team with other professionals to provide the holistic care so intrinsic to nursing's philosophy. Interprofessional team work requires that each discipline acknowledges one another with respect and compassion. No matter what role an individual fulfills on a team, the communication must be clear, direct, and respectful. This means being aware of one's own communication style and striving to adapt it to the needs of the team.

Physicians

Physicians invest many years of intense study and training. Typically, a person studying for a physician's license will spend 4 years as an undergraduate studying the biological sciences (JAMA, 2019). Once students complete the 4-year degree, they progress to medical school where more intense studying with practical training occurs. But it doesn't end with medical school. New physicians usually complete a residency program focusing on a specialty such as psychiatry, medicine, surgery, or a host of other specialties. Physicians may spend

---

Critical Thinking 17.2

Where do you rank with EI? Cherry (2018) provides a simple test to get an idea of your EI. To test your EI:

1. How did you rank?
2. What did you learn about yourself?
3. What can you improve?

Who is the "leader?" The leader is not always the person in charge and not always synonymous with the manager. The best leaders are those on the team who demonstrate the ability to engage others in supporting the mission and vision of the team/ organization. In general, the hope is that this person would be the designated person with the title of leader, such as the supervisor, manager, or director, but it could be the unit secretary, nursing assistant, or others in the nursing team that possess the skills to engage others. The concept of leader can be situation, official,

or unofficial. An effective leader/manager identifies these individuals (Jenson, 2013). An effective manager should quickly recognize those with experience in order to optimize team effectiveness. An example of this would be the manager who notes the leadership abilities of a new graduate and sends the nurse to class to learn how to become a charge nurse and offers them a position on the skin care team. Another example would be the manager who notices how the other members of the staff frequently refer to the unit secretary for advice and support on the unit. The unit secretary has gained the respect and admiration from the other team members. If the manager is planning change in a process for the unit, it would be a good idea to speak with the unit secretary and get buy-in to help the other members of the team actively engage in the change.

Evidence From the Literature

Source: Adapted from Golom, F. D., & Schreck, J. S. (2018). The Journey to Interprofessional Collaborative Practice: Are We There Yet? *Pediatric Clinics of North America*, 65(1), 1–12. https://doi.org/10.1016/j.pcl.2017.08.017

Discussion: **Interprofessional collaborative practice** (IPCP) is a service delivery approach that seeks to improve health care outcomes and the patient experience while simultaneously decreasing health care costs. The current article reviews the core competencies and current trends associated with IPCP, including challenges faced by health care practitioners when working on interprofessional teams. Several conceptual frameworks and empirically supported interventions from the fields of organizational psychology and organization development are presented to assist health care professionals in transitioning their teams to a more interprofessionally collaborative, team-based model of practice.

Implications for Practice:

Core competencies of IPCP give direction and scope to interprofessional teams. Even though competencies exist, we must continually look for ways to better the interprofessional teams to ultimately improve outcomes and decrease cost.

as long as 16 years training in their profession (JAMA, 2019). Physician Fellows spend an intense focused training within a specialty such as pulmonology. By virtue of their advanced medical training, the role of physician is indispensable when discussing various types of teams related to patient-centered care. On a hierarchical level, medical students perform exams and simple procedures, residents are MDs and prescribe orders, and fellows have completed residency and are specializing in a given field. Attendings are MDs that have completed their fellowship. Attendings have the final word on medical and surgical care of their patients.

Physician Assistant

Physician Assistants (PA) play a similar role as the nurse practitioner but with greater oversight by a physician. The PA is an extension of the physician role in clinics and hospitals. The advanced training of the PA can be a significant contribution to the health care team when physicians are not available. PA training consists of a master's degree in science and includes 2–3 years of didactic education combined with a minimum of 2000 hr of clinical experience in hospitals or clinics. Once the education component is completed, the graduate must be successful in a licensure exam (Healthcare Systems, 2019). In some states, PAs and **Nurse Practitioners** (NPs) are required to have a Collaborate Agreement with a physician to practice, while in other states they do not. A Collaborate Agreement is a legal binding agreement, passed by the state legislature, detailing the relationship between the PA or NP and becomes part of the scope of practice.

Nurse

The profession of nursing continues to grow as nurses expand their scope through research and education. The Nurse Practitioner is prepared to adapt to expanding access to care for all people, in particular those in rural or inner-city areas. The NP can relieve the heavy burden of too many patients per physician and introduces the nursing philosophy of holistic care to diagnosing and treating patients' medical conditions. A minimum education requirement for NPs is a master's degree with extensive clinical practice. In many universities, the NP education has been elevated to the Doctor of Nursing Practice level.

A CRNA practices in surgery under the supervision of an Anesthesiologist. CRNAs fill a critical role in preparing patients for surgical and other medical procedures in hospitals, in out-patient surgical clinics, and in many rural areas where there are few or no anesthesiologist (http://NursingLicensure.org, 2019).

Certified Nurse Midwifes (CNW) are registered nurses specifically trained in the care of women's reproductive systems and child birth, which include services such as gynecological services, reproductive health visits, regular gynecologic care, and post-menopausal care (ACNM, 2011). Nursing has some way to go before the **Advanced Practice Registered Nurse** (APRN) role is fully appreciated and supported but the data continues to support the APRN role as an IP (The Future of Nursing, 2010).

Nurse Managers, Directors, and Supervisors provide leadership and management within hospital teams and other healthcare organizations. These nurses bring leadership skills in building a team, negotiating, and resolving conflicts. Leadership is the road map to where the team is going; better healthcare for all. **Transformational leadership theory** (TLT) is the theory introduced by James Burns, a researcher, in his research on political leaders in 1978. The theory emphasizes the importance of the relationship between the leader and followers. TLT has a direct relationship to the concept of EI. Sullivan (2013) states "Transformation leaders inspire followers and uses power to instill a belief that followers also have the ability to do exceptional things" (p. 43). Leaders with strong EI rely on their ability to develop positive relationships with the people under their leadership.

Licensed Vocational Nurse

The role of the **Licensed Vocational Nurse** (LVN) or Licensed Practical Nurse is often minimized and yet these professionals contribute to the health and sanity of the patient care area. Their training is specific and practical or clinical, but no less valuable than any other health care team member. There is a place in health care and health care teams for all professionals charged with the care of people. LVNs are educated to care for patients with predictable outcomes. They excel in organizational skills and the care of multiple patients. They may administer medications and perform sterile procedures. Laws regarding intravenous medications and blood administration vary from state to state. They cannot perform initial assessments and initial care plans. RNs may delegate to LVN's.

Unlicensed Personnel

Unlicensed personnel (UP or UAP) such as clerical staff, medical technicians, and certified nursing assistants, also known as Patient Care Technicians, play vital roles in providing the basic needs of patients and support of the team. Training varies with the roles and between institutions. In general, UPs are unable to assess, plan, or evaluate care. They may only do what has been delegated to them and they have been trained to do so. They are often the eyes and ears on medical/surgical units and psychiatric units. Their service is vital to the health outcomes of patients and staff; therefore, their role on teams is very important.

Case Manager

The Case Manager is a trained individual certified in providing ancillary care for patients in clinics and post hospital discharge (AIHCP, 2006). The Academy of Case Management offers certification and fellowship programs to train healthcare professionals (AICHP, 2006). Case Managers play a vital role on health care teams, providing advanced knowledge navigating the health care systems for patients and family.

Other Members

Other members of the health care team are respiratory therapists and chaplains. **Respiratory Therapists** (RTs) are trained and licensed individuals in the care of the human respiratory system. Training for a respiratory therapist is a minimum of 2 years in an accredited college or community college (American Association for Respirstory Care (AARC), 2018). The respiratory technician, under the orders of an LIP and observations of a register nurse, provides care ranging from inhalation therapy to advanced mechanical ventilation for critical patients (AARC, 2018). Depending on the hospital or setting, RTs assess the pulmonary status, administer treatments, manage ventilators, and intubate and extubate.

Hospital Chaplains play an integral role on health care teams and care of patients. When people are ill, they face frightening and stressful moments. Chaplains support patients and hospital staff, helping them navigate religious and faith-based concerns and challenges (Donohue, et al., (2017). Chaplains are trained professionally according to their faith denomination or religious background. Chaplains often are able to assist in power of attorney and living will forms, as well as the spiritual needs of patients and families.

The members of the interprofessional team have been discussed, but the list is not complete and may differ from hospital to hospital. No matter what the composition of the interprofessional team, to understand their education and role within the team is paramount.

Advantages and Disadvantages of Teamwork

Teamwork has the potential to bring people closer, creating synergy in developing ideas and methods to accomplish a specific goal. Increased productivity can be enhanced when team members are cohesive in their purpose (Sullivan, 2013, p. 151). According the Sullivan, this is particularly true when the individuals share ". . . interests, values, attitudes, and back-

---

Real World Interview

As an RN in a surgical **intensive care unit** (ICU), interprofessional collaboration and teamwork are necessary to care for patients. To provide care to a patient we have to look at all aspects of patient care—what prescribed mobility limitations are in place (physical therapy), what medications the patient is receiving (pharmacy), how stable or unstable the patient is (medical team), the oxygen requirements they are on (respiratory therapy), and more, even before we step foot in a patient's room. This requires us to collaborate and communicate with all the health care professionals on the patient's team—including other nurses, physicians, respiratory therapists, occupational therapists, and pharmacists to name a few.

Nurses are in the center of the circle with the patient and their family as we communicate most closely with the other members of the team. Each of our professions interact with the same goals in mind: to provide the best available care and outcomes for our patients. I can't imagine an hour in a day without communicating with another professional regarding my patients and am so relieved I have so many other minds to collaborate with.

Janice Tazbir RN
Crown Point, IN

Table 17.2 **Members of the Team**

Title	Role & Expectations	Education & Training	Examples in a Team
Medical Student	Observe and assist physicians	Undergraduate degree, currently in medical school	Support and observation
Residents	Licensed Independent Practitioner (LIP) in advanced training program	Depends on the specialty. 2–5 years is normal	Function as LIP under the direction of an attending physician faculty
Physician Fellow	Advanced specialty training as an LIP	Intense specialty training under an attending physician faculty	Performs as a leader on a team with observation from the attending physician
Attending Physician	Primary medical lead in patient care issues	Has completed the above education May not have participated in a fellowship	Lead medical authority in patient care matters regarding medical decisions
Physician Assistant (PA)	LIP under the authority of an attending physician	Master's degree in science, 2–3 years didactic education and a minimum of 2000-hr clinical experience	Can function as a leader of a team providing medical advice and direction
Nurse Practitioner	Advanced Practice Registered Nurse. Consider an LIP with advanced nursing and medical contribution to patient care	Current license as a registered nurse plus master's or doctorate training in advance medical and nursing education. A minimum of 2000-hr clinical experience under the direct of an attending physician Collaboratory agree with an attending physician required in some states	Provide advanced nursing skills as member of a team. Can perform primary leadership role
Certified Registered Nurse Anesthetist (CRNA)	Advanced Practice Registered Nurse Consider an LIP with Provides advanced nursing contribution to patient care, anesthesia, pain management	Advance Practice Registered Nurse with master's or doctorate level training in Anesthesiology	Provide advanced nursing skills as member of a team Can perform primary leadership role
Certified Nurse Midwife (CNW)	Advanced Practice Registered Nurse Consider an LIP with Provides advanced nursing contribution to patient care, labor. and delivery and postpartum care	Advanced nursing care at the master's or doctorate level specializing in Labor, Delivery, and Postpartum care	Contributes advanced knowledge and skills within their specialty and leadership skills.
Nurse Managers, Directors, Supervisors, Clinical Nurse Specialist	Provide direct nursing care and leadership in a health care environment	Registered Nurse licensed by the state of residence Basic nursing education at the Diploma (3-year hospital-based training), Associate Degree (2-year program with some college training), Baccalaureate (4-year degree in nursing), master's or doctorate level.	Provides team building skills and leadership on healthcare teams
Licensed Vocational Nurse/Licensed Practical Nurse	Provide support role and patient care under the direction of a registered nurse	Licensed nurses at the 3-year basic hospital trained level The scope of practice is less than the degreed registered nurse	Participate in patient care teams as integral members of the nursing workforce.
Case Manager	Provides support to the medical, nursing, patient, and family in post-hospitalization needs	May be a registered nurse but not necessarily Advanced training and certification available	Provide expert advice to help patient and staff navigate post-discharge care and clinic management

(Continued)

Table 17.2   (Continued)

Title	Role & Expectations	Education & Training	Examples in a Team
Respiratory Therapist	Provides respiratory care for the patients	Respiratory therapist are licensed individuals trained in the care and management of patient respiratory status. The care may range from inhalation therapy to managing patient on respiratory devices such as ventilator assisted care	Respiratory therapist play an important role on various teams such Intensive Care and Cardio-pulmonary arrest teams
Hospital Chaplain	Hospital Chaplains have a significant role in assisting patients and families with emotional and spiritual support	Hospital Chaplains may be from any of the many denominations and religious groups. Training is based on the particular religion's requirements	Chaplains provide and spiritual and emotional perspective of the patient, families, and staff on health care teams

Source: Table created by P. Reed & B. Camus.

ground factors" (p. 151). Creating an effective team is paramount to effective teamwork.

On the other hand, when team members are not cohesive or have dissimilar goals, conflicts are sure to arise. The results can be delays in goal achievement, ill feelings among members, and/or some members not living up to their commitment to the team goals. The effects on the organization might be increased cost of projects and possible loss of employees.

Team leaders must be sensitive to the collective mood and atmosphere among the team members and take positive steps to intervene as quickly as possible when signs of diversity or other barriers arise. Effective leaders are skilled in the techniques of conflict resolution. A leader with a high level of EI may be more effective at using the concepts of Transformational Leadership to resolve conflicts and move forward with a common goal. The core of Transformational Leadership is goal oriented more strongly than rule orientation (Jacobs et al., 2013). The ability to perceive blatant on hidden barriers, be they system barriers or situational barriers, is a critical competency of individuals working in teams (QSEN, 2019). It is incumbent on the leaders and all team members to value and support the system that promotes the advancement of patient-centered care, the goal of health care teams.

Creating an Effective Team

Team building is a process. Cardinal (2015) lists five steps necessary to consider when building teams. These five stages are: (a) forming, (b) storming, (c) norming, (d) performing, and (e) adjourning. The team building process begins with a clear definition of the goals of the project/activity to be performed. Shoaib and Kohli's (2017) research on goal setting indicates that clarity increases team satisfaction and engagement. Their research further indicates the more challenging the goal, the greater the team members/employee's engagement. "Goals are related to affect in that goals set the primary standards for

---

Critical Thinking 17.3

Hospital Compare (www.medicare.gov/hospitalcompare) identifies your organization as falling below the national benchmark in communication with patients. Forming a team to address the deficiency, you ask one of the nurses to be on the team.

Describe the critical aspects of being part of a team that you need to know in being an active contributor to the team. Being part of team requires members to know their skills, their limits, their temperament. Team members are experts in their area of practice and should demonstrate respect for the professional knowledge of other disciplines on the team. Together, these characteristics provide a path to build trust and high-quality interpersonal communication.

Another quality of being part of a team is the ability to negotiate and compromise. Every member of a team has their own understanding and unique interpretation, as well as ideas to effect change. The roles are different and so the communications may be different, but each member must demonstrate advanced skill of good communication. The knowledge of a nurse is not that of a respiratory therapist, radiologist, or LIP and vice versa. Ultimately every team member has a unique role. Understanding, respecting, and supporting each role is critical to building an effective interprofessional team.

How will you better understand, respect, and support each role on the interprofessional teams you are a part of?

self-satisfaction with performance" (Shaib & Kohli, 2017, p. 1). Thus, Goal Setting Theory is applicable to the discussion of building teams. The leader sets the tone of the project for which the team is assembled by clearly delineating the goal and the individual roles for success.

Stages of a Team Process

There is a systematic process that enables teams to succeed in developing theories and actions to promote positive patient-centered care. In 1965, Bruce Tuckman initially developed the 5 Stages of Team Development and it was later updated by Tuckman and Jensen in 1977 (Tuckman, B. & Jensen, M. A., 1977). The five stages: (a) forming, (b) storming, (c) norming, (d) performing, and (e) adjourning, are shown in Table 17.3.

Forming Stage

In the forming stage, the individuals meet face-to-face for the first time. In this stage, the members meet one another, share information about themselves, and learn about others (Project Management, 2019). The leader has the responsibility to communicate the goals and objectives of the project and answer questions that arise. Through these discussions, the team member begins to find their place on the team and understand which roles are best suited to their particular skill and knowledge. The leader helps the team members in determining their roles and facilitating the team to establish the culture or norms for the project.

Storming Stage

During the storming stage, team members begin to share ideas and vie for roles. Storming is another step where the team members bounce ideas and strategies off each other (Project Management, 2019). This stage can be challenging, especially for members who are conflict-avoiders. In this stage, the role of the leader is a critical role in conflict resolutions, keeping the team on track and maintaining having the ultimate goal of the project as the focus of discussion (Project Management, 2019).

Norming Stage

The leader is instrumental in leading the team through this challenging period. In the norming stage, the conflicts are resolved, and a sense of team cohesiveness develops. The team focus develops and supersedes the individual focus on specific tasks. Through effective communication, a willingness to commit to the goals of the project overcome the narrower focus on individual priorities. The end result is a team focused on the original goal, both respectful and appreciative individuals.

Performing Stage

Having successfully navigated the challenging *norming stage*, the team has become a highly proficient and cohesive unit. Trust in each other and in the value of the project drives the team to completion of the project. In this stage, the team leader's role as decision maker is reduced as the team assumes this role. The leader continues to support, encourage, question, and strengthen the bond that has developed among the team members.

Adjourning Stage

Adjourning is a period of joy and pride in the work that has been accomplished but can produce feelings of sadness as the team dissolves and its members move on to new projects. Some members will stay in contact with each other and perhaps join again on other projects and the process will begin again. The final act of the team leader is to lead the team in celebration for accomplishing the goal. However, if the project did not meet the originally goal, the leader leads the team in the evaluation process to identify areas for improvement and the process may begin again at a later date.

Identify the Qualities of an Effective Team Leader

According to Sullivan (2013), leaders inspire, encourage, and empower others to excel to the maximum of their capability.

Table 17.3 Tuckman and Jensen's Stages of Team Process

Stage	Description
Forming	*Relationship development*: Team orientation, identification of role expectations, beginning team interaction.
Storming	*Interpersonal interaction and reaction*: Dealing with tension, conflict, and confrontation occurs.
Norming	*Effective cooperation*: Personal opinions are expressed and resolution of conflict with formation of solidified goals and increased group cohesiveness occurs.
Performing	*Group maturity and stable relationships*: Team roles become more functional and flexible and structural issues are resolved, leading to supportive task performance through group-directed collaboration and resource sharing.
Adjourning	*Termination and consolidation*: Team goals and activities are met, leading to closure, evaluation, and outcomes review. This may also lead to reforming when the need for improvement or further goal development is identified.

Source: Compiles with information from Tuckman & Jensen, 1977; Hall & Weaver, 2001; Poliko-Harris, 2003; Amos et al., 2005.

Sullivan (2013) identifies characteristics of an effective leader as ". . .exerts influence by using a flexible repertoire of personal behaviors and strategies" (p. 41). Leaders utilize personal and professional communication skills to build cohesive teams who work together to achieve a common goal. Communication with team members is transparent and clear. Employees are empowered to take initiatives and share their views and ideas with the team. Leadership is key to strong teams. Effective team leaders can make a difference between achieving the goal or missing the mark. This is a critical point in patient care. Health care workers work as teams. When there is a breakdown in the team leadership, the patient and the health care team is disadvantaged.

Concept of Teamwork Environment

Team work requires a level of communication and cooperation that enhances the skills and work of the team as a team. The sum of the parts (the members) together creates an environment conducive to achieving goals or missing the mark. This is a process of creating a positive working culture among the team members. Heathfield (2020) develops the critical concept of trust and respect among team members to build a strong and effective work environment and culture. Nursing is a caring discipline. Respect for diversity among nurses by nurses is key for building a cohesive and healing work environment.

Characteristics of a team identified in the definition from http://Bussinessdictionary.com (2019) include interdependence, common goals, and self-management. The skill sets of the members of a team help in defining the role of the members, but shared accountability by the team creates the synergy in applying those skill sets in achieving the goal/mission. The roles of a team are developed from clearly defined goal/mission. For example, let's consider the mission of ACLS to provide expert skill and knowledge in resuscitation efforts for people experiencing a life-threaten cardiopulmonary event. LIPs have advanced education and skill in the field of medicine, with additional training in ACLS to make them most often the appropriate person to lead the code team. Their licensed scope of practice is broader than the registered nurse. But if an LIP is not available or lacks training in ACLS, a registered nurse certified in ACLS would be the most qualified person to lead the team. A note of caution: nurses should always know their organizations policy in relation to nursing scope of practice. While certification in ACLS would permit a registered nurse to order and administer medications according to ACLS protocol, organizational policy limitations would take precedent over ACLS certification.

The point of the previous discussion is to demonstrate the critical role of each member of a team in accomplishing the mission/goal of the team. The provision of health care is not an individual endeavor but one that requires the orchestration of many different levels of knowledge and expertise. When assembling a team, a mission statement is key in defining and guiding the formation and function of the team. Teams are dynamic, living, breathing entities whose members have shared responsibilities and interdependence. Each member of the team is accountable for both their responsibilities and for the success or failure of the mission. The cohesive strength of the team is the synergy which enlivens the team as a single unit of combined expertise in accomplishing a goal or mission. New nurses will come to learn how to be part of a team and to lead a team.

New nursing graduates are the life blood of the nursing profession. Their role in the health care team is to learn and share their learning with the team. They are hands-on nurses eager to learn and grow in their profession and share their enthusiasm.

Crew Resource Management

While technical training assures proficiency in specific tasks, it does not address the potential for errors created by communication and decision making in dynamic environments. Experts in aviation have developed safety training focused on effective team management, known as **Crew Resource Management** (CRM). Improvements in the safety record of commercial aviation may be due, in part, to this training (Helmreich, 2017). Over the past 20 years, lessons from aviation's approach to team training have been applied to medicine (Pizzi, Goldfarb, & Nash, 2012), notably in the ICU [Shortell, et al., 1994], and anesthesia training [Howard, Gaba, Fish, Yang, & Sarnquist, 1992]. CRM training encompasses a wide range of knowledge, skills, and attitudes, including communication, assertiveness, situational awareness, problem solving, decision making, and teamwork.

Assertiveness is the willingness to actively participate, state, and maintain a position until convinced by the facts that other options are better. It requires initiative and the courage to act. Assertiveness differs from passive behavior, which is often submissive to avoid conflict and demonstrates a lack of initiative. Assertiveness also differs from aggressive behavior, which can be dominating, hostile, belligerent, and argumentative.

Situational awareness refers to the degree of accuracy by which one's perception of his or her current environment mirrors reality. Factors that reduce situational awareness include insufficient communication, fatigue/stress, task overload, task underload, group mind-set, a "press on regardless" philosophy, and degraded operating conditions.

CRM fosters a climate or culture where the freedom to respectfully question authority is encouraged. However, the primary goal of CRM is not enhanced communication, but enhanced situational awareness. It recognizes that a discrepancy between what is happening and what should be happening is often the first indicator that an error is occurring. This is a delicate area for many organizations, especially ones with traditional hierarchies, such as health care. Appropriate communication techniques must be taught to all nursing and medical practitioners so that they understand that the questioning of authority need not be threatening and so that all understand the correct way to question orders.

Todd Bishop, a CRM expert, developed a five-step assertive statement process that encompasses inquiry and advocacy steps (International Association of Fire Chiefs, 2003). The five steps are:

- Opening or attention getter—Address the individual as, for example, "Dr. Karen" or "Michelle", or whatever name or title will get the person's attention.

- State your concern—State what you see in a direct manner. "Mr. Jones has a pulse of 160."

- State the problem as you see it—"Mr. Jones is going into ventricular tachycardia."

- State a solution—"Mr. Jones needs an antiarrhythmic medication."

- Obtain agreement (or buy-in)—"Do you want to order an antiarrhythmic medication?"

The five steps are difficult but important skills to master, and they require a change in interpersonal dynamics and organizational culture.

As the largest group of health care workers, nurses are uniquely positioned and trained to be leaders. Developing a health care system responsive to the needs and desires of the patient for optimum patient outcome, nurses must be members of interprofessional teams, working across the health care continuum to meet the needs of all people.

In this chapter, we explored many aspects of teams and teamwork, including QSEN competencies, members, advantages and disadvantages, and creating an effective team. We also explored the stages of the team process, CRM, and the qualities of an effective leader within a team. With the knowledge gained from this chapter and self-reflection, you are on your journey to become an effective team member and soon to be a leader.

KEY CONCEPTS

- Effective teamwork and collaboration are essential to improving patient care outcomes.

- Teams and committees are formed for a variety of reasons, depending on the level of collaboration required or the specific purpose desired.

- The interprofessional team consists of many people with diverse training and backgrounds.

- Each team goes through the stages of a team process.

- An effective team member must be proactive, be motivated, have a certain personal sense of purpose or mission, and possess personal and time management skills.

- Teams are affected by team size, status differences, and psychological safety.

- Great teams have clear goals, well-defined role delineation, organized processes that are outcomes oriented, and open and honest interpersonal relationships.

- CRM training encompasses a wide range of knowledge, skills, and attitudes, including communication, assertiveness, situational awareness, problem solving, decision making, and teamwork.

KEY TERMS

| Team | Emotional Intelligence | Licensed independent practitioner (LIP) |

REVIEW QUESTIONS

1. You have arrived at the first meeting of an interprofessional committee on improving communication between nurses and physicians. Which stage of group process is this?
   a. Norming
   b. Storming
   c. Adjourning
   d. Forming

2. Based on the Tuckman and Jensen team process, what stage of team development is it when team members work harmoniously together, have open communication, take risks, and trust each other to complete assigned tasks?
   a. Forming
   b. Storming
   c. Norming
   d. Performing

3. A good leader does all, except which of the following?
   a. Encourages open communication and interpersonal relationship
   b. Uses only an authoritative leadership style
   c. Actively listens to team members' concerns and opinions
   d. Clearly identifies goals, roles, and the team process

4. Which of the following is not a characteristic of groupthink?
   a. Use of mind guards
   b. Illusion of unanimity
   c. Free discussion of ideas
   d. Pressure to conform

5. Which of the following communication roles is used to protect the team from outside pressures from those above them in the organizational hierarchy?
   a. Ambassador
   b. Task coordinator
   c. Scout
   d. Leader

6. Which of the following shows that an individual's performance is often determined in large part by the work group?
   a. Kaluzny study
   b. Dickson research
   c. Carnegie study
   d. Hawthorne experiments

7. Which of the following are characteristics of a successful team? Select all that apply.

   a. They socialize outside of the work environment.
   b. They understand the role of each team member.
   c. They communicate effectively.
   d. They possess identical expertise.
   e. They have an explicit purpose.

8. According to Miller et al., key nursing behavioral markers for interdisciplinary interaction include which of the following? Select all that apply.
   a. Having clear situational awareness
   b. Using a **situation, background, assessment, recommendation, response (SBARR)** communication method
   c. Being prompt for shift duty
   d. Using closed-loop communication
   e. Having a shared mental model

REVIEW QUESTION ANSWERS

1. Answer: D is correct.
   Rationale: (D) Forming is the initial stage of group process and best describes this situation. (A) Norming comes after forming, (B) storming is where members vie for positions within the group, and (C) adjourning is the conclusion of the group process.

2. Answer: D is correct.
   Rationale: (D) Performing is the stage of team development when team members work harmoniously together, have open communication, take risks, and trust each other to complete assigned tasks. (A) Forming is the initial stage, (B) storming is where ideas are gathered. and (C) norming is the beginning stage.

3. Answer: B is correct.
   Rationale: A good leader does all the following except (B) and uses only an authoritative leadership style. A good leader (A) encourages open communication and interpersonal relationship, (C) actively listens to team members' concerns and opinions, and (D) clearly identifies goals, roles, and the team process.

4. Answer: C is correct.
   Rationale: (C) Free discussion of ideas is not a characteristic of groupthink. Characteristics of groupthink include (A) use of mind guards, (B) illusion of unanimity, and (D) pressure to conform.

5. Answer: A is correct.
   Rationale: The communication role used to protect the team from outside pressures from those above them in the organizational hierarchy is Ambassador (A). The others, (B) task coordinator, (C) scout, and (D) leader, are incorrect.

6. Answer: C is correct.
   Rationale: The Carnegie study showed that an individual's performance is often determined by the work group (C). (A) The Kalunzy study, (B) Dickenson research, and (D) Hawthorne experiments did not.

7. Answers: B, C, and E are correct.
   Rationale: (B) They understand the role of each team member, (C) they communicate effectively, and (E) they have an explicit purpose. Incorrect responses include (A) they socialize outside of the work environment and (D) they possess identical expertise.

8. Answers: A, B, C, and D are correct.
   Rationale: According to Miller et al., key nursing behavioral markers for interdisciplinary interaction include (A) having clear situational awareness, (B) using a situation, background, assessment, recommendation, response (SBARR) communication method, (C) being prompt for shift duty, and (D) using closed-loop communication. The incorrect response is (E) having a shared mental model.

DISCUSSION POINTS

• What kinds of interprofessional teams do you see RNs as a part of in the hospital?

• What can you do to make yourself a better team member?

• How can you improve your emotional intelligence?

• How can you incorporate Crew Resource Management into your practice?

• Explain how you see the improvements in care related to interprofessional teams?

• Where should RNs be part of interprofessional teams in your institution where they currently are not? Why?

DISCUSSION OF OPENING SCENARIO

1. *How would you respond to this request?*

   It would be in the best interest for you, your patients, and your unit to accept this responsibility!

2. Would you be ready at this point to accept the responsibility?

   As an RN, even with only 6 months experience, you are equipped with the skills and abilities to accept this responsibility.

3. *How would you prepare yourself for this unfamiliar role?*

The best way to prepare yourself for committee membership is to find out the composition of the team members, your role in the committee, the objectives and goals of the committee and the timeline.

4. What qualities or skills do you need to possess to become a productive member of the team? As an RN, you possess all the skills necessary. Qualities to bring include active listening, critical thinking, ethical values, and patient advocacy.

EXPLORING THE WEB

Check these sites for information on teams (all accessed September 11, 2019):

- **American College of Health Care Administrators (ACHCA):** www.achca.org

- Belbin Team-Role Theory, products, conferences, and free online newsletter: www.belbin.com

- Free online newsletter on leadership: www.injoy.com

- Health care team's information: www.learningcenter.net

- Tuckman and Jensen stages of the team process: www.infed.org Search for Tuckman and Jensen.

- Like a Team www.likeateam.com Click on, "Like a Team" You Tubes.

- http://Nursezone.com for work and for life www.nursezone.com

- IHI site on teamwork and SBAR www.ihi.org Click on, Programs. Click on, Audio and Web Programs. Click on, On Demand: Effective Teamwork as a Care Strategy - SBAR and Other Tools for Improving Communication Between Caregivers.

INFORMATICS

Visit the AHRQ site on teamwork training at http://psnet.ahrq.gov Click on Patient safety primers. Click on Teamwork training. Complete the Teamwork Training. What did you learn from this module?

LEAN BACK

- How has nursing school prepared you (or not prepared you) to work in the interprofessional environment?

- How can you become a better team member?

- Did you realize when you went into nursing that most of your time would be working with other professionals other than registered nurses?

REFERENCES

ACNM. (2011). *Definition of midwifery and scope of practice of certified nurse-midwifes and certified midwives.* Retrieved from www.midwife.org/ACNM/files/ACNMLibraryData/UPLOADFILENAME/000000000266/Definition%20of%20Midwifery%20and%20Scope%20of%20Practice%20of%20CNMs%20and%20CMs%20Dec%202011.pdf.

American Association for Respirstory Care (AARC). (2018). *Position statement: Respiratory care scope of practice.* Retrieved from www.aarc.org/.../statement-of-scope-of-practice.pd.

American Heart Association. (2014). *Leadership roles resuscitation triangle roles [brochure].* AHA. Dallas, TX: American Heart Association, 21(1), 10–16

Amos, M., Hu, J., & Herrick, C. A. (2005). The impact of team building on communication and job satisfaction of nursing staff. *Journal for Nurses in Staff Development, 21*(1), 10–16.

Cardinal, R. (2015, June 23). 5 Steps to Building an Effective Team. Retrieved October 30, 2020, from https://www.huffpost.com/entry/5-steps-to-building-an-effective-team_b_7132406.

Cherry, K. (2018). *5 components of emotional intelligence. Very well mind.* Retrieved from www.verywellmind.com/components-of-emotional-intelligence-2795438.

Cronenwett, L., Sherwood, G., Barnsteiner, J., Disch, J., Johnson, J., et al. (2007). Quality and safety education for nurses. *Nursing Outlook, 55*(3), 122–131.

Donohue, P. K., Norvell, M., Boss, R. D., Shepard, J., Frank, K., Patron,

C. & Crowe T. Y. (2017). Hospital Chaplains: Through the Eyes of Parents of Hospitalized Children. Journal of Palliative Medicine. 2017 Dec; 20(12):1352–1358. doi: 10.1089/jpm.2016.0547. Epub 2017 Jun 26. PMID: 28650723.

Goleman, D. (2005). *Emotional intelligence* (10th ed.). New York: Bantam Books.

Hall, P., & Weaver, L. (2001). Interdisciplinary education and teamwork: A long and winding road. *Medical Education, 35,* 867–875.

Healthcare System Careers. (2019). *How to become a physician assistant.* Retrieved from www.healthcaresystemcareersedu.org/physician-assistant-2.

Heathfield, S. (2020, June). Top 10 Ways to Build Trust at Work. Retrieved October 30, 2020, from https://www.thebalancecareers.com/top-ways-to-build-trust-at-work-1919402

Helmreich, R. L. (2017). *Culture at work in aviation and medicine.* doi:10.4324/9781315258690

Helmreich, R. L., Merritt, A. C., & Wilhelm, J. A. (1999). The evolution of crew resource management training in commercial aviation. *The International Journal of Aviation Psychology, 9*(1), 19–32. doi:10.1207/s15327108ijap0901_2

Howard, S., Gaba, D., Fish, K., Yang, G., & Sarnquist, F. (1992). Anesthesia crisis resource management training: Teaching anesthesiologists to handle critical incidents. *Aviation, Space, and Environmental Medicine, 63,* 763–770.

International Association of Fire Chiefs. (2003). Crew Resource Management: A positive change for the fire service [Brochure]. Fairfax, VA: Author. Retrieved October 30, 2020, from https://www.nh.gov/safety/divisions/fstems/ems/training/documents/crewmgt.pdf

Jacobs, C., Pfaff, H., Lehner, B., Driller, E., Nitzsche, A., Stieler-Lorenz, B., Wasem, J. & Jung, J. (2013). The influence of transformation leadership on employee well-being: Results from a survey of companies in the information and communication technology sector in Germany. *Journal of Occupational and Environmental Medicine, 55*(7), 772–778. doi:10.1097/JOM.0b013e3182972ee5

JAMA. (2019). *A physician's education.* Retrieved from https://jamanetwork.com/journals/jama/fullarticle/2020375, doi:10.1001/jama.2014.16394.

Jenson, N. (2013). *How to recognize a leader.* Retrieved from www.huffingtonpost.com/neal-jenson/how-to-recognize-a-leader_b_3278536.html.

Lash, J. P. (1981). Chapter 1. In *Helen and teacher: The story of Helen Keller and Anne Sullivan Macy* (pp. 489). Harmondsworth, Middx, NY: Penguin.

Oakley, B., Felder, R., Brent, R.,. &., & Elhhajj, I. (2004). Turning student groups into effective teams. *Journal of Student-Centered Learning., 2*(1), 9–34. Retrieved from http://citeseerx.ist.psu.edu/viewdoc/download;jsessionid=D88A6AC11723A3D17EA0267BEF23DE7D?doi=10.1.1.422.8179&rep=rep1&type=pdf

Pizzi, L., Goldfarb, N., & Nash, D. (2012). Chapter 44 crew resource management and its applications in medicine. In S. Myers (Ed.), *Patient safety and hospital accreditation: A model for ensuring success.* New York: Springer Pub. Co.

Polifko-Harris, K. (2003). Effective team building. In P. Kelly-Heidenthal (Ed.), *Nursing leadership and management.* Delmar Cengage Learning: Clifton Park, NY.

Project Management. (2019). *The five stages of project team development.* Retrieved from https://project-management.com/the-five-stages-of-project-team-development.

Quality and Safety Education for Nurses. (2019). *Team work and collaboration.* Retrieved from http://qsen.org/competencies/pre-licensure-ksas/#teamwork_collaboration.

Shoaib, F., & Kohli, N. (2017). Employee engagement and goal setting theory. *Indian Journal of Health and Wellbeing, 8*(8), 877–880. Retrieved from www.ischolar.in/index.php/ijhw

Shortell, S. M., Zimmerman, J. E., Rousseau, D. M., Gillies, R. R., Wagner, D. P., Draper, E A.W., Knaus, A. & Duffy, J. (1994). The performance of intensive care units. Does good management make a difference? *Medical Care, 32*, 508–525.

Sullivan, E. J. (2013). *Effective leadership and management in nursing* (8th ed.). Upper Saddle River, NJ: Pearson Education Inc.

The Future of Nursing: Focus on Scope of Practice. (2010). Retrieved from www.nationalacademies.org/HMD/Reports/2010/The-Future-of-Nursing-Leading-Change.

Tuckman, B. W., & Jensen, M. A. C. (1977). Stages of small group development revisited. *Group and Organizational Studies, 2*(4), 419–427. doi:10.1177/105960117700200404

SUGGESTED READINGS

Agreli, H. F., Peduzzi, M., & Bailey, C. (2017). The relationship between team climate and inter professional collaboration: Preliminary results of a mixed methods study. *Journal of Interprofessional Care, 31*(2), 184–186. doi:10.1080/13561820.2016.1261098

American Academy of Case Management. (2006). American Academy of Case Management at AIHCP. Retrieved from https://aihcp.net/american-academy-of-case-management/?gclid=CjwKCAjwldHsBRAoEiwAd0JybfJKQB7qDuRCAapiMGAxR6nDKYbkTi8z3c6S4CnfnAw2__RSvur8ohoC33oQAvD_BwE.

Bedoya, P., Neuhausen, K., Dow, A. W., Brooks, E. M., Mautner, D., & Etz, R. S. (2018). Student Hotspotting: Teaching the Interprofessional Care of Complex Patients. *Academic Medicine : Journal of the Association of American Medical Colleges, 93*(1), 56–59. doi:10.1097/ACM.0000000000001822

Bentley, M., Freeman, T., Baum, F., & Javanparast, S. (2018). Interprofessional teamwork in comprehensive primary healthcare services: Findings from a mixed methods study. *Journal of Interprofessional Care, 32*(3), 274–283. doi:10.1080/13561820.2017.1401986

Dahlke, S., Meherali, S., Chambers, T., Freund-Heritage, R., Steil, K., & Wagg, A. (2017). The Care of Older Adults Experiencing Cognitive Challenges: How Interprofessional teams collaborate. *Canadian Journal on Aging = La Revue Canadienne Du Vieillissement, 36*(4), 485–500. doi:10.1017/S0714980817000368

Dahlke, S., Steil, K., Freund-Heritage, R., Colborne, M., Labonte, S., & Wagg, A. (2018). Older people and their families' perceptions about their experiences with interprofessional teams. *Nursing Open, 5*(2), 158–166. doi:10.1002/nop2.123

Darlow, B., McKinlay, E., Gallagher, P., Beckingsale, L., Coleman, K., et al. (2017). Building and expanding interprofessional teaching teams. *Journal of Primary Health Care, 9*(1), 29–33. doi:10.1071/HC16053

Duffy, P. A., Ronnebaum, J. A., Stumbo, T. A., Smith, K. N., & Reimer, R. A. (2017). Does including public health students on Interprofessional teams increase attainment of Interprofessional practice competencies? *The Journal of the American Osteopathic Association, 117*(4), 244–252. doi:10.7556/jaoa.2017.042

Feather, R. A., Carr, D. E., Garletts, D. M., & Reising, D. L. (2017). Nursing and medical students teaming up: Results of an interprofessional project. *Journal of Interprofessional Care, 31*(5), 661–663. doi:10.1080/13561820.2017.1322563

Fox, L., Onders, R., Hermansen-Kobulnicky, C. J., Nguyen, T.-N., Myran, L., Linn, B., & Hornecker, J. (2018). Teaching interprofessional teamwork skills to health professional students: A scoping review. *Journal of Interprofessional Care, 32*(2), 127–135. doi:10.1080/13561820.2017.1399868

Golom, F. D., & Schreck, J. S. (2018). The journey to Interprofessional collaborative practice: Are we there yet? *Pediatric Clinics of North America, 65*(1), 1–12. doi:10.1016/j.pcl.2017.08.017

Gould, K., Day, K. H., & Barton, A. T. (2017). Changing student attitudes through interaction: Findings from an interprofessional workshop. *Journal of Interprofessional Care, 31*(4), 540–542. doi:10.1080/13561820.2017.1287165

Grohmann, B., Espin, S., & Gucciardi, E. (2017). Patients' experiences of diabetes education teams integrated into primary care. *Canadian family physician Medecin de famille canadien, 63*(2), e128–e136.

Haque, F., Daniel, M., Clay, M., Vredeveld, J., Santen, S., & House, J. B. (2017). The Interprofessional clinical experience: Introduction to Interprofessional education through early immersion in health care teams. *MedEdPORTAL: The Journal of Teaching and Learning Resources, 13,* 10564. doi:10.15766/mep_2374-8265.10564

Housley, C. L., Neill, K. K., White, L. S., Tedder, A. T., & Castleberry, A. N. (2018). An evaluation of an interprofessional practice-based learning environment using student reflections. *Journal of Interprofessional Care, 32*(1), 108–110. doi:10.1080/13561820.2017.1356808

Hudak, N. M., Melcher, B., & Strand de Oliveira, J. (2017). Preceptors' perceptions of Interprofessional practice, student interactions, and strategies for Interprofessional education in clinical settings. *The Journal of Physician Assistant Education: The Official Journal of the Physician Assistant Education Association, 28*(4), 214–217. doi:10.1097/JPA.0000000000000168

Hustoft, M., Biringer, E., Gjesdal, S., Abetamus, J., & Hetlevik, O. (2018). Relational coordination in interprofessional teams and its effect on patient-reported benefit and continuity of care: A prospective cohort study from rehabilitation centres in Western Norway. *BMC Health Services Research, 18*(1), 719. doi:10.1186/s12913-018-3536-5

Institute of Medicine (IOM). (2010). *The future of nursing: Leading change, advancing health. Focus on scope of practice.* Retrieved from http://nationalacademies.org/hmd/reports/2010/the-future-of-nursing-leading-change-advancing-health.aspx.

Klein, C., Diaz Granados, D., Salas, E., Le, H., Burke, S., et al. (2009). Does team building work? *Small Group Research, 40,* 181–222. doi:10.1177/1046496408328821

Leclair, L. W., Dawson, M., Howe, A., Hale, S., Zelman, E., et al. (2018). A longitudinal interprofessional simulation curriculum for critical care teams: Exploring successes and challenges. *Journal of Interprofessional Care, 32*(3), 386–390. doi:10.1080/13561820.2017.1405920

Lockeman, K. S., Appelbaum, N. P., Dow, A. W., Orr, S., Huff, T. A., et al. (2017). The effect of an interprofessional simulation-based education program on perceptions and stereotypes of nursing and medical students: A quasi-experimental study. *Nurse Education Today, 58,* 32–37. doi:10.1016/j.nedt.2017.07.013

MacKenzie, D., Creaser, G., Sponagle, K., Gubitz, G., MacDougall, P., et al. (2017). Best practice interprofessional stroke care collaboration and simulation: The student perspective. *Journal of Interprofessional Care, 31*(6), 793–796. doi:10.1080/13561820.2017.1356272

McKibben, L. (2017). Conflict management: Importance and implications. *British Journal of Nursing (Mark Allen Publishing), 26*(2), 100–103. doi:10.12968/bjon.2017.26.2.100

Meyer, B. A., Seefeldt, T. M., Ngorsuraches, S., Hendrickx, L. D., Lubeck, P. M., et al. (2017). Interprofessional education in pharmacology using high-fidelity simulation. *Currents in Pharmacy Teaching & Learning, 9*(6), 1055–1062. doi:10.1016/j.cptl.2017.07.015

Mitchell, R., Boyle, B., O'Brien, R., Malik, A., Tian, K., et al. (2017). Balancing cognitive diversity and mutual understanding in multidisciplinary teams. *Health Care Management Review, 42*(1), 42–52. doi:10.1097/HMR.0000000000000088

Myers, S. (2012). *Patient safety and hospital accreditation: A model for ensuring success.* New York: Springer Pub. Co.

Patel, S., O'Brien, B. C., Dulay, M., Earnest, G., & Shunk, R. L. (2018). Team retreats for Interprofessional trainees and clinic staff: Accelerating the development of high-functioning teams. *MedEdPORTAL: The Journal of Teaching and Learning Resources, 14,* 10786. doi:10.15766/mep_2374-8265.10786

Peeters, M. J., Sexton, M., Metz, A. E., & Hasbrouck, C. S. (2017). A team-based interprofessional education course for first-year health professions students. *Currents in Pharmacy Teaching & Learning, 9*(6), 1099–1110. doi:10.1016/j.cptl.2017.07.006

Rousseau, C., Pontbriand, A., Nadeau, L., & Johnson-Lafleur, J. (2017). Perception of Interprofessional collaboration and co-location of specialists and primary care teams in youth mental health. *Journal of the Canadian Academy of Child and Adolescent Psychiatry = Journal de l'Academie Canadienne de Psychiatrie de l'enfant et de l'adolescent, 26*(3), 198–204.

Schug, V., Finch-Guthrie, P., & Benz, J. (2018). Interprofessional education and team-based learning in a research methods course. *Nursing Education Perspectives, 39*(6), 380–382. doi:10.1097/01.NEP.0000000000000264

Shortell, S. M., & Kaluzny, A. D. (2006). *Health care management* (5th ed.). Clifton Park, NY: Delmar Cengage Learning.

Smith, T., Fowler-Davis, S., Nancarrow, S., Ariss, S. M. B., & Enderby, P. (2018). Leadership in interprofessional health and social care teams: A literature review. *Leadership in Health Services (Bradford, England), 31*(4), 452–467. doi:10.1108/LHS-06-2016-0026

Sonke, J., Pesata, V., Lee, J. B., & Graham-Pole, J. (2017). Nurse perceptions of artists as collaborators in Interprofessional care teams. *Healthcare (Basel, Switzerland), 5*(3), 50. doi:10.3390/healthcare5030050

Stone, R. (2017). Interprofessional learning: Benefits for healthcare teams and patients. *British Journal of Nursing* (Mark Allen Publishing),, *26*(10), 571. doi:10.12968/bjon.2017.26.10.571

Team. (2019). In http://BusinessDictionary.com. Retrieved from www.businessdictionary.com/definition/team.html.

Ulrich, B., & Crider, N. M. (2017). Using teams to improve outcomes and performance. *Nephrology Nursing Journal: Journal of the American Nephrology Nurses' Association, 44*(2), 141–151.

Vogel, M. T., Abu-Rish Blakeney, E., Willgerodt, M. A., Odegard, P. S., & Johnson, E. L. (2018). Interprofessional education and practice guide: Interprofessional team writing to promote dissemination of interprofessional education scholarship and products. *Journal of Interprofessional Care,* 1–8. doi:10.1080/13561820.2018.1538111

Wellmon, R., Lefebvre, K. M., & Ferry, D. (2017). Effects of high-Fidelity simulation on physical therapy and nursing Students' attitudes toward Interprofessional learning and collaboration. *The Journal of Nursing Education, 56*(8), 456–465. doi:10.3928/01484834-20170712-03

Young, G. J., Cohen, M. J., Blanchfield, B. B., Jones, M. M., Reidy, P. A., & Weinstein, A. R. (2017). Assessing Interprofessional education in a student-faculty collaborative practice network. Education for Primary Care, . *28*(4), 223–231. doi:10.1080/14739879.2017.1298406

18

Delegation, Assignment, and Supervision of Patient Care

Ruth Hansten[1], Patricia Kelly Vana[2,3]

[1] Hansten Healthcare, Santa Rosa, CA, USA
[2] College of Nursing, Purdue University Northwest, Hammond, IN, USA
[3] Health Education Systems, Inc. (HESI), Houston, TX, USA

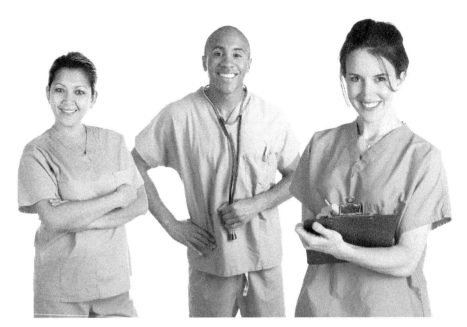

A collaborative and communicating team.
Source: jsmith/Getty Images

But again, to look to all these things yourself does not mean to do them yourself. . . if you do it, it is by so much the better, certainly, than if it were not done at all. But can you not ensure that it is done when not done by yourself? Can you ensure that it is not undone when your back is turned? This is what being "in charge" means. And a very important meaning it is, too. The former only implies that just what you can do with your own hands is done. The latter that what ought to be done is always done.

(Florence Nightingale, 1898, Notes on Nursing p. 40)

OBJECTIVES

Upon completion of this chapter, the reader should be able to:

1. Discuss the correlation of RN delegation, assignment, and supervision and optimal safe patient care.

2. Define delegation, assignment, accountability, authority, supervision, **Unlicensed Assistive Personnel (UAP)** or **Nurse Assistive Personnel (NAP)** or **Assistive Personnel (AP)**.

3. Review the 2016 National Guidelines for Nursing Delegation, **National Council of State Boards of Nursing (NCSBN)**.

4. List the Five Rights of Delegation.

5. Identify responsibilities of Employer/Nurse Leaders, Licensed Nurses, and Delegatees to support delegation.

6. Identify potential delegation barriers.

7. Outline three individual team member characteristics that could affect team communication.

8. Review a memory device used for hand-offs between shifts, departments, or points along the health care continuum, i.e., the 4 Ps, Purpose, Picture, Plan, and Part.

OPENING SCENARIO

Inappropriate delegation can be life threatening as in the following example.

*A patient was admitted to 3C with the diagnosis of **Transient Ischemic Attack (TIA)**. She required neurological assessments to be performed at the onset of every shift and whenever necessary as indicated by a change in the patient's condition. The night nurse assessed the patient at the beginning of her shift, noting that the patient's neurologic status was fully intact. During the night, the nurse periodically checked on the patient every 2 hr but did not awaken or re-assess the patient. The house supervisor had secured a UAP, working a double shift, as a sitter to keep the patient safe. The sitter had assured the nurse that the patient was "doing fine." The sitter did not report that when the*

patient had been assisted to the bathroom initially, she had no difficulty. Upon assisting the patient a second time, the sitter noted that the patient was leaning to one side so badly that she could not stand and required help from two additional UAPs. No one reported this to the nurse. When the nurse checked the patient at 6 a.m., she noted that the patient was not able to move her right side.

1. How could the nurse have avoided the delay in diagnosis and treatment?

2. What are the responsibilities of the nurse and the UAP sitter?

3. How would you find out their job responsibilities?

4. How could delegation and supervision have been appropriately performed in this situation?

Registered nurses, through the public trust embedded in their licensure, are expected to lead teams of health care workers to deliver optimal quality, safe nursing care. Throughout all practice sites, RNs delegate and assign tasks based on their knowledge of each patient's condition. They must also apportion and coordinate necessary work processes and supervise the completion of tasks while evaluating the patient's progress toward their intended outcomes. Managing care for more than one patient and working closely with other health care professionals and technicians has been a crucial part of nursing's role for more than a century. This chapter first presents a patient scenario that illustrates why delegation, assignment, and supervision skills are essential to optimal patient safety and quality of care. Key terms will be defined: delegation, assignment, accountability. Authority, supervision, UAP or NAP or AP (Assistive Personnel). As key terms are defined, further detail is provided, such as more in-depth description of the support personnel an RN assigns or delegates care to, and how to decide what to delegate. Further clarification of delegation and supervision decision-making includes a review of the National Guidelines for Nursing Delegation, National Council of State Boards of Nursing (NCSBN, 2016). Tools such as the five Rights of Delegation will be used to help describe the

thinking processes nurses use to make patient care decisions. An emphasis on the importance of teamwork and communication to promote patient safety and care quality will be maintained throughout the chapter, including the responsibilities of Employer/Nurse Leaders, Licensed Nurses, and Delegatees for best delegation and assignment practices.

Barriers to delegation and team communication on the part of both the RN and the UAP team members will be explored. A memory device used for hand-offs between shifts, departments, or points along the health care continuum will be reviewed, that is, the 4 Ps, Purpose, Picture, Plan, and Part. Real life examples gleaned from nurses' experiences will be used to illustrate key points.

The Correlation of RN Delegation, Assignment and Supervision and Optimal Safe Patient Care

Nurses must work closely with other health care personnel and use excellent team communication to get the necessary tasks completed for the best patient care. In our current world, it is essential for each person to work at the top of their skills

Table 18.1   Adverse Outcomes of Inadequate Delegation, Assignment, and Supervision

Inadequate Delegation, Assignment, and Supervision by the Nurse May Lead to:	Missed Care such as:	With Patient and Care Team Results such as:
	• Ambulation • Positioning • Turning • Hydration • Nutrition • Hygiene • Observation • Rounding • Toileting • Vital Signs • Oral Care	• Patient Deconditioning (loss of physical strength and/or function) • Extended length of stay • Pressure injuries/ulcers • Deep vein thrombosis and possible emboli • Pneumonia • Constipation • Falls • Urinary Tract Infections • Mouth Sores • Dehydration • Debilitation • Readmission to acute care • Admission to other care sites • Failure To Rescue (FTR) Deteriorating Patients • Poor Patient Satisfaction Scores • Poor RN and Care Giver Job Satisfaction • Possible Job and License Jeopardy

Source: Created by R. Hanstead & P. Kelly.

and abilities so that we don't misuse scarce financial and human resources that could be used for others in need of care. Competent entry-level workers performing routine, uncomplicated tasks can multiply the scope of an RN's in-depth global knowledge and ability to create care and healing for more persons overall, while amplifying scarce health care system resources. A well-led health care team also offers patients and their families additional, diverse individuals to observe, assist, and complete care tasks that would be left undone by an overwhelmed RN attempting to do all the care alone. Entry-level assistants may also grow into new health care roles with additional education.

Some novice nurses have believed that leading care teams is a skill best left for developing later in their practice, because it is difficult to assign tasks to others when one is learning the timing and difficulty of the tasks. However, expert delegation, assignment, and supervision are essential for patient safety. Employers of new graduates state that inexperienced nurses allow care to be omitted through ineffective delegation and supervision and that a lack of communication and teamwork skills create patient safety hazards (Diab & Ehrahim, 2019). Experienced RNs self report that these leadership abilities (delegation, assignment, and supervision) are some of the weakest of their professional practice skills, and that role confusion about which team member should be completing which task all contributes to job dissatisfaction (Hansten, Nurse Leader, 2014a).

Care omissions (sometimes called "missed care") due to inadequate RN delegation, assignment, and supervision are often a root cause of errors, health care acquired conditions, and lack of patient progress. When care is not done well or at all, the following negative outcomes can result: pressure injuries, dehydration, pneumonia, falls, urinary tract

infections, debilitation, deep vein thrombosis and emboli, constipation, extended patient lengths of stay, patients being sent to additional care sites due to lack of progress, hospital readmissions, and **Failure To Rescue** (**FTR**) deteriorating patients, etc. (Table 18.1) (Kalisch 2015; Mushta et al. 2018). If the RN doesn't delegate well to competent people such as UAP and make certain that nursing care tasks are being done consistently and well, patients suffer. Nurses and other caregivers often feel frustrated with a lack of teamwork and find themselves unhappy with their jobs. Nurses that delegate poorly can put their licenses at jeopardy as well (Brent, 2019; Brous, 2014). The Opening Scenario illustrates a situation in which an RN does not give thorough initial direction to a UAP to take vital signs and report immediately any changes, and has not made patient rounds for initial assessment. Perhaps the RN was involved with one patient and a change in another assigned patient went unheeded. Perhaps the RN merely expected to hear if abnormal signs had been noted. Late in the shift, the RN finally made rounds and finds that the patient has deteriorated and called a rapid response team. This FTR shows inadequate leadership, uncoordinated teamwork, and missed execution of task assignments. In a situation in which UAPs are left unsupervised and are unable to give care due to workload or other problems, the UAP may not report patient observations and care omissions to the RN. If the RN is unable to observe a patient by making rounds and/or direct observation, then a patient can swiftly develop a problem from missed care. Without adequate intervention, this missed care could result in hospital-acquired conditions that may be deadly, painful, expensive, and/or lengthen the patient's recovery.

The ability to lead a group of health care workers and manage the care that needs to be done using principles of delegation, assignment, and supervision, is such an important part of nursing, that in the National Council of State Boards of Nursing Licensure Examination (NCLEX) a student will often encounter test questions that assess the ability to delegate care. The **Quality and Safety Education for Nurses (QSEN)** Institute Prelicensure Competencies include knowledge, skills, and attitudes related to teamwork, communication, and collaboration, all of which are necessary competencies in leading teams and safeguarding patients. To ensure that these responsibilities are met, nurses are accountable under the law for nursing care rendered by both themselves and other personnel.

If these team leadership skills seem too hazardous or complex, remember that nurses rarely work alone without help from others. Mastering delegation, assignment, and supervision will not only enrich nurse's professional life but also those of their patients and team members. This chapter will help novice nurses feel safe and confident in performing the steps of delegation, assignment, and supervision correctly. Additionally, nursing care support roles are crucial to an environment of timely, safe, cost-effective, high-quality care. Significant demands on the health care system will likely see expansion of the types of nursing support workers and more rules related to their use, so the expert delegating nurse will be in high demand. (Maningo & Panthofer, 2018). Remember that UAPs are equipped to assist—not replace—the nurse. In order to assure that a competent UAP can safely assist the nurse within their own level of practice and job description, RNs must know what aspects of nursing can be delegated and what level of supervision is required to ensure that the patient receives safe, high-quality care.

Overview of Terms

In order for the student nurse to develop team leadership skills through expert allocation of work, a brief overview of terms is given in this section, necessary so that the student will not be confused by unfamiliar concepts (Table 18.2). Each term will be discussed more extensively in the appropriate following section of the chapter, along with information about how to implement that term in daily practice. These terms are closely linked: for example, a nurse that delegates or assigns care tasks must also supervise the personnel that were assigned the care and be certain that the care was done correctly and completely. The RN must also understand and differentiate team member roles. The RN has the authority within state nursing practice law to delegate tasks to competent other personnel delegates (sometimes referred to as "delegatees") such as UAPs. For this chapter we will most often use the term UAP for these unlicensed delegates. NAP is another term used for the same group of unlicensed delegates in some state nurse practice acts or advisory statements. The term, Assistive Personnel (AP), was adopted by the **American Nurses Association (ANA)** and NCSBN in their 2019 National Guidelines for Nursing Delegation to connote UAPs (ANA/NCSBN, 2019). The terms "delegates" or "delegatees" are used interchangeably as the personnel who have been delegated to do some work by another health care professional. A delegate or del-

egatee is described by the NCSBN as "one who is delegated a nursing responsibility. . . and is competent to perform it, and verbally accepts the responsibility" and could refer to an "RN, LPN/LVN or UAP" (NCSBN, 2016, p. 7). In this text we will most often use the term, "delegate" rather than "delegatee," unless quoting an organization that uses that terminology. RNs may also assign work to, direct, and supervise Licensed Practical Nurses/Licensed Vocational Nurses (LPN/LVNs). RNs who delegate and assign patient care are accountable for their professional decision making and for the nursing care of their patients, no matter which nursing support personnel (LPN/LVNs and/or UAPs) may be delivering some of the care. RNs may never delegate the nursing process or nursing clinical judgment (Anderson, 2018, p. 51).

Delegation Definition

Nursing delegation was discussed by Nightingale in the 1800s and has continued to evolve since then. The American Nurses Association (ANA) defined **delegation** as the "transfer of responsibility for the performance of a task from one individual to another while retaining accountability for the outcome" (ANA, 2014, p. 22).

Delegation was defined by the NCSBN in 2016 as, "Allowing a delegatee (NAP, for example) to perform a specific nursing activity, skill, or procedure that is beyond the delegatee's traditional role and not routinely performed." (NCSBN 2016, p. 6).

The ANA and National Council of State Boards of Nursing 2019 Joint Statement, National Guidelines for Nursing Delegation, states that, "The decision of whether or not to delegate or assign is based upon the RN's judgment concerning the condition of the patient, the competence of all members of the nursing team. and the degree of supervision that will be required of the RN if a task is delegated" (ANA, 2019, p. 1). The National Council of State Boards of Nursing states that, "The licensed nurse must determine the needs of the patient and whether those needs are matched by the knowledge, skills, and abilities of the delegatee and can be performed safely by the delegatee. The licensed nurse cannot delegate any activity that requires clinical reasoning, nursing judgment, or critical decision making. The licensed nurse must ultimately make the final decision whether an activity is appropriate to delegate to the delegatee based on the Five Rights of Delegation" Sources: National Council of State Boards of Nursing, 1995, 1996.

Who Are the Delegates? UAP or NAP or AP and LPNS/LVNS

State nurse practice acts define the legal parameters for nursing practice. Most states authorize RNs to thoughtfully delegate patient care activities, and all states expect RNs to be able to assign care. Individual state nurse practice acts may have different definitions and rules for delegation, assignment, supervision, and the roles permitted for various levels of personnel.

Table 18.2 Definition of Terms

Term	Definition
Delegation	Delegation is the transfer of responsibility for the performance of a task from one individual to another while retaining accountability for the outcome. (ANA, 2014, p. 22). Each state may have a different (similar) definition.
To assign (Verb)	To allocate "routine care, activities, procedures that are within the authorized scope of practice of the RN or LPN (LVN) or part of the routine functions" of the NAP (NCSBN 2016, p. 6, 7).
Assignment (noun)	The "routine care, activities, procedures that are within the authorized scope of practice of the RN or LPN/LVN or part of the routine functions" of the AP (NCSBN, 2016).
Supervision	Supervision is "the active process of directing, guiding, and influencing the outcome of an individual's performance of a task."
Accountability	Accountability is defined as "to be answerable to oneself and others for one's own choices, decisions, and actions as measured against a standard" (NCSBN, 2016, p. 7). Nursing accountability includes the preparedness and obligation to explain or justify to relevant others (including the regulatory authority) the relevant judgments, intentions, decisions, actions, and omissions, as well as the consequences of those judgments, intentions, decisions, actions, and omissions.
Authority	**Authority** is the right to act or to command the action of others; (NCSBN, 2016, p. 6). Authority occurs when a person who has been given the right to delegate based on the state nurse practice act also has the official power from an agency to delegate.
Competence	**Competence** is the "ability to accomplish specific skills safely and effectively under various circumstances" and true competency is confirmed as nurses "consistently display appropriate behaviors and sound judgments at the point of care" (Alfaro-LeFevre, 2017, p. 61).
Clinical judgment (or professional clinical judgment)	**Clinical judgment** is the "outcome of critical thinking or clinical reasoning, the conclusion, decision, or opinion you make after thinking about the issues" (Alfaro-LeFevre, 2017, p. 6).
LPNs/LVNs Licensed practical nurse or licensed vocational nurse	LPN/LVNs are licensed nurses that perform routine uncomplicated nursing care in a dependent role under the delegation (or "direction" depending on the state) and supervision of RNs or other licensed care providers such as nurse practitioners, physicians, dentists or others. Their roles vary depending on practice site and state.
UAP (Unlicensed assistive personnel) Or NAP (Nursing assistive personnel) Or AP (Assistive Personnel)	UAP job class is "an umbrella term to describe . . .paraprofessionals who assist individuals with physical disabilities, mental impairments, and other health care needs with their activities of daily living and provide care—including basic nursing procedures—all under the supervision of the registered nurse, licensed practical nurse (in some states), and other health care professionals (ANA, Duffy & McCoy, 2014)." AP (Assistive Personnel) is a term used to describe any assistive personnel trained to "function in a supportive role, regardless of title, to whom nursing responsibility may be delegated. This includes but is not limited to nursing assistants or aides (CNAs or certified nursing assistants), patient care technicians, CMAs (certified medication aides), and home health aides (formerly referred to as 'unlicensed' assistive personnel (UAP)" (ANA, 2019), www.nursingworld.org/globalassets/practiceandpolicy/nursing-excellence/ana-position-statements-secure/ana-ncsbn-joint-statement-on-delegation.pdf)
Delegates or delegatees	"Delegates" or "delegatees" are used interchangeably as terms for the personnel who have been delegated to do some work by another health care professional. A delegate, as described by the NCSBN, is "one who is delegated a nursing responsibility. . .and is competent to perform it, and verbally accepts the responsibility." A delegatee may be an RN, LPN/LVN or UAP (NCSBN, 2016, p. 7).

Source: Compiled by R. Hanstead & P. Kelly.

Unfortunately, research also shows that UAP are sometimes delegated tasks beyond their capabilities and that caregivers are also sometimes confused about their role boundaries (NCSBN 2016, Journal of Nursing Regulation, pp. 7–8). The ANA defines the **UAP** job class as

an umbrella term to describe . . . paraprofessionals who assist individuals with physical disabilities, mental impairments, and other health care needs with their activities of daily living and provide care—including basic nursing procedures—all under the supervision of

the registered nurse, licensed practical nurse (in some states), and other health care professionals. (ANA, Duffy & McCoy, Delegation and You, 2014).

In 2019, the ANA updated their term to Assistive Personnel (AP) to describe these same personnel trained to function in a supportive role, regardless of title, to whom nursing responsibility may be delegated. This includes but is not limited to nursing assistants or aides, Certified Nursing Assistants (CNAs), patient care technicians, CMAs (certified medication aides or Medication Aides-certified), and home health aides (formerly referred to as Unlicensed Assistive Personnel (UAP). (ANA, 2019, and NCSBN, 2019)

The Joint Statement of the ANA and NCSBN (2019) uses the term, Assistive Personnel (AP), to delineate unlicensed employees that aid the licensed nurse with nursing activities. The NCSBN has also stated that the term UAP can be used to identify the helpful unlicensed group that includes certified nursing assistants, patient care technicians of various types (i.e., psychiatric, rehabilitation), home health aides, certified medication aides, and certified medical assistants (CMA or MA) in ambulatory care (NCSBN, 2016, p. 7).

The term, UAP, also includes nurse aides, nurse technicians, patient care technicians, personal care attendants, unit assistants, and other non-licensed personnel. School nurses may work with school secretaries to deliver carefully-regulated care in the absence of the RN on-site; ambulatory nurses may supervise **Medical Assistants** (**MA**s); long-term-care or assisted-living nurses work with rehabilitation aides and Certified Medication Aides (CMAs) in some states; perioperative RNs may supervise surgical technicians; home health RNs delegate to home care aides with specific regulations and public health nurses coordinate and lead community health workers. Many of these roles are regulated separately within each state's practice regulations. In some states, medications and select injections can be given by Certified Medication Aides in long-term care or home care and Medical Assistants in ambulatory care (Beeber et al., 2018, p. 1–9; Maningo & Panthofer 2018, 1–2). All of these UAPs are considered unlicensed and their roles can vary from state by state.

Supportive unlicensed health care personnel may or may not hold various training certifications. Unlicensed personnel such as UAPs could be referred to as "delegates" or "delegatees" in state nurse practice acts or specialty nursing organization practice documents. LPN/LVNs are licensed, however, so these nurses are not considered a UAP, but an RN may be delegating to or directing them, assigning care to them, and supervising them. For novice nurses, role terminology can be confusing but this chapter will clarify how to apply the ideas of delegation and assignment to work with others in practical, daily nursing practice. The decision-making principles remain the same whether assigning or delegating, because an RN should not delegate or assign to a person any task beyond the RN's scope of practice, nor beyond the delegate's state-allowed practice or organization's job description, or beyond the delegate's competency. A competent RN would never assign nor delegate a task that does not match the individual patient's needs.

The nursing profession is responsible for determining the scope of nursing practice and may supervise the care given by such personnel as **Health Care Assistants** (**HCA**s) or Medical Assistants (MAs), even though they do not necessarily train them. The RN may also coordinate the care of a patient receiving care by other inter-professional health care team members and technicians such as respiratory therapists, physical therapists and technicians, and social workers, while not delegating, supervising, or assigning them care. The RN is in charge of nursing care and determines the appropriate utilization of any UAP involved in providing direct nursing care. The nurse who delegates to a UAP retains accountability for that patient and the completion and results of the task that was delegated. "The licensed nurse maintains accountability for the patient, while the delegatee (UAP, for example) is responsible for the delegated activity, skill, or procedure" (NCSBN, 2016, p. 11). A task delegated to a UAP cannot be re-delegated by the UAP.

Multiple levels of UAP give care to patients in various settings. LPN/LVNs may be able to delegate (or not) in certain states within some areas of practice and circumstances. Their scope of practice is also variable nationally.

In all cases, RNs must know the state practice statute, state rules, and State Board of Nursing advisory opinions for each team member's role in their state. The state practice statute may describe whether or not LPN/LVNs can delegate and in which setting. For example, the Washington State Nursing Care Quality Assurance Commission (the Washington State Board of Nursing's title) Advisory Opinion 13.01 clarifies the independent role of the RN and the interdependent and dependent role of the LPN. In that state, LPNs can delegate but only in certain settings: acute care, nursing homes, clinics, but not community settings or schools. (www.doh.wa.gov/Portals/1/Documents/6000/NCAO13.pdf). For an example of another state variance, in Texas, Licensed Vocational Nurses (as LPN/LVNs are titled there) are not allowed to delegate and their practice is "directed and supervised." (p. 2 of FAQ of Texas Board of Nursing Rule 224 Board Rule 224 at www.bon.texas.gov/faq_delegation.asp#t6).

State documents to guide your decisions are available online by visiting www.NCSBN.org, and linking to, Nursing Regulation. Then, click on, About U.S. Boards of Nursing, then scroll down to, Contact a nursing member, and find your state; and/or by visiting your state nursing board or quality assurance commission online. View not only the statute (law) but also the administrative code, rules, and advisory opinions that you will find at your state board's website.

How to Decide What to Delegate or Assign

As described by the ANA (Duffy & McCoy "Delegation and You," 2014), nurses must first know their patients, or perform an assessment of the needs of the patient/population. Secondly, a plan must be designed with the patient and his family before the RN can be certain about what tasks can and should be delegated, based on the patient/family's desired outcome. Thirdly, the nurse must analyze key factors before delegation, such as the scope of practice of the desired tasks, laws or regulations that guide nursing practice and the state practice guidelines for the UAP, the job description and policies of the employing organization, the competence of both the RN and the UAP, and the type and availability of supervision, given the circumstances. Next, the delegated tasks must be supervised, monitored, and evaluated, along with the patient's response to the tasks. The UAP must also be evaluated and feedback should be given. The RN is the final decision maker about delegation decisions because of their unique understanding of each particular patient, delegate, and situation and the RN should not be over-ridden by any organizational policies (ANA, 2014, Duffy& McCoy, Delegation and You, pp. 14–19.)

Accountability

Nurses are legally liable for their actions and are accountable for the overall nursing care of their patients. Professional nurses are accountable for their expert clinical leadership and decision,making, including decisions related to delegation, supervision, and assignment. **Accountability** is defined as, "to be answerable to oneself and others for one's own choices, decisions, and actions as measured against a standard" (NCSBN, 2016, p. 7). Being accountable as a nurse means being "answerable for what one has done" or said, or not done and "standing behind that decision or action" (Hansten & Jackson 2009 p. 79.)

Licensed nurse accountability involves compliance with legal requirements as set forth in the jurisdiction's laws and rules governing nursing. The licensed nurse is also accountable for the quality of the nursing care provided; for recognizing their own limits, knowledge, and experience, for asking for help or clarification when uncertain, and for planning for situations beyond the nurse's expertise (NCSBN, 2005). Nursing accountability includes the preparedness and obligation to explain or justify to relevant others (including the regulatory authority) the relevant judgments, intentions, decisions, actions, and omissions, as well as the consequences of those decisions, actions, and behaviors. Nurses are accountable for following their state nurse practice act (including rules and advisory opinions), the standards of professional practice from their board of nursing and/or their professional specialty, the policies of their health care organization, and nursing ethics. Nurses are also accountable for the full nursing process (assessment, nursing diagnosis, planning with the patient/family, implementation, and evaluation), monitoring changes in a patient's status, noting and implementing treatment for human responses to illness, and assisting in the prevention of complications.

The RN uses nursing judgment in all aspects of the nursing process. Professional **clinical judgment** is the "outcome of critical thinking or clinical reasoning, the conclusion, decision, or opinion you make after thinking about the issues" (Alfaro-LeFevre, 2017, p. 6). The monitoring of more stable patients cared for by the LPN/LVN and UAP may involve the RN's direct, continuing presence or the monitoring may be more intermittent. The assessment, nursing diagnosis, planning, and some parts of implementation such as teaching, and the evaluation stages of the nursing process may not be delegated to the UAP. Delegated activities or tasks usually fall within the implementation phase of the nursing process. Note that data collection such as taking vital signs or collecting intake and output information is not assessment. Assessment includes the interpretation of data for a particular patient. Remember that UAPs also have accountability to keep current in their particular certification, to communicate with the delegating nurse about their ability to accept and complete their assignment, and to complete the assignment they accepted.

Authority

The right to delegate duties and give direction to UAPs places the RN in a position of authority. **Authority** is the right to act or to command the action of others; it comes with the job and is required for a nurse to take action. The person to whom a task and authority have been delegated must be free to make decisions regarding the activities involved in performing that task. Without authority, the nurse cannot function to meet the needs of patients. In Washington State's administrative code, a definition of nursing supervision highlights that authority: **"Supervision** of licensed or unlicensed nursing personnel means the provision of guidance and evaluation for the accomplishment of a nursing task or activity with the initial direction of the task or activity; periodic inspection of the actual act of accomplishing the task or activity; and the authority to require corrective action." Source: Washington Administrative Code 246-840-010 Definitions. Public Domain. The fact that RNs possess this authority is sometimes surprising to practicing RNs, and questions about the RN's authority to require UAPs to correct their performance or task completion may be reflected in the NCLEX licensing examination.

Assignment

In 2016, the NCSBN updated the definition of delegation "to allow a delegatee (person to whom delegated tasks are allocated, a UAP, for example) to perform a specific nursing

---

Critical Thinking 18.1

No matter where RNs work in health care teams, they are busy. Delegating or assigning others some tasks could mean they could possibly miss changes in a patient's condition. How might nurses avoid omitting care or missing changes in patient's conditions that may have occurred in their delegated or assigned patients?

activity, skill, or procedure that is beyond the delegatee's traditional role and not routinely performed" (NCSBN, Journal of Nursing Regulation, 2016, p. 6). An **assignment** is the "routine care, activities, procedures that are within the authorized scope of practice of the RN or LPN/LVN or part of the routine functions" of the UAP (NCSBN, 2016, p. 6). This definition of assignment would clarify that when the RN is assigning care to another RN, it is not delegation, it is assignment. If the RN assigns routine care within the LPN/LVN job description, then the process is considered by the NCSBN as "assignment" rather than "delegation," although some states call this process "delegation" or "direction." of routine activities. Your state may or may not use the term "direction" but it may refer to task allocation when the delegate is licensed. The NCSBN also includes RN, LPN/LVNs, and UAP as "delegatees to whom the activity, skill or procedure has been delegated" thus inferring that "delegation" rather than "assignment" occurs when the task assigned is beyond the delegate's basic education level (NCSBN, 2016, p. 6). The ANA simplifies assignment with the definition that it is "the distribution of work that each staff member is responsible for during a given work period" (ANA, 2014, Delegation and You, p. 22). While this differentiation between assigning and delegating could be confusing to newly licensed nurses, the principles of delivering safe care through competent others remain the same. Whenever care performance is being transferred from the RN to another care provider, the assigning RN must ensure that the education, skill, knowledge, and judgment levels of the care provider being allocated to perform a task are commensurate with the assignment. In acute care settings, a charge nurse or manager may allocate care on an assignment sheet, taking into consideration the skill, knowledge, and judgment of the RNs, LPN/LVNs, and UAP. Assignments are given to team members that have the appropriate knowledge and skill to complete them. Assignments must always be within the legal scope of prac-

tice. Assignment sheets are used to identify patient care duties for RNs, LPN/LVNs, and/or UAP. Table 18.3 shows a basic concept of task assignment to help the student nurse think through the process.

An assignment designates those activities that a team member is responsible for performing as a condition of employment. This is consistent with the team member's job position and description, legal scope of practice, and education and experience. Scope of practice refers to the parameters of the authority to practice granted to a nurse through licensure (NCSBN, 2005). Experienced RNs are expected to work with minimal supervision of their nursing practice. The RN who assigns care to another competent RN who then assumes responsibility and accountability for that patient's care will not need to closely supervise that nurse's work unless the RN is a novice, a temporary float, or expresses concern about the assignment. The RN can assign or delegate or direct patient care (term used depends on the state) to the LPN/LVN or delegate or assign tasks to the UAP, but the RN retains accountability for the patient's nursing care. LPN/LVNs and UAP both work under the direction of the RN. LPN/LVNs could also work under the supervision of a dentist, MD, or advanced practice nurse, as well as an RN, for example in ambulatory care clinics. The LPN/LVN could be delegated, assigned, or directed specific tasks or patients for whom to perform care, but the RN remains responsible for supervising the nursing care of those patients. It is crucial to recognize that LPN/LVN roles are highly state and site specific. The LPN/LVN roles can vary from giving oral medications to administering intravenous fluids and intravenous medications (with special training and restrictions by state and site) and some standard treatments and data gathering based on state and organizational permissions. Blood product administration and total parenteral nutrition through central lines are often prohibited tasks for LPN/LVNs, but this can also vary by state and practice setting.

Table 18.3   **Assignment Sheet**

Unit Date Shift Charge nurse ———————— ———————— RN LPN/LVN UAP ———————— Breaks/Lunch	Room	Patient Name	Dx[a]	IV	Feed, I&O. Weight	Bath/ Type	Amb[b] X____	Code Status, Other

[a] Dx = Diagnosis.
[b] Amb = Ambulation.

Source: Created by R. Hanstead & P. Kelly.

Typical tasks that could be delegated or assigned to a UAP in acute care settings may include passing meal trays, feeding uncomplicated patients, assisting with transfers, positioning and ambulation, toileting, vital signs, transporting patients, hygienic care, and stocking supplies. The RN must know patients' conditions before delegating or assigning. The RN must understand patient circumstances, i.e., the patient's level of consciousness, vital signs, physical status, changing needs, complexity, stability, multisystem involvement, and technology requirements, such as the need for cardiac monitoring. The RN would also consider patient teaching and emotional support needs and plans for discharge or transfer as well as other family needs when delegating or making assignments. A key principle in nursing practice is that RNs are accountable for the nursing care of their patients, whether they do the care themselves, or delegate or assign these tasks to others (Table 18.4).

The student or novice nurse need not spend precious time learning whether they are "delegating" or "assigning" tasks to their co-workers while attempting to learn how to be a professional nurse themselves. The NCSBN has stated that asking personnel to do tasks within their basic educational program coursework is "assignment" rather than "delegation." However, novices and experienced nurses alike would have difficulty being current and cognizant of the basic educational competencies for the 100 or more UAP roles in use in the United States across the continuum of care. The process of nursing task allocation remains the same for safe, effective "delegation" and/or "assignment."

Five Rights of Delegation

Once nurses know what their own state board has promulgated related to rules for delegating, assigning, and supervising, and they are clear on the state role definitions or scopes of practice, each job description and role must be understood definitively. Then the nurse, with knowledge of the particular patients in their assignment and their intended outcomes, can match the competencies of the team members with the tasks that need to be done, delegate and/or assign these tasks, and then supervise appropriately. Remember that supervision is a multifaceted process of appropriate guidance, direction, oversight, and evaluation. An RN should never ask team members to perform a task that is not within the nurse's own competency or scope of practice, nor to step beyond the individual team member's role, competency, or approved job description, whether they are "delegating" or "assigning." Mental checklists such as the five Rights of Delegation (Table 18.5) apply to both processes of "delegating" and "assigning."

The five Rights of Delegation (NCSBN, 2016) is a memory tool for safety and confidence in delegating or assigning. Similar to the six Rights of Medication Administration checklist, this five Rights of Delegation checklist helps a nurse standardize their mental processes.

Right Task

Base all task assignments on the patient's desired outcome. What is the patient wanting to achieve from this episode of care? Two patients, one a new postop patient that would like to go home soon with a new hip, or another patient being allowed to die with dignity and comfort at a Hospice are very different desired patient outcomes. An RN's choices about who performs each patient's vital signs and what parameters an RN would give to the UAP for reporting vital signs would be very different. The task must fit with a particular patient's plan of care and should not be a "rote" choice, since there will be exceptions to tasks that are usually within the normal range of duties. For example, the task of "gathering vital signs" may not make sense for the dying patient or for a stable person that needs to sleep uninterrupted. Any task an RN would delegate or assign to a competent person must first be within the

---

Table 18.4   Key Delegation and Assignment Principles in Nursing Practice

RNs are accountable for the nursing care of their patients whether they:

- Do the care themselves or
- Delegate or assign and supervise tasks done by others

Once nurses are clear on:

- State board rules for delegating, assigning, and supervising
- State board role definition or scope of practice for each delegate
- Each delegate's organizational job description and role

Then the nurse, with knowledge of their patients' needs and their intended outcomes, can:

- Match the competencies of the team members with the tasks that need to be done, and
- Delegate, or assign these tasks appropriately.

When RNs delegate or assign a nursing task, they must also supervise, including:

- Appropriate initial direction,
- Monitoring the activity and its documentation,
- Periodic follow up,
- Evaluation of the results, and
- Feedback to the delegate.

Source: Adapted from: National Council of State Boards of Nursing (NCSBN), 2019. NCSBN and ANA National Guidelines for Nursing Delegation.

Table 18.5   The Five Rights of Delegation

Right task	The activity falls within the delegate's job description or is included in part of the established written policies and procedures of the nursing practice setting. The facility needs to ensure the policies and procedures describe the expectations and limits of the activity and provide any necessary competency training.
Right circumstances	The health condition of the patient must be stable. If the patient's condition changes, the delegate must communicate this to the licensed nurse and the licensed nurse must re-assess the situation and the appropriateness of the delegation.
Right person	The licensed nurse along with the employer and the delegate is responsible for ensuring that the delegate possesses the appropriate skills and knowledge to perform the delegated activity.
Right directions and communication	• Each delegation situation should be specific to the patient, the licensed nurse, and the delegatee. • The licensed nurse is expected to communicate specific instructions for the delegated activity to the delegatee; the delegatee, as part of two-way communication, should ask any clarifying questions. This communication includes any data that needs to be collected, the method for collecting the data, the time frame for reporting the results to the licensed nurse, and any additional information pertinent to the situation. • The delegatee must understand the terms of the delegation and must agree to accept the delegated activity. • The licensed nurse should ensure that the delegatee understands that she or he cannot make any decisions or modifications in carrying out the activity without first consulting the licensed nurse.
Right supervision and evaluation	The licensed nurse is responsible for monitoring the delegated activity, following up with the delegatee at the completion of the activity, and evaluating patient outcomes. The delegatee is responsible for communicating patient information to the licensed nurse during the delegation situation. The licensed nurse should be ready and available to help and intervene as necessary. The licensed nurse should ensure appropriate documentation of the activity is completed.
	Source: National Council of State Boards of Nursing (NCSBN), 2019. NCSBN and ANA National Guidelines for Nursing Delegation.

RN and UAP scope of practice, job description, and written policies and procedures of the facility. "The facility needs to ensure the policies and procedures describe the expectations and limits of the activity and provide any necessary competency training" Source: National Council of State Boards of Nursing (NCSBN), 2019. NCSBN and ANA National Guidelines for Nursing Delegation. The UAP must also be competent and willing to perform the assigned task.

Right Circumstance

Be aware that each practice arena (home health, long-term care, schools, acute care) may have different state rules related to delegation and assignment to team members. Also, each nurse must know that the patient's health condition is stable (NCSBN & ANA, 2019) and have enough knowledge of the patient's condition before knowing what can be delegated or assigned. How much supervision will be necessary and what are the number and type of personnel available? In home care, for example, a list of written, detailed instructions may be used to delegate or assign tasks to home health aides, since the RN is only available by phone or computer and/or on intermittent joint visits. "If the patient's condition changes, the delegatee must communicate this to the licensed nurse, and the licensed nurse must reassess the situation and the appropriateness of the delegation" Source: National Council of State Boards of Nursing (NCSBN), 2019. NCSBN and ANA National Guidelines for Nursing Delegation.

Right Person

The potential delegate must be competent as the organization's job descriptions and the delegate's skills checklist would spec-

ify. The task for each particular patient should match the UAPs abilities and willingness to perform the work.

"The licensed nurse along with the employer and the delegatee is responsible for ensuring that the delegatee possesses the appropriate skills and knowledge to perform the activity" Source: National Council of State Boards of Nursing (NCSBN), 2019. NCSBN and ANA National Guidelines for Nursing Delegation.

Consider the personalities and learning needs of each individual and use those criteria also. For example, think about whether the friendly and talkative nature of a UAP would match well with a patient needing extra socialization, or if a new LPN/LVN needs to get more comfortable with a particular skill and you or the nurse educator has time to teach them and evaluate their progress. Consider that the very hard-of-hearing patient may not communicate well with a soft-spoken, newly English-fluent UAP.

Right Direction and Communication

This is where supervision starts. When RNs delegate or assign patient care, they must supervise the delegates. Initial direction as a part of the supervisory process must be clear, concise, correct, and complete (ANA & NCSBN Joint Statement, 2006; Hansten, 2021 in Zerwekh and Garneau, p. 316).

"This direction and communication includes any data that need to be collected, the method for collecting the data, the time frame for reporting the results to the licensed nurse, and any additional information pertinent to the situation" Source: National Council of State Boards of Nursing (NCSBN), 2019. NCSBN and ANA National Guidelines for Nursing Delegation. Delegates must understand the instructions, ask any clarifying questions, and be willing and able to do the work as described. "The licensed nurse should ensure that the delegatee understands that she or he cannot make any decisions or modifications in carrying out the activity without first consulting the licensed nurse" Source: National Council of State Boards of Nursing (NCSBN), 2019. NCSBN and ANA National Guidelines for Nursing Delegation. Be certain to add parameters for reporting, for example, what patient conditions would mean "call me immediately," versus "wait to tell me when we huddle again before lunch." Best practices include offering initial direction to a UAP while making first rounds with them during the off-going shift report in acute care. This off-going/oncoming shift handoff report allows for the patient/family, RN, and UAP to understand the plan for the shift and may mean improved follow up and task completion. Check points along the shift must be planned early in the shift so that each team member can count on time to report patient care activity, patient condition changes, what's been accomplished, and variations in the shift's plan.

Right Supervision and Evaluation

Evaluation of the care and the UAP's work, along with offering and receiving feedback about how the work was done, is one of the lowest self-ranked professional leadership abilities and most in need of improvement in experienced RNs (Hansten Healthcare PLLC confidential database, 2019). Nursing evaluation (as a part of the supervision process) includes review of patient outcomes and response to care, sharing the information accrued by both the UAP and RN jointly throughout the care process, ongoing monitoring, evaluation, and follow up with the delegatee at the completion of the activity, review of how the care was completed by the UAP, and documentation of all completed patient activities in the organization's electronic health record or paper chart in accordance with the organization's standards. Ongoing checkpoints throughout the episode of care between RNs and delegates are essential to share patient and care progress information in order to update and change course when needed. A number of checkpoints or "catch up huddles" can be held before and after breaks, meals, and certainly before change of shift. For longer-term caseloads, these checkpoints may be weekly (e.g., in home care or assisted living settings).

Practical Application of the Five Rights of Delegation to a Legal Case

Because patient safety and care quality is a major emphasis of this chapter, practical application of the five Rights of Delegation to a legal case in which a patient died as a result of negligent task delegation or assignment will illustrate the importance of the five Rights of Delegation memory tool. Discussed in the *American Journal of Nursing* as an example of poor delegation contributing to an untimely death, an RN assigned an unfamiliar UAP (in this hospital, called a nursing assistant) to feed a patient with dysphagia. This patient with dysphagia was fed a sandwich without feeding precautions. The patient then choked, aspirated, and died (Brous, 2014).

1. **Right task?**

   No. The task of feeding a patient with dysphagia could possibly be delegated or assigned, but only if the RN was certain the delegate was competent and the patient was stable. "The facility needs to ensure the policies and procedures describe the expectations and limits of the activity and provide any necessary competency training" Source: National Council of State Boards of Nursing (NCSBN), 2019. NCSBN and ANA National Guidelines for Nursing Delegation. Many health care organizations will evaluate a UAP's competency on this feeding task with careful education and review and often record this evaluation on a competency check-list. This is a delegable or assignable task in a stable patient with a trained and experienced UAP, but not in this case, due to the fragility of the patient and the incompetence of the UAP.

2. **Right circumstance?**

   No. In this case, the RN had not assessed the patient's stability and ability to swallow, even though she had allegedly been told about his feeding plan and aspiration precautions by the patient's wife and physician. In the acute care hospital, it is possible that an RN could safely delegate or assign a competent UAP to feed a stable dysphagic patient if the RN knew that the UAP was competent and had possibly observed how well a particular UAP was able to feed a patient. When the RN does not know the patient's or team member's abilities well enough to safely assign tasks, no situation can be the "right" circumstance.

3. **Right person?**

   No. The UAP's competency was unknown to the RN. "The licensed nurse along with the employer and the delegatee is responsible for ensuring that the delegatee possesses the appropriate skills and knowledge to perform the activity" (NCSBN & ANA, 2019, p. 4). There could have been a lucky "near miss" situation had the UAP been trained and competent. The RN should never delegate or assign a task for which a person's competency is unknown.

4. **Right direction and communication?**

   No. If the RN had asked the UAP about their ability with feeding precautions, and asked, "what steps would you take to make sure Mr. T. doesn't choke?," she would have initiated two-way communication and discovery of the UAP's lack of understanding of feeding a dysphagic patient and aspiration precautions. Better direction and communication could have involved: rounding with the UAP to the patient's room to discuss the feeding steps, directing the UAP at the patient's bedside, and demonstrating feeding to the UAP during the first time this patient was fed. If the RN had never worked with the UAP before and then questioned the UAP before the task was delegated, and the UAP said, "Yes, I know how to do this," it would still be incumbent on the RN to further evaluate the situation and the UAP's ability and to supervise the feeding of this unstable patient, as needed. The UAP should not be pressured and should be encouraged to clarify her discomfort with procedures openly and honestly. "The licensed nurse should ensure that the delegatee understands that she or he cannot make any decisions or modifications in carrying out the activity without first consulting the licensed nurse"(NCSBN & ANA, 2019, p. 4).

5. **Right supervision and evaluation?**

No. "The licensed nurse is responsible for monitoring the delegated activity, following up with the delegatee at the completion of the activity, and evaluating patient outcomes" Source: National Council of State Boards of Nursing (NCSBN), 2019. NCSBN and ANA National Guidelines for Nursing Delegation. It is unclear whether or not the RN had set up routine times for the UAP to check in with her and receive ongoing clarification or whether the supervisory RN was making rounds to observe care being completed. The right supervision and evaluation could have saved this patient's life.

Safety errors are often multifactorial in origin and present multiple points at which the correct supervision and evaluation could stop the adverse event and save a life. Applying and using the five Rights of Delegation appropriately could have put a stop to a mistake that these RNs and UAPs will never forget. In the case of Mr. Travaglini, had the RN applied the five Rights of Delegation, the patient and his wife may have enjoyed more time together, rather than experiencing a harrowing death with a subsequent lawsuit.

Competence

Competence is the "ability to accomplish specific skills safely and effectively under various circumstances" and true competency is confirmed as nurses "consistently display appropriate behaviors and sound judgments at the point of care" (Alfaro-LeFevre, 2017, p. 61). All professionals would agree that maintaining competence is essential to expertly lead the care team, and expert clinicians grow not only in clinical knowledge but also emotional intelligence and ethical personal attributes. Licensed nurse competence is built upon the knowledge gained during a nursing education program, orientation to specific settings, learning experiences in their care specialty, reflection on their own strengths and challenges, and ongoing continuing education based on self-assessment, evaluation, and ongoing clinical changes.

UAP competence is built upon formal training and assessment, orientation to specific settings and groups of patients, interpersonal and communication skills, and the experience of the UAP in assisting the nurse to provide safe nursing care.

Chief nursing officers (**CNO**s) and managers are accountable for establishing systems to assess, monitor, verify, and communicate ongoing competence requirements in areas related to delegation and clinical issues (ANA &

NCSBN, 2006). Written documentation of these competencies is maintained in the employee's personnel file. Some organizations ask UAPs to carry laminated cards that show their completed task competencies or maintain a frequently updated online list. Most health care organizations require employees to undergo annual competency training for elements of care unique to their practice setting. Annual competency testing for RN, LPN/LVN, and UAP may include: patient safety, infection control, resuscitation, chain of command, privacy protection under **Health Insurance Portability and Accountability Act** (**HIPAA**), use of restraints, and a variety of other skills.

Supervision

Supervision is the provision of guidance or direction, evaluation, and follow up by the licensed nurse for accomplishment of a nursing task delegated to UAP (NCSBN, 1995). ANA (2014, Duffy & McCoy, Delegation and You) states that supervision is "the active process of directing, guiding, and influencing the outcome of an individual's performance of a task" (ANA, 2014, Duffy & McCoy, Delegation and You, p. 23). Supervision of licensed or unlicensed nursing personnel means:

- "the provision of guidance and evaluation for the accomplishment of a nursing task or activity with
- the initial direction of the task or activity;
- periodic inspection of the actual act of accomplishing the task or activity; and
- the authority to require corrective action" (Washington Administrative Code 246-840-010).

The type of clinical supervision discussed in this chapter does not include administrative supervision that is present in a managerial job description that allows for hiring and firing ability. Clinical supervision can be categorized as on-site, in which the nurse is physically present or immediately available while the activity is being performed, or off-site, in which the nurse has the ability to provide direction through various means of written, verbal, and electronic communication (ANA, 2005). On-site supervision generally occurs in the acute care setting where the RN is immediately available. Off-site supervision may occur in home care, group homes, or community settings such as schools. A nurse who is delegating, assigning, and supervising care will provide clear direction to the team about what tasks are to be performed for specific patients. The supervising nurse must identify when and how the care is to be done, what patient/family outcomes are expected from the care, what information must be collected and reported, the times for reporting information and results, and any other patient-specific information. The supervising nurse will also monitor patient status and staff performance and obtain feedback from staff and patients in an ongoing manner, intervening as necessary to ensure compliance with established standards of practice, policy, and procedure.

Feedback

Feedback is a part of the evaluation process that is required in supervision. If the LPN/LVN or UAP performs poorly, the RN should tell them about mistakes, privately as much as possible, in a supportive manner, with a focus on quality of patient care and learning from mistakes so that all can complete their work effectively. If a team member, whether an RN, LPN/LVN, or UAP (or with unsafe activity by any other professional), performs in an inappropriate, unsafe, or incompetent manner, the RN must intervene immediately and stop the unsafe activity, discuss it with the team member, document the facts, and report the situation to the nurse manager or nursing supervisor as soon as possible. It is important to note that regular feedback should be given to the team, both positive and negative when necessary. Frequent, detailed, specific feedback strengthens team motivation and reinforces positive traits in team members.

What to Assess Before Delegation or Assignment

Even though the development of working skills in delegation is an outcome expectation of baccalaureate nursing program graduates (AACN, 2019), as well as all nursing graduates, the new graduate nurse may feel overwhelmed by the amount of patient care required and the lack of time to complete the care. The new graduate may be consumed by feelings of inadequacy and failure. For instance, not knowing how to answer the phone or find supplies, as well as not finding time for a meal break, can be exhausting. All of these feelings and behaviors may be a result of trying to do it all and not asking for help. New graduate nurses may quickly realize that if they do not delegate, the patient's care will not be completed in a timely and effective manner. The consequences and likely effects must be considered when delegating patient care. Hansten (2020, in LaCharity) suggested assessment of a variety of factors that must occur before deciding to delegate:

- Potential for Harm and Dynamics of Patient Status: The nurse must first know the patients and the competencies of the available delegates. The RN should determine if there is a risk for the patient in the activity delegated or assigned based on the current circumstances. The highest priority in all factors for decisions about what can be delegated or assigned is patient safety.

- Complexity of the Task and the Overall Care: The RN can potentially delegate or assign simple tasks. These tasks often require psychomotor skills but should not include the need for nursing judgment or on-site readjustment of a complex task.

- Individual Safety or Infection Control Precautions: The RN must be aware of each patient's specific safety or infection control needs. These needs could preclude delegating or assigning the task completely or may mean two or more personnel would be more effective working together to meet the patient's needs.

- Special Technology or Skill Involved: The RN should fully understand the implications of care tasks, including if an unfamiliar technology is present. If personnel have not been fully in-serviced regarding unfamiliar technology's use, this would preclude delegating or assigning the task to a person who is not yet competent in the new unfamiliar technology.

- Amount of Problem Solving and Innovation Required: An RN must think through whether or not tasks might require creative problem solving and innovation in approach with special adaptation or special attention needed to complete the

---

Critical Thinking 18.3

Steve, RN, is working with a new RN, Nadia. Steve tells Nadia that when she assigns patient care to another RN, that RN assumes accountability for the care. Each licensed nurse is accountable for their own level of licensed practice. When Nadia delegates or assigns to a UAP, she delegates or assigns responsibility for the tasks but keeps the accountability for that patient's care. Each person on the team is accountable for being aware of their competencies and limitations, only accepting tasks and duties they are able to safely complete, and completing the tasks and duties they have accepted.

When Nadia asks Jill, the UAP, to give a bath, what does Nadia retain accountability for?

What is Jill accountable for?

Critical Thinking 18.4

The RN continuously monitors unstable, complex patients who have imminent threats to their airway, breathing, circulation, or safety. Examples of these unstable, complex patients might include a patient on a ventilator or an unconscious patient. The RN may be helped by UAPs for some tasks for these patients such as patient repositioning. The RN can delegate some of the care of stable patients to the LPN/LVN or UAP.

What are some other examples of unstable patients?

task. When the RN knows the patient's condition before delegating or assigning, the potential for unnecessarily putting delegates and the patient at risk during an unanticipated modification or interruption of a conventional task is decreased.

- Unpredictability of Outcome: An RN should avoid delegating tasks in which the outcome is not clear or the patient's response is unpredictable.

- How much Supervision will be Needed and RN Availability: The RN delegating and assigning must also consider the need for supervision and the current staffing level. If the RN must supervise five students or novice nurses at once, even the best supervisory efforts may be fragmented and the RN may have difficulty responding to all the questions in a timely fashion.

- Physical Location: The assigning RN must consider physical location of patients on the unit and the work traffic patterns. How close are the patients geographically? Does the assignment make sense in the allocated available time?

- Level of Patient Interaction and Continuity of Care: The supervisory RN should consider each patient's emotional needs and recognize the need for RN interaction and continuity of care time at the bedside with the patient and the patient's family. An RN making the best assignments also reviews the last shift's work plan, and notes how much time is saved with nurse-patient familiarity and continuity of care. The RN does not expect or encourage UAPs to perform teaching or counseling of patients/families, because this is beyond their scope of practice and requires use of professional nursing judgment.

Attention to the above factors will improve patient safety associated with delegation decision making. Additionally, the availability of a competent, willing delegate is essential to assess prior to decisions to delegate.

Employer/Nurse Leader Responsibilities

The employer and the nursing leader are accountable to set up a safe and effective positive culture/work environment for optimal teamwork. They must acknowledge that delegation is a professional nursing right and responsibility; provide training and education on delegation; communicate information about the delegation process and delegatee competence level; and develop and periodically evaluate the delegation process and delegation policies and procedures (ANA & NCSBN, 2019)

1. A nurse leader (possibly a Chief Nursing Officer [CNO]) must be identified for oversight at the health care organization, no matter what the setting.

2. A nurse leader will develop a group, committee, or task force to determine nursing responsibilities that can be delegated, to whom, and under what circumstances. A nurse leader will review delegation activities and job descriptions for each team member so that role confusion can be eased. In some organizations this would occur in a unit/department meeting or in a shared governance or professional practice council (NCSBN, 2016, pp. 9–10).

3. The nurse leader is responsible for orienting and helping all nurses develop their ability to delegate and assign. New graduates need guidance because they may want to be regarded favorably and may not ask UAPs to do many tasks. New graduate classes sponsored by a health care organization include such topics as delegation and assignment policies and procedures and health team members' roles. These classes or online modules are where graduate nurses learn the job descriptions of health care team members. This information is needed to determine what and to whom to delegate and assign tasks. The new graduate must also explore the state nurse practice act regarding delegation as well as their department's job descriptions.

4. The organization researches that each individual is licensed or certified by state agencies, as needed, prior to hire.

5. The organization is responsible to set up, communicate, and periodically evaluate delegation policies and procedures so that all caregivers are trained and educated in the specific skills they are required to perform and that they are checked for a basic level of competency. The organization must provide ongoing in-services and updates to help nurses hone their delegation and assignment skills and alert nurses to changes in professional roles, laws, or advisory opinions.

6. The nurse leader will determine the appropriate resources and staffing mix of personnel on a nursing unit. The nurse leader may have personnel with a variety of skills, knowledge, and educational levels. The acuity and needs of the patients usually determine the personnel mix. From this personnel mix, the new graduate nurse will begin to identify who can best perform assigned duties. The non-nursing duties are shifted toward UAP, clerical personnel, or housekeeping personnel to make the best use of individual skills.

7. The nurse leader is accountable to follow up with reported team member competency issues so that they are resolved in a manner that keeps patients safe and colleagues trustful.

Table 18.6 displays Employer/Nurse Leader responsibilities for efficient delegation and assignment.

Licensed Registered Nurse Responsibility

The Licensed RN is responsible and accountable for the protection of patients and the provision of nursing care. The RN is always responsible for patient assessment, diagnosis, care

Table 18.6 Employer/Nurse Leader Responsibilities for Efficient Delegation and Assignment

- Identify a Nursing Leader
- Follow professional standards for education, licensure, and competency in all hiring decisions, orientation, and ongoing continuing education programs.
- Have clear job descriptions and ongoing licensing and credentialing policies for nursing and medical providers, LPN/LVNs, UAP, and other health care staff. The organization must ensure that all staff members are safe, competent practitioners before assigning them to patient care. Orient staff to their duties, chain of command, and the job descriptions of RN, LPN, and UAP.
- Facilitate clinical and educational specialty certification and credentialing of all health care practitioners and staff.
- Provide standards for ongoing supervision and periodic licensure/competency verification and evaluation of all employees.
- Provide access to evidence-based, professional health care standards, policies, procedures, library, Internet, and medication information, with unit availability and efficient library and Internet access.
- Facilitate regular evidence-based reviews of clinical standards, policies, and procedures.
- Develop and regularly evaluate and communicate clear policies and procedures for delegation.
- Clarify nursing chain of command during nursing orientation and identify how to report patient care issues.
- Communicate nursing responsibilities that can be delegated, to whom, and under what circumstances.
- Communicate information about the competence level of all delegatees.
- Provide administrative support for supervisors and employees who delegate, assign, monitor, and evaluate patient care.
- Clarify health care provider accountability; e.g., if a health care provider, e.g., nursing or medical practitioner or physician assistant, delegates a nursing task to a UAP, the health care provider is responsible for monitoring that care delivery. This should be spelled out in hospital policy. If the RN notes that the UAP is doing something incorrectly, the RN has a duty to intervene and to notify the ordering health care provider of the incident. The RN always has an independent responsibility to protect patient safety. Blindly relying on another nursing or medical health care provider is not permissible for the RN.

- Try to provide for continuity of care by the same staff when possible, and consider the geography of the unit and fair, balanced work distribution among staff when assigning care.
- If delegates don't meet standards, talk with them to identify the problem. If this is not successful, inform the delegate that you will be discussing the problem with your supervisor. Document your concerns, as appropriate. Follow up with your supervisor according to your organization's policy.
- Develop a physical, mental, and verbal "no abuse" policy to be followed by all professional and health care colleagues. Follow up on any problems.
- Consider applying for ANA Magnet Recognition, ANA Pathways for Excellence Designation, or other designation for your facility. ANA Magnet Recognition is awarded by the American Nurses Credentialing Center to acute care nursing departments that have worked to improve nursing care, including the empowering of nursing decision making and delegation in clinical practice.
- Monitor patient outcomes, including nurse-sensitive outcomes, staffing ratios, and other patient, clinical, financial, and organizational quality outcomes.
- Develop ongoing clinical quality improvement practices.
- Benchmark with national groups.

- Maintain ongoing monitoring of incident reports, sentinel events, and other elements of risk management and performance improvement of the process and outcome of patient care.
- Develop Electronic Health Records (EHR), including systematic, error-proof systems for medication administration that ensure the six rights of medication administration, that is, the right patient, right medication, right dose, right time, right route, right documentation. Develop safe computerized order-entry systems and staffing systems.
- Provide documentation of routine maintenance for all patient care equipment.
- Maintain the National Patient Safety Goals (www.jointcommission.org).
- Develop intra-hospital and intra-agency safe transfer policies.
- Do not delegate if in a high-risk situation. The RN may be at risk if the delegated task can be performed only by the RN according to law, organizational policies and procedures, or professional standards of nursing practice; if the delegated task could involve substantial risk or harm to a patient; if the RN knowingly delegates a task to a person who has not had the appropriate training or orientation; or if the RN fails to adequately supervise the delegated activity and does not evaluate the delegated action by reassessing the patient (ANA, 2019).
- Develop a positive and just work culture and environment to help keep patients safe and employees supported in reporting near misses or other safety and quality issues.

Source: Kelly Patricia.

planning, evaluation, and teaching. The RN must identify patient needs and when to delegate. UAP may measure vital signs, intake and output, and other patient status indicators, but it is the RN who interprets this data for comprehensive assessment, nursing diagnosis, and development of the plan of care. UAPs may perform simple nursing interventions related to patient hygiene, nutrition, elimination, or activities of daily living, but the RN must ensure availability to the delegatee, evaluate the patient outcomes, maintain accountability for any delegated responsibilities, and is ultimately accountable for the patient's overall nursing care. Asking a UAP to perform

functions outside their roles is a violation of the state nursing practice act and is a threat to patient safety.

As the RN prepares to care for the patient, he or she should describe the health care team to the patient, ideally with the UAP present on first rounds and during shift report at the bedside. For example:

Hello Mrs. Jones, my name is Luke Ellingsen. I am a Registered Nurse, and I will be responsible for your care until 7 p.m. today. This is Thelma Marks, a nursing assistant, who will be working with me and will be in to take your vital signs and help you with your bath. Please use my cell phone number if you need me, or use your call light if you have any questions for Thelma or for me.

The below 8 points help clarify RN responsibilities:

1. The RN, based on their own practice setting, their state laws and regulations, and job descriptions, must have assessed and understand their patients well enough to be able to protect their patients and determine their needs and current condition in order to know what, when, and if to delegate.

2. The RN must then also delegate or assign tasks to competent persons who agree they are willing and able to do this RN-chosen task from their job descriptions for this particular patient.

3. The RN must use clear, two-way communication (written, oral, and/or demonstration) to describe what needs to be done and in what manner, and must be available to the UAP or delegate to answer questions that arise.

4. The RN must set up normal patient data parameters for the UAP to monitor, identify checkpoints for two-way feedback, and identify timelines for reporting back data and task completion to the delegating RN.

5. The RN must evaluate the outcomes of care and the manner in which the patient responds as frequently as needed within the RN's professional judgment.

6. The RN must offer feedback and evaluation to the caregivers they supervise. The best RN leaders also ask for feedback from their co-workers and the team members they supervise about their own communications and abilities.

7. If competency or education needs become apparent, the RN must follow up with the correct nurse manager or nursing supervisor to report the issues (NCSBN, 2016, pp. 10–11.)

8. The RN is accountable for reporting to a nursing supervisor or manager and using their organization's reporting chain of command if unit problems or conditions exist that inhibit optimal patient care. The RN should also participate in finding solutions to these identified issues that impact patient care or workplace effectiveness.

New Graduate RN Responsibility

Hansten (2019) reports that discrete competencies (such as making assignments, following up with UAPs, and offering feedback) within delegation, assignment, and supervision are self-reported by registered nurses as their least proficient leadership abilities (www.linkedin.com/pulse/another-look-rn-leadership-skill-level-patient-hansten-rn-mba-phd). New graduate nurses have a need to focus on the duties and

activities for which they are directly responsible while they develop clinical judgment abilities. They must accept duties and activities based on their own competence level and maintain their competence for delegated responsibilities. They must also maintain accountability for delegated activities and ask themselves, what duties can I delegate and to what extent? What do UAPs do? What do LPN/LVNs do? Reviewing the nurse practice act for a nurse's individual state is important and applies to all licensed nurses, regardless of whether the nurse is a new graduate or not. The nurse practice act is the legal authority for nursing practice in each state. In the individual states, the definitions, regulations, or directives regarding delegation may be different. The state nurse practice acts also determine what level of licensed nurse is authorized to delegate (NCSBN, 2005). The RN also reviews any other applicable state or federal laws; patient needs; job descriptions and competencies of the RNs, LPNs/LVNs, and UAPs; the agency's policies and procedures; the clinical situation; and the professional standards of nursing in preparation for delegation. Table 18.7 includes delegation or assignment suggestions for RNs. Table 18.8 (Kelly and Marthaler 2012) includes additional delegation and assignment suggestions for RNs.

Licensed Practical Nurse/Licensed Vocational Nurse (LPN/LVN) Responsibility

Licensed Practical Nurse/Licensed Vocational Nurse (LPN/LVN) are caregivers who have undergone a standardized training and competency and licensing evaluation. Their scope of practice varies in each state. Patient care may be assigned to an LPN/LVN, in keeping with their scope of practice as designated by state regulation. LPN/LVNs are able to perform duties and functions that UAPs are not allowed to do, and they are also responsible for their actions. LPN/LVNs usually care for stable patients with predictable outcomes, though they may assist the RN with seriously ill patients in **Critical Care Units** (**CCU**s). The LPN/LVN is not assigned initial patient assessment. After the RN has completed the patient's initial assessment and the plan of care, the LPN/LVN might be allowed to perform the ongoing head-to-toe assessments and monitor vital signs, Intravenous (IV) sites, IV fluids, breath sounds, etc. Duties of the LPN/LVN include the duties of the UAP and also may include, depending on state rules and job descriptions: passing medications; performing simple sterile dressing changes, colostomy irrigations, respiratory suctioning, and insertion of retention catheters; and in some states, teaching from a standard patient care plan under the direction of an RN.

If the LPN/LVN is certified in IV therapy and the policy of the state and the employing institution permits LPN/LVNs to provide IV treatment, LPN/LVNs may administer or start IV sites and fluids and monitor the IVs. The RN should not have an inordinate duty to supervise IV work by the LPN/LVN after the LPN/LVN skills in this area are verified. Note that prior competency certification of the LPN/LVN may have been done

Table 18.7 Delegation or Assignment Suggestions for RNs

Delegation or assignment suggestions	Examples
Be clear on the qualifications of the delegate, i.e., education, experience, and competency. Require documentation or demonstration of current competence by the delegate for each task. Clarify patient care concerns or delegation problems. Consult ANA and NCSBN position papers on delegation and your state board of nursing guidelines, as necessary. Know your job descriptions.	The charge nurse will assign a new graduate nurse a team of patients less complex than the assignment of an RN who has several years of experience.
Assess what is to be delegated or assigned and identify who would best complete the assignment.	The RN will ask a UAP to pick up specific equipment, e.g., a pediatric pulse oximeter from a stock room. The UAP has worked on this unit for 5 yr and is familiar with the type of equipment the nurse needs.
Communicate the duty to be performed and identify the time frame for completion. The expectations for personnel should be clear and concise.	The charge nurse tells another nurse, "While I am at lunch, Mr. Jones, the patient in bed 34-2 may ask for something for pain. Please make him comfortable, replace the ice pack, and tell him that it is too early for another pain medication for 60 more minutes."
Avoid changing tasks once they are assigned when team members request a change unless there are compelling reasons to disrupt plans already in progress. Changing duties should be considered when the task is above the level of the personnel, as when the patient's care is in jeopardy due to a change in status, or if there are other important reasons such as infection control or personnel developmental and learning needs.	The UAP was delegated the task of taking vital signs on a set of patients. One of the patients is receiving a blood transfusion and is very ill. The nurse may transfer the delegated task of taking vital signs on this patient to an RN.
Evaluate the effectiveness of the delegation of duties. Monitor care and check in with UAP frequently. Ask for a feedback report on the outcomes of care delivery.	After the patient was assisted to the bathroom, the nurse asked the UAP, what amount of assistance did the patient require? Is the patient safely back in bed?
Accept minor variations in the style in which duties are performed. Individual styles are acceptable as long as the duty is performed correctly within the scope of practice and all accepted ethical and/or scientific norms (such as sterile technique when necessary) and there is a good outcome.	Both of the following nurses are successful at providing care using different and acceptable methods. One nurse assesses the assigned patients, documents care, and then passes medications. Another nurse assesses the patients while passing medications and then documents care.
Take action when delegate does not carry out their assigned duties.	If a delegate does not carry out their assigned duties, the RN must take action to assure patient safety. Talk to the delegate and determine why the assigned duty was not carried out. Depending on the delegate's response, the RN may need to take one or more of the following actions: • Explain to the delegate the importance and method of performing assigned duties, • Report the incident to the nursing supervisor, and • Complete an evaluation form about the delegate's lack of performance if requested by the nursing supervisor. If any personnel continue with poor performance, the person may lose their position. The manager or supervisor is accountable for hiring and firing decisions.

Source: Kelly Patricia.

through evaluation on a skills day or through a competency validation under direct supervision of an RN, only in states where this IV therapy practice by an LPN/LVN is allowed.

In other states, LPN/LVNs are allowed to maintain existing IV lines and fluids under the supervision of an on-site RN but they are not allowed to start IVs. RNs should not rely on "word of mouth" information regarding LPN/LVN and UAP roles from other employees; instead the RN should review actual state rules and organizational documents such as job descriptions and competency checklists.

In Beeber et al. (2018) and Mueller et al.'s (2018) studies of the importance of nurse delegation policies in assisted living and residential care, it became clear that some nurses are confused about roles for RNs, LPN/LVNs, and medication technicians. As previously stated, the roles of LPNs/LVNs and some UAPs vary by state and by type of practice setting.

In some states, in nursing homes, the LPN/LVN may assume the charge nurse role with an on-site supervising RN. LPN/LVNs report their findings to the RN. The RN is still primarily responsible for overall patient assessment, nursing

Table 18.8   Additional Delegation and Assignment Suggestions for RNs

Consider prior to delegating

- Who has the time to complete the delegated task?
- Who is the best person for the task?
- What is the urgency of the task?
- Are there any time restraints?
- Who do you want to develop their skills?
- Who is the best person to meet the patient's needs?
- Who would enjoy completing the task?

Be clear on the qualifications of the delegate, that is, education, experience, and competency. Require documentation or demonstration of current competence by the delegate for each task. Clarify patient care concerns or questions about the delegated task. Find ANA position statements at www.nursingworld.org, the NCSBN at www.NCSBN.org and at your state board of nursing yearly to keep up to date with changes that may occur regarding delegation of nursing care.

Speak to your team members as you would like to be spoken to. There is no need to apologize for your need to have another team member perform a task. Remember that you are carrying out your professional responsibility. Assure the delegates that you will help them when you can. Be sure to do so.

Communicate the patient's name, room number, the task to be performed, and identify the time frame for completion. Best practices include the patient/family and the UAP in this discussion. Discuss any changes from the usual procedures that might be needed to meet special patient needs and any potential or expected changes that should be reported to the RN. The expectations for personnel before, during, and after task performance should be stated in a clear, pleasant, direct, and concise manner.

Identify the expected patient outcome and the limits on UAP authority.

Verify the delegate's understanding of delegated tasks, and have the delegate repeat instructions as needed. Verify that the delegate accepts the responsibility for carrying out the task correctly. Require regular, frequent mini-reports or check points of information about patients from the health care team including UAP, LPN/LVNs, etc.

Avoid removing tasks once assigned. This should be considered only when the task is above the level of the personnel, such as when the patient's care is in jeopardy because the patient's status has changed, or when time does not permit completion of previously assigned tasks.

Monitor task completion according to standards. Make frequent walking rounds to assess patient outcomes. Intervene as needed.

Accept minor variations in the style in which the tasks are performed. Individual styles are acceptable as long as patient standards and accepted scientific and ethical principles are maintained and good outcomes are achieved.

Try to meet team's needs for learning opportunities and consider any health problems and work preferences of the team members as long as they don't interfere with meeting patient needs.

If a delegate doesn't meet standards, talk with them privately to identify the problem. If this is not successful, inform the delegate that you will be discussing the problem with the supervisor. Document your concerns, as appropriate. Follow up with the supervisor according to your organization's policy.

Avoid high-risk delegation or assignment. Do not delegate or assign a task to a LPN/LVN or UAP if the task can be performed only by the RN according to law, organizational policies and procedures, or professional standards of nursing practice; or if the delegated task could involve substantial risk or harm to a patient. The RN should not knowingly delegate a task to a person who has not had the appropriate training or orientation; or fail to adequately supervise the delegated/assigned activity and must evaluate the delegated action by reassessing the patient and the results of the delegated or assigned activity. (ANA, 2005, 2014 in Duffy & McCoy)

Sources: Marthaler, M., & Kelly, P. (2012). Delegation of nursing care. In P. Kelly, Nursing leadership and management (3rd ed.). Clifton Park, NY: Delmar Cengage Learning,Boucher (1998); Zimmermann (1996); and ANA, (2005), ANA 2014 in Duffy and McCoy, ANA and NCSBN (2019).

diagnosis, planning, implementation, and evaluation of the quality of care delegated. Remember to consult your own state practice rules and organizational job descriptions about this highly variable role.

Unlicensed Assistive Personnel (UAP) Responsibility

UAP are delegatees and are trained to perform duties such as bathing, feeding, toileting, and ambulating patients or other tasks based on the state and their individual specialty education,

such as education related to Emergency, Psychiatric, or Perioperative, or Rehabilitation, HCAs of various levels, and Certified Medication Aides (CMAs). UAP are expected to document and report information related to patient care activities based on organizational guidelines. The RN will delegate or assign work to the UAP and is liable for those delegation decisions. According to the ANA (2005), if the RN knows that the assistant has the appropriate training, orientation, and documented competencies, then the RN can reasonably expect that the UAP will function in a safe and effective manner. However, each situation must be assessed based on the nurses' knowledge of the specific patient's condition and the individual abilities of the delegatee. Remember that state guidelines for UAP task roles vary.

An overview of basic UAP responsibilities would include:

1. Accepting only those activities or tasks they feel comfortable with and are able to perform competently.

2. Completing the tasks or activities successfully and as agreed upon, or update the RN promptly if unable to do so.

3. Maintaining competence levels for the UAP's delegated or assigned responsibility (NCSBN, 2016, p. 6).

4. Asking questions to clarify when unsure.

5. Maintaining open communication and feedback with all team members.

6. Maintaining accountability for delegated activities.

Health care organizations use UAP in all settings in order to ensure wise stewardship of health care costs; freeing RNs from duties that do not require an RN to do them; and allowing time for RNs to complete assessments of patients and RN-only care, as well as patient evaluation. It is more cost effective to have UAP perform non-nursing duties than to have nurses perform them. UAP can deliver supportive care; they cannot practice nursing or provide total patient care. The RN must be aware of the job description, skills, and educational background of the UAP prior to the delegation or assigning of duties. Delegation also allows entry-level workers to learn about the health care environment and provides a great stepping stone to a career in nursing and other health care roles after further education. Table 18.9 allows students to test themselves on delegation and assignment.

Table 18.9   Test Yourself

Questions	Yes	No
1. Do you recognize that you, as an RN, retain ultimate accountability for the nursing care of your assigned patients?		
2. Do you spend most of your time completing tasks that require an RN and that could not be done by someone else on your team?		
3. Do you trust the ability of your team to complete assignments successfully?		
4. Do you allow UAPs sufficient time to solve their own problems before intervening with advice (if this is reasonable, considering patient safety)?		
5. Do you clearly outline expected outcomes when delegating and hold your team accountable for achieving these outcomes?		
6. Do you support your team with an appropriate level of feedback and follow up?		
7. Do you use delegation and challenging work assignments as a way to help your team develop new skills?		
8. Does your team know what you expect of them?		
9. Do you take the time to carefully select the right person for the right job?		
10. Do you feel comfortable asking for feedback on your own performance as a leader?		
11. Do you clearly identify all aspects of an assignment to your team when you delegate?		
12. Do you assign tasks to the most entry level team member capable of completing them successfully?		
13. Do you support your team when they are learning?		
14. Do you allow your team reasonable freedom to achieve outcomes?		

Source: Created by R. Hanstead & P. Kelly.

Real World Interview

"I have been a nursing assistant for years so as a new RN I am very careful to include my team in our shift report, patient rounding, and I make sure we have checkpoint huddles before and after all breaks and meals. I 'get my hands dirty' in that I help with messy tasks so that no one thinks I consider myself better than them. If they need help when I am on the phone, I explain later what I was doing that was so important, like, 'I was on the phone with the son telling him about Mrs. Joan's sepsis.' I make sure to ask for feedback from my team as well as offer a feedback discussion at the end of the shift. 'What could I have done better? What could we have done better as a team?' and I point out what we achieved together for the patients. 'We saved Mr. Peterson and he is doing better in the Critical Care Unit (CCU)! And look how happy Mr. Jackson was with his new hip and ambulation!' I always get a hand from my team because they know we are together in all of this."

Name Withheld, RN, in Midwest.

Under-Delegation and Over-Delegation

Personnel in a new job role such as a new nursing graduate, new charge RN, or new nurse manager, often under-delegate. Believing that older, more experienced staff may resent having someone new delegate to them, a novice nurse may simply avoid delegation or assigning care tasks. New nurses may seek approval from other staff members by demonstrating their ability to complete all assigned duties without assistance. In addition, new nurses may be reluctant to delegate or assign because they do not know or trust individuals on their team or are not clear on the scope of all their duties or what they are all allowed to do. New nurses can become frustrated and overwhelmed if they fail to delegate and assign appropriately. They may fail to establish appropriate controls such as failing to offer initial direction, failing to set up checkpoint times to regroup with their team, failing to clarify expectations with staff, or failing to evaluate care and follow up properly. They also may not delegate the appropriate authority to go with assigned responsibilities. Perfectionism and a fear of a delegate not doing their work can lead new nurses to feel they are overwhelmed with patient care responsibilities. More experienced nursing staff members can help new nurses by intervening early on, assisting in the delegation and assignment process, and clarifying responsibilities.

Over-Delegation

Over-delegation or assigning too many duties to others can also place the patient at risk. The reasons for over-delegation or assignment are numerous. Personnel may feel uncomfortable performing duties that are unfamiliar to them, and they may depend too much on others. They may be unorganized or inclined to either avoid responsibility or immerse themselves in details. Over-delegation leads to delegating or assigning duties to personnel who are not educated for the tasks, such as expecting LPN/LVNs and UAP to perform RN-only work. Delegating or assigning duties that are inappropriate for personnel to perform because they have been inadequately educated is dangerous and against the state nurse practice act. Over-delegating duties can overwork some personnel and underwork others, creating obstacles to appropriate delegation or assignment of tasks. Table 18.10 reviews some obstacles to team leadership and excellence in delegation, assignment, and supervision. Table 18.11 (Kelly and Marthaler 2012) is a review of the elements to consider when delegating or assigning care.

Critical Thinking 18.5

It was just about 8:30 p.m. on the 7 p.m. to 7 a.m. shift on 2 East. Most of the practitioners had made their rounds, so the evening was calming down. The UAP, Jill, was picking up the dinner trays from the patient's rooms. Steve, the RN, had just sat down to document his patient assessments when he heard UAP Jill yell, "I need some help in Room 2510! Mr. Olson is not breathing." As several of the nurses ran to Room 2510, the UAP ran for the emergency crash cart. The cart was wheeled into the patient's room during the overhead announcement by the operator, "CODE BLUE, Room 2510." The nurses initiated **Cardiopulmonary Resuscitation (CPR)**. The UAP plugged the cart into the wall, turned the suction machine on, and then assisted the family out of the room and stayed with them until the nurse was able to talk with them.

How does completion of these tasks by the UAP contribute to patient care?

In what ways does the UAP relieve the pressure on the nurse to provide acute patient care?

Table 18.10 Obstacles to Delegation

- Fear of being disliked
- Inability to give up any control of the situation
- Fear of making a mistake
- Inability to determine what to delegate and to whom
- Inadequate knowledge of the delegation or assignment process
- Past experience with delegation that did not turn out well
- Poor interpersonal communication skills
- Lack of confidence to move beyond being a novice nurse
- Lack of administrative support for nurses delegating to LPN/LVN and UAP
- Tendency to isolate oneself and choose to complete all tasks alone
- Inappropriate number and skill or competency mix of personnel for the individual patient population
- Lack of confidence to delegate to staff members who were previously one's peers
- Inability to prioritize using Maslow's hierarchy of needs and the nursing process
- Thinking of oneself as the only one who can complete a task the way "it is supposed" to be done
- Inability to communicate effectively
- Inability to develop working relationships with other team members
- Lack of knowledge of the capabilities of staff, including their competency, skill, experience, level of education, job description, and so on

Source: Kelly Patricia.

Table 18.11   Elements to Consider when Delegating or Assigning

• Federal, state, and local regulations and guidelines for practice, including the state nurse practice act, Board of Nursing Rules and Advisory opinions • Specialty Nursing Organization standards or policies (e.g., Emergency Nurses Association)	• Job description of registered nurse, licensed practical nurse/licensed vocational nurse, nursing assistive personnel • Nursing professional standards • Health care agency policy, procedure, and standards, job descriptions	• Five Rights of Delegation (ANA and NCSBN, 2019) • Knowledge and skill of personnel • Documented personnel competency, strengths, and weaknesses (select the right person for the right job) • NCSBN/ANA Joint Statement, Employer/Nurse Leader Responsibility, Licensed Nurse Responsibility, and Delegatee Responsibility (2019)

RN is accountable for Application of the Nursing Process and KNOWING the Patient
Assessment and Clinical Judgment
Nursing Diagnosis
Planning Care
Implementation and Teaching
(Parts of Implementation, e.g., Some Tasks, Can Be Delegated or Assigned)
RN Delegates or Assigns, As Appropriate
RN retains Accountability
(Note that LPN/LVNs and UAP are also Responsible and Accountable for Their Actions)
Evaluation

RN	LPN/LVN	UAP
RNs assess, plan care, monitor, and evaluate all patients, especially complex, unstable patients with unpredictable outcomes. Intervene quickly to assure patients' physiological, safety, and psychological needs. Administer medications, including IV push. Start and maintain IVs and blood transfusions. Perform sterile or specialized procedures, for example, Foley catheter and nasogastric tube insertion, tracheostomy care, suture removal, and so on. Educate patient and family. Maintain infection control. Administer Cardiopulmonary Resuscitation (CPR). Interpret and report laboratory findings. Triage patients. Prevent adverse nurse-sensitive patient outcomes, for example, cardiac arrest, pneumonia, and so on. Monitor patient outcomes.	LPN/LVNs care for stable patients with predictable outcomes. They work under the direction of the RN and are responsible for their actions within their scope of practice. Gather patient data. Implement patient care. Maintain infection control. *Provide and reinforce teaching from standard teaching plan as directed by RN.[a]* *Depending on the state and with documented competency, may do the following:[a]* *Administer medications.* *Perform sterile or specialized procedures, for example, Foley catheter and nasogastric tube insertion, tracheostomy care, suture removal, and so on.* *Perform blood glucose monitoring.* *Administer CPR (most states)* *Perform venipuncture and insert peripheral IVs, change IV bags for patients receiving IV therapy, and so on.*	UAP assist the RNs and the LPNs and give technical care to stable patients with predictable outcomes and minimal potential for risk, and assist with close RN supervision of those patients that are higher risk. UAP work under the direction of an RN and are responsible for their actions and task completion. Assist with activities of daily living. Assist with bathing, grooming, and dressing. Assist with toileting and bed making. Ambulate, position, and transport. Feed and socialize with patient. Measure intake and output (I&O). Document care. Weigh patient. Maintain infection control. *Depending on the state and with documented competency, may do the following:[a]* • *Perform blood glucose monitoring.* • *Collect specimens.* • *Administer CPR.* • *Take vital signs (most states).*

RN uses Clinical Judgment and is Responsible for Evaluation of all Patient Care.
Clinical judgment is "outcome of critical thinking or clinical reasoning, the conclusion, decision, or opinion you make after thinking about the issues." Alfaro-LeFevre, 2017, p. 6

Source: Developed with information from Kelly & Marthaler (2012) and National Guidelines for Nursing Delegation Effective Date: April 29, 2019.NCSBN—ANA Jointly, available at www.ncsbn.org/NGND-PosPaper_06.pdf (2019). Accessed August 31, 2019.
[a]State practice acts differ: Check your own state nurse practice regulations.

Chain of Command

The chain of command identifies the order in which nurses report problems that impact their practice or patient care. The chain of command is used when a nurse cannot solve a prob-lem on their own, as barriers exist that prevent the nurse from doing their best for a patient in a given situation. These bar-riers are reported by the nurse to the next supervisory person above them in the chain of command. All health care person-nel serve the patient and their family and are accountable to them and to the community. Nursing Assistive Personnel and Licensed Practical Nurses are accountable to the RN, including new graduate RNs. The RN is accountable to the charge nurse who is accountable to the nursing managers/directors, who are responsible to the house shift administrators or supervisors. The house shift administrators or supervisors are accountable to the Chief Nursing Officer who is accountable to the **Chief Executive Officer** (**CEO**). The CEO is responsible to the Board of Directors, who is ultimately accountable to their patients, the community they serve, the accrediting organizations, and federal and state regulators. (Figure 18.1).

From a practical standpoint, a nurse encountering patient care problems would first talk with their charge nurse and the patient's attending physician in a community setting. In a university setting, the nurse would first talk with their charge nurse and the medical resident on call, then the medical fellow, then the attending physician. The Rapid Response Team or the Code Blue Team is utilized first in critical situations that warrant immediate patient attention. If a problem is not resolved, the nurse and charge nurse will assess the situation, and, if needed, contact the patient's physician and other nursing and medical groups and hospital administrators who would best handle or solve the problem, for example, the Chief Nursing Officer, Medical Director, Chief of the Medical Staff, Chief Executive Officer, etc. Groups that may be called to address an issue could be unit or organizational shared governance or

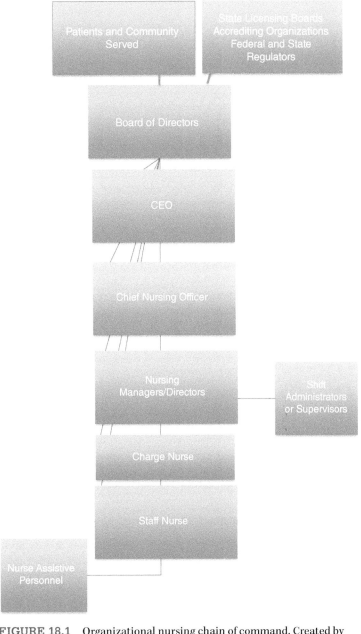

FIGURE 18.1 Organizational nursing chain of command. Created by R. Hanstead & P. Kelly.

shared decision-making professional councils or committees such as Patient Safety and Quality, Compliance, Ethics, Pharmacy and Therapeutics, Risk Management, or various other Medical and Nursing Committees, including Union representatives or Bargaining Units in a union environment.

Examples of instances for implementing the chain of command include but are not limited to instances where:

- Impairment of a practitioner is suspected.

- The patient's physician is unable to be reached.

- The physician is acting outside the scope of his/her privileges.

- The physician's orders instruct the nurse to perform something outside the scope of his/her practice and the issue was unable to be resolved between them.

- There is progressive deterioration of a patient's clinical condition and the nurse believes the patient requires medical intervention that cannot be provide by a nurse

- The nurse's assessment of the patient varies significantly from the physician's assessment and the nurse believes that the discrepancy places the patient at serious risk of harm.

Accurate, factual documentation of the facts in the patient's medical record of all contacts with individuals through the chain of command should be done by the person who placed the call/made the contact. The nurse caring for the patient should document initial physician notification, discussion, any refusals, the reason for any refusals of an order, notification of the charge nurse and other people in the chain of command, and specific information given to the physician and others in the chain of command concerning the patient. Documentation of all contacts with individuals through the chain of command should be done by the person who placed the call/made the contact. Every nurse, no matter the practice setting, should clearly understand the chain of command where they are employed. Not knowing the chain of command or not following it can cause serious repercussions to the patient, the nurse, and the institution.

The Nursing Process and Delegation

Ultimately, some professional activities involving the specialized knowledge, judgment, or skill of the nursing process can never be delegated (NCSBN, 2016). Some of these activities could include patient assessment, triage, nursing diagnosis, nursing plans of care, extensive teaching or counseling, telephone advice, outcome evaluations, and patient discharges. Delegated tasks are typically those tasks that occur frequently, are considered technical by nature, are considered standard and unchanging, have predictable results, and have minimal potential for risks (ANA 2014, 5–7). As a professional standard for all nurses in all states, the assessment, nursing diagnosis, planning, and evaluation stages of the nursing process may not be delegated. Delegated activities usually fall within the implementation phase of the nursing process.

State Boards of Nursing

State Boards of Nursing exist to protect the public, not to protect RN licenses. The best way for nurses to protect their licensure has to do with understanding their state regulations and standards of practice and abiding by them. Some states specify nursing tasks that may be delegated in their rules, regulations, standards of care, or advisory opinions. It is crucial that every RN remember: because a task can be delegated, this does not mean you must delegate it, nor does it mean you should delegate that task if your clinical judgment dictates that this task for this particular patient is not wisely delegated or assigned to a UAP. For example, a nurse can assign postoperative ambulation. However, if the patient has been unstable, hypotensive, and this is the first time the patient will sit up and ambulate postoperatively, the nurse can be liable for assigning a UAP to do a task that they are not able to safely complete, given the patient's state. The UAP may try to get the patient up the first time postoperatively alone, and the patient could fall. Although the tasks in the examples in Table 18.12, and Table 18.13 of "tasks that can possibly be delegated or assigned" and "which tasks can be delegated or assigned" are similar to tasks listed in some UAP state guidelines or rules, the nurse must always assess the situation and the patient, as well as check for interstate variation regarding delegation.

Note that state websites offer not only the statute (law), but also administrative codes and/or rules and advisory opinions that provide you with guidelines for practice. Be certain you are checking the correct site for your practice arena; for example, there may be a special portion of the administrative code or rules for home health that are different from acute care, or for such specialized roles as Certified Medication Aide, Surgical Technician, Medical Assistant, and others. Review your nursing specialty website for guidelines regarding what and when to delegate or assign. Some of these nursing specialties include psychiatric, emergency, perioperative, perinatal, rehabilitation, ambulatory care, schools, or public health nursing. Check state requirements with your state board of nursing or link to more suggestions about how to access assistive personnel role information at www.ncsbn.org

Teamwork and Collaboration

Teamwork and collaboration are essential for the best communication. All people communicate and do their work better if leaders respect individual differences in the way the team learns and in the way their brains process information. Communication or work habit differences such as voice, speaking style, and sense of time all may impact teamwork and collaboration effectiveness. For example, patient information can be difficult or simple for team members to understand based on the manner in which it is given and whether the individual being instructed is a visual, auditory, or kinesthetic or tactile learner. If the UAP tends to learn more by visual cues, instructions and work assignments should be printed or be otherwise visual. When a patient discussion is essential because the

Table 18.12 Delegation or Assignment Task Examples

Nursing Tasks Never Delegated or Assigned
- Patient assessment (physical, psychological, and social assessment, which requires professional nursing judgment, intervention, referral, or follow up). Data collection without interpretation is not assessment.
- Planning of nursing care and assessment of the patient's response
- Implementation that requires judgment
- Health teaching and health counseling other than reinforcement of what the RN has already taught
- Evaluation of the patient's response
- Medication administration (In many states, some medication administration can be assigned to LPN/LVNs. In some states, simple medications and some injections can be delegated to certified medication aides, home health aides, and medical assistants with specific training and certification. Refer to your current state nursing practice act to determine is delegation or assignment of medications are allowed or prohibited.)

Nursing Tasks Not Routinely Delegated or Assigned
- Note that the below tasks may sometimes be delegated if the staff has received special credentialing such as education and competency testing and are certified.
- Sterile procedures
- Invasive procedures, such as inserting tubes in a body cavity or instilling or inserting substances into an indwelling tube
- Care of broken skin other than minor abrasions or cuts generally classified as requiring only first aid treatment (without topical medication)
- Intravenous therapy (in some states can be delegated or assigned to LPN/LVNs with limitations)

Nursing Tasks Most Commonly Delegated or Assigned: the RN can decide NOT to delegate any task, no matter how routine, based on the RN's nursing judgment, if the patient or delegate situation dictates.
- Noninvasive and non-sterile treatments
- Collecting, reporting, and documenting data such as vital signs, height, weight, intake and output
- Ambulation, positioning, and turning
- Transportation of the patient within the facility
- Personal hygiene and elimination, including cleansing enemas (no medicated enemas)
- Feeding (depending on patient situation and delegate's competency), cutting up food, or placing meal trays
- Socialization activities
- Activities of daily living

Source: Kelly Patricia.

Table 18.13 Which Tasks Can Be Delegated or Assigned?

Identify which members of the health care team could potentially perform each of the following nursing activities. *NONE of these tasks may be delegated or assigned if the RN has not performed the 5 Rights of Delegation and knows the patient's condition and stability as well as the competence of the caregiver first. Delegation and Assignment should NEVER be a rote "always" activity. This table is only for the student's use to determine what* <u>could</u> *be delegated or assigned if the patient care situation was perfectly stable and all team members were competent.*

Nursing activity	RN	LPN/LVN	UAP/NAP/AP
Administer blood to a patient			
Assess a patient going to surgery			
Develop a teaching plan for a patient newly diagnosed with diabetes			
Measure a patient's intake and output			
Provide a bath to an immobilized patient			
Change a dressing			
Give patient report when transferring a patient from ICU to a step-down unit			
Give insulin			
Evaluate a patient's Do Not Resuscitate (DNR) status			
Give an oral medication			
Assist a patient with ambulation			
Give an intramuscular (IM) pain medication			
Give an intravenous (IV) pain medication			

6/23/19

Source: Created by R. Hanstead & P. Kelly.

(Note: check your state practice act in the particular state where you work, and the facility's job descriptions, in order to be certain regarding administering IV fluids, blood, insulin, IM and IV pain medications.)

patient is an auditory learner and processes information best by hearing it, then verbal instructions may need to be repeated and backed up with written assignments. If language proficiency is a barrier or when the UAP is a kinesthetic or tactile processor of information, showing them how to perform a task through action and movement is a good option to set the stage for best task completion. Kinesthetic or tactile UAPs learn best by doing. Individual types of information processing differences will be useful to keep in mind when the RN offers initial direction or instructions for assignments or when the RN perceives that tasks are not being understood or done appropriately. The RN may need to help the UAP organize and understand assignments by creating additional methods to keep track of work assigned and work completed through personalized written notes or voice-recording instructions or videotaped demonstrations.

Family of origin issues such as how fast or how slow people speak, how conflict or questions are handled, and how much space or physical closeness people maintain between themselves can be a barrier to best teamwork and collaboration results. For example, ineffective delegation can take place when an individual's space is violated. Some delegators stand too close when speaking. Conversely, some members of a group may feel left out if they are not sitting close to the delegator. They may not feel included or important. The RN can learn how issues such as voice speed and physical space work best for each person by simple observation, asking, and listening. If the RN has observed the delegate often speaking animatedly at close proximity to others, a few quiet words of instruction or being handed an assignment sheet without further discussion may not be well-understood or appreciated by the delegate. At times, the RN may interpret the individual characteristics of their team members incorrectly and assign blame or think the UAP is "not listening." Asking for feedback about how best to communicate with each individual is helpful.

> *How do you like to receive your assignments? What did your "best team leader ever" do to communicate with you? Would you like more clearly written instructions? Would it be useful to make rounds to discuss patients? What works best for you so we communicate most effectively?*

The above are a few questions that can be used to develop clear communication.

Another individual difference affecting delegation is the concept of time. Some people tend to move slowly and may be perceived as late, whereas other people move quickly and are prompt in meeting deadlines or completing tasks early and volunteering to assist others. The RN must be very clear related to instructions so that the RN's idea of "prompt" or "right away" meets the other person's understanding of expectations, for example, "I need those vital signs by 0900 so I can give the medication." RNs sometimes assume that UAPs or LPN/LVNs are not industrious or don't care, when in fact individual differences in communicating or work habit issues need to be addressed with excellent RN leadership, teamwork, and collaboration.

Teamwork and Collaboration Routines

Engaged and enthusiastic teamwork and collaboration is initiated by the RN who is clear on intended patient outcomes and the plan for the day, shift, episode of care, and/or longer-term results. RNs must lead this teamwork and collaboration for the right care to be completed by the team in an efficient manner. A patient's daily or most emergent needs are foremost. For example, "Mr. Jones would like to focus on improving his pain level today; he can start moving more when he feels he is at a 4." Longer-term and/or discharge plans are also imperative to share for putting the picture of care into place for the team: "Mr. Jones plans to go to a rehabilitation center, probably tomorrow" or "Mr. Jones is going to hospice as soon as this round of chemotherapy has been completed." Clarity about the intended patient results allow the team members to be an engaged part of the process of helping the patient rather than producing a few limited, boring disconnected tasks without context.

One of the most effective ways of solving some of the team's role or task confusion is by offering clear instructions during shift hand-off report at the patient's bedside in acute and long-term care, thus allowing for clarity about the team's plan for the shift. For home health care, an on-site discussion with the patient/family and caregivers would be similar to a shift hand-off report discussion. Holding shift or case updates, checkpoints, or and/or huddles during a shift help clarify plans for the rest of the patient care episode.

Another leadership method an RN can use to make sure the team is clear on the patient care plan and shares expectations of each other, is by debriefing, or reviewing and evaluating the shift or episode of care toward the end of the shift so that each individual can quickly discuss what worked and what didn't. Questions such as, "What worked this shift/case, and what didn't?" and "What would you suggest we do differently if we had the same situation tomorrow?" will help RNs receive feedback and allow for an open team atmosphere for improving safety and quality.

The new graduate RN can use feedback to learn how to better lead the team. Ask, "Because I am trying to learn how to be a better RN, I would really truly appreciate what you would suggest for me to do differently." Then wait. Leave time for others to feel comfortable giving feedback on what they think. The new graduate can also ask, "What were the attributes of those RNs you love working with?" if the team is not forthcoming with feedback at first. Open communication will foster growth of the team's efficiency, effectiveness, and ability to flex with the changes that occur so suddenly in both patients and organizations.

Appreciation of each other and the work that was accomplished and celebrating the outcomes enjoyed by the patients

Case Study 18.1

During your next clinical rotation, review the NCSBN and ANA National Guidelines for Delegation available at www.ncsbn.org/NGND-PosPaper_06.pdf, Accessed October 26, 2019. How does this guide help you decide what to delegate or assign? Identify the patient's needs, and identify what an RN could safely delegate. What did you decide?

is a great way to offer feedback and solidify a team. The more clear, detailed, appreciative feedback offered, the more that RNs find that their team members understand the authenticity of comments, such as,

> *I really appreciate how well the two of you worked together in the isolation room when the incontinent patient needed changing. It was so important to get that done quickly to avoid skin breakdown! You two make such a great part of our team and I appreciate you pitched in and helped while I was working with the case conference for Mrs. Peterson's discharge.*

Delegation, Omitted Care, and Patient Safety: The Swiss Cheese Safety Model

Bittner and Gravlin (2009) first identified the impact of delegation and critical thinking on missed or omitted but necessary nursing care. Nurses don't always know what other people's roles are and don't always feel confident in their clinical judgment and their delegation skills. Bittner, Gravlin, Hansten, and Kalisch (2011) studied the necessity of better teamwork to avoid the negative impact of poor delegation on patients and health care professionals. Kalisch and others have published international studies related to missed care (Kalisch, 2015; Kalankova, Gurkova, Zelenikova, & Ziatova, 2018), noting similar issues in all countries studied. Although health care administrators attempt to supply the very best personnel for the patients' needs, it is impossible to guarantee the right number and type of employees on every shift and every case. However, RNs can augment their delegation and assignment skills so that the personnel available can be utilized in an optimal manner, so that care is not denied or left unfinished on a regular basis. Hansten proposes a Swiss Cheese Safety Model (Figure 18.2) based on James Reason's iconic 1990 model in *Human Error* (1990, Cambridge University Press), to avoid Errors or Health Care Acquired Conditions (Hansten, 2014a,b). The Swiss Cheese Safety Model illustrates that the following safety defenses must occur to ensure best teamwork and avoid errors and negative impacts on patients.

1. RN knowledge of accountability. This includes understanding of how to make safe delegation and assignment decisions.

2. UAP knowledge of their role.

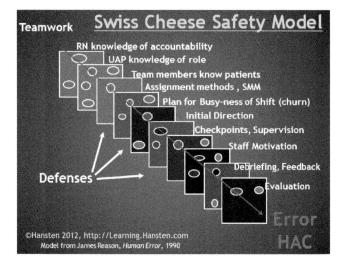

FIGURE 18.2 Swiss cheese safety model to avoid errors and health care acquired conditions.
Source: © Hansten, 2012, http://learning.hansten.com/. Model from James Reason, Human Error, 1990.

3. Team members knowledge of patients and their needs and planned outcomes.

4. Clear patient assignment methods and a **Shared Mental Model (SMM)** or plan for patient care. An SMM is a shared understanding, language, or mental roadmap that allows teams to flourish because everyone on the team understands what to expect of each other and how they will proceed with their work.

5. Plan for busy-ness of the shift and churn (churn is a term for changes in patient census with many admissions, transfers, discharges).

6. Clear initial direction of assignments and delegation.

7. Carefully planned checkpoints and supervision throughout the shift.

8. Staff motivation to get their jobs done with a focus on meeting each patient's needs and planned outcomes.

9. Debriefing and feedback completed by the RN and UAPs mutually so that patient care improvements can occur in the future.

10. Evaluation of patient care as is required by principles of expert delegation, assignment and supervision. (Hansten 2014a,b).

The Swiss Cheese Model illustrates that, although many layers of safety defenses lie between potential errors and Health Care Acquired Conditions (HAC), there are flaws in each layer that can allow an error to occur if the flaws are lined up with each other.

Nurses must be aware of the negative impacts of missed care and avoid Errors, Health care Acquired Conditions (HACs), team de-motivation, and burnout by applying these 10 safety defenses to their nursing practice.

Case Study 18.2

You are working with an RN, an LPN/LVN, a UAP, and a sitter. Your patients include the following:

1. 2501/Ms. J. D.: 68-year-old female, post-op day 1, post-shoulder repair, confused; fall risk; half side rails up, fall alarm on bed.

2. 2502/Mr. D. H.: 45-year-old male diabetic, post-op day 1, amputation just below the knee; Insulin sliding scale, complaining of pain; restlessness; diaphoretic.

3. 2503/Mr. H.M.: 35-year-old male, history of alcohol abuse: complaining of abdominal pain; new hematemesis of

coffee-ground fluid; IV of 0.9% normal saline at 125 cc/hour; alert.

4. 2504/Mr. J. K.: 20-year-old male college student, just admitted, threatening to commit suicide; alert and oriented.

Which tasks from the list in Table 18.13 would you give to each of them, i.e., the RN, the LPN/LVN, the UAP, and the sitter, if each patient were stable?

Who would you ask to perform afternoon care for all patients, pass water, answer call lights, and pick up supplies?

Who would give the medications and change dressings?

Evidence from the Literature

Source: Adapted from Diab, G., & Ehrahim, R. (2019) Factors leading to missed nursing care among nurses at selected hospitals. *American Journal of Nursing Research, 7*(2), 136–147.

Discussion: In research related to the concept of missed care, or care that should have been done but was not completed, nurses with less than five years of experience were more apt to not only report care omissions, but were also more likely to actually not complete necessary care. Care omissions were linked to a lack of sufficient staff and other resources, as well as problems with communication. Delegation abilities and whether or not care was completed meant that nurses tended to be more dissatisfied with their jobs. These findings are compatible with the confidential Hansten Healthcare nursing professional practice skill self-assessment database (Hansten Healthcare PLLC, 2019).

Implications for Practice: Nurses can feel uncomfortable with their ability to apply their delegation, assignment, and supervision skills. New graduate nurses identified that they needed to learn how to lead, delegate, assign, and supervise well—all skills that are more readily taught in the clinical area as opposed to a classroom. Therefore, it should be a priority for students and novice nurses to learn how to lead a team of UAPs and to begin to use delegation, assignment, and supervision skills. The impact of poor team leadership means missed nursing care, which leads to patients being harmed and nurses being dissatisfied with their work. When competent UAP and adequate supplies are present, excellent RN team leadership skills can result in better patient results and health care worker job satisfaction.

Case Study 18.3

A new nursing graduate, Jamilla, has been assigned to work with Abdul, a UAP, and five patients. Jamilla introduces herself to Abdul and asks him what types of patient care he usually performs. He tells Jamilla that he gives baths and takes vital signs. Jamilla asks Abdul to get all of the vital signs and give them to her written on a piece of paper. She asks Abdul if he documents them. He states that he does document them. Later that morning, Dr. Kent is making rounds on his patients, two of whom are Jamilla's patients. He asks Jamilla for the most recent vital signs. She then asks Abdul for the vital signs on all the patients. Abdul tells her he has not taken them yet. Dr. Kent then asks Jamilla to get the vitals

herself. By the time Jamilla returns with the vital signs, Dr. Kent has gone and has written orders she cannot read.

There are several factors in this delegation situation that should have been handled differently. Name them.

Do you think the new graduate was ready to delegate to the UAP? Why or why not?

Were the duties that were delegated or assigned appropriate for the UAP?

Would review of the job description for each health care personnel identified in this case study help solve this problem in the future?

Critical Thinking 18.7

The Joint Commission Sentinel Event Alert of September 2017 highlighted serious patient safety problems with communication, in particular, inadequate hand-off communication between shifts, between departments of the hospital (e.g., perioperative areas, critical care, emergency departments, medical surgical), and between patient transfer stops along the health care continuum (i.e., from acute care to home care or ambulatory care clinics and vice versa) (Joint Commission 2017). Similar serious patient safety problems with communication can occur during inadequate hand-offs between care providers on any team. Clear information about individual patients and their potential safety concerns and desired patient outcomes must occur in shift hand-offs with off-going RNs and oncoming RNs and UAPs. When patient information that is shared from team member to team member is insufficient, delayed, confusing, or inconsistent with patient conditions or needs, patients are at high risk for errors, delays, or omissions. How is patient information shared from team member to team member on the clinical units that you have been on as a student?

The 4 PS, Purpose, Picture, Plan, Part

One template or memory device used for hand-offs between shifts, departments, or points along the health care continuum includes the 4 Ps, Purpose, Picture, Plan, Part (Hansten, *Relationship & Results Oriented Healthcare Planning & Implementation Manual*, 2014b). This memory device helps health care workers focus on what the patient wants, not only what the treatment team would like to achieve with their standardized treatment plan. The 4 Ps are:

- **Purpose**: **Why is this patient here?** "Mr. Jones has probable bacterial pneumonia. He wants to be able to breathe well for his daughter's wedding, which is next weekend."

- **Picture**: **What does he look like now and what does he want to look like later?** "He's reddish blue, respirations 26/min, sputum green/gray, wheezing, pulse oximeter 84%, fever 101.4 F., BP 96/60, awaiting labs." **What is his picture of success?** "He wants to be able to go home as soon as possible to rest up for his daughter's wedding."

- **Plan**: **What is the plan for this patient for the short term (shift) and the longer term?** "We will follow the standard plan of care for a patient with pneumonia. We are using X and Y antibiotics IV until the sputum culture and sensitivity results are back. He's been hypovolemic due to the fever and dehydration but his BP is improving as we replace fluids. Mr. Jones would like to be discharged as soon as possible, with home care support if necessary, because of his daughter's impending wedding."

- **Part**: **What will each person do? What part does the patient/family play as well as the health care professionals?** "He and his wife are going to a pulmonologist after he improves. He's agreeing to update all vaccinations also, as he hadn't had his pneumonia and flu vaccinations. This shift, I would like you to. . ." The RN can then give instructions to the UAP about assigned tasks. Other members of the inter-professional team, such as respiratory therapists, might be included during hand-offs in a discussion of what each shift needs to complete.

Critical Thinking 18.8

1. During your clinical laboratory experiences, have you observed or received hand-off reports of patient care that were clear?

2. If you have had excellent hand-offs, what were the key data that were emphasized?

3. If you were not given sufficient information during hand-offs to do your job effectively, what other data would have been useful to you?

4. Think about what information you want to be certain to include when offering information and guidance to UAPs. How might you find out whether or not the information you shared was sufficient or too extensive?

Critical Thinking 18.9

Nurses are leaders. When they get a high-risk patient, they move quickly to follow high risk evidence-based patient guidelines, keep the patient warm (95 F (35 C)), stop their bleeding, and give Cardiopulmonary Resuscitation (CPR) when needed. Nurses assure their high-risk patients receive oxygen and are intubated quickly, as needed. Nurses check their high-risk patients' vitals (TPR and BP, Pulse Ox), put the patient on a cardiac monitor, start a large bore IV, give warm IV fluids, and draw labwork, as part of their nursing delivery of caring, safe, high-quality, patient-centered, evidence-based patient care. Have you seen a nurse assume this type of nursing leadership during your clinical experiences? How will you prepare to assume this leadership role upon graduation?

KEY CONCEPTS

- If RNs delegate, assign, and supervise poorly and care is omitted or done inadequately or with errors, patients and nurses suffer negative consequences.

- The RN must have a clear understanding of the definitions of delegation, assignment, supervision, and accountability.

- Unlicensed Assistive Personnel (UAP) or Nurse Assistive Personnel (NAP) or Assistive Personnel (AP) are those personnel trained to function in a supportive role to the RN and who have been assigned or delegated a task.

- LPN/LVNs are licensed individuals that perform routine uncomplicated nursing care in a dependent role under the supervision of RNs or other licensed care providers such as nurse practitioners, physicians, dentists, or others.

- The NCSBN and ANA National Guidelines for Delegation is a useful tool when developing skill in delegating patient care.

- State nurse practice acts differ so the RN must be familiar with their own state regulations, rules, advisory opinions, as well as their organization's job descriptions.

- The Five Rights of Delegation are the Right task, the Right circumstance, the Right person, the Right direction and communication, and the Right supervision and evaluation.

- Nurses must know the competencies of delegates.

- Accountability is being responsible and answerable for the actions or inactions of self or others.

- Authority occurs when a person who has been given the right to delegate based on the state nurse practice act also has the official power from an agency to delegate.

- The RN is accountable for decisions to delegate and assign and for the performance of the delegated or assigned nursing duties.

- To assign is when a nurse directs an individual to do something the individual is already authorized to do by state regulations.

- Supervision is the provision of guidance or direction, evaluation, and follow up by the licensed nurse for accomplishment of a nursing task delegated to a UAP.

- Feedback within the team is a necessary part of supervision.

- An assignment is the distribution of work that each staff member is responsible for during a given shift or work period.

- Key elements must be in place in an organization for efficient nursing delegation and assignment to occur.

- Professional clinical judgment is the mental process that a nurse exercises, based on the presenting situation, when forming an opinion and reaching a clinical decision based upon an analysis of the available evidence.

- One template or memory device used for hand-offs between shifts, departments, or points along the health care continuum is the 4 Ps, Purpose, Picture, Plan, Part.

- The Swiss Cheese Safety Model is helpful in visualizing defenses against errors and avoiding Healthcare Acquired Conditions.

KEY TERMS

Accountability	Competence	Unlicensed Assistive Personnel (UAP)
Assignment	Delegation	or Nurse Assistive Personnel (NAP) or
Authority	Supervision	Assistive Personnel (AP).
Clinical judgment		

REVIEW QUESTIONS

1. What issues can occur if the RN does not delegate or assign work effectively and care is not completed? Select all that apply.
   a. Pressure ulcers or injuries from lack of turning the patient
   b. Team members unhappy due to care being done inadequately or poorly organized
   c. Blood transfusion reaction
   d. Deep vein thrombosis
   e. Pneumonia
   f. Dehydration

2. When a nurse considers delegating a task, what five rights should be utilized?
   a. Right patient, right chart, right physician, right results, right information

   b. Right person, right patient, right task, right documentation, right time frame
   c. Right task, right circumstance, right person, right direction/ communication, right supervision and evaluation
   d. Right room, right time, right person, right documentation, right directions

3. The nurse has become incredibly busy with discharging two patients and expecting a new patient any second. The following are tasks that need to be completed right away. What task can the nurse delegate to a UAP to help out with managing the nurse's time with patients?
   a. Remove sutures from an incision and apply dressing to the patient's left wrist.

b. Provide tracheostomy care to the patient.

c. Sit with a patient who was recently diagnosed with Crohn's disease who is crying.

d. Perform patient assessment.

4. The staff working on the unit includes four RNs, two LPNs, and a UAP for 25 patients. What assignment is the most appropriate for one of the LPNs?

a. Assess a newly admitted patient.

b. Pass medications to a group of patients.

c. Pass water to all of the patients on the unit.

d. Ambulate stable patients.

5. What is the most appropriate task for the RN to delegate to the UAP?

a. Silence the IV pump until the RN arrives.

b. Notify the family of a patient who has died.

c. Administer a soapsuds enema to a patient who has requested it for constipation.

d. Reinforce teaching to a patient who has had an above the knee amputation.

6. What part(s) of the nursing process is/are usually delegated to a UAP? Select all that apply.

a. Assessment

b. Nursing diagnosis

c. Planning

d. Implementation

e. Evaluation

f. Clinical judgment

7. The charge nurse working with an RN, an LPN, and a UAP is very busy with the group of patients on the unit. One patient's intravenous line has just infiltrated, a practitioner is on the phone waiting for a nurse's response, a patient wants to be discharged, and the UAP has just reported an elevated temperature on a new surgical patient. Who should be assigned to restart the intravenous line?

a. LPN

b. UAP

c. RN

d. Charge nurse

8. A new graduate nurse is assigned a patient who is two days postoperative who has had a colostomy. The patient has an order to have a nasogastric tube inserted immediately. The new graduate has never inserted this type of tube in a patient. How should the new graduate nurse proceed in this situation?

a. Delegate the task to a UAP.

b. Read over the procedure, and then insert the tube.

c. Notify the practitioner of the new graduate's inexperience.

d. Ask an experienced RN for assistance with the procedure.

9. When a nurse considers delegating a task, which of the following are individual personal characteristics of the delegate that should be considered? Select all that apply.

a. Method of processing information (auditory, visual, kinesthetic, or tactile)

b. Competence

c. Length of work experience

d. Willingness to complete work

10. When nurse A asks another nurse B to observe his or her group of patients while at lunch, and one patient falls out of bed, which nurse is responsible?

a. The nurse A originally assigned to the patient who went to lunch is responsible.

b. The nurse B who was observing the group of patients is responsible.

c. Neither nurse is responsible.

d. The actions of both nurses will be reviewed.

REVIEW QUESTION ANSWERS

1. Answers A, B, D, E, and F are correct.

Rationale: Blood checking or administration should not be delegated to anyone, so the RN would be monitoring the blood transfusion (C). However, in a few states LPNs could be involved in blood administration. Check your state. If patients are not cleaned, turned, toileted, with excellent perineal and skin care and receive inadequate hydration and nutrition and movement, pressure ulcers can occur (A), as can deep vein thrombosis, and possible emboli from the thrombus (D). Lack of turning or repositioning and ambulation can predispose a patient to pneumonia (E). Dehydration (F) from lack of attention to feeding and administering fluids can occur in patients without IVs or nasogastric fluids. Team members are dissatisfied when care is done inadequately or poorly organized (B).

2. Answer: C is correct.

Rationale: Right task, right circumstance, right person, right direction/communication, right supervision and evaluation is correct; refer to the 5 Rights as included in the chapter (C). All of the other answers (A, B, and D) may be useful for patient comfort and safety but they are not the Five Rights of Delegation.

3. Answer: C is correct.

Rationale: If the UAP is kind and helpful, he could sit with the Crohn's patient (C) once the RN has talked with the patient initially. A UAP cannot remove sutures (A), or apply dressings to an incision (A), or provide tracheostomy care (B). Patients can only be assessed by the RN (D), although data such as vital signs can be retrieved by others.

4. Answer: B is correct.

Rationale: LPNs pass medications in most states (B). Some medications will be RN-only such as IV push, central line, antiarrhythmics, pressors, etc. Check your state and organization. Admission assessment (A) is in the RN role, although data collection assistance for that assessment could be from either an LPN or UAP. Passing water (C) would be appropriate for the UAP. Ambulating stable patients (D) could be a possible task for the UAPs.

5. Answer: C is correct.

Rationale: UAPs can administer non-medicated enemas (C). Silencing pumps by UAPs (A) is risky since there is often an important reason the pump is beeping and will need RN intervention to resolve. Notification of death (B) would be an RN-only process and would require astute nursing judgment. UAP are not usually allowed to reinforce teaching (D) (check your area of practice regarding reinforcement of standardized teaching plans, as this could be allowed in some states and in some areas, such as home health, clinics, long-term care).

6. Answer: D is correct.
   Rationale: Some interventions (D) or tasks selected by the RN can be delegated if appropriate for that patient. Assessment (A), Nursing Diagnosis (B), Planning (C), and Evaluation (E) cannot be delegated. Clinical judgment (F) is a part of nursing but is not considered a distinct part of the nursing process in that clinical judgment is used throughout the entire process of nursing, so cannot be delegated.

7. Answer: C is correct.
   Rationale: An RN (C) can be assigned to restart the IV. The charge RN (D) could restart the line if the RN is responding to the practitioner on the phone. The patient with a fever is also an important priority but either the charge RN or the RN should soon perform additional assessment (B). In some states, LPNs (A) can start IVs, but in some states this is not allowed. If in a state where LPNs can start IVs, the LPN could also restart the line (A). LPNs are not always allowed to take physician orders over the telephone so that choice is eliminated.

8. Answer: D is correct.
   Rationale: When in doubt, ask an experienced RN for assistance (D). Inserting an NG tube by someone new to the procedure

is not permitted (A, B) without assistance. The experienced RN should be able to assist with the tube insertion. There is no need to notify the ordering practitioner (C) unless another problem emerges.

9. Answer: A, B, C, and D are correct.
   Rationale: All of the above answers (A, B, C, D) show that the RN is thinking about not only whether or not the delegate is competent, but also how well they may do the job and how best to communicate instructions to that individual understands well and can follow through.

10. Answer: D is correct.
    Rationale: The actions of both nurses will be reviewed (D). Did Nurse A leave the patient highly medicated with the bed in high position without bed railings up? Did Nurse A toilet the patient before leaving for her break? Did Nurse B let the patient cry for help to the bathroom before falling? A review of all factors leading up to the fall will be reviewed to determine how to best avoid this kind of problem in the future. Nurse A (A) and Nurse B (B) both have responsibility and accountability for care of the patient and for patient safety so both are responsible (C). In organizational cultures that use just practices, the situation would be assessed and the action of each nurse would be reviewed as well as all the health care system issues that allowed for a fall to occur. Unless the nurses had willful patterns of leaving patients at risk intentionally, the nurses should not fear termination or other counseling but should participate in review of the situation so that falls can be avoided in the future.

REVIEW ACTIVITIES

1. Have you had any clinical opportunities to delegate or assign duties? If so, identify what you delegated or assigned and to whom. Discuss how your delegation or assignment affected the patient and your work. What would you do differently next time? Use the Five Rights of Delegation to help walk through your decision.

2. Observe the delegation and assignment process at your organization. How is the unit, department, or organizational delegation or assignment process set up so that each person on a team communicates well with the rest of the team? What suggestions would you make to improve their delegation procedures or communication process?

3. You are caring for a new patient in Room 2510. You are trying to decide whether to delegate his care to UAP Jill or to UAP Penny. Jill is not certified and is not always easy to work with but usually does her fair share of the work. Penny is certified. She always does her fair share and is easy to work with. She is able to perform dressing changes. Which individual will

you choose based on their individual strengths, certifications, competence level, and collaborative or industrious attitude? Which personal factors are most important? What is fair to both Jill and Penny and the patient?

4. Look at the assignment sheet for the shift your clinical day is on. Who is listed on the assignment sheet? What assignments are made on the sheet? During the shift, did you observe an RN ask another RN to do a job for them? If yes, could the UAP have done it?

5. Discuss with a UAP and an RN their preparation in regard to delegation, supervision, and teamwork. How much education or training has each of them received? How long ago did they receive it? What type of education or training did they receive? Is the RN familiar with the "Five Rights of Delegation?" How is the education of the RN and the training of the UAP different?

6. Talk with UAPs regarding how the RNs could better lead their teams and how you could best prepare yourself to be a great team leader.

DISCUSSION POINTS

1. What can you learn from the negative and positive nursing delegation qualities you have noticed in the RNs you have worked with as a student?

2. Did you see care being omitted in your student experiences resulting in hospital acquired conditions?

3. How aware were you of your authority as an RN in delegation, assignment, and supervision?

4. How well did the RNs supervise you in your student experiences and make certain that delegated or assigned work was completed?

5. Do you think the organizations where you have had student experiences are fulfilling their organizational responsibilities for delegation?

DISCUSSION OF OPENING SCENARIO

1. How could the nurse have avoided the delay in diagnosis and treatment?
    a. In order to avoid the patient deteriorating without immediate attention, several initial safeguards would have been useful. First of all, both the RN and the UAP must know their job descriptions: what are the expectations of the UAP working as a "sitter?" Certainly, the RN could not expect the UAP/sitter to perform neurological assessment. If the RN had given adequate initial direction to the UAP, directing her to report any change in movement or mentation immediately, the UAP may possibly have alerted the RN more quickly when the weakness first occurred. If the RN had asked the UAP to perform vital signs every 2 hours, changes may have been identified more quickly. The RN also should have observed the patient more closely and completed a neurological assessment every 2 hours rather than allowing the patient to sleep.

2. What are the responsibilities of the nurse and the sitter (a UAP)?
    a. RNs, Sitters, and/or UAPs job descriptions are usually available in either a policy/procedure manual or online in the health care organization's human resources job

descriptions. The RN is accountable to delegate and/or assign responsibilities to the UAP and to supervise the care and the RN is also accountable for the overall nursing care of the patient. The UAP is responsible to keep the patient safe and to report any patient changes in a timely manner. Other tasks such as vital signs may have been assigned to the UAP and should have been reported to the RN.

3. How would you find out their job responsibilities?
    a. As mentioned above, most health care organizations usually keep job descriptions in either a policy/procedure manual or in the online human resources job descriptions, with job responsibilities and competency checklists in an online format searchable all shifts.

4. How could delegation and supervision have been appropriately performed in this situation?
    a. Clear initial delegation and direction to the UAP, identification of the UAP's need to report changes immediately, along with better ongoing observation and supervision by the RN would have speeded up the assessment and treatment of this patient and might have even prevented further neurological damage.

EXPLORING THE WEB

- Log on to www.nursingworld.org the American Nurses Association (ANA) site, to view safety and quality of care issues. Look for delegation policy under nursing practice:

    ○ www.nursingworld.org/practice-policy/nursing-excellence/official-position-statements/id/joint-statement-on-delegation-by-ANA-and-NCSBN (accessed February 12, 2019).

    ○ www.nursingworld.org/practice-policy/scope-of-practice (accessed February 14, 2019).

- Go to the www.NCSBN.org website:

    ○ Search for delegation: www.ncsbn.org/search.htm?q=delegation (accessed February 14, 2019).

    ○ Find www.ncsbn.org/4516.htm Medication Administration in Nursing Homes: RN Delegation to UAP and review the research (accessed February 14, 2019).

    ○ Having trouble locating your own state's nurse practice act? Go to the link from the NCSBN.org website to your own state practice website. /www.ncsbn.org/contact-bon.htm (accessed February 142,019).

- Check out these references and online education related to delegation and supervision:

- www.amazon.com/Ruth-I.-Hansten/e/B001IR3H1S (accessed April 8, 2019).

- Online CE including 10 Steps for Professional Practice: at http://learning.hansten.com https://nurse.freecelms.education/by/ms-ruth-hansten-bsn-phd-mba-rn-fache (accessed April 8, 2019).

- Part 1: Delegation, Supervision, and Teamwork: https://nurse.freecelms.education/by/ms-ruth-hansten-bsn-phd-mba-rn-fache/ms-ruth-hansten-bsn-phd-mba-rn-fache/165678/leadership-at-the-point-of-care-part-1-delegation-supervision-and-teamwork (accessed April 9, 2019).

- Blueprint for Successful Clinical Supervision and Teamwork: https://nurse.freecelms.education/by/ms-ruth-hansten-bsn-phd-mba-rn-fache/ms-ruth-hansten-bsn-phd-mba-rn-fache/165677/leadership-at-the-point-of-care-part-2-blueprint-for-successful-clinical-supervision-and-teamwork (Accessed April 9, 2019).

- Making Assignments: https://nurse.freecelms.education/by/ms-ruth-hansten-bsn-phd-mba-rn-fache/ms-ruth-hansten-bsn-phd-mba-rn-fache/165676/leadership-at-the-point-of-care-part-3-effective-assignments-for-rns-and-assistive-personnel-acute-care (Accessed April 9, 2019).

- www.RROHC.com (Relationship & Results Oriented Healthcare resources including videos, accessed April 8, 2019).

INFORMATICS

1. Search the web for your own state's nurse practice act and your board of nursing or state nursing care quality assurance commission. Search for delegation and supervision policies and standards of nursing practice. Look for LPN/LVN scope of practice and note what the parameters of LPN/LVN intravenous treatment or therapy are. Look for Advisory Opinions on your state board website if anything is unclear.

2. Search the QSEN website, http://qsen.org/teamwork-collaboration Look at the question posed for students related to teamwork and collaboration. The question is: "What are some examples of teamwork and collaboration you have seen in health care? These examples can be at a clinical site, in the workplace, or even during a hospital stay?" (accessed February 15, 2019).

LEAN BACK

- When you read this chapter about delegation, what were your thoughts and/or fears about how well you would be able to delegate and lead a team?

- What discrepancies have you have seen in actual care settings as a student that conflict with what is taught here about excellent delegation and supervision?

- What could you as a new graduate do to develop a higher level of teamwork than what you are seeing in your clinical settings?

- How can you guard against errors of omission or commission related to delegation?

- What guidelines or memory assists will you use to help delegate and supervise others effectively?

- What guidelines or memory assists will help you in your NCLEX-RN Examination with questions related to delegation and teamwork?

REFERENCES

Alfaro-LeFevre, R. (2017). *Critical thinking, clinical reasoning, and clinical judgment* (6th ed., pp. 61). Philadelphia, PA: Elsevier.

American Association of Colleges of Nursing. (2019). *The essentials of baccalaureate education for professional nursing practice*. Retrieved from www.aacnnursing.org/Education-Resources/AACN-Essentials.

American Nurses Association. (2014). In M. Duffy & S. F. McCoy (Eds.), *Delegation and you: when to delegation and to whom.* Silver Springs, MD: American Nurses Association. (ANA's You Series: Skills for Success)

American Nurses Association. (2019). National guidelines for nursing delegation. Effective January 4, 2019, by ANA Board of Directors/NCSBN Board of Directors. www.nursingworld.org/practice-policy/nursing-excellence/official-position-statements/id/joint-statement-on-delegation-by-ANA-and-NCSBN (file available only members at www.nursingworld.org/globalassets/practiceandpolicy/nursing-excellence/ana-position-statements-secure/ana-ncsbn-joint-statement-on-delegation.pdf This file can also be accessed at www.ncsbn.org/NGND-PosPaper_06.pdf.

American Nurses Association (ANA) and National Council of State Boards of Nursing (NCSBN). (2006). *Joint statement on delegation.* Retrieved from www.ncsbn.org/Delegation_joint_statement_NCSBN-ANA.pdf.

American Nurses Association (ANA). (2005). *Principles for delegation.* Retrieved from www.safestaffingsaveslives.org/WhatisSafeStaffing/SafeStaffingPrinciples/PrinciplesforDelegatiotml.aspx#Definitions.

Anderson, A. (2018). Delegating as a new nurse. *American Journal of Nursing, 118*(12), 51–55.

Beeber, A., Zimmerman, S., Mitchell, C., & Reed, D. (2018). Staffing and service availability in assisted living: Importance of nurse delegation studies. *Journal of the American Geriatric Society, 9*, 1–9.

Bittner, N., & Gravlin, G. (2009). Critical thinking, delegation, and missed care. *Journal of Nursing Administration, 39*(3), 142–146.

Bittner, N., Gravlin, G., Hansten, R., & Kalisch, B. (2011). Unraveling care omissions. *Journal of Nursing Administration, 41*(12), 510–512.

Boucher, M. A. (1998). Delegation Alert. *American Journal of Nursing, 98*(2), 26–32.

Brent, N. (2019). Delegating in nursing continues to be a legal minefield. *Nurse.com Blog.* Retrieved from www.nurse.com/blog/2019/01/28/delegating-in-nursing-continues-to-be-legal-minefield.

Brous, E. (2014). Lessons learned from litigation: The case of Bernard Travaglini. *American Journal of Nursing, 114*(5), 68–70.

Diab, G.,. &., & Ehrahim, R. (2019). Factors leading to missed nursing care among nurses at selected hospitals. *American Journal of Nursing Research, 7*(2), 136–147.

Hansten Healthcare Confidential Database. (2019). *Database of 2000 nurses self assessment of patient care leadership professional practice skills.* Santa Rosa, CA: Hansten Healthcare.

Hansten, R. (2014a). Coach as chief correlator of tasks to results through delegation skill and teamwork development. *Nurse Leader, 12*, 69–73.

Hansten, R. (2014b). *The master coach manual for Relationship & Results Oriented Healthcare.* Port Ludlow, WA: Hansten Healthcare PLLC.

Hansten, R. (2019, April). Another look at RN leadership skill level and patient outcomes. *Linked In Pulse.* www.linkedin.com/pulse/another-look-rn-leadership-skill-level-patient-hansten-rn-mba-phd.

Hansten, R. (2020). Introductory chapter. In L. LaCharity, C. Kumagai, & B. Bartz (Eds.), *Prioritization, delegation and assignment* (4th ed.). St. Louis, MO: Elsevier.

Hansten, R. (2021). Guidelines for Prioritization, Delegation, and Assignment Decisions. In J. Zerwekh & A. Garneau (Eds.), *Nursing today: Transitions and trends* (9th ed., pp. 316). St. Louis, MO: Elsevier.

Hansten, R., & Jackson, M. (2009). *Clinical delegation skills: A handbook for professional practice* (4th ed.). Boston, MA: Jones & Bartlett.

Kalankova, D., Gurkova, E., Zelenikova, R., & Ziatova, K. (2018). Application of measuring tools in the assessment of the phenomenon of rationing/missed/unfinished care. *KONTAKT/Journal of nursing and the social sciences related to health and illness,* (Kont.zsf.jcu.cz) http://doi.org/10.32725/kont.2018.1. October: 1–9

Kalisch, B. (2015). *Errors of omission: How missed nursing care imperils patients.* Silver Spring, MD: ANA.

Maningo, M., & Panthofer, M. (2018). Safety corner: Appropriate delegation in ambulatory care nursing practice. *AAACN Viewpoint, 40*(1), 14–15.

Marthaler, M., & Kelly, P. (2012). Delegation of nursing care. In P. Kelly (Ed.), *Nursing leadership and management* (3rd ed.). Clifton Park, NY: Delmar Cengage Learning.

Mueller, C., Vogelsmeier, A., Anderson, R., McConnell, E., & Corazzini, K. (2018). Interchangeability of licensed nurses in nursing homes: Perspective of directors of nursing. *The End to End Journal, 1*, 1–27.

Mushta, J., Rush, K., & Anderson, E. (2018). Failure to rescue as a nurse-sensitive indicator. *Nurs Forum, 53*, 84–92.

National Council of State Boards of Nursing (NCSBN). (2005). *Working with others: A position statement.* Chicago, IL: National Council of State Boards of Nursing.

National Council of State Boards of Nursing (NCSBN). (2019). *NCSBN and ANA national guidelines for nursing delegation.* Retrieved from www.ncsbn.org/NGND-PosPaper_06.pdf.

National Council of State Boards of Nursing. (2016). National guidelines for nursing delegation. *Journal of Nursing Regulation, 7*(1), 5–14.

National Council of State Boards of Nursing (NCSBN). (1995). Delegation concepts and decision-making process. *NCSBN position paper.* Retrieved from https://ncsbn.org/1625.htm.

NCSBN. (1995). Delegation decision-making process. National Council of State Boards of Nursing 1995 Annual Meeting Business Book. August 1995 - St. Louis, Mo.

Nightingale, F. (1898). *Notes on nursing.* New York: Appleton & Co. iBooks. Accessed February 5, 2019. Retrieved from. https://itunes.apple.com/us/book/notes-on-nursing/id506604714?mt=11

Reason, J. (1990). *Human Error.* Cambridge, UK: Cambridge University Press.

The Joint Commission. (2017). Inadequate Hand-off Communication. *Sentinel Event Alert* (Issue 58).

Washington Administrative Code 246-840-010 Definitions. (2019). Supervision. Accessed February 7, 2019. Retrieved from https://app.leg.wa.gov/wac/default.aspx?cite=246-840-010

Washington State Department of Health Nursing Care Quality Assurance Commission Advisory Opinion 13.01. (2019). Registered Nurse and Licensed Practical Nurse Scope of Practice, 3-8-2019. Page 4(1–12). Accessed April 3, 2019. Retrieved from www.doh.wa.gov/Portals/1/Documents/6000/NCAO13.pdf

Zimmerman, P. G. (1996). Delegating to assistive personnel. *Journal of Emergency Nursing, 22*(3), 206–212.

SUGGESTED READINGS

American Nurses Association. (2014). In M. Duffy & S. F. McCoy (Eds.), *Delegation and you: when to delegation and to whom.* Silver Springs, MD: ANA. (ANA's You Series: Skills for Success)

Anderson, A. (2018). Transition to practice: Delegating as a new nurse. *American Journal of Nursing, 118*(12), 51–55.

Ayello, E., & Sibbald, R. G. (2019). Pressure injuries: Nursing-sensitive indicator or team- and systems-sensitive indicator? *Advances in Skin and Wound Care, 32*, 5), Suggested Reading:, 199–200.

Ballard, K., Haagenson, D., Christiansen, L., et al. (2016). Scope of nursing practice decision-making framework. *Journal of Nursing Regulation, 7*(3), 19–21.

Bittner, N., Gravlin, G., Hansten, R., & Kalisch, B. (2011). Unraveling care omissions. *Journal of Nursing Administration, 41*(12), 510–512.

Bittner, N. P., & Gravlin, G. (2009). Critical thinking, delegation, and missed care in nursing practice. *Journal of Nursing Administration, 39*(3), 142–146.

Hansten, R. (2008). *Relationship & results oriented health care planning and implementation manual.* Port Ludlow, WA: Hansten Healthcare PLLC.

Hansten, R. (2014). Coach as chief correlator of tasks to results through delegation skill and teamwork development. *Nurse Leader, 8*, 69–73.

Hansten, R. (2014). *The master coach manual for relationship & results oriented healthcare.* Port Ludlow, WA: Hansten Healthcare PLLC.

Hansten, R. (2019). Delegation and Assignment in the Clinical Setting. In L. LaCharity, C. Kumagai, & B. Bartz (Eds.), *Prioritization, delegation and assignment* (4th ed.). St. Louis, MO: Elsevier.

Hansten, R. (2019, April). Another look at RN leadership skill level and patient outcomes. *Linked In Pulse.* www.linkedin.com/pulse/another-look-rn-leadership-skill-level-patient-hansten-rn-mba-phd.

Hansten, R. (2019, Auguest). New ANA/NCSBN delegation and assignment regulations for nurses and nurse leaders. *LinkedIn Pulse.* www.linkedin.com/pulse/new-anancsbn-delegation-assignment-regulations-nurses-ruth/?trackingId=bjgIHNpJHcz8SlqLOAzsTg%3D%3D

Hansten, R. (2021). Delegation and Assignment in the Clinical Setting. In J. Zerwekh & A. Garneau (Eds.), *Nursing today: Transitions and trends* (9th ed., pp. 316). St. Louis, MO: Elsevier.

Hansten, R., & Jackson, M. (2009). *Clinical delegation skills* (4th ed.). Boston, MA: Jones & Bartlett.

Kelly, P., & Tazbir, J. (2014). *Essentials of Nursing Leadership & Management* (3rd ed.). Clifton Park, NY: Delmar Cengage Learning.

19

Time Management and Setting Patient Care Priorities

Patrick J. Joswick

Kalamazoo Valley Community College, Kalamazoo, MI, USA

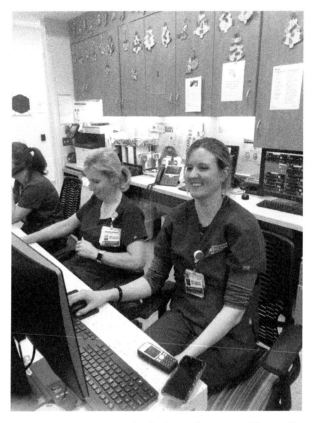

Nurses use time management and priority setting to provide excellent care within the restraints of time.
Source: Photo used with permission

> Lost time is never found again.
> Benjamin Franklin (1900).

OBJECTIVES

Upon completion of this chapter, the reader should be able to:

1. Apply principles of priority setting to patient care situations.

2. Apply time management strategies to the reality of delivering effective nursing care.

3. Relate time management strategies to enhance personal productivity.

Kelly Vana's Nursing Leadership and Management, Fourth Edition. Edited by Patricia Kelly Vana and Janice Tazbir
© 2021 John Wiley & Sons Ltd. Published 2021 by John Wiley & Sons Ltd.
Companion Website: www.wiley.com/go/kelly-Nursing-Leadership

OPENING SCENARIO

Inez has just completed her medical-surgical orientation as a new graduate registered nurse. This evening is her first solo shift, but she is frightened and feels like she is holding up the world on her new graduate shoulders. Although she feels that all rests on her, she is not really alone. Inez and Carole, the other RNs, are responsible for 12 possible patients on this section of the unit along with one certified nursing assistant. Currently, there are 10 patients in this section, but a new admission is on the way, another patient is returning from surgery, the dinner trays are arriving, and Inez has medications to pass. Just as the dinner trays arrive, a patient's family member runs out to Inez and states that her mom is confused and incontinent and has pulled out her IV.

1. *How can Inez figure out what to do first?*

2. *What tools do you have to organize your care?*

3. *How can using prioritization help in managing time?*

Introduction

The domain of health care is dynamic with ever-evolving system processes and complex methods of logistics. The use of time effectively and efficiently is essential to achieve optimal patient outcomes. **Time management** can be defined as aligning personal goals with the time that is readily available interrelated to the likes, dislikes, and preferences of the individual (Kelley, 2017). Nurses are continuing to inherit increasing roles and responsibilities and must perceive time as an asset rather than a burden (Henry, 2014). Regardless of the area of specialty, nurses must remain resilient, adaptive, and proactive with the resource of time to achieve affordable, accessible, quality care. Patient safety and satisfaction are interrelated to time management by the health care team. Effective and efficient time management will facilitate proper prioritization of patient care, combat burnout, and increase job satisfaction of the nurse. In this chapter we will apply principles of priority setting to patient care situations and time management strategies to the reality of delivering effective nursing care as well as relate time management strategies to enhance personal productivity.

Outcome Orientation

It is important to recognize that more is achieved through an outcome orientation than through an emphasis on the process of task completion. Long-term goals must be determined. It is best to break long-term goals down into achievable outcomes that are the steps toward long-term goals. Such goals cannot be achieved overnight. Long-term goals and outcomes should be written down in a traditional planner or device. Even though these goals are written, they should remain flexible and reviewed often. Flexibility should be built into any outcome orientation. There may come a time when the outcome is no longer realistic or should be shifted to a more realistic goal as circumstances change (Donohue & Crenshaw, 2015). With this concept in mind, we will explore the Pareto Principle later in this chapter.

Time Analysis

Another time management concept is analysis of time to effectively use it. Nurses cannot possibly know how to better plan time without knowing how they currently use it. When keeping track of time, it is important to consider the value of a nurse's time as well as the use of time. Today the tracking of time is easier than ever due to the electronic name badges that many facilities use. Additional benefits of the electronic badges include tracking of time spent with patient encounters, frequency of hand washing, radiation exposure, and even location history within and outside of the clinical unit (Pong, Holliday, & Fernie, 2018). Refer to Table 19.1 Activity Log.

Valuing Nursing Time

Nurses often undervalue their time. Consider salary and benefits. Benefits are frequently forgotten, but they raise employer costs by 15–30% of salary. If a nurse is making $38.00 an hour, benefits add $5.70–$11.40 to the hourly cost of a nurse's time. The value of nursing time in this example, excluding what the organization is paying in worker's compensation and payroll taxes, is $43.70–$49.40 an hour. The organization has also invested in nurse recruitment, orientation, and development, which can easily exceed $40,000 per nurse. Nursing time is an expensive commodity. Keeping this in mind when considering what tasks can be delegated to personnel who receive less compensation, or when considering what tasks are busy work and do not support achieving an outcome, is invaluable.

Use of Time

Numerous studies have shown how nurses use their time. Many studies have been done on acute care nurses, because they comprise the majority of nurses. An estimated one-third of nursing time is spent on direct patient care (Higgins et al., 2017). A significant portion of a nurses' time is spent on charting and reporting, and the remainder of time is spent on admission and discharge procedures, professional communication, personal time, and providing care that could be provided by unlicensed personnel, such as transportation and

Table 19.1   Work Activity Log

Time	Name of activity (Medication administration, vital signs, bed-making, patient transport, and so on)	Time required and feelings (Energetic, bored, and so on)	Could be better done by someone else? Who? (LPN, nursing assistant, housekeeper, and so on)	Toward what outcome achievement? (Increase in patient's functional status, prevention of complications, and so on)
0500	Treadmill	30 min—energetic	Keep for self	Fitness
0530	Shower and breakfast	45 min—energetic	Keep for self	Health
0630	Drive to work	10 min—alert	Keep for self	Get to work
0700	Hand-off shift report	15 min—alert	Keep for self	Patient identification
0730	Patient rounds/planning	15 min—alert	Keep for self	Prioritize patients
0800				
0830				
0900				
0930				
1000				
1030				
1100				
Etc.				

Source: Table created by P. Joswick.

housekeeping (Higgins et al., 2017). Lavander, Meriläinen, and Turkki (2016) performed a systematic review of time among nurses. Six categories of time management were considered including direct care, indirect care, documentation, unit-related work, personal time, and non-nursing duties. RNs spend about one-third of their time on direct patient care, defined as activities performed in the presence of the patient or family; 42–45% of time on indirect care activities, which include all activities done for an individual patient but not in the patient's presence; 15% on unit-related activities, which include all unit general maintenance activities; and 13–20% on personal activities, which include activities that are not related to patient care or unit maintenance (Lavander, et al., 2016). Documentation accounted for the largest proportion of time at approximately 25%, followed by care coordination and

patient care activities, each accounting for 14% (Lavander et al., 2016) (Figure 19.1).

Given such a distribution of nurses' time, shifting the use of time could have a major impact on outcomes. If non-nursing activities could be performed by non-nursing personnel instead of nurses, more time could be redirected toward essential nursing responsibilities.

How do you use your time? Memory and self-reporting of time have been found to be unreliable. Staff are often unaware of time spent socializing with colleagues, making and drinking coffee, snacking, time spent using cell phones and other electronic devices for personal use to include social media, and other nonproductive time. Self-reporting of time is not recommended for estimating the total number of activities or the average time an activity takes to complete (Barrero et al., 2009).

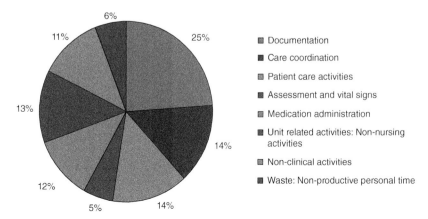

FIGURE 19.1   Use of nursing time. Figure created by P. Joswick, Data Citation: Lavander, Merilainen and Turkki (2016).

Activity Log

An **activity log** is a time management tool that can assist the nurse in determining how time is used. The activity log (Table 19.1) should be used for several days. Behavior should not be modified while keeping the log. The nurse should record every activity, from the beginning of the shift until the end, as well as periodically noting feelings while doing the activities—alert, energetic, tired, bored, and so on. Review of this log will illuminate time use as well as time wasted. Analysis of the log will allow the separation of essential professional activities from activities that can be performed by someone else (Grohar-Murray & Langan, 2011; Sullivan, 2018)

Many nurses become nurses out of idealism. They want to help people by meeting all their needs. Unfortunately, most new graduates find it impossible to meet all or even most of their patients' needs. Needs tend to be unlimited, whereas time is limited. In addition to the direct patient care responsibilities, there are shift responsibilities, charting, practitioners' orders to be transcribed or checked, medication supplies to be restocked, and reports to be given.

New graduates often go home feeling totally inadequate. They wake up remembering what they did not accomplish. One young nurse shared with tears in her eyes that once, when she answered a call bell late in her shift, the patient requested a pain medication. She went to the narcotics cabinet to get the medication but was interrupted by an emergent situation. When she arrived home, she was so exhausted that she fell asleep rapidly, only to awaken with the realization that she had not returned with her patient's medication. Her guilt was tremendous. She had gone into nursing to relieve pain, not to ignore it.

Time management allows the novice nurse to prioritize care, decide on outcomes, delegate appropriately, and perform the critical interventions first. Time management skills are important, not just for nurses on the job, but for nurses in their personal lives as well. They allow nurses to make time for fun, friends, exercise, and professional development.

General Time Management Concepts

Time management has been defined as "a set of related common-sense skills that helps you use your time in the most effective and productive way possible" (Mind Tools, n.d.). Another way to say this is that time management allows us to achieve more with available time. Four valuable time management concepts to master are understanding: the relative effectiveness of effort (the Pareto Principle), the importance of outcome versus process orientation, the value of analyzing how time is currently being used, and what can be safely delegated and what the nurse must do. It is important to analyze and manage time to achieve key outcomes effectively and efficiently.

The Pareto Principle

Time management requires a shift from wasting time on the process of being busy to organizing time to achieve desired outcomes and get things done. Often, a busy frenzy of activity is reinforced with sympathy and assistance. Too often, this frenzied behavior is accomplishing very little, because it is not directed at the right outcome. The **Pareto Principle** states that 20% of focused effort results in 80% of outcome results, or conversely that 80% of unfocused effort results in 20% of outcome results (Figure 19.2).

Pareto's Principle, named after Vilfredo Pareto, was invoked by the **total quality management** (TQM) movement and is now reemerging as a strategy for balancing life and work through prioritization of effort (Hughes & Wilson, 2017). Effective time management requires that a shift be made from doing unfocused efforts that require 80% of time for achieving 20% of desired outcome results to doing planned and focused efforts that use only 20% of time or input to achieve 80% of desired outcome results. It is important to analyze how your time is being used to manage time and achieve desired outcomes.

If time management achieves more outcomes, why do so many people continue at a crazy, hurried pace? There are several explanations for this. They do not know about time management, they think they do not have time to plan, they do not want to stop to plan, or they love crises (Mind Tools, n.d.).

Prioritizing Use of Time

To plan effective use of time, nurses must understand the big picture, decide on desired outcomes, and do first things first. One concept frequently used by nurses in understanding the big picture of patient needs is Maslow's hierarchy of needs pyramid. The base of which is physiological needs, above which is safety, then love and belonging, esteem or respect, and on

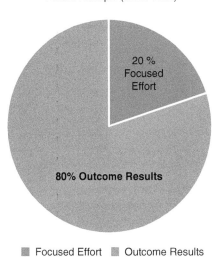

Pareto Principle (80/20 Rule)

20 %
Focused
Effort

80% Outcome Results

■ Focused Effort   ■ Outcome Results

Figure 19.2   The Pareto principle.
Source: Figure created by P. Joswick, adapted from The Pareto Principle.

Critical Thinking 19.1

Four of Jose's patients were discharged today by 10:00 a.m. The nursing supervisor asked Jose to help out in the **emergency room** (ER). Jose agreed and was assigned to help the triage nurse. Identify the order in which patients should be seen in the ER.

Group I

* A two-year-old boy with chest retractions

* A one-year-old girl choking on a grape

* A five-year-old boy with a knee laceration

How about Group II? Which patient would you see first?

* Group II

* A 60-year-old female who is nonresponsive and drooling

* A 30-year-old male trauma patient who has absent breath sounds in the right side of his chest

* A 15-year-old female who cut her wrist in an attempted suicide

---

top of the pyramid is self-actualization. Alfaro-Lefavre (2017) builds on Maslow by suggesting three levels of prioritization. The base or first level prioritization is airway, breathing, circulation to include cardiac status, and life-threatening vital signs and lab values, the next level includes those things that are immediately subsequent to the first level such as mental status changes, acute pain, acute elimination issues, and any imminent risks. The third level refers to longer-term problems, education, coping, sleep, and like issues (Alfaro-Lefavre, 2017).

Understand the Big Picture

Before priorities are set, the big picture must be examined to include, but not limited to, the purpose for care, the current clinical picture (situation), and picture of the desired outcomes (Hansten, 2018). No nurse works in isolation. Nurses should know what is expected of their co-workers, what is happening on the other shifts, and what is happening beyond the unit. If nurses know what is expected of their co-workers, they can offer assistance during co-workers' busy times and in turn receive assistance during their own busy times. If the previous shift was stressed by a crisis, a next shift may not get started as smoothly (Hansten, 2018). If areas outside the unit are overwhelmed, someone might be moved from one unit to assist on the overwhelmed unit elsewhere in the hospital. When nurses take the big picture into consideration, they are less likely to be frustrated when asked to assist others on their unit or on other units in the hospital. They can also build into their time management plan the possibility of giving and receiving assistance.

Decide on Optimal Desired Outcomes

When nurses begin their shifts, they need to decide what outcomes can be achieved. **Desired optimal outcomes** are the best possible objectives to be achieved given the resources at hand.

As nurses decide on desired optimal outcomes, they must consider what can and should be achieved given less-than-optimal circumstances and limited resources. These circumstances could include a rough start to a busy shift; personnel late, absent, or uncooperative; and a patient crisis. It is hard for nurses to give themselves permission to do less-than-optimal work, but sometimes achievement of these outcomes is the best that can be expected. These outcomes should be achieved given less-than-optimal circumstances and limited resources.

Do First Things First

To decide what is reasonable to accomplish, a nurse has to come to terms with the resources that are available and the outcomes that must be achieved. If someone has called in sick and no replacement is available, it might be unreasonable for a nurse to plan to reinforce teaching or discuss the home environment with a patient scheduled to leave the next day. However, there would be no question that interventions that prevent life-threatening emergencies or save a life when a life-threatening event occurs are priorities (Hansten, 2018). They must be done no matter how short the staffing. It is imperative that nurses protect their patients and maintain both patient and staff safety as well as perform the activities essential to the nursing and medical care plans.

First Priority: Life-Threatening or Potentially Life-Threatening Conditions

Life-threatening conditions include patients at risk to themselves or others and patients whose vital signs and level of consciousness indicate potential for respiratory or circulatory collapse (Hansten, 2018). A patient whose condition is life threatening is the highest priority and requires monitoring until transfer or stabilization. Life-threatening conditions can occur at any time during the shift and may or may not be anticipated. Patients must be monitored to prevent the occurrence of adverse nurse-sensitive patient outcomes, such as a cardiac arrest from an inadvertent airway occlusion, etc.

A quick guide to assessing life-threatening emergencies is as simple as ABC. A stands for Airway. Is the airway open and patent or in danger of closing? This is the highest priority of care. B stands for Breathing. Is there respiratory distress? C stands for Circulation. Is there any circulatory compromise? This is a way of prioritizing actions. Although there is clearly an order of importance, ABC is often assessed simultaneously while observing the patient's general appearance and level of consciousness (Table 19.2). Patients with life-threatening conditions usually have an IV access line and receive continuous monitoring of their cardiac rhythm, blood pressure, pulse, respiration, and oxygen saturation level. Their temperature and urinary output and their potential for other life-threatening conditions is monitored closely as well.

Table 19.2   Top Priority Patients with Potential Threats to Their ABCs

Patient	Potential threats
Respiratory patients	• Airway compromise • Choking • Asthma • Chest trauma
Cardiovascular patients	• Cardiac arrest • Shock • Hemorrhage
Neurological patients	• Major head injury • Unconscious • Unresponsive • Seizures
Other patients	• Major trauma • Traumatic amputation • Major burn, especially if airway involvement • Abdominal trauma • Vaginal bleeding • Anaphylaxis • Diabetic with altered consciousness • Septic shock • Child or elder abuse

Source: Adapted from the *Canadian Pediatric Triage and Acuity Scale: Implementation Guidelines for Emergency Departments.* Retrieved August 7, 2010, from www.caep.ca

Second Priority: Activities Essential to Safety

Activities that are essential to safety are very important and include those responsibilities that ensure the availability of life-saving monitoring, medications, and equipment, and that protect patients from infections and falls. They include asking for assistance or providing assistance during two-people transfers or turning and movement of heavy patients (Hansten & Jackson, 2009). They also include monitoring the patient for the prevention of adverse nurse-sensitive outcomes. Nurse-sensitive patient outcomes are those outcomes that are most affected by or sensitive to nursing care (Mastal, Matlock, & Start, 2016). These include skin injury, falls, and infections.

Third Priority: Comfort, Healing, and Teaching

Activities that include comfort, healing, and teaching are essential to the plan of care and lead to outcomes that relieve symptoms and/or lead to healing. They are the activities that, if omitted, will hinder the patient's recovery. These essential activities include those that relieve symptoms—pain, nausea, and so on—and those that promote healing, such as nutrition, ambulation, positioning, medication administration, and teaching (Figure 19.3 Prioritization Triangle). If an activity is neither important nor urgent, then it becomes the lowest priority (Figure 19.4 Determining Priorities).

Some activities that are often thought of as important may not be. Sometimes laboratory data, vital signs, and intake and outputs are ordered to be monitored more frequently than the status of the patient indicates. Frequent monitoring of these parameters may make no significant difference in patient outcomes. When nurses begin their shifts, they should question the activities that make no difference in outcomes (Hansten & Jackson, 2009). If a practitioner orders these activities, a nurse should work to get the order changed. If there is a nursing order that does not make a difference, the nurse should change

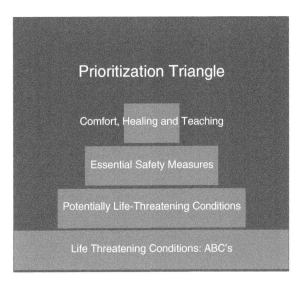

FIGURE 19.3   Prioritization triangle.
Source: Figure created by P. Joswick.

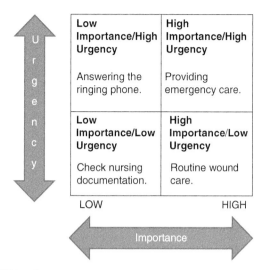

FIGURE 19.4   Determining priorities.
Source: Figure created by P. Joswick.

it. Nurses should give priority to the activities that they know are going to make a difference in patient outcomes.

Application of Time Management Strategies to the Delivery of Care

After priorities are set, nurses know which the most important activities are to accomplish first. Time management strategies can be used in all areas of care delivery to maximize the effectiveness of the nurse's time and minimize lost time and efforts.

Estimate Activity Time Consumption

Nurses need to estimate how much time each activity will take and plan accordingly. The previously discussed activity log may help estimate how much time many activities will take. Perhaps a patient tends to need more time for medication administration than do other patients, so the wise nurse will save that patient's medication administration until last. By estimating the time of activities, nurses can schedule the best time to perform activities. Nurses may notice when passing 6 p.m. medications that water pitchers are empty and juice cups dry. Scheduling the nursing assistant to fill water pitchers and pass refreshments prior to medication administration will be a prudent response to such an observation.

Create an Environment Supportive of Time Management and Patient Care

Often in the frenzy of giving care, nurses forget the obvious. Where are the linens, supplies, medications, and so on located? Are there optimal locations? Is stocking things a priority in order to make them available? Do nurses really stop and think before going to a patient's room with pain medications or for a treatment?

How many trips does one treatment take? It should take only one trip, but if a nurse hurries in and leaves something at the nurse's station, then the nurse will have to return to retrieve it. These are simple things that take time. The nurse should consider all aspects of the unit environment and get together with co-workers to make a difference. Do specialty carts, such as those for intravenous infusion, isolation, laboratory collections, routine wound care, and so on, need to become more efficient and effective?

USE Shift Hand-Off Report

Prior to planning for the shift of duty, the end of shift hand-off report at best can lead to an efficient, effective, and safe start to the shift. At worst, it can leave the oncoming shift with inadequate or old data on which to base their plan. In 2005, the **Joint Commission** (JC) reported that communication breakdowns were correlated with adverse outcomes, and it included a standardized approach to shift hand-off communication as one of its patient safety goals (Riesenberg, Leisch, & Cunningham, 2010). So, the day of haphazard shift hand-off reporting has ended. There are various ways to conduct an end of shift hand-off report—for example, a face-to-face meeting, walking rounds, and bedside report in the patients room (Table 19.3).

Evidence supports rounds in the patient room as the ideal way to do hand-off reporting (Gregory, Tan, Tilrico, Edwardson, & Gamm, 2014). The information has to be transmitted and time must be provided for questions and answers. This allows time for both transmission of information and for questions and answers to facilitate safe, effective, and efficient care and most importantly involves the patient in the report. If the outgoing nurse fails to cover all pertinent points, the oncoming shift must ask for the appropriate information. See Table 19.4 for a tool for taking and giving shift hand-off reports.

Formulate the Plan for the Shift

Having received pertinent information from the shift report, nurses can consider the big picture; decide on optimal and reasonable outcomes; and set priorities based on life-threatening conditions, safety considerations, and activities essential to comfort, healing, and teaching. The nurse can then develop an assignment sheet (Figures 19.5 and 19.6) after considering nursing standards, patient care routines, and several other factors that must be considered in planning for a shift (Table 19.5).

Make Assignments

Because nurses cannot accomplish patient objectives by themselves, they must delegate and make assignments to other team members. This can be challenging and requires understanding of delegation principles, which are discussed in Chapter 18. The assignment sheet should identify who will perform the intervention. Figures 19.5 shows an assignment sheet excerpt and Figure 19.6 shows the entire blank assignment sheet with

Table 19.3   Methods of End-of-Shift Hand-Off Report: Advantages and Disadvantages

Method	Advantages	Disadvantages
Face-to-face report	• Nurses get clarification and can ask questions. • Nurse giving report has actual audience and tends to be less mechanical. • Nurses are more likely to give pertinent information than they would to a tape recorder.	• It is time consuming. • It is easy to get sidetracked and gossip or discuss non-patient-related business. • Both oncoming and departing nurses are in report. • Patients are not included in planning.
Walking rounds	• Provides the prior shift and incoming shift staff the opportunity to observe the patient while receiving report. Staff can address any assessment or treatment questions. • Information is accurate and timely. • Patient is included in the planning and evaluation of care. • Accountability of outgoing care provider is promoted. • Patient views the continuity of care. • Incoming shift makes initial nursing rounds. • Departing nurse can show assessment and treatment data directly to oncoming nurse.	• It is time consuming. • There is a lack of privacy in discussing patient information.

Source: Table created by P. Joswick.

Table 19.4   Tool for End-of-Shift Hand-Off Report

	Notes
Demographics	• Room number • Patient name • Sex • Age • Practitioner
Diagnoses	• Primary • Secondary • Nursing • Medical • Surgery Date
Patient status	• Do Not Resuscitate (DNR) status • Current vital signs • Problem with ABCs, level of consciousness, or safety • Oxygen saturation • Pain score • Skin condition • Ambulation • Fall risk • Suicide risk • Presence/absence of signs and symptoms of potential complications • New orders/changes in treatment plan
Fluids/tubes/oxygen, laboratory tests and treatments	• IV fluid, rate, site • Tube feedings—type of tube, solution, rate, and toleration • Oxygen rate, route, other tubes (e.g., chest tube, NG tube, Foley, and so on), type of tube and type of drainage • Abnormal lab and test values • Labs and tests to be done on oncoming shift • Treatments done on your shift, including dressing changes (times, wound description) and procedures • Identify treatments to be done during next shift
Expected shift outcomes	• Priority outcomes for nursing diagnoses • Patient learning outcomes
Plans for discharge	• Expected date of discharge • Referrals needed • Progress toward self-care and readiness for home
Care support	• Availability of family or friends to assist in ADL/IADL (activities of daily living/instrumental activities of daily living)
Priority interventions	• Interventions that must be done this shift

Source: Table created by P. Joswick.

ASSIGNMENT SHEET EXCERPT   Unit 2   South _____

_____

Date <u>February 2,</u>   Notify RN

_____   immediately if:

Shift ____<u>Days</u>_____   T   <97 or >100

Charge nurse __<u>Mary</u>_____   P   <60 or >110

_____ R   R   <12 or > 24

RNs Breaks/Lunch   SBP <90 or >160

<u>Steve 0900 and 1100</u>   DBP <60 or >100

<u>Lakeisha 0930 and 1130</u>   BS <70 or >200

<u>Colleen 1000 and 1200</u>   <u>Pulse</u>

_____   <u>oximetry</u>

_____   <u><95%</u>

_____   _____

UAPs   Urine output <30

Breaks/Lunch   cc/hour

<u>Juan 0900 and 1100</u>   Narcotic count <u>Steve</u>_____

<u>Pat 0930 and 1130</u>   _____

                                                 Glucometer check <u>Colleen</u>____

                                                 _____

                             Notify RN one hour Stock pyxis <u>Lakeisha</u>_____

                             prior to end of shift: _____

                              I and O   Pass water <u>Juan</u>_____

                              Patient goal   _____

                              achievement   Stock linen <u>Pat</u>_____

                                                 _____

                                                 Other <u>Colleen attend in-</u>

                                                 <u>service at 1300</u>_____

FIGURE 19.5   Assignment sheet excerpt.
Source: Figure created by P. Joswick.

Unit _____

Date _____

Shift _____	Notify RN immediately if:	Narcotic count
Charge nurse	T <97 or >100	_____
_____	P <60 or >110	Glucometer check
Breaks/Lunch	R <12 or > 24	_____
RN	SBP <90 or >160	Stock Pyxis _____
_____	DBP <60 or >100	_____
_____	BS <70 or >200	Pass water
_____	Pulse oximetry <95%	_____
LPN _____	Urine output <30 cc/hour or 240cc/8	Stock linen
_____	hours	_____
UAP	Notify RN one hour prior to end of shift:	Other _____
_____	I and O	
_____	Patient goal achievement	

Room/Pt Initials Staff AM/PM Wt/I&O IVs Activity Accucheck Tests NPO Comment

FIGURE 19.6   Blank assignment sheet.
Source: Table created by P. Joswick.

columns. Assignments should be part of the planning process and should include delegation of nursing and non-nursing tasks to others, with specific reporting guidelines and deadlines for accomplishment of the tasks. Many factors are considered in making assignments (Table 19.6).

Timing the Actions

Identifying the time by which an intervention should be completed is important. If the time is flexible, then that should also be noted. Assigning a completion time for the intervention makes it more likely for the intervention to be completed during the shift. This makes the outcome more likely to be accomplished (Hansten & Jackson, 2009).

Make Patient Care Rounds

If for some reason the end-of-shift hand-off report did not include walking rounds, the oncoming nurse needs to first make initial rounds on the patients at risk for life-threatening conditions or complications. As the nurse makes rounds, he

or she performs rapid assessments. These assessments may vary from the information given during the shift hand-off report, so the information gathered on rounds may change the shift plan. A patient with asthma that has been calm and without respiratory distress on the previous shift may have experienced a visitor who wore perfume and/or brought bad news. As the oncoming nurse makes initial rounds and uses the quick ABC assessment, the nurse may quickly determine that the patient has suddenly developed respiratory distress. The patient may have been initially prioritized as requiring only supportive activities directed at healing, but now the patient is experiencing a life-threatening reaction and requires appropriate nursing interventions as well as continuous monitoring. While assessing the patient, the nurse also checks all the patient's IV lines to make sure that the correct fluid is infusing and the infusion site is without a complication. The nurse checks all the patient's drains, tubes, and continuous treatments. The nurse also listens to the patient's concerns and desires. It is important to remember that plans are just that, plans, and have to be flexible based on ever-changing patient care needs. Times for treatments and medications

Table 19.5   Factors to Consider in Planning for a Shift

Concern	Considerations
Plan:	
What is the big picture?	How many patients? Any staffing issues? Any environmental concerns? Is unit geography conducive to patient care delivery?
What are the desired outcomes?	If everything goes well and as expected, what does the nurse hope to accomplish? If unexpected setbacks occur, what can the nurse, staff, and patients really accomplish?
What are the priorities, nursing standards, and nursing routines?	Who is at greatest risk for potential life-threatening complications? Has all emergency equipment been checked? Are patients who are at a high risk for falls or suicide identified and measures taken? Who are the patients suffering from significant symptoms—airway, breathing, circulation? Are there any other complex patient or family needs? What nursing standards and patient care routines are needed by patients?
Intervene:	
What are the parts to be accomplished?	Monitoring? Medication administration? Treatments? Teaching? Counseling? Physical and functional care? Unit support, e.g., stocking, maintenance?
Who is available to do the work, and what skills and attributes do the personnel have?	RN? LPN? UAP? What are the other responsibilities of staff? What is staff's attitude and dependability? Do any patients need continuity of care by same staff? Is there a fair work distribution among staff? Do any patients need isolation or protection? Do staff need to be protected from some patients? What is the skill, education, and competency of staff, i.e., RN, LPN, UAP?
What can the RN do? What about the LPN? What can the UAP do? There is much variation in the titles of nursing assistive personnel (UAP), e.g., unlicensed nursing personnel, nursing assistant, nurse aide, patient care attendant, patient care aide, etc. Besides those titles, some states use the term *unlicensed assistive personnel* (UAP) (National Council of State Boards of Nursing [NCSBN], 2016)*.	RN identifies standards and patient care routines and teaches, counsels, and supervises all nursing care. LPN can do medication administration and treatments. UAP can complete physical care such as bathing, performing oral care, and obtaining vital signs. Assign and delegate accordingly.
When should the actions be completed by? What are the guidelines for completion?	Give a set time for completion of all tasks.
Evaluate:	
Are the shift outcomes achieved?	How will you check throughout the shift and at the end of the shift? Is your team in need of assistance? Has anything unexpected happened to change your plan? Has patient status changed? At the end of the shift, did you accomplish outcomes?

Source: Table created by P. Joswick.

Table 19.6   Factors Considered in Making Assignments

- Priority of patient needs
- Geography of nursing unit
- Complexity of patient needs
- Other responsibilities of staff
- Attitude and dependability of staff
- Need for continuity of care by same staff
- Agency organizational system
- State laws, e.g., state nurse practice act
- Required continuing education
- Need for fair work distribution among staff
- Need for lunch/break times
- Need for isolation
- Need to protect staff and patients from injury
- Skill, education, and competency of staff, that is, RN, LPN, UAP
- Hospital policy and procedure
- Patient care standards and routines for surgical, medical, maternal, child, and/or mental health patients
- Environmental concerns
- Equipment checks, medication checks
- Accreditation regulations
- Needs of other units in hospital, number of staff, problems left over from earlier shifts, etc.
- Desired patient outcomes

Source: Table created by P. Joswick.

may have to be changed. Often, nurses believe that the times for administering medication are inflexible, yet practitioners usually write medication orders as daily, twice a day, three times a day, or four times a day. These kinds of orders give nurses flexibility in administration times. Although unit pol- icy dictates when these medicines are given, unit policy is under nursing control. Rounding at the beginning of the shift is not enough; periodic rounding by nursing staff should be done hourly checking for the 3 Ps: pain; potty (need to toi- let); positioning (Manges & Groves, 2019).

Evaluate Outcome Achievement

At the end of the shift, the nurse reexamines the shift action plan. Did the nurse achieve the outcomes? If not, why? Were there staffing problems or patient crises? What was learned from this for future shifts?

Avoid Priority Traps

Bing-Jonsson et al. (2016) state that prioritizing has several traps that nurses should avoid. These are:

- Doing whatever hits first
- Taking the path of least resistance
- Responding to the squeaky wheel
- Completing tasks by default
- Relying on misguided inspiration

A frequent trap for nurses is acting upon the "doing whatever hits first" trap. This nurse typically responds to things that happen first. For example, a nurse at the beginning of the day shift chooses to fill out the preoperative checklist for a patient going to surgery the next day rather than assess the rest of the patients first.

The second trap is the "taking the path of least resistance" trap. Nurses in this trap may make a flawed assumption that it is easier to do a task themselves, whereas the task could have been delegated, and the nurses could be completing another task that only a nurse can complete. For example, the nurse admitting a patient needs to take the vital signs, weigh the patient, get the patient settled, complete the baseline assessment, and call the practitioner for orders. Weighing the patient and getting the patient settled are tasks that can be delegated to **unlicensed assistive personnel** (UAP) so the nurse may complete the baseline assessment of the patient and then call the practitioner for orders.

The third trap is the "responding to the squeaky wheel" trap, where the nurse feels compelled to respond to whatever need has been vocalized the loudest. In this case, the nurse may choose to respond to a family member who has come to the nursing station every half hour with some concern. To appease the family, the nurse may take time to focus on one of their many verbal concerns and overlook a more pressing patient care need elsewhere.

The fourth trap is called the "completing tasks by default" trap. This trap occurs when the nurse feels obligated to complete tasks that no one else will complete. A common example is emptying the garbage when it is full instead of asking housekeeping to complete the task.

The last trap is the "relying on misguided inspiration" trap. A classic example of this trap is when the nurse feels "inspired" to document findings in the chart and avoids tackling a higher-priority responsibility. Unfortunately, some tasks will never become inspiring. These tasks need discipline, conscientiousness, and hard work to complete them.

Strategies to Enhance Personal Productivity

Time management applies not only to work but also to the nurse's personal life. Too often, nurses feel that they have no personal life because of rotating shifts, weekend work, and stressful work experiences. Proper time management will allow nurses to take control of both their work life and their personal life. Use a variation of the activity log in Table 19.1 to review how you spend your personal time. It will help to determine your most energetic time of day. Activities that take focus and creativity should be scheduled at high-energy times, and dull, repetitive tasks at low-energy times. Scheduling time for proper rest, exercise, and nutrition allows for quality time.

Create More Personal Time

There are three major ways to create time. One is to delegate work to others or hire someone else to do work. Another is to eliminate chores or tasks that add no value. The last way is to get up earlier in the day. When you delegate a task, you cannot control when and how the task is completed. Initially, it may take more time to get others to do the chore than to just do it yourself, but this investment of time should save you time and energy in the future. If a chore is boring and

Case Study 19.1

You are working the day shift on a medical-surgical unit. You are responsible for six patients with the assistance of UAP and an LPN. What are the outcomes you want to achieve? Please use the criteria previously given for prioritizing, i.e., ABC, safety, etc. Which patients will you give to each care provider? Make out an assignment sheet, building on the format in Figure 19.6. Discuss your rationale.

Patient	Priority nursing assessments
Ms. JD is a 68-year-old patient who is postop day 1 after a total shoulder replacement following a traumatic fall. She is confused and on multiple medications and has a history of hypertension and multiple falls. She is anxious and frightened by the "visiting spirits."	ABCs, level of consciousness, vital signs, safety, distal pulse, incision/dressing check, breath sounds. See this patient second during rounds.
Mr. DB is a 55-year-old patient with insulin-dependent diabetes mellitus, juvenile onset at age 12. He is postop day 2 after a right below-the-knee amputation. He complains of severe right leg pain and is restless. Mr. DB has a history of noncompliance with diet and is on sliding scale insulin administration.	ABCs, symptoms of hypoglycemia, glucoscan at 4 p.m. and 9 p.m., vital signs, safety, incision/dressing check, pain, diabetic teaching. See this patient third during rounds. You may need to check his glucose level STAT.
Mr. JK is a 35-year-old patient with a history of alcohol abuse, admitted for severe abdominal pain. He is throwing up coffee-ground-like emesis.	ABCs, level of consciousness, seizure and shock potential, hematemesis, DTs, safety, vital signs, CBC, hematocrit, type and cross-match, 16-gauge IV line for possible blood transfusion, oxygen, cardiac monitor. See this patient first during rounds.

Now, identify the priority nursing assessments for this next group of patients.

Priority Patient Assessments, Group II

Patient	Priority nursing assessments
Ms. HM is an 85-year-old patient who was transferred from a nursing home because of dehydration. She is vomiting and has abdominal pain of unknown etiology. Intravenous hydration continues and a workup is planned. Ms. HM is alert and oriented.	
Mr. AB is a 72-year-old patient who is status post cerebrovascular accident. He is to be transferred to rehabilitation. He needs his belongings gathered and a nursing summary written.	
Ms. VG is an 82-year-old patient who is postop day 5 after an open reduction of a femur fracture. She has a history of congestive heart failure, hypertension, and takes multiple medications. Her temperature is elevated. She is confused.	

mundane, it makes more sense to work an hour more at a job you enjoy to pay for someone else to do the unrewarding, boring work.

Getting up one hour earlier in the day for a year can free up 365 hours, or approximately two weeks a year, of extra time that can be used to enrich life. After several days of rising an hour earlier, an individual may feel tired and respond to the fatigue by going to bed a little earlier (Vanderkam, 2016). This may be a good strategy for many people, especially those who are not productive in the evening and spend time doing activities that are minimally rewarding, such as watching television. If a person does not try to get to bed earlier, however, and the end result of getting up early is fatigue, the strategy is not beneficial.

Use Downtime

During any day, there is time available that is seldom used, often referred to as "downtime." When waiting at appointments, in lines, or for others, people often have time available. Wait time can sometimes be avoided by calling ahead to verify appointments and arriving no more than 5 min early. During unavoidable waits, the time can be put to good use by having reading and writing materials handy.

Traveling or commuting time as a passenger is frequently frittered away. Listening to books on tape is a good way to catch up on reading. Many libraries have a collection of books on tape. If privacy is not an issue, phone calls can be initiated

Critical Thinking 19.2

Throughout the day shift, nursing and unit staff communicate and work together to deliver quality patient care according to standards. The nursing standards and routines that the nursing staff will apply to these patients reflect the ANA Standards of Nursing Practice and include routines of care such as:

   Bedfast patients—Turn Q2H, intake and output, etc.

   All patients—Q4H vital signs, hygiene, fresh water, etc.

   Depending on the type of patient care unit, the day shift routine might go like this:

7:00 a.m.	Charge nurse reviews patient care assignments with all nurses and unit staff. Day shift takes hand-off shift report from night shift. Patient rounds and assessment begin and continue every half hour and as needed.
7:30 a.m.	UAP obtain **vital signs** (VS). Patient breakfast served.
7:45 a.m.	Patient assessment, including ABCs, VS, lab work, medications, IV fluids; a.m. hygiene care begins following nursing care standards; turn and reposition patients Q2H.
8:00 a.m.	Health care providers make rounds; patients sent for diagnostic tests; regular patient rounds and assessments.
8:30 a.m.	VS reassessment as needed; patient rounds.
9:00 a.m.	Medications given; patient rounds continue; 15-minute breaks begin for all staff.
9:30 a.m.	Patient rounds continue; documentation begun.
10:00 a.m.	Patient rounds; turn and reposition patients.
10:30 a.m.	Patient rounds.
11:00 a.m.	Patient rounds; lunch breaks start for all staff.
11:30 a.m.	Patient rounds; reassessment of VS of those patients with 7:30 a.m. abnormal VS.
12:00 p.m.	Patient rounds; turn and reposition patients. Patient lunch served.
12:30 p.m.	Patient rounds.
13:00 p.m.	Medications given; patient rounds.
13:30 p.m.	Patient rounds.
14:00 p.m.	Patient rounds. Intake and output reports completed; documentation completed. Turn and reposition patients.
15:00 p.m.	Patient rounds. Hand-off shift report from day shift to evening shift.

   Is this patient care routine similar to one you have seen on a patient care unit where you have worked? Make out a day shift routine for a unit you are familiar with. Make up an assignment sheet like the one in Figure 19.6 for the same unit.

and returned during commutes when you are a passenger. Don't make phone calls while driving.

Sometimes it is important just to sit back and enjoy the scenery or the company. Time management principles aim at creating more enjoyable time, not filling every moment with chores.

Critical Thinking 19.4

The relationship between personal lifestyle and the incidence of several diseases has been demonstrated. Many health promotion programs include the expectation that people invest in themselves. Do you invest in yourself with your daily activities to promote higher education; planned savings; healthy eating; regular exercise; deferred gratification; avoidance of smoking, tanning booths, drugs, excessive alcohol consumption; and regular physical checkups? Do you know people who seem to live only from one day to the next because their perspective of time is in the immediate and they do not seem to recognize the benefits of setting priorities and doing long-term planning?

Critical Thinking 19.3

Nurses set priorities fast when they "first look" at a patient. As you approach your patient, get in the habit of observing the following:

First look:
- Eye contact as you approach
- Speech
- Posture
- Level of consciousness

  Airway
- Airway sounds or secretions
- Nasal flare

  Breathing
- Rate, symmetry, and depth
- Positioning
- Retractions

  Circulation
- Color

- Cyanotic
- Presence of IV or oxygen
- Pain
- Vital signs (TPR and BP)
- Pulse oximetry
- Cardiac monitor

  Drainage
- Urine
- Blood
- Gastric
- Stool
- Sputum
- Wound

Practice your "first look" the next time you approach a patient. Does this improve your assessment skills?

Control Unwanted Distractions

Personal life is not immune from distractions that get in the way of accomplishing personal goals. These may include such distractions as visitors, unplanned phone calls, low-priority tasks, and requests for assistance (Tables 19.7 and 19.8).

Find Personal Time for Lifelong Learning

Finding time for lifelong learning is a struggle for recent graduates and even more-seasoned nurses. The complexity of health care demands an educated workforce. So as soon as one degree is completed, it is time to start thinking about the next.

There are ways to achieve your dreams of more education and work and still have a personal life. Henry (2014) offers tips for balancing school, family, and work in Table 19.9.

Returning to school is certainly a challenge, but with time management skills, the return to school can result in the accomplishment of personal outcomes, a degree, and new knowledge.

Table 19.7 Strategies for Avoiding Personal Time Distractions

Distraction	Strategies
Casual visitors	Let visitors know that you only have a short amount of time to address and concerns Remain standing.
Unplanned phone calls	Use voice mail. Set a time to return calls. Don't call when driving.
Unwanted/low-priority jobs	Say no to jobs that have little value or in which you have little interest. Leave low-priority tasks undone. If an unwanted job must be done, pay or ask for assistance.
Requests for assistance	Encourage others to be more independent. Give them encouragement but send them back to complete the job. Decisions to help should be conscious decisions, not drop-in distractions.
Clutter	Clear your work area of clutter and keep it clean. Organize your work area and take a few minutes at the end of your shift to prepare your area for the next shift.
Interruptions	Open your mail over the garbage can. Respond, delegate, or throw it out. Organize your papers. Keep your notebooks, calendar, and phone lists in one three-ring binder so that you have your essentials together.
Procrastination	Break a task down into manageable segments and return to it again and again until it is complete.
Perfectionism	Become a pursuer of excellence, not a perfectionist, as you pursue your goals (Table 19.8).
Texting	Turn your phone off and check at scheduled intervals; let your friends and family know this.
Social media	Check social media no more often than once a day. It is a way of communicating but should not take over your life.
E-mails	E-mails should be checked at scheduled intervals and responded to appropriately.

Source: Table created by P. Joswick.

Table 19.8 Behaviors of Perfectionists vs. Pursuers of Excellence

Perfectionists	Pursuers of excellence
• Hate criticism	• Welcome criticism
• Are devastated by failure	• Learn from failure
• Get depressed and give up	• Experience disappointment but keep going
• Reach for impossible goals	• Enjoy meeting high standards within reach
• Value themselves for what they do	• Value themselves for who they are
• Have to win to maintain high self-esteem	• Do not have to win to maintain high self-esteem
• Can only live with being number one	• Are pleased with knowing they did their best
• Remember mistakes and dwell on them	• Correct mistakes and then learn from them

Note. Courtesy of White, Duncan, and Baumle (2011) © Reprinted with permission of Cengage.

Table 19.9 Personal Time Management when Returning to School

- Let your employer know that you are interested in returning to school. Most employers are supportive of additional education and will be flexible with your schedule. But they will continue to expect a competent, dedicated employee.
- Develop technological skills. By using a computer, you can e-mail professors and classmates at any time. You can do online research. You can easily incorporate constructive criticisms into papers and build on previous work. Technology is the working student's friend.
- Discover a flexible educational program. Many programs offer several classes in a row on a single day, weekend and night classes, or immersion classes for a week at a time. Some programs offer distance learning opportunities.
- Do not be surprised by the demands of school. Courses will be difficult and demanding of time. Remember that you have faced difficult demands and challenges before. Use the same techniques that helped you in the past and develop some new ones.
- Solicit support from family and friends. They may offer emotional support, financial assistance, household assistance, child care, and so forth.
- Use all available resources at school and at work. Develop mentors and role models. Establish relationships with faculty. Discover and use academic support services such as writing centers and tutors. Read syllabi and course instructions carefully.
- Focus on the outcome. Keep the end in sight, and do not give up. Take it one course at a time. Reward yourself along the way. When a course is completed, celebrate.
- Be careful of the sacrifices. You may replace some hobbies with school. But save some time for the things that are really meaningful to you and your family.
- Manage time. Ten minutes spent on planning saves time and energy later. Keep your sense of humor.
- Take care of yourself and your responsibilities. Set aside a day to take care of personal chores and errands.
- If you need a break, take one. Take time to reflect on what you are accomplishing. If you are feeling overwhelmed, take only one course or take a semester off.
- Study on the run. Taping lectures and listening to them as you commute is a great way to study on the run.

Source: Adapted from Purdue University Global Academic Support Centers. Retrieved on August 20, 2019 at www.purdueglobal.edu/blog/student-life/time-management-busy-college-students

Summary

In this chapter, you have been challenged to review not only concepts, but to apply time management and prioritization in your practice and in your life. You have applied principles of priority setting to patient care situations and time management strategies to delivering effective nursing care. Time management strategies to enhance personal productivity have also been shared. Time management and prioritization are skills that need to be practiced and honed. Having effective time management and prioritization skills will make your career less stressful, more organized, and this will relate to better patient outcomes and maintaining patient safety.

KEY CONCEPTS

- General time management strategies include an outcome orientation, analysis of time cost and use, focus on priorities, and visualizing the big picture.
- Shift planning begins with developing both optimal and reasonable outcomes.
- Priority setting considers what is life threatening or potentially life threatening, what is essential to safety, and what is essential to the plan of care.
- The shift action plan assigns activities aimed at outcome achievement within a time frame.

- End-of-shift hand-off reports include face-to-face meetings and walking rounds.

- The shift action plan is evaluated at the end of the shift by asking if optimal or reasonable outcomes have been achieved.

- Time wasters that might interfere with outcome achievement include procrastination, inability to delegate, inability to say no, management by crisis, haste, indecisiveness, interruptions, socialization, complaining, perfectionism, and disorganization.

- Time management applies to personal life as well as the job.

- Quality time can be achieved by analyzing time use and energy patterns.

- Delegation and getting up 1 hr earlier can create time.

- Additional time can be found by productive use of travel time and waiting time.

- Distractions can be controlled by making your environment less inviting, by using voice mail or an answering machine, by saying no, and by encouraging others to be independent.

- It is possible to balance work, family, and school.

KEY TERMS

Activity log

Desired optimal outcomes

Pareto Principle

Time management

REVIEW QUESTIONS

1. The nurse has just finished the change-of-shift report. Which patient should the nurse assess first?
   a. A postoperative cholecystectomy patient who is complaining of pain but received an IM injection of morphine five minutes ago.
   b. A postoperative appendectomy patient who will be discharged in the next few hours.
   c. A patient with asthma who had difficulty breathing during the prior shift.
   d. An elderly patient with diabetes who is on the bedpan.

2. The staff RN's assignment on the 7 a.m. to 3 p.m. shift includes a newly admitted patient with pneumonia who has arrived on the unit, a new postoperative surgical patient requesting pain medication, and a patient diagnosed with nephrolithiasis who is complaining of nausea. What should the nurse do first after shift report?
   a. Assess the newly admitted pneumonia patient.
   b. Give morphine to the new postoperative patient.
   c. Set up the 9 a.m. medications.
   d. Administer Zofran (Ondansetron hydrochloride) to the patient complaining of nausea.

3. The nurse has been assigned to a medical-surgical unit on a stormy day. Three of the staff can't make it in to work, and no other staff is available. How will the nurse proceed? Select all that apply.
   a. Prioritize care so that all patients get safe care.
   b. Provide nursing care only to those patients to whom the nurse is regularly assigned.
   c. Have the patients' families and ambulatory patients take care of the other patients.
   d. Refuse the nursing assignment, as the increased number of patients makes it unsafe.

   e. Quickly make rounds on all assigned patients to assess needs.
   f. Decide on desired outcomes.

4. The nurse has just completed listening to the morning report. Which patient will the nurse see first?
   a. The patient who has a leaking colostomy bag.
   b. The patient who is going for a bronchoscopy in two hours.
   c. The patient with a sickle cell crisis and an infiltrated IV.
   d. The patient who has been receiving a blood transfusion for the past 2 hours and had a recent hemoglobin of 7.2 grams/dL.

5. A new graduate RN organizing her assignment asks the charge nurse, "Of the list of patients assigned to me, who do you think I should assess first?" What is the best response the charge nurse could make?
   a. "Check the policy and procedure manual for whom to assess first."
   b. "Assess the patients in order of their room number to stay organized."
   c. "I would assess the patient who is having respiratory distress first."
   d. "See the patient who takes the most time last."

6. Of the following new patients, who should be assessed first by the nurse?
   a. A patient with a diagnosis of alcohol abuse with impending delirium tremens (DTs).
   b. A patient with a newly casted fractured fibula, complaining of pain.
   c. A patient admitted 2 hours ago who is scheduled for a nephrectomy in the morning.
   d. A patient diagnosed with appendicitis who has a temperature of 37.8°C (100.2°F) orally.

7. The nurse has just come on duty and finished hearing the morning report. Which patient will the nurse see first?
   a. The patient who is being discharged in a few hours.
   b. The patient who requires daily dressing changes.
   c. The patient who is receiving continuous IV Heparin per pump.
   d. The patient who is scheduled for an IV Pyelogram this shift.

8. A nurse can enhance personal productivity by doing which of the following? Select all that apply.
   a. Analyzing time, getting up an hour early, and delegating unwanted tasks.
   b. Getting up an hour early, answering the phone, and inviting a friend in to talk.
   c. Analyzing use of time, getting up early, and waiting patiently.
   d. Avoiding working and going to school at the same time.
   e. Controlling unwanted distractions such as texts, e-mails, and unplanned phone calls.
   f. Using downtime by having reading and writing materials available.

9. You have received a report on the following patients. Who would you make patient care rounds on first?
   a. Patient who is concerned that he has had no bowel movement for two days.
   b. Patient who has suffered several acute asthmatic attacks within the last 24 hours.
   c. Patient who is now comfortable but has had several episodes of breakthrough pain since yesterday.
   d. Patient who is severely allergic to peanuts who just ate potato chips fried in peanut oil.

10. With reference to the same patients as in question 9, which patient has the second highest priority to be seen by the nurse?
   a. Patient who is concerned that he has had no bowel movement for two days.
   b. Patient who has suffered several acute asthmatic attacks within the last 24 hours.
   c. Patient who is now comfortable but has had several episodes of breakthrough pain since yesterday.
   d. Patient who is severely allergic to peanuts who just ate potato chips fried in peanut oil.

REVIEW QUESTION ANSWERS

1.

Answer: A is correct.

Rationale: Complications from the cholecystectomy could be occurring due to unresolved pain after administration of morphine (A). (B) is incorrect because the patient is stable. (C) is incorrect because the patient could be potentially unstable but the presentation of troubled breathing was from the last shift, and other patients require more immediate attention. (D) is incorrect because the patient has a potential need for assistance but other patients require more immediate attention.

2.

Answer: A is correct.

Rationale: Assessment is a priority for a newly admitted patient who has just arrived on the unit, to rule out unstable possibility (A). (B) is incorrect because ABC takes priority in comparison to pain. (C) is incorrect, as all other actions are a priority, and (D) is incorrect as nausea is an expected side effect of their condition.

3.

Answers A, E, and F are correct.

Rationale: Prioritization is essential (A). (B) is incorrect as all patients must be cared for and (C) is incorrect as nurses are responsible for patient safety. (D) is incorrect as the nurse must go to the unit to ensure safe and effective. Quickly making rounds on all assigned patients is a process of prioritizing care (E) and desired outcomes are warranted (F).

4.

Answer: C is correct.

Rationale: The patient with the infiltrated IV has a circulation issue which could be a complicated from the sickle cell crisis (C). (A) is incorrect as the leaking colostomy bag could be dealt with after seeing patient (C). (B) is incorrect as the patient is stable.

(D) is incorrect as the hemoglobin count is expected as the patient is receiving a blood transfusion due to the low hemoglobin level.

5.

Answer: C is correct.

Rationale: Assessing the patient who is having respiratory distress first is followiong ABC priorization for patient care (C). Patient priorization is not bound by policies and procedures (A). Assessing the patients in order of their room number is inappropriate (B). and time of care does not incorporate all aspects of patient prioritization (D).

6.

Answer: A is correct.

Rationale: Inpending delirium (DTs) is a life threatening condition, so must this patient must be seen first (A). Pain after a newly casted fractured fibula is an expected find with this condition (B). The patient scheduled for a nephrectomy is stable (C) and a raised temperature is an expected with appendicitis.

7.

Answer C: is correct.

Rationale: The patient who is receiving continuous IV Heparin per pump is a circulation issue with the potential for significant bleeding complications (C). The patient being discharged, the patient requiring daily dressing changes. and the patient scheduled for an IV Pyelogram are all stable (A, B, and D).

8.

Answers C, E, and F are correct.

Rationale: Use appropriate strategies to enhance personal productivity (C, E, and F). It is inappropriate to delegate unwanted tasks (A), personal productivity can be impeded by talking on the phone (B), and both working and going to school can have an effect on productivity (D).

9.

Answer: B is correct.

Rationale: Acute asthmatic attacks within the last 24 hours are a breathing issue and the patienty is unstable and must be seen first (B). (A) and (C) are stable. Peanut oil is refined and safe for those with a peanut allergy (D).

REVIEW ACTIVITIES

1. For the next three days, complete an activity log (Table 19.1) for both your personal time and your work time. On what activities are you spending the majority of time? When is your energy level the highest? Is your energy level related to food intake?

2. Compare your use of nursing time to Figure 19.1. Are there any distractions that you can eliminate? What time management concepts might assist you in improving your time management?

3. You go to work one day and there are too many staff members on the unit. Several patients have been discharged. The nursing supervisor asks you to float to another medical-surgical unit. Note the example of the use of priority setting in caring for a group of three patients on this unit (see box).

Priority assessments, Group I	
Patient	**Priority nursing assignments**
Ms. JD is a 68-year-old who is postop day one after a total shoulder replacement following a traumatic fall. She is confused and on multiple medications, with a history of hypertension and multiple falls. She is anxious and frightened by the "visiting spirits." Her daughter stays with her at all times.	Vital signs, safety, distal pulse, incision/dressing check, and breath sounds. See this patient third during rounds. Safety is a prime concern with this confused patient, as well as watching for any postoperative concerns.
Mr. DB is a 55-year-old with insulin-dependent diabetes mellitus, juvenile onset at age 12. He is postop day two after a right below-the-knee amputation. He complains of severe right leg pain and is restless. Mr. DB has a history of noncompliance with diet and is on sliding scale insulin administration.	Vital signs, Glucoscan at 4 p.m. and 9 p.m., safety, incision/dressing check, pain, DB teaching. See this patient second during rounds. He has pain, restlessness, and a relatively new amputation. He is a diabetic and could have a postoperative complication or an insulin reaction. If in doubt, check Glucoscan.

10.

Answer: A is correct

Rationale: After addressing the asthmatic patient first, the second priority would be (A) the patient that has not had a bowel movement in two days. Though not an emergency, this is a patient concern that should be addressed. (C) is stable. Peanut oil is refined and safe for those with a peanut allergy (D).

Priority assessments, Group I	
Patient	**Priority nursing assignments**
Mr. JK is a 35-year-old patient with a history of alcohol abuse, admitted for severe abdominal pain. He is throwing up coffee-ground-like emesis.	Level of consciousness, seizure and shock potential, hematemesis, DTs, safety, vital signs, CBS, hematocrit, type and cross-match, 16-gauge IV line, pulse oximeter, cardiac monitor. See this patient first during rounds. He is a candidate for the development of shock.

Now, identify the priority nursing assessments for this next group of patients back on your regular unit.

Priority assessments, Group II	
Patient	**Priority nursing assignments**
Mrs. Hohman, a 61-year-old with a hypertensive crisis three days ago, blood pressure decreasing daily, now 180/102. She periodically complains of headache.	
Mrs. Glusak, a 67-year-old transferred two hours ago from ICU, with a recent brain attack/CVA, responsive to painful stimuli, and has right-sided paralysis. Family at bedside.	
Mrs. Zurich, a 78-year-old with cellulitis of the right toe and a history of diabetes mellitus, needs teaching.	

1. What are your distractions from outcome achievement? Develop a plan to minimize your distractions.

2. Use Table 19.4, Tool for End-of-Shift Hand-Off Report, to organize your patient care report.

DISCUSSION POINTS

- How can you use this information to improve your practice tomorrow? Five years from now?

- Have you ever worked with an RN with amazing time management skills? How does the information from this chapter help you understand how those skills are developed?

- Prioritization is necessary for nursing and to be successful on NCLEX. How can you apply prioritization in the clinical setting to help you in the testing setting?

DISCUSSION OF OPENING SCENARIO

1. *How can Inez figure out what to do first?* Inez should follow the recommended avenues for prioritization of care by focusing on immediate physiological and life-threatening conditions to begin her process. Additional consideration must be made about the optimal desired outcomes of the patients being cared for by Inez. In addition, applying the primary, secondary, and tertiary prioritization of care will guide Inez to provide safe and effective care to her patients and embody the role as a Registered Nurse.

2. *What tools do you have to organize your care?* There are many tools to help with the organization of patient care. Time analysis, use of time, and understanding the big picture for desired patient outcomes are useful. The SBAR format for report is universally understood by all nurses and can facilitate a streamlined and effective report.

3. *How can using prioritization help in managing time?* Time management and prioritization are interrelated and contingent on each principle. Nurses must create an environment that is supportive for time management, formulate the plan for prioritization of patients, make succinct patient care rounds, and evaluate outcome achievements while avoiding priority traps.

EXPLORING THE WEB

- Find a free online calendar or download an app that you can access from any device:http://apple.com/ical

  http://calendar.yahoo.com
  http://calendar.google.com

- Look at all the hints and free tools on time management at the Mind Tools website. Can you put any of the ideas to use?www.mindtools.com

- If you find time management an impossible challenge, you can find professional assistance at the Professional Organizers website.www.organizerswebring.com

- Check out this University of Michigan site for time management tips.www.umich.edu

- Take a look at the personal time management guide atwww.time-management-guide.com

INFORMATICS

Visit the QSEN site: http://qsen.org/faculty-resources/courses/learning-modules/module-two

Complete the Learning Module 2 Managing the Complexity of Nursing Work: Cognitive Stacking. How do nurses manage the complexity of their work? In this module, you will learn about stacking, a continuous process of organization and prioritization embedded in RN work that occurs as care situations evolve. Currently stacking is learned primarily after graduation from a pre-licensure program. Explain the cognitive work of RNs during actual care delivery.

LEAN BACK

- How has poor time management or prioritization caused problems in your personal and professional life?

- After evaluating your time management skills, what are your barriers to improvement.

- Consider the lifetime of worth knowing and applying time management skills. How can this skill translate to a happier life?

REFERENCES

Alfaro-Lefavre, R. (2017). *Critical thinking, clinical reasoning, and clinical judgment* (6th ed.). Philadelphia, PA: Elsevier.

Barrero, L. H., Katz, J. N., Perry, M. J., Krishnan, R., Ware, J. H., & Dennerlein, J. T. (2009). Work pattern causes bias in self-reported activity duration: A randomised study of mechanisms and implications for exposure assessment and epidemiology. *Occupational and Environmental Medicine, 66*(1), 38–44.

Bing-Jonsson, P. C., Hofoss, D., Kirkevold, M., Bjørk, I. T., & Foss, C. (2016). Sufficient competence in community elderly care? Results from a competence measurement of nursing staff. *BMC Nursing, 15*(1), 5.

Donohue, M. T., & Crenshaw, J. T. (2015). Self-management: Stress and time. In P. S. Yoder-Wise (Ed.), *Leading and managing in nursing* (6th ed., pp. 518–543). St. Louis: Mosby.

Franklin, B. (1900). Poor-Richard's Almanac: Benjamin Franklin. New York, NY: Caldwell.

Gregory, S., Tan, D., Tilrico, M., Edwardson, N., & Gamm, L. (2014). Bedside shift reports: Wht does the evidence say? *The Journal of Nursing Administration [JONA], 44*(10), 541–545.

Grohar-Murray, M. E., & Langan, J. C. (2011). Managing resources: Time. In M. E. Grohar-Murray & J. C. Langan (Eds.), *Leadership and management in nursing* (4th ed., pp. 286–296). Stanford, CT: Appleton & Lange.

Hansten, R. I. (2018). Guidelines for prioritization, delegation and assignment decisions. In L. A. LaCharity & C. K. Kumagai (Eds.), *Prioritization, delegation, and assignment: Practice exercises for the NCLEX examination* (4th ed., pp. 1–10). St. Louis: Mosby.

Hansten, R. I., & Jackson, M. (2009). *Clinical delegation skills: A handbook for professional practice* (4th ed.). Sudbury, MA: Jones & Bartlett Publications.

Henry, B. J. (2014). Nursing burnout interventions. *Clinical Journal of Oncology Nursing, 18*(2), 211–214.

Higgins, L. W., Shovel, J. A., Bilderback, A. L., Lorenz, H. L., Martin, S. C., Rogers, D. J., & Minnier, T. E. (2017). Hospital nurses' work activity in a technology-rich environment. *Journal of Nursing Care Quality, 32,* 208–217.

Hughes, G., & Wilson, C. (2017). From transcendence to general maintenance: Exploring the creativity and wellbeing dynamic in higher education. In F. Reisman (Ed.), *Creativity, Innovation and Wellbeing. London: KIE Conference Publications* (pp. 23–65).

Kelley, C. B. (2017). Time management strategies: purposeful rounding and clustering care. *MedSurg Nursing, 26*(1), S1+.

Lavander, P., Meriläinen, M., & Turkki, L. (2016). Working time use and division of labour among nurses and health-care workers in hospitals–a systematic review. *Journal of Nursing Management, 24*(8), 1027–1040.

Manges, K. A., & Groves, P. S. (2019). Exploring the hidden functions of nursing bedside shift report: A performance, ritual, and sensemaking opportunity. *Journal of Nursing Care Quality, 34*(3), 256–262.

Mastal, M., Matlock, A. M., & Start, R. (2016). Capturing the role of nursing in ambulatory care: The case for meaningful nurse-sensitive measurement. *Nursing Economics, 34*(2), 92–98.

Mind Tools. (n.d.). *What is time management: Working smarter to enhance productivity?* Retrieved from www.mindtools.com/pages/article/newHTE_00.htm.

National Council of State Boards of Nursing (NCSBN). (2016). National guidelines for delegation. *Journal of Nursing Regulation, 7*(1), 1–14. Retrieved from www.ncsbn.org/Working_with_Others.pdf

Pong, S., Holliday, P., & Fernie, G. (2018). Effect of intermittent deployment of an electronic monitoring system on hand hygiene behaviors in health care workers. *American Journal of Infection Control, 47*(4), 376–380. doi:10.1016/j.ajic.2018.08.029

Riesenberg, L. A., Leisch, J., & Cunningham, J. (2010). Nursing handoffs: A systematic review of the literature. *American Journal of Nursing, 110*(4), 24–34.

Sullivan, E. J. (2018). *Effective leadership and management in nursing* (9th ed.). New York: Pearsong.

Vanderkam, L. (2016). *Simple ways to add 2 hours more hours to your day.* Retrieved from http://fortune.com/2016/03/05/productivity-time-management-tips

White, L., Duncan, G., & Baumle, W. (2011). *Foundations of basic nursing* (3rd ed.). Clifton Park, NY: Delmar Cengage Learning.

SUGGESTED READINGS

Barker, A. M., Sullivan, D. T., & Emery, M. J. (2006). *Leadership competencies for clinical managers.* Sudbury, MA: Jones & Bartlett Publishers.

Brafman, O., & Beckstrom, R. A. (2006). *The starfish and the spider.* New York: Penguin Group.

Carrick, L., & Yurkow, J. (2007). A nurse leader's guide to managing priorities. *American Nurse Today, 2*(7), 40–41.

Childre, D. (2008). *De-stress kit for the changing times.* Boulder Creek, CA: Institute for Heartmath.

Cohen, S. (2005). Reclaim your lost time with better organization. *Nursing Management, 36*(10), 11.

Emmett, R. (2009). *Manage your time and reduce your stress: A handbook for the overworked, overscheduled, and overwhelmed.* New York: Walker Publishing Company, Inc.

Jackson, M., Ignatavicius, D. D., & Case, B. (2006). *Conversations in critical thinking and clinical judgment.* Sudbury, MA: Jones & Bartlett Publishers.

Kaplan, R. S. (2007). What to ask the person in the mirror. *Harvard Business Review, 84,* 86–95.

Morgenstern, J. (2005). *Never check e-mail in the morning. And other unexpected strategies for making your work life work.* New York: Fireside.

Robinson, J., & Godbey, G. (2005). Time in our hands. *The Futurist, 39*(5), 18–22.

Vestal, K. (2009). Procrastination: Frustrating or fatal? *Nursing Leadership, 7*(2), 8–9.

Change, Clinical Decision Making and Innovation

20

Patricia A. Keresztes
Department of Nursing Science, Saint Mary's College, Notre Dame, IN, USA

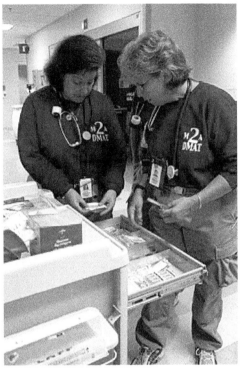

Nurses collaborate to make clinical decisions every day.
Source: Photo used with permission from S. Paturalski and S. Stewart.

Without change there is no innovation, creativity, or incentive for improvement. Those who initiate change will have a better opportunity to manage the change that is inevitable.

William Pollard (1828–1893)

OBJECTIVES

Upon completion of this chapter, the reader should be able to:

1. Explain change from personal, professional, and organizational perspectives.

2. Identify models of change used in health care.

3. Plan, implement, and evaluate a change project using a change model.

4. Relate change strategies.

5. Explain the role and characteristics of a change agent in the change process.

6. Apply the concept of innovation to health care.

7. Apply decision making to clinical situations.

Kelly Vana's Nursing Leadership and Management, Fourth Edition. Edited by Patricia Kelly Vana and Janice Tazbir
© 2021 John Wiley & Sons Ltd. Published 2021 by John Wiley & Sons Ltd.
Companion Website: www.wiley.com/go/kelly-Nursing-Leadership

8. Explain how problem solving, critical thinking, reflective thinking, and intuitive thinking relate to decision making.

9. Examine clinical reasoning and the benefits of clinical reasoning.

10. Identify different clinical decision support tools available for nursing.

11. Examine limitations to effective decision making.

12. Apply strategies to strengthen the nurse's role in decision making for patients.

OPENING SCENARIO

Jesus is a new graduate nurse working on a step-down unit. One of his patient's "just isn't right."

1. *He needs to organize his thinking to clearly understand what the whole clinical picture is, but how? In the past*

he has had the support of clinical faculty, but now he is functioning as an independent RN.

2. *How can he use clinical reasoning to help him in the real world?*

3. *What steps in the critical thinking process will help him in this situation?*

Change is the only constant we have in life. Living organisms must constantly adapt to changes in their environment or die. In this same way, human beings must also successfully adapt and manage change in order to maintain homeostasis and equilibrium. Rapid changes and innovations occurring in the world today require continuous human responses. How these changes and innovations are perceived by the individual can mean the difference between successful adaptation and maladaptation, survival, and extinction. A quote by Henry Ford (AZ Quotes), "We do not make changes for the sake of making them, but we never fail to make a change when once it is demonstrated that the new way is better than the old way" can still be applied today in health care. In order for changes to be successful there needs to be a reason and need for the change. Nurses don't change the way they provide patient care because of a whim, but only because there is a need or reason for the change. In this chapter we will explore how change impacts nursing, models for change, and how best to adapt to the changing health care environment. Also, we will define and examine **critical thinking** and **clinical judgment** and how to apply those to clinical situations. Last, we will examine nurses as innovators and discuss opportunities for nurses to be innovators in health care.

Changes in technology, economic factors, and global influences have made it impossible for hospitals to remain in the "status quo." Swaim (2014) identified several factors as to why change is needed. These include new technology, new opportunities, new leadership in the organization, and new ways for work performance. The rising costs of health care have caused hospitals and health care organizations to examine new organizational and partnership models to be able to save money but continue to provide high-quality patient care. Mergers of health care organizations often lead to a reorganization of nursing and a possible reduction in nursing staff. Options of health insurance are changing, and premiums are constantly rising for those consumers who are fortunate enough to have

health care insurance. The cost of Medicare and Medicaid also continues to rise, and the nation must grapple with payment. For those without any access to health care, the costs continue to soar. Delays in seeking care because of an individual's inability to pay for services and medications often result in nurses caring for sicker patients with multiple diagnoses.

Change is occurring in the rates of diseases within populations and how these diseases are treated. The numbers of people diagnosed with diabetes, cancer, and heart disease continue to rise with changing diets, sedentary lifestyles, and an aging population. People can learn more about their own disease risks with the widespread availability and access to genetic testing. Changing demographics within the population has resulted in a diversity of cultures and languages as well. Challenges continue for nursing and others involved with health care delivery to understand these cultures and to communicate effectively.

Nurses are learning new technology at a rapid pace. The explosion of technology into the area of health care means that how nurses provide care to patients will continue to change. Nurses must continuously learn new systems of patient care documentation, monitoring devices, and changes in diagnosis and treatment of disease. This includes nurses adapting to changing documentation systems to nurses in telehealth. The use of telehealth means nurses are assessing patients through a webcam or remotely monitoring a patient through a smart device. The use of telemedicine and remote access monitoring helps in early detection and treatment of disease. Access to the internet is practically universal and increases the involvement and knowledge level of patient's as they participate in their own health care.

Evidence-based practice is changing the way decisions are made regarding health care treatment and how nursing care is delivered. Interventions such as surgery and diagnostic testing that once required lengthy and costly stays in hospitals are often provided now in outpatient settings. The length of stay in hospitals has been shortened, both by the impact of enhanced technology and the requirements of managed care.

Change

There are many definitions of *change*, and there are many types of change. Merriam-Webster (2018) defines change as "to make different in some particular way," "to make radically different," or "to give a different position, course, or direction." Each separate meaning has various implications. The first definition can be a very simple change in just making something different. This could be changing your furniture in your house or changing the way you drive into work. The second definition is a more drastic change in making something radically different. This could be moving to a different state and working in a new hospital, becoming a travel nurse, or going back to school for an advanced degree. These definitions of change help us understand that change can be very simple or can be more complicated. The level of the degree of change influences how well we respond and adapt to the change.

Benefits of Change

While much of the literature focuses on the stress of change and how to adapt to change, it is also important to consider the benefits of the change. The changes in health care are mostly associated with cost savings. However, much of the change that has occurred over the last decade has also improved patient safety and access to health care. The transition from a hand-written medication administration record to an electronic version has decreased the number of medication errors. Also, the transition to barcode scanning of patient's identification bands and scanning of medications prior to administration has also drastically reduced the number of medication errors. McQuerrey (2018) also points out many other advantages to changes in the workplace. These factors include fresh approaches, new challenges, updated policies and procedures, and increased opportunities. These factors have many implications for staff nurses. Nurses have opportunities to be on policy and procedure committees to enact change for the improvement of patient care by updating and creating new policies and procedures. The new procedures help educate and guide the practice of nursing staff members. Opportunities for staff nurses to be involved in not only policy changes but patient care issues, hiring of new staff nurses and managers, submitting ideas for cost savings and improvements of patient care, and choosing new technologies. Staff nurses are often on unit practice councils to provide input on these issues. For example, staff nurses have developed creative ways for self-scheduling to support those who are going back to school for advanced degrees. Nurses have also been involved in units where there has been significant remodeling of the unit or being involved in the development of a completely new building. Nurses also have opportunities to be involved in implementing evidenced-based practice guidelines for their units.

Types of Change

Nurses experience change in a variety of ways. The different types of change can be found in Table 20.1. For purposes of discussion, **personal change** is a change made voluntarily for your own reasons, usually for self-improvement. This may include changing your diet for health reasons, taking classes for self-improvement, or removing yourself from a destructive or unhealthful environment or situation. **Professional change** may be a change in position or a job or obtaining education or credentials that will benefit you in a current position or allow you to be prepared for a future position. Professional change is often planned and involves extensive alterations in both personal and professional lives. Although either personal or professional change may be stressful, if it is voluntary and carries intrinsic or extrinsic rewards, it is often considered important and worth the stress. Realize that choosing not to choose to have professional change is a choice in itself, perhaps with benefits or with stress and burnout.

There are also different types of changes nurses experience that occur in organizations. Organizations may initiate change from the top down or from the lower level up. If the hospital administration develops a new policy on dress code, then that filters down to all staff members at the unit level. This is an

Table 20.1   Types of Change, Definition, Examples

Type of change	Definition	Examples
Personal	Change made by the individual to improve their health, appearance, lifestyle	Change in hairstyle Change in diet Change in activity/exercise
Professional	Change made by an individual to improve their career, potential job opportunities, advancement, and income	Going back to school Working in a different hospital Working in a different specialty
Organizational	Change that occurs in an organization in administration, operational procedures, mission	Mission and values Mergers with other institutions New leadership teams Policies and procedures Organizational structure

Source: Patricia A. Keresztes.

Real World Interview

A planned leadership succession change gave me distinct opportunities to broaden my leadership knowledge base before stepping into the role of Vice-President for Nursing. I had to learn operations, metrics, and regulations of various nursing departments throughout the hospital system. Then I worked closely with ancillary operators such as lab, pharmacy, nutritional services, and PT/OT. The concerted effort in the planned organizational change was to provide me with the operational foundation for the broad scope of my new role. The planned organizational change was very effective because of this opportunity to develop the arsenal of what I needed to lead nursing in the organization. Planned organizational change is a gift because you get the opportunity to do the planning and forethought into the change.

Sarah Paturalski, RN, MBA, Vice President of Nursing & Clinical Services at Memorial Hospital of South Bend, IN

---

example of change from the top down. An example of change that would occur from the lower level upward is the initiation of self-scheduling. In the beginning, some nursing units began experimenting with self-scheduling. As this model of scheduling became popular and successful for the staff, it became part of hospital-wide scheduling policies.

Many health care organizations now engage in **planned organizational change**. Rasel (2014) defines planned change as "any kind of alteration or modification which is done in advance and differently for the improvement of present position into brighter one." Organizational change that is planned and purposeful is generally better accepted by all employees. It is used to improve efficiency or improve financial standing or for some other organizational purpose. Change is planned to meet organizational goals. One of the goals most organizations have is to maintain a positive financial balance. Change to ensure a healthy financial standing maintains jobs and increases the organization's capability to meet its mission. Improved efficiency is good for the organization's capability to get goods and services to the customer. Improved efficiency in health care provides better-quality care for patients and improves the workload of the employees.

There are levels and types of organizational change. The three levels of change are an increasing intensity of change within the organization. These levels are **developmental change, transitional change**, and **transformational change** (MBA Knowledge Base, 2019). All three of these have an impact on nursing. In **developmental change**, nurses are involved in improving skills or processes to meet standards of care. An example of this is annual competencies in the hospital setting, where nurses practice skills or care standards as they improve and refine with the best available evidence. In **transitional change**, nurses leave old ways of doing patient care and implement new procedures and technologies. An example of this is that at many institutions they are removing the second nurse verification for blood administration and relying on a multiple bar code system; having two nurses check blood is an ingrained practice. These types of changes may be very uncomfortable with seasoned nurses and may cause multiple questions and discussions. Nurses use evidenced-based practice to examine new ways of patient care and provide a rationale for adopting the change. **Transformational**

change involves major shifts in the vision, strategy, or structure of an organization and usually occurs at an administrative level. Organizations may adopt a new strategic vision or strategic plan as a result of new leadership (MBA Knowledge Base, 2019). A common occurrence in health care in the merging of hospitals into one health care system. Smaller hospitals in more rural areas are joining with larger community hospitals in order to stay financially sound. This creates a completely different environment for the staff nurses as they become part of a different organization. This can lead to staffing and scheduling changes and radical difference in how patient care is done. Additionally, the larger community hospital or university-based hospital may have a vastly different vision and value systems. Hospital may also use one of many theories of change. Table 20.2 compares different change theories and their uses.

Models of Change

Health care organizations may follow one of the many models of change. In order for organizational change to be successful these models emphasize the importance of each individual as a key contributor to the success of the change. When nurses are consulted and are a part of change within the hospital there is a greater chance that the change will be successful. The models for change used by health care organizations include the **Institute for Healthcare Improvement** (IHI) Psychology of Change Framework (Hilton & Anderson, 2018), Kotter's (Kotter, 2012) eight-step change model, and the Deming's (2018) **Plan-Do-Check-Act** (PDCA) model. The change models can also be used by nurses to guide changes in nursing practice. Evidenced-based practice is another example of a model of change that is used by all health care professions to change patient care practices. These change models are also used in nursing to design and implement **continuous quality improvement** (CQI) projects.

The IHI Psychology of Change Framework

The IHI Psychology of Change Framework (Hilton & Anderson, 2018) is designed to advance and sustain improvement particularly within health care and the health care organizations. The objective is "to create the conditions that enable

Table 20.2   Comparison Chart of Change Theories and Their Uses

	Lewin	Lippitt	Havelock	Rogers
Theorist and year	Lewin (1951)	Lippitt (1958)	Havelock (1973)	Rogers (1983)
Title of model	Force-field model	Seven phases of change	Six-step change model	Diffusion of innovations theory
Steps in model	1. Unfreeze. 2. Move. 3. Refreeze.	1. Diagnose problem. 2. Assess motivation and capacity for change. 3. Assess change agent's motivation and resources. 4. Select progressive change objectives. 5. Choose appropriate role of change agent. 6. Maintain change. 7. Terminate helping relationship.	1. Build relationship. 2. Diagnose problem. 3. Acquire resources. 4. Choose solution. 5. Gain acceptance. 6. Stabilize and self-renew.	1. Awareness 2. Interest 3. Evaluation 4. Trial 5. Adoption
Use in change projects	General model for most situations and organizations.	Good for changing a process and general change.	Often used for educational change or cultural change.	Used in organizational change, individual change, and group change.

Sources: Compiled with information from Lewin (1951); Lippitt (1958); Havelock (1973); Rogers (1983).

Evidence from the Literature

Citation: Henry, L. S., Christine Hansson, M., Haughton, V. C., Waite, A. L., Bowers, M. et al., (2017). Application of Kotter's Theory of Change to Achieve Baby-Friendly Designation. *Nursing For Women's Health, 21*(5), 372–382.

This article shows how the use of a change model can be helpful in guiding a proposed change to improve patient care. There is also the focus on the importance of the interdisciplinary approach when planning for a change in patient care.

McHugh, C., Krinsky, R., & Sharma, R. (2018). Innovations in Emergency Nursing: Transforming Emergency Care Through a Novel Nurse-Driven ED Telehealth Express Care Service. *Journal of Emergency Nursing: JEN: Official*

Publication of the Emergency Department Nurses Association, 44(5), 472–477.

This article describes the development and initiation of an ED-based telehealth express care service. This was developed by a multidisciplinary ED team consisting of nurses, physicians, physician assistants, and nurse practitioners. The implications for practice include the use of a multidisciplinary team and use of technology with telehealth. The use of this technology decreased the length of stay in the ED waiting room which increased patient satisfaction. The use of this telehealth program also increased the efficiency and use of the ED staff while continuing to provide safe and high-quality patient care.

individuals and groups across systems to exercise power and courage in order to advance and sustain improvements in health and health care" (p. 8). The framework is designed around five interrelated domains of practice:

1. unleash intrinsic motivation

2. co-design people-driven change

3. co-produce in authentic relationship

4. distribute power

5. adapt in action.

This model of change is important for nurses, as it emphasizes the value of each person in an organization. It also

recognizes that each person in an organization will be affected by a change but that each person can also contribute in a meaningful way to that change. These factors are crucial to the successful implementation of change in a health care organization.

Kotter's Eight-step Model

Kotter (2012) developed his model so that organizations can be successful when implementing a change. Change can be successful when it is planned carefully and started with a solid foundation. The eight steps in Kotter's model are: create urgency, form a powerful coalition, create a vision for change, communicate the vision, remove obstacles, create short-term wins, build on the change, and anchor the changes in corporate culture. When this model is used by health care

Critical Thinking 20.1

A. You are caring for an 80-year-old female who has had a total knee replacement. She is widowed with two children. She lives by herself as her children live about 2 hr away. She will be discharged to a rehabilitation facility.

1. In planning for her discharge, what are the resources that will be needed for her to go back to her home?
2. Identify the disciplines that will be involved in her post-operative care and rehabilitation.

3. What are the priorities the nurse must consider when planning for her discharge?

B. You are caring for a 64-year-old Hispanic male who is two days post-operative from having coronary artery bypass grafts. You are to begin working with him for discharge planning.

1. What implications does the patient's ethnic background have on his post-operative discharge teaching in regard to diet?

What is the priority of care for this patient in the post-operative phase?

---

organizations, nurses are valued because their input is sought during every step. Burden (2016) used this model to implement a quality improvement initiative designed to reduce the risk of surgical site infections in breast surgery patients. The changes made through this change model resulted in a significant reduction in surgical site infection in breast surgery patients (Burden, 2016). This model can easily be adapted by nurses to guide changes in practice that can lead to improvements in quality of patient care and cost savings. Table 20.3 summarizes Kotter's eight-step change process with strategies (Figure 20.1).

Deming PDCA

The four steps described by Deming (2018) in the PDCA model are Plan, Do, Check, Act. This is represented as a circle where the cycle should always be repeating itself. The PDCA model is useful when organizations are starting a new improvement project, designing new products or services, planning data collection and analysis in order to evaluate problems, and when implementing any change. In the plan stage the individual or organization recognizes the need or opportunity to make a change. The next step involves doing or testing out a potential change. Next the check is reviewed and results are analyzed. Lastly, the individual or organization will act and take action on what is learned through the first three steps. The change may be implemented or rejected based upon the findings. The cycle then starts all over.

Rand et al. (2018) used the PDCA change model in their study on **Human Papillomavirus** (HPV) vaccination rates in primary care. The "Plan" for the study was to send questionnaires to the identified practices on giving the HOV vaccine and develop a training session on the guidelines for giving the vaccine. The "Do" was providing the information training sessions. The "Check" was sending a follow-up questionnaire to identify current rates of giving the vaccine to those who should receive the vaccine. The "Act" was to continue to monitor the rates at which the vaccine was appropriately given and continue with education. The study found that vaccination rates increased from 53% to 73%. Using the PDCA model, these authors were able to change behavior and make a difference in patient care (Figure 20.2).

Table 20.3   Kotter's Eight-Step Process and Strategies

Steps	Strategies
1. Create urgency	Examine opportunities Identify threats Develop scenarios Start honest discussion
2. Form a powerful coalition	Identify the leaders Work on team building Identify stakeholders Include a mixture of staff from all departments
3. Create a vision for change	Determine values essential for change The vision should match the need for change Create strategy for success Vision should be easy to communicate
4. Communicate the vision	Frequent conversations Keep communication simple and straightforward Address concerns, questions Have consistency with communication
5. Remove obstacles	Recognize and reward those who help with the change Identify those resisting change
6. Create short-term wins	Make the easiest changes first Communicate the successes
7. Build on the change	Continue to set goals Re-evaluate change and make necessary adjustments Look at new ideas
8. Anchor the changes in the culture	Educate new staff on the changes Recognize those key to the change

Source: Adapted from Kotter, J. (2012).

Steps for Effective Change

In order for change to be effective, there are several steps that are recommended. Organizations have to recognize that there is a need for a change. Maintaining the "status quo" for health care organizations and in nursing and delivering nursing care is no longer an option. Once the need for a change has been determined then the organization can follow certain steps that will help the change be effective.

Kotter's 8-Step Change Model

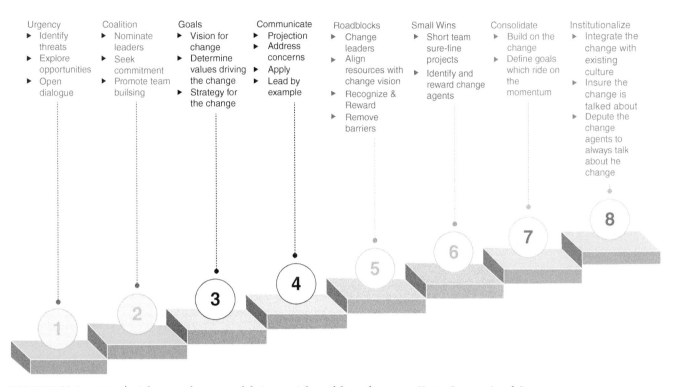

FIGURE 20.1   Kotter's eight-step change model. *Source:* Adapted from the source Kotter International, Inc.

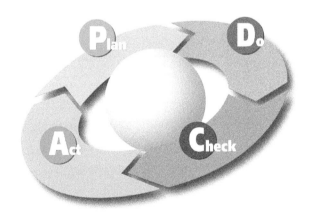

FIGURE 20.2   PDCA model. Adapted from: Vasić, M., Potkonjak, A., Stanojevic, Darko & Dimitrijevic, M. (2015).

Courtney (2016) identified six steps to be taken if change is going to be effective. First, the organization needs to clearly define the change and align it with the mission. One of the first questions you may ask is "Why is this change occurring?" If you understand the reason why the change is occurring and exactly what the change is will make the change acceptable. This is also the first question that may be asked by the staff nurse "Why are we changing what or how we are doing patient care?" If this first step is never addressed, then it is unlikely that the change will be successful.

Second, Courtney (2016) advises to determine the impact of the change on those affected. If a nursing unit will change from 8-hr shifts to 12-hr shifts, how will this impact the staffing of the unit. This change will impact every nurse in the hospital. Maybe some of the nurses are not able to do 12-hr shifts because of physical limitations. How will this affect those nurses? Understanding the impact of the change on those directly impacted will make a difference in the acceptance and implementation of the change.

The next step that Courtney (2016) identified for successful change is communication of the change. If you go into work and suddenly find that you will be taking on more patients as part of your assignment, you will be angry and resistant to that change. Part of adapting to the change is knowing what changes will be happening.

The fourth step identified by Courtney (2016) for successful change is providing training and education on that change. This could include training on new equipment, education on a new policy or procedure, or education on new medications. It is essential for the staff nurse to receive adequate training on new equipment, such as a glucometer or a new protocol for patient care.

The fifth and last step for effective change is implementing a support structure. Knowing that you have access to staff who have been trained on a new glucometer or **electronic health record** (EHR) decreases anxiety when the change is implemented.

The Change Agent

Throughout this discussion of change, the term **change agent** has been used instead of manager, leader, or administrator. The change agent leads and manages change. From this perspective, all nurses are change agents. Change agents may be from inside or outside an organization, and may have become a leader or manager because he or she is an innovator and likely to enjoy change. No matter the title or place of employment, the change agent is the person who is ultimately responsible for the success of the change project, large or small. The role of the change agent is to manage the dynamics of the change process. This role requires knowledge of the organization, knowledge of the change process, knowledge of the participants in the change process, and an understanding of the feelings of the group undergoing change. Probably the most important role of the change agent is to maintain communication, momentum, and enthusiasm for the project, while still managing the process. Table 20.4 identifies change agent approaches.

The change agent should possess some important characteristics. These include trust and respect from the recipients of change, as well as from the chief executives in the organization. The recipients of change must trust not only the change agent's interpersonal skills to provide information and manage change, but also the change agent's personal integrity and standing as an honest, ethical, and principled individual. The executives in the organization must trust that the change agent will accomplish the established goals given the proper support. Credibility and flexibility are also important characteristics for the change agent to possess. The change agent cannot be temperamental or rigid. The ability of the change agent to compromise and negotiate is also important.

An essential characteristic of the change agent is the ability to maintain and communicate the vision of the change. No matter how small or large the project is, the vision or picture of that change must be maintained and kept in the forefront of everyone's memory. The ability to articulate the vision and to mold disparate concepts into that vision is paramount to success. The astute change agent recognizes that those affected by the change may not have the same vision, so the change agent must paint a vivid mental picture of the change and how it will work during change implementation. The change agent will also have to recognize that those developing the project have some definite inclusion concepts that must be folded into the vision for success. Inclusion concepts are those ideas or concepts that the affected parties believe are absolutely necessary for their peace of mind or for moral value. Including these concepts in the change process helps people feel ownership and value, that is, a piece of them or their idea is in the plan.

Perhaps the most outstanding skill the change agent needs is the ability to communicate and have good interpersonal skills. Communication throughout the change process cannot be emphasized enough. Each stage must be communicated to all who want or need to know about the project. The ability to establish trusting relationships, interact with others, and manage conflict is of utmost importance to the success of the project. Honesty is the key to truly excellent communication. People are better able to deal with the truth than with a half-truth or a lie. If a project team member's idea is not acceptable for whatever reason, let them know immediately so there are no misunderstandings later. Communication includes using positive, concise, clear words that communicate accurately and responsibly. Ambiguity in communication is an error that leads to conflict and distrust later in the project. Credible communication maintains open communication lines and helps to manage the process. The change agent must be sensitive to the project team members' feelings and involvement with the way things were. Do not denigrate or disrespect what was. Concentrate on how much better things can be.

Another important characteristic of the change agent is the ability to empower people to control the change project as it affects their lives. Those most affected by the change must be

Table 20.4 Change Agent Approaches

1. Begin by articulating the vision clearly and concisely. Use the same words over and over. Constantly remind people of the goals and vision.
2. Map out a tentative timeline and sketch out the steps of the project. Have a good idea of how the project should go.
3. Plant seeds with, or mention some ideas or thoughts to, key individuals from the first step through the evaluation step so that some idea of what is expected is under consideration.
4. Select the change project team carefully. Make sure it is heavily loaded with those who will be affected and other experts as needed. Select a variety of people. For example, an innovator, someone from the late majority group, a laggard, and a rejector are probably good to include. These people provide insight into what others are thinking.
5. Set up consistent meeting dates and keep them. Have an agenda and constantly check the timeline for target activities.
6. For those not on the team but affected by the project, give constant and consistent updates on progress. If the change agent does not, someone on the project team will, and the change agent wants to control the messages.
7. Give regular updates and progress reports both verbally and in writing to the executives of the organization and those affected by the change.
8. Check out rumors and confront conflict head on. Do not look for conflict, but do not back away from it or ignore it.
9. Maintain a positive attitude, and do not get discouraged.
10. Stay alert to political forces both for and against the project. Get consensus on important issues as the project goes along, especially if policy, money, or philosophy issues are involved. Obtain consensus quickly on major issues or potential barriers to the project from both executives and staff.
11. Know the internal formal and informal leaders. Create a relationship with them. Consult them often.
12. Having self-confidence and trust in oneself and one's team will overcome a lot of obstacles.

Source: Adapted from Lancaster, J. (1999). *Nursing issues in leading and managing change.* St. Louis, MO: Mosby.

involved in assessing, planning, implementing, and evaluating the change. Without this support, the change cannot be successful. The change agent needs to be open and empowering about the selection of people to work on the project. Empowerment and participation in the project help people own the project and support its successful implementation. It is important for the change agent to respond appropriately to people's responses to change and not dismiss or be disrespectful of those reactions. Empowerment is a powerful tool in helping people realize that although something is changing, they have some control and input into that change. The change agent needs to use that empowerment to move the change along and to help people respond positively to the change.

The change agent must have some intuition during the evaluation steps, so that he or she can bow out of the change and allow those affected to accept ownership of the change. This is a matter of timing and insight into when the staff are ready to accept and incorporate the change as its own. During evaluation, the change agent must support modifications and revisions that help transfer project ownership.

As has been reiterated previously, change is an inevitable part of life and will continue to affect the health care system for several years to come. It is important to maintain an attitude that change is preferable to stagnation. This will help leaders identify opportunities for change and embrace those changes for a better quality of work life or for better care for the patient. Inevitably, change will and does occur. As we hone our change agent skills, change becomes easier, expected and understood as necessary to better our profession and improve patient outcomes.

Responses to Change

Stark (2017) identified several responses that people have in response to change. These include both negative and positive behaviors. Maybe you can identify with some of these behaviors when you have faced a change. Anger, gossip, job security, panic, quit, enthusiasm, accept a challenge, look at the bigger picture. The two main responses to change can be either acceptance and **adaptation to change** or resistance and rejection to change.

Adaptation and Acceptance

For nurses dealing with the continuous change in the workplace can be very stressful. Part of the stress of change is the fear of the unknown. This includes learning how to use new equipment, changes in policies and procedures, and changes in leadership and management. Nurses are constantly learning new equipment, changes in documentation, and changes in workplace flow of patients. However, there are several helpful tips for nurses to use to help decrease the stress and anxiety of changes in the workplace. The best way to adapt to change is to acknowledge that change is occurring (Weston, 2015). Once a staff nurses acknowledges that a new glucometer is going to be used, the better the ability to learn how to operate this new piece of equipment. Another tip for dealing with change

is to be a part of the change (Weston, 2015). If the nursing unit is going to implement doing a change-of-shift report at the bedside, being a part of the change process can help the nurse provide valuable insights into how that can be done in the most effective manner. Being a part of the change helps the nurse give the input from the nursing perspective, which can help assist other staff nurses accept the change as well. One aspect of change that is essential is communication. The staff nurses need to be active in reading communication from managers and hospital leadership. This includes participating in unit staff meetings, reading emails from administration, and keeping up with latest trends in health care so that when a change is being implemented the nurses have some familiarity with it from reading journals or attending conferences. Lastly, Weston (2015) also suggests that continuing to be a part of the team by doing your work and seeing the bigger picture is also helpful in adapting to change. The staff nurse may want to continue to provide high-quality care to patients while simultaneously acknowledging the change that is occurring but not letting it cause stress in the workplace. A staff nurse may know that a new EHR will be introduced over the next few months, but will attend classes as needed while continuing to use the old documentation system. Adapting these habits and mindsets can effectively help the staff nurses reduce the stress and anxiety of change in the workplace.

A study by Andre and Sjovold (2017) focused on examining and comparing the work cultures in a nursing unit that had a successful implementation of change versus a unit that had an unsuccessful implementation of a change. The authors found that in the unit which had a successful change, the personnel working in that unit felt they had higher influences in ruling, caring, loyalty, engagement, task orientation, and acceptance compared to the personnel in the unsuccessful change unit (Andre & Sjovold, 2017). This study has many implications for staff nurses and health care organizations involved with change. Many of the factors for successful change focus on workplace environment culture such as caring, engagement, and empathy. Organizations that promote a positive workplace culture by valuing these qualities in staff nurses may be able to bring about change in a more effective manner. Additionally, when staff nurses feel that the organization values these characteristics, it leads to a better adaptation to change.

Resistance and Rejection

No matter how carefully the organization has planned and implemented a change, there will always be those who are resistant to the change or reject the change itself. It is up to the managers and supervisors to identify this as early on as possible and work with these individuals to get them to come on board with the change. Fortunately, there are strategies that managers can use to help with this process. The Hayes Management Group (2019) state that it is very important to help the person resistant to the change identify the reasons for the resistance and then find ways to resolve them. Communication with those resistant to change is essential. The manager should sit down with those individuals resistant to change and have an open conversation about why that staff member is resistant to the change. Is it fear of the unknown? Is it a lack of knowledge? Weston (2015) suggests that many resist change simply because of fear. Fear of the unknown is very common. Weston (2015) suggests a few strategies to overcome fear of change and decrease the resistance to change. He suggests that managers help staff acknowledge the change. This again goes back to the need for communication. If staff are informed about the change, it gives them time to acknowledge and realize that the change is occurring. Weston (2015) also suggests that managers get the staff who are resistant to change to be a part of the change process. Get the staff members involved in the education and training of other staff members and involved in the planning and implementation of the change. Lastly, Weston (2015) suggests that managers help staff identify their fear of the change and replace those fears with something positive. If a staff member is fearful of a new electronic health care record, replace that fear with helping the staff member understand that this new EHR may decrease the time for documentation which increases the amount of time spent in direct patient care. Replacing a fear with a positive can be effective in decreasing the resistance to a change.

Maintaining the Change

The last part of the change process may be the most difficult, that is, maintaining the change. It is well documented that nurses giving reports at the bedside of patients can reduce errors. Nursing units will implement a change to giving bedside reports and monitor the effectiveness and compliance of staff nurses. Several months after this change has been implemented, the nursing units no longer monitor compliance and make the assumption that this is now a standard for the nurses. However, often nurses may go back to the "old" way of giving reports outside the patient's room. In this case the change has not been maintained. In order to maintain a change, it is important that those change agents who brought about the change remain committed to maintaining that change. It is also important that continued follow up with measurements of compliance with the change continues to happen. Another strategy to help maintain the change is to develop leaders for the future that will stay committed to the change.

Critical Thinking

Scenario

You received a report from the night shift on a patient that was involved in a motor vehicle accident. The patient suffered two fractured ribs on the left side of the chest. The patient has been stable overnight with stable vital signs and an oxygen saturation of 96%. The patient has been receiving morphine intravenous for pain every 2–3 hr. When you go in to assess the patient, you notice the patient appears to be having trouble breathing. The oxygen saturation level is 88% and the patient's heart rate has gone from 80 to 110, respiratory rate is 18–26/min, and blood pressure is now 148/82. In questioning the patient about the pain, the patients rates the pain as a five for most of the night. The patient is on 2 l nasal cannula. This situation requires the nurse to make judgments about the current situation of the patient. Why has this patient's condition differed from the report received from the night nurse? The nurse must make clinical decisions on what further information is needed to be collected in this situation and then, based upon that information, what interventions are needed. The nurse listens to the patient's breathing and notices a decrease on the side of the broken ribs. Based upon this information, the nurse increases the oxygen to help increase the oxygen saturation levels and notifies the physician to get an order for an X-ray for a possible pneumothorax. The nurse understands that a main complication of fractured ribs is a pneumothorax. The chest X-ray confirms the patient has developed a pneumothorax and the nurse prepares for the insertion of a chest tube.

Critical Thinking

In order for nursing to survive in the constant changing health care environment, nurses need to learn and apply critical thinking skills and clinical judgment. The rapid turnover of patients in hospitals, the need to multitask, and the higher levels of acuity of patients have made it necessary that nurses develop different types of thinking and apply these different types of thinking into making sound clinical judgments and decisions.

Types of Thinking

There are many different types of thinking that we all do as individuals without realizing it. Thinking about planning a vacation is much different than thinking about a career change. Many are creative thinkers when they look at scenery and determine the best light and angles to take pictures. As nurses, thinking about patient situations and performing patient care requires "multi-thinking" to provide safe and effective nursing care. Different types of thinking that are more specific to nursing include **reflective thinking**, **intuitive thinking**, **analytic thinking**, **holistic thinking**, and **critical thinking**. With experience, the nurse may do all these types of thinking at the same time.

Reflective Thinking

Pesut and Herman (1999) describe **reflective thinking** as watching or observing ourselves as we perform a task or make a decision about a particular situation. We have two selves, the active self and the reflective self. The reflective self watches the active self as it engages in activities. The reflective self acts as observer and offers suggestions about the activities. To be a good critical thinker, practice reflective thinking. Reflection upon a situation or problem after a decision is made, allows one to evaluate the decision. Nurse educators assist students to become better reflective thinkers through the use of clinical journals, examinations, simulations, and Socratic questioning, to name a few. Using journals helps students reflect on clinical activities and improve their clinical decision-making abilities. The use of simulations with nursing students is a very effective way to help students utilize reflective thinking. The debriefing sessions that are done after a simulation help the student reflect upon the decisions made about the patient during the scenario and how that decision impacted the patient. Reflection upon a situation or problem after a decision is made allows the individual to evaluate that decision. New nurses should continue to use reflective thinking throughout their practice to build their confidence in the clinical decisions they make.

Intuitive Thinking

Intuitive thinking is a type of discernment or insight that nurses develop that helps them to act in certain situations. Intuitive thinking, or intuition, is "the perception and understanding of concepts without the conscious use of reasoning" (Papathanasiou, Kleisiaris, Fradelos, Kakou, & Kourkouta, 2014). Intuitive thinking may result from unconscious assessment and analysis of data based on an individual's past experience. Alfaro-LeFevre (2017) contends that expert thinking is usually the result of using intuition and drawing on evidence at the same time to make well-reasoned decisions. Nurses often make decisions about patient care based in part on intuitive thinking. For example, the nurse is caring for a patient who has had a cardiac catheterization. The patient is scheduled to be discharged to go home. When the nurse is performing discharge teaching the patient "does not seem right." The nurse notes that although the patient is awake, alert, and oriented, the patient is taking a long time to answer questions as compared to earlier in the day. Sensing something is not right, the nurse does not complete the discharge but places the patient back to bed for a further assessment and evaluation. The nurse calls the physician to report the concern and upon further investigation it is determined the patient has suffered a small cerebrovascular accident as a complication of the cardiac catheterization. Although intuitive thinking may seem contrary to using the logical, evidenced-based reasoning that is so prevalent in nursing literature, it is based upon clinical knowledge and experience. The saying, "trust your gut instinct" is a truism in nursing.

Analytical Thinking

Interested in problem-solving or solving mysteries? This is analytical thinking. Analytical thinkers look at a situation in a logical, step-by-step manner and may break down a situation into various parts or analyze facts to make a clinical judgment. Analytic thinking can be described as logical and coherent. Nurses use analytical thinking to look at different aspects of objective assessment data, such as physical assessment findings, patient symptoms, laboratory data, and medical history to develop a nursing plan of care.

Holistic Thinking

The term "holistic thinking" refers to a big picture mentality, in which a person recognizes the interconnectedness of various elements that form larger systems, patterns, and objects." What is holistic thinking? Holistic thinking in nursing means that we assess, plan, implement, and evaluate care for patients, not only from a physical aspect but also from a psychological, cultural, racial, and religious perspective. For the nurse caring for a woman with breast cancer, nursing care goes far beyond administration of chemotherapy. How do we help the woman cope with a diagnosis of breast cancer? How do we help the woman manage the side effects of chemotherapy such as hair loss? In applying holistic thinking, the nurse begins to help the woman with breast cancer to order a wig before her hair falls out or refer her to a support group to help with the psychological and emotional ups and downs she will face. The nurse may also have to make adjustments in the diet based upon religious beliefs to help this woman maintain adequate nutrition. This type of thinking is what separates nursing from many other health care professionals.

Critical Thinking

There is no more important type of thinking that nurses must learn and cultivate than critical thinking. The Foundation for Critical Thinking has defined critical thinking as "the intellectually disciplined process of actively and skillfully conceptualizing, applying, analyzing, synthesizing, and/or evaluating information gathered from or generated by observation, experience, reflection, reasoning or communication" (www.criticalthinking.org/pages/defining-critical-thinking/766). Though a very long definition, if you look at certain words within this definition, it is very specific to nursing. A simpler way to put it is, you think about your thinking to make your thinking better. Nurses are always gathering information from observations, communicating with patients and families, and drawing on their past patient care experiences—this is the first step of the nursing process. After the nurse gathers the data, the information is analyzed and conceptualized and formed into a nursing diagnosis and a plan of care for the patient. The information obtained also helps in implementing nursing care. The last step of the nursing process is evaluation, which is also included in the definition of critical thinking.

Often in the nursing school faculty, they say they want you to "think like a nurse." At that time in your career you may not have understood what this means. As you apply knowledge learned in the classroom to the clinical setting, critical thinking begins. For example, you are taking care of a patient with Type 2 Diabetes Mellitus. During your assessment, the patient complains of a headache, is shaky and sweaty. You notice that the patient has not eaten any of their breakfast. In the report, the night nurse stated the patient's morning blood glucose was 73/dl. The patient is scheduled to receive their morning oral hypoglycemic medication. Based upon the information from the patient, your assessment, and the laboratory data, you make the decision to not administer the oral hypoglycemic and recheck the patient's blood glucose value which is now 52 mg/dl. This demonstrates your ability to apply and analyze

Real World Interview

Critical Thinking

I learned good decision-making skills from the preceptors I had in critical care, which has helped me make decisions in my leadership role. Good critical thinkers make really strong leaders. Critical thinkers can very quickly break down situations by assessing the situation, thinking about what is happening and what

caused it and based upon the nurse's decision what is the result to the patient. In all decision making, nurses must always keep the patient at the center of the decision. Nurses must make the best decision in the moment with what information is available.

Sarah Paturalski, RN, MBA Vice President of Nursing & Clinical Services at Memorial Hospital of South Bend, IN

data, come to a conclusion about the information obtained (the patient may be hypoglycemic), and determine your next course of action (check another blood glucose).

Characteristics of Critical Thinkers

Some have an inherent ability to think critically, while for others it is a skill that must be learned and developed over time. Alfaro-LeFevre (2017) identified several qualities that are present in critical thinkers. These qualities include being self-aware, curious, reflective, logical, confident, open-minded, and responsible. To help develop critical thinking skills it is important to identify your own learning, personality, and communication styles. This is being self-aware. A good critical thinker is able to examine decisions from all sides and take into account varying points of view. A good critical thinker does not say "We've always done it this way" and refuse to consider alternate ways. The critical thinker generates new ideas and alternatives when making decisions. The critical thinker asks "why" questions about a situation to arrive at the best decision. Critical thinkers need to be effective communicators in different forms of communication. Critical thinkers are good listeners which allows them to develop a deeper understanding of the meaning of others' speech or feelings. They must also be able to write clearly and speak clearly in their communication with others. Lastly, critical thinkers must be fair and open-minded, showing tolerance for those with different viewpoints, cultures, and lifestyles.

As you begin to apply critical thinking to nursing, use these qualities when you are reading material from a textbook, listening to an oral presentation, writing a paper, answering test questions, presenting ideas in oral form, or caring for a patient. Ask yourself whether the ideas are clear or unclear, precise or imprecise, accurate or inaccurate. Are they relevant or irrelevant, broad-minded or narrow-minded, logical or illogical, deep or superficial, or fair or unfair? Critical thinking skills develop over time and with practice.

Learning to Think Critically

In nursing school, it is important to not only learn the sciences such as anatomy, physiology, and microbiology, as well as diseases, pharmacology, and nursing care, but also to learn to think critically. A part of learning to critically think is to develop clinical reasoning. Alfaro-LeFevre (2017) defines

clinical reasoning as "the process you use to think about issues at the point of care—for example, deciding how to prevent and manage patient problems" (p. 6). For some people, critical thinking comes naturally while some need to learn and develop critical thinking skills. Clinical reasoning is like critical thinking, yet clinical reasoning is clinically based, active, and lets clinicians use science to develop plans of care in the real world. Nursing professors utilize various techniques to help students begin to develop both clinical reasoning and critical thinking. The use of simulations helps experience different types of patients and responses to the patients in the scenario in a safe environment. The simulations help with the development of clinical reasoning as nurses actively make decisions at the bedside of the "patient" during the simulation. As described earlier, the debriefing sessions that are done after a clinical simulation help you reflect and learn how to improve your clinical reasoning and critical thinking abilities. Many nursing professors also use the method of Socratic questioning. The Socratic method of questioning is a form of critical thinking which uses six distinct types of question to help you question your question (Intel Teach Program).

These types of Socratic questions with examples can be found in Table 20.5.

Concept Mapping

Another method that may be helpful in learning how to critically think and reason is using concept maps. Concept mapping involves creating a visual picture that links data together. The data are clumped together and referred to as concepts. For example, in the middle of the map is a diagnosis of a patient. Around the diagnosis are concepts that pertain to that diagnosis, such as assessment data, laboratory values, symptoms of the diagnosis, pathophysiology, and nursing diagnosis. The ability to understand the links between the concepts is beneficial in developing critical thinking.

Case Study

Use the following scenario to develop your own concept map. Consider the following questions:

1. What is the priority problem for this patient?

2. What data supports your priority problem?

3. What are appropriate goals and interventions for this patient? (Figure 20.3)

Table 20.5 Socratic Questioning

Socratic type question	Examples
Questions for clarification:	Why do you say that? What do you mean by_____? How is this related? Could you explain this in more detail?
Questions which produce assumptions	What can we assume from this lab data? What does those symptoms mean? Can you verify your assumption?
Questions which necessitate reason or evidence	What is the evidence in the literature to support your finding? What has caused you to come to this conclusion? Why do you think this happened?
Questions regarding perspectives.	Is there another way to look at this? Have you thought of the other person's point of view when faced with this diagnosis? How can this patient manage their disease?
Questions on implications or consequences.	What is the implication of this? Does this relate to previous knowledge? How does administering this drug effect the patient?
Questions on the question or an issue	What does this mean? How can you apply this to your patient? What was the point of this enquiry?

Source: List created by P. Keresztes.

Concept Map Example

The patient is a 77-year-old Hispanic female who lives alone in a two-story house and is able to manage herself independently. She states that she has not been feeling well for days. She has been feeling tired and short of breath. She was admitted yesterday with a diagnosis of pneumonia and congestive heart failure. She has shortness of breath, a nonproductive cough, and bibasilar crackles/rales in lower lobes. Her chest X-ray shows infiltrates. She has a temperature of 100.5 °F. She has a history of hypertension, peripheral vascular disease, and frequent urinary tract infections. Her ejection fraction is 28%.

VITALS: T: 100.5 °F, P = 92 and regular, R = 24 and rapid, B/P = 98/52. She has been placed on 2 l of oxygen via nasal cannula with a saturation of 92% at rest, and 89% during activity.

She is alert and oriented. And has diminished sensation to her feet. Her weight is 176 lb, which is a 15-lb gain since her last visit to the doctor's office one month ago.

ABDOMEN: abdomen is large and soft with positive bowel sounds.

INTEGUMENT: Skin warm and dry. Lower legs are smooth and shiny and have a cellophane like appearance. She has pitting edema to her feet and extends to 3 in above her ankle. The skin of the lower legs is red with a shiny appearance. Right heel ulcer 2×2 cm, center with white-yellow drainage, and surrounding area red.

LABS ON ADMISSION:

Blood sugar 135
(80–110 mg/dl)

WBC 22.3 (5–10.0/mm³)   BUN 50 (7–18 mg/dl)

Sodium 135 (136–142 mEq/l)   Creatinine 2.0 (0.6–1.2 mg/dl)

Potassium 3.6 (3.5–5.0 mEq/l)   Chloride 99 (98–106 mEq/l)

BNP 525 (<100 pg/ml)

ODRERS:	MEDS:
Low sodium diet	Lasix drip at 3 cc/hr.
Oxygen @ 2 l/nasal cannula	ASA 81 mg every day
Daily weight	Norvasc 10 mg in am
Fluid restrictions – 1,200 cc/day	Protonix 40 mg IV push every day
Wet to dry dressing change right heel BID	Ceftriaxone 2 g every 12 hr IVPB
	KCL 20 mEq BID
	Lopressor 25 mg BID
	Albuterol treatments every 6 hr
	Percocet 5/325 mg 1 every 6 hr prn pain

Example Concept Map

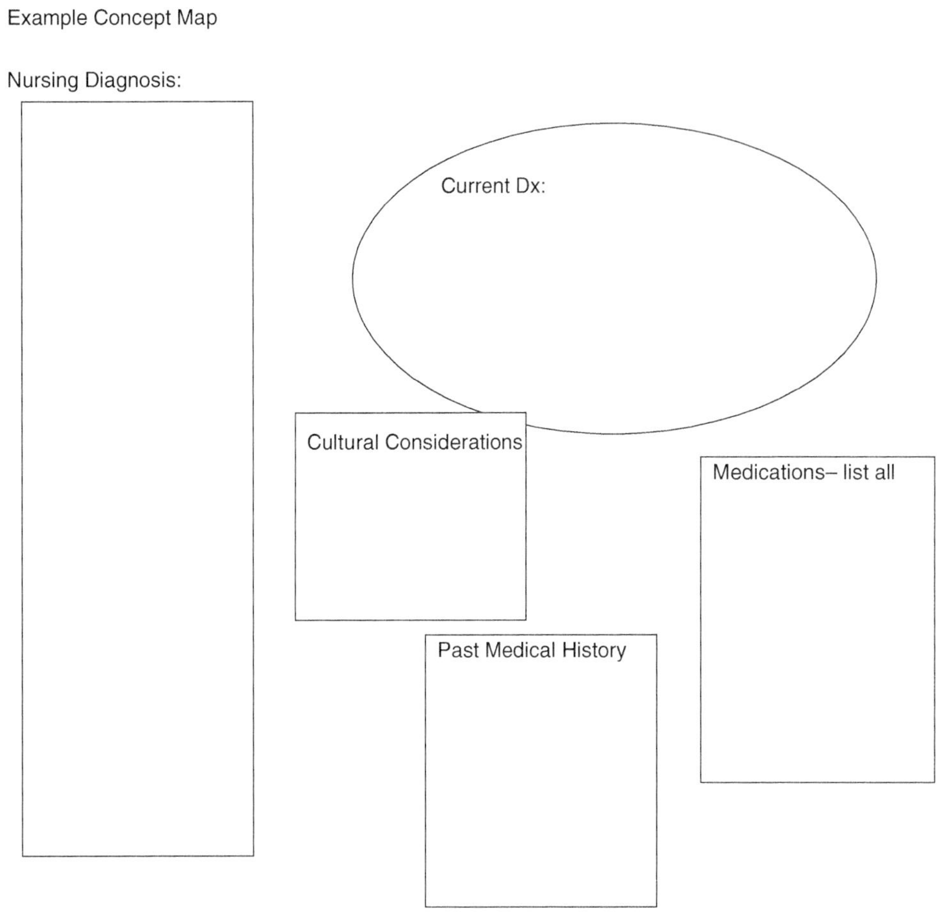

Example Concept Map

Nursing Diagnosis:

Current Dx:

Cultural Considerations

Medications– list all

Past Medical History

FIGURE 20.3   Concept map.
Source: P. Keresztes.

The National Council Licensure Examination (NCLEX)

Critical thinking is essential in order to be successful on the nursing licensure examination. The **National Council of State Boards of Nursing** (NCSBN) develops and oversees the national nursing licensure examination (NCLEX). The current licensure examination assesses the knowledge, skills, and abilities that are essential for the entry-level nurse to use in order to meet the needs of clients requiring the promotion, maintenance, or restoration of health. Candidates may be administered multiple choice items as well as items written in alternate formats. These formats may include but are not limited to multiple response, fill-in-the-blank calculation, ordered response, and/or hot spots. Also included within the questions can be multimedia such as charts, tables, graphics, sound, and video clips (www.ncsbn.org/2019_RN_TestPlan-English.pdf). The licensure examination contains questions that require critical thinking and the ability to examine a set of data and make determinations about the priority focus of care for the patient. The questions on the licensure examination are written using **Bloom's taxonomy** for the cognitive domain (Bloom, et al., 1956; Anderson & Krathwohl, 2001). Anderson and Krathwohl (2001) made revisions to Bloom's

taxonomy, which resulted in the levels of cognition found in Table 20.6.

It is important to understand Bloom's taxonomy because the National Council of State Boards of Nursing (NCSBN) develop the licensure examination questions based upon this taxonomy. Since the practice of nursing requires application of knowledge, skills, and abilities, the majority of items are written at the application or higher levels of cognitive ability, which requires more complex thought processing. Developing critical thinking skills is essential to being able to successfully pass the licensure examination.

Clinical Judgment

The NCSBN is developing a next generation licensure examination with a further emphasis on clinical judgment. This is because nurses are responsible for advanced levels of assessment of sicker and more complex patients and making clinical judgments and decision making about appropriate interventions is essential to providing high-quality and safe patient care. The end point of both clinical reasoning and critical thinking is clinical judgment. Clinical judgment requires that the nurse makes decisions as to what to do with the information gathered about a patient situation. Nurses who have learned to be

Table 20.6 Revised Bloom's Taxonomy

Level of cognition	Definition	Example
Remembering	The ability to recall information	Identifying the bones in the body
Understanding	The ability to understand information	How the kidneys work
Applying	The ability to use information in a new way	The signs and symptoms in patients with kidney failure
Analyzing	The ability to break down information into its essential parts	The reason why lab values are abnormal in renal failure
Evaluating	The ability to judge or criticize information	Determining the effectiveness of a medication
Creating	The ability to create something new from different elements of information	Identifying new ways to treat a pressure ulcer

Source: Adapted from Anderson, L., Krathwohl, D., & Bloom, B. (2001).

critical thinkers will also develop the clinical judgment skills that are necessary to identify, associate. and interpret the clinical signs and symptoms that patients present to them on an everyday basis (Dickison et al., 2016). This includes subjective data nurses receive directly from the patient and objective data received from the EHR, physical assessment, other members of the inter-professional team and observation. The ability to put all this data together into a meaningful clinical picture involves being able to critically think. Basing treatments and interventions on the data obtained leads to the use of clinical judgment. The nurse is continuously gathering and making sense of data in providing safe and high-quality patient care. The NCSBN's (2018b, Summer) operational definition of nursing clinical judgment is "an iterative decision-making process that uses nursing knowledge to: observe and assess presenting situations; identify a prioritized client concern; and generate the best possible evidence-based solutions in order to deliver safe client care." This definition can be closely related to the nursing process steps of assess, diagnose, and implement.

After defining the construct of clinical judgment, a **Clinical Judgment Model** (CJM) was developed to identify the steps of the process of clinical judgment. The CJM examines what happens when the nurse enters the patient's room and begins obtaining more information about the patient. The CJM states that as the nurse begins their encounter with the patient, the nurse will form one or more hypotheses, prioritize each hypothesis, generate solutions, and take the necessary actions (NCSBN, 2018a,b). The focus for the NCSBN on the next generation licensure exam is how to measure the CJM. This ability to actually measure the construct of clinical judgment is something new to the licensure exam. The licensure exam must measure more than knowledge and the ability to apply knowledge to a specific patient situation. The next generation of the licensure examination strives to measure the unique ability of the nurse to generate hypotheses from the data and make the appropriate responses. The nurse must not only have the knowledge required but also the ability to translate that knowledge into appropriate clinical judgments (NCSBN, 2018a,b).

Decision Making

In everyday practice, nurses make decisions about patient care. As the nurse gains experience in clinical practice, decision making will become somewhat automatic in certain circumstances, but other decisions will remain complex. Nurses also make decisions about patient care along with other members of the inter-professional team.

Clinical Decision Support (CDS) Tools

The expansion of information technology has enabled the entire inter-professional team access to **clinical decision support** (CDS) tools to help provide safe and high-quality patient care. The use of CDS tools can provide timely and relevant information to all members of the health care team to aid in making better informed clinical decisions. The CDS tools can include physician orders created for particular conditions or types of patients, such as for the prevention of venous thromboembolism or blood clots during a hospital stay. In the office and clinic setting, the CDS can provide reminders for preventive care, such as vaccinations, mammograms, and colonoscopies. The use of CDS in the EHRs can also alert the nurse to potential drug–drug interactions and other avoidable medication errors.

There are many advantages to using CDS tool. The goal for these technological tools is to improve the quality and safety of patient care. The CDS tools are also helpful in improving patient outcomes, gathering all data within one database for easy access, alerting to potential interactions or errors, and saving time and money.

Nurses also must make continual decisions on the flow of patients through the hospitals. Patients are continuously being admitted, transferred, and discharged. A CDS tool of virtual tracking is used by hospitals and helps with the flow of patients throughout the hospital. There are many virtual patient tracking software systems available. These systems provide real-time data on all patients throughout the hospital. Information on length of stay, physicians, and assigned nurses can all be monitored through one screen. Also, admissions, transfers, and discharges are also updated regularly to inform units of the flow of patients. This information helps nursing supervisors, charge nurses, and staff nurses understand the workload of units and make effective and timely decisions on the flow of patients. This information also helps other departments, such as environmental services, to quickly clean and turnover patient rooms to minimize delays of patients waiting to be transferred.

One of the main duties of nurse managers is staffing and scheduling. Many units have now gone to a self-scheduling system. CDS software is frequently used by nursing staff to do their own scheduling. The use of self-scheduling can improve the job satisfaction of nurses. Scheduling software is also used throughout the hospital, so that nursing supervisors and central staffing units can make better informed decisions as to where to place staff members.

Group Decision Making

Certain situations call for group decision making. There are occasions when it is more appropriate for a group to make the decision rather than the individual nurse. Each situation is different, and an effective manager adopts the appropriate mode of decision making—group or individual. Today's leadership and management styles include people in the decision-making process who will be most affected by the decision. Decisions affecting patient care should be made including the groups implementing the decision and the patient and support systems.

The effectiveness of groups depends greatly on the groups' members. The size of a group and the personalities of group members are important considerations when choosing participants. More ideas can be generated with groups, thus allowing for more choices. This increases the likelihood of higher-quality outcomes. Another advantage of groups is that when followers participate in the decision-making process, acceptance of the decision is more likely to occur. Additionally, groups may be used as a medium for communication. The old saying, "more minds, the better," illustrates this point.

Today's leadership and management styles include people in the decision-making process who will be most affected by the decision. Decisions affecting patient care should be made, including the groups implementing the decision.

The effectiveness of groups depends greatly on the groups' members. The size of a group and the personalities of group members are important considerations when choosing participants. More ideas can be generated with groups, thus allowing for more choices. This increases the likelihood of higher-quality outcomes. Another advantage of groups is that when followers participate in the decision-making process, acceptance of the decision is more likely to occur. Additionally, groups may be used as a medium for communication.

Delphi Group Technique

The Delphi technique differs from nominal technique in that group members "are not meeting face to face." Questionnaires are distributed to group members for their opinions, and these

are then summarized and disseminated with the summaries to the group members. This process continues for as many times as necessary for the group members to reach consensus. An advantage of this technique is that it can involve a large number of participants and thus a greater number of ideas.

Consensus Building

Consensus is defined by *Merriam-Webster's Collegiate Dictionary* (2018) as "a general agreement; the judgment arrived at by most of those concerned; group solidarity in sentiment and belief." A common misconception is that consensus means everyone agrees with the decision 100%. Contrary to this misunderstanding, **consensus** means that all group members can live with and fully support the decision, regardless of whether they totally agree. Building consensus is useful with groups, because all group members participate and can realize the contributions each member makes to the decision. A disadvantage to the consensus strategy is that decision making requires more time. This strategy should be reserved for important decisions that require strong support from the participants who will implement them. Consensus decision making works well when the decisions are made under the following conditions: all members of the team are affected by the decision; implementation of the solution requires coordination among team members; and the decision is critical, requiring full commitment by team members. Although consensus can be the most time-consuming strategy, it can also be the most gratifying with optimal outcomes.

Limitations to Effective Decision Making

What are obstacles to effective decision making? Obstacles to effective decision making can be related personal, interpersonal or professional experience, and background. Restricted knowledge, limited alternatives, and the cost of alternatives may also affect a decision's quality. Incorporating critical thinking into the decision-making process helps to prevent these factors from distorting the decision-making process. Muntean (2012) identified factors that can influence nurses in making clinical decisions. These include age and educational level, experience and knowledge base, communication with others in the interdisciplinary team, and environmental factors such as the pressure of time, interruptions, and area of specialty. Comfort with decision making improves with experience. Early in the nurse's career, the nurse is commonly indecisive or uncomfortable with decisions. Alfaro-LeFevre (2017) has identified several strategies that help to improve critical thinking, which in turn will also help to improve decision making.

- Do I have all the facts that I need to make a decision?

- Have I explored the alternatives and the pros and cons of each alternative?

At times, delaying a decision until more information is obtained may be the best approach. Asking "why," "what else," and "what if" questions will help you to arrive at the best decision. When more information becomes available, decisions can be revised. Very few decisions are final. Another helpful strategy for improving decision making is to anticipate questions and outcomes. For example, when calling a practitioner to report a patient's change in condition, the nurse will want to have pertinent information about the patient's vital signs and current medications readily available.

Nurses who practice strategies to promote their own critical thinking will in turn be good decision makers. A foundation for good decision making comes with experience and learning from those experiences. By turning decisions with poor outcomes into learning experiences, nurses will enhance their decision-making ability in the future.

Innovation

This is an exciting time to be a nurse, as the health care industry is looking more than ever before to nurses to provide new ideas and innovation for health care. This includes ways to improve patient-centered care, create cost-effective ideas, and enhance safety of patient care. Merriam Webster (2020) defines innovation as "a new idea, device, or method, the act or process of introducing new ideas, devices, or methods". It is especially important in health care today that nurses become innovators because of the focus of cost saving and the overall cost of health care. The **American Nurses Association** (ANA) has collaborated with key partners to develop a three-part innovation framework to: cultivate and inspire future nurse innovators; ignite nursing innovation; and highlight and celebrate nursing innovation.

Characteristics of Innovators

Who are nurse innovators? Who can be a nurse innovator? Innovators can be nurses at the bedside, nurses in administrative positions, nurses in the community, or nurse educators. All nurses have the ability to be innovators. Newquist (2015) identified several characteristics of those people who are successful innovators. These include being a divergent thinker, having curiosity, being passionate, having stamina, being a leader, having respect for other innovators, and having courage. These characteristics may also be applied to nursing. As discussed above, nurses are "multi-thinkers" looking at situations in different ways to come to a conclusion about how to provide care. Nurse are always curious as to how patient care can be done differently. This includes how to provide patient care in a more timely and efficient manner and how to provide care in a more cost-effective manner. Most importantly, nurses are always wanting to know how to provide patient care that is most satisfying to the patient and family. Nurses are involving the patient and the family in patient-centered care. Nurses work with patients to establish daily goals during the hospitalization. Family members are involved in the care of their loved ones while in the hospital. This includes providing family members with the opportunity to stay in the patient's room

overnight or be in the room while their family member is being resuscitated. Clearly, anyone who wants to be a nurse has to be courageous. It takes courage to provide care for the people who are at a very vulnerable time of their life. This includes patients experiencing illness, pain, and death. Nurses do not shy away from these stressful and demanding situations, but actively take the lead in the care of the patient.

Nurse Innovators

Nurses may not think of themselves as innovators, but nurses have designed and developed new techniques, equipment, and treatments to improve patient care. Of course, nursing started with one of the greatest innovators, Florence Nightingale. In the early 1850s, Nightingale took a nursing job in a Middlesex hospital for an ailing governess. Soon after starting there, Nightingale was promoted to superintendent within just a year of being hired. The position proved challenging as Nightingale had to deal with a cholera outbreak and unsanitary conditions that led to the rapid spread of the disease. Nightingale made it her mission to improve hygiene practices, significantly lowering the death rate at the hospital in the process. What Nightingale is most known for is how she changed the way in which care was provided to wounded soldiers during the Crimean War. She collected data in order to identify reasons for the excessively high mortality rates of soldiers at the Scutari military barracks. She was able to demonstrate that the primary cause of death of these soldiers was from poor environmental conditions, not battle wounds. Her evidence demonstrated that excessively high mortality rates were related to inadequate nutrition, poor sanitation, lack of clean drinking water, and shortages of supplies such as clean clothing and warm blankets. Nightingale was able to advocate for change to improve the way necessary supplies were distributed. She enhanced sanitation and nutrition standards in the hospital environment, improved health outcomes, and decreased the mortality rate. Nightingale is also credited with developing documentation notes as a way to communicate more effectively with physicians (www. history.com/topics/womens-history/florence-nightingale-1) (Figure 20.4).

The list of nurse innovators just begins with Florence Nightingale. Table 20.7 gives an example of nurse innovators throughout history.

Opportunities for Innovation

There are many opportunities where there is a need for innovation in health care. The Cleveland Clinic (2018) identified several areas where there is a strong potential for innovations that can transform health care. Many of these innovations have strong implications for nursing. The top predicted innovation will be in the area of pain management and the development of alternatives therapy to the use of opioids. A major crisis in the United States is the overuse and misuse of opioids. According to the Department of **Health and**

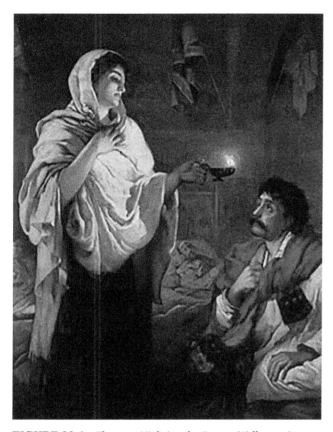

FIGURE 20.4 Florence Nightingale. *Source:* Wellcome Images

Human Services (HHS) (2019), 130 people died every day in 2017 from opioid-related drug overdoses. Additionally, 11.4 million people misused prescription opioids. These numbers are astounding, and nurses are in a position to help with creating and using innovative ways to manage patient's pain. Nurses have already been using alternative pain management therapies such as guided imagery, music therapy, and therapeutic touch. Nurses will continue to have a significant role in the area of pain management.

In the area of nursing and medical education, the Cleveland Clinic (2018) predicts further innovations in the use of virtual and mixed reality. As a student, you have already been a part of doing simulations. The advances in the mannequins used in simulations has dramatically changed the education of nurses. Mannequins can move, talk, heave breath sounds, heart sounds, and bowel sounds. Pupils on mannequins can constrict to a penlight. As technology continues to advance there will be more opportunities to create virtual reality situations to help faculty teach the next generation of nurses and for nurses to practice care in a safe environment.

Lastly, The Cleveland Clinic (2018) predicts further innovations in genetic testing and prediction of disease. Nurses will be responsible for teaching and providing counseling to patients based upon their genetic code. Nurses must be aware of resources available to patients to make adequate referrals for prevention and management of disease.

The advances within health care continue at a rapid speed. It is up to each individual nurse to not only keep up with these advances but also influence and create them.

Innovation creates change in systems. Nurse leaders are instrumental in pinpointing the need for change in systems and for guiding the change process. Student nurses who are learning about the change process and innovation can develop leadership projects during their educational experiences that

Table 20.7 List of Nursing Innovators

Nurse innovator	Innovation	Source
1800s Florence Nightingale	Hygiene protocols	www.history.com/topics/womens-history/florence-nightingale-1
1881 Clara Barton	Founded the American Red Cross	www.redcross.org/about-us/who-we-are/history/clara-barton.html
1920s Elizabeth Kenney	Treatment of polio-passive range of motion	www.britannica.com/biography/Elizabeth-Kenny
1940s: Bessie Blount Griffin	Invented a special feeding tube for paralyzed veterans	www.blackpast.org/african-american-history/bessie-blount-griffin-1914-2009
1950s: Sister Jean Ward	Neonatal Phototherapy by exposing the babies to sunlight	https://nursing.jnj.com/nursing-news-events/nurses-change-makers-throughout-history
1960s: Anita Dorr	Invented the crash cart. First executive director of the National Emergency Department Nurses Association	https://nf.ena.org/eweb/DynamicPage.aspx?webcode=ENACOEFoundationList&pager=10&listcategory=endowments
2000s: Teri Barton-Salina and Gail Barton-Hay	Designed color-coded IV lines	www.nurse.com/blog/2012/06/18/mothers-of-invention-california-rns-debut-color-tinted-iv-lines
2012 Rebecca Koszalinkski	Speak for Myself®, a mobile app specifically developed to help patients who are unable to communicate, express their needs more quickly and precisely	https://nursing.jnj.com/nursing-news-events/nurses-change-makers-throughout-history

Source: List compiled by P. Keresztes.

Real World Interview

Innovation

"I saw a need in the lower socioeconomic community for access to fresh produce and locally grown, nutritious foods. Prompted by some of the homeless in our area, I started an urban free pick garden. Now, ten years later, there are more than 40 gardens providing a uniquely dignified free food experience where everyone is welcome to gather, harvest the free and nutritious food while enjoying the green space. As a nurse innovator, I advocate for the most vulnerable in our society creating environments conducive to health and wellness".

SARA L. STEWART, RN, MSN
Executive Director Unity Gardens Inc.

enhance their abilities to become leaders of effective change in the future. These change projects can serve to demonstrate the leadership potential of students who are interviewing for a nursing position after graduation. Employers are very interested in candidates who have the ability to manage a project that brings about effective and innovative change to a health care setting.

Summary

Health care continues to change at a rapid pace. In order for nursing to continue to provide high-quality and safe patient care, nurses must be able to adapt to the rapid changes. Nurses can adapt to change by accepting that change is necessary, educating themselves on the change, and participating in planning and implementing change. Nurses must also learn to develop and enhance their critical thinking and clinical judgment skills to provide patient-centered care. The next generation NCLEX exam will focus on testing the nurse's ability to make sound clinical judgments when given patient care scenarios. Nurses also have an opportunity to be innovators in the delivery of patient care. Being an innovator may include implementing a new model for providing patient care, designing new hospital units, or implementing new technologies into patient care.

KEY CONCEPTS

- Health care continues to change at a rapid pace.

- Change can occur in your personal or professional life and in the organization you work.

- Models of change used in health care include the IHI, PDCA, and Kotter's eight-step model.

- The change agent is critical to a change being successful.

- Critical thinking is an essential skill for the nurse to provide high-quality and safe patient care.

- Nurses can develop and enhance their critical thinking skills.

- Nurses are "multi-thinkers," using critical thinking, reflective thinking, and intuitive thinking in making decisions about patient care.

- The NextGen NCLEX will focus on clinical judgment using patient case studies.

- Group decision making is essential in health care.

- Nurses are innovators in today's health care.

- The current health care environment provides an excellent opportunity for nurses to be innovative.

KEY TERMS

Adaptation to change	Consensus building	Innovation
Analytic thinking	Continuous quality improvement	Intuitive thinking
Bloom's taxonomy	Critical thinking	Kotter's eight-step change model
Change	Delphi group technique	Personal change
Change agent	Deming's Plan-Do-Check-Act	Planned organizational change
Clinical decision support tools	Developmental change	Professional change
Clinical judgment	Group decision making	Reflective thinking
Clinical reasoning	Holistic thinking	Transformational change
Concept mapping	IHI Psychology of change framework	Transitional change

REVIEW QUESTIONS

1. Which of the following patients has a higher priority need?
   a. A newly diagnosed diabetic needs to be taught how to give himself an insulin injection.
   b. A patient, who is post parathyroidectomy, has a critically low calcium level.
   c. A patient has asked for assistance with AM care.
   d. A bedridden patient needs to be turned and positioned.

2. Which of the following clients has a higher priority need?
   a. A patient asks for pain medication.
   b. A patient who has had surgery and needs a dressing change.
   c. A patient who has been discharged asks for their discharge instructions.
   d. A patient who needs to have their Foley discontinued.

3. The nurse is establishing an ongoing quality improvement program. For it to be successful, what must be present?
   a. Administrative support for all managers.
   b. Health care providers must be able to determine treatment options.
   c. Bedside nurses must contribute to the quality improvement process.
   d. Patient education is provided to increase consumer knowledge about what is quality care.

4. Change occurs throughout life. What is a major factor that influences a successful change from school to practice?
   a. Level of new knowledge and skills required in a new environment.
   b. Amount of class work required to obtain a degree.
   c. Personal history of previous developmental transitions.
   d. Influence of classmates and their transitional experiences.

5. A rural hospital was switching to computerized charting. Many of the senior nurses were starting to feel inwardly anxious about the coming change because of the new technology involved. What is an effective strategy to decrease anxiety with a change?
   a. Threaten to dismiss the nurses if they do not accept the change.
   b. Provide education to the nurses on the new computerized system.
   c. Allow the nurses to continue to use the old system of charting.
   d. Transfer those nurses to another unit.

6. The nurse has finished receiving morning change of shift report. Which patient should the nurse assess first?
   a. The patient diagnosed with pneumonia who has bilateral crackles.
   b. The patient on strict bedrest who is complaining of calf pain.
   c. The patient who complains of low back pain when sitting in a chair
   d. The patient who is upset because the food is cold all the time.

7. The nurse is preparing to administer medications after receiving the morning change of shift report. Which medication should the nurse administer first?
   a. The IV PPI to a patient who is to NPO for an endoscopy.
   b. The insulin Humalog to a patient who has the breakfast tray in the room.
   c. The loop diuretic to a CHF patient with a serum potassium of 3.2 mEq/l.
   d. The laxative to a patient who has not had a bowel movement in 3 days.

8. What is a growing concern with health care as it exists today in the United States?
   a. The increased number of those with health insurance.
   b. The higher costs of health care in the United States.
   c. Decreased hospital visits and stays for patients.
   d. Better quality of health care.

9. A staff registered nurse is leading a multidisciplinary clinical pathway team in the development of care for a patient with total knee replacement. Which of the following statements would exemplify leadership behaviors in a clinical pathway team meeting?
   a. Only nursing is responsible for pain control of the patient.
   b. Our pharmacist has provided some excellent pain control literature.
   c. Physical therapy's expertise is in rehabilitation, rather than pain control.
   d. All departments should work together to provide optimal pain control.

10. The nurse is preparing to administer a unit of packed red blood cells to an elderly patient diagnosed with anemia. What is needed for a blood transfusion? (Select all that apply)
    a. Obtain the unit of blood from the blood bank.
    b. Start an IV access with D5W at a keep-open rate.
    c. Have the patient sign the consent to receive blood products after the transfusion is started.
    d. Check the unit of blood with another nurse at the bedside.
    e. Initiate the transfusion at a slow rate for 15 minutes.

REVIEW QUESTION ANSWERS

1. Answer: B is correct.
   Rational: A complication following a parathyroidectomy is lowered calcium levels, which can lead to tetany, hypotension, and irregular heart rhythms (B). The newly disagnosed diabetic patient is stable and only requires discharge teaching (A). Assistance with AM care and turning and positioning of a patient does not require a nurse and can be delegated (C, D).

2. Answer: A is correct.
   Rational: A request for pain medication is a high priority and must be addressed immediately. A dressing change if low priority (B). The patient who has been discharged is stable and can wait for discharge instructions (C). Discontining the patient's Foley is low priority and can be delegated (D).

3. Answer: C is correct.
   Rational: If bedside nurses contribute to the ongoing quality improvement program, they will be investing in the change (C). Administrative support for all managers is not necessary for the process to be successful (A). Treatment options determined by health care providers are not part of the quality improvement process (B). Consumer knowledge about quality care is not related to the question (D).

4. Answer: A is correct.
   Rational: Learning knowledge and skills will help with the change process (A). The amount of class work required to obtain a degree, one's personal history of previous developmental transitions, and influence of classmates' transitional experiences will not influence a successful change (B, C, D).

5. Answer: B is correct.
   Rational: Education and training help to ease the anxiety of change (B). Threats are not helpful with adaptation to change (A). Nurses must adapt to change and will not do so if continuing in the old ways (C). Transferring nurses to another unit will not help them to adapt (D).

6. Answer: A is correct.
   Rational: Rales are a sign of fluid build-up in the lungs and needs to have an immediate response and intervention by the nurse (A). A patient on strict bedrest complaining of calf pain and a patient complaining of low back pain when sitting in a chair do not require immediate intervention (B, C). Complaints about the food are not a high level of priority (D).

7. Answer: B is correct.
   Rational: A patient needs to have insulin given with the meal (B). The IV PPI is not necessary mediation prior to endoscopy (A). The loop diuretic may cause further reduction in serum potassium levels (C). Administering a laxative is not a high priority (D).

8. Answer: B is correct.
   Rational: A growing concern is that health care costs continue to rise in the United States (B). There is a decrease in the number of people without health insurance (A). Decreased hospital visits and stays for patients is not a concern (C). Better quality of health is a concern but less than the rise in health care costs (D)

9. Answer: D is correct.
   Rational: All departments working together to provide optimal pain control is an interdisciplinary issue and a good leader will involve all disciplines (D). This issue requires input from all disciplines so A, B, and C are incorrect.

10. Answers A, D, and E are correct.
    Rational: The unit of blood from the blood bank is required for this procedure (A). Hospital policies require that two nurses check the blood at the patient's bedside (D). The transfusion should be initiated at a slow rate for 15 minutes, because of the likelihood of a transfusion reaction occurring will be during the first 15 minutes of the transfusion (E). Blood transfusions can only be administered with IV fluids of 0.9 normal saline (B) and the consent form must be signed prior to the transfusion being started (C).

REVIEW ACTIVITIES

1. You are asked to implement a change to giving the change of shift report at the patient's bedside.

   a. Who would ask to get involved with the change and why?
   b. How would you communicate this change to the staff?
   c. What do you perceive as barriers to this change?
   d. How would you introduce this change to the staff nurses?

2. You are wanting to go back to school to be a nurse practitioner.

   a. What factors would you consider when making this professional change?
   b. How would this change impact your personal life?
   c. Who else would be impacted by your decision?

3. You are beginning your orientation as a new nurse on a medical-surgical unit.

   a. What can you do to help with your ability to make clinical judgments about your patients?
   b. What clinical experiences do you want to help you develop your critical thinking skills?
   c. Who can you identify as nurses that have good critical thinking skills?

4. As a staff nurse you see a need for additional teaching for patients who have been newly diagnosed with diabetes?

   a. How can you be a nurse innovator to help with this issue?
   b. What ways can you think of to help with the education of these patients?
   c. What innovative ways, including the use of technology, can be used in the education of patients?

DISCUSSION POINTS

1. How have you made changes in your life since you started nursing school?

2. What are changes that you have seen occur in the health care system?

3. What change have you seen occur in any of your clinical rotations?

4. What does critical thinking in patient care mean to you as a nurse?

5. How have you developed critical thinking in patient care?

6. What can you do to develop your critical thinking skills?

7. How can you be an innovator in nursing?

8. How can hospitals encourage and support nurses to be innovators?

DISCUSSION OF OPENING SCENARIO

Jesus is a new graduate nurse working on a step-down unit. One of his patient's "just isn't right".

1. *He needs to organize his thinking to clearly understand what the whole clinical picture is, but how? In the past he has had the support of clinical faculty, and now he is functioning as an independent RN.*
   a. *Jesus needs to trust his instincts and use all his skills concurrently to "put it together." He also has to remember he has the support of the inter-professional team.*

2. *How can he use clinical reasoning to help him in the real world?*

   a. *The "real world" does not present information in a clear and logical order. Clinical reasoning lets nurses use information available to draw conclusions and implement care accordingly.*

3. *What steps in the critical thinking process will help him in this situation?*
   a. *All of the steps will help. Review the definition: "the intellectually disciplined process of actively and skillfully conceptualizing, applying, analyzing, synthesizing, and/or evaluating information gathered from or generated by observation, experience, reflection, reasoning, or communication."*

EXPLORING THE WEB

- Access the Foundation for Critical Thinking website. Critical Thinking. www.criticalthinking.org Accessed February 17, 2019. Find the Nursing and Health Care section. Read one of the articles on the topics listed.

- Access Creating and Sustaining Change in Nursing Care Delivery. http://healthcare.mckinsey.com/sites/default/files/MCK_Hosp_Nursing.pdf Accessed February 17, 2019. Read the article.

- Access Change Theories in Nursing. https://bizfluent.com/about-5544426-change-theories-nursing.html Accessed February 17, 2019.

- Access Adopt an Evidence-Based Practice Model to Facilitate

Practice Change. https://voice.ons.org/news-and-views/adopt-an-evidence-based-practice-model-to-facilitate-practice-change Accessed February 17, 2019. How do these models compare to the change models in the chapter?

- Access Issues and Trends in Nursing: Essential Knowledge for Today and Tomorrow. www.nursing.jbpub.com/issues/critical_thinking.cfm Accessed February 17, 2019. Complete one of the critical thinking exercises.

- Access The American Nurses Association Innovation. www.nursingworld.org/practice-policy/innovation Accessed February 18, 2019.

INFORMATICS

- Go to, http://qsen.org Accessed February 18, 2019. Click on, qstudent, and then click on, QStudent 6 teamwork and Collaboration. Click "Continue Reading" and learn more about this content.

- Access the Foundation for Critical Thinking website. Critical Thinking, www.criticalthinking.org Accessed February 17, 2019. Find the Nursing and Health Care section. Read one of the articles on the topics listed.

LEAN BACK

- What do you see in practice that reflects a change or planned organizational change?

- What change do you think could be made in your clinical rotations that would improve your learning?

- How have you changed your thinking process over the course of your clinical rotations?

- How does the content on critical thinking and reasoning change the way your think about patient care?

- How do you see nurses as innovators in patient care or in health care overall?

- How can you be an innovator in your nursing career?

REFERENCES

Alfaro-Lefevre, R. (2017). *Critical thinking, clinical reasoning, and clinical judgment: A practical approach* (6th ed.). Philadelphia, PA: Elsevier.

Anderson, L. W., & Krathwohl, D. R.. (Eds.) (2001). *A taxonomy for learning, teaching and assessing. A revision of Bloom's taxonomy of educational objectives*. New York: Addison Wesley Longman, Inc.

Andre, B., & Sjovold, E. (2017). What characterizes the work culture at a hospital unit that successfully implemented change-a correlation study. *Health Services Research.*, *17*(486), 1–7.

Bloom, B. S., Engelhart, M. D., Furst, E. J., Hill, W. H., & Krathwohl, D. R. (1956). *Taxonomy of educational objectives: The classification of educational goals. Handbook I. cognitive domain*. New York: David McKay.

Burden, M. (2016). Using a change model to reduce the risk of surgical site infection. *British Journal of Nursing, 25*(17), 949–955.

Courtney, F. (2016). *6 steps to effective organizational change management.* Retrieved from www.pulselearning.com/blog/6-steps-effective-organizational-change-management.

Deming PDCA cycle: A clear and concise reference. (2018). 5STARCooks.

Dickison, P., Luo, X., Kim, D., Woo, A., Muntean, W., & Bergstrom, B. (2016). Assessing the higher-order cognitive constructs by using an information-processing framework. *Journal of Applied Testing Technology, 17*(1), 1–19.

Havelock, R. G. (1973). *The change agent's guide to innovation in education.* Englewood Cliffs, NJ: Educational Technology.

Hayes Management Consulting. (2019). *White paper. 5 steps to healthcare change management.* Retrieved from www.hayesmanagement.com/thought-leadership/white-papers.

Hilton, K., & Anderson, A. (2018). *IHI psychology of change framework to advance and sustain improvement.* IHI White Paper, Boston, MA: Institute for Healthcare Improvement.

Kotter, J. (2012). *Leading change.* Boston, MA: Harvard Business Review Press.

Lancaster, J. (1999). *Nursing issues in leading and managing change.* St. Louis, MO: Mosby.

Lewin, K. (1951). *Field history in social science.* New York: Harper & Row.

Lippitt, R. (1958). *The dynamics of planned change.* New York: Harcourt Brace.

MBA Knowledge Base. (2019) Levels and types of organizational change. Retrieved.

McQuerrey. (2018). *Benefits from change in the workplace.* Retrieved from https://smallbusiness.chron.com/benefits-change-workplace-13255.html.

Merriam-Webster's Online Dictionary. (2018). Retrieved from https://www.merriam-webster.com/dictionary/change.

Muntean, W. (2012). Nursing clinical decision-making: A literature review. Paper commissioned by the National Council of State Boards of Nursing.

NCSBN. (2018a). *Measuring the right things.* In Focus. Available at: https://ncsbn.org/InFocus_Winter_2018.pdf

NCSBN. (2018b). Item development for the next generation NCLEX (NGN) summer. Available at: www.ncsbn.org/12720.htm

Newquist, E. (2015). *7 characteristics of highly successful innovators.* Retrieved from www.innovationexcellence.com/blog/2015/03/13/7-characteristics-of-highly-successful-innovators.

Papathanasiou, I., Kleisiaris, C., Fradelos, E., Kakou, K., & Kourkouta, L. (2014). Critical thinking: The development of an essential skill for nursing students. *Acta Inform Med, 22*(4), 283–286.

Pesut, D. J., & Herman, J. (1999). *Clinical reasoning: The art & science of critical & creative thinking.* Clifton Park, NY: Delmar Cengage Learning.

Pollard, W. (1828–1893). William Pollard Quotes. Retrieved November 05, 2020, from https://www.brainyquote.com/quotes/william_pollard_163245

Rand, C. M., Tyrrell, H., Wallace-Brodeur, R., Goldstein, N. P., Darden, P. M., Humiston, S. G., Albertin, C. S., Stratbucker, W., Schafer, S.J. & Szilagyi, P. G. (2018). A learning collaboration model to improve papillomavirus vaccination rates in orimary care. *Academic Pediatrics, 18*(2), S46–S53. doi:10.1016/j.acap.2018.01.003

Rasel. (2014). Definition of planned change in organization. Retrieved from http://bankofinfo.com/definition-of-planned-change.

Rogers, E. M. (1983). *Diffusion of innovations* (3rd ed.). New York: Free Press.

Stark, P. (2017). Employee responses to organizational change. Retrieved from https://peterstark.com/employee-responses-change#.

Swaim. (2014). Nine reasons organizations need to change. Retrieved from www.processexcellencenetwork.com/organizational-change/columns/why-organizations-change-and-what-they-can-change

Webster, M. (2020). Innovation. Retrieved October 30, 2020, from https://www.merriam-webster.com/dictionary/innovation

The Cleveland Clinic Advisory Board. (2018, October 26). The top 10 health care innovations for 2019, according to Cleveland Clinic. Retrieved November 05, 2020, from https://www.advisory.com/daily-briefing/2018/10/26/innovations

Vasić, M., Potkonjak, A., Stanojevic, Darko & Dimitrijevic, M. (2015). Quality implications on the business of logistic companies. Istrazivanja i projektovanja za privredu. 13. 87-92. 10.5937/jaes13-8389.

Weston, B. (2015, February 23). 10 Tips for Dealing with Change Positively in Your workplace. Retrieved November 05, 2020, from https://www.linkedin.com/pulse/10-tips-dealing-change-positively-your-workplace-ban-weston

SUGGESTED READINGS

Adib-Hajbaghery, M., & Sharifi, N. (2017). Effect of simulation training on the development of nurses an nursing students' critical thinking: A systematic literature review. *Nurse Education Today, 50*, 17–24.

Alamrani, M. H., Alammar, K. A., Alqahtani, S. S., & Salem, O. A. (2018). Comparing the effects of simulation-based and traditional teaching methods on the critical thinking abilities and self-confidence of nursing students. *The Journal of Nursing Research: JNR, 26*(3), 152–157.

Albert, N. M. (2018). Operationalizing a nursing innovation center within a health care system. *Nursing Administration Quarterly, 42*(1), 43–53.

Chapman, C., Barker, M., & Lawrence, W. (2015). Improving nutritional care: Innovation and good practice. *Journal Of Advanced Nursing, 71*(4), 881–894.

Chisholm, L., Zimmerman, S., Rosemond, C., McConnell, E., Weiner, B. J., Lin, F.-C., & Hanson, L. (2018). Nursing home staff perspectives on adoption of an innovation in goals of care communication. *Geriatric Nursing (New York), 39*(2), 157–161.

Eines, T. F., & Vatne, S. (2018). Nurses and nurse assistants' experiences with using a design thinking approach to innovation in a nursing home. *Journal of Nursing Management, 26*(4), 425–431.

Garwood, J. K., Ahmed, A. H., & McComb, S. A. (2018). The effect of concept maps on undergraduate nursing Students' critical thinking. *Nursing Education Perspectives, 39*(4), 208–214.

Gilissen, J., Pivodic, L., Gastmans, C., Vander Stichele, R., Deliens, L., Breuer, E., & Van den Block, L. (2018). How to achieve the desired outcomes of advance care planning in nursing homes: A theory of change. *BMC Geriatrics, 18*(1), 47.

Glogovsky, D. (2017). How can policy change guide nursing practice to reduce in-patient falls? *Nursing, 47*(12), 63–67.

Leach, V., Tonkin, E., Lancastle, D., & Kirk, M. (2016). A strategy for implementing genomics into nursing practice informed by three behaviour change theories. *International Journal of Nursing Practice*, *22*(3), 307–315.

Lee, D. S., Abdullah, K. L., Subramanian, P., Bachmann, R. T., & Ong, S. L. (2017). An integrated review of the correlation between critical thinking ability and clinical decision-making in nursing. *Journal of Clinical Nursing*, *26*(23–24), 4065–4079.

Orr, P., & Davenport, D. (2015). Embracing change. *The Nursing Clinics of North America*, *50*(1), 1–18.

Sloane, D. M., Smith, H. L., McHugh, M. D., & Aiken, L. H. (2018). Effect of changes in hospital nursing resources on improvements in patient safety and quality of care: A panel study. *Medical Care*, *56*(12), 1001–1008.

Small, A., Gist, D., Souza, D., Dalton, J., Magny-Normilus, C., & David, D. (2016). Using Kotter's change model for implementing bedside handoff: A quality improvement project. *Journal of Nursing Care Quality*, *31*(4), 304–309.

Sportsman, S. (2018). Next generation NCLEX (NGN): A brief summary. Retrieved from https://collaborativemomentum.com/2018/11/13/next-generation-nclex-ngn-a-brief-summary.

The US Department of Health and Human Services. (2019). *The opioid epidemic by the numbers*. Retrieved from www.hhs.gov/opioids/about-the-epidemic/index.html.

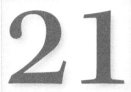

Power and Politics

Richard J. Maloney[1,2], Patsy L. Maloney[3,4]

[1] University of Washington, Tacoma, Washington, USA
[2] Policy Governance Associates, Tacoma, Washington, USA
[3] University of Washington, Tacoma, Washington, USA
[4] Pacific Lutheran University, Tacoma, Washington, USA

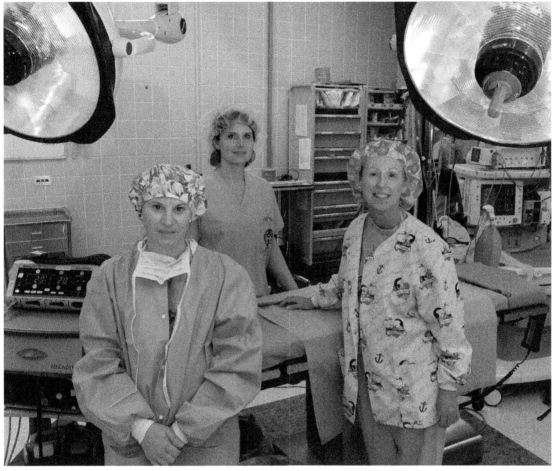

Source: U.S. Air Force

The sole advantage of power is that you can do more good.

(Baltasar Gracian, 1892, p. 101)

OBJECTIVES

Upon completion of this chapter, the reader should be able to:

1. Describe the following sources of power and analyze each in the context of an entry-level nurse: expert, legitimate, referent, reward, coercive, connection, and information.

2. Define power at the personal, professional, and organizational levels.

Kelly Vana's Nursing Leadership and Management, Fourth Edition. Edited by Patricia Kelly Vana and Janice Tazbir
© 2021 John Wiley & Sons Ltd. Published 2021 by John Wiley & Sons Ltd.
Companion Website: www.wiley.com/go/kelly-Nursing-Leadership

3. Explain why nurses have a professional responsibility to increase their power and analyze how new nurses can increase their personal and professional power.

4. Summarize the history of collective bargaining and related legislation.

5. Explain the role of nurse as advocate and nursing as political force.

6. Describe how power can be used in various settings, i.e., at the bedside; in the workplace; in nursing, hospital, and community committees; on boards of directors, and on public policymaking bodies to more effectively meet nursing responsibilities.

OPENING SCENARIO

Pat, a new graduate who has just finished a medical-surgical nursing residency program, is working with a patient for whom a surgical consult has been written. Dr. Killian, who will be doing the surgical consultation, is referred to as "Dr. Killjoy" by the unit clerk and senior nurses on the unit because she takes the joy out of a nurse's life by "putting nurses in their place." Pat knows Dr. Killian has the reputation of being demeaning and inappropriately demanding when interacting with new nurses. Pat knows that in a couple of hours, Dr. Killian will be on the unit and will ask to see the nurse who did the surgical admission sheet.

If you were Pat, how would you prepare for the meeting?

What would be your approach as you begin your meeting with Dr. Killian?

Where could you go to seek support, should the meeting not go well?

Effective nurses are powerful. Skillfully employing leadership, objectivity, creativity, and a specialized body of knowledge, they influence others as part of their professional practice. They develop and exert power from multiple sources and in a variety of situations. They intentionally employ an understanding of power to influence others, accomplish organizational goals, and ensure safe, competent patient care. Collectively, effective nurses protect and advance the interests of nursing staff. On a broader stage, nurses take part in the political process to advocate for patients' interests, promote nursing values, and achieve desired public policy goals.

This chapter discusses power, its sources and its uses at the personal, professional, and organizational levels. Understanding the need to hold and wield power as a professional responsibility, new nurses can learn how to increase their personal and professional power. Also included is a history of collective bargaining and related legislation, with an emphasis on nursing and health care. Readers will understand the role of nurse as advocate, and how nursing acts as a political force in shaping the future of health care in the United States. Understanding and using power will benefit the new nurse throughout a career in nursing, in various settings: at the bedside; in the workplace; on nursing, hospital, and community committees; on Boards of Directors, and public policymaking bodies, and allow them to more effectively meet their nursing responsibilities.

Power

Power is the ability to acquire and use influence to achieve one's goals. Power, regardless of level, is derived from an ability to influence others' thinking or behavior, a capacity which effective nurses nurture. Effective nurses strive to gain knowledge of the distribution of power in their organization, the circumstances under which power can be used, and strategies associated with recognizing, increasing, and using power.

Nursing differs significantly from the too-commonly-held image of "nurse as handmaiden." Nurses cannot afford to sustain a submissive social image of nurses doing only what they are told. They must develop and use power. Patients' needs are more complex than ever, so effective nurses are needed who can advocate for their patients as well as for themselves. Nurses must assert well-informed opinions and stand up for what is best for patients, exercising professional power where the nurse's judgment is key. The work place benefits when nurses support one another, and in a larger setting, society benefits when nursing speaks as a profession. Since its earliest days, this has been so. Florence Nightingale was no pushover, and her use of power changed health care.

A Professional Responsibility

Inherent in the role of the nurse are both professional responsibility and accountability for decisions made and actions rendered. As members of a profession, nurses assume responsibility for defining their role and providing service to society. Typically, professions are distinguished by certain specific characteristics; these include, but are not limited to formal educational requirements, autonomy of practice, adherence to an established code of ethics, expansion of the level of knowledge, and a common culture and values present among

Critical Thinking 21.1

The work and contributions of some nurses are so significant that they change the world. When we consider the relevance and significance of nursing history, we realize the contributions made by nurses who saw themselves as powerful and acted on that empowered self-image to improve the lives of others. Such an empowering self-image begins for many entry-level nurses on day one, while a lack of historical awareness within the nursing profession empowers others to discount nursing's importance to society.

Ultimately, this can limit our future as nurses and our potential for making even greater contributions to the future of health care.

Can you name two nurses who were powerful figures in modern history and tell why their contributions are so significant? See Exploring the Web in this chapter for ideas.

Can you identify some obstacles they experienced because they were nurses?

members (Joel & Kelly, 2002). Professions progress through an expected evolutionary process. This consists of expanding the scientific base, creating technical workers to share in the essential mission of the field, standardizing and up-grading education for entry into practice, and moving forward with specialization (Joel, 2002). With professional responsibility comes accountability and the need for sufficient power to ensure that the responsibility is fulfilled.

A person's orientation to power often takes one of two forms. One form is that people are motivated by a desire for ego reinforcement and personal gain, while another form promotes power as a means to achieve the common good. Concern that power is an inherently bad thing, and therefore something to be avoided, is reflected in the following observation from Lord Acton (Seldes, 1985, p. 234): "Power tends to corrupt, and absolute power corrupts absolutely." People with this view of power

tend to worry that those given power ultimately should not have it because of its potential for harm. According to this view, those who are motivated to acquire power are not to be trusted—they seek power for their own personal gain and at any cost.

The other point of view is that power can be considered a good thing, a force for good as reflected in Gracian's (1892, p. 172) saying: "The sole advantage of power is that you can do more good." Effective nurses see and employ power as a positive force, something that helps them fulfill their professional responsibility to patients, coworkers, the nursing profession, and themselves. They accept a professional obligation not to view power negatively and not to shun the drama of "power struggles" by avoiding its use altogether. Instead, effective nurses see power as a positive force, and are more inclined in their professional capacity to acquire and use power so they can promote the common good.

Evidence from the Literature

Citation: Buresh, B., & Gordon, S. (2013). *From Silence to Voice*. Ithaca, NY: Cornell University Press.

Discussion: This book argues that not enough nurses are willing to talk about their work, particularly the application of nursing knowledge, without somehow downplaying its value. When nurses and nursing organizations do talk about their work, they project an inaccurate picture of nurses using a script that emphasizes virtue over knowledge. They discuss the virtuous and caring acts of nurses, but not the expert knowledge nurses bring to patient care. Also, when giving voice to nursing, nursing groups sometimes downplay or devalue the bedside nursing that occurs in direct care of the sick while elevating the elite status of advanced practice nurses, nurse

administrators, or nurse academics. Both portrayals contribute to social stereotypes of a nurse who is "just a nurse." Ironically, the deemphasizing of bedside nursing contrasts with the message of advocates for patient safety, including physicians Lucian Leape, Michael Leonard, and Michael Woods, who explain why we need assertive nurses and why physicians should listen to them.

Implications for Practice: If nursing is misunderstood by the public or by those with influence, it will continue to be vulnerable to the budget axe, and new resources for nursing education and practice won't surface. A focus on the virtues of nurses is an invitation to seek not the best and brightest nurses but rather the most virtuous, meekest, and self-sacrificing.

Real World Interview

I try to use power in a positive manner in the pain management clinic that I manage. I attempt to get people to move without them necessarily knowing they are being helped. I think that power at the bedside is a personal thing. Confidence, authenticity, and genuineness are qualities I most value and I see these as empowering

nurses in practice. I feel that the middle manager in nursing gets power by developing staff, building self-confidence on a personal level, and delegating authority in a way that supports others. In higher levels of nursing management, I found through my military experience that the best leaders almost give power away, with the only caveat being that the persons being delegated to represent the leader are accountable for the decisions they make. I believe that the tighter a person holds onto power, the less powerful she or he becomes. I also believe that nurses run the risk of losing power when they look for power outside nursing to direct them. New graduates should seek experiences and input from a variety of people and glean what they can from each experience. It is somewhat like a smorgasbord. Ultimately, the new nurse has to decide what she or he wants because there is no one answer or approach to power. No one really has *the* answer; instead, they have *an* answer.

Nancy Safranek, MSN, RN
Director, Outpatient Services, PACU, SP, PMC
Puyallup, Washington

Sources of Power

Most researchers agree that sources of power are diverse and vary from one situation to another. Sources of power are categorized as expert, legitimate, referent, reward, coercive, and connection. More recently, another power source—information—has been added to the typology (Raven, 2008). Generally speaking, nurses acquire and exert influence as a result of one or a combination of these power sources. Some of these power sources are found in an organizational context, while other power sources are more personal. Power that an organization confers on a new nurse—for example, the authority inherent in assignment as a staff RN by virtue of assigned duties—is not necessarily available in another setting in which the nurse has different assigned duties.

Expert Power

Power derived from the knowledge and skills nurses develop over time is called expert power. There are special considerations to keep in mind about expertise and power. The more knowledge and skill the nurse has, the more the nurse is perceived as an expert. The geometric explosion of knowledge has made expertise more valuable and technological advances making information more accessible have enabled more people to acquire expertise on any given subject. Knowing more than others do about a subject, combined with the legitimacy of holding a position that is recognized as requiring expertise, gives an individual a decided advantage in any situation. But the less known an individual's expertise is within a given group, the less effective that individual's expert power becomes. Visible reciprocal acknowledgment of expertise among co-workers in a group balances power and enhances group productivity, whereas lack of reciprocal acknowledgment has the opposite effect. Combining expertise with high authority is most powerful if the person in a high position of authority consistently demonstrates the expertise associated with the position. Entry-level nurses enhance their expert power and their ability to get the patient care mission accomplished if they add to their current knowledge through professional reading and professional development and seek additional opportunities to improve their clinical skills.

Legitimate Power

Power derived from the position of authority that a nurse holds in a group is called legitimate power. Examples include legitimate power derived from an academic degree, licensure, certification, experience in the role, and job title. The more comfortable nurses are with legitimate power, the easier it is for them to fulfill the potential of their role. Nurses with legitimate power are expected to use what authority they have to get the job done, and they may even be punished for not doing so. Sometimes, too little legitimacy or authority is delegated to nurses when they are given leadership responsibility. People generally follow legitimate leaders with whom they agree. Although legitimacy is a significant factor in influencing others, it is not universally effective and it is generally insufficient as one's only source of power. New nurses may be placed in positions of authority with inherent legitimate power relatively quickly after orientation. For example, they may be assigned as charge nurses, supervising licensed practical or vocational nurses on a shift. Appropriate and timely use of legitimate power enables the nurse to assure positive patient care outcomes. Nurses must, however, be aware of the limits of legitimate power and use power available to them from all sources.

Referent Power

Power derived from how much others respect and like an individual, group, or organization with which one is associated is called referent power. Nurses who are identified with respected, trustworthy individuals or groups will benefit from referent power by virtue of such identification. A nurse identified as a graduate of a respected university enjoys the benefit of prestige-based referent power from such identification. New nurses often start the job with a blank slate as far as referent power is concerned but can quickly gain influence among co-workers by identifying with other individuals or groups that co-workers respect. Through identification with their university, church, or some other association, for example, the entry-level nurse can tap into referent power. Dressing and communicating professionally and looking like a nurse worthy of respect can confer additional referent power. Because it is based on being liked and respected, referent power can be harmed if power from other sources, such as legitimate, reward, or coercive power is abused or poorly exercised.

Reward Power

Power that comes from the ability to give others something they value in response to their behavior is called reward power. Meaningful rewards exist in addition to, and often in preference to, money, such as informal acknowledgment for good work or formal recognition before one's nursing peers at an awards ceremony. The manner in which rewards are distributed is also important. For example, when everyone receives rewards, or they are given in an arbitrary or unpredictable manner, their power to motivate is greatly diminished. Rewards are not likely to permanently affect behavior. Once given, rewards stimulate a desire for more rewards, but this effect can be short-term. New nurses often lack the formal ability to give rewards, but they can informally exercise reward power by giving appropriate positive feedback about the performance of others with whom they work. Withholding rewards can result in resentment and a less collegial relationships with nurses you work with. Consistent and fair use of reward power enhances one's overall power base.

Coercive Power

Power that comes from the ability to punish others for their behavior is called coercive power. This type of power is often considered the least desirable tactic to be used by people in positions of authority. It can be immediately effective in forcing short-term behavior but is demotivating over a longer term. A new nurse indirectly exercises coercive power when reporting incidents that could result in disciplinary action and sometimes unknowingly be perceived as a "tattle-tale." Sometimes a nurse's duty to patients requires it, but coercive power should be used sparingly, for it can damage working relationships. In any event, this source of power demands careful thought, and appropriate use.

Connection Power

Power that comes from personal and professional connections with others is called connection power. Nurses can dramatically increase their influence by understanding that people are not only very aware of those with power, they also are aware of their associates. A new nurse visiting the office of the Director of Nursing Services or the Vice President for Patient Care Services should not forget that clerical workers in the outer office have a relationship with their boss and thus have connection power. If you try to go around them, take their power lightly, insult or patronize them, you have risked your own power base in relation to the Director or Vice President. Similarly, if an entry-level nurse bypasses a person who is directly responsible for a situation, such an attempt reflects negatively on the nurse. Nurses should work to resolve issues at the lowest appropriate level before they take their concerns to a higher level of authority. Nurses are expected to understand the chain of command and policies of the organizations (both formal and informal "rules of the road") in which they work. Nurses who are on nursing, hospital, and community committees and boards of directors have the opportunity to meet and connect with other people and build power. As with other sources of power, connection power can be misused, so nurses should be both fully aware of its existence and thoughtful about its use, or they may suffer a loss of overall power and influence.

Information Power

Power based on information that someone can provide to the group is called information power. Information power is especially important because, to be functional, health care teams and organizations require accurate, timely, and shared information. Regardless of a nurse's leadership style, information plays an increasingly critical role. Legitimate power, reward power, and coercive power are bestowed on individuals by virtue of their position in the organization. They tend to be effective only for a short period of time unless they are accompanied by other forms of power, such as information power. To be perceived as having information power, nurses must have access to and share knowledge that is both accurate and useful. Membership on nursing, hospital, and community committees and boards of directors can enhance the information power of nurses. Information power can improve patient care, increase collegiality, enhance organizational effectiveness, and strengthen one's professional role and connections. New nurses who value team membership will empower coworkers and themselves by giving and receiving information with which to do the job more effectively. See Table 21.1 for a summary of the different sources of power and examples of each for nursing.

Power in Nursing

Power in nursing can be applied in various ways (personal, professional, and organizational) and can be seen in various contexts as it is derived from numerous sources (expert, legitimate, referent, reward, coercive, connection, and information). The nurse is encouraged to understand power in order to appropriately use it to carry out job tasks effectively and efficiently. A person can hold power as an individual in several contexts: personal power, professional power, and organizational power.

Personal Power

Power based on characteristics within the individual make up **personal power**. For example, parents and teachers are often seen as personally powerful because of the special relationships they have with their charges and the knowledge they possess. Power at the personal level is closely linked to how one perceives power, how others perceive an individual, and the extent to which someone can influence events. Nurses who use power at a personal level are likely to manifest a high level of self-awareness and self-confidence and carry that power with them in various settings.

As a new nurse, you will encounter situations requiring that you develop and use your personal power to influence outcomes for your patients. It is essential that new nurses have the values and attitudes that predispose them to capable and ethical use of power, the knowledge to understand it, and the skills to acquire and employ personal power throughout their careers. Sources of power commonly associated with personal power include expert, referent, connection, and information power.

Table 21.1   Examples of Power for Nursing

Type	Source	Examples for nursing
Expert	Power derived from the knowledge and skills nurses develop over time. The more knowledge and skill the nurse has, the more the nurse is perceived as an expert	Communicating information from current evidence-based journals and bringing expert skill to patient care
Legitimate	Power derived from the position of authority that a nurse holds in a group (e.g., degree, licensure, certification, experience in the role, and job title)	Wearing or displaying symbols of professional standing, including licensure and certification
Referent	Power derived from how much others respect and like an individual, group, or organization with which one is associated	Gaining power by affiliating with nurses and others who have power in an organization
Reward	Power that comes from the ability to give others something they value in response to their behavior	Using a hospital award to motivate behavior
Coercive	Power that comes from the ability to punish others for their behavior	Using the hospital disciplinary evaluation system to alter another's behavior
Connection	Power that comes from personal and professional connection with others	Developing good working relationships and mentoring with your boss and other powerful people
Information	Power based on information that someone can provide to the group.	Sharing useful knowledge gleaned from the Internet and other sources with coworkers.

NIST (2013) Developed with information from Hersey, Blanchard, & Natemeyer (1979); French & Raven (1959); and Raven (2008).

Professional Power

Power conferred on members of a profession by others with whom they work and by the larger society to which they belong is called **professional power**. Such power assigns status based on trust in specialized knowledge and skills and a position of acknowledged authority within the scope of a professional role. In return, professional nurses offer a service that society values. Requirements for a vocation to be considered a profession include: (a) a long period of specialized education, (b) a service orientation, and (c) the ability to be autonomous (Jacox, 1980). Jacox defines autonomy as a characteristic of a profession in which its membership is self-regulating and has publicly recognized control of its own functioning in the work situation. Sources of power commonly associated with professional power include expert, referent, and information power.

People who are professionals and are perceived as experts in health care have a significant amount of authority and influence, which makes them more effective than those not perceived as experts. There are at least two ways to wield professional power. The first way is to be introduced and promoted to a group as a professional with professional expertise. This establishes credibility, but if not validated in actual practice, such credibility can fade. The second way is to actually demonstrate professional knowledge and skill, so that these attributes are consistently on display in a clinical setting. Remarkably, nurses sometimes are reluctant to be identified as experts or to assert their expertise to patients, practitioners, administrators, other nurses, other health care workers, and the public in general. Such reluctance and lack of self-assuredness must be addressed if the individual nurse, or the nursing profession, for that matter, is to become more visible and achieve the status and degree of empowerment needed to fulfill nursing's fullest potential.

Organizational Power

Power based on an organizational hierarchy, one's position in that hierarchy, and one's understanding of the organization's structures and functions is called **organizational power**. Organizational power is enhanced by the exercise of personal and professional power in the decisions nurses make and the actions they take to organize their work, accomplish their goals, and obtain necessary resources for themselves and their patients. Development of leadership and political skill (including its use in "office politics" and on nursing, hospital, and community committees and boards of directors) also enhances a nurse's organizational power, by extending influence through others in the organization and community. Sources of power commonly associated with organizational power are legitimate, reward, coercive, connection, and information power.

Critical Thinking 21.2

Think about the challenges you will face as a new nurse on a busy medical-surgical unit. How will you fit into the professional work group? Who can you rely on among your new co-workers? What is the status of nursing vis-à-vis medical practitioners, pharmacists, and food service workers? What sources of power do you bring into the work setting? How might you establish awareness of and enhance your knowledge and skills as a competent member of the team? Are you able to appropriately assert yourself in this new environment? What additional assets do you need to bring to the job? What nursing, hospital, or community communities or boards of directors can you join?

Real World Interview

Ms. Cox is 38 years old and has been hospitalized four times. She underwent surgery this past spring and has encountered nursing care and nurses in various roles throughout the health care system. Ms. Cox is articulate and reflective, having earned a degree in English and holding a position at a selective liberal arts university as an admissions counselor. She states,

"I don't think nurses know they are powerful. Nurses can take on more than they think they can. They have the power to change the system in which they work. Yet I also see nurses as the most overworked, underpaid, and underachieving profession. There is so much more they could be doing if they didn't spend so much time railing against the machine. They are telling the wrong people—each other—that they are frustrated. They should be telling the ones with real power, or, better yet, more of them should become the ones in power. Instead, they suffer with each other and stay angry. It appears almost passive-aggressive how nurses deal with power. My concern is that it can affect patient care in a negative way. Believe me when I say patients value nurses, but the people writing the paycheck for nurses must value nurses. Patients need nursing far more than they need anything else. The better nurses that have cared for me have been instrumental in my healing. Beyond knowing when I need medication or performing some procedure, it is the smile, the touch, and the well-placed word of encouragement that has gotten me through. This is where nurses have power, because no one but a real nurse can provide it. It comes from the heart."

Audrey Cox
Patient
University Place, Washington

Nurse Empowerment

In the nursing literature, empowerment is usually viewed as something positive or highly desirable. Linnen and Rowley (2014) describe structural empowerment as an organizational strategy such as supportive and empathetic team relationships that have a positive effect on individual nurses, who become empowered in the workplace and in turn enhance productivity, quality of patient care, patient safety, staff morale, retention, and overall nursing job satisfaction. Using the sources of power described by Raven (2008), we can conceive of nurse empowerment as capacity building, in which one's capacity to influence others is enhanced by an increase in any of the six sources of power.

Nurses disempower themselves if they see themselves or the nursing profession as powerless. On the other hand, nurses empower themselves and others in many ways. Interpersonally, they empower others if they perceive them to be able to use power. If an individual, a group, or an organization is perceived as being powerful, that perception can by itself empower the individual, group, or organization. Kennedy, Hardiker, and Staniland (2015) describes how empowered nurses contribute to clinical learning and the work environment. Joining together to advocate for patients in the workplace or form a collective bargaining unit to give voice to employee concerns, and accessing professional nursing associations to advocate for broad, social goals, are ways to empower nurses for collective action.

Understanding power in all its forms and from a variety of perspectives is not just important for nurses personally, it is important for them professionally, and for their nursing organizations as well. Understanding power helps the novice nurse make better decisions, become more effective, and enhances the delivery of patient care. It allows nurses to gain more control of their personal lives and their work lives. Table 21.2 presents a framework for developing personal, professional, and organizational power.

Case Study 21.1

Maria and Haley work on the same nursing unit in a large, metropolitan hospital. Both predominantly work the evening shift and have less than 1 year's experience since graduating from nursing school. Maria has been offered increasingly more difficult patient assignments, including assignment of charge nurse duties, and recently was selected for a two-week leadership training program. Haley has not adapted as well and has withdrawn from what was once a close relationship with Maria. Haley seeks consolation from the nurses she and Maria claimed they would never emulate. Haley takes her breaks and eats dinner with two nurses who complain that the best nurses are undervalued in the organization, yet these same nurses were not supportive of Maria or Haley or any other new nurses oriented to their unit. Maria seeks out others she perceives to be knowledgeable and more successful in their professional roles. She strives to participate in nonmandatory meetings as well as clinical rounds, using them as an opportunity to ask questions. Thus, she is beginning to increase her personal level of power by connecting with the other staff and gathering information. One night after a difficult shift, Haley accuses Maria of abandoning her and playing up to administration, saying that Maria is being used by the unit's nurse manager. Haley tells Maria that the other nurses are planning to file a complaint against the unit supervisor for selecting Maria, over the nurses that have been on the unit longer, to attend the leadership training program.

What does Haley's behavior tell you about her personal orientation toward power?

How should Maria react to Haley in this situation?

Apply your understanding of power to suggest how Maria can help Haley develop power.

Table 21.2   A Framework for Empowerment

Type of power	Steps to empowerment
Personal power	Find a mentor.
	Notice who holds power in your personal, professional, and organizational life. Introduce yourself to them.
	Find and maintain good sources of evidence-based information.
	Seek answers to questions.
	Make a plan to develop all sources of personal, professional, and organizational power.
	Regularly evaluate the plan.
Professional power	Assess patient's condition using relevant, objective measurements.
	Collaborate with administrators and other nursing and medical practitioners and health care workers involved in the care of your patients.
	Join your professional nursing organization.
	Consult with significant others, friends, and members of the patient's family.
	Monitor and improve patient care quality.
Organizational power	Get involved in the organization beyond direct patient care.
	Volunteer for committee assignments that will challenge you to learn and experience more than what is expected of you in a staff nurse role.
	Think about the following when involved with committees:
	• What is the committee trying to do? • What specific information does the committee use to operate and make decisions? • How does the committee apply to my practice, to my colleagues, to my patients, to my organizational unit, and to the organization as a whole?
	Continually improve and add to the knowledge you have in relation to your patients, your colleagues, your organizational unit, the organization as a whole, and the profession of nursing.
	Readily share appropriate knowledge with others who will value it and use it to a good end.
	Evaluate your plans regularly. Did you achieve the expected outcomes? If not, why? Were there staffing problems or patient crises? Were the activities that were necessary for outcome achievement carried out?
	How can you apply lessons learned from this evaluation to the future?
	Continue to develop all your sources of power.
	Volunteer to be involved with health care at the local, state, and national levels.

Source: Richard J. Maloney & Patsy L. Maloney.

The Power of Professional Nursing Organizations

Where do nurses turn when they have concerns but no power to change the situation? Both new and experienced nurses can turn to their professional organizations. Alone, a nurse is only one voice, but collectively, nurses are powerful. Professional nursing organizations play a major role in advocating for issues impacting nurses and their patients. Their role includes but is not limited to developing policy statements, lobbying for regulations and legislation that serve and protect the consumers of nursing care, and advocating for both nurses and patients.

There are times when tension exists between a professional organization's duty to advocate for its members and its duty to advocate for the welfare of the public. The organization must balance this tension while continuing to promote patient safety.

Representing the interests of the nation's 4 million registered nurses through its 50 constituent state affiliates, the **American Nurses Association (ANA)** is the largest association of registered nurses in the United States. ANA is at the forefront of improving the quality of health care for all. Founded in 1896,

and with members in all 50 states and U.S. territories, ANA is a strong voice for the profession. ANA is not focused on a specific nursing specialty. It represents nurses from all specialties, all work sites, and all levels of nursing education. ANA has many goals, but one of them is to assure safe, quality care for patients (American Nurses Association, 2018). To achieve its patient safety goal, ANA develops and disseminates documents such as *Nursing's Social Policy Statement* (ANA, 2010) and the *Code of Ethics for Nurses* (ANA, 2015). These documents define nurses' contract with society and each nurse's obligation to act ethically. Patient safety is part of this contract as well as the ethical responsibility of nurses. ANA lobbies for regulations and legislation that ensure patient safety. This is done largely through state nursing associations, state nursing boards, and state legislatures, which define nursing practice in each state. ANA advocates for the consumers of health care by pushing for evidence-based patient outcome data and encouraging nursing certification and credentialing. Educated consumers can choose facilities with improved patient outcomes and well-prepared nurses.

Many professional organizations speak for nurses. Most are specialty organizations with small memberships. Some specialty organizations, such as Emergency Nurses Association and the Association of Critical Care Nurses, have larger memberships (Table 21.3).

Union Power

A **union** is a formal and legal group that acts as a collective bargaining agent to formally present worker desires to management. Collective bargaining is subject to Federal labor law administered under the purview of the **National Labor Relations Board** (**NLRB**). In collective bargaining, an employee group bargains with management for protections and benefits the group desires. If the group cannot achieve its goals through informal bargaining with management, the group may decide to work with a collective bargaining agent and form a union. In January 2004, after a 12-year campaign by the **California Nurses Association** (**CNA**), California became the first, and to date only, state to implement mandatory nurse-to-patient ratios. The CNA later merged in 2009 with the United American Nurses and Massachusetts Nurses Association to form the

Table 21.3 **Nursing Organizations**

Organization	Web site
Academy of Medical-Surgical Nurses	www.amsn.org/
Academy of Neonatal Nursing	www.academyonline.org
Air & Surface Transport Nurses Association	www.astna.org
American Academy of Ambulatory Care Nursing	www.aaacn.org
American Academy of Nurse Practitioners	www.aanp.org
American Association for Men in Nursing	www.aamn.org
American Association for the History of Nursing	www.aahn.org
American Association of Colleges of Nursing	www.aacnnursing.org
American Association of Critical-Care Nurses	www.aacn.org
American Association of Heart Failure Nurses	www.aahfn.org
American Association of Legal Nurse Consultants	www.aalnc.org
American Association of Managed Care Nurses	www.aamcn.org
American Association of Neuroscience Nurses	http://aann.org
American Association of Nurse Anesthetists	www.aana.com
American Association of Nurse Life Care Planners	www.aanlcp.org
American Association of Occupational Health Nurses	aaohn.org/
American Association of Spinal Cord Injury Nurses	www.aascin.org
American College of Nurse-Midwives	www.midwife.org
American Association of Nurse Practitioners	www.aanp.org
American Forensic Nurses	www.amrn.com
American Holistic Nurses Association	www.ahna.org
American Nephrology Nurses' Association	www.annanurse.org
American Nurses Association	www.nursingworld.org
American Nursing Informatics Association	www.ania.org
American Organization of Nurse Executives	www.aone.org
American Pediatric Surgical Nurses Association	www.apsna.org
American Psychiatric Nurses Association	www.apna.org
American Society for Pain Management Nursing	www.aspmn.org
American Society of Ophthalmic Registered Nurses	http://asorn.org
American Society of Peri Anesthesia Nurses	www.aspan.org
Association of Camp Nurses	www.campnurse.org
Association of Child Neurology Nurses	www.childneurologysociety.org
Association of Nurses in AIDS Care	www.nursesinaidscare.org
Association of Nursing Professional Development	www.anpd.org

(Continued)

Table 21.3   **(Continued)**

Organization	Web site
Association of Operating Room Nurses (same as Association of Perioperative Registered Nurses)	www.aorn.org
Association of Pediatric Gastroenterology and Nutrition Nurses	apgnn.org
Association of Pediatric Hematology/Oncology Nurses	http://aphon.org
Association for Radiologic and Imaging Nursing	www.arinursing.org
Association of Rehabilitation Nurses	www.rehabnurse.org
Association of Women's Health, Obstetric and Neonatal Nurses	www.awhonn.org
Chi Eta Phi Sorority, Inc.	chietaphi.com
Dermatology Nurses' Association	www.dnanurse.org
Developmental Disabilities Nurses Association	ddna.org
Emergency Nurses Association	www.ena.org
Family Medicine Residency Nurses Association	www.fmrna.org
Gerontological Advanced Practice Nurses Association	www.gapna.org
Home Health care Nurses Association	www.nahc.org
Hospice and Palliative Nurses Association	https://advancingexpertcare.org
Infusion Nurses Society	www.ins1.org
International Association of Forensic Nurses	www.forensicnurses.org
International Organization of Multiple Sclerosis Nurses	http://iomsn.org
International Society of Nurses in Cancer Care	www.isncc.org
International Society of Nurses in Genetics	www.isong.org
International Society of Plastic and Aesthetic Nurses	ispan.org/
National Association of Clinical Nurse Specialists	www.nacns.org
National Association of Hispanic Nurses	www.nahnnet.org
National Association of Neonatal Nurses	www.nann.org
National Association of Nurse Practitioners in Women's Health	www.npwh.org
National Association of Orthopedic Nurses	www.orthonurse.org
National Association of Pediatric Nurse Practitioners	www.napnap.org
National Association of School Nurses	www.nasn.org
National Association of School Nurses for the Deaf	www.nasnd.net
National Black Nurses Association	www.nbna.org
National Council of State Boards of Nursing	www.ncsbn.org
National League for Nursing	www.nln.org
National Organization of Nurse Practitioner Faculties	www.nonpf.com
Nurses Organization of Veterans Affairs	vanurse.org
Oncology Nursing Society	www.ons.org
Pediatric Endocrinology Nursing Society	www.pens.org
Preventive Cardiovascular Nurses Association	pcna.net
Sigma Theta Tau International	www.sigmanursing.org
Society of Gastroenterology Nurses and Associates, Inc.	www.sgna.org
Society of Otorhinolaryngology and Head-Neck Nurses, Inc.	sohnnurse.com
Society of Pediatric Nurses	www.pedsnurses.org
Society of Trauma Nurses	www.traumanurses.org
Society of Urologic Nurses and Associates	www.suna.org
Transcultural Nursing Organization	www.tcns.org
Wound, Ostomy and Continence Nurses Society	www.wocn.org

Source: Compiled by Richard J. Maloney & Patsy L. Maloney.

National Nurses United (**NNU**). Currently, the NNU is the largest union and professional association of registered nurses in the U.S., with more than 150,000 members nationwide. NNU promotes collective action for nurses with campaigns to promote the economic and professional interests of all direct care RNs, the expansion of the voice of direct care RNs and patients in public policy, and the enactment of patient advocacy rights and safe nurse-to-patient care ratios, similar to California. The California Department of Health currently mandates the following nurse-to-patient staffing ratios:

- 5 : 1 patient-to-nurse in medical-surgical units

- 1 : 1 in trauma

- 2 : 1 in labor and delivery; and

- 2 : 1 in intensive care units (SEIU Local 121RN, 2018).

NNU also works to strengthen the voice of RNs in the national health care reform debate and in electoral campaigns from coast to coast, available at, www.nationalnursesunited. org/about, accessed September 17, 2019.

The main purpose of most nursing collective bargaining units is to give nurses a voice in the larger work setting in which they are employed (Roux & Halstead, 2018). Many nurses belong to numerous collective groups, including specialty nursing organizations, church organizations, clubs, community groups, and so on. The reasons most people belong to these collective groups is to promote and support the interests of a group and to better themselves and their communities. Another type of nursing collective group action besides collective bargaining formalized by a union contract, is workplace advocacy, a less structured process by which nurses' voice can be heard. Workplace advocacy is discussed later in this chapter. Shared governance, still another type of collective action, is discussed in Chapter 5.

Collective Bargaining

Collective bargaining, the practice of employees bargaining as a group with management for wages, benefits, and working conditions, has existed in the United States in one form or another since as early as the 1790s. Historically, people who did this were highly skilled artisans who found that by working collectively they could set wages and standards for their skills. By the end of the nineteenth century, unions grew as a means of strengthening worker protections and advocating for worker rights. This union growth accelerated during the 1930s. The Erdman Act, passed in 1898, was the first federal legislation to deal with collective bargaining. Rights that many workers enjoy today came from the struggles of others who had the fortitude to stand up for what they believed was right. Numerous legislative acts have been passed to ensure the rights of workers (see Table 21.4). Table 21.5 shows terminology useful in understanding the collective bargaining process. The decision about whether or not to participate

Table 21.4 Summary of Selected Legislation Affecting Workers

Year and title of legislation	Summary
1898: Erdman Act	Outlawed discrimination by employers against union activities
1935: National Labor Relations Act (Wagner Act)	Gave private employees the right to organize unions to demand better wages and safer work environments
1938: Fair Labor Standards Act	Set minimum wage and maximum hours that can be worked before overtime is paid
1947: Taft-Hartley Act	Restored some management powers that had been reduced or taken away by the Wagner Act; intent was to restore balance between unions and management
1962: Kennedy Executive Order 10988	Amended National Labor Relations Act to allow public employees to join unions
1964: Civil Rights Act	Set equal employment standards such as equal pay for equal work
1965: Executive Order 11246	Set affirmative action guidelines
1967: Age Discrimination Act	Protects against forced retirement due to age
1973: Rehabilitation Act	Protects rights of disabled people
1973: Vietnam Veterans Act	Ensures reemployment rights to veterans
1974: Taft-Hartley Amendments to the Wagner Act	Allows employees of nonprofit organizations to form unions
1986: False Claims Act	Allows whistle-blowing without fear of retribution
1993: Family Medical Leave Act	Allows up to 12 weeks of job-protected leave based on medical reasons
2004: California State Hospital RN to Patient Staffing Law	Legislates minimum staffing ratios in acute care setting
2008: American with Disabilities Act	Prohibits discrimination and assures equal opportunities in the workplace for those with disabilities
2010 Patient Protection and Affordable Care Act	Increases the number of Americans with access to health care; guarantees access for those with pre-existing conditions; expands Medicaid; creates pool for the self-insured.

Source: Adapted from National Labor Relations Board. (2000). *Our history.* Retrieved November 02, 2020, from https://www.nlrb.gov/about-nlrb/who-we-are/our-history

Table 21.5 Collective Bargaining Terminology

Term	Definition
Agency shop	Synonymous with "open shop." Employees are not required to join the union but may join it.
Arbitration	Last step in a dispute. Indicates a nonpartial third party will be involved in the dispute and may make the final decision. Arbitration may be voluntary or imposed by law.
Collective bargaining	The practice of employees bargaining as a union group with management for wages, benefits, and working conditions.
Collective bargaining agent	Entity that works on behalf of employees to formalize collective bargaining through union activity.
Contract	A set of guidelines and rules voted and agreed upon between union and management that guides work practices, wages, and other benefits.
Dispute	A disagreement between management and the union. A dispute may go through (a) mediation and conciliation, (b) arbitration, and possibly, (c) a strike. A dispute may be settled at any stage.
Employee at will	An employee working without a contract. The employee agrees to work under given rules and may be terminated if the employee breaks any rules imposed by management.
Fact finding	Fact finding is used in labor management disputes that involve government-owned companies. It is the process in which claims of labor and management are reviewed. In the private sector, fact finding is usually performed by a board of inquiry.
Grievance	A grievance occurs when a union member believes that management has failed to meet the terms of the contract or labor agreement and communicates this to management.
Grievance proceedings	A formal process in which a union member believes that management has failed to meet the terms of a contract. The steps usually include (a) communication of the grievance to management, (b) mediation between a union representative and a member of management, and possibly, (c) arbitration. The grievance may be settled at any step.
Lockout	The closing of a place of business by management in the course of a labor dispute to attempt to force employees to accept management terms.
Mediation and conciliation	A step in the grievance process in which a nonpartial third party meets with management and the union to assist them in reaching an agreement. In this step, the third party has no actual power in decision making.
National labor relations board (NLRB)	The National Labor Relations Board (NLRB) was formed to implement the Wagner Act. The two major functions of the NLRB include (a) determining and implementing the free democratic choice of employees as to whether they choose to be or choose not to be in a union and (b) preventing and remedying unfair labor practices by employers or unions.
Professional	A person who has knowledge and skills gained from extensive formal study and preparation and has autonomy to practice within a society in exchange for the benefits received by a society.
Self-expression	"The expressing of any views, argument, or opinion, or the dissemination thereof, whether in written, printed, graphic or visual form [,] if such expression contains no threat or reprisal or force or promise of benefit" (National Labor Relations Act, 1994).
Strike	An act in which union members withhold the supply of labor for the purpose of forcing management to accept union terms.
Supervisor	A person with the authority to (a) impart corrective action and (b) delegate to an employee.
Union	A formal and legal group that brings forth desires to management through a collective bargaining agent and within the context of the National Labor Relations Board.
Union dues	Money required of all union employees to support the union and its functions.
Union shop	A place of employment in which all employees are required to join the union and pay dues. Union shop is synonymous with the term closed shop.
Whistle-blowing	Whistle-blowing is the act by which an individual discloses information regarding a violation of a law, rule, or regulation, or a substantial and specific danger to public health or safety.

Source: Adapted from National Labor Relations Board. (2018). *Employer/union rights and obligations.* Retrieved from www.nlrb.gov/rights-we-protect/employerunion-rights-and-obligations.

in collective bargaining by joining a union is a personal one but may be dictated by the existence of union contracts in available job opportunities within a geographical area. Table 21.6 summarizes the pros and cons of unionization.

Why Nurses Seek Unionization

RNs, whether employed as salaried workers or on an hourly basis, have a legal right to participate in collective bargaining in the majority of health care facilities in the country. In 1989,

Table 21.6   Pros and Cons of Unionization

Pros	Cons
The union contract guides standards.	There is reduced allowance for individuality.
Members are able to be a part of the decision-making process.	Other union members may outvote your decisions.
All union members and management must conform to the terms of the contract without exception.	All union members and management must conform to the terms of the contract without exception.
A process can be used to question a manager's authority if a member feels something was not right. More people are involved in the decision-making process.	Disputes are not handled directly between individual and management; there is less room for personal judgment.
Union dues are required to make the union work for you.	Union dues must be paid even if individuals do not support unionization.
Unions give a collective voice to employees.	Employee may not agree with the collective voice.
Employees are able to voice concerns to management without fear of losing job security	Unions may be perceived by some as not professional.

Source: Richard J. Maloney & Patsy L. Maloney.

the NLRB identified eight types of collective bargaining units, including one for RNs that they consider appropriate in the hospital setting. Other collective bargaining units in the hospital may include **licensed practical nurses** (**LPN**s), secretaries, and housekeepers. Excluded from representation are nurses, even LPNs, who serve as supervisors and may not be eligible under labor law for representation by a collective bargaining agent.

When nurses feel powerless, they may attempt to unionize. Some nurses believe that they need to be represented by a strong collective voice so that management will listen to them and changes will be instituted. Nurses are also motivated to join unions when they feel the need to voice concerns and complaints to management without fear of jeopardizing their jobs. Other motivations for forming unions include job stress, abusive or neglectful management, and physical demands or hazards encountered in the work environment.

Many nurse managers believe that it is best to deal quickly and effectively with work-related issues as they arise, thus avoiding the necessary formalities of the collective bargaining process, with their added costs to the hospital, and the possibility that further restrictions might be imposed on managers. A new nurse or a nurse changing his or her place of employment should review any union contract as part of their orientation.

Often nurses' attraction to union power is prompted by the failure of the organization to lead employees and protect their rights. Issues that are commonly the subject of collective bargaining include wages, work environment, workload, job dissatisfaction, and nurse turnover (Arnold, Blankenship, & Hess, 2017).

If Your Workforce Unionizes

The process of forming a collective bargaining unit and negotiating a contract may take anywhere from 3 months to 3 years. A collective bargaining agent is an agent that works on behalf of employees to formalize collective bargaining through unionization. An example of steps to follow in organizing a local unit of a labor union is presented in Table 21.7.

Table 21.7   Steps in Organizing a Collective Bargaining Unit

How to form a union	
Step 1	Nurses that are interested in forming a union need to come together and discuss the interest.
Step 2	Have the group meet with a union organizer to understand the union, to help strategize and organize.
Step 3	Build internal support for the union by sharing information from the organizer with other nurses.
Step 4	Illustrate support by an election or vote to determine if the majority is interested. Once majority is determined, leaders may be chosen and a contract negotiated.

Source: Adapted from 4 Steps to Form a Union: AFL-CIO. (n.d.). Retrieved February 24, 2020, from https://aflcio.org/formaunion/4-steps-form-union

The manager's role in collective bargaining is complex, because the manager could find themselves working with as many as eight different contracts for various categories of employees. The unionization process may result in increased costs for the hospital and may limit the authority of its managers. Table 21.8 lists some ways managers can legally respond to a call for collective bargaining (National Labor Relations Board, 2018).

Nurses wishing to organize for the purpose of collective bargaining must be sure they carefully follow the laws pertaining to unionization. It is important to carefully select the collective bargaining agent. It is useful to find out about the former success of the union, details of how nurses will be supported, and where and how the union dues are spent. Spend time talking to other nurses in union settings to see how their contract is structured and if collective bargaining has helped with the issues that led them to unionize in the first place. Table 21.9 lists suggestions for the nurse during the process of unionization (NLRB, 2018).

Table 21.8 A Manager's Role During a Unionization Drive

Do:

- Know the law; make sure the rights of nurses as well as the rights of management are clearly understood.
- Act clearly within the law, no matter what the organization delegates to you as manager.

Don't:

- Threaten employees with loss of jobs or benefits if they join or vote for a union or engage in protected activity.
- Threaten to close the hospital if employees select a union to represent them.
- Question employees about their union sympathies or activities in ways that tend to interfere with, restrain or coerce employees in the exercise of their rights under the NLRA.
- Promise benefits to employees to discourage their union support.
- Transfer, lay off, terminate, assign employees more difficult work tasks, or otherwise punish employees because they engage in union activity.
- Transfer, lay off, terminate, assign employees more difficult work tasks, or otherwise punish employees because they file unfair labor practice charges or participate in an investigation conducted by NLRB.

Source: Data from National Labor Relations Board (2018). Employer/union rights and obligations.

Table 21.9 A Nurse's Role During a Unionization Drive

Do:

- Know your legal rights and the rights of the manager.
- Act clearly within the law at all times.
- Report to the NLRB if a manager acts unlawfully, such as firing an employee for organizing.
- Keep all nurses informed with regular meetings held close to the hospital.
- Set meeting times conveniently around shift changes and assist with child care during meetings.

Source: National Labor Relations Board (2018).

Nursing Collective Bargaining Agents

Many unions act as collective bargaining agents for millions of workers, including nurses, other health care workers, laborers, and specially trained workers such as actors and fire fighters in the United States. Some examples include: The Teamsters Union; the General Service Employees Union; the National Union of Hospital and Health Care Employees; the **Service Employees International Union** (**SEIU**); the United Autoworkers of America; and the United Steelworkers of America. The two most recognized national associations that have served as collective bargaining agents for registered nurses include the ANA and NNU. Another powerful union with nurses as a small part of their membership is the SEIU.

The ANA represents the nation's entire RN population, whether they are members or not. The ANA no longer considers itself a collective bargaining agent but remains a staunch public advocate for all nurses. The ANA's mission is "Nurses advancing our profession to improve health for all" (ANA, 2018). The ANA represents the interests of nurses in healthy work environments and in unhealthy areas as well. The ANA advances the nursing profession by fostering high standards for nursing practice and lobbies Congress and regulatory agencies on health care issues affecting nurses and the general public. The ANA initiates many policies involving health care reform. It also publishes its positions on issues ranging from whistle-blowing to patients' rights. The ANA recently launched a major campaign to mobilize nurses to address the staffing crisis, to educate and gain support from the public, and to develop and implement initiatives designed to resolve the staffing crisis. ANA has created the National Database of Nursing Quality Indicators (NDNQI) that helps show, with the use of data, the link between nursing care and patient health. The American Nurses Credentialing Center, a subsidiary of the ANA, created the Magnet Recognition Program to recognize health care organizations that provide the very best in nursing care. Since 1994, more than 480 organizations have received this award (ANA, 2018). ANA's Bill of Rights for Registered Nurses supports workplace advocacy, asserting that nurses have the right to negotiate employment terms and conditions, and to have letters of employment that set forth wages, work schedules, how work performance will be evaluated, and orientation information. In addition to union advocacy, ANA points out that non-union employees, as a group, may advocate employment concerns, and that the principles contained in the Bill of Rights for Registered Nurses are applicable to group negotiations.

In 1995, the CNA separated from the ANA at a time when CNA was pushing for laws mandating safe patient to nurse staffing ratios. In 2009, CNA, the National Nurses Organizing Committee, the Massachusetts Nurses Association, and United American Nurses formed NNU to represent their common interests on a national level. NNU is the only exclusively nurses' union that is affiliated with the American Federation of Labor and Congress of Industrial Organizations (AFL-CIO). NNU represents more than 150,000 nurses through collective bargaining in 15 states. It is also a professional association of registered nurses (National Nurses United, 2018). Its goal is for nurses to improve practice and have a greater voice in decisions that affect patient safety. NNU is considered to be an aggressive union that has initiated and supported striking for nurses' rights.

Managing in a Union Environment

Managers are well advised to work with the union to enforce rules within the context of contract agreements. In some ways,

Evidence from the Literature

Citation: The Pros and Cons of Joining a Nurses Union. 2016. Nurse Advisor. Available at, http://nurseadvisormagazine.com/tn-exclusive/the-pros-and-cons-of-joining-a-nurses-union, retrieved September 24, 2019.

Discussion: This article discusses the pros and cons of joining a nursing union. According to the U.S. Bureau of Labor Statistics in 2016, only 18% of RNs belong to a union.

The **Pros are:**

- **Better Pay:** Some sources claim that unionized nurses can earn from $200 to $400 more per week than nurses who don't belong to a union.
- **Job Security**: Union contracts often forbid cuts in hours and employment and forbid the dismissal of employees for arbitrary reasons. Some union contracts also feature guaranteed pay raises.
- **Improved Workplace Conditions**: Most unions fight for the improvement of the conditions in the workplace, including better nurse-to-patient ratios, better safety protocols, access to appropriate safety and hygiene equipment, and the dismissal of mandatory overtime.
- **Legal Representation**: Unions often provide representation to address grievances for when a nurse is mistreated, either physically or verbally, in the workplace.

Cons

- **Union Fees**: Most unions charge a percentage of the nurse's salary as "union dues" for their representations.
- **Job Risks**: Some employers do everything in their power to dismiss an employee for joining or trying to organize a union, which is illegal but difficult to prove. Also, if the union calls for a strike, the nurse is at risk of being permanently replaced by other individuals willing to cross the picket line.
- **Unpaid Strikes**: Whenever a union calls for a strike, the nurse is forced to skip work without pay, though a few unions have a strike fund for when this happens.
- **Difficult to Remove Troublesome Employees**: It's particularly difficult to fire an underperforming unionized employee due to their contracts.
- **Seniority-based Promotions**: In most cases, unionized workers are promoted due to their seniority, instead of their performance.

Nursing Implications:

It is important for the beginning nurse to know the pros and cons of unions when making a decision whether to join or not.

Evidence from the Literature

Citation: Wenzler, D. T. (2015). *Magnet Recognition Program®* *Status: Impact on HCAHPS Patient Satisfaction*. Retrieved December 10, 2018 from https://idea.library.drexel.edu/islandora/object/idea%3A6569

Discussion: This dissertation study examined the relationship between hospital recognition by the **American Nursing Credentialing Center (ANCC)** Magnet Recognition Program and patient satisfaction scores on the **Hospital Consumer Assessment of Health Care Providers and Systems (HCAHPS)**. The study found a significant relationship between Magnet status and patient satisfaction as measured by response to the question "Would you recommend this hospital to your friends and family?"

Implications for Practice: This study reinforces the idea that nurses have a significant impact on patient satisfaction. Nurses on units scoring higher inpatient satisfaction can describe the features of the patient care model, leveraging inter-professional relationships, being patient advocates, and exercising autonomy in practice. These qualities are the drivers of positive scores on the HCAHPS patient satisfaction survey items, e.g., "Willingness to recommend the hospital to family and friends." Nursing leaders should monitor these items and educate nurses about the components of patient satisfaction surveys for their units. Regular discussions, huddles, and patient care rounding should be implemented to discuss patient satisfaction as a measure of quality. Nurses need to incorporate patient- and family-centered care into their daily management of patients.

managing after a union is in place is less difficult because of the explicit language in most union contracts that provides a supportive structure for decision-making. Corrective actions, rules concerning allowed absences, etc. are agreed upon, voted on, and documented in the union contract.

Nurses may experience a conflict between their identity as a professional and their needs as a represented union employee. When analyzing nursing's status as a profession, nurses agree that specialized education and a service orientation are necessary to become a nurse, but nurses disagree on the extent to which they have sufficient autonomy in their practice. Many

nurses argue that autonomy cannot be achieved as individuals, and therefore unionization is necessary. Other nurses see the raw use of power for work stoppages or strikes as antithetical to a service orientation. The debate about whether it is professional to be a part of a nurses' union continues.

The Future of Nursing: Leading Change, Advancing Health

The Robert Wood Johnson Foundation (RWJF) partnered with the Institute of Medicine (IOM) in 2010 and released a Report on The Future of Nursing: Leading Change, Advancing Health

(Institute of Medicine, 2011). This Report offered a series of recommendations to advance nursing's contributions to the health care environment. Following this report, the American Association of Retired Persons (AARP) and RWJF launched the Future of Nursing: Campaign for Action to shepherd the implementation of the Report's recommendations. The Future of Nursing: Campaign for Action coordinated through the Center to Champion Nursing in America (CCNA), works nationally and through state Action Coalitions to advance its goals. The Future of Nursing: Campaign for Action Dashboard 2017 yearly progress report on the 2010 IOM Recommendations on The Future of Nursing: Leading Change, Advancing Health Report notes the following progress on the goals:

- Goal: Increase the proportion of nurses with a Baccalaureate Degree to 80% by 2020. 2017 Dashboard reports 56% of employed nurses hold a Baccalaureate (or higher) Degree in nursing.

- Goal: Double the number of nurses with a doctorate by 2020. 2017 Dashboard reports 28,004 employed nurses have a doctoral degree

- Goal: Advanced Practice Registered Nurses should be able to practice to the full extent of their education and training. 2017 Dashboard reports Advanced Practice Registered Nurses are able to practice to the full extent of their education and training in approximately one-third of U.S. states.

- Goal: Expand opportunities for nurses to lead and disseminate collaborative improvement effort. Unfortunately, the 2017 Dashboard reports the number of health professions courses that include both RN students and graduate students of other health professions has decreased.

- Goal: Health care decision-makers should ensure leadership positions are available to and filled by nurses. 2017 Dashboard reports 6,532 nurses have reported serving on non-Nursing Boards

(Future of Nursing: Action Dashboard, available at, https://campaignforaction.org/wp-content/uploads/2019/07/Dashboard-Indicator-Updates_7.9.19.pdf, and The Nurses on Boards Coalition, available at www.nursesonboardscoalition.org).

Advocacy and Politics

Advocacy is the process of exercising voice to communicate issues of concern and the need for action. Advocacy promotes both self-interest and the interest of others, whether in the work setting, throughout the organization, or in the larger society.

Politics is the process of forming alliances, exercising power and protecting and advancing particular ideas or goals. Generally, this includes anything affecting one's daily life, such as the way an office or household is managed, or how one person or group exercises influence over another. Politics

inherently involves the use of power at various levels of competition, negotiation, and collaboration for getting what is needed to achieve desired outcomes, as well as to protect and enhance the interests of patients, groups, and individuals.

Politics exist because resources are limited, and some people control more resources than others. Resources include people, money, facilities, technology, and rights to properties, services, and technologies. Power is itself a limited resource, but it can be increased. Politically empowered individuals, groups, or organizations have the ability to provide or control the distribution of desirable resources. The consumer movement in health care is a political movement to improve health care resources and health care outcomes. It reflects consumer perceptions and values, and influences patient care delivery.

In the public arena of politics, nurses are the largest health care group and need to be politically active for the good of patients and the overall viability of the health care system. A major force intersecting with nursing politics is the consumer movement in health care. Nurses can exercise political power to advance nursing services and give all patients and potential patients a stronger voice as informed consumers of their health care. Nurses are encouraged to develop strong political skills and partner with their professional nursing organization and consumer groups to take the lead in improving health care.

Nurse as Advocate

Nurse advocates speak out from a desire to have a say within their work setting for patient welfare as well as for themselves. Nurse advocates study the issues, garner political support, and contact policy makers such as the chairperson of the hospital board or key legislators through phone calls, letters, and e-mail messages. Nurses join professional organizations and actively participate to ensure a more collective, unified voice that supports health care issues and policies that have value for consumers and nursing. Nurse advocates who are most involved will be seen supporting political activities and candidates, assisting during political campaigns, helping to draft legislation, and even running for political office.

Nurses enter the nursing profession with a certain amount of credibility by virtue of their education and training. This credibility is symbolized by the nursing license. To do their job well, nurses need the greater power that comes with credibility. To increase their credibility, effective nurses demonstrate professional competence. Nurses who are most effective assert professional credibility in several ways. They are lifelong learners and grow professionally throughout their careers in nursing. They approach their vocation as a mission of service to the public and to the nursing profession, and as an honorable way to make a living. These nurses take ownership of situations in which they find themselves and work to resolve problems and overcome obstacles to providing the best possible patient care. Nurses strengthen their position on the job by sharing accountability for health care problems with other health care providers. Pointing fingers at others, such as supervisors, administrators, politicians, or practitioners, for health care problems, or looking to others for solutions, only serves to weaken nurses' power.

Nursing's accountability to the public is part of its professional responsibility. This means that nurses must work closely with colleagues to assure quality care as patient advocates. Patient advocacy includes preserving and protecting the ability of patients to make decisions regarding their care. Patients look to nurses for this kind of advocacy, but in the workplace, nurses are often too busy to serve as a patient advocate, which causes both nurses and patients distress.

Nurses in many hospitals serve on professional practice councils. These councils may be part of a shared governance organization within the hospital that works to improve patient care and the work environment of staff. (See Chapter 5, Organization and Staffing of Patient Care at the Unit Level.)

Workplace advocacy refers to the actions nurses take to address problems or make changes in their everyday workplace setting. This type of advocacy is probably the most common in nursing. Many workplace advocacy issues involve patient care, but some of these issues involve working conditions. Examples of workplace advocacy include forming a committee to address problems in the assignment of work, devising alternatives to achieve optimal care, and coming up with new ways to improve clinical practice. Note that a supportive management will view workplace advocacy as a means of strengthening staff and promoting teamwork. An authoritarian management, however, may prefer rigid adherence to policy, and thus would not be likely to encourage workplace advocacy. As patient advocates, nurses protect patients from known harm. Nurses may become aware of procedural or legal violations that endanger public health or safety or result in health care fraud. However, some nurses who are aware of such wrongdoing do nothing because of fear of retribution. Fraud and other instances of wrongdoing are costly to health care payers and ultimately the taxpayer.

Within the workplace, nurses who can effectively compete, negotiate, and collaborate with others to get what they want or need develop and use strong political skills. They have the greatest ability to build strong bases of support for themselves, patients, and the nursing profession. Nurses consistently are rated number one in consumer opinion polls asking who are considered to be the most trusted professionals (https://news.gallup.com/poll/245597/nurses-again-outpace-professions-honesty-ethics.aspx, accessed May 9, 2019). Nurses can garner consumer support for professional nursing positions to help patients and in the process help the profession of nursing by tapping into this strong support.

Patient and Consumer Advocacy

From the beginning of the profession, nurses have served as patient advocates. This role of nurse as patient advocate has changed as the profession of nursing and society itself have evolved, and nurses act more proactively today, operating within an assertive framework of expertise to ensure respect for the rights of patients as directors of their own care. Advocacy can now be seen as representing patient needs to others in the health care organization or interpreting the health care environment for patients. There is, therefore, a strong argument that advocacy means increasing patient power both as an individual and as a consumer force to be reckoned with, rather than coping with lack of power or vulnerability, as some authors have implied (Choi et al., 2014). For this reason, if a nurse is to act as a patient advocate, interpret the health care environment to the patient, and guide the patient through the health care maze, the nurse needs to know the health care system.

Sometimes advocating for a patient's rights places a nurse in conflict with another health care provider or the organization as a whole. This can be risky for the nurse. Nurses must therefore acquire the necessary power to take on such risk. Entry-level nurses benefit from the modeling of expert nurses and the support of team-based learning approaches to successfully act as patient advocates.

Historically, patients have been assigned the role of passive recipient of health care, but with the consumer movement, this patient-provider relationship is changing. No longer do health care providers have a monopoly on all the answers. Information is readily available through Internet resources. Three examples are Healthline (www.healthline.com), PubMed (www.ncbi.nlm.nih.gov/pubmed, and WebMD (www.webMD.com). These resources have facilitated the move from patient passive recipient to patient as active consumer of health. Patients with chronic diseases can become active members in organizations that educate and advocate for those with the disease. In addition to greater understanding of health care and its risks, consumers increasingly expect greater involvement in health care decisions. But there remain challenges. Federal regulations defining a patient's right to access their health data has failed to ensure access. Although the Health Insurance Portability and Accountability Act (HIPAA) requires health care organizations to provide patients with access to any data that are "readily producible," organizations have been slow to respond, some ironically citing HIPAA patient privacy requirements as a reason. More remains to be done to take advantage of the capabilities of available technology. Silicon Valley has initiated some efforts. For example, Apple (HealthKit) provides a simple interface for computer devices under patients' control; We Are Curious is a company that creates communities of people seeking answers to health questions such as "How much sleep is the right amount for me?" or "Which diet gives me sufficient energy and keeps me at a healthy weight?" Amazon, Microsoft, and Alphabet (Google) are collaborating with health care systems to store data in the cloud so patients can access and share medical records, especially between providers (Mandl & Kohane 2016).

Evidence from the Literature

Citation: McDonald, L. (2018). Florence Nightingale, Nursing, and Health Care Today (2018). New York: Springer Publishing Co. LLC.

Discussion: The purpose of this historical research on the work of Florence Nightingale is to illuminate her work as a social reformer of a public health system. She advocated health promotion and disease prevention based on evidence. Nightingale extended the use of nurses that she had trained in hospitals to the care of the poor in what were termed workhouses. She not only placed nurses in these workhouses, but she lobbied powerful key figures for passage of laws for the poor. She persuaded these key figures to support her ideas for reform. Due to her hard work, the Metropolitan Poor Bill was passed by Parliament in 1867 and was followed by other reforms that improved the lot of poor people in Britain. Nightingale was able to obtain the support of powerful and influential people due to her meticulous attention to detail and careful, methodical preparation. Nightingale used what is now dubbed "Nightingale methodology." First, study the best information in print, especially government reports and statistics.

Second, interview experts, and if the available information is inadequate, survey others with a questionnaire. When you have a proposed plan, test it at one institution, consult with the practitioners that implemented it, and send out the draft reports for comment before sending the final report out for publication and dissemination to the influential. She was ahead of her time in setting out core principles of the nursing profession, including setting high ethical standards and promoting continuing education to maintain professional practice knowledge and skills.

Implications for Practice: New nurses often believe that their responsibilities begin and end at the bedside. But historical research demonstrates that from the very beginning of modern nursing, nurses have not only given care but partnered with others to influence public opinion and to change legislation for the benefit of the health care consumer, especially the vulnerable—the poor, the mentally ill, soldiers, and children. As a new nurse, view yourself as a patient advocate who is willing to join with others through professional associations or consumer groups to improve health care and the system within which it is delivered.

Critical Thinking 21.3

Political conflict occurs when people hold significantly different or conflicting opinions about any policy issue. Consumers often disagree about what health care should be, who should provide it, how much it should cost, and/or who should pay for it. As a new nurse, you have a professional responsibility to promote consumer dialogue and offer creative, thoughtful, and evidence-based solutions to health care problems. But nurses may disagree with one another on some of the same issues consumers have about health care.

What do you think your responsibility is as a consumer of health care?

What is your responsibility as a health care provider?

Can your responsibility as a consumer sometimes conflict with your responsibility as a provider?

Give an example of such a conflict.

Health Care Consumer as Partner

Informed consumers are important partners with nurses in ensuring safe care. Efforts to elicit effective participation by patients in health care are called by many names, including patient-centered, patient engagement, and patient experience. Such improvement initiatives often resemble the efforts of manufacturers to engage consumers in designing and marketing products. Health care services, however, are fundamentally different from other products. They are "coproduced" by both clinician and patient, who work together on patient outcomes (Batalden, Batalden, Margolis, Seid, & Armstrong, 2015). Failure to recognize this unique character of a health care service and its implications could limit nurses' success in partnering with patients to improve health care. Coproduction is a model of health care service, with specific roles, relationships, and aims of interdependent work. Implications and challenges exist for patients and health care professional development, for service delivery system design, and for understanding and measuring benefit in health care services.

Working through their professional organizations, nurses collaborate with consumer groups by creating formal partnerships that promote the role of nurses as consumer advocates in health policy arenas and strengthen the political position of both partners. These partnerships create a stronger political voice than either group has alone. The partners gain power when interacting with any policy-making body, because they represent: (a) a larger voting block (a group that represents the same political position or perspective); (b) a broader funding base (a source of financial support); and (c) a stronger political voice (an increase in the number of voices supporting or opposing an issue). Increasingly, professional organizations in nursing recognize the value of partnering with consumers to build a better health care system.

In a coproduction service model of health care practice, good outcomes are more likely if:

• The patient can and does seek and receive help in a timely way;

- The clinician and patient communicate effectively;

- They develop a shared understanding of the health care problem; and

- They generate a mutually acceptable evaluation and management health care plan.

Since both patients and health care professionals are responsible for coproduced outcomes, health outcomes are a result of the dispositions, competencies, and actions of both parties (Batalden, Batalden, Margolis, Seid, & Armstrong, 2015).

Consumer demands also affect nurse advocacy. Increasingly, consumers are becoming more educated. As discussed earlier, we have more access to information via various media (radio, television, print), but especially the Internet. Armed with information, consumers are demanding positive results and are holding those in the health care system accountable for better health care outcomes. If the trend toward increased litigation related to professional negligence and medical malpractice is any indication, just having an ethical process for providing care will not satisfy the consumer who experiences negative health outcomes. The strongest potential for litigation in health care comes from too few health care professionals accepting personal responsibility for ensuring that health care services are provided in a safe, competent manner, at a system level as well as at a personal level.

Interestingly, in a role reversal, some patients as consumers of health care have begun advocating for nurses. Perceiving nurses as overextended by the nature of the work environment, those patients have contended that something must be done to improve the working conditions of nursing. Nurses in California used consumer support to build the case for opposing significant staffing cuts affecting nursing practice in their state. With strong consumer support, California nurses in 1999 drafted a proposal that was enacted into state law, mandating a minimal staffing level of registered nurses per patient in acute care hospitals, the intent of which was to protect patients from dangerous staffing levels while receiving nursing services (Mark, Harless, Spetz, Reiter, & Pink, 2013).

Professional Associations as Advocates for Health Care Consumers

Nurses, working through professional organizations such as the ANA, have been strong, early supporters for patients' rights, regardless of the patient's ability to pay. In a 2016 document entitled ANA's Principles for Health System Transformation, (2016), the first principle advocates for universal access to a standard package of essential health care services for all citizens and residents. Other professional groups, such as the American Medical Association (AMA) and the American Hospital Association (AHA), have received far more media recognition for their support of patients' rights. This is an indication that the AMA and AHA are better funded, wield more political power, and may do a better job than the ANA in presenting their positions on consumer issues to the media. However, in 2008, a study of nursing's future conducted by the Institute of Medicine (now called the National Academies of Sciences, Engineering and Medicine), the future of nursing was described in which nurses are full partners, with physicians and other health care professionals, in redesigning health care in the United States. (IOM, 2008).

Any political vision to make health care more consumer friendly and service oriented must address cost, access, choice, and quality. Perhaps the vision starts with this formula: the highest quality of care for all people at the least cost. Yet defining, much less evaluating, quality is culturally bound and very complicated. Many people cannot afford minimal health care services. Other people are increasingly unwilling to subsidize the care of other patients by paying increased costs for their health care.

Most people understand that responsibility requires being held accountable for one's behavior, decisions, and affiliations with others. Like all professions, nursing engages in a social contract, with society giving nurses certain recognition and privileges and requiring in return that nursing be accountable to the public (ANA, 2018). Individual nurse practice acts of each state address these concepts.

Stakeholders and Health Care

A vision for high-quality, low-cost care is spread among a number of vested interest groups, or stakeholders, such as patients, nursing and medical practitioners, administrators, pharmacists, physical therapists, dieticians, pharmaceutical and insurance companies, and so on, collaborating with one another to develop a workable philosophy, to include a mechanism for checks and balances to minimize abuse and misuse, and to encourage intelligent, ethical decisions on behalf of patients by those wielding the most political power.

Similarly, control of health care resources has multiple stakeholders. Everyone is a stakeholder in health care at some level, but some people are far more politically active about their stake in health care than others. Lobbyists represent these stakeholder groups, including insurance companies, consumer groups, professional organizations such as the ANA, and other health care groups such as nursing and medical practitioners, pharmacists, dieticians, physical therapists, administrators, and educational groups. Stakeholders exert political pressure on health care policymakers—local, state, and federal legislative bodies—in an effort to make the health care system work to the economic advantage of the stakeholders.

The vigilance of government, payers, and even attorneys regarding health care is understandable. Some health care providers focus on "What's good for my agency, good for my interest group, or good for me?" rather than on "What is going to work for the patients and all the other health care stakeholders over the long run?"

When such health care stakeholders are motivated and directed solely by their own perceived needs, competitive political strategies replace more collaborative approaches to addressing the consumer's health care needs. Accountability becomes a serious issue, because the goal of overtaking the

Critical Thinking 21.4

Consider these health care stakeholders:

- Patients
- Insurance companies
- State health authority
- Hospital administrators
- Hospital staff nurses
- Nurse aides
- Medical practitioners
- Nurse practitioners
- Pharmacists
- Dieticians
- Physical therapists
- Social workers

How might each of these stakeholders see the importance of efficient, high-quality care to patients on a clinical unit?

Identify how each of them might define the need for patient access to services differently?

Who will pay for such care?

Of the following, who will be in favor of payment: Insurance company? Patient? Unemployed person? Taxpayer?

Case Study 21.2

Juan and Casey are study partners in the final semester of a nursing program. Juan has served as a medical corpsman and worked as an emergency medical technician for several years, whereas Casey entered college right out of high school, starting as a business major. One of their class assignments is to develop a strategy for reducing malpractice risks in a hospital setting. Casey proposes redefining the patient as the customer of health care services, arguing that adopting a more customer-oriented approach to health care services in hospitals would improve patient satisfaction and subsequently reduce malpractice claims. He adds that in interviews conducted with residents at a senior rehab center about their experience in health care facilities, they complained about not being treated as an adult, being called by their first name, and similar slights that communicate a patronizing institutional bias against the elderly and a lack of consumer-orientation exhibited

by providers' in the system. Juan opposes this customer-oriented strategy. He thinks that health care providers are just adopting the culture of corporate America when they define patients as customers. He believes patients should be treated as something more than customers. He also argues that patients do not know what is best for them in most health care situations.

Do you think patients should be defined as health care customers?

How would you help Juan and Casey seek agreement by reconsidering each of their arguments, acknowledging its valid points from one perspective but considering it from another viewpoint?

How can both arguments be used to improve the overall patient experience?

competition supersedes the goal of offering the highest-quality services. People who will own the future of health care must address this growing problem of accountability. They will have to establish and sustain their credibility during a time when more people are distrustful of the health care system, its providers, insurance companies, other third-party payers, and legislators.

The Politics of Health Care

Health care in the United States depends on a continuous and growing supply of resources from both the public and private sectors and stimulates competition for such resources with other priorities. Such resources include people, such as the providers of health care services, and the money to pay for these people, as well as pay for facilities, technology, administration, and equipment, among others. With health care requiring so many resources on such a large economic scale, thousands of people in and out of government are involved in resource allocation—hence, the politics of health care. Most people have good intentions, but many of these people often disagree about how resources can best be acquired and distrib-

uted to support health care.

The public is aware that access to health care resources may not continue to meet their health care needs, especially as they age and become more dependent on related services. They are often frightened by media reports of increasing health care expenditures. Although most consumers of health care do not directly pay for the majority of their health care costs, their portion of health care expenses incurred as individuals is rapidly increasing.

Health policy is formulated, enacted, and enforced through political processes at the local, state, or federal levels. For example, at the local level, policies are established and implemented by an individual hospital's leadership or by management of a regional health care system regarding whether or when flu injections are made available to high-risk populations. At the state level, policies affect nurses by defining nursing practice, nursing education, and nursing licensure. These policies are often governed by a state nurse practice act designating a state nursing commission or health professions board as the administrative authority for enforcing these policies. Federal policies are evident in the rules and regulations governing Medicare and Medicaid funding, and other health insurance policies such as those resulting from the **Affordable Care Act** (**ACA**). All these examples of health policy and resources accentuate the need for nurses to be tuned in politically.

Nursing's Role in Health Care Policy

Advocacy enters the formal world of politics as the setting for health care advocacy expands, and the need increases. Nurses must therefore set political goals as individual nurses, nurse citizens, nurse activists, and nurse politicians for the future (Table 21.10). Many nurses want to avoid the political nature of their work, believing that a human service like health care should not be impacted by politics. They may also ignore the business aspects of health care until they find themselves in a leadership position responsible for a budget. But all health care is inextricably linked to politics and economics as well as to accessibility of health services and providers. As a human service, health care has yielded remarkable returns in terms of improving overall quality of life as well as in extending life spans. As a business, health care affords millions of people, including nurses, with economic opportunities and lifelong careers.

Entering health care politics need not be complicated. When bills affecting health care are initiated in state and federal legislative bodies, nurses should learn about these bills, obtaining copies and studying them. In this very practical way, nurses add to their political knowledge base with regard to health care policy and can enter the politics of health care policy.

Ultimately, health care is defined and controlled by those wielding the most political influence. If nurses fail to participate in the process and exert political pressure on health care policymakers, they inevitably lose ground to others who are more politically active. It is unrealistic to believe that other stakeholders will take care of interests advocated by nursing as competition for health care resources increases. Historically, some stakeholders in health care have never supported nursing as a profession or even acknowledged a professional role for nurses. Therefore, like other health care providers, nurses must compete, negotiate, and collaborate with others to ensure the future of health care includes nursing interests and concerns.

Table 21.10   Political Roles for Nurses

Role	Activities	Example
Nurse individual	• Highlights important role of nurse to prevent nursing-sensitive outcomes, for example, pneumonia, cardiac arrest, and so on • Sets goals to strengthen nursing as a profession. Participates in local and state professional meetings. Obtains certification in nursing specialty areas • Highlights the essential dimensions of nursing (Table 21.11) • Participates as a member in health care consumer groups, for example, the AARP, and so on	**You**—as a new graduate have a political role as a nurse individual
Nurse citizen	• Votes and writes members of Congress and state legislators on issues of interest • Educates patients on how to evaluate Website sources of health care information	**You**—as a new graduate have a political role as a nurse citizen. Be informed, vote, and participate
Nurse activist	• Participates as a member of a professional organization that lobbies and influences state and federal legislation • Notifies hospital Board of Trustees of any quality issues	**Mary Wakefield, RN, PhD**—Dr. Wakefield was an advocate for rural health care. She was appointed as Administrator for Health Resources and Services Administration (*HRSA*) by President Barack Obama from 2009 to 2015 and acting United States Deputy Secretary of Health and Human Services from 2015 to 2017. (www.grandforksherald.com/news/4189928-devils-lake-native-mary-wakefield-looks-life-after-top-dc-job, accessed December 10, 2018)
Nurse politician	• Runs for a political office and serves society as a whole • Collaborates with other health care professionals to improve care at the local/state	**Lois Capps, RN, MA**—Congresswoman Capps was first sworn into Congress in 1998. She represented California's 24th Congressional District from 1998 to 2017. She spent her life working to improve access to quality health care. Her experiences as a registered nurse influenced her as she played a key role in many of the major health policy debates in Congress (https://en.wikipedia.org/wiki/Lois_Capps accessed December 10, 2018)

Source: Richard J. Maloney & Patsy L. Maloney.

Case Study 21.3

Sahra is a maternity support nurse for First Steps, a specific state-funded program designed to provide care to underserved and underinsured pregnant women. Sahra is in her third year of professional practice and has become highly resourceful and able to work in new situations with minimal supervision. Many of her patient case referrals come through a partnership with the local hospital's Teen Parent Resource Center, which targets girls under 20 who have dropped out of school during their pregnancy. Many of Sahra's patients are from families at high risk for domestic violence and substance abuse. Recently, Sahra was informed that the Teen Parent Resource Center will be discontinuing its partnership with First Steps because of funding issues.

> What does Sahra need to know to continue serving her high-risk population?
>
> What are her options?

Political Strategy for Nursing

The need for political strategy must be fully understood as nurses develop politically. The purpose of developing political strategy is to find different ways to achieve the goals one is advocating for, while identifying and working with the other stakeholders and their goals. Political strategy attempts to shape opinion, formulate a policy, or take action in support of a particular objective. To be feasible, a political strategy requires commitment and awareness of the needs of other stakeholders. Effective political strategy involves considerable forethought and clarity of purpose in even the most ambiguous situations. Nurses who are most likely to wield political influence operate with strategy in mind before taking political action, such as voicing concerns, making demands, or advocating for others.

Every nurse should be cognizant of what other involved groups think regarding any relevant political health issue. It is also essential to study political issues and major stakeholders' positions prior to becoming involved, then to seek opportunities for collaboration with potential allies on common goals. It is important that nurses listen to other policy perspectives and understand as many facets of an issue as possible when making health policy proposals. Proposals should include purpose, rationale, arguments in favor, and carefully crafted responses to opposing views. This reduces the amount of unnecessary political fights and encourages more collaboration with other political groups prior to submitting any policy proposal to policymakers. The more support obtained from the various stakeholders in any policy arena, the better chance that a workable health care policy will be developed and implemented.

To be most effective politically, nurses must be able to clearly explain nursing to any audience or stakeholder: what nursing is; why nursing is important to society; what distinctive services nurses provide; how nursing benefits consumers, including the prevention of nursing-sensitive outcomes such as pneumonia, cardiac arrest, and so on; and what nursing services cost in relation to other health care services. Although anecdotal stories and emotional appeals may be effective with certain audiences, it is far more powerful to present research-based evidence to support the political positions of nursing professionals. Table 21.10 details political roles for nurses, while Table 21.11 describes the essential dimensions of nursing, including influencing public policy for social justice.

Table 21.11   Essential Dimensions of Nursing

- Providing a caring relationship that enhances healing and health
- Focusing on the full range of experiences and human responses to illness and health within both physical and social environments
- Appreciating the subjective experience and the integration of such experience with objective data
- Diagnosing and intervening in care by using scientific knowledge, judgment, and critical thinking
- Advancing nursing knowledge through scholarly inquiry
- Influencing social and public policy to promote social justice
- Assuring safe, quality, and evidence-based care

Source: Richard J. Maloney & Patsy L. Maloney.

Changes in Patient Population

Certainly not all consumers of health care agree about what health care should be, who should provide it, and how it should be paid for. The social, cultural, economic, psychological, and demographic characteristics of consumers largely determine their attitudes and inclination toward the health care system, its providers, and its services. Consumers experience some level of personal risk when changes are made in the health care system, especially changes involving payment for services and providers. If consumers such as elderly persons perceive that their out-of-pocket cost for health care will extend beyond their capacity to pay or will increase in the future, they are highly motivated to exert political pressure on policymakers to reverse the perceived trend.

The fastest-growing consumer group now and for years to come is the elderly—persons 65 and older (Colby & Ortman, 2018). An estimated 51 million Americans turned 65 by 2017. The number of elderly people (65 years of age and older) is growing at an explosive rate and is expected to reach 87 million by 2050 (Colby & Ortman, 2018). People over age 50 control approximately one-half of the country's disposable income as well as three-quarters of its financial assets and 80% of its savings. Yet most elderly Americans are not wealthy. Over 7 million elderly are projected to qualify for Medicaid benefits as of 2020 (Medicaid.gov, 2020).

Without doubt, this aging of the U.S. population will profoundly affect health care at every level. Studies of voting behavior of U.S. citizens show that the elderly have no predictable political orientation toward anything except obvious threats to their perceived entitlements such as Medicare or Social Security, the most widely recognized entitlement being Social Security benefits.

Many elderly persons join consumer groups to have a greater political voice, most hoping to influence health policy decisions so that they receive the health care services they will need in the future. A growing number fight social isolation, a historically prominent and persistent problem, through involvement in consumer groups and the Internet. In this way, they establish closer contact with the outside world and strengthen their relationships with other health care stakeholders.

The AARP (formerly known as the American Association of Retired Persons), with more than 15 million members, constitutes a growing political powerhouse and potential consumer partner for nursing in many ways. A large percentage of nurses are 50 years of age or older and qualify for membership in the AARP. Because of growth in the population of their members, few other consumer groups appear to have the potential that the AARP has for defining the health care system of the future.

Not all involved in health care represent the interests of consumers, who have an arguably dominant role in health care politics. This situation exists for a variety of reasons. Some contend that consumers do not necessarily know what is best for them. They say that health care experts such as nursing and medical practitioners are better able to direct health care policy. Others maintain that only those who pay for the services should make policy decisions, that health care is not necessarily a right, and that health care services should be based on ability to pay. There is evidence that when informed of the goal of health reform efforts to contain costs, people are more likely to agree that cost information should be a significant factor in decision-making by providers, or patients themselves, about treatment. Significantly influencing the development of trust in such decisions is the degree of transparency of information that enables the patient to become a knowledgeable consumer (Richmond et al., 2017).

The need for greater transparency of information has led to increasing political activism by third-party payers, including the government, business, and health insurance companies. Exposure of Medicare/Medicaid fraud (e.g., billing for services that weren't provided in the form of phantom billing and upcoding; performing unnecessary tests; or giving unnecessary referrals) has led to questioning by many about the very nature of professional practice and the power society assigns to professionals.

Nurses have come to understand how the control and distribution of resources in health care can drastically affect their incomes, workloads, work environments, and patients. Nurses across the country have reported that patient load per nurse provider has increased significantly. However, without political influence, these nursing concerns do little to change health care at any level.

Nurses must work to strengthen the long tradition of pulling together various practitioners within health care: nurses and physicians, administrators, pharmacists, physical therapists, dieticians, and so on. The evolution of the role of nurse navigator, for example, empowers patients by coordinating inter-professional teams to work toward patient-centered care by giving patients timely, seamless, culturally appropriate guidance and support. Results include improvements in access, equity, efficiency, effectiveness, and sustainability of health services, particularly during transitions from acute to continuing care (McMurray & Cooper, 2017). Although unknown by many of today's practicing nurses, a tradition of practices similar to those of a nurse navigator began with Florence Nightingale and her "Nightingale Methodology" (McDonald, 2018). As discussed earlier, new nurses who recognize their critical role in addressing the major issues in health care delivery at the bedside will ensure that nursing enters into a partnership with hospital executives who have control in the wider health care system of which the hospital is a part. As partners, they can then compete, negotiate, and collaborate with other stakeholders at the system level to be more politically effective. These nurses must also be concerned with the price of health care at the system level and understand that resources are controlled and distributed through health policy decisions.

Nurses' involvement in political arenas such as policy-making committees and hospital boards of directors includes advocating for the recipients of health care when those in need have little or no voice and who need a stronger voice. The professional nurse should understand and be able to articulate the relevance of politics to nursing practice. Making a difference in health care arenas is the goal of political involvement in policy making. As Margaret Mead said, "Never doubt that a small group of thoughtful committed citizens can change the world, indeed it's the only thing that ever has."

The Problem of Health Care Reform

Health care in the United States is an issue of great concern to the public, and one that has been at center stage for national and state policy makers. It is one in which the nursing

Critical Thinking 21.5

Many hospitals have a Board of Directors, made up of key health care and community representatives. This Board of Directors exercises power and helps develop the goals for the hospital. Does your hospital have any nurses on its Board of Directors? Do your career goals include joining a Board of any hospital, nursing, or community Board of Directors?

profession not only has an interest but has special knowledge and a professional duty to express its views.

In the United States (U.S.), many stakeholders play a role in the political process affecting health care delivery. Increasing demand for reform has been prompted by many flaws in the U.S. health care system. A 2018 study published in the International Journal of Health Services found 28 million Americans uninsured and 18 million elderly adults with a gap in their coverage (Himmelstein, 2018). Millions more cannot afford high cost-sharing provisions in their health insurance policies. Only 19% of low income insured (less than $24,000 annual income) used any preventive care in 2017, compared with 38% of the wealthy (more than $70,000 income). Twenty three percent of seniors reported having "problems getting care because of costs."

Spending on health care in the U.S. is the highest in the world, yet is often rated lowest in quality among countries with advanced economies. The 2016 per capita health care expense was $8,788, while that of comparable countries is roughly half that amount. The three largest payers for health care remain Medicare for people age 65 and over and some people with disabilities (22.1%), Medicaid for people of all ages in need of public assistance (17.8%), and personal out-of-pocket (12.4%). Medicare alone enrolled more than 56 million Americans in 2016 (National Center for Health Statistics, 2018).

Health care expenditures are highly concentrated, with a tiny but expensive portion of the population, those who are chronically, seriously, or terminally ill, accounting for half of aggregate health care spending, while half of the population, healthy individuals with little current health care needs, account for a tiny portion of the total expense. This means that insurers' gains to be had from avoiding serving the sick greatly outweigh any possible gains from managing their care. As a consequence, insurers' resources have been devoted to such avoidance, which is in opposition to the interests of the insured (Blumberg & Holahan, 2017). An estimated 530,000 families turn to bankruptcy each year because of medical issues and bills (retrieved May 2019 from www.cnbc.com/2019/02/11/this-is-the-real-reason-most-americans-file-for-bankruptcy.html). The effect of insurance caps, exclusions, and inability to fund or continue **Consolidated Omnibus Budget Reconciliation Act** (**COBRA**) coverage led to their financial distress. Medical impoverishment is almost unheard of in other advanced countries, either because the state covers everyone, or everyone is obliged by law to have insurance.

Opinions regarding the U.S. insurance-based health care system have shifted, with 56% of physicians (up from 42% in 2008) favoring a single-payer system, and 62% of adults in the general population (up from 52% in early 2017) believing that health care coverage is "the responsibility of the Federal government" (Himmelstein, 2018). The underlying question in the debate on health care reform remains whether health care coverage should be viewed as a basic right (payable by society at large) or, on the opposite end of the continuum, a privilege (payable by the individual with or without the coverage of purchased insurance plans) (Bauchner, 2017) (Table 21.12).

The Patient Protection and Affordable Care Act

The Patient Protection and ACA was passed in 2010 with the intent of improving the health of the nation by increasing the number of insured and plugging holes in coverage for those who are underinsured. The ACA provided for the phased introduction over 4 years of a comprehensive system of expanded health insurance, including mandated insurance enrollment for all, with a penalty for anyone failing to buy insurance. Provisions were included to eliminate some of the worst practices of the insurance companies, including exclusion of those with existing preconditions, premium loading (additional cost added to premiums for higher-risk individuals to ensure profits for the insurance company), policy cancelation due to technicalities or when illness seems imminent, and annual or lifetime coverage caps. ACA also instituted a minimum ratio of direct health care spending to premium income, price competition through establishment of pools for the uninsured and underinsured, standard insurance coverage levels to enable like-for-like comparisons by consumers, and a web-based health insurance exchange where consumers could compare prices and purchase plans. The ACA preserved private insurance and private health care providers and provided government financed subsidies to enable the poor to buy insurance (Kantarjian, 2016).

Table 21.12 Selected History of Policy Actions to Reform Health Care

Date	Policy action
1965	Medicare, which covers both hospital and general medical insurance for people 65 or older and poor and certain younger people with disabilities, paid for by a Federal employment tax; and Medicaid, which permits the Federal Government to partially fund a health care program for the poor, with the program managed and co-financed by individual states.
1985	The Consolidated Omnibus Budget Reconciliation Act of 1985 (COBRA), which amended the Employee Retirement Income Security Act of 1974 (ERISA) to give some employees the ability to continue health insurance coverage after leaving employment.
1997	The State Children's Health Insurance Program (SCHIP) was established by the federal government in 1997 to provide health insurance to children in families at or below 200% of the federal poverty line.
2010	Patient Protection and Affordable Care Act

Source: Adapted from Kaiser Family Foundation. (2010). Timeline: History of Health Reform in the U.S. [Brochure]. Oakland, CA: Author. Retrieved 2010, from https://www.kff.org/wp-content/uploads/2011/03/5-02-13-history-of-health-reform.pdf

> ## Critical Thinking 21.6
>
> An entry-level nurse is empowered by not only by using information for providing patient care, but also by using information in areas beyond direct patient care. Think about the following for a new nurse involved with a committee:
>
> What is the committee trying to do?
>
> What specific information does the committee use to make decisions?
>
> How does the committee's work apply to the new nurse's practice, their colleagues, their patient care unit, and the organization as a whole?
>
> What is the strength of the information a new nurse has in relation to patients, colleagues, the patient care unit, and the organization as a whole?
>
> Is a new nurse serving on a committee readily sharing information (allowable by law) with others who will value it and use it to good end?

Attempts to repeal ACA include an effort early in 2017 to repeal and replace the original bill, then an attempt to pass a "repeal only" bill, which would be followed later by a replacement bill. Both attempts failed to win approval in Congress, but the Congress did repeal the unpopular individual mandate, which coerced individuals into buying insurance they did not want or did not think they needed. A report from the Urban Institute (Blumberg et al., 2017) shows that repeal of the ACA would result in more than a 100% increase in the number of uninsured, representing a nearly 30% increase in cost and the near collapse of the individual insurance market, those self-employed individuals or employees of small companies who do not have group purchasing power, such as is available to employees of large companies.

The Limits of Power

It would be naive to think that one can necessarily expect easy acceptance, understanding, or even support for what one is attempting to do. Machiavelli, an early authority on power, is reported to have said:

> *There is nothing more difficult to take in hand, more perilous to conduct than to take a lead in the introduction of a new order of things, because the innovation has for enemies all those who have done well under the old conditions, and lukewarm defenders in those who may do well under the new.*
> **(Machiavelli & Rebhorn, 2003)**

The nurse will do well to heed this warning. Machiavelli recognized that the power to innovate even small changes should be employed thoughtfully. Nurses should carefully study and understand power, how it is developed, and its uses, in order to accomplish and contribute what they can as a professional responsibility to society.

In summary, this chapter discussed the importance of nurses acquiring and wisely using power. We explored sources you can tap into and how power can benefit others—your patients, your colleagues, and society as a whole. As Gracian observed, you are and should be empowered to "do more good." Power is not used to lord over others, but to serve, to do good. Effective nurses understand, acquire, and use power at personal, professional, and organizational levels to ensure safe quality care. Now you may be tempted to ask "How can I as a new nurse do all this?" The answer is simple. It is your professional responsibility to make a difference, and you do this one step at a time. Begin by focusing on yourself; proceed to your work, you organization, your profession, and the society; one step at a time. You can do this.

KEY CONCEPTS

- Power can be described as the ability to get and use resources to achieve goals.

- Effective nurses understand power from multiple perspectives.

- Effective nurses have a positive orientation toward power and feel comfortable discussing the expert knowledge that nurses bring to patient care.

- Sources of power include expert, legitimate, referent, reward, coercive, connection, and information power.

- Power is used at personal, professional, and organizational levels.

- The personal power of effective nurses is evident in the decisions they make.

- Effective nurses increase their own power sources and use power for safe, competent care.

- Nurses have a critical role in addressing the major system-level issues in health care delivery.

- Collective bargaining through unionization is a collective action model that is formal and legally based. It uses a written contract to guide nursing and workplace issues.

- Political, economic, and social changes such as aging, cultural diversity, and the costs of technology and medications in the United States are transforming the health care system.

- When a consumer group forms a political coalition with other groups, such as nurses, in a given community, the political influence of both is strengthened.

- The ANA is a full-service professional organization that represents the nation's entire registered nurse population. The ANA is politically active and lobbies on issues affecting nursing and the general public.

KEY TERMS

Advocacy	Information power	Professional power
Coercive power	Legitimate power	Referent power
Collective bargaining	Organizational power	Reward power
Collective bargaining agent	Personal power	Union
Connection power	Politics	Workplace advocacy
Expert power	Power	

REVIEW QUESTIONS

1. Which of the following sources of power should a new nurse expect to increase during the first few months on the job?
   a. Expert power
   b. Legitimate power
   c. Referent power
   d. Coercive power

2. When a person fears punishment enough to act or behave differently than he or she would otherwise, the source of the other person's power is called which of the following?
   a. Coercive power
   b. Reward power
   c. Expert power
   d. Connection power

3. How can a new nurse's personal power be enhanced? Select all that apply.
   a. Collaborating with colleagues on special projects outside the work setting.
   b. Taking part in gossip on the nursing unit.
   c. Volunteering to serve on organizational committees led by non-nurses.
   d. Getting to know one's coworkers off duty and sharing recreational activities together.
   e. Becoming more self-aware of personal nursing knowledge and skills.
   f. Identifying a competent coworker and learning from him or her.

4. Three levels of power include all but which of the following?
   a. Personal
   b. Professional
   c. Organizational
   d. Unit

5. Which of the following can most interfere with a new nurse's base of personal power?

   a. Wearing a badge that indicates the nurse's name and professional license.
   b. Hesitating when giving instructions to unlicensed assistive personnel.
   c. Introducing oneself to patients by giving first and last name.
   d. Explaining a nursing procedure by citing the evidence that supports it.

6. How can a new nurse gain power on a nursing unit within a few weeks on the job? Select all that apply.
   _____ a. Identify a mentor on the unit and ask for guidance.
   _____ b. Associate with competent and respected coworkers.
   _____ c. Suggest improvements in unit routines that seem unclear.
   _____ d. Consult appropriate websites, unit policies and procedures, and other resources for more information about patients' diagnoses and treatment.
   _____ e. Steer clear of physicians and other nurses in daily nursing activities.
   _____ f. Seek information about patients from their family members and friends.

7. Which statements concerning unions are true? Select all that apply.
   a. Unions work through a collective bargaining agent.
   b. Unions represent only hourly employees.
   c. Unions represent only salaried employees.
   d. Unions formally present a group's desires to management.
   e. Nurse managers are part of the union.
   f. All union agreements support striking.

8. Which are correct concerning collective bargaining? Select all that apply.
   a. Collective bargaining is formal and only occurs through unionization.
   b. Collective bargaining agents represent the interests of the nurses.

c. Collective bargaining is done by a group acting with a single voice.

d. Workplace advocacy is a type of collective action.

e. Collective bargaining status can be attained with the NLRB.

9. Which large collective bargaining agents do nurses commonly belong to? Select all that apply.

a. National Nurses United

b. Service Employees International Union

c. International Nurses Union

d. California Nurses Association

e. Health Care Union of Ohio

10. Which of the following is true regarding the consumer movement in the United States?

a. It is a passing fad.

b. It challenges nurses to be more professionally accountable.

c. It is sustainable only through partnerships with the nursing profession.

d. It is encouraged by all health care systems and providers.

REVIEW QUESTION ANSWERS

1. Answer: A is correct.

Rationale: Learning occurs from day 1 on the job, and is likely to be continuous in increasing the new nurse's expert power. Knowledge and competence are growing from the first day on the job, so expertise is likely to increase right away and continue over time as new knowledge and experience is gained. (A). Legitimate and coercive power are primarily acquired with the assignment of authority to accompany increased responsibility. However, this requires a delay for a new nurse, until that authority is earned (B). Referent power is immediate for a new nurse, based on that which the nurse has already. But it is not likely to grow quickly (C). As mentioned above, coercive power is not gained without the authority that more experience may bring. A new nurse does not expect to increase coercive power quickly (D).

2. Answer: A is correct.

Rationale: Coercive power is gained by the ability to punish (A). Reward power is based on the ability to grant rewards, so is not based on the ability to punish (B). Expert power is based on acquired knowledge and capability/skills, and is not based on the ability to punish (C). Similarly, connection power is also not based on the ability to punish, but is based on connection to someone with power (D).

3. Answers A, C, D, E, and F are correct.

Rationale: Collaborating with colleagues adds to one's referent and expert power, because people tend to identify with and like a new nurse who is willing to collaborate, and the new nurse gains knowledge through such collaboration with more experienced nurses (A). Gossip has a tendency to reduce one's referent power, because of the likelihood that the individual's reputation is thereby diminished (B). Volunteering adds referent power because, once again, people tend to like someone who volunteers, and also potentially adds to one's connection power because of the increased relationship that develops with other who have their own power (C). Getting to know one's co-workers off duty and sharing recreation tends to increase the referent power of someone whom others get to like (D). Becoming more self-aware of their own knowledge and skills enables a new nurse to increase their expert power, because self-assessment facilitates growth (E). Identifying a competent co-worker and learning from him or her tends to increase a new nurse's expert power when that new nurse learns from their more experienced colleagues (F).

4. Answer: D is correct.

Rationale: All three levels (Personnel, Professional, and Organizational) are described in the text as different ways (levels) at which a new nurse can develop and use power (A, B, & C). Unit power is not mentioned in the text, and would only be a subset of organizational power (D).

5. Answer: B is correct.

Rationale: Hesitating when giving instructions to a nursing aide, can diminish the confidence of others in how much a nurse knows and is able to do, so the expert power can thereby be interfered with (B). Wearing a badge might indicate to others the level of expertise a nurse has, so if the perception of others about that expertise is impacted, then one's expert power is enhanced. Introducing oneself to patients by giving first and last name is a method of increasing one's referent power. Also, explaining a nursing procedure by citing the evidence that supports it not only increases the knowledge of a patient, but enhances the nurse's expert power. So (A), (C), and (D) enhance power, rather than interfere with it, and only (B) interferes with a new nurse's power.

6. Answers A, B, C, D, and F are correct.

Rationale: (A) is a correct answer because having (and using) a mentor increases the likelihood that you will grow in expert power as you learn from your mentor; your connection to a well-chosen mentor increases your connection power; your friendship with that mentor increases your referent power; and your ability to acquire and use helpful information will also be increased. (B) is correct because your connection power, your expert power, and your information power will be enhanced through association with competent and respected coworkers. (C) is correct because the inquiries and research and learning you have to go through to come up with suggested improvements (if you have indeed done this kind of preparation) will enhance your expert power. (D) is correct because increasing knowledge through reliable resources will increase your expert power. Finally, (F) is correct because seeking such information about patients from family and friends will increase your information power. (E) is not correct because steering clear of physicians and nurses in your daily nursing activities will decrease several sources of power: referent (because you will lose friendships that you should be developing); expert (because you will not be learning from such interactions); and connection (because you will leave undeveloped your connection with others).

7. Answers A and D are correct.

Rationale: (A) is correct because, as stated in the text, a collective bargaining agent is defined as the one channel through which individual union members collectively exercise their "voice." (D) is correct because unions are formed to "speak" to management on behalf of their members. (B) is not correct because unions represent a variety of employee groups; in some cases different unions serve salaried and hourly employees, in other cases the category of work (such as registered nurses) may include both salaried and hourly workers. (C) is similarly not correct because unions represent a variety of employee groups; in some cases different unions serve salaried and hourly employees, in other cases the category of work (such as registered nurses) may include both salaried and hourly workers. (E) is not correct because the National Labor Relations Act (as administered by the NLRB) has differentiated and defined nurse managers as part of "supervisory" employees who are not entitled by law to representation by the union. (F) is not correct because most union agreements contain a provision (usually one of the first provisions in the contract) called a "no strike" clause, declaring that the agreement explicitly states that employees will not resort to strikes.

8. Answers A, B, C, D, and E are correct.
Rationale: (A) is correct because unionization (the process of forming a union) is a protected right of employees under the federal National Labor Relations Act. Such a process culminates in recognition of a union which then serves as the formal channel for collective bargaining between represented employees and management. (B) is correct because, once a union of nurses is formed, the union becomes the recognized agent for collective bargaining in representing the interests of its membership. (C) is correct because the culmination of a unionization process is the forming of a union for the purpose of collective bargaining with management, and the agent of such collective bargaining (the union) operates as a single voice on behalf of all represented employees. (D) is correct because (as described in the section "Union Power") workplace advocacy is a process by which "nurses' voices can be heard in a less structured process" (than a union contract). Also, since 2003 the ANA has provided support for workplace advocacy as an alternative to collective bargaining, and "the ANA position is that workplace advocacy can be an alternative to unionization in promoting collaboration and communication among nurses." (E) is correct because part

of union recognition as protected by the NLRB is acting as formal agent of collective bargaining on behalf of its members when bargaining with management. (F) is incorrect because, as described in the text, the "ANA strives for excellence with initiatives such as magnet status certification and the National Database of Nursing Quality Indicators."

9. Answers A, B, and D are correct.
Rationale: (A) is correct because National Nurses United is listed under the section "Nursing Collective Bargaining Agents" as one of the collective bargaining agents commonly representing nurses. (B) is correct because although nurses are not a large part of their membership, the SEIU represents a very large number of health care workers nationwide and thus has a powerful voice. (D) is correct because "the California Nurses Association separated from the ANA and in 2009 formed the National Nurses United." NNU is the only exclusively nurses' union that is affiliated with the American Federation of Labor and Congress of Industrial Organizations (AFL-CIO). (C) and (D) are incorrect because there is no mention of an "International Nurses Union" or a "Health Care Union of Ohio."

10. Answer: B is correct.
Rationale: (B) is correct because informed consumers will demand greater accountability as they gain more information about what they can expect from health care providers. (A) is incorrect because there is no sign that the consumer movement is doing anything but gathering momentum. (C) is incorrect because the consumer movement has a life of its own, with or without the support or involvement of nursing. The only motivation that connects the interests of health care consumers and those of nursing professionals is when their interests overlap. It is through such overlapping interests that past and future cooperation can be expected and encouraged. (D) is incorrect because not all health care systems and providers want nurses (a significant proportion of health care providers) and consumers (a much larger body of people) to unite; doing so makes for a very potent political force, which might advocate against some of the interests of health care systems and providers.

REVIEW ACTIVITIES

- Identify a nursing leader. Observe the nurse and note what type of power the nurse uses to meet objectives.

- Watch a television show that portrays nurses. Note how nurses use or do not use the different types of power available to them. What do you observe?

- Observe our national leaders. What examples of the use of power do you see? Is power used in helpful or unhelpful ways? Explain.

- Observe a nursing unit during a shift. How do nursing co-workers use various types of power to influence one another?

- In current health care legislation, whose interests are being promoted?

- You are hired in a hospital that is a union shop. How does unionization differ from other collective action models such as workplace advocacy?

DISCUSSION POINTS

- During your last clinical experience, did you notice any nurses exhibiting expert power? Explain.

- Were there any physical manifestations of power on the unit, such as a physician lounge with snacks provided?

- Consider the sources of power presented in the chapter. How do you anticipate accessing and using each?

- Which sources of power would you feel the most comfortable using in your setting as you delivery care?

- Does the collective power of a specialty nursing association appeal to you? Which specialty nursing association would you like to join?

- How can power be used to improve patient care?

DISCUSSION OF OPENING SCENARIO

- If you were Pat, how would you prepare for the meeting?

    You may wish to talk with the charge nurse to get advice. Then carefully review each entry in the surgical admission sheet, clarifying your understanding not only of <u>what</u> was entered, but <u>why</u> the information is needed. Take note of potential alternative interpretations that could be made for each entry, and questions that might be asked about what you observed and what you did. Then prepare a short summary of information obtained as the patient was being admitted and your actions using the **Situation – Background – Assessment – Recommendations (SBAR)** format.

- What would be your approach as you begin your meeting with Dr. Killian?

    Approach the meeting knowing what you recorded earlier. Be prepared to give a brief summary. Be prepared to push back, in the event Dr. Killian says or does anything that is not in keeping with a professional conversation; in effect, be prepared to speak up if something in the interaction is unacceptable.

- Where could you go to seek support, should Dr. Killian act inappropriately and the meeting not go well?

    Visit the charge nurse and/or nurse manager to seek their support. With the support of the nurse manager, seek a collegial relationship with Dr. Killian that includes respectful communication.
    If in a bargaining unit, inform your union steward.

EXPLORING THE WEB (ALL ACCESSED FEBRUARY 20, 2019)

- The Truth About Nursing. This site critiques and advocates for accuracy in the media's portrayal of the role of nursing and of nurses. www.nursingadvocacy.org

- NursingPower. This site has a funny, not scholarly, synopsis of nursing power. www.NursingPower.net

- NursingWorld. This site, published by the American Nurses Association, discusses a variety of nursing resources and issues, including collective power. www.nursingworld.org

- On the site for the American Nurses Association (www.nursingworld.org), find your state nurses' association. What did you learn about your state nurses' association?

- Google. On the Google search engine, perform a search using the term "nursing leaders." www.google.com

- Distinguished Nurses. Find two nurses identified on the following site: www.distinguishedwomen.com

- Identify some Web sites for consumer groups:

    - AARP (American Association of Retired Persons): www.aarp.org

    - Citizen's Council on Health Care: www.cchconline.org

    - Consumer Reports. Search for health information on this site: https://advocacy.consumerreports.org/issue/health

    - National Labor Relations Board. Learn about the history of collective bargaining in the United States: www.nlrb.gov

INFORMATICS

- Go to the website for the National Labor Relations Board (www.nlrb.gov) Accessed March 15, 2019.

- Conduct a case search using the search terms "nursing" and "supervisor" and click on the box for "Representation" to review cases in which the NLRB had to decide who is considered a nursing Mt issue. What was the basis of the board's decision? What was its effect?

- Go to the QSEN website: (http://qsen.org) Accessed March 15, 2019.

- Click on RESOURCES, and then click on BOOKS, REPORTS & TOOLKITS. Look for tags along the right-hand side of the page. Click on the TEAMWORK AND COLLABORATION tag. Look for subjects that explore the dynamics encountered by the new nurse working in an inter-professional setting. What did you learn?

LEAN BACK

- How can a comprehensive understanding of power and politics impact your ability to succeed as a beginning nurse?

- How can you use this knowledge of power and politics to improve not only your own career, but also your ability to deliver excellent patient care?

- Would you consider working in a hospital with a union? Why or why not?

REFERENCES

American Nurses Association. (2010). *Nursing's social policy statement: The essence of the Profession* (3rd ed.).

American Nurses Association. (2015). *Code of ethics for nurses with interpretive statements* (2nd ed.).

American Nurses Association. (2018). www.nursingworld.org

Arnold, M. F., Blankenship, L. V., & Hess, J. M. (2017). *The Administration of Health Systems: Comparative perspectives*. New York: Routledge.

Bauchner, H. (2017). Health Care in the United States: A right or a privilege. *Journal of the American Medical Association*, *317*(1), 29.

Blumberg, L., & Holahan, J. (2017). Strengthening the ACA for the long term. *The New England Journal of Medicine*, *377*(22), 2105–2107.

Buresh, B., & Gordon, S. (2013). *From silence to voice*. Ithaca, NY: Cornell University Press.

Choi, S., Cheung, K., & Pang, S. (2014). A field study of the role of nurses in advocating for safe practice in hospitals. *Journal of Advanced Nursing*, *70*(7), 1584–1593.

Colby, S. L., & Ortman, J. M. (2018). *U.S. Census Bureau report - projections of the size and composition of the U.S. population: 2014 to 2060*. Washington, DC: U.S. Government Printing Office. Retrieved from http://wedocs.unep.org/bitstream/handle/20.500.11822/20152/colby_population.pdf

French, J. P. R., Jr., & Raven, B. (1959). The bases of social power. In D. Cartwright & A. Zander (Eds.), *Group dynamics* (pp. 607–623). New York: Harper & Row.

Gracian, B. (1892). *The art of worldly wisdom*. (J. Jacobs, Trans.). Boston, MA: Dover Publications, 2005. (Original work published 1647)

Hersey, P., Blanchard, K., & Natemeyer, W. (1979). Situational leadership, perception and impact of power. *Group and Organizational Studies*, *4*, 418–428.

Himmelstein, D., Woolhandler, S., Almberg, M., & Fauke, C. (2018). The ongoing U.S. health care crisis: A data update. *International Journal of Health Services: Planning, Administration, Evaluation*, *48*(2), 209–222. Retrieved from https://journals-sagepub-com.offcampus.lib.washington.edu/doi/abs/10.1177/0020731418764073

Jacox, A. (1980). Collective action: The basis for professionalism. *Supervisor Nurse*, *11*(9), 22–24.

Kantarjian, H. (2016). The affordable care act, or Obamacare, 3 years later: A reality check. *Cancer*, *123*(1). Wiley Online Library. Retrieved from https://onlinelibrary.wiley.com/doi/full/10.1002/cncr.30384

Kennedy, S., Hardiker, N., & Staniland, K. (2015). Empowerment an essential ingredient in the clinical environment: A review of the literature. *Nurse Education Today*, *35*((3)).

Linnen, D., & Rowley, A. (2014). Encouraging clinical nurse empowerment. *Nursing Management*, *45*(2), 44–47. Retrieved from www.nursingcenter.com/journalarticle?Article_ID=1690253&Journal_ID=54013&Issue_ID=1690119

Machiavelli, N., & Rebhorn, W. A. (2003). *The prince and other writings*. New Providence, NJ: Barnes & Noble.

Mandl, K. D., & Kohane, I. S. (2016). Time for a patient-driven health information economy? *The New England Journal of Medicine*, *374*, 205–208. Accessed from www.nejm.org/doi/full/10.1056/NEJMp1512142

Mark, B. A., Harless, D. W., Spetz, J., Reiter, K. L., & Pink, G. H. (2013). California's minimum nurse staffing legislation: Results from a natural experiment. *Health Research and Education Trust*, *48*(2 Pt 1), 435–454. Retrieved from www.ncbi.nlm.nih.gov/pmc/articles/PMC3626342

McDonald, L. (2018). *Florence nightingale, nursing, and health care today*. New York: Springer Publishing Co. LLC.

McMurray, A., & Cooper, H. (2017). The nurse navigator: An evolving model of care. *Collegian*, *24*(2), 205–212.

National Center for Health Statistics, Health, United States. (2018). *With special feature on mortality (2018)*. Hyattsville, MD: U.S. Department of Health and Human Services, Centers for Disease Control and Prevention. Retrieved from www.cdc.gov/nchs/hus/index.htm

National Labor Relations Act. (1935). Retrieved from www.nlrb.gov/resources/national-labor-relations-act-nlra.

National Labor Relations Board. (2018). *Employer/union rights and obligations*. Retrieved from www.nlrb.gov/rights-we-protect/employerunion-rights-and-obligations

National Nurses United. (2018). *About NNU*. Retrieved from www.national-nursesunited.org/about.

Raven, B. (2008). The bases of power and the power/interaction model of interpersonal influence. *Analyses of Social Issues and Public Policy*, *8*((1)).

Richmond, J., Powell, W., Maurer, M., Mangrum, R., Gold, M., et al. (2017). Public mistrust of the U.S. health care system's profit motives: Mixed-methods results from a randomized controlled trial. *Journal of General Internal Medicine*, *32*(12), 1396–1402.

Roux, G., & Halstead, J. A. (2018). *Issues and trends in nursing: Practice, policy and leadership*. Burlington, MA: Jones & Bartlett Learning.

SEIU Local. (2018, January 9). *Did you know that California law sets nurse-to-patient ratio requirements for hospitals?* Retrieved from www.seiu121rn.org/2018/01/09/did-you-know-that-california-law-sets-nurse-to-patient-ratio-requirements-for-hospitals.

Seldes, G. (1985). *The great thoughts*. New York: Ballantine Books.

Wenzler, D. T. (2015). *Magnet recognition program® status: Impact on HCAHPS patient satisfaction*. Retrieved from https://idea.library.drexel.edu/islandora/object/idea%3A6569.

AFL-CIO. (n.d.). *4 steps to form a union: AFL-CIO*. Retrieved from https://aflcio.org/formaunion/4-steps-form-union.

American Nurses Association. (2016). *ANA's principles for health system transformation*. American Nurses Association. Retrieved from https://qualitysafety.bmj.com/content/25/7/509 (IOM, 2008).

Batalden, M., Batalden, P., Margolis, P., Seid, M., Armstrong, G., et al. (2015). *Coproduction of health care service*. BMJ Publishing Group. Retrieved from https://qualitysafety.bmj.com/content/25/7/509

Institute of Medicine. (2011). *The future of nursing: leading change, advancing health*. Washington, DC: The National Academies Press. doi:10.17226/12956

Joel, L. A. (2006). *The nursing experience: Trends, challenges, and transitions*. New York: McGraw-Hill, Medical Pub. Division.

Joel, L. A., & Kelly, L. Y. (2011). *Kelly's dimensions of professional nursing*. New York: McGraw-Hill Medical Publishing Division.

Medicaid.gov. (2020). *Seniors and medicare and medicaid enrollees*. Medicaid.gov. Retrieved from www.medicaid.gov/medicaid/eligibility/seniors-medicare-and-medicaid-enrollees/index.html

SUGGESTED READINGS

Benner, P. E. (2000). *From novice to expert: Excellence and power in clinical nursing practice* (Commemorative ed.). Upper Saddle River, NJ: Prentice Hall.

Cherry, B., & Jacob, S. R. (2017). *Contemporary nursing: Issues, trends, & management* (7th ed.). St. Louis, MI: Elsevier.

Hart, C. (2015). The elephant in the room: Nursing and nursing power on an interprofessional team. *Journal of Continuing Education in Nursing*, *46*(8), 349–355.

Mason, D., Gardner, D., Outlaw, D. B., Hopkins, F., & O'Grady, E. E. T. (2016). *Policy & politics in nursing and health care* (7th ed.). St. Louis, MI: Elsevier.

Nurse, N. (2016). Charting nursing's future. *The American Journal of Nursing*, *116*(9), 61–62.

Yoder-Wise, P. (2018). *Leading and managing in nursing* (7th ed.). St. Louis, MI: Elsevier.

22 Legal Aspects of Nursing

Carol L. Wallinger[1,2]

Rutgers Law School, Rutgers School of Nursing, Camden, NJ, USA

Cooper Medical School, Camden, NJ, USA

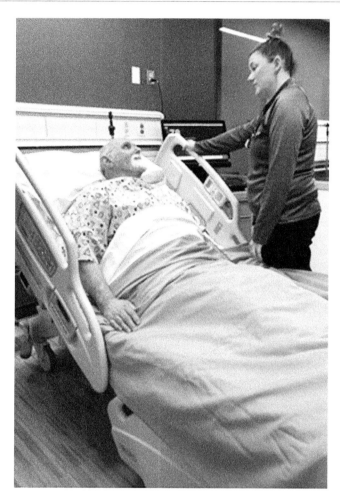

Patient and nurse discussing patient's current symptoms and the possibility of a delay.

Photo used with permission.

"Nurses have the best chance of explaining the wisdom of their clinical decision-making with an accurate and comprehensive patient record."

(A. Starr, Personal communication, July 5, 2019)

OBJECTIVES

Upon completion of this chapter, the reader should be able to:

1. Identify the sources and types of federal and state laws, regulations and case law, and recognize their impact on nursing practice.

Kelly Vana's Nursing Leadership and Management, Fourth Edition. Edited by Patricia Kelly Vana and Janice Tazbir

© 2021 John Wiley & Sons Ltd. Published 2021 by John Wiley & Sons Ltd.

Companion Website: www.wiley.com/go/kelly-Nursing-Leadership

2. Explain the importance of a nurse knowing what is contained in the Nurse Practice Act enacted in the state in which the nurse is practicing.

3. Analyze common errors of nursing practice that lead to malpractice actions, and outline actions a nurse can take to minimize committing these errors.

4. Relate legal protections for nursing practice, including Good Samaritan laws, and the importance of excellent communication skills for nurses.

5. Discuss the role of excellent nursing documentation in patient care and identify strategies nurses can use to optimize use of electronic health records.

6. Analyze the nurse's role as a patient advocate and in the duty to both be vigilant in assisting patients to communicate their health needs and protecting the patient's safety and legal rights.

OPENING SCENARIO

You are working on a post cardiac surgery unit and have been given an order to discharge a 58-year-old male who had cardiac bypass surgery 4 days ago. Before discharging you review the morning vital signs taken by the nurse's aide under your supervision. The patient's temperature is 100.9 °F (38.3 °C), and upon assessing the patient, he tells you that he feels a bit "chilled." You notify the surgical resident of the elevated temperature and the patient's comments, but you are told to continue with the discharge.

1. *After notifying the surgical resident about the elevated temperature, do you need to gather additional information about the patient's condition before you discharge him?*

2. *What do you do if the patient appears to be too ill for discharge? Is there anyone else you can contact?*

3. *If you discharge the patient and he develop sepsis or a serious illness, who of the following might be held responsible: you, the nurse's aide, the surgical resident, the surgeon who performed the surgery?*

A law is any custom or practice that a community decides should control the action of that community's members. We are each members of many communities, including our nation, our state of residence, the city or town where we live, and the community of professionals with whom we practice nursing. This chapter reviews how laws in the United States are enacted and implemented and how the various types of law affect nursing practice. Then, the chapter discusses common errors nurses make that can lead to a malpractice claim and provides strategies for avoiding those errors. One of those strategies discussed is developing excellent communication skills and a practice of thorough, careful, and detailed documentation. Finally, the chapter recognizes the importance of the nurse's role as a patient advocate. Nurses must advocate on behalf of patients to protect patients' legal rights and, whenever necessary, promote patient safety.

Sources of Law

The United States Constitution grants its citizens the authority to enact, implement, and interpret laws. A **constitution** is a set of basic laws that specifies the powers of the various branches of government and how these branches interact with each other. Our constitution authorizes three branches, all of which have the power to make law. These are the Legislative, Executive, and Judicial branches.

Generally, it is the role of the Legislative branch, both at the federal and state levels, to listen to the members of the community and propose bills that enforce the collective community's preferred behaviors. These proposed bills become enforceable when the Chief Executive signs the bill into law, at which point it becomes a **statute**. At the federal level, the President is the Chief Executive, and at the state level, the Chief Executive is the Governor. Thereafter, the Executive branch and its agencies (e.g., the Department of Health and Human Services, or the Environmental Protection Agency) are required to draft the rules and regulations that will be used to implement the statute. Finally, when petitioned by parties in a particular court case, the judicial branch interprets both the statute itself, and the agency's rules and regulations, and decides if they correctly and fairly represent the community's and the legislature's wishes, and if so, whether they were correctly applied in that particular case. The judicial branch issues its law in the form of judicial opinions from one or more judges who heard the parties' case. Law that originates from these opinions from a particular case is referred to as case law. Table 22.1 identifies the three branches of government and gives examples of these relationships.

Table 22.1   The Three Branches of Government

	Legislative branch	Executive branch	Judicial branch
Example at Federal Level	Americans with Disabilities Act (ADA) (1990)	The Equal Employment Opportunity Commission (EEOC) publishes rules specifying what employers must do to help a disabled employee.	In 1999, the U.S. Supreme Court interpreted the law to require that to be protected by the law, an individual must have an impairment that limits a major life activity and that is not corrected by medicine or appliances (e.g., glasses, blood pressure medicine). *Sutton v. United Airlines* (1999); *Murphy v. United Parcel Service, Inc.* (1999).
Example at State Level	Nurse Practice Act	The state board of nursing develops rules specifying the requirements for licensure of a registered nurse in that state.	A state court can determine whether the board of nursing's rules comply with the scope and purpose of the nurse practice act in that state.

Source: Created by C. Walliger.

Types of Law: Statutes and Case Law

There are two types of law that govern nursing practice, statutes and case law. As noted above, statutes originate with the legislature. For example, the Patient Protection and Affordable Care Act, often shortened to the Affordable Care Act or nicknamed "Obamacare," is a federal statute that was enacted by the 111th United States Congress and signed into law by President Barack Obama on March 23, 2010. In contrast, case law originates with the judicial branch. Case law develops over time, one case and judicial opinion at a time. In addition to dividing law into statutes and case law, law can also be divided into the various specialties, such as torts and contracts, just as medicine is divided into specialties such as neurology, cardiology, and orthopedics. For example, tort law, the specialty that covers accidents and injuries, including malpractice, has mostly developed case by case, and in the absence of a governing law. When a court is faced with a subsequent case with the same legal issue and similar facts, the court is required to follow all prior decisions, or precedents. This requirement to follow precedent transforms an individual case into case law.

Federal and State Statutes that Impact Nursing Practice

The **Health Insurance Portability and Accountability Act (HIPAA)** was enacted to, among other things, safeguard certain private health care information. Under the HIPAA Privacy Rule, disclosure of certain protected health information, such as a patient's medical diagnosis or plan of care, can result in civil and/or criminal penalties, if the patient has not given written consent to the disclosure of that information (HHS Office of the Secretary, Office for Civil Rights, 2017).

Nurses in all practice areas and of all experience levels face HIPAA issues each day. For example, imagine a busy nurse who is called to the nurse's station to take a phone call from a patient's family member the nurse has not met. Under HIPAA, the nurse may not release any protected health information to the caller unless the nurse is certain that the caller has the patient's permission to receive that information. If the nurse has any doubt about the caller's permission, the nurse must end the call and confirm with the patient that the caller is allowed access to the patient's information. Having to end the call without answering the caller's questions may result in temporary frustration for the caller, but the nurse must be certain the patient has given permission.

Occupational Safety and Health Administration (OSHA)

The **Occupational Safety & Health Administration (OSHA)**, works to establish a safe workplace for employees. This includes enacting regulations concerning storage of hazardous substances, protection of employees from infection, and protection of employees from violence in the workplace. Hospitals are subject to numerous OSHA regulations designed to protect the health and safety of nurses and other health care workers. From the minute the new nurse joins the hospital staff, he or she is likely to come into contact with OSHA-mandated products or programs every day. For example, any unvaccinated nurse joining the staff of a hospital will be offered Hepatitis B vaccination pursuant to OSHA regulations. Additionally, nurses working with patients who may have tuberculosis will be issued special OSHA-approved respirators to prevent the nurse from becoming infected. Every day, nurses will utilize OSHA-mandated and approved "sharps" containers that hold used needles, and personal protective equipment such as gloves, gowns, and surgical face masks. New nurses should review hospital policies and procedures to ensure that they are using these safety devices properly.

State Nurse Practice Acts

Under each state's nurse practice act, state boards of nursing are given the authority to define the practice of nursing within certain broad parameters specified by the legislature, mandate the requisite preparation for the practice of nursing, and discipline members of the profession who deviate from the rules governing the practice of nursing. Other professions such as medicine and dentistry have similar practice acts established in state law.

An important issue to nurses is the transferability of their nursing license from one state to another. A license to practice nursing is generally valid only in the state where it is issued. In most cases, a nurse wanting to practice in a state other than where his or her license was issued must apply for a license in that state. For nurses who frequently move from one state to another, this can be a burdensome process. There is an ongoing movement to allow nurses licensed in one state to automatically receive licensure to practice in another state. The Nurse Licensure Compact, a project of the National Council of State Boards of Nursing, is an agreement among some states to allow nurses licensed in other states who are parties to the agreement to practice without applying for a new license. As of January 2015, 25 states had joined this agreement, meaning that half of the states still required nurses to apply for a license in the state where they want to practice. However, there were state-level differences in background check requirements that caused some states to decline to join the Compact. The Council spent the period between 2015 and January 19, 2018 addressing these issues, and then created an enhanced and up-to-date version, named **Enhanced Nurse Licensure Compact** (eNLC). After a period of transition to the new Compact, after July 1, 2019, 31 states will be participating, and 4 other states (Indiana, Massachusetts, Michigan, and New Jersey), have legislation pending to join the Compact. You can check at www.ncsbn.org/compacts to determine if your state is a member of the Compact (last accessed February 10, 2019). Of course, nurses should always contact the Board of Nursing in any state where they intend to practice, to determine eligibility and licensure requirements.

Tort Issues that Impact Nursing Practice

Remember from above that the law can be divided into various specialties, and that tort law is the specialty that includes injuries, accidents, and malpractice.

A **tort** can be any of the following:

- The denial of a person's legal right
- The failure to comply with a public duty
- The failure to perform a private duty that results in harm to another.

There are two types of torts: intentional and unintentional. Assault, battery, false imprisonment, defamation, invasion of privacy, and fraud are all intentional torts, because they require intentional, deliberate behavior on the part of the nurse (Table 22.2). By contrast, malpractice is an unintentional tort, in that the nurse's behavior was an unintentional mistake.

Assault and Battery

Assault is a threat to touch another in an offensive manner without that person's permission. The threat is an intentional act that creates fear of harm in another person. Threatening a patient verbally, or "pretending" to strike a patient, for example raising your arm over your head with an open palm with your hand aimed in the patient's direction would be an example of an assault.

Table 22.2   Selected Intentional Torts

Tort	Definition	Example
Assault	Threat to touch another person in an offensive manner without that person's permission.	Nurse who threatens to strike a patient, or to give a patient a treatment against his will.
Battery	Actually touching another person without that person's consent.	Nurse who actually strikes a patient, or gives a treatment against the patient's will, or in the absence of informed consent to that treatment.
False imprisonment	Physically preventing or leading the patient to incorrectly believe the patient is prevented from leaving a place.	Nurse who restrains a patient who is of sound mind and is not in danger of injuring himself or others.
Defamation, including libel and slander	Intentionally communicating or publishing false information, including written (libel) or verbal (slander) remarks that may cause damage to a person's reputation.	Nurse who makes a false statement that damages the patient's reputation, such as stating that a patient who is slurring his words is "inebriated" when that may not be true.
Invasion of privacy	Public revelation of true, nondefamatory but private information about another.	Nurse fails to secure the computer on which the nurse just charted patient information, and a passer-by reads the patient's diagnosis, when the patient did not give permission for the diagnosis to be public information.
Fraud	Criminal deception for the purposes of personal or financial gain.	Nurse assists a provider to bill for services that were not rendered or accepts payments (kickbacks) for referring patients to providers.

Source: Adapted from Black's Law Dictionary. (2014) Thomson West, 10th Ed.

Battery is the touching of another person without that person's consent. In the health care arena, complaints of this nature usually pertain to whether the individual consented to (or subsequently withdrew consent to) the treatment administered by the health care professional. All states have a requirement that health care providers inform patients about the risks and benefits of a proposed treatment so that patients make informed decisions about their treatment and can withdraw themselves from care when they desire.

False Imprisonment

False imprisonment is the act of physically preventing or leading a patient to incorrectly believe the patient is prevented from leaving a place. A claim of false imprisonment may be based on the inappropriate use of chemical restraints, such as medications, or physical restraints. Federal law mandates that health care institutions employ the least restrictive method of ensuring patient safety. Physical or chemical restraints are to be used only, if necessary, to protect the patient from harm when all other methods have failed. If the nurse uses restraints on a competent person who is refusing to follow the practitioner's orders, the nurse can be charged with false imprisonment or battery. If restraints are used in an emergency situation, the nurse must contact the practitioner immediately after restraint application to secure an order for the restraints. Also, the nurse must check the institution's policies regarding the type and frequency of assessments required for a patient in restraints and how often it is necessary to secure a reorder for the restraints. For example, usually adults in restraints are checked by the registered nurse every 2 hr or more frequently, as needed. Some patients in restraints may need continuous observation. These policies ensure the patient's safety and must be consistent with state law.

Defamation

Defamation is intentionally communicating or publishing false information, including written (libel) or verbal (slander) remarks that may cause damage to a person's reputation. Defamation is governed by state law, and in a Virginia case, a patient was awarded $100,000 for defamation when a doctor falsely told co-workers during a procedure that the patient had syphilis and tuberculosis. (Anesthesiologist trashes sedated patient—and it ends up costing her, T. Jackman, Washington Post, June 23, 2015. www.washingtonpost.com/local/anesthesiologist-trashes-sedated-patient-jury-orders-her-to-pay-500000/2015/06/23/cae05c00-18f3-11e5-ab92-c75ae6ab94b5_story.html?utm_term=.9c7cadf998b9) (last accessed March 23, 2019).

Invasion of Privacy

The nurse is required to respect the privacy of all patients, and the confidentiality of all patient information. **Invasion of privacy** is the public revelation of private information about another in an objectionable manner; even if the information is true and nondefamatory, a cause of action may arise (and damages may be awarded) (Blacks Law Dictionary, 10th edition, 2014). The nurse may be privy to very personal patient information and must make every effort to keep it confidential. This often necessitates policing conversations with co-workers that have the potential for being overheard by others, so that no patient information is accidentally revealed. Nurses must also remember to log off from the computer before leaving a patient's room and be mindful that other people may be able to see both computer screens and paper records if their security is not assured.

Sometimes the protection of a patient's privacy conflicts with the state's mandatory reporting laws for the occurrence of specified infectious diseases such as syphilis or **Human Immunodeficiency Virus** (HIV). The need to protect an individual's privacy may also conflict with the state's mandatory reporting laws on suspected patient abuse. For example, all states have statutes that require certain "mandatory reporters," such as health care providers, to notify local authorities whenever elder abuse is suspected. Such a requirement could conflict with the patient's wishes, if the patient does not want the potential abuse or abuser investigated. Other information that state or federal law may require to be revealed includes a patient's blood alcohol level, incidences of rape, gunshot wounds, and adverse reactions to certain drugs. Failing to strictly follow reporting laws could lead to criminal liability, civil liability, or disciplinary action, including the loss of license and the suspension or termination of employment. Nurses must consult the institution's reporting policies and confer with its risk management department to ascertain their responsibilities and course of action.

The **American Nurses Association**'s (ANA) Code of Ethics states that nurses must protect the patient and the public when incompetence or unethical or illegal practice compromises health care and safety (Code of Ethics, Provisions 3 & 6, 2015). Many states have adopted this concept in their nurse practice acts, thereby creating a legal obligation to report. Nurses who observe unethical behavior in a hospital should report this through the chain of command and as directed in the institution's policies and procedures manual or by the laws of the state.

Fraud

Health care fraud results in losses to private insurers and the government, via Medicare and Medicaid, in the tens of billions of dollars each year (NHCAA, 2020). Health care fraud is committed typically by a very small minority of health care providers, but the types of fraud are wide ranging. Examples include: billing for services that were never rendered, or for more expensive services than were actually provided; performing medically unnecessary services or testing, solely for the purpose of billing; "unbundling" or billing each step of a procedure as if it were a separate procedure; and accepting payments (kickbacks) for patient referrals. In 2018, a nurse was sentenced to 1 year in jail for accepting payment of more than $390,000 from Medicaid over a 5-year period. The nurse submitted false claims for private-duty nursing services that the nurse never provided to two severely disabled home care patients (Attorney General Press Release, 2018).

Patient Confidentiality in the Age of Social Media

Given the reality that most nurses carry a smartphone that is capable of taking pictures and can easily access the Internet, nurses must be especially vigilant about protecting patient confidentiality and ensuring that no patient information is ever posted on any social media site. Nurses should never take any pictures of patients on the nurse's smartphone or post any stories or comments about patients on any social media sites, even if the patient (or the patient's family) verbally agrees to the post. Such a post would likely violate both federal laws regulating health care institutions and HIPAA, as well as generate intentional tort claims of breach of confidentiality, defamation, and invasion of privacy, and might well result in the nurse being disciplined or fired. State criminal laws also could be violated, and the nurse could be the subject of a disciplinary action by the state board of nursing.

The National Council of State Boards of Nursing published a "Nurses Guide to the Use of Social Media" brochure that discusses the common myths and misunderstandings of social media (National Council of State Boards of Nursing, 2018).

The brochure advises of the potential consequences for a nurse's inappropriate use of social media. Depending on the laws of the jurisdiction, the Board of Nursing could investigate the nurse for:

- Unprofessional conduct,
- Unethical conduct,
- Moral turpitude,
- Mismanagement of patient records,
- Revealing a privileged communication, and,
- Breach of confidentiality.

Unintentional Torts: Negligence and Malpractice

Negligence is the failure to provide the care a reasonable person would ordinarily provide in a similar situation. If you tailgate the car in front of you, and the cars collide when that driver brakes suddenly, you were driving negligently, that is, below the standard that a reasonable driver would use in that situation. But your behavior was unintentional because you did not mean to cause an accident. When a professional commits negligence, it is called malpractice. More specifically, the term **malpractice**, which is a form of negligence, refers to a professional's wrongful conduct in the discharge of his or her professional duties or failure to meet standards of care for the profession, which results in harm to another individual entrusted to the professional's care. If a nurse fails to meet the standard of care, the patient, if harmed by this failure, can initiate a malpractice action against the nurse for damages. In a malpractice lawsuit, the nurse can be sued because of something the nurse did incorrectly, (commission) or because the nurse failed to do something that was required (omission).

Steps of a Malpractice Lawsuit

In order for a patient to succeed at proving malpractice, the patient must prove all of the following four elements or steps of a malpractice lawsuit:

1. A duty or obligation created by law, contract, or standard practice that is owed to the patient by the professional;

2. A breach of this duty by the professional, either by omission or commission;

3. Actual harm suffered by the patient, which can be physical, emotional, or financial; and

4. Causation—proof that the breach of duty caused the alleged harm.

Critical Thinking 22.1

You are a new nurse working on the obstetrical unit of your local hospital. Your close nurse colleague, George Nurse also works on this unit. George has a reputation as a smart, likeable, and hardworking nurse who also knows how to let loose and have a good time when work is out. However, lately George has been coming to work late and appears "out of it." You spoke with George, who told you that he is having a difficult time at home and has not been as focused at work as he needs to be. He promises that he will try to leave his personal life at home.

For a month after your discussion with George, everything seems fine. However, in the past 2 weeks, you have noticed that George has bloodshot eyes and that his speech seems slurred at times. He looks unkempt and unclean, and the narcotic count for Vicodin has been off for three separate shifts that he worked. You are concerned that George may be using drugs or alcohol and that it may be impacting his nursing care.

What professional obligation do you have in this situation? What action do you take? Who can you go to for help in this situation? What is the definition of a "professional?"

A recent Louisiana appellate court case described both the patient's burden of proof and the "reasonable care" standard by which a nurse would be judged:

> *"In a medical malpractice action, the plaintiff must prove by a preponderance of the evidence the applicable standard of care, a violation of that standard of care, and a causal connection between the violation of the standard of care and the claimed injuries. A nurses' duty is to exercise the degree of skill ordinarily employed under similar circumstances, by members of the nursing profession in good standing in the same community or locality, and to use reasonable care and diligence, along with his or her best judgment, in the application of his or her skill to the case." Myles v. Hospital Serv. Dist. 248 So. 3d 545, 549 (2018).*

Step 1, proving that a duty or obligation created by law, contract, or standard practice was owed to the patient by the professional nurse, is not difficult. If the patient was under the nurse's care at the time of the incident, then the nurse owed the patient a professional duty, as described in the above quote from the <u>Myles</u> case.

Step 2, the court determines if there was a breach of duty by the professional, either by omission or commission, using a "reasonable person" standard, asking what a reasonable nurse would do in a similar situation. At trial, both parties would present nursing expert testimony and other evidence (the institution's policies and procedures and other sources of evidence (Table 22.3)) about whether the care that was rendered adhered to accepted nursing standards and whether the patient suffered actual physical, emotional, or financial harm (Step 3), and whether the harm was caused by the nurse's breach of duty or actions (Step 4).

Table 22.3   Selected Sources of Evidence Regarding the Standard of Care

- Evidence-based health care literature
- Nursing and medical textbooks, articles, and research
- State professional practice acts, such as nurse practice act, physician practice act
- Standards of professional associations, e.g., American Nurses' Association Standards
- Equipment manufacturers manuals, e.g., cardiac monitoring equipment manuals
- Written policies and procedures of a facility, such as Foley catheter insertion procedures
- Nurse, practitioner, or other health care professional expert testimony
- Professional health care accreditation agency criteria, for example, The Joint Commission criteria
- Medication textbooks, such as *Physicians' Desk Reference*, *American Society of Health-System Pharmacists Drug Information* Handbook, and so on.

Source: Created by C. Wallinger.
Note: Not all sources of evidence are used in all states.

The institution's policies and procedures describe the performance expected of nurses in its employ and a nurse deviating from them can be liable for malpractice. Occasionally, such failure to adhere to institutional protocol can result in the employer denying the nurse a defense in a lawsuit. Therefore, as discussed in more detail below, nurses should always consider carrying their own personal malpractice insurance which would cover the nurse if the nurse's employer declined coverage.

Practicing nurses must also adhere to the standards of care for the nursing profession in the community. These standards include, for example, checking the six "rights" of medication administration or repositioning the bedbound patient at regular intervals.

As noted above, in Step 3, the patient must prove that the patient suffered some actual physical, emotional, or financial harm damages, and in Step 4, the patient must prove causation, that is, that the breach of duty directly caused the patient's alleged harm. The patient must submit evidence supporting the allegations in Steps 3 and 4. This is usually presented through the patient's testimony and the reports and testimony of expert witnesses. The defendant, the health care provider, also submits expert witness testimony in defense of the malpractice allegation. In order for there to be a finding of malpractice, the judge or jury must weigh the evidence submitted by both parties and be convinced that the nurse's actions actually caused the alleged harm to the patient. For example, even if it is proved that a nurse made a medication error, if the error was not the cause of the patient's harm, the patient will not win in recovering damages from the nurse. In a 1997 case, a patient with sickle cell anemia died after suffering a cardiopulmonary arrest attributed to an aspiration that was witnessed by a visitor. The visitor immediately called for and obtained help. Although revived, the patient never regained consciousness and was eventually taken off life support. At trial, the patient's family was able to prove that the nurse assigned to this patient did not follow the institution's policy of documenting frequent observations, which were mandated because the patient was receiving a blood transfusion at the time of the cardiac arrest. However, in reviewing the case on appeal, the appellate court noted the following:

> *"[T]he record contains no evidence which suggests what could have been done even if the nurse had been seated at his bedside prior to the arrest. Plaintiff has failed to offer any proof that more immediate assistance would have prevented the catastrophic results of his aspiration. Based on the evidence in this record, we conclude that more frequent monitoring would have made no difference." (Webb v. Tulane Medical Center Hospital [1997])*

Thus, even though the plaintiff successfully proved a breach of a duty, the breach was not found to be the cause of the patient's death and the nurse was not found to be liable for malpractice.

In 2009, CNA Insurance Company published a study examining the types and frequency of nursing malpractice actions throughout the United States. The study found that:

> *"the role of the nurse in medical malpractice litigation has experienced a paradigm shift over the last several years. In the past, nurses were considered by many plaintiffs' lawyers and some judges to be mere 'functionaries' or 'custodians' who played a limited role in the care and treatment of patients." (CNA Financial Corporation, 2009. p. 35).*

"While nurse as custodian claims continue to be asserted, plaintiffs' lawyers have now begun to pursue claims that focus on the nurse as clinician, responsible for using professional judgment in the course of treatment." (p. 36).

> *"The following are examples of the new paradigm of nursing claims: (p. 36).*

> - *Following a fall by a geriatric patient, the nurse is sued for failure to change the service plan despite increasing patient problems with gait and behavior.*
> - *A child is born with profound brain damage and the nurse is alleged to have failed to properly interpret fetal monitoring strips.*
> - *A lawsuit charges the nurse with failure to appreciate a patient's risk for skin breakdown and to take appropriate preventive measures.*
> - *After a patient experiences an adverse drug reaction, the family alleges that the nurse failed to properly administer and provide the correct dosage.*

> - *A patient in the emergency department has a cardiac arrest, and a lawsuit is filed alleging that the triage nurse failed to appreciate acute cardiac symptomatology."*

CNA Financial Corporation. (2015). CNA HealthPro Nurse Claims Study: An Analysis of Claims with Risk Management Recommendations 1997–2007. Hatboro, P. A.: Author. PDF of report available at www.nso.com/nursing-resources/claim-studies.jsp Accessed April 18, 2011.

CNA's most recent report, issued in 2015, studied nursing liability claims from 2010 to 2014. (Nurse Professional Liability Exposures: 2015 Claim report Update, by CNA Insurance Company and Nurses Services Organization. Available at www.nso.com/Learning/Artifacts/Claim-Reports/Nurse-Professional-Liability-Exposures-2015-Claim (last accessed March 18, 2019). Table 22.4 represents a compilation of both the 2009 and 2015 reports of Nursing Malpractice Cases. CNA's 2015 study noted that "many of the medication administration errors involve nurses using 'workarounds' to bypass the facility's established safety procedures" (p. 25). On February 20, 2019, a former Vanderbilt University Medical Center nurse was indicted for reckless homicide after giving a patient the wrong drug and the patient died. The nurse bypassed the medication cabinet's automatic setting and mistakenly administered the paralytic agent vecuronium, instead of Versed, a sedative often given for procedural sedation. Versed is not a paralytic. After the indictment, the American Nurses Association (ANA) issued a statement expressing condolences to the patient's family and calling for a "full and confidential peer

Table 22.4 Nursing Malpractice Cases

Treatment

- Failure to treat symptoms/illness/disease in a timely manner in accordance with established standards/protocols/pathways
- Failure to implement established treatment protocols or established critical pathways in a timely manner
- Delay in implementing ordered, appropriate treatment
- Improper/untimely nursing technique or negligent performance of treatment resulting in injury
- Premature cessation of treatment

Communication

- Failure to report complications of pregnancy, labor or delivery to physician/licensed independent practitioner in a timely manner
- Failure to respond to patient's concerns related to the treatment plan in a timely manner
- Failure to notify physician/licensed independent practitioner of patient's condition and/or lack of response to treatment in a timely manner
- Failure to report complications of post-operative care to physician/licensed independent practitioner in a timely manner
- Failure to obtain physician/licensed independent practitioner orders to perform necessary additional treatment(s) in a timely manner

Medication Errors

- Wrong dose, route, rate or medication given to patient
- Infiltration of intravenous medication into tissue and/or sensory injury
- Medication not covered under state scope of practice
- Failure to immediately report and record the incorrect or improper administration of medication/prescription
- Wrong patient
- Wrong/delayed time of medication administration
- Missed dose

Table 22.4 (Continued)

Monitoring/Observing/Supervising

- Abandonment of patient, including checking patient's status and vital signs at appropriate intervals
- Improper/untimely nursing management of patient or medical complication
- Improper/untimely nursing management of pre-operative, peri-operative, or post-operative treatment or complication
- Improper application of restraints, or ordering or management of physical or chemical restraints, and/or failure to remove restraints at proper increments of time, in violation of the institution's procedures
- Improper/untimely nursing management of behavioral health/mental health patient or behavioral health complication
- Improper/untimely nursing management of patients in need of physical restraints, including 1:1 supervision, timed release of restraints, comfort breaks, fluids and nourishment.

For additional information about malpractice cases, see The National Practitioner Data Bank (NPDB) which is a web-based repository of reports containing information on medical malpractice payments and certain adverse actions related to health care practitioners, providers, and suppliers. www.npdb.hrsa.gov/topNavigation/aboutUs.jsp accessed 5/8/2019.

Critical Thinking 22.3

Review the nursing malpractice cases in Table 22.4. Have you ever seen a similar case or any case that might result in a malpractice claim? What do you think would be your first action if you saw a fellow nurse's care fall below the standard of care and that nurse potentially committing malpractice? Would you speak to the nurse directly? What would you say? Would you speak to the nurse's supervisor, in addition to speaking to the nurse?

---

review process in which medical errors can be examined and system improvements and corrective plans can be established to ensure that errors such as this do not occur in the future." Further, the ANA advised that "the criminalization of medical errors could have a chilling effect on reporting and process improvement." (ANA February 19, 2019).

Nursing Advocacy: Required as Part of the Nursing Process

The ANA Code of Ethics and many state nurse practice acts require nurses to serve as patient advocates (ANA Code, Provision 3, 2015). A patient's illness, combined with the institutional nature of hospitals, often results in patients becoming passive recipients of health care instead of active partners. Nurses must be vigilant in both assisting patients to communicate their desires and needs to the health care team, and in protecting the patient's safety and even legal rights. For example, occasionally a provider's order may appear suspect or clearly contrary to accepted medical practice. In such situations, the nurse must exercise professional judgment and be a patient advocate, refusing to carry out the order if it

would put the patient in danger. Most hospitals have policies and procedures to assist the nurse in carrying out this advocacy function. These procedures often require the nurse to take the issue up the chain of command, from the nursing manager up through the hospital administration and medical staff if necessary. Nurses are increasingly being held liable for malpractice in failing to question potentially dangerous provider orders.

Nurses also serve as advocates by safeguarding patient legal interests, such as the right to make informed health care decisions. In this role, nurses frequently collaborate with other members of the health care team and provide patient education to ensure that patients understand the risks and benefits of procedures, medication regimens, or laboratory tests. Additionally, nurses may help patients express their desires regarding end-of-life decisions to the medical team. Advanced directives are discussed in detail later in this chapter.

It is not uncommon for a nurse to find conflicts between an employer's expectations and the nursing standard of care. A nurse working in a medical-surgical unit, for example, may be asked to take care of an unsafe number of patients, or a surgical nurse with no experience working in the Emergency Room may be asked to "float" to this unit. In these situations, nurses

Case Study 22.1

You are working the night shift. The practitioner for one of your patients has ordered a dose of a medication to be given to the patient. The medication dose ordered is too high for this particular patient. You are unable to locate the practitioner to check the order. Who would you consult with next? What would you do to ensure safe care for your patient?

must advocate on behalf of their patients and their profession and consider how best to take on such an assignment, without being accused of "patient abandonment" or threatening the nurse's employment. Because most nurses are employed as "at will" employees, a nurse would run the risk of being fired for refusing to float, especially if a unit is desperately short staffed due to illness. However, the floating nurse could negotiate to be assigned to the less complex patients, and then notify the supervisor if one of those patients needed a procedure for which the nurse was not adequately trained. Ultimately, however, if the nurse determines that he or she cannot safely carry out the hospital's order, the nurse must not do so. A nurse in this situation would be wise to maintain patient safety and notify the supervisor of the patient safety concerns. (Frequently asked legal questions, C. Buppert, 2015) (Nurses Services Organization, 2019).

Informed Consent

Informed consent is the process of communication between a doctor or advanced practice nurse and a patient that apprises the patient of the nature, risks, and alternatives of a medical procedure or treatment. It is more than a signature on a form (Joint Commission, 2016). The patient has the right to receive sufficient information to make an informed decision about whether to consent to or refuse a procedure. The doctor or advanced practice nurse that will be performing the medical procedure or treatment has the responsibility to explain to the patient the nature of the procedure or treatment, and its benefits, alternatives, and risks and complications. The nurse who witnesses the patient sign the consent is certifying only that the nurse observed the patient sign the consent. The nurse is not certifying as to the content of the discussion between the doctor or advanced practice nurse and the patient. Nurses frequently witness the patient's signature on the consent

---

Critical Thinking 22.2

You are assigned to a medical-surgical unit, working the night shift. Your supervisor calls and says that one of the RNs assigned to the critical care unit has called in sick and you must work that unit instead of your usual assignment. You have never worked in the critical care setting before and have received no orientation to this unit. You are now asked to work there when it is short of staff.

Can you outright refuse? What information should you convey to the supervisor, and what accommodations should you ask for?

Real World Interview

Nursing practice in today's health care environment is multifaceted and complex. Our patients and communities expect quality care from nurses at all levels of practice. The responsibility to keep abreast of current practices is an integral component of a nurse's licensure requirements. Nursing professionals must understand their scope of practice and the legal requirements necessary to maintain their license in good standing. As a former member of a State Board of Nursing, I assure you that this is important for all nurses, experienced or novice. We begin to discuss these legal implications with our nursing students in our Transition to Professional Nursing course to prepare them for the nursing practice environment.

Increased emphasis is being placed on patient safety through regulatory agencies, the Joint Commission, and other national nursing organizations. Quality and Safety in Nursing Education (QSEN) competencies are embedded into our nursing curriculum and our high-fidelity simulations. The QSEN competencies are patient-centered care, teamwork and collaboration, evidence-based practice, quality improvement, safety, and informatics. QSEN is a national initiative to align nursing education and nursing clinical best practices in both quality and safety to continually demonstrate improvement in these areas.

There needs to be a commitment through a variety of initiatives to improve overall patient outcomes, such as reduction in medication errors or improvement in patient outcomes and nursing sensitive indicators. Nurses have a significant impact and contribution to overall positive outcomes in the current health care environment.

As a sustained focus is placed on improvement of care and patient safety, evidence-based practice must be integrated into the daily practice patterns of patient care. Proven evidence-based policies and procedures need to dictate how patient care is administered, rather than "this is how we have always done it." Failure to adhere to best practices within your scope of practice can result in negative patient outcomes and ultimately lead to licensure problems or legal action. Above all, staying current in skills, knowledge, and education helps nurses to meet the practice standards that are expected in today's health care environment.

Marsha King DNP, RN, MBA, NEA-BC, CNE
Dean, Associate Professor
University of Saint Francis-Crown Point site
Past President of the Indiana State Board of Nursing

form, and as part of the nursing process, must ascertain that the patient understands the procedure/treatment the patient is scheduled to undergo. If the patient states that the patient does not understand the procedure/treatment, the nurse must take immediate steps to ensure the patient is not sent for the procedure or treatment and must inform the doctor or advanced practice nurse about the patient's lack of understanding. The nurse should also report the incident up the chain of command, and notify the immediate supervisor on duty (charge nurse, nurse manager, etc.) about the situation. The nurse should be sure to document each of these conversations in the electronic health record, using the patient's actual words, if possible.

For a consent form to be legal, a patient, in most states, must be at least 18 years of age; be mentally competent; have the procedures with their risks and benefits explained in a manner he or she can understand; be aware of the available alternatives to the proposed treatment; and consent voluntarily. The nurse must also be familiar with which other people are allowed by state law to consent to medical treatment for another when that person cannot consent for himself or herself. Frequently, these include the person possessing medical power of attorney, a spouse, adult children, or other relatives, if no one is available in one of the other categories listed.

Advanced Directives: Living Wills and Powers of Attorney

Federal law requires that a hospital ask the patient, upon admission, whether he or she has a living will. If not, the hospital must ask the patient whether he or she would like to enact one. A **living will** is a written advance directive voluntarily signed by the patient that specifies the type of care he or she desires if and when he or she is in a terminal state and cannot sign a consent form or convey this information verbally. It can be a general statement, such as "no life-sustaining measures," or specific, such as "no tube feedings or respirator." A **power of attorney** is a legal document executed by an individual (principal) granting another person (agent) the right to perform certain activities in the principal's name. It can be specific, such as "sell my house at the closing on X date," or general, such as "make all of my decisions for me, including doing my banking, paying my bills every month, and making all my health care decisions related to treatment." In most states, a power of attorney is voluntarily granted by the individual and does not take away the individual's right to exercise his or her own choices. Thus, if the principal (the patient) disagrees with his agent's decisions, the patient's wishes are the ones that prevail. If a situation occurs in which an agent, acting on a power of attorney, disagrees with your patient regarding discharge plans, contact your supervisor for further assistance in deciding an action consistent with your patient's wishes and best interests. The supervisor will meet with the parties, and then decide what other hospital resources need to be involved, including pastoral care, the ethics committee, risk management, and the hospital's general counsel.

The authority to make health care decisions for another may be granted in a general power of attorney document or in a specific document limited to health care decisions only, such as a health care power of attorney. The requirements for a health care power of attorney vary from state to state, as do most legal documents. Note that a nurse could face an allegation of battery for failing to honor an advance directive such as a living will, medical power of attorney, or durable power of attorney.

Sometimes the patient's family has difficulty allowing health care personnel to follow the wishes expressed by the patient in a living will, and conflicts arise. These should be communicated to the nurse manager, and the patient's physician, as well as the hospital ethics committee, pastoral care department, risk management department, or whichever hospital department is responsible for handling such issues. If the patient verbalizes wishes regarding end-of-life care to the family, difficult situations can sometimes be avoided, and the patient should be encouraged to do this, if possible. The nurse should be familiar with the requirements for the implementation of a living will in the state where the nurse practices.

Do Not Resuscitate (DNR) Orders

The attending medical practitioner may write a Do Not Resuscitate (DNR) order for an inpatient, directing the staff not to perform the usual CardioPulmonary Resuscitation (CPR) in the event of a sudden cardiopulmonary arrest. The practitioner may write such an order without evidence of a living will on the medical record, and the nurse should be familiar with the institution's policies and state law regarding when and how a practitioner can write such an order in the absence of a living will. Often, a DNR order is considered a medical decision that the practitioner can make, preferably in consultation with the family, even without a living will executed by the patient. If the nurse feels such a DNR order is contrary to the patient's or family's wishes, the nurse should consult the policies and procedures of the institution. These may include going up the chain of command until the nurse is satisfied with the course of action. This may entail notifying the nursing supervisor, the medical director, the institution's chief operating officer, state regulators, or the Joint Commission (JC). Often, an institution has an ethics committee that examines such issues and makes a determination on the appropriateness of the DNR order.

Medical Aid in Dying/Death with Dignity

In 2014, 29-year-old Californian Brittany Maynard was diagnosed with glioblastoma, the same brain cancer that ended the lives of, among many others, Senators Edward Kennedy (2009) and John McCain (2018). Brittany's brain cancer was uncurable but because her body was relatively healthy, she worried about the prospect of many long months in hospice, with seizures and unknown pain and suffering. Rather than have her family experience many months of her suffering, she chose to move to Oregon and establish residency in order to access that state's Death with Dignity law for help with medical aid in dying. Brittany chose to take her lethal dose of medication on November 14, 2014.

The advocacy organization Compassion & Choices (2019) defines medical aid in dying as a:

> "safe and trusted medical practice in which a terminally ill, mentally capable adult with a prognosis of 6 months or less to live may request from his or her doctor a prescription for medication which they can choose to self-ingest to bring about a peaceful death." https://compassionandchoices.org/about-us; last accessed March 19, 2019.

Currently, nine jurisdictions authorize medical aid in dying: California, Colorado, Hawaii, New Jersey, Montana, Oregon, Vermont, Washington state and Washington, D.C. Oregon was the first state to enact its Death with Dignity law in 1994, and California's statute took effect on June 9, 2016. Brittany Maynard's husband and mother were instrumental in convincing the California legislature to pass the law. Most recently, New Jersey's medical aid in dying statute was signed into law on April 12, 2019.

Medical aid in dying is different from either assisted suicide or euthanasia in that with medical aid in dying, the patient retains the control over who administers the lethal dose of medication. Euthanasia, by which another person administers the lethal dose of medication, is contrary to the ethical codes of both the American Nurses Association and the American Medical Association. Also, because another person administers the lethal dose of medication, euthanasia also is illegal in every state, because it meets the definition of murder/manslaughter.

Legal Protections in Nursing Practice

As discussed earlier in this chapter, nursing practice is guided by state nurse practice acts and agency policies and procedures. Other resources for the nurse include Good Samaritan laws, skillful communication, and risk management programs.

Good Samaritan Laws

Good Samaritan laws have been enacted to protect the health care professional from legal liability. The essential elements of commonly enacted Good Samaritan law are as follows:

- The care is rendered in an emergency situation.

- The health care worker is rendering care without pay.

- The care provided did not recklessly or intentionally cause injury or harm to the injured party by providing inappropriate care outside the scope of practice.

Note that these Good Samaritan laws are intended to protect the volunteer who stops to render care at the scene of an accident. They would not protect emergency medical technicians (EMTs) or other health care professionals rendering care at the scene of an accident as part of their assigned duties and for which they receive pay. In performing these duties, these paid emergency personnel would be evaluated according to the standards of their professions.

Skillful Communication

The nurse must communicate accurately and completely both verbally and in writing. In the nursing malpractice cases detailed earlier in Table 22.4, note how many of the malpractice cases were the result of a failure to communicate by the nurse. For example, the nurse may have failed to notify the practitioner of a change in the patient's status, or the nurse failed to document the assessments performed. It is essential that the nurse document everything related to the patient accurately and thoroughly. Often, a lawsuit involving medical malpractice will take several years to come to trial. By that time, the nurse may have no memory of the incident in question and must rely on the written record prepared at the time of the incident. This record is frequently in the courtroom and may be projected onto a large screen for everyone to see, as the nurse is questioned by the patient's attorney. All errors are apparent, and omissions stand out by their absence, especially if they are data that should have been recorded per institutional policy. The old adage "if it isn't written, it wasn't done" will be repeated to the jury numerous times. Therefore, each nurse needs to develop a personal system to ensure that documentation is done in timely manner. Sometimes events intervene, and charting must be done later in the day. But as a general practice, events should be recorded as soon as possible after an occurrence, even if it is something as routine as taking the patient's vital signs. Bedside computer terminals greatly facilitate this type of documentation.

Documenting Nursing Care

In general, nursing documentation should follow the nursing process, and should include the tasks/work performed with the patient, such as vital signs, medications, treatments, interventions, and reassessments. Document patient symptoms using the patient's own words. When teaching a patient, document the patient's questions, and that the patient understands what has been taught. Document objective observations (who, what, where, when), but not opinions or speculation as to why an event occurred. Observations should include specific details, such as the amount, color, and consistency of drainage. Avoid words such as "a lot" and instead use precise terms as "50 ccs" or "an area the size of a quarter." If an adverse event occurs, use an objective description, stating what was directly observed, what statements were made, and what information was given to the patient/family. Include the assessments, interventions, and follow-up care. The following is an excellent resource on documentation:

www.nursingcenter.com/clinical-resources/nursing-pocket-cards/nursing-documentation (2019) last accessed March 22, 2019. Also: Principles for Nursing Documentation: Guidance for Registered Nurses, American Nurses Association (2010)

Electronic Health Records/Electronic Medical Records

Computerized health information systems are now used routinely by many hospitals and doctor's offices. These can take the form of Electronic Medical Records (EMR) that are kept only at that doctor's office, or Electronic Health Records (EHR) that typically collect information from all of a patient's providers, store it centrally, and allow for mass data collection, evaluation, and research. In either case, these clinical data repositories have fundamentally changed how nurses document the care they provide to patients. If not used properly, the EHR and EMR can create communication gaps. In 2018, Pagulayan, Eltair, and Faber described a retrospective patient-chart audit that was prompted by a series of human errors and near misses. The authors found that because of a number of design gaps in the electronic records system, combined with nurses' time constraints, nurses had resorted to work arounds, leading to less-than-complete documentation, less critical thinking, and communication gaps. The authors' solution was to integrate the critical thinking inherent in the nursing process (assess, plan, intervene, evaluate) with the electronic record system to give the nurses a better system for documentation. One year later, an audit showed improved documentation in multiple areas, including medication reconciliation and documenting patient chief complaints and comorbidities. See Table 22.5 for Tips for Working with Electronic Health Records.

SBAR: A Useful Tool for Patient Handoffs to Other Professionals

Situation, Background, Assessment, Response (SBAR) is a verbal tool that was developed to increase the quality of interprofessional communication, whether during an acute event, or when handing off a patient from one care area to another. A systematic review (meta-analysis) of 14 studies that implemented SBAR noted that "the Joint Commission reported that poor communication is a contributing factor in more than 60% of a hospital adverse events they reviewed" and concluded that "there was moderate evidence for improved patient safety through SBAR implementation, especially when used to structure communication over the phone. However, there is a lack of high-quality research on this widely used communication tool." Müller et al. (2018) (Table 22.6),

Table 22.5 Tips for Working with Electronic Health Records

Tips for Working with Electronic Health Records:

- Complete all basic software training and be sure to participate in all updates.
- When the physical location of the computer forces the nurse to face away from the patient, explain the electronic documentation procedure to patients and let them know they can interrupt with questions or concerns.
- Consider reading back the information to the patient as you type it into the system.
- Do not rush when entering data—be accurate and consistent.
- Remember that each patient encounter should be recorded as a stand-alone record—avoid using "cut and paste" versions of old notes or pre-written notes.
- Be sure you understand your health care agency's process for addendums, corrections, and deletions, as well as the time deadline that is set by the software for you to "lock" the patient's EHR. Corrections, amendments, clarifications, and additions are a normal part of clinical documentation, but they must be completed within the time allotted by the agency and the software.

Source: Balestra, M. (2017) and Gawande, A. (2018)

Table 22.6 SBAR – A Useful Tool for Patient Handoffs to Other Professionals

S = Situation: Identify yourself, and then briefly describe the problem.	**"Dr. Smith, this is Lisa Jones from the ER. Mr. Baker's wheezing is suddenly worse."**
B = Background	"He is the 54-year-old man with COPD who is in the ER awaiting a bed upstairs. While receiving a respiratory treatment, he became acutely short of breath."
A: Assessment	"His wheezing got substantially worse right after the respiratory treatment started. I think he is having an unusual reaction to the treatment."
R: Recommendation	"I stopped the treatment and I think you need to see him right away. I think he needs IV steroids."

Source: Data from Müller, Jürgens. & Redaèlli (2018).

Risk Management Programs

Risk management programs in health care organizations are designed to identify and correct systemic problems that contribute to errors in patient care or to employee injury. The emphasis in risk management is on quality improvement and protection of the institution from financial liability. Institutions usually have reporting and tracking forms that record incidents that may lead to financial liability for the institution. When an incident occurs, risk management will assist in identifying and correcting the underlying problem that may have led to the incident, such as faulty equipment, staffing concerns, or the need for better orientation for employees. If a systemic problem is identified, the risk management department may revise polices and develop educational programs to address the problem.

The risk management department will also investigate and record information surrounding a patient or employee incident that may result in a lawsuit. This helps personnel remember critical factors if they are asked to testify at a later time. The nurse should complete a risk management incident report and notify the risk management department of all reportable incidents as mandated by institutional policies and procedures. Note also that employee complaints of harassment or discrimination can expose the institution to significant liability and should promptly be reported to supervisors and the risk management, human resources, or whichever other department is specified in the institution's policies. See Table 22.7 for a checklist of actions to decrease the risk of nursing liability.

Malpractice/Professional Liability Insurance

Nurses should strongly consider carrying their own malpractice insurance. Nurses often think their actions are adequately covered by the employer's liability insurance, but this is not necessarily so. If, in giving care, the nurse fails to comply with the institution's policies and procedures, the institution may deny the nurse a defense, claiming that because of the nurse's failure to follow institutional policy or because of the nurse working outside the scope of employment, the nurse was not acting as an employee at that time. Also, nurses are being named individually as defendants in malpractice suits more frequently than in the past. It is important to remember that the hospital's attorney is not the nurse's attorney. The hospital's attorney represents the hospital and its interests, which may be adverse to the nurse's interests. Consequently, it is advantageous for the nurse to be assured of a defense independent of that of the employer. Professional liability insurance provides that assurance and covers the cost of an attorney to defend the nurse in a malpractice lawsuit. Such insurance is available through the American Nurses Association at www.nursingworld.org and various commercial providers.

In addition, an employer's policy will not insure a nurse should there be a complaint filed against the nurse's license with the state board of nursing. Individual professional liability insurance policies provide coverage for assault, HIPAA confidentiality violations, libel or slander accusations, depositions and property damage (Pohlman, 2015).

Table 22.7   Actions to Decrease the Risk of Liability

- Always treat patients and their family with kindness and respect. Communicate with your patients by keeping them informed and listening to what they say.
- Acknowledge unfortunate incidents, and express concern about these events without either taking the blame, blaming others, or reacting defensively.
- Chart and time your observations immediately, while facts are still fresh in your mind, especially when something adverse has occurred with the patient.
- Take appropriate actions to meet the patient's nursing needs. Be assertive and professional.
- Acknowledge and document the reason for any omission or deviation from agency policy, procedure, or standard.
- Maintain clinical competency and professional certifications.
- Acknowledge your limitations. If you do not know how to do something, ask for help.
- Promptly report any concern regarding the quality of care, including the lack of resources with which to provide care, to a nursing administration representative.
- Delegate patient care based on the documented skills of licensed and unlicensed personnel.
- Communicate the patient's name, room number, and expectations for staff before, during, and after duty performance in a pleasant, direct, and concise manner when delegating patient care.
- Identify realistic, attainable outcome standards for the completion of any task that is delegated. Make frequent walking rounds to assure quality patient outcomes after delegation.
- Follow evidence-based standards of care and the facility's policies and procedures for administering care and reporting incidents. Document the reason for any omission or deviation from agency policy, procedure, or standard.
- Avoid taking telephone and verbal orders. If needed, repeat the order back to the practitioner to assure clarity. Document that you did this with the statement, Verbal Order Repeated Back (VORB).
- Encourage the development of clearly written and/or computerized orders from all practitioners.
- Document the time of nursing actions and changes in conditions requiring notification of the practitioner. Include the response of the practitioner. Use the chain of command at your agency to report any concerns.
- Complete incident reports immediately after incidents occur. Discuss critical factors with the risk manager to increase your retention of the facts. Keep a copy of the incident report, and your charting/documentation if your facility's policies allows it.
- Follow professional guidelines for safe transfer of all patients both inside and outside the agency.

Source: Created by C. Wallinger.

Evidence from the Literature

Citation: Reising, D. L. (2012). Making your nursing care malpractice-proof. *American Nurse Today, 7*(1), 24–28.

Discussion: This article provides a wealth of practical information on how to reduce your risk of being sued for malpractice and what to do if you are named in a malpractice lawsuit. The article defines the elements of a malpractice suit, which are based on the traditional four-step malpractice test, and provides two case examples, one where the four malpractice factors are met, and one where they are not met. According to the article, the most common malpractice claims against nurses are for failure to follow standards of care, failure to use equipment in a responsible manner, failure to assess and monitor, failure to communicate, failure to document, and failure to act as a patient advocate or follow the chain of command. The article explains these claims and then provides a case example for each. The article provides 11 recommendations to reduce a nurse's chances of being named in a malpractice claim, including that nurses know and follow the state's nurse practice act as well as following your facility's policy and procedures, and staying up to date in your field or specialty area. The article also emphasizes the crucial importance of communicating openly and factually with patients, families, and reporting abnormal assessments in a timely fashion to the patient's health care providers.

Implications for Practice: The expansion of the nurse's responsibilities, along with the public recognition that a nurse's role has evolved from a custodian to a full member of the clinical treatment team, means that a nurse is more likely than ever to be faced with a lawsuit for malpractice.

Real World Interview

There is no magic potion that can fix the various industry-wide problems that are present in modern-day nursing practice. Nurses must always keep up to date in their clinical practice and take care to document all care provided. Even with those best practices, it is inevitable that mistakes will happen and regretful that patients are injured by those mistakes. When that occurs, it is important to determine the root cause and respond by taking legitimate steps to improve the delivery of care. This starts with an honest review of a complete and comprehensive medical record.

Documentation is second only to safe, competent nursing practice when protecting oneself from the risk of being the subject of a professional malpractice case. By the time nurses complete their schooling, creating a clear and concise record should be second nature. However, modern "advances" such as the EMR and charting by exception have largely replaced the art of writing a colorful narrative that paints a detailed clinical picture for anyone reviewing the chart in the future.

While the EMR can sometimes look cleaner than the handwritten notes of years gone by, it rarely tells the complete story or provides a reliable clinical picture, particularly several years later when memories fade and the chart is the only record of events. When combined with the time constraints resulting from all-too-common issues with poor staff-to-patient ratios and higher patient acuities, even the best nurse can find him or herself in the sights of a nursing malpractice attorney. If that happens, nurses have the best chance of explaining the wisdom of their clinical decision making with an accurate and comprehensive patient record. Nurses should not shy away from writing a narrative note if that is the best way to document what occurred with the patient on a particular day. Indeed, nurses should insist upon having the time and resources to do so. Failing in this regard does a disservice to patients and increases the risk of a nurse finding him/herself on the wrong side of a lawsuit.

The job is difficult, but the rewards are great. There are precious few careers that allow a person to return home from a day's work knowing that they did something to save or improve a person's quality of life. From a medico-legal perspective, nurses must keep their skills current, and assure that every day's work doesn't end until a full picture of that day's events is charted in the medical record.

**Adam M. Starr, RN, JD,
medical malpractice attorney**

Nurse/Attorney Relationship

Despite the nurse's best intentions, a nurse may be named as a defendant in a lawsuit and need to retain the services of an attorney. LaDuke (2000) made the following suggestions for consulting and collaborating with an attorney:

1. Retain a specialist. Generalists are competent to handle many matters, but professional malpractice, professional disciplinary proceedings, and employment disputes are best handled by specialists in those areas.

2. Be attentive. Read the documents the attorney produces and attend court proceedings to observe the attorney's performance.

3. Notify your insurance carrier as soon as you are aware of any real or potential liability issue. Inform your agent about the status of your case every few months, even if it is unchanged.

4. Keep costs sensible. Your attorney should explain initially verbally and then in writing, in your fee agreement, how

Real World Interview

Most nurses are familiar with the phrase, "If it was not documented, it was not done." Insofar as this phrase is used to encourage thorough documentation, it reflects good nursing practice. Timely, accurate, and complete documentation is an excellent way to protect oneself from litigation. However, lawyers who represent plaintiffs in medical malpractice cases are aware of this "rule" and often attempt to use it against nurses in health care liability claims.

Imagine the following scenario: A patient is admitted to the hospital, and Nurse A performs an initial assessment of the patient. Nurse A notes in the patient's chart that the patient has good capillary refill. Nurse A proceeds to take the patient's vital signs, including capillary refill, hourly throughout Nurse A's 8-hr shift. The patient's capillary refill remains good, and the nurse makes no further documentation in the chart relating to the patient's capillary refill. After Nurse A's shift, Nurse B takes over the patient's care. One hour into Nurse B's shift, the patient codes and expires. The patient's family sues Nurse A. The plaintiffs' lawyer is cross-examining Nurse A.

LAWYER :   "Nurse A, are you familiar with the phrase, 'If it wasn't charted, it wasn't done'?"

NURSE A :   "Yes."

LAWYER :   "That's a common rule in nursing practice, isn't it?"

NURSE A :   "Yes."

LAWYER :   "You were taught that in nursing school, weren't you?"

NURSE A :   "Yes, I was."

LAWYER :   "And after you documented that the patient had good capillary refill upon admission, you did not document anything relating to the patient's capillary refill for the next 8 hours, did you?"

NURSE A :   "Well, no."

LAWYER :   "So if we use your rule, 'If it wasn't documented, it wasn't done', we can assume you never checked the patient's capillary refills during your shift after the initial assessment, right?"

NURSE A :   "No. I checked, but it hadn't changed, so I didn't chart anything."

Do you see what just happened? Nurse A provided competent nursing care, but the lawyer made it appear as if Nurse A was negligent. A nurse involved in litigation should not blankelty agree with this documentation rule. You simply cannot document everything noted in an assessment of a patient. Moreover, most nurses would agree that patient care takes priority over charting. This rule ignores that. Bad charting looks bad. Good charting protects you. Even lapses in charting do not correlate with bad nursing care. Nurses should not lose sight of that when faced with litigation.

Robyn D. Pozza Dollar, JD
Austin, Texas

the fee will be computed and how you will be billed. The attorney may require you to pay a retainer fee.

5. Keep informed. The attorney should address your questions and concerns promptly. You are entitled to be kept informed about the status of your case. You are entitled to copies of all correspondence, legal briefs, and other documents.

6. Weed through writing. Your attorney needs to explain all facts and options. Examine all relevant documents, and do not hesitate to make corrections in the same way you would correct a medical record by drawing a line through the incorrect or misleading information, writing in the correction, and signing your initials after it.

7. Set your own course. Insist on a collaborative relationship with your attorney for the duration of your case.

KEY CONCEPTS

- Nursing practice is governed by federal and state statute, regulations, and case law.

- Nurses are legally responsible for their actions and can be held liable for negligent care.

- Nurses have an ethical and legal obligation to advocate for patients.

- Every health care institution has its own policies and procedures designed to help nurses carry out their professional responsibilities.

- Nurses need to be familiar with their institution's policies and procedures for giving care and for reporting variances, illegal activities, or unexpected events.

- HIPAA legislation was enacted to safeguard private health care information.

- Many sources of evidence are used to identify the standard of care.

- Nursing malpractice examples include treatment problems, communication problems, medication problems, and monitoring/observing/supervising problems.

- The ANA Code of Ethics, and many state Nurse Practice Acts requires nurses to serve as advocates for patients.

- Legal protections in nursing practice include Good Samaritan laws, skillful communication, and risk management programs.

- Torts that can occur in health care include malpractice, assault, battery, false imprisonment, defamation, invasion of privacy, and fraud.

- Nurses need to be familiar with their state nurse practice act to understand the scope of practice permitted in that state.

- Good Samaritan laws exist in many states.

- Risk management programs improve the quality of care and protect the financial integrity of institutions.

KEY TERMS

Advanced directive	Fraud	Negligence
Assault	Good Samaritan laws	Power of attorney
Battery	Informed consent	Risk management programs
Constitution	Invasion of privacy	Statute
Defamation	Living will	Tort
False imprisonment	Malpractice	

REVIEW QUESTIONS

1. You are given a written order by a provider to administer an unusually large dose of pain medicine to your patient. In this situation, which of the following is an appropriate nursing action?
   a. Administer the medication because it was ordered by a provider.
   b. Refuse to administer the medication and move on to another patient.
   c. Select a dose that you feel comfortable with and administer that dose.
   d. Clarify with pharmacy as to the correct dose, then speak with the provider about your concerns and the information you learned from pharmacy about the correct medication dose.

2. A practitioner has ordered you to discharge Mr. Jones, a post-surgery patient, from the hospital, despite a new temperature of 102.0 °F (38.8 °C). The practitioner refuses to talk with you about the patient. In this situation, which of the following is an appropriate nursing action?
   a. Administer an antipyretic medication and discharge the patient.
   b. Discharge the patient with instructions to call 911 if he has any problems.
   c. Do not discharge the patient until you have discussed the matter with your nursing manager and are satisfied regarding patient safety.
   d. Discharge the patient and tell the patient to take Tylenol when he gets home.

3. A practitioner has issued a Do Not Resuscitate (DNR) order for your patient, a 55-year-old man with cancer. You spoke with the patient this morning, and he clearly wishes to be resuscitated in the event that he stops breathing. What is the most appropriate course of action?
   a. Attempt to talk the patient into agreeing to the DNR.
   b. Ignore the patient's wishes because the practitioner ordered the DNR.
   c. Contact the medical licensing board to complain about the practitioner.

   d. Consult your hospital's policies and procedures, speak to the practitioner, and discuss the matter with your nurse manager.

4. The Health Insurance Portability and Accountability Act (HIPAA) protects which of the following types of information?
   a. The nurse's right to take her health insurance with her if she leaves the employer.
   b. The confidentiality of certain protected health information.
   c. The hospital's right to disclose protected health information.
   d. A patient's right to be insured, regardless of employment status or ability to pay.

5. Which of the following elements is not necessary for a nurse to be found negligent in a court of law?
   a. A breach of the nurse's duty or obligation to provide competent care.
   b. The nurse's intention to be negligent.
   c. A duty or obligation for the nurse to act in a particular way.
   d. Physical, emotional, or financial harm to the patient.

6. Which type of law authorizes state boards to enact rules that govern the practice of nursing?
   a. State Statutes.
   b. State Case law.
   c. State Legislative history.
   d. State Criminal law.

7. You are a new nurse working on a medical-surgical unit. One of your patients, an elderly woman, has an advanced directive that requests that no CPR be done in the event that she stops breathing. One day she stops breathing, and someone on your unit calls a "code" and begins resuscitative efforts. You go along with the team and help to resuscitate the patient. She regains a pulse but never regains consciousness. She is now ventilator dependent and her family is very angry with you and the staff. Which of the following is a potential legal allegation you could face?
   a. Battery and malpractice.
   b. Violation of patient privacy.
   c. Criminal recklessness.
   d. Revoked nursing license.

8. Which of the following is not an essential element of a Good Samaritan law?
   a. The care is rendered in an emergency situation.
   b. The health care worker is rendering care without pay.
   c. The health care worker is concerned about the safety of the victims.
   d. The care provided went beyond the legal scope of practice for that health care worker, and the party suffered an injury or harm because of that care.

9. In which of the following situations could a nurse not be accused of false imprisonment? Select all that apply.
   a. Restraining a competent person without a provider's order

   b. Inappropriate use of physical restraints
   c. Inappropriate use of chemical restraints
   d. Using restraints in an emergency situation to protect the patient from harm

10. The goal of a risk management program in an institution is to do which of the following? Select all that apply.
    a. Identify and correct systemic problems in the facility.
    b. Identify when better orientation is needed for staff.
    c. Identify issues with equipment and staffing.
    d. Punish the person responsible for the error.
    e. Reduce legal and financial liability for the institution.
    f. Reduce the number of errors made in patient care.

REVIEW QUESTION ANSWERS

1. Answer: D is correct.
   Rational: (A) is contrary to the nurse's role as a patient advocate. (B) is inappropriate because the patient's pain must be treated. (C) is incorrect because the RN is not licensed to prescribe medicine; it is outside the scope of the RN's practice. (D) ensures the patient's pain is treated with a correct dose of medicine.

2. Answer: C is correct.
   Rational: All of the other choices put the patient at risk for injury, and therefore are contrary to the nurse's role as a patient advocate. Also, the nurse must act because nurses can be held liable for malpractice in failing to question potentially dangerous provider orders.

3. Answer: D is correct,
   Rational: The patient's wishes are paramount and must take precedence here. Only (D) ensures that the patient's wishes will be followed. The first 2 choices (A, B) are both contrary to the nurse's role as patient advocate. (C) could potentially expose the nurse to an accusation of defamation if the physician's reputation is negatively affected without a legal basis.

4. Answer: B is correct.
   Rational: HIPAA specifically protects the confidentiality of certain protected health information, and provides for significant penalties for violation (B). (A) is not about information. (C) is incorrect because HIPAA specifically prohibits a hospital from disclosing protected health information without the patient's permission. (D) is wrong because HIPAA does not involve a patient's insurance or employment status.

5. Answer: B is correct.
   Rational: Negligence is an unintentional tort; the nurse's intention is irrelevant (B). (A, C, and D) are all required for a patient to prove a nurse was negligent.

6. Answer: A is correct.
   Rational: Each state has a statute that authorizes the state Board of Nursing to enact such rules (A). (B, C, and D) are important but they do not impact the practice of nursing.

7. Answer: A is correct.
   Rational: A "code" would be a battery, i.e., an unwanted touching. The "code" also could be malpractice because the nurse's care fell below the prevailing standard of care in that the nurse failed to abide by the patient's wishes (A). (B) is incorrect because no patient information was disclosed. (C) is incorrect because there was no criminal behavior by the nurse. (D) is incorrect because the civil malpractice system is separate from licensure by the state.

8. Answer: D is correct.
   Rational: If the health care worker provides care beyond that worker's scope of practice and the party suffered an injury or harm because of that care, the worker is not covered by the Good Samaritan law (D). (A, B, and C) are the requirements that must be met if the worker is to be protected by the Good Samaritan Act.

9. Answer: D is correct.
   Rational: D is not false imprisonment because there was a patient emergency. (A, B, and C) could all lead to such charges because the actions put the patient in jeopardy of injury, rather than protecting the patient from injury, and the patient was not free to leave the situation.

10. Answers A, B, C, E, and F are correct.
    Rational: The risk management system is not designed to punish the person responsible for the error, but instead is designed to prevent future errors (D).

REVIEW ACTIVITIES

1. Talk to the risk manager at the hospital in which you have your clinical assignments. Ask the risk manager how he or she handles an incident report. Is it used for improving the hospital's care in the future? If so, how? Ask if the hospital or facility uses some form of the CANDOR system to explain medical errors to patients and their families.

2. Identify the various ways in which nurses you observe in your clinical rotations discuss orders and treatments with practitioners

and other nurses. How do nurses address incorrect or dangerous medication orders? Talk with nurses you encounter about how they handle these situations.

3. Research the various companies that offer nursing malpractice insurance, and determine the cost and coverage associated with a nursing malpractice policy. Go to an Internet search engine, such as www.google.com Search for nursing malpractice insurance. What did you find? Note the Nurses Service Organization (NSO) Web site at www.nso.com Recent legal cases are reported there.

DISCUSSION POINTS

- Consider the common errors of nursing practice that lead to malpractice actions, as outlined in Table 22.4. What actions can a nurse can take to minimize these committing these errors?

- Consider the communication errors outlined in Table 22.4. What specifically would you say to a provider who is "too busy" to come to see your patient prior to you sending the patient for a procedure when it is clear to you that the patient does not understand the procedure and its risks?

- Review the story of the Vanderbilt nurse who used a "work around" to bypass the medication system's safeguards, leading to the death of a patient. During your recent clinical experiences, have you seen nurses perform a "work around?" Was there an emergency at that time?

- Documentation should follow the nursing process and should include the tasks/work performed with the patient, such as vital signs, medications, treatments, interventions, and reassessments. In particular, it is imperative to document the patient's response to clinical treatments. During your recent clinical experiences, when you have reviewed the nurse's notes, have you seen documentation of the patient's response to clinical treatments or pain medication?

DISCUSSION OF OPENING SCENARIO

1. After notifying the surgical resident about the elevated temperature, do you need to gather additional information about the patient's condition before you discharge him?

   Discussion: Yes, you would want to do a full physical assessment, including listening to lung sounds and checking the patient's wounds for drainage, and his skin color for temperature and mottling, etc.

2. What do you do if the patient appears to be too ill for discharge? Is there anyone else you can contact?

   Discussion: yes, you should follow the chain of command by first speaking with your charge nurse and nurse manager. Second, call the patient's attending surgeon directly and use SBAR to relay your findings, and relate who you have spoken to. If necessary, contact the nursing supervisor and the risk management department. Be sure to document all of these conversations.

3. If you discharge the patient and he develops sepsis or a serious illness, who of the following might be held responsible: you, the nurse's aide, the surgical resident, the attending surgeon who performed the surgery?

   Discussion: The nurse's aide would not be held responsible because the aide is unlicensed and working under your direction. You, the surgical resident and the attending surgeon could be held responsible, because you all had a duty to the patient to provide competent care. (Step 1). If the patient can later prove the remaining 3 steps of a malpractice claim, that is that treatment (discharging the patient with an elevated temperature) fell below the prevailing standard of care (Step 2), that the patient suffered harm (Step 3), and that the harm was directly caused by the treatment (Step 4), then the patient could be successful in a malpractice case.

EXPLORING THE WEB

- You have a patient who is to be transferred to a nursing home for recuperation. Visit this site to see where you could refer a family that is looking to evaluate the local nursing homes regarding their adherence to the federal regulations for nursing homes, HTTPs Accessed June 19, 2019.

- Visit this site to learn about the Modules used to implement the CANDOR system for explaining medical errors: www.ahrq.gov/professionals/quality-patient-safety/patient-safety-resources/resources/candor/introduction.html. Accessed June 3, 2019

- Use Google to research "living wills" and "power of attorney." What did you find there? Google "Five Wishes" or visit the Individuals and Families tab at, https://fivewishes.org Accessed June 19, 2019, to see a simple, easy-to-use advance directive document written in plain English. For more information about advance directives/powers of attorney, visit the Financial and Legal tab at the American Association of Retired Persons' (AARP) Family Caregiving website www.aarp.org/caregiving Accessed June 19, 2019. or polst.org/advance-care-planning/polst-and-advance-directives/ Accessed June19, 2019.

- Go to this site to find the impact of the HITECH Act on the privacy and security concerns associated with the electronic transmission of health information: www.hhs.gov/hipaa/for-professionals/regulatory-initiatives/index.html Accessed June 3, 2019.

- Visit the Quality and Safety Education for Nurses website for more information about the use of the SBAR tool and teaching strategies in the clinical setting,

- http://qsen.org/teaching-pre-licensure-nursing-students-to-communicate-in-sbar-in-the-clinical-setting Accessed June 3, 2019.

- http://qsen.org/Improving-communication with SBAR in the clinical setting. Accessed June 3, 2019.

- Here are other web sources about SBAR:

  o www.ihi.org/resources/Pages/Tools/SBARToolkit.aspx Accessed June 3, 2019.

  o www.jointcommission.org/at_home_with_the_joint_commission/sbar_%E2%80%93_a_powerful_tool_to_help_improve_communication Accessed June 3, 2019.

INFORMATICS

1. Review this article to learn how a registered nurse and an emergency physician created a computerized algorithm/early warning system that automatically alerts providers to the clinical signs of sepsis, and how they regularly track patient data to evaluate the impact of their efforts. The article is, Preventing Sepsis by Reimagining Systems and Engaging Patients, www.healthaffairs.org/doi/10.1377/hlthaff.2019.00339 Accessed 5/8/2019. Have you encountered these types of computer-based warnings in your acute care clinical sites?

2. While reviewing that article, review footnote 5, which describes the Rory Staunton Foundation. Visit the Foundation's site at https://rorystauntonfoundationforsepsis.org/sepsis-protocol Accessed 5/8/2019. See how this Foundation's advocacy with state legislatures is changing the treatment of sepsis across the country by advocating for mandatory sepsis protocols. Have you encountered these types of sepsis protocols at your acute care clinical settings?

LEAN BACK

- Now that you understand the importance of excellent nursing documentation in the defense of a malpractice claim, how will that affect your practice as a student nurse?

- How will it affect your practice as a graduate nurse?

REFERENCES

American Nurses Association. (2010). *Principles for nursing documentation: Guidance for registered nurses.* Silver Springs, MD: American Nurses Assocation.

American Nurses Association. (2015). *Code of ethics for nurses with interpretive statements.* Silver Springs, MD: American Nurses Assocation.

American Nurses Association. (2019). Retrieved from www.nursingworld.org/news/news-releases/2019-news-releases/ana-responds-to-vanderbilt-nurse-incident.

Attorney General Press Release. (2018, June). A.G. Underwood Announces Sentencing Of Registered Nurse Who Stole Over $390,000 From Medicaid. Retrieved November 05, 2020, from https://ag.ny.gov/press-release/2018/ag-underwood-announces-sentencing-registered-nurse-who-stole-over-390000-medicaid

Balestra, M. (2017). Electronic health records: Patient care and ethical and legal implications for nurse practitioners. *The Journal for Nurse Practitioners, 13*(2), 105–111.

Black's Law Dictionary. (2014) 10 Thomson West.

Buppert, C. (2015). *Frequently asked legal questions keeping nurses awake at night.* Boulder, CO: Law Office of Carolyn Buppert, P.C. Nurses Services Organization. Retrieved from /www.nso.com/Learning/Artifacts/Articles/when-to-refuse-an-assignment.

CNA Financial Corporation. (2009). *CNA HealthPro nurse claims study: An analysis of claims with risk management recommendations 1997–2007.* Hatboro, PA: CNA Financial Corporation. PDF of report available at www.nso.com/nursing-resources/claim-studies.jsp.

CNA Financial Corporation. (2015). *CNA insurance company and nurses services organization: Nurse professional liability exposures: 2015 claim report update.* Retrieved from www.nso.com/Learning/Artifacts/Claim-Reports/Nurse-Professional-Liability-Exposures-2015-Claim.

Communication and Optimal Resolution (CANDOR) Toolkit. (n.d.). *Agency for healthcare research and quality.* Rockville, MD. Retrieved from www.ahrq.gov/professionals/quality-patient-safety/patient-safety-resources/resources/candor/introduction.html.

Compassion & Choices. (2019). *Our Mission. Our Work. [Brochure].* Portland, OR: Compassion and Choices. Retrieved from https://compassionandchoices.org/wp-content/uploads/Our-Mission-Our-Work-FINAL-2-19-19.pdf.

HHS Office of the Secretary, Office for Civil Rights. (2017, June). HIPAA for Professionals. Retrieved from www.hhs.gov/hipaa/for-professionals/index.html

Huff, C. (2019). Preventing sepsis by reimagining systems and engaging patients. *Health Affairs, 38*(5), 704–708. doi:10.1377/hlthaff.2019.00339

Jackman, T. (2015, June). Anesthesiologist trashes sedated patient-and it ends up costing her, *Washington Post.* Retrieved from www.washingtonpost.com/local/anesthesiologist-trashes-sedated-patient-jury-orders-her-to-pay-500000/2015/06/23/cae05c00-18f3-11e5-ab92-c75ae6ab94b5_story.html?utm_term=.9c7cadf998b9.

Joint Commission. (2016). Informed consent: More than getting a signature. *QuickSafety.* p. 21. Retrieved from www.jointcommission.org/issues/article.aspx?Article=5kmqmwV14ugGGireNakQqaCw1iqenpbl1IjAYdRsubU%3D.

LaDuke, S. (2000). What should you expect from your attorney? *Nursing Management, 31*(1), 10.

Müller, M., Jürgens, J., & Redaèlli, M. (2018). Impact of the communication and patient hand-off tool SBAR on patient safety: A systematic review. *BMJ Open, 8*, e022202. doi:10.1136/bmjopen-2018-022202

Murphy v. United Parcel Service, 527 U.S. 516 (1999).

Myles v. Hospital Serv. Dist, 248 So. 3d 545, 549 (2018).

National Council for State Boards of Nursing. (2020). *Facts about the NLC [Brochure].* Chicago, IL: National Council of State Boards of Nursing. Retrieved from www.ncsbn.org/NLC_Facts-FINAL.pdf.

National Council of State Boards of Nursing. (2018). *A nurses guide to the use of social media.* Chicago, IL: National Council of State Boards of Nursing. Retrieved from www.ncsbn.org/NCSBN_SocialMedia.pdf.

National Health Care Anti-Fraud Association. (2020). The Challenge of Health Care Fraud. Retrieved from www.nhcaa.org/resources/health-care-anti-fraud-resources/the-challenge-of-health-care-fraud/.

New York Attorney General's Office. (2018). Retrieved from https://ag.ny.gov/press-release/ag-underwood-announces-sentencing-registered-nurse-who-stole-over-390000-medicaid

Nurses Services Organization. (2009). *CNA HealthPro nurse claims study: An analysis of claims sith risk management recommendations 1997–2007* (pp. 1–54). Chicago, IL: CNA. Retrieved from www.nso.com/Learning/Artifacts/Articles/when-to-refuse-an-assignment.

Pagulayan, J., Eltair, S., & Faber, K. (2018). Nurse documentation and the electronic health record. *American Nurse Today, 13*(9), 48–54.

Pohlman, K. J. (2015). Why you need your own malpractice insurance. *American Nurse Today, 10*(11), 28–30.

Reising, D. L. (2012). Making your nursing care malpractice-proof. *American Nurse Today, 7*(1), 24–28.

Sutton v. United Airlines, 527 U.S. 471 (1999).

Webb v. Tulane Medical Center Hospital. (2019). 700 So. 2d 1141, 1145 (La. 1997). Retrieved fromwww.nursingcenter.com/clinical-resources/nursing-pocket-cards/nursing-documentation.

SUGGESTED READINGS

Berwick, D., & Gaines, M. (2018). How HIPAA harms care, and how to stop it. *Journal of the American Medical Association, 320*(3), 229–230.

Fink, S. (2016). *Five days at Memorial: Life and death in a storm-ravaged hospital.* New York: Broadway Books.

Gawande, A. (2018, November). Why doctors hate their computers. *New Yorker.*

Jacoby, S. R., & Scruth, E. A. (2017). Negligence and the nurse: The value of a code of ethics for nurses. *Clinical Nurse Specialist* (July/August), *31*(4), 183–185.

Potter, K. A. (2018, Winter). *The dark side of social media: When its misuse violates a person's privacy rights, Trial Advocate Quarterly.* p. 16.

Ethical Aspects of Nursing

23

Joan Dorman
Purdue University Northwest, College of Nursing, Hammond, IN, USA

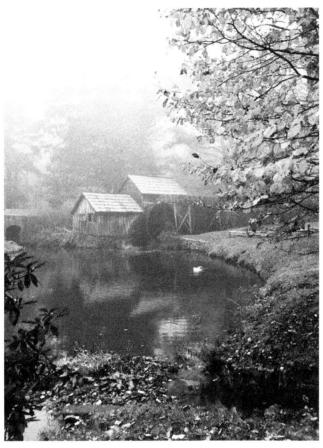

When the fog lifts and things come into focus, we are able to reflect.
Source: Joan Dorman

It is curious that physical courage should be so common in the world and moral courage so rare. **Mark Twain, 1907**

OBJECTIVES

Upon completion of this chapter, the reader should be able to:

1. Define ethics.
2. Identify historical and philosophical influences on nursing practice.
3. Devise a personal philosophy of professional nursing.

Kelly Vana's Nursing Leadership and Management, Fourth Edition. Edited by Patricia Kelly Vana and Janice Tazbir
© 2021 John Wiley & Sons Ltd. Published 2021 by John Wiley & Sons Ltd.
Companion Website: www.wiley.com/go/kelly-Nursing-Leadership

4. Analyze ethical theories, virtues, principles, and values as the basis for professional nursing practice.

5. Support participation on ethics committee in health care organization.

6. Explain values clarification.

7. Apply an Ethical Positioning System (EPS) Model to an ethical dilemma.

8. Discuss ethical issues related to patients' rights.

9. Support ethical nursing leadership and management's responsibility in professional practice.

10. Develop an ethical workplace.

11. Review the International Council of Nursing's Code of Ethics for Nurses and the American Nurses Association Code of Ethics for Nurses.

OPENING SCENARIO

In a large teaching hospital, a patient you are caring for says he does not want to go on living. He has had cancer for several years and states he is tired of being sick. When you ask him whether he has shared these feelings with his family, he says that he does not want them to think he is giving up. You report the patient's statements to the nurse on the next shift and explain how you encouraged him to talk with his family and his practitioner. That evening, the patient suddenly has a cardiac arrest and a code is called. The patient

ends up on a ventilator, receives five units of blood, and is comatose. The patient did not have advance directives and Do Not Resuscitate (DNR) orders had not been signed.

1. *What are your thoughts about maintaining the patient's life in this situation?*

2. *Who should make the decision about the patient's situation while he is comatose?*

3. *How can you act as an advocate for the patient and the family?*

Introduction

Throughout its history, nursing has relied on ethical principles to serve as a guideline in determining care. Nurses are confronted with ethical dilemmas in all types of practice settings. This chapter provides an overview of the nursing profession's challenges related to ethical theories, virtues, principles, and values in today's health care environment. Some of the terms used in this chapter might be confusing, but they are all related to each other. In the following discussion, you can see their relationships and that these terms are connected. Ethical leadership and management's responsibility in professional practice and organizations is explored. The chapter goes on to discuss developing a personal philosophy of professional nursing and the value of ethics committees, ethical workplaces, and values clarification. An EPS Model is applied to an ethical dilemma as well as to ethical issues related to patients' rights. Finally, the International Council of Nursing's Code for Nurses and the American Nurses' Association Code for Nurses is discussed.

Historical and Philosophical Influences on Nursing Practice

Nursing practice evolved from the needs of society and has been strongly influenced by religions and women. Society created the profession of nursing for the purpose of meeting specific, perceived health needs (Burkhardt & Nathaniel, 2014).

Nursing fulfilled the need to care for people with these needs. A strong instinct for the preservation of humanity gave people the motivation to help one another. The concern for the health of the community was evident in antiquity and continued as civilizations developed (Donahue, 2011). A relationship between nursing and the community evolved as social needs and individual motivation to care for others developed.

In the early Christian era, workers who were engaged in nursing, usually women, were often trained in the doctrines of the church, including unquestioning obedience, humility, and sacrificing oneself for the good of others. An individual nurse did not make independent decisions, but followed instructions given by a priest or practitioner. Donahue states that nursing has its origin in a mother's care of helpless infants and must have coexisted with this type of care from earliest times (Donahue, 2011). Mothers cared for family members when they were helpless and sick. During the Christian era, women were selected by Jesus to care for those in need because of the compassion they showed as they ministered to the poor and sick. Thus, Christianity greatly enhanced women's opportunities for useful social service (Donahue, 2011).

Ethics

Ethics is a branch of philosophy dealing with what is morally right or wrong. The study of ethical behavior has resulted in different ethical theories that apply to nursing practice and form a framework for ethical decision making. Table 23.1 describes

Table 23.1 **Selected Ethical Theories**

Ethical theory	Interpretation
Deontology	Actions are based on moral rules and unchanging principles, such as "do unto others as you would have them do unto you." An ethical person must always follow the rules, even if doing so causes a less desirable outcome. Theory states that the motives of the actor determine the goodness or value of the act. Thus, a bad outcome is acceptable as long as the intent was good.
Teleology	A person must take those actions that lead to good outcomes. The theory states that the outcome of an act determines whether the act is good or of value and that achievement of a good outcome justifies using a less desirable means to attain the end.
Virtue ethics	Virtues such as truthfulness and trustworthiness are developed over time. A person's character must be developed so that by nature and habit, the person will be predisposed to behave virtuously. Living a virtuous life contributes both to one's own well-being and to the well-being of society.
Justice and equity	A "veil of ignorance" regarding who is affected by a decision should be used by decision makers, because it allows for unbiased decision making. An ethical person chooses the action that is fair to all, including those persons who are most disadvantaged.
Relativism	There are no universal ethical standards, such as "murder is always wrong." Ethical standards are relative to person, place, time, and culture. Whatever a person thinks is right, is right. This theory has been largely rejected.

Source: J. Dorman

Critical Thinking 23.1

Most ethical concerns simply deal with doing the right thing. In some cases, however, there is also a legal component. Examples may be stealing or assault. With this in mind, which of the following behaviors are Ethical and Legal? Ethical and Illegal? Unethical and Legal? or Unethical and Illegal?

- Reporting an abuse victim to law enforcement officers against his wishes
- Honoring a terminally ill patient's request to have "no heroic" actions taken
- Discontinuing a comatose patient's life support at the request of the family
- Diverting medications from a patient for your own use

---

some of these theories. Ethics governs professional groups and provides a framework for determining the right course of action in a particular situation. For nurses, the actions they take in practice are primarily governed by the ethical principles of the nursing profession. These principles influence practice, conduct, and the relationships that nurses are held accountable for in the delivery of care. Health care ethics, also called **bioethics**, are ethics specific to health care and also serve as a framework to guide behavior. An **ethical dilemma** occurs when there is a conflict between two or more ethical principles and there appears to be no "correct" decision. **Morality** refers to the distinction between right and wrong or good and bad behavior. **Laws**, in contrast, are state and federal government rules that govern all of society. Laws mandate behavior.

Philosophy

Philosophy is the rational investigation of the truths and principles of knowledge, reality, and human conduct. Personal philosophies stem from an individual's beliefs and values. These beliefs and values develop based upon a person's experiences in life, cultural influences, and education. These beliefs and values, in turn, become one's ethical compass, pointing the way

to right or wrong. A professional nurse's personal philosophy affects that nurse's philosophy of nursing. Throughout the nursing educational process, students begin forming their philosophy of nursing. This philosophy is influenced significantly by a student's personal philosophy and past experiences. One's personal philosophy should be compatible with the philosophy of the nursing department where the nurse works. This helps the future nurse develop into an effective leader and practitioner. An example of a personal nursing philosophy is the following:

> *I believe professional nursing care promotes an optimal level of wellness in body, mind, and spirit to those being served. I believe professional nurses must hold themselves to the highest standards of the profession and honor the profession's Code of Ethics in all aspects of practice.*

Many health care centers have addressed ethical concerns by developing professional practice models. The American Nurses Association Nursing Code of Ethics (ANA, 2015a,b), Nursing Scope and Standards of Practice (ANA, 2015a,b), and Quality and Safety Education for Nurses competencies (Cronenwett et al., 2007) are useful in developing these

---

Critical Thinking 23.2

Mr. Johanssen smokes three packs of cigarettes a day and is seen in a free clinic for chronic obstructive pulmonary disease. All attempts to get him to stop smoking have failed. Mr. Johanssen tells you that smoking is the one pleasure he has in life and he does not want to give it up.

Do you respect Mr. Johanssen's wishes?

Does he have a right to the free treatment and medications?

Are limits to Mr. Johanssen's treatments justified?

Critical Thinking 23.3

New graduates should formulate a philosophy of nursing based on personal beliefs and values. Reflections on the following questions can assist in the development of a philosophy:

What do I believe about nursing practice?

Should nurses be patient advocates?

How should professionals conduct themselves when patient values differ from a nurse's personal values?

How can I influence patient care based on my nursing philosophy?

Are the virtues of compassion, discernment, trustworthiness, and integrity important both personally and professionally?

---

models. Professional nursing models of care are shared with employees and consumers to illustrate an organization's philosophy and commitment to excellence. A Nursing Model of Care can be viewed in Chapter 5. Other nursing models of care can be viewed at www.bing.com/images/search?q=nursing+model+of+care&id=A3CCDDB8AE80CE6CE15 E2EDB366BD6B809F8510B&FORM=IQFRBA, accessed May 13, 2019.

Virtue is a quality considered morally good or desirable in a person. Beauchamp and Childress (2019) list four focal virtues that are more significant than others and that are illustrative of a virtuous person: compassion, discernment, trustworthiness, and integrity. Compassion, so valuable in nursing, is the ability to imagine oneself in the situation of another. Discernment is possession of acuteness of judgment and understanding which can then result in decisive action. Trustworthiness is present when trust is well-founded or deserving. It is accounted for in the reputation of the nurse among co-workers. Integrity may be considered firm adherence to a code of conduct or an ethical value and means soundness and reliability as well as consistency of convictions, actions, and emotions. Trustworthiness and integrity are virtues expected in all people but are especially necessary for professional nurses. These virtues form the foundation for an ethically principled discipline and have been endorsed throughout the profession's history (Burkhardt & Nathaniel, 2014).

Ethical principles also provide a basis for nurses to determine the appropriate action when faced with an ethical dilemma in the practice setting. A **Principle** is a fundamental truth that serves as the foundation for a system of beliefs or behavior. A **Value** is the regard that something is held to deserve due to its importance, worth, or usefulness Table 23.2.

Ethics Committees

In this time of incredible technological advancement, health care institutions find themselves increasingly faced with ethical dilemmas. These ethical dilemmas span the age continuum from pre-birth and birth to death and post-death. Most health care institutions have ethics committees to help deal with these ethical dilemmas. An ethics committee is comprised of an interprofessional group representing medicine, nursing, pastoral care, pharmacy, nutritional services, social services, quality management, legal services, and/or the community. On any given occasion, there may also be guests, for example, members from a specialty area such as obstetrics or oncology. Family members may also be invited to an ethics committee meeting Figure 23.1.

The mission of a hospital's ethics committee is to provide thoughtful and timely consultation when an ethical issue arises. This might involve an emergency meeting of some or all of the members. There is generally a written policy guiding the consultation process. The committee needs to know the background of the ethical issue and all pertinent information. They need to explore the options, along with the risks and benefits of these options, and review the ethical theories and principles involved. They need to examine the possibilities for resolution and the potential outcomes of those resolutions. The committee does not make a decision. The ethics committee consults, gives guidance, and provides any resources needed for ethically sound decision making. In the case of the patient

Table 23.2 **Ethical Principles**

Ethical principle	Definition	Example
Beneficence	The duty to do good to others and to maintain a balance between benefits and harms	• Provide all patients, including the terminally ill, with caring attention. • Become familiar with your local, state, and national laws regarding organ donations. • Treat every patient with respect and courtesy.
Nonmaleficence	The principle of doing no harm	• Always work within your current American Nurses Association Nursing: Scope and Standards of Practice. • Never give information or perform duties you are not qualified to do. • Observe all safety rules and precautions. • Keep areas safe from hazards. • Perform procedures according to facility protocols. • Ask an appropriate person about anything you are unsure of. • Keep your education and skills up to date with competency building and life-long learning.
Justice	The principle of fairness that is served when an individual is given that which he or she is due, owed, deserves, or can legitimately claim	• Treat all patients fairly, regardless of economic or social background. • Learn the local, state, and national laws and your facility's policies.
Autonomy	Respect for an individual's right to self-determination; respect for individual liberty	• Be sure that patients have consented to all treatments and procedures. • Become familiar with local, state, and national laws and facility policies dealing with advance directives. • Respect patient privacy and confidentiality.
Fidelity	The principle of promise keeping; the duty to keep one's word if possible, to be trustworthy. It refers to loyalty within the nurse–patient relationship.	• Be sure that necessary contracts or promises have been completed. • Be committed to providing safe, quality care for your patients. • Be your patient's advocate.
Respect	Consider others to be of high regard. The right of people to make their own decisions	• Provide all persons with information for decision making. • Avoid making paternalistic decisions for others.
Veracity	Refers to loyalty within the nurse-patient relationship.	• Admit mistakes promptly. Offer to do whatever is necessary to correct them. • Refuse to participate in any form of fraud.
Accountability	The obligation to accept responsibility and account for actions	• Assure all documentation is thorough, accurate, and timely.
Confidentiality	Refers to nondisclosure of private information.	• Assure there is not discussion of patients in public areas. • Keep all electronic or written records private.

on the ventilator in the opening scenario, the ethics committee may invite family members of the patient on a ventilator, as well as other members of the inter-professional team who care for the patient, to assist the ethics committee with the review.

Values and Values Clarification

Value is the regard that something is held to deserve due to its importance, worth, or usefulness. If you were told that you must pack a bag for a special trip but you may bring only three items from your belongings, what items would you choose? The items selected are what you value.

Values Clarification is the process of analyzing one's own values to better understand what is truly important. In their classic work—*Values and Teaching*—Raths, Harmin, and Simon (1978, p. 47) formulated a theory of values clarification and proposed a three-step process of valuing, i.e., choose a value, prize the value, and act on the value,

1. *Choosing*: Beliefs are chosen freely (i.e., without coercion) from among alternatives. The choosing step involves analysis of the consequences of various alternatives.

2. *Prizing*: The beliefs that are selected are cherished (i.e., prized).

3. *Acting*: The selected beliefs are demonstrated consistently through behavior.

Nurses must understand that values are individual rather than universal; therefore, nurses should not try to impose their own values on patients.

Guides to Ethical Decision Making

Nurses have long sought guidance in the face of ethical dilemmas. The differences in knowledge and skill between novice and expert nurses is measurable, but the ease or torment with which

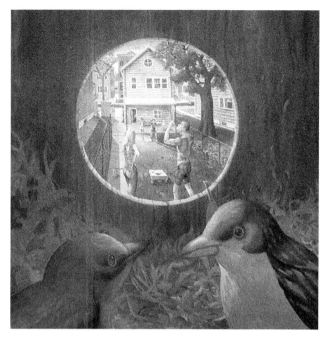

FIGURE 23.1   One must try to see things from various perspectives, especially with ethical issues. J. Dorman.
Source: Tom Torluemke.

these same nurses make ethical decisions is often virtually the same. For that reason, it seems that a specific ethical decision-making tool is helpful. Just as most of us rely on some sort of Global Positioning System (GPS) navigation device when traveling into "uncharted waters," nurses often find themselves looking for the route that might lead them to an ethical decision.

Jonsen, Siegler, and Winslade (2015) have published a practical approach to ethical decision making in clinical ethics. Their model is directed not only to physicians and medical students, but to hospital administrators, ethics committees, and other health care workers. Their model consists of four topics:

- Medical indications: How might this patient benefit?

- Patient preferences: Is the patient's right to choose being respected?

- Quality of life: What are the prospects for a meaningful life?

- Contextual features: What other issues need to be considered?

In examining each of these four topics, the authors ask that we consider the ethical principles inherent in the decision we ultimately make.

The Ethical Positioning System Model

The EPS Model follows the format of the nursing process, with a few additions. It is a helpful tool for ethical decision making (Table 23.3, Figures 23.2 and 23.3).

An Ethics Test

A practical way of improving ethical decision making is to run decisions that you are considering through an ethics test when any doubt exists. The ethics test presented here (Bowditch & Bruno, 2007) has been used to promote ethical behavior in organizational training programs. Decision makers are taught to ask themselves:

- Is it right?

- Is it fair?

- Who gets hurt?

- Would you be comfortable if the details of your decision were reported on the front page of your local newspaper or through your hospital's e-mail system?

- Would you tell your child or young relative to do it?

- How does it smell? This question is based on a person's intuition and common sense.

Critical Thinking 23.4

Gary was a "frequent flyer" in a local Emergency Department (ED). He would show up late at night in the ED, very intoxicated, at least five times a month. He was always alone, and, at times, he was homeless. The staff would bathe him, start an IV with vitamins and Thiamine, and tuck him in for a good night's sleep. In the morning, they would order him breakfast, find clothing for him in the special stash they kept, and send him on his way. He was always polite and grateful for their care. He knew all the nurses by name, and they all knew Gary. They had tried to get him into rehab on various occasions, but he was not ready to quit drinking. One night, the paramedics brought Gary in after someone had slit his throat. He died in surgery that night. The ED nurses were devastated. Gary was only 46 years old and should have had a whole life ahead of him. They felt that all they had done was for naught. They had not been able to help him.

About 3 weeks later, the ED staff received a letter from a woman that identified herself as Gary's sister. She lived in California. She said she was writing on behalf of her brother because she knew he would want the staff to know how important they were in his life. He often said that they were the only ones that treated him with dignity and respect, and that he felt like they were his family. The nurses realized that you do not always recognize how or when you are helping people, but the impact of their care is profound, nonetheless.

Did the ED nurses help Gary?

Should they have done something differently?

Evidence From the Literature

Citation: Peter, E. (2018, January 31). Overview and Summary: Ethics in Healthcare: Nurses Respond. *Online Journal of Issues in Nursing, 23* (1). Retrieved November 28, 2018.

Discussion: The author discusses the many ways in which nurses can advocate for nursing actions that demonstrate ethical awareness in small ways, not just those that garner public awareness. Connecting patients to resources and supporting patients and team members when misunderstandings or injustices occur are just a few examples. Ethics education at the workplace can have a tremendous impact. Nurses, in the workplace, can emphasize the ethical implications of interpersonal, technological, and social issues in their professional lives.

Implications for Practice: Nurses empowered to promote ethical behaviors in the workplace will enhance patient care, teamwork, and, most certainly, professional satisfaction.

Critical Thinking 23.5

Select a patient care ethical issue of your choice in class. Have the class split into two groups, one on each side of the issue. Have each group discuss the ethical issues involved. Instruct the groups to consider all pertinent ethical theories and principles; any conflicts between them; any relationship to the people involved and impacted; and any relevant sociocultural, political, or religious aspects that may influence this ethical issue. Then ask a volunteer from each group to state the group's position. Share any references that the group may have found.

What were the pros identified? What were the cons?

Did any of the group's comments alter your own position on this ethical issue?

Table 23.3 The Ethical Positioning System (EPS) Model

1. <u>Assessment</u>: In this step, the nurse gathers all available data. This includes identifying all people involved in the decision-making process and exploring everything pertinent to the context of the situation (Figure 23.3).
2. <u>Nursing Dilemma</u>: This is a simple statement of the problem.
3. <u>Planning</u>: In this step, the nurse examines all possible choices of actions and identifies pros and cons for each choice. Ethical principles and the American Nurses Association Code of Ethics for Nurses with Interpretive Statements (2015) are reviewed for consideration in the case.
4. <u>Diagram</u>: This is a visual image of the planning process described above. This is a one-page picture of all the considerations, making the appropriate ethical decision clearer.
5. <u>Implementation</u>: One choice is selected and implemented.
6. <u>Evaluation</u>: The choice is evaluated. Did it work? What was the outcome? What was learned?

Source: Dorman, J. (2009). *EPS model.* Unpublished Manuscript.

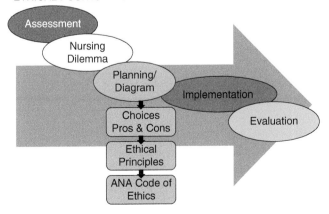

ETHICAL POSITIONING SYSTEM DIAGRAM

FIGURE 23.2 The Ethical Positioning System Model.
Source: Dorman, J. (2009). *EPS model.* Unpublished Manuscript.

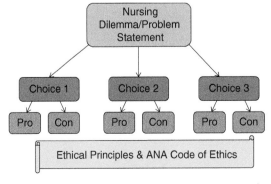

ETHICAL POSITIONING SYSTEM MODEL

FIGURE 23.3 The Ethical Positioning System Diagram (Step 4 of the EPS Model).
Source: Dorman, J. (2009). *EPS model.* Unpublished Manuscript.

Case Study 23.1

Tom, a nursing student, was doing a clinical rotation in the ED. He was faced with the following ethical dilemma and he decided to apply the EPS Model to aid in ethical decision making.

STEP 1. ASSESSMENT

- Tom, a nursing student, was doing a clinical rotation in the ED.

- He was seriously considering ED nursing, and hoped to learn as much as possible from this one-day experience.

- Suddenly, the ambulance doors open, and the paramedics bring in a woman with schizophrenia. She is struggling to leave and screaming obscenities. Security is called and the woman is placed in full leather restraints.

- Many of the other patients are disturbed by this patient's behavior.

- The nurses at the nurses' station are laughing and making fun of the woman.

- This patient apparently has a history of coming into the ED in crisis.

- The woman's distress seems to be exacerbated by the lack of care and, perhaps, by the nurses' behavior.

STEP 2. NURSING DILEMMA

- Tom recognizes the nurses' behavior as non-ethical and certainly non-therapeutic.

- He recognizes this as an ethical dilemma, and he is not sure how he should respond.

Choice 1. Tom could do nothing and ignore the situation.
- *Pro*: The nurses will not think Tom is a know-it-all.
- *Pro*: This will take no time or effort from Tom.
- *Con:* The nurses will think Tom agrees with them.
- *Con*: The patient will continue to be distressed.
- *Con*: The other patients will be disturbed.
- *Con*: Tom will feel guilty for not acting as a patient advocate.

Choice 2. Tom could suggest to the nurses that they help this patient.
- *Pro*: Tom will feel he is a patient advocate.
- *Pro:* They may go help the patient.
- *Con*: The nurses might resent his interference.
- *Con*: It might make the school look bad.
- *Con*: The nurses might ignore him and do nothing.

Choice 3. Tom could report the nurses to a manager.
- *Pro*: The manager might offer educational review to the nurses.
- *Pro*: Tom would feel he had advocated on behalf of mentally ill patients.
- *Pro*: There could be a change in attitude and behavior.

- *Con*: The staff might resent the school and students.
- *Con*: Any changes would not be immediate.

Choice 4. Tom could sit with the patient and calm her down.
- *Pro:* Tom would feel he was a patient advocate.
- *Pro:* The patient and others would be calmed.
- *Con*: This would not help in future situations.
- *Con*: The nurses would not learn from this.

ETHICAL PRINCIPLES

- *Accountability*: As a nurse, you are accountable for your actions. The nurse must show respect for human dignity.

- *Fidelity:* You have a duty to and a relationship with your patient.

- *Beneficence:* You want to do good and prevent harm.

- *Justice:* Each patient deserves fair and equitable treatment.

ANA CODE OF ETHICS

- 1.1 *Respect for human dignity:* nurses should respect the dignity of every patient.

- 1.2 *Relationships to patients:* nurses have a duty to advocate and care for their patients.

- 2.1 *Primacy of the patient's interests*: the nurse's primary commitment should be to the patient.

- 4.2 *Accountability for nursing judgments, decisions, and actions*; the nurse is accountable for actions grounded in respect for human dignity.

STEP 4. DIAGRAM (FIGURE 23.4)

STEP 5. IMPLEMENTATION

- Tom selected choice 4. He sat down with the patient, spoke quietly to her, and was able to calm her down.

- Within a short time, Tom was able to engage her trust.

- The other patients in the ED were able to relax.

- The nurses in the station were mostly oblivious to Tom's efforts.

- Within a short time, some of the restraints were removed. The patient was transferred to Behavioral Health.

STEP 6. EVALUATION

- The patient responded well to Tom's care and concern. She calmed down, and the staff was able to start an IV and administer IV medication.

- The other patients were grateful for the quiet.

- Unfortunately, the other nurses did not seem to recognize the importance of this therapeutic intervention.

- Tom decided that if he were to face this situation again, he would make a point of calling attention to his intervention and to the therapeutic results. He felt he could have accomplished this in a non-confrontational manner.

PROBLEM STATEMENT: WHAT SHOULD THE NURSE DO?

1. Do nothing	2. Ask nurses to help	3. Report nurses	4. Calm patient
Pro: Not know-it-all	Pro: Pt. advocate	Pro: Education	Pro: Pt. Advocate
Pro: No effort	Pro: They may help	Pro: Advocate	Pro: Pt. calmed
Con: Think Tom agrees	Con: Nurses resent	Pro: Maybe change	Pro: Help other pts.
Con: Patient no better	Con: School looks bad	Con: Resent school	Con: No future help
Con: Other pts bothered	Con: Nurses ignore	Con: Not immediate	Con: No learning
Con: Tom feels guilty			

Ethical Principles:
Accountability
Fidelity
Beneficence
Justice

ANA Code of Ethics:
1.1 Respect for human dignity
1.2 Relationships to patients
2.1 Primacy of patient interests
4.2 Accountability for nursing action

FIGURE 23.4   Application of The Ethical Positioning System Diagram.
Source: J. Dorman.

Patient Rights

A Patient's Bill of Rights was first adopted by the American Hospital Association (AHA), in 1973 and was revised in 1982 and 1992. This Bill of Rights was developed to assure that the health care system would be fair and meet patient needs. It provides patients with a guide to addressing problems with their care and encourages them to participate in staying healthy or getting well. In 2003, the AHA replaced the Bill of Rights with the Patient Care Partnership. The Patient Care Partnership is a booklet informing patients of what to expect during their hospital stay. It discusses their right to high-quality hospital care; a clean, safe environment; involvement in their care; protection of their privacy; help when leaving the hospital; and help with billing claims. The Patient Care Partnership can be found on the AHA Web site (www.aha.org), accessed January 2, 2019.

The U.S. Department of Health and Human Services, in partnership with the AHA, published Five Steps to Safer Health Care for Patients. These steps include:

- Asking questions if you have doubts or concerns

- Keeping an up-to-date list of medications

- Obtaining results of tests or procedure

- Talking to your doctor about which hospital best fits your needs

- Making sure you understand what will happen if you need surgery.

These five steps were originally published in 2004, last reviewed in 2014, and can be found on the Agency for Healthcare Research and Quality Web site (www.ahrq.gov), accessed January 2, 2019.

Real World Interview

One of my most difficult cases involved a man in his early forties who was in a coma, ventilator dependent, and declared brain dead. The patient was from a different culture, and when the family arrived 6 weeks later from his country abroad, they refused to allow him to be removed from the ventilator. His parents said they were told by the gods that their son would be well several months in the future. After 2 months in the hospital, the administration began to put pressure on the family to transfer the patient. (Note from the author: At the time of this interview, the outcome was yet to be determined. Situations such as this, as well as cases involving disposition of undocumented immigrants that are ready for discharge from the hospital, but who require on-going care, are becoming common in our current health care arena. There are no easy answers to these situations, but one would hope that compassion would be one of the considerations.)

Emily Davison, RN
Case Manager
Pleasant Hill, Missouri

Nursing Leadership and Management

Nurse leaders and managers are in a position to assure that the professional environment in which they practice is ethically principled and that it accepts accountability for the American Nurses Association Code of Ethics (2015a,b) set by the profession of nursing. The professional environment can empower nurses and can foster autonomy and an appreciation of the diversity of persons and opinions. By treating others with fairness, dignity, and respect, nurse leaders and managers can influence the decisions made by the organization.

Organizational Benefits Derived from Ethics

Health care institutions are increasingly faced with making decisions based on the financial bottom line which might ultimately affect the quality of care provided. Ethically and socially responsible decisions are sometimes compromised in the name of financial concerns. At the same time, hospitals have suffered financial losses when ethics were cast aside. There have been numerous health care errors, often leading to malpractice suits, which can be traced back to cutbacks in staff or other resources. Quality and safety issues in health care have increasingly come under scrutiny. The

AHA, the National League of Nursing, the National Institutes of Health, and the American Association of Colleges of Nursing have all designated quality and safety initiatives as the highest priority. Additional information is available on their websites (www.aacn.nche.edu, www.nursingworld.org, www.nih.gov, www.aha.org, and www.nln.org), accessed January 3, 2019.

Creating an Ethical Workplace

An ethical workplace is dedicated to the well-being of all patients. Quality and safety are the foundations of patient care, enabling the nurse to be beneficent, to do good, to be non-maleficent, and to prevent harm. Considerations of quality and safety help nurses design an ethical work environment dedicated to caring for patients. *The* following suggestions for an ethical work environment are useful in an organization concerned with quality and safety:

1. Develop formal mechanisms for monitoring ethics, such as an ethics program or ethics hotline.

2. Develop written organizational elements to support an ethical workplace (Table 24.4).

Evidence From the Literature

Citation: Rushton, C. H. & Stutzer, K. (2015, June). Addressing 21st Century Nursing Ethics: Implications for Critical Care Nurses. AACN Advanced Critical Care, 26 (2), 173–176.

Discussion: The authors discuss how there are internal and external pressures that are threatening the integrity of nurses. Some of these pressures are disparities in access to health care, determining goals at the end of life, and distribution of resources that threaten the respect, dignity, quality, and safety of the patients. In August of 2014, Johns Hopkins sponsored a national summit on Nursing Ethics for the twenty-first century. The goal of the summit was to determine a blueprint for the future. Participants concentrated on ways nursing and ethics intersect in four domains: clinical practice, research, education, and public policy.

Some of the recommendations that came from the Nursing Ethics summit are:

- Become familiar with the ANA Code of Ethics.
- Become a member of your hospital's Ethics Committee.
- Courageously advocate when there is an ethics concern.
- Share the blueprint and vision of an ethical environment with nursing leadership.
- Embed ethical practice questions in patient daily care rounds.

Implications for Practice: One of the intentions of the national summit on Nursing Ethics was to raise awareness of ethical issues and be a catalyst for action. The hope was to engage others in exploring ethical issues that keep nurses up at night and to identify innovative solutions.

Evidence from the Literature

Citation: Kennedy, M. S. (2018, November). To be a nurse: What does it really mean? American Journal of Nursing, 118 (11), 7.

Discussion: The author is a retired nurse who still identifies as a nurse. She wonders what it means to be a nurse in the current social and political climate. Are nurses compassionate to vulnerable populations, regardless of social or legal status? Nurses have long been dedicated to non-judgmental patient care. How can a nurse support policies that may cause irreparable harm to children, or object to providing care to vulnerable people? The author

cites Provisions 1, 8, and 9 of the ANA Code of Ethics, available at www.nursingworld.org/practice-policy/nursing-excellence/ethics, accessed November 30, 2018.

Implications for Practice: As nurses, we are called upon to care for all kinds of people. How do we deal with caring for patients that may have different beliefs or values, or even a patient that is a criminal? Nurses need to do a self-assessment, so that they can be sure that they do justice to their patients based on their individual needs.

3. Develop widespread communication strategies in the hospital to reinforce ethically and socially responsible behavior.

4. Show leadership by example: If people throughout the organization believe that behaving ethically is "in" and behaving unethically is "out," ethical behavior will prevail.

5. Encourage confrontation about ethical deviation: Unethical behavior may be minimized if every employee confronts anyone seen behaving unethically.

6. Develop training programs in ethics and social responsibility, including messages about ethics from managers, classes on ethics at colleges, and exercises in ethics (DuBrin, 2016) Table 23.4.

Nurse-Physician Relationships

Nurses working in organizations often confront ethical dilemmas in working with patients and their families. To resolve these dilemmas, the nurse must often work closely with the medical practitioner. Nurses often find that medical practitioners hold beliefs different from theirs about values, communication, trust and integrity, role responsibilities, and organizational politics and economics. These beliefs affect both nurses and medical practitioners' ethical beliefs, which in turn affect their decisions about treatment, which may lead to conflicts between nurses and medical practitioners. These conflicts can be limited with clear ethical guidelines and policies, established by inter-professional teams, and overseen by an ethical administration. When an ethical issue arises, resolution might be tedious and riddled with resentment without clear guidelines and policies.

The Gallup Organization's 2017 annual poll on professional honesty and ethical standards ranked nurses as number one. Of the 22 professions tested, 5 have high ethical ratings: nurses (82%), military officers (71%), grade school teachers (66%), medical doctors (65%), and pharmacists (62%). For more information, see: https://news.gallup.com/poll/224639/nurses-keep-healthy-lead-honest-ethical-profession.aspxEthical Codes, accessed January 3, 2019.

Table 23.4   Organizational Elements to Support an Ethical Workplace

- Follow professional standards for education, licensure, and competency in all hiring decisions, orientation, and ongoing continuing education programs.
- Have clear job descriptions and ongoing licensing and credentialing policies for nursing and medical practitioners, LPN/LVNs, nursing assistants, and other health care staff. The organization must ensure that all staff are safe, competent practitioners before assigning them to patient care. Orient all staff to each other's roles and job descriptions.
- Facilitate clinical and educational specialty certification and credentialing of all health care practitioners and staff.
- Provide standards for ongoing supervision and periodic licensure/competency verification and evaluation of all staff.
- Provide access to professional health care standards, policies, procedures, library, and medication information. Assure unit and hospital availability and efficient Internet access.
- Facilitate regular evidence-based review of critical health care standards, policies, and procedures.
- Have clear policies and procedures for delegation and chain-of-command reporting lines for all staff from RN to charge nurse to nurse manager to nurse executive, to risk management, the hospital ethics committee, the hospital administrator, medical practitioners, the chief of the medical staff, the board of directors, the state licensing board for nursing and medicine, and the Joint Commission (JC).
- Provide administrative support for supervisors and staff who delegate, assign, monitor, and evaluate patient care.
- Clarify nursing and medical practitioner accountability. For example, if a medical practitioner delegates a nursing task to nursing assistant, the medical practitioner is responsible for monitoring that care delivery. This must be spelled out in hospital policy. If an RN notes that the nursing assistant is doing something incorrectly, the RN has a duty to intervene and to notify the ordering practitioner of the incident. The RN always has an independent responsibility to protect patient safety. Blindly relying on another nursing or medical practitioner's judgment is not perm issible for the RN.
- Provide standards for regular RN evaluation of nursing assistants and LPN/LVN; reinforce the need for nursing assistant and LPN/LVN accountability to RNs. RNs must delegate and supervise; they cannot abdicate this professional responsibility.
- Develop physical, mental, and verbal "No Abuse" policy, to be followed by all professional and nonprofessional health care staff.
- Consider applying for Magnet status for your facility. This status is awarded by the American Nurses Credentialing Center to nursing departments that have worked to improve nursing care, including the empowering of nursing decision making and delegation in clinical practice.
- Support the development of a strong ethics committee with an inter-professional team. Make it available to all staff.
- Monitor patient outcomes, including nurse-sensitive outcomes, staffing ratios, and other clinical, financial, and organizational quality indicators. Develop ongoing clinical quality improvement practices.
- Maintain ongoing monitoring of incident reports, sentinel events, and other elements of risk management and performance improvement of the process and outcome of patient care.
- Develop systematic, error-proof systems for medication administration that ensure the six rights of medication administration—that is, the right patient, right medication, right dose, right time, right route, and right documentation. Include computerized order entry.
- Provide documentation of routine maintenance for all patient care equipment.
- Attain Joint Commission Patient Safety Goals for the current year. These can be retrieved at www.jointcommission.org/assets/1/6/2018_HAP_NPSG_goals_final.pdf (Retrieved November 8, 2018)
- Develop safe intra-hospital and intra-agency transfer policies.

Source: J. Dorman

Case Study 23.2

As you receive a hand-off report at the start of your shift, the nurse informs you not to tell Mrs. Sun, Room 240, of her diagnosis. Mrs. Sun is being treated with chemotherapy for ovarian cancer and she is not aware of her diagnosis. The family does not want her to know, because they say she will not be able to handle it. The physician spoke with the family and decided to respect their wishes.

When you make patient care rounds on Mrs. Sun, she asks you to stop her medication. She states it is making her sick. She says she was not sick when she came into the hospital, and she wants to know what this medicine is for. What will you say to Mrs. Sun? Use the EPS Model to analyze this case.

Step 1. Assessment: Consider all the information you know about this case. Who are the people involved? Are there additional factors such as cultural considerations? Mrs. Sun is receiving chemotherapy for ovarian cancer, but she is not aware of her diagnosis. Her family does not believe she could handle it, so they have convinced the physician not to discuss the diagnosis with Mrs. Sun. The medicine is making Mrs. Sun ill, and she asks the nurse what this medication is supposed to be for.

Step 2. Nursing dilemma: What should you tell Mrs. Sun?

Step 3. Planning: Consider your choices and the pros and cons.

Choice 1: Tell Mrs. Sun the truth, that she is being treated for ovarian cancer.

- *Pros*: You will be telling the truth and respecting your patient's autonomy.
- *Cons:* You do not know what her reaction will be. There is concern about her being able to handle the news. Also, you may not be able to answer questions about her options or prognosis. The physician and the family may be angry.

Choice 2: Tell Mrs. Sun that you do not have any additional information about her case and that you are unable to give her any additional information.

- **Pros**: It lets you off the hook, and she may be pacified for the moment.
- **Cons**: She will probably refuse treatment at this time. Your comment is a lie and is in opposition to several ethical principles and the ANA Code of Ethics.

Choice 3: Tell Mrs. Sun that you are going to look into her situation and that you will be back to speak with her. Phone the physician and the family and let them know the current situation. Suggest to them that they reconsider their decision and give Mrs. Sun the correct information. Suggest a consultation with the hospital ethics committee.

- **Pros**: You are being honest with all involved.
- **Cons**: The family or physician may still not agree to discuss the diagnosis with the patient. They may blame you for the dilemma. The patient may not be able to handle hearing about her diagnosis.

Ethical Principles of autonomy, respect, beneficence, nonmaleficence, and veracity apply to this case.

The ANA Code of Ethics for Nurses: 1.4, the right to self-determination; 2.3, collaboration; and 6.3 responsibility for the health care environment

Step 4. Diagram (Figure 23.5)

What will you decide?

Step 5. Implementation: You notified the physician and family of the dilemma and they agreed to come in for a meeting with the patient. All of the options for treatment were discussed with the patient along with the risks and benefits.

Step 6. Evaluation: Mrs. Sun was able to ask questions and had time to deliberate. She decided to continue treatment for the time being, but knew she had options. Using the EPS Model worked well in this case.

PROBLEM STATEMENT: WHAT SHOULD THE NURSE DO?

1. Tell Mrs. Sun the truth	2. Tell patient you do not have any information	3. Phone physician and family
Pro: Rexpect patient's autonomy	Pro: Lets you off the hook	Pro: Pt. advocate
Pro: You wan't have to lie	Pro: She may be pacified	Pro: You are being honest
Con: Unsure of her reation	Con: They may not agree to tell the truth	Con: They may not agree to tell the truth
Con: You may not be able to answer questions	Con: May refuse treatment	Con: They may blame you
Con: The physician and family may be angry	Con: You are lying	Con: In they do tell the patient, she may be upset

Ethical Principles:	ANA Code of Ethics:
Beneficence	1.1 Right to self-determination
Nonmaleficence	2.3 Collaboration
Veracity	6.3 Responsibility for the healthcare environment
Autonomy	

FIGURE 23.5 Problem statement, What shold the nurse do?

Source: J. Dorman

Codes of Ethics for Nurses

One mark of a profession is the determination of ethical behavior for its members. Several nursing organizations have developed codes for ethical behavior. The International Council of Nurses Code of Ethics for Nurses (2012) is discussed in Table 24.5.

The ANA Code of Ethics for Nurses with Interpretive Statements (2015) may be viewed in its entirety at the site listed at www.nursingworld.org/practice-policy/nursing-excellence/ethics, accessed January 3, 2019. Read the ANA Code of Ethics for Nurses nine provisions, which are summarized below. Following each provision, there is a real-life situation. Ask yourself after each provision and situation, how could the nurse meet this ANA Code of Ethics for Nurses provision in this situation?

Provision 1 is concerned that the nurse treats everyone with respect.

Ann Smith, RN is caring for John T., a patient on the orthopedic unit of a local community hospital. John is 1 day post op from a left total knee replacement. He was up in a chair for lunch today but did not tolerate it well and refuses to get up for dinner. John weighs 300 lbs. and has several co-morbidities. Ann feels disgusted with John's morbid obesity and has been very impatient with John.

Provisions 2 assures that the patient is the nurse's number one concern.

Sarah Norman, Nurse Practitioner, has been working with a group of physicians in their private practice for several years. Recently, the physicians have become partners in a business that promotes multivitamins for such things as arthritis, energy level, and overall health. They have offered Sarah a portion of the profits for every patient she signs up for the vitamin program. Sarah is not sure these vitamins are appropriate for many of the patients.

Provision 3 encourages the nurse to advocate for, and protect the safety of, the patient.

Meredith Henry, RN is working on a busy medical surgical unit. On this particular evening, she has been spending a great deal of time in the room of a loud and confused patient. When Alice, the nursing assistant, informed Meredith that a new patient had arrived in room 3808 and was complaining of severe back pain, Meredith told Alice to go and start the assessment on this new patient.

Provision 4 assures that the nurse accepts responsibility and accountability for nursing actions.

Alyssa Adams is an RN on an intermediate care unit of an urban teaching hospital. She has been on this unit for 2 years and is quite proud of the care they provide. Recently, however, Alyssa has been concerned about her co-worker, Margaret. Margaret has been an RN for 25 years and has been on this unit for 7 years. Lately, Margaret has been impatient and intolerant of even the slightest inconvenience or stray from the norm. She is snappy to her co-workers and less than caring with her patients. Alyssa suspects Margaret may have an issue with drugs.

Provision 5 states that the nurse must practice self-care along with care for others and must maintain competence and professional growth.

Charles O'Brien has been an RN for 2 years and realizes he still has a great deal to learn. He does not think his manager or the institution place education in high regard. He is beginning to wonder if this is the right work environment for him.

Provision 6 reminds the nurse to be sure the work setting is an ethical environment.

Adam Martin, RN has been working at Sunshine Manor, Extended Care Facility, for almost 8 months and has become increasingly concerned about safety issues at the facility. He thinks the staffing is minimal for the number of patients, and the policies and procedures are inaccessible. As one of only three RNs on the unit, Adam has been trying to improve

Table 23.5 International Council of Nurses Code of Nursing Ethics

An International Code of Ethics for Nurses was first adopted by the International Council of Nurses (ICN) in 1953. It has been revised and reaffirmed at various times since, most recently with the review and revision completed in 2012.

Preamble

Nurses have four fundamental responsibilities: to promote health, to prevent illness, to restore health, and to alleviate suffering. The need for nursing is universal. Inherent in nursing is a respect for human rights, including cultural rights, the right to life and choice, to dignity, and to be treated with respect. Nursing care is respectful of and unrestricted by considerations of age, color, creed, culture, disability or illness, gender, sexual orientation, nationality, politics, race, or social status. Nurses render health services to the individual, the family, and the community and coordinate their services with those of related groups.

The International Council of Nursing Code of Ethics for Nurses

www.icn.ch/ code-of-ethics-for-nurses/ Retrieved March 13, 2019

The ICN Code of Ethics for Nurses has four principal elements that outline the standards of ethical conduct: Nurses and people, Nurses and practice, Nurses and the profession, and Nurses and co-workers.

Source: International Council of Nurses.

conditions and make sure policies are visible and up-to-date. He has had very little success.

Provision 7 states that the nurse should participate in research, scholarly inquiry, and the development of professional standards for both nursing and health policy.

Mandy Paris is in her last semester of nursing school, and works as a nurse intern in a local hospital. She has noticed that there are several quality improvement initiatives taking place in regard to decreasing falls, pressure ulcers, and catheter associated urinary tract infections. Mandy is working on an evidence-based practice project at school and believes in their value. She wishes the quality improvement staff would open these projects to nurses on the various units.

Provision 8 assures that the nurse collaborates to protect human rights and reduce health disparities.

Mike Cummings, RN has been working at a community hospital for 3 years on a cardiac step-down unit. As Mike is discharging Charles, a 53-year-old male with severe hypertension and a recent transient ischemic attack. Charles shares that he does not have money for his medications and does not know how to check his blood pressure. When he asks Mike if he can help him find resources in the area, Mike states he is not from around here and really does not know what is available.

Provision 9 states that the nurse must promote nursing values, maintain the integrity of the profession, and integrate principles of social justice into nursing and health policy.

Angela Updike has accepted an RN position at a small community hospital in a Hispanic area of a major city. Angela studied Spanish in high school and is able to translate on some occasions. She is worried, however, because many of her patients are concerned about recent immigration practices. Angela agrees that some of these practices are inhumane, and she is trying to find a professional nursing position on this.

The Future

Ethical issues in the future that will challenge nursing practice include the allocation of resources, use of advanced technologies, an aging population, and an increase in behavior-related health problems, such as alcohol or drug addiction or diseases related to obesity. These issues all magnify the importance of professional nurses providing leadership and emphasizing ethical behavior in all practice settings.

This chapter has provided an overview of the nursing profession's challenges related to ethical theories, virtues, principles, and values in today's health care environment. The terms used in this chapter have been clarified, yet now is the time to actualize these in your nursing practice. Case studies have

---

Critical Thinking 23.5

The nurse is caring for a patient in the surgical Intensive Care Unit (ICU) who is connected to a ventilator. He is on a sedation protocol with continuous intravenous infusion of Versed, a powerful sedative that requires constant monitoring and titration to maintain the required level of sedation. During the night shift, the nurse discovers that the medication bag is almost empty and the pharmacy, which is closed, did not send up another medication bag. The nurse looks up the medication and mixes the medication herself, inadvertently mixing a double-strength dose. The night charge nurse was busy supervising a cardiac arrest situation outside the ICU and was unavailable to double check how the medication was mixed.

Thirty minutes after the nurse hung the new IV bag of medication, the patient's blood pressure dropped significantly. The

family was notified that their loved one had taken a turn for the worse and that they should come to the hospital immediately. The physician was notified, and she ordered a medication to raise the blood pressure. In backtracking for the cause of the hypotension, the nurse realized that she had mixed the sedative double-strength, and she reduced the dose by half.

When the patient's family arrives, the patient's blood pressure had started to return to normal. They ask the nurse what happened and why their mother was on the new IV medication to raise the blood pressure.

Should the family be told about the error? If so, who should tell them? The nurse? The physician? What approach should be used? What ethical principles enter into the decision? Table 23.5.

Case Study 23.3

Source: The Patient Care Partnership, American Hospital Association. (2003) site at www.aha.org/aha/issues/Communicating-With-Patients/pt-care-partnership.html, accessed June 1, 2019, This document has replaced the Patient Bill of Rights. Note what The Patient Care Partnership says about the following:

- High-quality hospital care
- A clean and safe environment

- Involvement in your care
- Protection of your privacy
- Help when leaving the hospital
- Help with your billing claims

How can you use this information to help patients?

helped you can see their relationships and that these terms are connected. Ethical leadership and management's responsibility in professional practice and organizations has been stressed. Hopefully this chapter has helped you develop and/or strengthen your personal philosophy of professional nursing and the value of ethics committees, ethical workplaces, and values clarification is evident. An EPS Model was introduced

and applied to an ethical dilemma and can and should be used in clinical practice. Finally, the International Council of Nursing's Code for Nurses and the American Nurses' Association Code for Nurses has been discussed and applied in clinical situations. As nurses, keeping aware of ethics in all situations is part of our caring profession and guides us in our care.

KEY CONCEPTS

- Ethics is a branch of philosophy dealing with what is morally right or wrong.

- Historically, nursing practice evolved from the needs of society and has been strongly influenced by religions and women.

- A person's personal philosophy and past experiences will influence their philosophy of nursing.

- Teleology, deontology, virtue ethics, justice and equity, and relativism are examples of ethical theories that influence nursing practice.

- Ethical principles include beneficence, non0maleficence, fidelity, justice, autonomy, respect for others, and veracity.

- Ethics committees provide thoughtful and timely consultation

when an ethical issue arises in the hospital.

- Values clarification is the process of analyzing one's own values to better understand what is truly important.

- The EPS Model is a helpful tool for ethical decision making.

- Numerous ethical issues face today's nurses.

- Nurses have the responsibility to uphold ethical nursing leadership and management in professional practice.

- Nurses who are dedicated to ethical principles will work to develop an ethical workplace.

- The ANA Code for Ethics in Nursing and the International Council of Nurses' Code of Ethics for Nurses provide guidance for ethical nursing practice.

KEY TERMS

Autonomy	Fidelity	Respect for others
Beneficence	Justice	Values
Bioethics	Morality	Values clarification
Ethical dilemma	Nonmaleficence	Veracity
Ethics	Philosophy	

REVIEW QUESTIONS

1. When the nurse is obtaining a patient's consent, the patient states that the surgeon did not give the patient information on the risks of surgery. The nurse should do which of the following?
   a. Tell the patient the risks.
   b. Report the surgeon to the ethics committee.
   c. Report the surgeon to the unit manager.
   d. Inform the surgeon that the patient is unaware of the risks of surgery.

2. The nurse notices that a co-worker has been drinking and is not able to practice safely. The nurse should do which of the following?
   a. Inform the manager or shift director immediately.
   b. Warn the co-worker that black coffee is in order.
   c. Discuss the situation with the other nurses working.
   d. Do nothing, but keep an eye on the nurse.

3. The nurse demonstrates accountability by doing which of the following?
   a. Accepting an assignment, even if it appears unsafe.

   b. Reviewing practitioner orders for accuracy and completeness.
   c. Striving to improve patient satisfaction.
   d. Finding the person to blame for errors.

4. Which of the following represents a teleological theory?
   a. The goodness of an action is based on the intent.
   b. The end justifies the means.
   c. There are no universal ethical standards.
   d. Do unto others as you would have them do unto you.

5. The primary role of a hospital ethics committee is which of the following?
   a. Decide what should be done when ethical dilemmas arise.
   b. Prevent the practitioner from making the wrong decision.
   c. Provide guidance for the health care team and family of the patient.
   d. Prevent ethical dilemmas from occurring.

6. Ethical dilemmas may be referred to the hospital ethics committee by which of the following?
   a. Medical practitioners only

b. Lawyers only

c. Hospital administration only

d. Nursing and medical practitioners, lawyers, and the health care team members and/or families of patients

7. Mrs. Jones rides the elevator to the fifth floor, where her husband is a patient. While on the elevator, Mrs. Jones hears two nurses talking about Mr. Jones. They are discussing the potential prognosis and whether Mr. Jones should be told. The nurses are violating which of the following ethical principles?

a. Autonomy

b. Veracity

c. Justice

d. Confidentiality

8. The nurse realizes that neglecting to inform the patient about the plan of care is a violation of which of the following?

a. The Patient Care Partnership

b. The patient's right to privacy

c. The patient's right to confidentiality

d. The fifth amendment of the constitution

9. During morning report, the night nurse tells you that Mr. P., who is admitted for pancreatitis, is a drug addict and an alcoholic and caused all his own problems. You realize that this nurse is exhibiting a lack of which of the following focal virtues?

a. integrity

b. compassion

c. discernment

d. trustworthiness

10. A nurse caring for a cancer patient demonstrates paternalism when she cannot decide if she should give the patient discouraging lab results. Which ethical principle would be compromised if the nurse decided not to report the results?

a. Justice

b. Autonomy

c. Confidentiality

d. Fidelity

REVIEW QUESTION ANSWERS

1. Answer: D is correct.

Rationale: The nurse should give the physician the benefit of the doubt and collaborate to assure that the patient receives the information and that the physician has the opportunity to make things right. You would not (B) report this to the Ethics Committee. It is not an ethical issue at this point. You would not (C) report this to the unit manager unless it became an ongoing issue. You would not (A) take it upon yourself to tell the patient the risks. This is a physician responsibility as part of obtaining the consent.

2. Answer: A is correct.

Rationale: The nurse recognizes that an action must be taken emergently to prevent harm to a patient. Telling the manager is an immediate action that can result in that nurse being relieved of her responsibilities at that time. Black coffee (B) would not help at this time, nor would taking a chance and (D) keeping an eye on the nurse. Discussing the situation with other nurses (C) would accomplish nothing.

3. Answer: B is correct.

Rationale: When receiving orders from a practitioner, the nurse is responsible and accountable for assessing the orders for accuracy and completeness. This is a necessary crosscheck to prevent errors. Patient satisfaction (C) is a concern for all hospital employees but not a measure of accountability. Blaming others (D) is not accepting accountability, and accepting (A) an assignment that is not safe can lead to disaster.

4. Answer: B is correct.

Rationale: Teleological theory claims that an action is judged by the outcome and that the intent of the action (A) is not a concern. Ethical standards (C) are not a concern to teleology, nor is (D) the golden rule which may, or may not, have a positive outcome.

5. Answer: C is correct.

Rationale: The hospital ethics committee provides guidance in cases where the right decision is not clear. They do not decide the appropriate action (A) nor can they prevent an ethical dilemma from occurring (D). An ethics committee can make suggestions but they would not be able to prevent a practitioner from making a wrong decision (B).

6. Answer: D is correct.

Rationale: Any member of the health care team, family members, physicians, lawyers, etc. could request an ethics committee consult. The request is not limited to medical practitioners (A), lawyers (B), or hospital administration (C).

7. Answer: D is correct.

Rationale: Any and all patient information is confidential. It is a HIPAA violation to discuss patient information in a public place. This would not have an effect on the patient's autonomy (A). Truthfulness or veracity (B) is not an issue here, nor is justice (C).

8. Answer: A is correct.

Rationale: The Patient Care Partnership clearly states that the patient has the right to be informed of all information regarding his/her case. The patient's right to privacy (B) would not apply here, not would (C) the right to confidentiality. The fifth amendment of the Constitution (D) is concerned with protection against self-incrimination, which has no place here.

9. Answer: B is correct.

Rationale: The nurse in this case is displaying a lack of compassion or empathy for the situation of the patient. If the nurse acted on this lack or caring, he/she could compromise his/her (A) integrity or (D) trustworthiness. The nurse has used discernment (C) to examine the implications of the case, but chooses to blame the patient for his own demise.

10. Answer: B is correct.

    Rationale: Autonomy is our right to self-determination, and without all the necessary information, this patient could not make an informed decision. Justice (A) would not be compromised by withholding information, nor would (D) fidelity, provided the nurse was worrying about the reaction of the patient. Confidentiality (C) would not be breeched by giving the patient information about her own condition.

REVIEW ACTIVITIES

1. An elderly woman, age 88, is admitted to the ED in acute respiratory distress. She does not have a living will, but her daughter has Power Of Attorney (POA) for health care and is a health care professional. The patient has end-stage renal disease, end-stage Alzheimer's disease, and congestive heart failure. Her condition is grave. The doctors want to intubate her and place her on a ventilator. The sons agree. The daughter states that their mother would not want to be on a machine just to prolong her life.

   Divide into groups and apply the EPS Model to this case.

2. As a hospice nurse, you are involved with pain management on a regular basis. Many of the medications prescribed for the management of pain also depress respirations.

   Determine a protocol for the use of these medications, keeping in mind that the purpose of hospice is to promote comfort. Support your decisions with ethical theories and principles.

DISCUSSION POINTS

• Can you think of an ethical dilemma in today's world that is causing polarization and divisiveness? Divide into groups and discuss this issue.

Do you believe that lying for benevolent motives is ever justifiable? Can you give examples of when lying may have been beneficent?

DISCUSSION OF OPENING SCENARIO

1. *What are your thoughts about maintaining the patient's life in this situation?*

   Discussion: As the nurse, you know the patient's wishes, so it would be difficult to see the patient being kept alive. At this point medical futility and quality of life become major issues.

2. *Who should make the decision about the patient's situation while he is comatose?*

   Discussion: The family will be faced with making the decision, but the nurse can share what the patient said before the code was called.

3. *How can you act as an advocate for the patient and the family?*

   Discussion: The nurse could arrange a meeting with the physician and the family to discuss the prognosis and the patient's wishes.

EXPLORING THE WEB

• See what this website, www.nursingworld.org, says about nursing competencies, ethics, and health care policy. Accessed January 3, 2019.

• Go to the following site to view the American Hospital Association's Patient Care Partnership, www.aha.org. Accessed January 3, 2019.

   Search for, **Ethics**, at the following websites:

• National League of Nursing, www.nln.org. Accessed January 3, 2019.

• National Institutes of Health www.nih.gov. Accessed January 3, 2019.

• American Association of Colleges of Nursing, www.aacn.nche.edu. Accessed January 3, 2019.

INFORMATICS

Return to the area of this chapter that dealt with the ANA Code of Ethics. Search the Code for the specific interpretive statements that best apply to each scenario. www.nursingworld.org/practice-policy/nursing-excellence/ethics.

Go to the QSEN website, http://qsen.org/competencies and choose 2 of the 6 competencies. Discuss how the study of Nursing Ethics applies to each of those competencies.

LEAN BACK

- Think of a time when you were faced with an ethical dilemma as a student. How did you resolve the dilemma?

- Think of a political situation that is discussed regularly on the news. Examples might be immigration, the economy, or relationships with other countries. What ethical principles apply to your view of these situations?

REFERENCES

American Hospital Association Patient Care Partnership. (2003). What to expect during your hospital stay. Retrieved 2020, from https://www.aha.org/system/files/2018-01/aha-patient-care-partnership.pdf

American Nurses Association. (2015a). *Code of ethics for nurses with interpretive statements*. Retrieved from www.nursingworld.org/practice-policy/nursing-excellence/ethics

American Nurses Association. (2015b). *Nursing: Scope and Standards of Practice* (3rd ed.). Retrieved from www.nursingworld.org/practice-policy/scope-of-practice

Beauchamp, T. L., & Childress, J. F. (2019). *Principles of biomedical ethics*. New York: Oxford University Press.

Bowditch, J. L., & Bruno, A. F. (2007). *A primer on organizational behavior* (7th ed.). New York: Wiley.

Burkhardt, M. A., & Nathaniel, A. K. (2014). *Ethics & issues in contemporary nursing* (3rd ed.). Clifton Park, NY: Delmar Cengage Learning.

Cronenwett, L., Sherwood, G., Barnsteiner, J., Disch, J., Johnson, J., Mitchell, P., Sullivan, D. T. & Warren, J. (2007). Quality and safety education for nurses. Nursing Outlook, 55(3), 122–131. doi:10.1016/j.outlook.2007.02.006

Donahue, M. P. (2011). *Nursing, the finest art* (3rd ed.). St. Louis, MO: Mosby.

Dorman, J. (2009). *EPS model*. Unpublished Manuscript.

DuBrin, A. (2016). *Leadership: Research findings, practice, and skills* (8th ed.). Boston, MA: Cengage Learning.

International Council of Nurses. (2012). *Code for nurses*. Geneva: Switzerland.

Jonsen, A. R., Siegler, M., & Winslade, W. J. (2015). *Clinical ethics* (8th ed.). New York: McGraw Hill.

Kennedy, M. S. (2018). To be a nurse: What does it really mean? *American Journal of Nursing, 118*(11), 7.

Mark Twain Quotes. (n.d.). *BrainyQuote.com*. Retrieved from BrainyQuote.com website: www.brainyquote.com/quotes/mark_twain_104717

Peter, E. (2018). Overview and summary: ethics in healthcare: nurses respond. *Online Journal of Issues in Nursing, 23*(1). *QSEN Competencies*. Retrieved from http://qsen.org/competencies/pre-licensure-ksas

Raths, L. E., Harmin, M., & Simon, S. B. (1978). *Values and teaching: Working with values in the classroom*. Columbus, OH: Charles E. Merrill.

Rushton, C. H., & Stutzer, K. (2015). Addressing 21st century nursing ethics: Implications for critical care nurses. *AACN Advanced Critical Care, 26*(2), 173–176.

Twain, M. (1907). Mark Twain Quotes. Retrieved November 05, 2020, from https://www.brainyquote.com/quotes/mark_twain_104717

SUGGESTED READINGS

Agency for Healthcare Research and Quality. (2014). *Five steps to safer health care for patients*. Retrieved from www.ahrq.gov/consumers

Bell, J., & Breslin, J. M. (2008). Healthcare provider moral distress as a leadership challenge. *JONA's Healthcare, Law, Ethics, and Regulation, 10*(4), 94–97.

Butts, J. B., & Rich, K. L. (2020). *Nursing ethics across the curriculum and into practice* (4th ed.). Burlington, MA: Jones & Bartlett Learning.

DeMarco, J. P., & Jones, G. E. with Daly, B. J.(2019). *Ethical & legal issues in nursing*. Ontario, Canada: Broadview Press.

Dewey, A., & Holecke, A. (2019). *The nurse's healthcare ethics committee handbook*. Indianapolis, IN: Sigma Theta Tau International.

Engel, J., Salfi, J., Micsinszki, S., & Bodnar, A. (2017). Informed strangers: Witnessing and responding to unethical care as student nurses. *Global Qualitative Nursing Research, 4*, 1–9.

Fowler, M. D. (2016, September/October). *Nursing's code of ethics, social ethics, and social policy*. Hastings Center Report.

Fry, S. T., & Johnstone, M. J. (2008). *Ethics in nursing practice* (3rd ed.). New York: Blackwell Publishing.

Robichaux, C. (2016). Developing ethical skills: From sensitivity to action. *Critical Care Nurse, 32*(2), 65–72.

Rushton, C. H. (2016, September/October). *Creating a culture of ethical practice in health care delivery systems*. Hastings Center Report.

Stephens, T. M. (2017). Situational awareness and the nursing code of ethics. *American Nurse Today, 12*(11), 56–59.

The Patient Care Partnership. (2018). Retrieved from www.aha.org/system/files/2018-01/aha-patient-care-partnership.pdf

Wood, D. (2016a). *The top ethical challenges for nurses*. American Mobile. Retrieved from www.americanmobile.com/nursezone/nursing-news/the-top-ethical-challenges-for-nurses/#sthash.jlj6Aaq0.dpuf

Wood, D. (2016b). *4 Common nursing ethics dilemmas*. Nursechoice. Retrieved from www.nursechoice.com/traveler-resources/4-common-nursing-ethics-dilemmas/

Culture, Generational Differences, and Spirituality

24

Amanda Kratovil

Purdue University Northwest, College of Nursing, Hammond, IN, USA

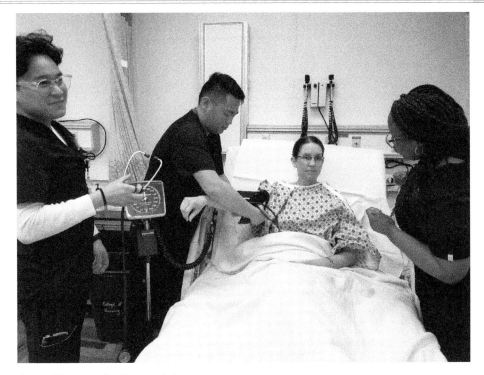

Source: Photo used with permission.

If we are to achieve a richer culture, rich in contrasting values, we must recognize the whole gamut of human potentialities, and so weave a less arbitrary social fabric, one in which each diverse human gift will find a fitting place.

(Margaret Mead, 1935)

OBJECTIVES

Upon completion of this chapter, the reader should be able to:

1. Apply cultural considerations to the role of a nurse leader.

2. Compare and contrast the demographics of the U.S. population and U.S. nurses.

3. Identify factors contributing to health disparities and health care disparities.

4. Describe how organizational culture can influence leading a team.

5. Describe the current generations and their behaviors that influence leading and managing patient care.

6. Identify methods of assessment and meeting spiritual needs of patients.

7. Apply knowledge of spirituality to problem solving in the nurse leader role.

Kelly Vana's Nursing Leadership and Management, Fourth Edition. Edited by Patricia Kelly Vana and Janice Tazbir
© 2021 John Wiley & Sons Ltd. Published 2021 by John Wiley & Sons Ltd.
Companion Website: www.wiley.com/go/kelly-Nursing-Leadership

OPENING SCENARIO

A woman, Mrs. Ahmad, entered the emergency department (ED) at 3:30 a.m., holding her abdomen and crying. Her school-aged son, Asad, followed closely behind, but no other family was present. Upon assessment by nurse Heather, it was determined that the patient was pregnant, but did not appear to be very far along. However, very little maternal or fetal history could be collected from the woman because she only spoke Arabic. Since her son spoke some English, Heather began questioning him about the pregnancy. Asad translated what the nurse said in English, to his mother. Asad then translated what his mother told him, to Heather. He said that the baby was about 25-weeks old, but out of respect for his mother, omitted the complaint that his mother verbalized about vaginal bleeding with large clots for the last several hours. The nurse, knowing that the hospital did not have an Arabic interpreter available at the hospital at this time of night, continued to gather crucial information about the mother and unborn baby through Asad. When the ultrasound technician, Mr. Rugness, entered the room to perform the ultrasound of Mrs. Ahmad, both mother and son started yelling in Arabic. Quickly, Heather recognized that the male ultrasound technician may pose a cultural conflict for Mrs. Ahmad, and asked Mr. Rugness to step into the hall. While discussing Mrs. Ahmad's case with the physician and Mr. Rugness, Asad frantically entered the hallway, crying and saying that his mother had blood dripping from her.

1. *Describe the concerns and risks associated with having the son continue to interpret for his mother?*

2. *List alternatives to having the son interpret for his mother that the nurse could employ.*

3. *Explain how culture and language barriers may affect the patients' outcomes and some strategies the nurse could use to overcome these barriers.*

We live and work in a multicultural society defined by diversity. **Diversity** is the individual differences we encounter among people regarding age, race, ethnicity, **socioeconomic status** (SES), education, religion, gender and sexual orientation, generation, and health status. In the United States, there are nearly 329 inhabitants who speak at least 350 different languages and identify with nearly 50 religious groups and subgroups (Pew Research Center, 2015; U.S. Census Bureau, 2015). Additionally, a child is born approximately every 8 seconds and two international migrants enter the border nearly every minute (U.S. Census Bureau, 2018a). It is inevitable that as nurses we will be expected to work with colleagues and care for patients whose culture and preferences are different than our own. As nurses we must be deliberate about acknowledging and addressing the individual differences of not only our patients, but also the intra- and inter-professional health care team members with whom we collaborate to ensure the delivery of culturally competent care to our patients.

Providing culturally competent care is a major goal of health care but is challenging as the demands greatly differ both within and between cultural groups (Marion et al., 2017; Murcia & Lopez, 2016). Developing a basic knowledge of cultural groups and norms can provide clues to people's behaviors and needs, and improve health outcomes. However, it is important to remember that despite our patients, colleagues, and ourselves being members of a cultural group, we must individualize our approach to meet the needs of the person, not merely a culturally group. This chapter will provide the nurse with the knowledge necessary to understand and incorporate cultural considerations needed to competently assess, plan, provide, and evaluate care for diverse populations in preparation to pass the **National Council Licensure Examination** (NCLEX-RN exam). Health disparities, organizational culture, spirituality, and current generation behaviors are discussed as well.

Culture

There are many definitions of culture. It is important to recognize that everyone has a culture regardless of their racial or ethnic background. Nevertheless, some people do not strongly associate with a specific culture and may fail to realize they are part of some culture (Mendez, 2015). Traditionally, **culture** refers to the learned patterns of human behavior that are passed down from one generation to the next and include the language, thoughts, communication, actions, customs, beliefs, values, and institutions of groups of individuals interacting with one another (Burkhard & Nathaniel, 2014; Leininger, 2006). Although people from all cultures share most human characteristics, the general study of culture highlights the ways in which individuals differ and are similar to individuals in other cultures. Individuals from one culture may think, solve problems, perceive, and structure the world differently from individuals of another culture.

Culture incorporates the experience of the past and influences the present and future. In other words, culture is learned and then shared. People learn about their culture from parents, teachers, religious and political leaders, and respected peers. This cultural knowledge is then transmitted to future members of a culture and the next generation. Culture influences what we eat, the language we speak, our values, behaviors, and our perception of the world; culture serves as a mostly unconscious point of reference that has a strong influence on health and illness. As children grow up, they gradually internalize the values and beliefs of their culture, and they, in turn, share these values and beliefs with their children.

Cultural Diversity and Sensitivity

It is important to recognize the diversity within cultures as much as between cultures. For example, if you have different values and beliefs than your family or peers, does that mean you do not belong to that cultural group? Cultural diversity can be influenced heavily by spirituality, religion, SES, acculturation, age, gender, sexual orientation, generation, and country of origin; it is not limited to race or ethnicity (Garneau & Pepin, 2015). It is important not to view people solely as their culture. In other words, culture is dynamic and the characteristics of individuals belonging to a specific cultural group may be different than those commonly associated with that culture.

When interacting with members from your own culture, it may be instinctual to assume that the norms of your culture are applicable to that individual. This **ethnocentric bias,** that is judging the behaviors or beliefs of another person based on our own cultural standards, can impair our judgment and ability to provide culturally sensitive care to patients (Burkhard & Nathaniel, 2014; De Chesnay, 2016). Consider being assigned to care for a patient who just underwent a voluntary procedure to have their pregnancy terminated. Although you may not agree with this patient's health care choices, you must strive to not allow your own cultural standards or biases interfere with your care.

Cultural sensitivity is demonstrated when the nurse understands the values and behaviors of another culture and strives to meet the individual needs of that person without imposing their own cultural values on others. Cultural sensitivity is a precursor for developing cultural competency in nursing care and is a key component of the **Quality and Safety Education for Nurses** (QSEN) competency of patient-centered care (Cronenwett et al., 2007). Nurses can begin to develop cultural sensitivity by recognizing that they *are* part of a culture and have certain values, beliefs, and behaviors based on that culture (Burkhard & Nathaniel, 2014; De Chesnay, 2016). Personal reflection on one's own cultural values will improve the recognition and acceptance of others' diversity. Culturally sensitive nurses also avoid stereotyping. **Stereotyping** occurs when we categorize people into groups and expect that their behaviors, perspectives, and thoughts will follow a prescribed pattern based on preconceived ideas (Burkhard & Nathaniel, 2014). Nurses can minimize stereotyping by adhering to the **American Nurses Association** (ANA) Code of Ethics with Interpretive Statements (Fowler, 2015). Specifically, Provision 1 of the Code of Ethics with Interpretive Statements requires that nurses practice with compassion and respect for inherent dignity, worth, and unique attributes of every person. If we respect others and treat others with dignity, we will arguably be providing culturally sensitive and patient-centered care. Developing cultural sensitivity also means that we understand the various dimensions of culture, including population groups and subcultures.

Population Groups

It is important to recognize that within each of the broad statistical categories of population groups, there are numerous cultural groups. The diverse characteristics of these groups are reflected in their lifestyles, values and beliefs, health-related and illness-related practices, preferences for care, and family member patterns of interaction. For example, many cultural groups are included in the category of *White* (also referred to as Anglo-American or Caucasian). Individuals in these groups may trace their heritage to a European nation, Australia, North

---

Critical Thinking 24.1

Think about your own values and behaviors.

1. What is important to you and how do you express this to others?
2. How do your values and behaviors compare to those with whom you associate in your family, work, school, or community?

3. Can you identify any health behaviors that may originate or differ from the groups with whom you associate? What does it mean if you can or cannot?

Real World Interview

Being born in the Middle East and raised in the states, essentially my entire life (immigrated at 18 months) has given me the best of both worlds. I feel that I can fully relate to my Palestinian/Middle Eastern heritage and concurrently I can fully relate to being an American raised in the states as a proud child of the 1980s. I have had so many experiences that encompass both heritages. While I feel that they are different in many ways, to me they are essential parts of who I am as an individual.

Laila Atieh, RN
Tinley Park, IL

America, or many other nations and regions. Among U.S. residents, a large group of approximately 43 million people have a German heritage. Another 31.5 million Americans trace their heritage to Ireland, and more than 23 million Americans have an English heritage (U.S. Census Bureau, 2017) (Table 24.1).

There is also great diversity among the individuals who are included in the Hispanic population category. Hispanics may trace their heritage to different countries of origin, different dialects spoken, and to different customs and beliefs, including practices related to health and illness. Hispanics may include people from the Caribbean, Cuba, El Salvador, Guatemala, Puerto Rico, Mexico, Central and South America, and Spain (Murcia & Lopez, 2016; Lee, Martin & Hall, 2017).

The term *Black* is similarly very inclusive and can refer to individuals who may trace their heritage from African nations such as Eritrea and Kenya; those from the Caribbean, Haiti, and the Dominican Republic. Furthermore, the term *Native American* includes members of more than 573 federally recognized Native American and Alaska Native tribes (e.g., Cherokees, Navajo, Chippewa, Sioux, Choctaw, American Indian/Athapaskan, Aleuts, and Eskimos) who reside in North America (National Conference of State Legislatures, 2016). Likewise, the term *Asian* can refer to Japanese, Chinese, Indochinese, Filipino, Korean, Vietnamese, Cambodian, Laotian, Thai, Indonesian, Pakistani, Hmong, and Indian populations, each of which contains numerous, diverse subcultures.

Now that we have looked at groups in the larger context of populations, let us examine some of the characteristics of smaller subcultures.

Subcultures

Another way to explore differences in individuals is in the context of smaller groups within a culture called subcultures. Subcultures may be based on the following:

- Professional and occupational affiliations (e.g., nursing)
- Nationality, ethnicity, or race (a shared historical and political past)
- Age groups (adolescents, older adults)
- Gender (feminists, men's groups)
- Socioeconomic factors (income, education, occupation)
- Political viewpoints (Democrat, Republican)
- Sexual orientation (gay, lesbian, bisexual, or transgendered groups)

The Nursing Profession

When you started nursing school, you became a part of the subculture of nursing. Many of the norms, behaviors, and customs of the "nurse" were unfamiliar, and initially you probably suffered from some degree of culture shock. **Culture shock** develops when someone is being exposed to values and beliefs of an unfamiliar culture. As a nursing student you had to learn a whole new culture. During your years of study, you gradually internalized many of the values and beliefs taught by your instructors. Eventually, you became comfortable with the values and beliefs you learned in your school of nursing, and by the time you graduate, you are assimilated into the professional nursing subculture. Successful assimilation into a new culture occurs when new members of a culture learn and internalize that culture's important values.

At the completion of your nursing program it is expected that you will become a registered nurse and encompass all the rights, privileges, and responsibilities associated with the culture of nursing. These include having entry level knowledge to pass the NCLEX-RN exam; demonstrating a standard level of care that adheres to the American Nurses' Association

Table 24.1 Ten Most Common Heritages

Reported ancestry	Estimate	Margin of error
German	43,093,766	+/− 133,481
Irish	31,479,232	+/− 126,360
English	23,074,947	+/− 96,420
American	20,024,830	+/− 114,083
Italian	16,650,674	+/− 100,388
Polish	9,012,085	+/− 64,795
French (except Basque)	7,673,619	+/− 59,457
Scottish	5,399,371	+/− 43,591
European	5,321,714	+/− 46,235
Norwegian	4,295,981	+/− 47,318
Hispanic or Latino	56,510,571	+/− 1,541

Source: U.S. Census Bureau, 2013–2017 American Community Survey 5-Year Estimates. Hispanic or Latino Origin by Specific Origin. (2019b) Retrieved from https://factfinder.census.gov/faces/tableservices/jsf/pages/productview.xhtml?pid=ACS_11_5YR_B03001&prodType=table

(ANA) Standards of Practice (2015) and the Code of Ethics with Interpretive Statements (Fowler, 2015); and promoting the safety and quality of health care systems by adhering to the QSEN Competencies (Cronenwett et al., 2007). Nevertheless, each of you will demonstrate these standards in a unique fashion based on your personal values, history, experiences, gender, age, sexual orientation, and your social, political, and religious beliefs. Just because you are a nurse, you would not want your patients to label or define you solely as "the nurse," devoid of any individual characteristics, would you? Likewise, it is important we do not define our patients solely by their culture.

Upon admission to a hospital, patients become members of a new culture. In this world filled with strange sights, unfamiliar sounds, and strangers, many patients experience culture shock. Ideas about health and illness, proper communication, right and wrong, and death and dying are all founded in one's culture. Culture provides a lens through which patients view their health care experiences. Even under the best of circumstances, culture shock intensifies for patients who are recent immigrants, who do not speak the native language, or whose culture is different than the nurse (Mendez, 2015). When nurses, families, patients, and health care members have different cultural beliefs within the context of the health care setting, cultural issues may arise and can negatively affect patient outcomes and satisfaction with the health care. In situations of cultural incongruences in the health care setting, the nurse can act on behalf of the patient as an advocate. As a patient advocate, the nurse and the inter-professional team can ensure they are providing culturally sensitive care to their patients.

Race and Ethnicity

Race describes a geographical or global human population distinguished by genetic traits and physical characteristics such as skin color or facial features. Race and ethnicity are different. The U.S. Census classifications for race are (U.S. Census Bureau, 2018b):

- White

- Black or African American

- American Indian or Alaska Native

- Asian

- Native Hawaiian or Other Pacific Islander

- More than one race

Similarly, cultural ethnicity identifies a person or group based on a racial, tribal, linguistic, religious, national, or cultural group—for example, Jewish or Irish. People of a common race sometimes, but not always, share a common culture. The U.S. Census Bureau relies on self-identification for the collection of data related to the race and ethnicity of the United States population (see Figure 24.1 for current U.S. population by race data).

Race and ethnicity data are collected from U.S. residents every 10 years. In 2010, the census questionnaire asked two separate questions about residents' race and Hispanic ethnicity to capture the most accurate data. For example, residents were first asked about their Hispanic, Latino, or Spanish Origin followed by a second question about their race (i.e., White, Black, American Indian/Alaska Native, Asian, and/or Hawaiian/Pacific Islander). These classifications are expected to remain unchanged for the 2020 census, despite previous recommendations of the U.S. Census Bureau with the hope of improving the response rate (Fontenot, 2018; Parker, Horowitz, Morin, & Lopez, 2015; Wang, 2018). However, the final decision for the 2020 census was to keep the questions on race and ethnicity as two questions.

The ethnic and racial composition of the population of the United States has been changing dramatically since the 1990s. According to the 2017 population projections for the United States, children, including past and present immigration and births, will greatly contribute to the future racial and ethnic diversity anticipated for the country. By 2020, it is projected that minority youths (under 18 years old) will outnumber White youths, and by 2027, 18–29-year-old Whites will be the new minority (Census Bureau, 2018a). In all age categories, the White population will become the new minority in the United States by 2045 (Frey, 2018). To reflect the changing ethnic and racial landscape of the United States, increasingly diverse languages, beliefs, lifestyles, and practices can be seen among residents throughout the country.

Likewise, the outlook for a more diverse nursing workforce is promising. In 2015, nearly 20% of registered nurses identified themselves as being from a racial and/or ethnic minority population, with newly licensed nurses ranking highest in racial and ethnic diversity (National State Boards of Nursing, 2016). According to the **Health Resources and Services Administration** (HRSA 2017), the estimate of the diversity in nursing through 2030 is expected to be generally consistent with the expected changes in the U.S. population projected by the U.S. Census Bureau. See Figure 24.2 for future

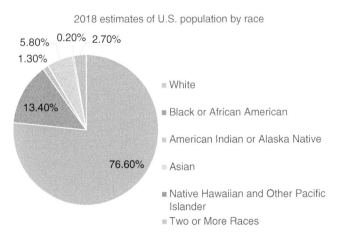

FIGURE 24.1 2018 U.S. population by race.
Source: U.S. Census Bureau, 2019a. Quick Facts United States.

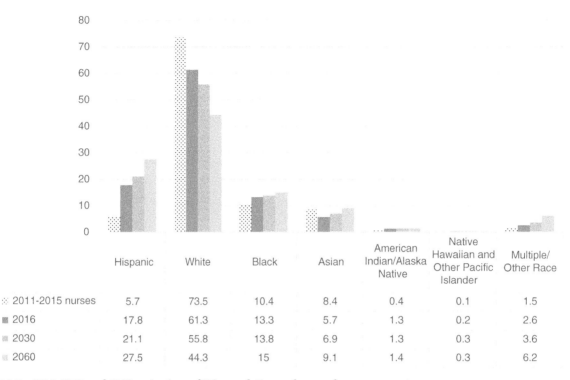

	Hispanic	White	Black	Asian	American Indian/Alaska Native	Native Hawaiian and Other Pacific Islander	Multiple/ Other Race
2011-2015 nurses	5.7	73.5	10.4	8.4	0.4	0.1	1.5
2016	17.8	61.3	13.3	5.7	1.3	0.2	2.6
2030	21.1	55.8	13.8	6.9	1.3	0.3	3.6
2060	27.5	44.3	15	9.1	1.4	0.3	6.2

FIGURE 24.2   2016, 2030, and 2060 projections of U.S. population and nurses by race, percentages.
Source: Vespa, Armstrong, & Medina, 2018. (U.S. Department of Commerce). U.S. Department of Health and Human Services (2017). Sex, Race, and Ethnic Diversity of U.S. Health Occupations (2011–2015). Retrieved from https://bhw.hrsa.gov/sites/default/files/bhw/nchwa/diversityushealthoccupations.pdf

estimates of nursing diversity. This congruency between the nurse and patient is important for improving patient satisfaction with their health care as well as patient outcomes (Meyer & Zane, 2013; Shepherd et al., 2018).

Gender and Sexual Orientation

The profession of nursing has historically been dominated by females. However, this trend is changing. According to the National Nursing Workforce study, the number of newly licensed male nurses has increased from 8% in 2015 to 9.1% in just 2 years (Smiley et al., 2018). This indicates that the rate at which males are entering the nursing profession is improving, but the proportion of males to females is still well below the general population. Regarding their employment profile, men entering the nursing workforce generally move into leadership roles earlier and more frequently than women (Arndt, 2015; Berkery, Tiernan, & Morley, 2014). Also, a greater proportion of men are employed in hospitals and in the subspecialty of nurse anesthetists than women (Munnich & Wozniak, 2017).

Gender diversity is important in nursing to minimize disparities that can occur in care when patients experience differences in care based on the gender of the nurse. Historically, women have exhibited a greater overall empathetic response to physical and verbal demonstrations of suffering. In a 2017 study, Vigil et al. (2017) re-confirmed that the gender of nurses and patients affects patients' assessment and nurses' prioritization of patient

care in U.S. emergency departments. Read the Evidence from the Literature to learn about how gender may impact patient care.

While most people identify as either male or female, there is a subculture that must be acknowledged. The transgender population is part of the **lesbian, gay, bisexual, transgender, and queer or questioning** (LGBTQ+; the "+" encompasses other sexual and gender minorities; ANA, 2018) population. It is estimated that LGBTQ+ nurses comprise a large minority group in nursing, although the exact number is unknown (Gates, 2017). Gates (2017) estimated approximately 10 million (4.1%) adults identify as LGBTQ+. Both LGBTQ+ nurses and patients experience a distinct set of challenges in the health care system including stigma, discrimination, poor health insurance, and unequal access to care (Kates, Ranji, Beamesderfer, Salganicoff, & Dawson, 2017). Because of the ongoing challenges they face, many LGBTQ+ populations may avoid or delay medical treatment.

The American Nurses Association (ANA, 2018) recently published the Nursing Advocacy for LGBTQ+ Populations, a position statement openly condemning discrimination based on sexual orientation and/or gender identity and acknowledging the societal stigma, discrimination, and bias that continues to contribute to disparate care and negative health outcomes for the LGBTQ+ populations. The ANA Position Statement affirms the need for the LGBTQ+ populations to "receive culturally congruent, competent, sensitive, safe, inclusive, and ethical care." Additionally, one of the goals of the *Healthy People 2020* is to "Improve the health, safety, and well-being

Evidence From the Literature

Citation: Vigil, J. M., Coulombe, P., Alcock, J., Stith, S. S., Kruger, E., & Cichowski, S. (2017). How nurse gender influences patient priority assignments in U.S. emergency departments. *Pain*, 158(3), 377–382.

Discussion: The authors of this article conducted research to investigate if the pain intensity of patients presenting to the emergency department (ED) was measured differently by male and female nurses. An additional goal of the researchers was to compare how male and female nurses prioritize patients' care based on the nurses' perception of patients' pain intensity, heart rate, and respiratory status using a standardized methodology called the **Emergency Severity Index** (ESI). The following findings were identified:

- Patients' pain intensity, heart rate, and respiratory rate measurements were not affected by the nurse's gender.

- The nurses' gender impacted how pain intensity and respiratory rate measurements influenced the priority of care (the ESI) for male patients.
- Higher perceived pain intensity scores were considered a higher priority (higher ESI) by female nurses, but less of a priority (lower ESI) by male nurses.
- Male patients with high respiratory rate received more of a priority (higher ESI) by male nurses, but nurse gender did not influence the priority of care for female patients.

Implications for Practice: Disparate patient care, including unreliable assessment and subsequent treatment of patients, may be provided by nurses based on the gender of the nurse, even when a standardize tool is used for evaluating patients and prioritizing their care.

Critical Thinking 24.2

After reading about the impact of gender on nursing care, think about the following questions:

1. Do you think that the increasing number of male nurses will help or hurt the gender disparity in patient care?
2. Discuss why or why not.

Real World Interview

I believe being a gay woman has made me more cognizant of other marginalized groups and more aware of how institutionalized medicine can further marginalize these individuals, despite best intentions of individual providers. It's made me aware of how I talk to my patients, especially kids and teens, when using pronouns or asking about relationships.

Regarding my own identify, I really did feel like I had to hide that I am a lesbian from my patients and their families, especially in neonatal and pediatric intensive care. You never know how people will react to it, and I never wanted families to doubt my ability to care for their children. It was just easier to dodge questions about whether I was dating anyone or label a significant other as a "friend" when making conversation with patients and their parents, particularly early in my career. I started to be more open about it over the last couple years, but I still am very cautious about sharing that part of my life.

I've never felt discriminated against—not outrightly so. I've been very fortunate to have worked primarily in large academic centers. When I first was coming out to coworkers, there were a couple offhanded comments, not directed at me and I don't believe intended to be hurtful. I remember one of my fellow nurses talking about the Pride Parade, a conversation she initiated. I wasn't out to her yet. She said something along the lines

of the parade being so fun, how she loved going and watching the dancing cowboys, seeing the floats, but feeling really anxious around lesbians—"especially the ones you don't know are lesbians." I knew this nurse fairly well, so I still came out to her shortly after and talked to her about how that comment made me feel. But it reinforced that I needed to be aware of who I was sharing my personal life with.

I struggle with this because I think it's important for gay, lesbian, bisexual, and transfolk to be visible, especially in such an important field. It really doesn't do any service by hiding that piece of our identities, but I've always been worried that a parent would request that I didn't care for their child if I came out to the "wrong" person—that would absolutely devastate me. I also think it's important for kids and teens to know that there are gay, lesbian, bisexual, and transfolk out in the world, and that we are successful people, saving lives, every day. When I knew kids were hospitalized because of issues related to their sexuality (depression or self-harm attempts, for example), I always made a point of casually mentioning my girlfriend or asking if they were dating anyone, rather than asking about a boyfriend or girlfriend specifically, so they knew I was sort of a "safe space" for them to talk.

Claire Sorenson, PhD, RN

Chicago, IL

of **lesbian, gay, bisexual, and transgender** (LGBT) individuals" (Healthy People 2020, 2019). Still, most research indicates that LGBTQ+ populations remain marginalized and vulnerable in health care (Nhamo & Macleod, 2018).

Health Care Disparities

The factors that contribute to the health and illness of individuals are complex. For example, there are modifiable and non-modifiable risk factors that influence health and illness. Some of the factors that individuals can modify to reduce their risk of illness are diet, exercise, exposure to pollutants (e.g., smoking), and level of stress (to some degree). Other factors are non-modifiable and cannot be changed, including genetic predisposition to disease, heredity, race, ethnicity, age, and biological gender. Additional factors also play into health and illness that are influenced by other things such as social, economic, and/or environmental factors (e.g., access to health care, poverty level, sexual identity, disability, SES, and geographical location). When social, economic, and/or environmental disadvantages lead to differences in health, a **health disparity** is said to exist, Healthy People 2020, (2019). These health disparities include differences in the occurrence of illness, disease, and death among minorities and other vulnerable populations in the United States (U.S. National Library of Medicine, 2018). Health disparities are often linked with race and ethnicity, geography, socioeconomic status (income, education, or occupational status) of populations. Although there has been significant improvement in the general health of the United States, ongoing disparities in morbidity and mortality are experienced by minority populations like African Americans, Hispanics, American Indians, Alaskan Natives, Native Hawaiian, and other Pacific Islanders compared to the entire U.S. population (Xu, Murphy, Kochanek, Bastian, & Arias, 2018). For example:

- In 2016, for all causes of death, individuals from non-Hispanic Black populations were 1.2 times more likely to die than those from non-Hispanic White populations, and 1.4 times more likely to die than those from Hispanic populations.

- In 2016, non-Hispanic Blacks were 1.4 times more likely to die from cerebrovascular diseases than non-Hispanic Whites, and non-Hispanic Whites were 1.1 times more likely than Hispanics to die from the same cause (Xu et al., 2018).

- In 2016, non-Hispanic Blacks were 2 times more likely to die from diabetes mellitus than non-Hispanic Whites (Xu et al. 2018).

- In 2016, non-Hispanic Blacks were 2.2 times more likely to die from essential hypertension and hypertensive renal disease than non-Hispanic Whites (Xu et al., 2018).

- In 2016, the infant mortality rates were highest among babies born to non-Hispanic Black mothers; non-Hispanic Black babies were 1.2 times more likely to die than American Indian or Alaska Native babies (11.4 deaths per 1,000 live births vs 9.4 per 1,000), and 1.5 and 1.27, respectively, times more likely to die than Native Hawaiian or Other Pacific Islander (7.4 per 1,000) (Center for Disease Control, 2019, 2019a).

- Between 2013 and 2015, infants who lived in rural counties were 2.4 times more likely to die from sudden infant death syndrome than those who lived in large urban counties (5.5 and 2.78% respectively) (Ely & Hoyert, 2018).

The cause of health disparities is multi-factorial and not easily explained solely by biological traits of ethnic populations. These health disparities are believed to arise from a complex mix of biology and genetics (e.g., sex and family history), individual behavior (e.g., smoking, alcohol, and drug use), social environment (e.g., SES and discrimination), physical environment (e.g., cleanliness, location), and health service (e.g., access to high-quality care).

Socioeconomic Disparities

Health disparities affect those of lower SES, whether measured by income, education, or occupational status, independent of race or ethnicity. For example, both Black and non-Hispanic White men with less than 12 years of education are almost 3 times more likely to die from cancer than Black and non-Hispanic White male college graduates (American Cancer Society, 2018). Additionally, the prevalence of diabetes varies based on education level, with 12.6% of adults with less than a high school education having a diagnosis of diabetes versus 9.5% of those with a high school education and 7.2% with more than a high school education (CDC, 2017).

Both culture and health disparities are dynamic. In other words, health disparities are likely caused by not only one condition like income, but rather many factors that influence the health of individuals in varying ways. For example, people with lower SES are more likely to smoke, be obese, have a higher exposure to harmful environmental toxins, have less access to preventive care and early treatment, and have inadequate health insurance (American Cancer Society, 2018). Furthermore, the highest rates of poverty are associated with race and ethnicity. In 2016, Blacks had the highest poverty rate (22%), followed by Hispanics (19.4%), Asians (10.1%), and non-Hispanic Whites (8.8%) (Semega, Fontenot, & Kollar, 2017). It is likely that the causes of health disparities are intertwined, making it difficult to point to only one cause.

Differences in the Quality of Health Care

As we have seen, individuals can modify some of their risk factors for illness (e.g., smoking, activity level, and diet). In other cases, the ability to modify risk factors lies outside of the individual. Leaders of the health care system, the government, and to some extent health care providers, control some of the factors that put individuals or populations at risk of illness. Lack of equal access to quality care is one example of a risk factor

Evidence From Literature

Citation: Rider, G. N., McMorris, B. J., Gower, A. L., Coleman, E., & Eisenbery, M. A. (2018). Health and care utilization of transgender and gender nonconforming youth: A population-based study. *Pediatrics*. doi: https://doi.org/10.1542/peds.2017-1683

Discussion: The authors of this study sought to examine the mental and physical health characteristics and utilization of health care services among high-school students who identified as **transgender and gender nonconforming** (TGNC) as compared to cisgender (a person who identifies with their designated birth sex) students. This is important because previous research with TGNC populations has been limited to small and nonrepresentative samples. The current study included data from 80,929 high school students, 2,168 of whom identified as TGNC. It was determined that TGNC students reported significantly poorer physical and mental health, including poorer use of preventative services, and more nurse office visits than cisgender students. The authors of the study hypothesized that TGNC youths may perceive that society views them as "wrong" or that they are somehow "wrong" when they present differently than what society expects based on their birth sex. As a result of the societal message, TGNC youths experience stress and invalidation that negatively impacts their health. When seeking health care, TGNC youths may fear that they will be seen as "different" and as a result, fear they may be treated differently by health care providers (e.g., mistreatment, refused care, or health care providers not using their preferred pronouns). Fear of a physical exam may also contribute to underutilization of health care services.

Implications for Practice: As health care providers, we must ensure that the health care environment is welcoming and comfortable. We can do this by asking people how they identify and if they have experienced any forms of victimization like bullying or discrimination. Asking these questions will help convey a sense of inclusivity and caring. Additionally, the results of the study show that school nurses are in a unique position to start conversations with youths about sexual identity, offer support on a day-to-day basis, provide preventative and other medical services for youths, and promote anti-bullying programs and programs that improve school acceptance of TGNC youth.

that has been shown to negatively affect the health outcomes of populations but is outside the control of individuals. Disparities in access to quality health care are influenced by factors like SES, race, ethnicity, and sexual/gender orientation. Lack of health insurance coverage contributes to this disparity. In 2016, the U.S. Hispanics population had the highest rate of uninsured people (16%), followed by Blacks (10.5%), Asians (7.6%), and non-Hispanic Whites (6.3%). Likewise, non-Hispanic Black and Hispanic children are nearly twice as likely than non-Hispanic White children to have untreated tooth decay, suggesting a disparity in the access to care (National Institute of Health, 2015).

The introduction of the **Affordable Care Act** (ACA) in 2015, commonly known as Obama Care, provided hope for reducing disparities in access to affordable and equitable health care (Adepoju, Preston, & Gonzales, 2015). However, researchers continue to identify disparities in access to health care due to lack of insurance coverage. Additionally, under the Trump administration, anti-immigrant sentiments have significantly impaired immigrants' access to health care, especially immigrants who have illegally entered the U.S. Immigrants may not legally have access to health care and/or may be too fearful to seek it due to the recent hardship they have faced coming to and remaining in the United States.

It is also important to consider that the children (who are largely U.S. born) of immigrants may be exposed to "toxic stress" as a result of opposition related to their parents' or their own immigration into the United States. Toxic stress has been shown to result in short- and long-term negative health effects and is another example of how individuals can be exposed to factors outside of their control that increase their risk of illness (Artiga & Urbi, 2017). Although the government and policy makers in the U.S. may be responsible for some of the disparities in access to health care, health care providers also play an important role in the disparate treatment of patients.

A large body of literature suggests that unconscious or implicit biases by health care providers in clinical decision making can lead to patients being treated differently based on their race, gender, weight, age, language, income, and

---

Critical Thinking 24.3

Think about how you would respond to a person who did not speak your language, did not have insurance, or proof of citizenship, but who was seeking care for an illness or injury at the facility in which you work. Would you turn them away? Would you treat them?

1. How do you feel about equal access to health care for all humans?

2. Do you believe that everyone should have an equal opportunity to maintain their health and wellness?

3. What would you do if your facility required health insurance or a social security number to provide care and a patient who did meet those qualifications needed health care?

insurance status (ANA, 2018; Quinn-Szcesuil, 2018; The Joint Commission, 2016). The LGBTQ+ population is one that has experienced differential treatment directly as a result of either conscious or unconscious health care provider biases. In a 16-article international literature review, Nhamo & Macleod (2018) found members of the LGBTQ+ population consistently felt that their health care providers did not treat them with respect, did not provide patient-centered care, and were undereducated on the LGBTQ+ population. Consequently, LGBTQ+ patients often avoided seeking health care, when needed in the future.

Eliminating Health Disparities

The elimination of health disparities is a significant world priority and public health concern. Among the many advocates for reducing disparities in health care are Healthy People 2020 (2019), the **World Health Organization** (WHO), The National Academy of Medicine (formerly the Institute of Medicine), The U.S. Department of Health and Human Services, **American Hospital Association** (AHA), The **Center for Disease Control** (CDC), The ANA and The Joint Commission. Nurses must recognize, respect, and incorporate patients' cultural beliefs into their care to help reduce the disparities that occur in health care. Nurses from all backgrounds as well as nurses from racially and ethnically diverse backgrounds can help reduce health care disparities. One way that nurses can help reduce disparities is to strive to understand the diverse needs, customs, and behaviors of the patients for whom they provide care. Improving the diversity of the nursing profession may also help reduce disparities in health care as patients may feel more comfortable receiving care from nurses with whom they share a common race or culture. As we learned in this chapter, the diversity of nurses is improving; there are more ethnic and racial populations represented in nursing, more men, and more LGBTQ+ nurses than ever before. However, nurses also need to work together to decrease health care disparities through interventions focused on policy change and acknowledgement of one's own prejudices and biases that may affect the care of patients. Such interventions primarily lie with health care providers, health care organizations and institutions, academics, community organizations, payers, and government (Aurilio, 2017; Thornton et al., 2016). Other interventions for nurse leaders include:

- Increase the diversity of the nursing staff to enhance patient and provider relations and reduce problems in cross-cultural communication (ANA, 2018; Aurilio, 2017).

- Utilize culturally and linguistically appropriate approaches to nursing care that can be flexible to patient needs while still identifying and addressing potential barriers that are specific to the individual patient (Center for Disease Control, 2019b).

- Demonstrate a model of respect, including a zero tolerance to discriminatory practices (ANA, 2018).

- Conduct research in and implement evidence-based practices that are inclusive in nature (ANA, 2018).

- Examine the organization's culture, policies, conditions, and training needs and then advocate for changes that reduce disparities (ANA, 2018; Aurilio, 2017).

- Practice a patient-centered approach to health care that accounts for individual cultural needs (Cuevas, O'Brien, & Saha, 2017).

- Provide future nurses with the "**knowledge, skills, and attitudes** (KSAs) to continuously improve the quality and safety of the health care system in which they work" (QSEN, 2018).

- Utilize the National Standards for **Culturally and Linguistically Appropriate Services** (CLAS) in Health and Health Care to improve health equity, quality, and reduce health disparities (Think Cultural Health, 2018).

Cultural Congruence and Cultural Competence

As you may recall, providing culturally competent or culturally congruent care begins with cultural sensitivity. **Culturally congruent practice** is applying evidence-based nursing care that aligns with the cultural values, beliefs, behaviors, and perspectives, of the patient and other stakeholders (ANA, 2015). Similarly, **cultural competence** is how nurses provide culturally congruent practice to the patients for whom they care (ANA, 2015). Culturally competent nurses embrace a culture of diversity, respect for others, and commit to a lifelong journey of professional development. Inherent in the development of cultural competence is self-awareness, continual evaluation of current competence, continual professional growth, and the use of evidence-based tools to assess and critically appraise cultural competence (Marion et al., 2017).

As we learned, unconscious or implicit biases of health care workers can promote unequal or disparate care for patients. Our personal culture has a meaningful impact on the care we deliver as nurses. The way we view ourselves is often reflected in the nurse-patient interactions. Engaging in self-assessments of our personal cultural values and beliefs, unconscious or implicit biases, religious beliefs, personality, and communication style allows us to identify our personal values that can impair the delivery of equitable care to our patients. It also sets the stage for integrating new cultural knowledge about our patients into our professional role and health care interventions. Self-awareness requires a conscious effort of the nurse to better understand one's own self. In other words, if you want to improve your nursing care by becoming more self-aware, you must dedicate time and effort to this task; self-awareness does not happen by chance. There are a variety of self-assessment tools that nurses can use to better understand their knowledge, feelings, and attitudes toward people of different cultures. For example, Santos, Goldstein, & Tracey (2017) developed an assessment tool that nurses and health care providers can use to assess their own attitudes toward transgender patients. This 24-item survey requires users to self-reflect on their attitudes and beliefs about statements like "I think it is critical for all transgender clients to participate in activities that are traditional for their assigned sex" and "All transgender clients should choose a male or female pronoun that is consistent with their affirmed gender" (Santos et al., 2017, p. 372). Self-Assessment tools also exists for nurses and nursing students to evaluate their cultural competence and cultural awareness (see Table 24.2 for some common cultural competence self-assessment tools).

After assessing our own cultural values, we are ready to assess the patient's culture and the impact it may have on our interactions with them. Cultural assessment of the patient during the nursing process (i.e., assessment, diagnosis, outcomes identification, planning, implementation, and evaluation) can ensure we deliver quality care that is also culturally congruent (Marion et al., 2017). Many nursing schools added curricula in the 1990s to ensure that nurses have adequate preparation for cultural competence. In addition, all nurses need to commit themselves to enhancing their knowledge of different cultures by doing such things as reading about various cultures and their traditional health practices, seeing films about different cultures, talking with patients and coworkers about their cultural backgrounds, or acting as a participant observer in a cultural setting such as an ethnic community celebration or gathering. Nurses also have opportunities to participate in continuing education for cultural competency. For example, the **Office of Minority Health** (OMH), U.S. Department of Health and Human Services (Think Cultural Health, 2018), offers a free online continuing education program titled "Culturally Competent Nursing Care: A Cornerstone of Caring"

(see the Informatics Exercise at the end of the chapter). Note that every new person you meet who is from another culture will also give you the opportunity to broaden your appreciation of different cultures and improve your cultural competence.

Nurse leaders are often asked to work with people who are different from themselves because of their ethnicity, race, culture, religion, generation, or sexual orientation. This can result in workplace problems, including difficulties with communication. To manage and understand these potential difficulties, cultural nursing theories and conceptual models offer some direction. Table 24.3 reviews several of these: Leininger's Transcultural Nursing (2006), Purnell's Model for Cultural Competence (2008), Campinha-Bacote's Process of Cultural Competence in the Delivery of Health Care Service (2003), Giger and Davidhizar's Transcultural Assessment Model (2008), and Spector's Health Traditions Model (2009). Each of these models offers the nurse insight into examining the cultural beliefs and needs of culturally diverse patients. Using a model to provide care will help nurses integrate culturally competent care into the nursing process.

The native or preferred language of a patient must also be considered when providing culturally congruent and culturally competent care. Consider how you might feel if you were ill and in need of medical assistance. You enter the hospital and you are unable to read or understand anything that is said or given to you. Do you think you would feel safe, comfortable, or confident in the care you were going to receive? Today, there are many tools and resources available to ensure patients are provided with information in their preferred language. It is also important to recognize when patients express that they understand what you are saying to them, but their behaviors and actions do not reflect their understandings.

Table 24.2   Cultural Competence Self-Assessment Tools

Tool	Tool characteristics
Cultural Awareness Scale (CAS), (Rew et al., 2003)	36-item, Likert-type scale, questionnaire with 5 subscales designed to measure cultural awareness of nursing students.
Cultural Competence Assessment (CCA), (Schim et al., 2003)	25-item, Likert-type scale, with subscales designed to measure the cultural competency of hospice nurses.
Cultural Self-Efficacy Scale (CSES) (Bernal & Froman, 1993)	30-item, Likert-type scale, designed to test one's perception of cultural competence self-efficacy.
Inventory for Assessing the Process for Cultural Competency (IAPCC and IAPCC-R) (Campinha-Bacote, 2009)	The original Inventory has 20-items, and the revised has 25-items, Likert-type scale, designed to measure cultural competency of health care providers.
Nurse Cultural Competence Scale (NCCS), (Perng & Watson, 2012)	41-item, Likert-type scale, designed to measure cultural awareness, knowledge, sensitivity, and skills of nurses.
Transcultural Self-Efficacy Tool (TSET) (Jeffreys & Smodlaka, 1996)	83-item, Likert-type scale, with 3 subscales designed to assess nursing students' perceived self-efficacy for cultural competency.
Ethnic Competency Skills Assessment Inventory (ECSAI), (Napholz, 1999)	23-item, Liker-type scale, designed to assess self-reported cultural competency of nursing students.
Cultural Competency Instrument (CCI) (Kosoko-Lasaki et al., 2006)	20-items, Likert-type scale, designed to assess cultural knowledge, attitudes, and sensitivity of health care providers and investigators.
Cross-Cultural Evaluation Tool (CCET) (Hughes & Hood, 2007)	20-items, Likert-type scale, designed to measure the cultural sensitivity of nursing students.

Source: Complied by A. Kratkovil.

Table 24.3   Cultural Nursing Theories and Models

Theory, author (year)	Characteristics	Basic tenets	Application to beginning nurse leader
Leininger (2006) Culture Care Theory	Formal approach to the study and practice of comparative holistic cultural care and health and illness patterns while respecting differences.	All cultures have caring behaviors that may vary from culture to culture. Each culture identifies what it values for care. An understanding of each culture is important for providing care and meeting patient needs. Need to evaluate world view, social structure, language, ethnohistory, environmental context, and folk and professional systems.	Initial theory was created in the 1960s and is frequently updated and edited. Seeks to provide culturally congruent nursing care that is meaningful to the recipient.
Purnell (2008) Purnell Model for Cultural Competence	An organizing framework for assessing culture across disciplines. States that cultural competence is a process, not an endpoint.	The model is represented by a circle with rims moving from the global society to the community, to the family, and to the individual. The inner circle has 12 pie slices representing 12 domains of culture—i.e., overview/heritage, communication, family roles and organization, workforce issues, biocultural ecology, high-risk behaviors, nutrition, pregnancy, death rituals, spirituality, health care practices, and health care practitioners.	This grand theory offers direction for practice. Analyzing the patient belief system in each of the 12 domains gives direction to the nursing process.
Campinha-Bacote (2003) Process of Cultural Competence in the Delivery of Health Care Service	Cultural competence is a process where in the nurse works to effectively meet needs within a cultural context.	*Cultural desire* leads the nurse to engage in developing cultural competence. *Cultural awareness* is a self-examination and exploration of one's own cultural background. *Cultural knowledge* is learning about diverse groups and understanding beliefs and values specific to the patient. *Cultural skill* is the ability to collect data and complete a cultural assessment. *Cultural encounters* occur when the nurse is engaged in interactions with diverse patients, meeting their needs in a culturally sensitive manner.	This process reflects the need for the nurse to have an awareness of patient needs and then to actively seek to meet those needs. The model serves as a guide for becoming culturally competent.
Ginger and Davidhizar (2008) Transcultural Assessment Model	Method for completing and evaluating the outcomes of cultural assessment.	Has five concepts that focus on transcultural nursing and the provision of culturally diverse nursing care, provision of culturally competent care, identification of the cultural uniqueness of individuals, development of culturally sensitive environments, and development of culturally specific illness and wellness behaviors.	Consider communication, space, social organization, time, environmental control, and biological variations when assessing culture.
Spector's (2009) HEALTH Traditions Model.	Based on the concept of holistic health (i.e., physical, mental, and spiritual health) and personal ways to maintain, protect, and restore health.	Has three main components including heritage consistency, HEALTH traditions, and Ginger and Davidhizar's theory (Ginger, 2012) about the relationship between culture and health. *Heritage consistency* describes how closely a person's lifestyle reflects their tribal culture or traditional cultural background (i.e., German, Irish Asian).	Nurses must understand that some patients have a more traditional approach to health and healing while others will adhere less to those traditional practices. Understanding patients' heritage consistency is important for providing patient-centered care.

Source: Compiled by Amanda Kratovil.

Critical Thinking 24.4

During your discharge teaching of a postpartum woman who gave birth to an 8 lb., 7 oz baby 3 days ago, you become concerned that she does not fully understand everything you are saying to her. You were told by the previous nurse that she speaks "some English" and stated that her preferred language is English. However, when you watch her interact with her baby, she is not able to follow the instructions you provided her.

1. How do you address this concern with her?
2. What action should you take to ensure her and the newborn's safety?
3. What can you do if she insists she understands?

On-site medical interpreters and translators are available in most hospitals for an increasing number of languages. Although you may have to wait for the arrival of a medical interpreter, this option offers the advantage of face-to-face communication with the patient. Other forms of interpreter or translator services include:

- Multi-language printing of medical information, discharge instructions, consent forms, medical records, and other patient documents.

- On-Demand Phone Interpreting available via calling a toll-free number on the phone.

Video Remote Interpreting offers videoconferencing technology over the internet. Common modalities of this technology include smart phones, tablets, and/or computers on wheels (see Figure 24.3). This type of interpreting can be especially helpful for those patients who are deaf or hard of hearing.

To ensure that we are delivering culturally competent care, we must evaluate the impact our care has on patients. Unfortunately, there are not many cultural competence assessment instruments that have undergone rigorous reliability and validity testing and that use objective patient data as the outcome measurement (Shen, 2015). As an alternative, the ANA (2015) recently developed a new standard and corresponding competencies for the delivery of culturally congruent nursing practices. The 13 competencies included in Standard 8 (ANA, 2015) provide guidelines that, when used appropriately, will promote cultural congruent and culturally competent nursing care.

Many **cultures, subcultures, races, ethnicities, and population groups** exist within the United States, each person adding to the diversity of the nation. Globally, it is unknown just how many **different groups** make up the world's population. What is certain, is that as nurses we will be required to collaborate with and care for people who are different from ourselves. Although it is not realistic to learn every nuance of every culture, it is essential to learn as much as possible about the cultures represented in our community. Table 24.4 provides an overview of cultural norms, health care beliefs, and religious beliefs often seen in the United States. The content in this table provides information for beginning a dialogue between the nurse and patient. Note that the norms and beliefs may not be valid for all individuals within a cultural group. Furthermore, you should never assume you know someone's values or cultural norms because of their stated **culture.** To best achieve cultural congruence and cultural competence, you must be aware of your own personal cultural values, be sensitive to and accepting of the influence of culture, have a commitment to continual learning about different cultures, and provide care that is in harmony with the cultural beliefs and lifestyles of patients.

Organizational Culture

Before leaving the concept of culture, it is important to discuss organizational culture. We have discussed the culture of the nurse and the patient, now we must understand how the culture of the organization influences the health care team and ultimately patient outcomes. **Organizational culture** is the system of shared values and beliefs that actively influences the behavior of organization members. The term *shared values* is important, because it implies that many people are guided by the same values and that they interpret them in a similar way. Organizational values develop over time and reflect an organization's history and traditions. The culture of an organization is important because it has been shown to influence nurses in many ways such as being helpful and supportive toward new members, job satisfaction, nurses' willingness to report errors, bullying and incivility, and patient outcomes.

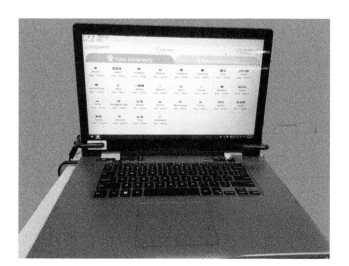

FIGURE 24.3 Computer on wheels with Video Remote Interpreting.
Source: Used with permission.

The culture and values of an organization impact the workplace environment, and ultimately the nurse. For example, think about working for an organization that values equity and an inter-professional model of health care (i.e., shared governance). On the other hand, think about an organization that values a top-down approach to health care (i.e., where the decisions are made from the leaders of the organization). The workplace environment will be different for the nurse working in each of those organizations. The nurse working in the organization that values shared governance may be encouraged to

Table 24.4   Cultural Norms, Health Care Beliefs, and Religious Beliefs

Cultural group	Cultural norms	Health care beliefs	Religious beliefs
Hispanic	• Maintaining eye contact is valued. • A pat on the back or arm is considered friendly. • Treating others with respect is valued. • Cakes and sweets may be a regular part of the diet. • Children are highly valued and loved. • May have different perception of time; for example, may have a problem being on time for appointments.	• Fatalistic and may view illness as a punishment from God. • View health as the ability to rise in the morning and go to work. • May or may not follow medical advice. • May consult a folk healer, for example, curandero. • Will use Western medications but will stop when they feel they can no longer afford it.	• Are often Roman Catholic but may be member of other Christian group; may light candles, attend mass, pray to God, Jesus, the Virgin Mary, and saints. • Traditional men view religion as a preoccupation of women. • May have statues of saints at home.
Muslim	• Have modest lifestyles for both men and women. Women wear loose-fitting clothing that includes a head covering called a *hijab*. • Immediate and extended family needs are very important, often above the needs of the individual. • Eye contact and physical touch are prohibited by the opposite sex except by family members. • There is a focus on cleanliness; right hand considered clean. Must wash hands before prayer.	• Often have a fatalistic view of health. • Disease is often viewed as "God's will," a test of an individual's conviction or as retribution for transgressions. • Due to issues of modesty, having a health care provider and interpreter of the same sex is generally preferred. • Avoidance of eye contact	• Commonly of the Islamic faith. • Pray 5 times daily (dawn, midday, midafternoon, sunset, night). While praying, often face southeast toward Mecca. • Have a restrictive diet similar to that of Orthodox Judaism that prohibits alcohol, pork, and any animal that has not been slaughtered according to Islamic customs. • Will fast during Ramadan between sunrise and sunset. Teach about pre-dawn and post-evening meals for diabetic patients. • Believe the Qur'an to be the book of divine guidance and direction for humanity and consider the text in its original Arabic to be the literal word of God. • Gather for communal prayer on Friday afternoons.
Black and African American	• Dominant language is English • Have tradition of involving many in raising children. • Many households are headed by women. • May be frank, direct and expressive in speech. • Facial expressions may be demonstrative. • Unrelated persons often live in the home. • High incidence of poverty. • Oriented to the present.	• Often distrust or have discomfort with majority group and health care system. • Older people, especially grandmothers, are respected and should be included when teaching and supporting patients. • Most prefer to be greeted formally as Mr. Mrs., Ms., or surname. • May try self-care first and use all forms of pharmacological and some nonpharmacological alternatives and complimentary medicines prior to seeking care. • View health as being in harmony with nature, and view illness as disharmony. • Some have fatalistic attitude about illness.	• Are heavily involved in church religious groups. • Black minister is strong influence in community. • May use faith healers or herbalists. • Are active in singing and praying. • Illness is between the individual and God; illness may be viewed as punishment from God. • May see illness as the will of God.

Table 24.4 (Continued)

Asians	• Work hard, have respect for elders and nature, have esteem for self-control and loyalty to all family and extended family. • Are traditionally patriarchal. • Have respect for elders. • May not consider shaking hands to be polite. • Submissive to authority. • Pride and honor are extremely important.	• Prefer a same-sex health care practitioner. • Expect health care to include an injection or prescription. • May not make important decisions without checking with an astrologer or almanac for a lucky day.	• Have broad group of practices from Christianity to Buddhism, Taoism, ancestor worship, Muslim, and many others, depending on the geographic area. • Prayer and offerings are dominant in many groups. • May use faith healers or herbalists.
Pacific Islanders	• May ascribe to a holistic world view – interconnectedness of family, environment, self, and spiritual world. • Family and community play an important role and often live in close proximity or tightly knit communities. • Interpersonal and social behavior is based on mutual respect and sharing.	• Illness thought be due to an imbalance of physical, mental/emotional, and spiritual anchors. • Often distrust Western style of health care. Rarely respond positively to health education and treatment based on scare tactics. • Stoic; do not complain. • May use Western medication but choose over-the-counter drugs for minor ailments. • Massage is a method to achieve harmony. • Family is important and should be involved in health care decision making.	• Have deeply rooted spiritual connections. • Hold belief in unity, balance, and harmony. • Use traditional healers. • Some may be Christian.
Native Americans	• Family and tribal affiliations are part of daily life. • May have extended family structure and live with relatives from both sides of the family. • Have a holistic view of life and health. • Often suffer from poverty, poor nutrition, and inadequate access to health care. • Avoid eye contact. • Elders often assume leadership role. • Share goods with others. • Cooperate with others. • Work for good of the group.	• Physical illness may be due to violation of a taboo or being out of harmony. • Skeptical regarding the benefit and habit-forming properties of medications. • Holistic orientation to health. • May wait to see Western practitioner until seen by a healer. • Oriented to the present. • Accept nature rather than try to control nature.	• Religion or spiritual affiliation is based on personal choice. • May have Christian beliefs and traditional beliefs. • Have spiritual orientation. • May fear witchcraft as cause of illness and use a medicine bag received from a healer, which should be kept with the patient at all times. • May carry object at all times to guard against witchcraft.

The information presented is from multiple sources and is meant to serve as a starting point to understanding. All people are individuals and these norms and beliefs may not be valid for all within a cultural group identified in the table.

Source: Compiled with information from Attum (2019);Ko & Turner (2017); and The State of Queensland. Multicultural Health (2013).

join committees where participation in nurse-driven initiatives is expected. The other nurse will likely not have the opportunity to participate in decision making. To help nurse leaders develop and maintain a healthy working environment, the AACN recommends the following:

- *Skilled Communication:* Nurses must be as proficient in communication skills as they are in clinical skills.

- *True Collaboration:* Nurses must be relentless in pursuing and fostering true collaboration.

- *Effective Decision Making:* Nurses must be valued and committed partners in making policy, directing and evaluating clinical care, and leading organizational operations.

- *Appropriate Staffing:* Staffing must ensure the effective match between patient needs and nurse competencies.

- *Meaningful Recognition:* Nurses must be recognized and must recognize others for the value each brings to the work of the organization.

- *Authentic Leadership.* Nurses leaders must fully embrace the imperative of a healthy work environment, authentically live it, and engage others in its achievement. Source: American Association of Colleges of Nursing, Nursing Excellence, Healthy Work Environments. Reproduced with permission from © American Association of Colleges of Nursing.

These AACN standards are oriented toward both the individual nurse and the organization. It is also important to understand how the organizational values can influence communication, collaboration, and decision making among nurses. For example, if the organization does not invest in or properly staff translators or tools for communicating with culturally diverse patients, then it is sending a message to the nursing staff that communication with various cultures is not a priority. To help guide health care organizations to meet the needs of culturally diverse populations, The OMH (Think Cultural Health, n.d.-a) developed standards to improve the quality of health care by ensuring the delivery of effective, equitable, understandable, and respectful health care to patients with diverse cultural beliefs and practices, languages, and health literacy. These standards provide a structure for organizations to provide CLAS and to reduce health care disparities (Table 24.5).

Organizational Socialization

As a new member of a team or work group, it is important to be socialized into the organization. In most organizations, this socialization begins as part of the new employee's orientation process. This allows the organization to promote the organization's values to the new employee from the beginning. The individual responsible for a new hire's orientation is often also responsible for enhancing the socialization process. When

Table 24.5   National Standards for Culturally and Linguistically Appropriate Services (CLAS) in Health and Health Care

Principal Standard:

1. Provide effective, equitable, understandable, and respectful quality care and services that are responsive to diverse cultural health beliefs and practices, preferred languages, health literacy, and other communication needs.

Governance, Leadership, and Workforce:

2. Advance and sustain organizational governance and leadership that promotes CLAS and health equity through policy, practices, and allocated resources.

3. Recruit, promote, and support a culturally and linguistically diverse governance, leadership, and workforce that are responsive to the population in the service area.

4. Educate and train governance, leadership, and workforce in culturally and linguistically appropriate policies and practices on an ongoing basis.

Communication and Language Assistance:

5. Offer language assistance to individuals who have limited English proficiency and/or other communication needs, at no cost to them, to facilitate timely access to all health care and services.

6. Inform all individuals of the availability of language assistance services clearly and in their preferred language, verbally and in writing.

7. Ensure the competence of individuals providing language assistance, recognizing that the use of untrained individuals and/or minors as interpreters should be avoided.

8. Provide easy-to-understand print and multimedia materials and signage in the languages commonly used by the populations in the service area.

Engagement, Continuous Improvement, and Accountability:

9. Establish culturally and linguistically appropriate goals, policies, and management accountability, and infuse them throughout the organization's planning and operations.

10. Conduct ongoing assessments of the organization's CLAS-related activities and integrate CLAS-related measures into measurement and continuous quality improvement activities.

11. Collect and maintain accurate and reliable demographic data to monitor and evaluate the impact of CLAS on health equity and outcomes and to inform service delivery.

12. Conduct regular assessments of community health assets and needs and use the results to plan and implement services that respond to the cultural and linguistic diversity of populations in the service area.

13. Partner with the community to design, implement, and evaluate policies, practices, and services to ensure cultural and linguistic appropriateness.

14. Create conflict and grievance resolution processes that are culturally and linguistically appropriate to identify, prevent, and resolve conflicts or complaints.

15. Communicate the organization's progress in implementing and sustaining CLAS to all stakeholders, constituents, and the general public.

Source: Think Cultural Health (n. d.). National Standards for Culturally and Linguistically Appropriate Services (CLAS) in Health and Health Care. Public Domain.

there is a good fit of ethics, values, and behaviors between the preceptor and a new individual, the socialization process goes smoothly and often occurs rapidly. To ensure socialization that meets the organizational goals, it is important that nurse leaders monitor the orientation process. Frequent evaluation by both the preceptor and the new hire are critical to the success of the new employee and the organization.

Socialization is beneficial to the organization when employees are a good fit—that is, the employee has a high commitment to the organization, little intention to leave, a high level of job satisfaction, and little work-related stress. This is important as the national nursing turnover rate is rising, creating high costs for organizations. Things to consider when entering a new work environment in any culture are the organizational behavior style for greetings, titles, punctuality, body language, and dress (Table 24.6).

These organizational behavior styles are important to the workplace environment. Additionally, it is important for employees to avoid assumptions about how other individuals think, act, or speak. New employees should consider these workplace behavior guidelines to ensure organizational cohesiveness (Table 24.7).

Most organizations have a workplace culture that has a strong mission and vision and is dedicated to safety. However, there will be organizations that can only be described as toxic. In these organizations, the staff and/or leadership is dysfunctional. Instead of problem solving, the goal of these organizations is faultfinding and placing blame. Staff may observe excessive control on the part of the leader or a unit or worker in a constant state of crisis. This dysfunctional toxic environment may be a unit within a hospital or the entire organization. Choosing your workplace environment wisely will make your work life more satisfying. The following is a list of signs that indicate the workplace and/or organization is toxic (Source: Lockhart, 2018):

- top-down leadership
- an inequitable system of reward and recognition
- abuse of position and power
- lack of respect

Table 24.6 United States' Organizational Behavioral Styles

Concepts	Things to consider
Greetings	• Americans usually acknowledge each other with a smile, nod of the head, and/or verbal greeting such as "Hello" or "Hi." • When greeting someone in a business situation, a firm handshake is appropriate, such as when greeting a manager of nursing or human resources.
Titles	• When introducing yourself or others, give your first name followed by your last name. • Use the appropriate title the first time you address an individual, such as Mrs., Dr., Ms., or Mr. Wait to be directed to call them by their first name.
Time	• Punctuality is highly respected in nursing, so be on time to interview appointments and work. • Know where you are going, and plan to be on time.
Body language	• Use of direct eye contact is expected in all work situations and when working with patients. However, some patients may not respond to direct eye contact, depending on their culture. • In conversation, keep a distance of approximately one arm length from the speaker; closer proximity is often considered rude.
Dress	• When in doubt, use a professional business attire, i.e., a professional suit with white blouse or dress shirt for meetings and interviews, a professional nursing uniform for working with patients, etc. • For your work environment, ask what traditional dress is in a particular work area or nursing unit before starting a new job or purchasing new uniforms. • Even in areas where daily dress is casual, business situations should be considered formal.

Source: Amanda Kratovil.

Table 24.7 Workplace Behavior Guidelines

- To be successful in health care, work to adapt to your organization's culture.
- People from other cultures often may not think and behave the way that you do. What might be normal behavior in your culture may be inappropriate in another culture and vice versa.
- Communication requires listening and clarifying meaning to ensure understanding. It is often a good idea to rephrase what you have heard to test your understanding.
- When seeking clarification, go to the source of the communication. Do not ask other coworkers to clarify work requests that originated from a third party or from your leadership personnel.
- Observe for cultural differences in the workplace and attempt to understand and accommodate those differences.
- In health care, holidays and weekends are considered part of the work requirements for nurses. If you need time off to celebrate a cultural or religious holiday, make arrangements early with your manager. Also, realize that health care is a 24/7 business.

Source: Amanda Kratovil.

Evidence from the Literature

Citation: Campione, J., & Famolaro, T. (2018). Promising practices for improving hospital patient safety culture. *The Joint Commission Journal on Quality and Patient Safety*, 44(1), 23–32. doi: https://doi.org/10.1016/j.jcjq.2017.09.001

Discussion: The purpose of the study was to gain knowledge about successful strategies used by hospitals to improve patient safety culture. The authors of this study retrospectively reviewed 536 hospitals' data from the Agency for Healthcare Research and Quality (AHRQ) Surveys on Patient Safety Culture (SOPS) from 2007 to 2014. They identified the "top-improving" hospitals and conducted semi-structured interviews with up to three leaders from six of the top institutions. Three common best-practices that improved patient safety culture were identified: (a) involving staff and leadership in quality improvement goals and action planning; (b) implementing multifaceted patient safety initiatives and programs; and (c) improving methods for administering and disseminating culture measurement surveys.

Implications for Practice: Nurse leaders should recognize that successfully creating a culture of safety requires the involvement of both leadership and all levels of staff. Additionally, it is important that event reporting is viewed as an opportunity for change rather than for blame.

- unmotivated and disengaged staff
- tolerance for antisocial behavior
- poor mentoring and coaching
- lack of honest transparency in communication
- no value placed on work-life balance and personal needs
- reactivity not proactivity

It can be difficult to know if an environment is toxic before you become part of it. However, if you find yourself in a workplace exhibiting many of the above-mentioned characteristics, you will have to decide if you want to leave or stay and try to make improvements to the culture. There is no right or wrong answer, only what you determine is best for you. You can weigh the pros and cons of staying and leaving to help you make your decision.

A Culture of Safety

Organizations create a culture of safety by taking a systems approach to identifying, understanding, and preventing potential and real errors that occur in the health care setting. The National Patient Safety Foundation (2015) describes a strong culture of safety as one in which members of the health care team and leaders are accountable for unprofessional conduct and mistakes but the culture is not punitive in nature. Rather, the goal in a strong culture of safety is to create a system of identifying and correcting errors by learning from previous errors to prevent reoccurrences. This can be achieved by exploring the contextual factors associated with errors including staff behaviors, perceptions, attitudes, and their commitment to the culture of safety. The ANA adopted a position statement in 2010 supporting the *Just Culture* initiatives that originated from the aviation industry to promote the reporting of mistakes as the foundation of a strong culture of safety. Organizations with a strong culture of safety encourage health care providers to report errors and potential errors that will be examined with a non-punitive approach to identify how these errors can be prevented in the future.

Working with Staff from Different Cultures

Staff nurses from different cultures may have different perceptions of staff responsibilities to each other, different perceptions of the nurse's role in patient care, a different locus of control, a different time orientation, and speak a different language.

Different Perceptions of Staff Responsibilities

Cultural values deeply influence what a person feels is most important, that is, the welfare of the individual or the welfare of the group. Individualism emphasizes the importance of individual rights and rewards. Collectivism emphasizes the importance of group decisions and places the rights of the group as a whole above the rights of any individual in the group. For example, some nurses tend to accept difficult assignments without complaint. They also may be more willing to do what other nurses might consider demeaning, for example, cleaning cabinets. Because nurses from some cultures value the group's rights first, they believe that a nurse's individual duties have less value than the combined work of all the nurses on the unit. Maintaining face and ensuring harmony are Eastern cultural values that may be more important to some nurses than upsetting a supervisor to get an easier assignment. An emphasis on minimizing conflict and maintaining harmony, teamwork, and commitment to group and family loyalty typifies most Eastern cultures (Chen et al., 2017).

In contrast, nurses educated in Western cultures often place value on individualism and independence. Individualistic cultures are commonly achievement oriented. In other words, people from individualistic cultures may be more likely to feel that success is something that is achieved by individual work rather than teamwork. Likewise, Western nurses may complain to the supervisor if they feel assignments are unfair or involve menial work. This assertive behavior is consistent with ingrained values of equitable work distribution. In a work setting, most employees will tend toward either individualistic or collectivist values (Choi, Colbert, & Oh, 2015). Organizations and nurse leaders need to ensure that they orient their new staff to the culture of the organization and/or unit to ensure the staff recognize the workplace behaviors that are expected.

Different Perceptions of the Nurse's Role

The nurse wears many hats in the health care setting. Accordingly, nurses' time is spent on different tasks. Nurses spend their time providing direct patient care at the bedside (e.g., patient assessments, nursing procedures, administering medications, and communicating with patients), in-direct patient care away from the patient (e.g., planning care, checking results, reviewing patient information, documenting, collaborating with other health care professionals), and engaging in quality improvement projects is the 3rd category of ways nurses spend their time. Many factors determine how much time a nurse spends providing direct patient care. In health care settings where documentation is required for reimbursement, nurses must spend a considerable amount of time documenting (Gomes, Hash, Orsolini, Watkins, & Mazzoccoli, 2016). Often, there is a conflict between the time spent documenting and the time spent in direct patient care (O'Brien, Weaver, Settergren, Hook, & Ivory, 2015).

The time a nurse spends in direct patient care may also be impacted by the patients' heritage and/or culture. In some heritages and/or cultures (e.g., African Americans, Greeks, and Puerto Ricans), it is common for the family to assume the responsibility of providing basic care (i.e., bathing and feeding) to a sick family member (Purnell, 2014). Accordingly, the role of the nurse will be different than for heritages and/or families who assume this is the role of the nurse.

Differences in Dress

The vast majority of health care agencies have a policy statement regarding clothing and accessories worn by employees in the organization. This is often referred to as a "dress code."

Today, nurses are usually required to wear a specific color or style of uniform to allow patients to easily distinguish them from other health care providers (e.g., patient care technicians, physicians, respiratory therapists, and physical/occupational therapists). Additional dress code requirements regarding hair, nail polish, and jewelry are often part of the organizational culture to reduce rates of infection and improve patient outcomes. However, nurse leaders need to examine these policy statements regularly from a cultural standpoint. The dress code may need to be revised to accommodate traditional dress such as saris worn by Hindu, turbans worn by Sikh men, and head coverings such as the hijab or veil worn by Muslim women. Dress code accommodations should be made so long as patient safety is not jeopardized.

Differences in Locus of Control

Locus of control refers to the degree of control that individuals feel they have over events. People who feel in control of their environment have an internal locus of control. People who believe that luck, fate, or chance controls their lives have an external locus of control.

Health care providers who are trained in the United States often have an internal locus of control. American medical and nursing practitioners feel that it is their duty to exercise control of the health care environment to assure quality patient care and diagnose disorders, plan interventions, carry out procedures, and do everything possible to save the patient's life.

Conversely, health care providers from cultures that have an external locus of control may have a more fatalistic attitude toward their patients and thus feel that they cannot control matters. Differences in locus of control may be revealed when staff from differing cultures are late, take excessive break periods, or fail to complete work on time. In other words, those who feel their success or ability to affect certain situations is outside of their control may not value deadlines or obligations for work the same as those who feel they are in control of the outcome of the situation (by being on-time). Differences in locus of control are often correlated with the cultural values and significance of work; with spiritual beliefs and practices (e.g., a higher being is in control); as well as with issues in language and communication. As a nurse leader, it is essential to give clear work expectations regarding shift schedules, promptness, break schedules, and time allocations for job related duties.

Critical Thinking 24.5

You are a nurse manager in a level-3 **neonatal intensive care unit** (NICU). The dress code for your unit requires nurses to wear hospital administered scrub tops and bottoms without any additional clothing or jewelry, no artificial nails, no nail polish, and long hair must be pulled back. The strict dress code is necessary for infection control in the NICU. A new nurse is hired and due

to her culture, requests to be allowed to wear long sleeves and a hijab on her head.

1. How can you respect her culture and maintain infection control in the NICU?
2. Who might you collaborate with to make the most culturally competent decision?

Differences in Time Orientation

Cultural groups are either past-, present-, or future-oriented. Time orientation is helpful for understanding how individuals think about and use their time. In Western countries like the United States, people generally value the future over the present, suggesting a tendency to plan for the future in anticipation of needs and goals. Southern Blacks and Puerto Ricans value the present over the future. Asian countries vary greatly in their time orientation. Western Europe and countries that speak Germanic languages in Northern Europe are more future oriented than those in the Mediterranean region or those who speak Romance languages such a Greece and Italy (Lee, Liu, & Hu, 2017).

The ways in which different cultural groups value time can create challenges in the health care workplace. For example, in India, deadlines are viewed more loosely than in Western cultures, with the focus being on doing things the *right* way rather than for the sake of meeting the deadline (Pant, 2016). It is important that during the orientation of a new nurse, the expectations for time-management are clearly outlined. Setting goals for the development of time management skills during the orientation process can help a new nurse be successful.

Educational Differences

The educational preparation, the regulation of nursing education, and the practices of nurses across the world are very diverse. For example, in Britain, the nursing curriculum is focused on prophylactic and pharmacology medicine with many basic science courses and few practical courses (Deng, 2015). In China, the primary focus of nursing courses is on clinical nursing. Although theory is taught, a significant disconnect remains between theory and practice in China. In Australia, there is a large emphasis on nursing as a profession, including a curriculum focusing on humanities and life science courses. In the Unites States, nursing theory, nursing process, evidence-based practice, and psychosocial aspects of nursing create the framework of the curriculum (Deng, 2015).

The lack of standardization in nursing curriculums across the world makes it difficult for nurse leaders to validate the competencies of nurses who were educated in a different part of the world than where they are seeking employment. The National Council of State Boards of Nursing (2015) provide Boards of Nursing standardized criteria for ensuring all nurses

licensed in the United States, regardless of their place of education, are safe and qualified to practice.

Communication Differences

Culturally competent communication between nurses, patients and nurses, and among members of the inter-professional health care team is crucial for improving health outcomes across the increasingly diversified population. Today, large health care centers in the United States may be primarily staffed by nurses and practitioners for whom English is a second language. For example, in urban medical centers on the East Coast, it is not unusual to hear a Filipino nurse and a Haitian nurse attempting to communicate with a resident practitioner who has been educated in India. Unless these caregivers take the time to clarify their communications, serious errors may result. Effective communication has become a competency standard across the world (U.S. Department of Health and Human Services, Office of Minority Health, 2018).

Even when the nurse leader is working with staff from the same cultural background, it requires astute leadership skills to decide whether to speak with a staff member face to face, send an e-mail, or contact the person via telephone about a particular issue. The nurse leader exercises substantial judgment when making choices about successful communication methods with all staff and patients, including staff and patients from differing cultural backgrounds. Things to consider when planning communications with others include: the timing and medium (e.g., open forums, workshops, special interest groups, in-services) of the communication, voice tone and pitch, and the location for face-to-face exchanges (Henderson, 2015).

Language and cultural differences may also be a source of friction between nurses and health care providers from different cultures. Our culture provides a lens through which we see patients, their diagnoses, the context of their illness, and it creates a basis for understanding inter-professional communications about the patient and the plan of care. Differences in language and cultural beliefs and practices can create miscommunications in the health care setting that impact not only inter-professional job satisfaction, but also patient outcomes (Kreps, 2016).

Errors in communication between health care providers is the second highest cause of sentinel events in the United States (Ellison, 2015). Sometimes you may need to work with

---

Critical Thinking 24.6

You are orienting a new nurse to your unit. The new nurse is an immigrant from India. His patient assessments are thorough and accurate but have remained exceptionally slow (i.e., over an hour on average) throughout his 6-week orientation. He does not seem to notice or mind that his lengthy assessments are constantly putting him behind schedule.

1. How should you address this concern with the new nurse?
2. What actions should you take to ensure this new nurse is successful after orientation?

a foreign practitioner who is difficult to understand because of language differences or a strong accent. In this case, do not take verbal orders, particularly over the telephone. Even when an order is written, take the time to clarify the order with the practitioner. De Meester, Verspuy, Monsieurs, & VanBogaert (2013) found that using the **Situation-Background-Assessment-Recommendation** (SBAR) framework (Rosenthal, 2013) significantly improved nurse-physician communication. See Table 24.8 for an SBAR example.

The nurse should also act as a patient advocate in the event that the patient finds it difficult to understand a foreign practitioner. Clarifying the plan of care, discharge instructions, and even the informed consent process can be very helpful for patients and can encourage their autonomy in decision-making. Communication practices of nurse leaders should include strategies to improve communication and good working relationships.

Improving Communication in the Team

If you are assigned to work with a nurse or staff member who is from a different culture and who speaks English as a second language, try these techniques to facilitate communication:

- Recognize that your co-worker probably has an educational background in nursing that may be very different from your own.

- Acknowledge that the coworker's value system and perception of what constitutes good patient care may differ from your own.

- Try to assess your co-worker's level of understanding of verbal and written communication. For example, ask a coworker to explain a practitioner's order to you in his or her own words. It also helps to assess a patient with the coworker and note what terms the person uses to describe the patient's signs and symptoms.

- Avoid the use of slang terms and regional expressions. For example, Chinese, Japanese, and Filipino nurses may not understand such expressions as "piggybacking," "doing a double," or "rigging" something to work.

- Provide your coworker with resources, such as written procedures and protocols, that may help to reinforce your verbal communication.

- Remember to praise your coworker's competency in technical skills being careful to not inadvertently be offensive. An example of an unintentional offense is: "You navigate the electronic medical record well for a Filipino."

- Appreciate the knowledge that you can gain by working alongside a skilled nurse from another culture. Observe how nurses from a different culture relate to patients who are from their culture.

- When offering constructive criticism use *I* statements instead of *you* statements. For example: "I feel that the time you spend on breaks is more than our allowed time." is better than "You take breaks that are longer than we are allowed."

Managerial Responsibilities

Nurse managers have a crucial role in ensuring the organizational culture remains safe for patients and health care providers. Recall, one way in which nurse managers can improve the culture of safety within their organization or unit is to implement the CLAS standards. Additionally, the **Comprehensive Unit-based Safety Program** (CUSP) is an evidence-based method that nurse managers and health care leaders can use to help improve the culture of safety in health care organizations (Agency for Healthcare Research and Quality, 2015). The CUSP program can help organizational leaders improve health care safety by aligning the unit's goals with the organization's goals for cultural competency; mentoring nurses to care for diverse patients by exemplifying cultural competency; encouraging and monitoring the delivery of patient-centered care; hiring a diverse workforce; listening and addressing concerns of patients related to quality of care and satisfaction; and monitoring and enforcing unit-based safety initiatives. Miller et al. (2016) found that by implementing the CUSP program into a community-based academic health care system, the rates of **central line-associated blood stream infections (CLABSIs)**, **catheter-associated urinary tract infections (CAUTIs)**, and

---

Table 24.8   Example SBAR Communication between Nurse and Physician

Situation	Hello Dr. Jones. This is Desiree, the nurse caring for patient Mr. Mahammad in Room 25 on 9 West.
Background	Mr. Mahammad was admitted yesterday with **Diabetic KetoAcidosis** (DKA). He began the new dose of Lantis you prescribed at 0200 this morning and is stable. However, Mr. Mahammad is Muslim and tomorrow is Ramadam. He is stating that he will fast from sun rise to sun set.
Assessment	Mr. Mahammad's most recent glucose was 126 at 2200. But he is very clear that he will not be able to eat anything after sunrise, which is at 0623 tomorrow morning. He will fast until sunset, which is at 1943 tomorrow night. I am concerned that he will become hypoglycemic without food during his fasting.
Recommendation	I recommend that Mr. Mahammad be allowed to eat a special high protein diet just before sunrise. I also recommend that I use a short acting insulin after the early breakfast and hold the Lanus for the day. I will check his glucose levels Q2 until his fast is complete.

Source: Amanda Kratovil.

ventilator-associated pneumonias (VAPs) were significantly reduced in two intensive care units.

Another consideration for nurses in a managerial and leadership role is their personal style of leadership. If a nurse leader is to be successful in creating change or improving the culture of safety, they need the right tools (e.g., CLAS and CUSP) as well as the right leadership style. Mannix, Wilkes, & Daly (2015) found that the use of avoidance in making decisions can have a negative effect on the workplace. Have you ever worked in an environment where an issue in the workplace has been identified by several employees but despite bringing it to the manager's attention, the issue continues? That is an example of avoidance in leadership. Likewise, passive leadership has been linked to behavioral incivility in the workplace (Harold & Holtz, 2015). In other words, when managers and leaders fail to provide leadership to their employees or do not take an active role in leading change, the workplace environment becomes toxic, which can lead to employee distress, mental health issues, and a poor work attitude (Barling & Frone, 2017). Nurse managers might consider using the following approaches to promote a more positive organizational culture, especially when the staff is diverse:

- Be attentive to the physical and mental needs of your staff (Akerjordet, Furunes, & Haver, 2018).

- Plan informal meetings for nurses to discuss their cultural values. For example, it may benefit both groups of nurses for Asian nurses to share with American-born nurses their cultural values concerning respect for authority and vice versa.

- Empower nurses with shared governance, autonomy, and professional development (Akerjordet, Furunes, & Haver, 2018).

- Create health care teams that are adequately staffed with a mix of skills.

- Facilitate collegial relationships by providing cultural workshops and ask knowledgeable individuals to present information about the values, behaviors, and communication patterns of the different cultural groups that are represented on staff.

Generational Perceptions

In the United States, there are currently five generations delivering and receiving health care. Like culture, each generation brings with it a new set of values, beliefs, perceptions, and behaviors. A **generation** is a group that shares common contextual factors including economic, social, and cultural conditions (Rickes, 2016). Many definitions include specific dates to define generations; however, there remains some debate over this, especially with the newest generation, Generation Z (Seemiller & Grace, 2016). In any case, a generation is approximately 15–20 years in length and has a different value system from the preceding generation and later generations. Various historical events define generations. For example, our newest and most diverse generation, Generation Z, cannot remember a time without internet and mobile communication (Christensen, Wilson, & Edelman, 2018). As nurses, we take our generational differences with us into patient care and the

Table 24.9 **Generational Characteristics**

Generation	Year of birth	Common characteristics
Generation Z (iGeneration)	1996 to present	<ul><li>Newest and most diverse generation to hit the workforce.</li><li>Have been exposed to terrorism, natural disasters, bullying, and a financial recession.</li><li>Social media, smartphones, and technology have always been a part of their life.</li></ul>
Generation Y (Millennials)	1980–1995	<ul><li>"Helicopter parents."</li><li>First generation educated on sustainability of the environment.</li><li>Culturally diverse and optimistic.</li><li>Value mentorship</li><li>Technologically savvy.</li></ul>
Generation X (Gen Xers)	1965–1979	<ul><li>Latch-key kids.</li><li>Self-reliant and independent.</li><li>Can remember life without personal computers.</li><li>Prefers direct communication, to understand the reasoning for decisions, and dislikes micromanagement.</li><li>Seeks work-life balance</li></ul>
Baby Boomers	1946–1964	<ul><li>Near the age of retirement</li><li>Experienced great educational and economic expansion during their youth.</li><li>Will work long hours but enjoys recognition.</li><li>Are among the largest population requiring nursing care.</li></ul>
Veteran (Silent Generation)	1922–1945	<ul><li>Largely retired</li><li>Raised during the Great Depression and World War II</li><li>Value hard work, dedication, job benefits</li><li>Loyal to their employers</li></ul>

Source: Compiled by Amanda Kratovil.

work environment. We often assume that those around us are like us and think like us. This is not always true.

The nursing workforce is more age diverse today than ever before in history. The current five generations in the United States are the Veteran or Silent Generation, born between 1922 and 1945; the Baby Boomers, born between 1946 and 1964; Generation X (Gen Xers), born between 1965 and 1979; Generation Y (Millennials), born between 1980 and 1995, and the newest generation to hit the workforce, Generation Z (iGeneration), born between 1996 to now (Table 24.9).

The Veteran or Silent Generation, born between 1922 and 1945, was raised in difficult times, including the Great Depression and World War II. They value consistency, hard work, and dedication, are team oriented, and are loyal to their employers (Christensen, Wilson, & Edelman, 2018). Nurse leaders should know that this generation values one-on-one coaching, job benefits including visible rewards and recognition, and consistency. The Veteran or Silent Generation is now largely retired; it was followed by the Baby Boomers, born between 1946 and 1964, who came of age during a time of much available education and economic expansion. They work for self-worth, are competitive, and are process oriented. In other words, Baby Boomers view success as something that is a result of their hard work, and they feel proud about achieving that goal. Nurse leaders should know that this generation will work long hours, enjoy teamwork and committees, and recognition. Baby Boomers are the largest generation and they are approaching retirement when they will increasingly need nursing care as they age. Furthermore, this generation of nurses are among the rapidly retiring, contributing to the nursing shortage (Christensen, Wilson, & Edelman, 2018).

The Generation X (Gen Xers), born between 1965 and 1979, are often called latch-key kids, as their parents were often away working. They learned to be self-reliant and independent. They experienced an increased rate of parental divorce, witnessed the advent of personal computers and feel comfortable with them, and are an outcome-oriented generation. In other words, the Generation X values the end product of a goal over the process of achieving that goal; the goal and the fastest way to get there are always in view. Nurse leaders should know that this generation prefers direct communication including individual feedback, works independently, dislikes micromanagement, and prefers to understand the reasoning behind requirements. The Generation Xers often observed their parents going through multiple changes in their work organizations, such as downsizing and rightsizing. Therefore, they tend to be skeptical, independent workers who seek a balance between work and leisure (Christensen, Wilson, & Edelman, 2018).

Generation Y (Millennials), born between 1980 and 1995, grew up at the end of the Cold War. Generation Y were raised during more uncertain and less predictable times than their parents. Accordingly, as children, this generation had parents who were very involved in their lives (i.e., helicopter parents) and who affirmed their academic and personal achievements.

Additionally, Generation Y grew up with the Internet, texting, and social media, terrorism, a speak-your-mind philosophy, and were the first generation educated about the sustainability of the environment (Sherman, 2015). This generation is a culturally diverse and optimistic generation that is focusing on early retirement. Nurse leaders should recognize this generation's proficiency in technology, their desire for constant and immediate feedback, need for interpersonal skill development and instant gratification, and their team-oriented nature (Christensen, Wilson, & Edelman, 2018).

Generation Z (iGeneration), born between 1996 to now, are the most diverse generation yet. They have never known a life without Internet, smartphones, and social media. This has led to a need for instant gratification and answers. They have watched terrorism and natural disasters occur live on television and social media, have experienced bullying, and are familiar with the suffering of financial recessions. They are visual communicators and hands-on learners who value realism and thrive in teams. However, since this generation is just entering college, the information about this generation is preliminary (Christensen, Wilson, & Edelman, 2018).

With at least three generations in the health care workforce, and the fourth now starting to enter it, intergenerational differences will undoubtedly arise and cause challenges. While intergenerational differences can be challenging, they can also improve the strength of health care teams. The following approaches can be used to address the challenges of a multigenerational workforce (Christensen, Wilson, & Edelman, 2018):

- Customize rewards systems to accommodate generational differences (i.e., instant rewards like gift cards for Generation Y (Millennials) and Generation Z, public recognition for Baby Boomers, and letting the Generation X go home early).

- Use the strength of each generation to create a stronger team:

  - Pairing Baby Boomer's with Generation Y may satisfy the desire for Baby Boomers to mentor and Generation Y to be mentored.

  - The Generation X are skeptics so encourage them to participate in quality initiatives

  - Trial new incentive programs with Generation Y since they are the most difficult to retain

  - Encourage Y and Generation Z to be technology champions and help those with less experience.

- Vary communication strategies and mediums (e.g., post flyers or notices, use email, and verbal methods) to reach the communication preference of each generation (Chicca, 2018).

Creating an environment of inclusion and embracing the diversity of the generations can create a rich health care environment that promotes organizational excellence and improves patient outcomes.

Real World Interview

Some of the generational changes I see among my older nurses in reference to education is they do not seem to have a desire for advanced degrees, although they do put time and effort into other areas of professional development (certification, webinars, seminars, etc.). I do remind the older nurses to listen more and talk less with the newer nurses. I have learned a lot from my younger nurses. Older nurses sometimes think they always know more than the younger nurses. That is not always the case. The younger nurses will quickly return to school for a graduate degree, many not long after completing their undergrad. Both our older and younger nurses are involved in committees. I do see more involvement from our older nurses related to childcare/family obligations of the younger nurses. In relation to work-ethic, our younger nurses seen to have a better understanding of work-life balance. I see many times during the interviewing process that new grads will wait to take a vacation prior to taking the NCLEX. This is not the case with our older nurses. Many of them took their NCLEX immediately after graduation and started their position shortly after that.

Some of my changes in leadership to accommodate generational differences include the way we communicate. We do group texting, my newsletter is electronic, we have a closed Facebook page, just to name a few. I still communicate the conventional way for my older nurses. In relation to workload, our older nurses are sometime challenged by all the documentation that is required, and the newer nurse simply goes with the flow most of the time. Both young and old nurses complain about the same things—too much documentation and not enough time with the patients. The advice I would give to any manager is to learn the strengths and weakness of both young and older nurses and try to create a collaborative relationship between them. Always avoid stereotyping, as this can be very demeaning and dangerous. Make sure to always be a forward thinker that practices inclusion at all times.

Lorian Williams-Willis, MSN, RNC, APN
Dolton, Il

Religion and Spirituality

The meaning of spirituality is different to everyone. For some, spirituality means that they participate in organized religion (e.g., going to a church, synagogue, mosque, etc.). For others, spirituality is a non-religious experience that can take many forms (e.g., private prayer, yoga, meditation, quiet reflection, a belief in the supernatural, or long walks). And similar to culture, the religious and spiritual climate of the United States is changing. According to the Public Religion Research Institute, the major changes include (Cox & Jones, 2017):

- Less than 43% of Americans identify as White Christians, significantly less than the nearly 81% of Americans identifying as such in 1976.

- Catholics (16% in 2006 and 11% in 2017) and White Evangelical Protestants (23% in 2006 and 17% in 2017) are declining.

- Jewish, Muslims, Buddhists, and Hindus religions are growing and increasingly represented by young generations.

- The Catholic Church is becoming more diverse with only 36% of White, non-Hispanic Catholics being under 30 years old.

- Asian and Pacific-Islander Americans have a more diverse religious profile than other racial or ethnic groups (i.e., Asian and Pacific-Islander Americans identify with a variety of religions).

- Almost half of the LGBTQ+ populations do not identify a religious orientation.

- Young adults are more likely (38%) than seniors (12%) to not identify a religious affiliation.

Figure 24.4 shows the top 8 religions by race in the United States, and Figure 24.5 shows religious affiliation by generation in 2016.

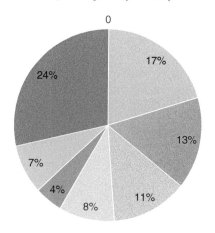

Top 8 Religions by Ethnicity

- White evangelical Protestant
- White mainline Protestant
- White Catholic
- Black Protestant
- Hispanic Protestant
- Hispanic Catholic
- Unaffiliated
- Other nonwhite Protestant

FIGURE 24.4   Top 8 religions by race in the United States.
Source: Pew Research Center (2019). Religious Landscape Study. Retrieved from www.pewforum.org/religious-landscape-study

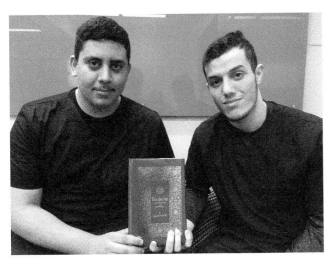

FIGURE 24.5 Men respectfully holding the Qur'an.
Source: Photo used with permission.

Religion and spirituality are important to both nurses and patients. In nearly every culture, spirituality is a component of healing but commonly gets overlooked in the health care setting. This often leaves both patients and nurses facing moral distress. Understanding a patient's religion and/or spirituality can help the nurse empathize with the patients, provide patient-centered care by offering faith-based interventions, and influence hospital policies and procedures (Zaidi, 2018). Here are some practical nursing considerations for different religious groups:

- Roman Catholics may want to have religious relics in their hospital room, some of which can be large.

- Muslims pray five times per day and may request their bed to be moved to face southeast, toward Mecca.

- Muslims have a restrictive diet that prohibits pork and any meat not slaughtered according to Islamic customs.

- Muslims may be required to fast (no food, water, or IV fluids) from sunrise to sunset on Ramadan. Diabetic patients may require additional precautions and teaching to prevent complications.

- The Qur'an is considered the literal word of God when written in Arabic. Handling of the Qur'an should only be done after one's hands have been washed or using a clean barrier such as a cloth.

Spiritual Assessment

Providing holistic patient care includes assessing the spiritual needs of the patient in addition to the biophysical and psychosocial needs. To provide spiritual care, an understanding of the patient's beliefs can be used to plan appropriate interventions and promote autonomy. In contemporary nursing, spirituality has become an important area of assessment during hospitalization, especially during the end of life. However, asking the questions, "What is your religion?" or "What religious needs can we meet during your hospitalization?" leaves the nurse with only descriptive labels. To meet the spiritual needs of patients, nurses need to understand more than these labels. Integrating spirituality into our everyday practices can help us become more comfortable with the concept of spirituality. As our comfort increases, we will become less likely to regard spirituality as a private or personal issue and more willing to address patients' concerns. Recommendations for integrating spirituality into health care to better help patients achieve health include a three-step process (Giske & Cone, 2015):

- Step one is *turning in on spirituality*, which encompasses the nurse being sensitive to the patients' readiness and willingness to open to spirituality (in any form).

- Step two, *uncovering deep concerns*, is a time sensitive process where nurses identify patients, and allocate time to those who need their attention. During the nurse-patient interaction, great care must be taken to respect the patients' privacy and understand where inter-personal boundaries exists, while demonstrating active and therapeutic communication skills to encourage patients to open up about deep spiritual concerns.

- Step three, *facilitating the healing process*, occurs when the patient begins to share with the nurse, and the nurse follows the lead of the patient by engaging in active listening. This process also requires the nurse to engage with the patient's family and in inter-professional collaboration (i.e., chaplains, social work, etc.).

Additionally, the Joint Commission of Accreditation of Healthcare Organizations (JCAHO) (2018) outlines the Rights and Responsibilities of the Individual Standards that require hospitals to accommodate patients' spiritual and religious needs. JCAHO suggests health care providers take an interdisciplinary approach to meeting that standard on spirituality by incorporating chaplains into the care of patients.

Assessing spirituality and meeting those needs of the patient is the responsibility of all health care providers. This responsibility can be led by chaplains. Chaplains are specifically trained to assess and fulfill the religious and spiritual needs of the patient and their family. Professional chaplains are increasingly becoming part of the inter-professional health care team along with physicians, nurses, and pharmacists. Many inpatient health care facilities have professional chaplains that can assist the health care team in multiple ways, such as helping patients make difficult health care decisions using a patient-centered approach; determining the most appropriate spiritual interventions for individual patients; visiting the patient and family; facilitating prayer or meditation; providing referrals to support groups; as well as aiding in end-of-life issues (Marin et al., 2015). The involvement of the chaplain in the holistic care of patients also improves patients' satisfaction with their health care (Marin et al., 2015).

In some care settings, however, chaplains are not readily available, and nurses may be expected to help meet the spiritual needs of patients. Conducting a spiritual assessment is a vital step to determine the specific spiritual concerns that the patient may have. There are many simple spiritual assessment mnemonics that can be used to help nurse remember what to address with patients when conducting a spiritual assessment. Jenkins, Wikoff, Amankwaa, and Trent (2009, p. 35) developed a mnemonic assessment tool for nurses titled "FAITH." The tool assesses five areas:

- **F**amily, friends, or the patient's support network
- **A**ffiliations, e.g., religious denomination, church membership, clubs
- **I**llness consequences for the patient's life, e.g., employment, education, and parental role consequences
- **T**reatment concerns of the patient
- **H**ow the nurse can assist with meeting the spiritual needs of the patient, e.g., prayer, facilitating clergy visitation, etc.

Puchalski's (Puchalski & Romer, 2000) process for spiritual assessment within routine interactions with patients is the FICA Spirituality History Tool. The pneumonic FICA stands for:

- **F**aith, belief, meaning—whatever is meaningful to the person
- **I**mportance and influence of others; support
- **C**ommunity—spiritual groups to which the person belongs
- **A**ddress/action in care—approach care in a patient-centered manner.

Additionally, Parsian and Dunning's (2009) spirituality questionnaire evaluates several components of patients' spirituality that the nurse can assess:

- Self-awareness (e.g., attitude, self-confidence, compassion)
- The significance of spiritual beliefs in one's life
- Spiritual practices (e.g., meditation, involvement in ecological programs)
- Spiritual needs (e.g., the importance of relationship maintenance and searching for life purpose).

Carson and Koening's (2008) spiritual assessment involves five broad questions that the nurse can utilize while caring for the patient to respond to both verbal and nonverbal patient indicators that communicate the presence of a spiritual need. The questions help identify the follow for the patient:

- Are there any conflicts between spiritual beliefs and medical care (e.g., the receipt of blood products)?
- What impact do spiritual beliefs have on decision making?
- Are involvement and support from any religious communities (e.g., churches, mosques, synagogues) desired?
- Are feelings of comfort or stress associated with the spiritual beliefs?

- Is there a need for additional referrals? When deciding which spiritual assessment framework the nurse will use, the patient needs, the environment in which care is being provided, and the individual nurse's ability to implement the assessment during care, should all be considered. Regardless of the assessment tool chosen, assessing the spiritual needs of patients is an important component of providing holistic health care to patients of different cultures.

Spiritual Distress

Spiritual distress is a **North American Nursing Diagnosis Association** (NANDA) term used to identify when an individual has an impaired ability to integrate meaning and purpose in life through the individual's connectedness with self, others, art, music, literature, nature, or a power greater than themselves (Herdman, Kamitsuru, & NANDA, 2018). To decrease or eliminate spiritual distress, it is expected that an individual will connect with the elements he or she considers important to arrive at meaning and purpose in life. These elements may include meditation; prayer; participating in religious services or rituals; communing with nature, plants, and animals; sharing of self; and caring for self and others.

Once spiritual needs have been identified, the nurse must develop interventions to help patients. Nursing interventions for spiritual needs could include the nurse requesting a visit from a patient's spiritual leader, turning the direction of the bed to promote ritualistic prayer, or offering the patient uninterrupted quiet time to allow the patient time for personal prayer or reading of spiritual and religious material. Many religious groups (e.g., Christians, Jews, Muslims, Buddhists, etc.) communicate spiritually through prayer or meditation. The nurse can act as a patient advocate and facilitate the interventions necessary to promote this spiritual communication. For example, a Muslim patient may need to have their bed turned southeast, toward Mecca.

Barriers to Spiritual Care

Barriers to providing spiritual care may often be experienced more commonly for nurses than barriers to providing any other type of care or service. Atashzadeh-Shoorideh, Zakaryaee, and Fani (2018) conducted a qualitative study aimed at understanding the barriers and facilitators in providing spiritual care for parents whose children were battling cancer. They found that lack of resources (i.e., social and emotional support) was a main barrier, while multiple support structures (i.e., emotional, health care, social, and spiritual education) facilitated spirituality. Additionally, the nurse may be uncomfortable or embarrassed by his or her own spirituality and find it upsetting to deal with the issues that bring up personal spiritual distress, such as death and dying or suffering and grief.

These barriers to spiritual care sometimes cause nurses to legitimatize a reason to avoid the necessary spiritual assessment of the patient's needs; spiritual needs are often ignored and forgotten. As a result, patients experience even more distress and suffering. This distress can be avoided by supporting and spending time with the patient, assessing the patient's spiritual needs, and collaborating with the chaplain for patient care.

Incorporating Spirituality into Patient Care

The nurse leader who incorporate spirituality into patient care and encourages other nurses to do the same ensures that this component of holistic nursing is not forgotten or marginalized. For example, a Sunni Muslim man is required to attend the local mosque on Fridays. This employee may therefore request time off on all Fridays. Another Catholic may request off on Sundays to attend other religious services. This can create a scheduling issue for the nurse leader. A possible solution is to pair two nurses, where one works every Friday and the other works every Sunday. Both nurses are then able to meet their spiritual needs without a negative impact on staffing the nursing unit.

There are religious holidays and celebrations that have spiritual and cultural significance. An understanding and empathetic approach to requests for time off and vacation will help to ensure contented staff and minimize turnover. It is also important to consider important markers of life such as weddings, births, and deaths. There are many cultural and spiritual overtones to these life events that need to be respected by nursing leadership practices. Sensitivity to the spiritual practices of the staff will enable the nurse manager to provide a compassionate and caring leadership.

Developing Spiritual Leadership

Spiritual leadership involves using values and beliefs as the basis for dealing with all staff and patients within an organization. It is using compassion, caring, and nurturing to create an environment that reflects the values and beliefs of the leaders, patients, and staff. Spiritual leaders develop trust and connect with their staff on both a personal and professional level. This connection is then the basis for change and growth within the organization. The ability to connect and build relationships among staff and leadership, inspire others, and spot problems early on results in a cohesive and positive workplace.

The nurse has an obligation to provide culturally competent care to patients. Providing culturally competent care is important for reducing health disparities and improving the outcomes of all patients regardless of their race, ethnicity, culture, SES, gender, religion, sexual orientation, age, or generational group. As the demographic landscape of the U.S. is becoming more diverse, the nurse must be open to self-reflection to identify their feelings and attitudes toward people of other cultures and religions. Through this self-reflection, nurses will be better able to meet the needs of a diverse patient population. With four generations of nurses now in the workforce, nurse leaders are faced with an added challenge of ensuring the organizational culture reflects a culture of safety for patients and contentment for staff. Nevertheless, it is crucial that organizational leaders strive to meet the challenge. The well-being of our patients and nurses depend on it.

KEY CONCEPTS

- Culture affects both the nursing staff and the patient.

- Cultural competence is an important component of nursing.

- Each culture has its own values.

- Health care disparities continue to exist for members of minority populations.

- Various population groups and subpopulation groups in nursing are growing.

- Organizations in which nurses work have distinct cultures.

- At least three distinct generations make up the current workforce population, i.e., the Baby Boomers, the Generation X, and Generation Y (Millennials), with Generation Z just entering the workforce. Each generation has different values, goals, and expected outcomes from its work and life experiences.

- Spirituality may include religion and reflects one's values and beliefs.

- Spiritual assessment is a requisite of holistic nursing.

- Many barriers can interfere with meeting a patient's spiritual needs.

KEY TERMS

Culture	Diversity	Organizational culture
Culturally Congruent Practice	Ethnocentric bias	Race
Cultural sensitivity	Generation	Spiritual distress
Culture shock	Health disparity	Stereotyping

REVIEW QUESTIONS

1. Stephanie, born in 1972, the night shift charge nurse, is requesting more time off than any other charge nurse. Which of the following is most likely the reason for her requests based on her generation?
   a. Prefers to work the day shift and is hoping for a schedule change
   b. Believes that there are other nurses just as capable to fill her role
   c. Wants to increase her leisure time to balance with work
   d. Seeks to be rewarded for time spent at work

2. Nurses may fail to meet spiritual needs because of which of the following?
   a. Lack of compassion
   b. Lack of knowledge regarding the patient's illness
   c. Lack of understanding of the patient's spiritual beliefs
   d. Lack of chaplains in the care area

3. During orientation to work on a new unit, the nurse experiences a sense of isolation from his preceptors. Which of the following actions will best increase his socialization into the preceptor group?
   a. Ask as many questions as he can
   b. Request that his orientation be increased for two more weeks
   c. Study the differences between his values and his preceptor group's values
   d. Arrive late for duty frequently

4. An organization's workplace culture reflects which of the following?
   a. The cultural affiliations of the staff
   b. The religion practiced by the hospital's leadership group
   c. The culture of its preceptors
   d. The values and beliefs of the organization

5. You hear loud voices coming from your African American patient's room where you were just informed that several visitors arrived. Which of the following would be an appropriate action?
   a. Call the behavioral response team (BART); it is likely there is an altercation in the room
   b. Ask the visitors to leave because they are disrupting your patient's rest
   c. Ask the visitors to speak "at indoor levels" because they are disrupting other patients
   d. Explain that you are going to close the door to the room for their privacy

6. Strategies to improve cultural competency skills include which of the following? Select all that apply.

   a. Participation in continuing education offerings about culturally congruent care
   b. Development of culturally competent approaches to care
   c. Talking with patients about their cultural views on health care
   d. Assessing your own skill level and seeking improvements
   e. Talking with staff and colleagues about their cultural views on health
   f. Identifying and reducing ethnocentric bias

7. Causes of health care disparities include which of the following? Select all that apply.
   a. Patient health behaviors
   b. Conscious bias
   c. Institutional discrimination
   d. Unconscious bias
   e. Diverse health care workers
   f. Biological variation

8. After shift report, the nurse is preparing to enter the room of patient, Guadalupe González. While reviewing the patient's chart, the nurse notes that the patient is listed as of "Hispanic/Latino origin." What is the best way for the nurse to determine which culture Mrs. González identifies with?
   a. Ask the patient which culture she identifies with
   b. Determine her culture by her hair color and skin complexion
   c. Determine her culture by her accent
   d. Determine her culture by her body shape and size

9. You arrive at the care conference for your patient and realize that an interpreter is not present, even though the patient's preferred language is Spanish. The inter-professional team is all present and the conference is starting. What actions can you take to best advocate for your patient?
   a. Encourage the patient to pray
   b. Request an interpreter
   c. Encourage the patient to leave the conference
   d. Start the meeting and explain the information to the patient later through an interpreter
   e. Explain to the health care team the need for an interpreter prior to starting

10. A practicing Muslim nurse requests to wear her hijab while on duty. Which of the following actions would be most appropriate?
   a. Decline the request
   b. Advocate for modification of the organization's dress code
   c. Review the organization's dress policy
   d. Make the accommodation

REVIEW QUESTION ANSWERS

1. Answer: C is correct.
   Rational: Generation X seeks work-life balance. (A) is incorrect because Generation X are direct communicators and would express a desire to work the day shift directly. (B) and (D) are incorrect because self-reliance and independence are traits of Generation X.

2. Answer: C is correct.
   Rational: Nurses commonly lack an understanding of the spiritual needs of their patients related to lack of knowledge or embarrassment, not lack of compassion (A). (B) is not related to the spiritual needs of the patient. (D) would not restrict the nurse from conducting her own spiritual assessment of the patient.

3. Answer: C is correct.
Rational: Self-reflection can help the new nurse understand his own values as well as those of the group. (A) and (B) are incorrect because without an exploration of values for both himself and the group, he will not find answers to his questions by asking more or increasing his orientation. (D) is incorrect because it is not professional to arrive late.

4. Answer: D is correct.
Rational: Organizational culture is the system of shared values and beliefs that actively influences the behavior of it member. (A, B, C) are all part of the organization, but individually they do not influence the organizational workplace culture.

5. Answer: D is correct.
Rational:It is common in the African American culture to speak loudly. (A, B, C) do not reflect cultural congruent care, as the "loud voices" are cultural norms.

6. Answers A, B, C, D, E, and F are correct.
Rational: All are ways to improve cultural competency skills.

7. Answers A, B, C, D, and F are correct.
Rational: Health disparity occurs when social, economic, and or environmental disadvantages lead to differences in health. When members of the health care team or the organization consciously or unconsciously discriminate or provide different care to different people, disparities occur. The biological nature of a person's genetics or their health behaviors may also influence the occurrence of disease and illness. A diverse health care workforce helps eliminate health care disparities.

8. Answer: A is correct.
Rational: The best way to determine with which culture Mrs. González identifies is to ask her. (B, C, D) will lead the nurse to categorize Mrs. González into a culture based on her physical appearance.

9. Answers B and E are correct.
Rational: Halting the meeting until the interpreter arrives and helping the health care team understand the need for the interpreter are ways to advocate for the patient that requires an interpreter. (A, C, D) will not advocate for a patient who needs an interpreter.

10. Answer: C is correct.
Rational: Reviewing the dress code policy is the first step to meeting the cultural needs of this patient. The dress code may not restrict the nurse from wearing her hijab and therefore answers (A, B, D) may not be necessary.

REVIEW ACTIVITIES

1. You are called to problem-solve a situation between a patient and a staff nurse. The patient is refusing to allow the nurse to take care of him because the nurse is wearing a headscarf. How will you handle the situation?

2. You live in a small community with little diversity. A patient that you are scheduled to take care of is visiting from a large city. This patient is from India and speaks only Hindi, a language unfamiliar to the staff. When you walk into the room, there are no visitors and no one to translate. How will you approach your care in a culturally competent manner?

3. You are hiring several new graduate nurses to work on a unit that has had little turnover in the past 10 years. Many of the current staff are Baby Boomers and from Generation X and have been in this organization for the entire length of their career. How will you go about integrating the Y and Z Generations of nurses into this group?

4. You are taking care of a trauma patient in the ER. The patient has burns over 70% of his body. The likelihood of the patient's survival is unknown. There is a lot of noise and distraction in the ER as well as many family members within earshot. The patient asks you to pray for him and his family. How will you respond?

5. Tom Swan is a 34-year-old who suffered a biking accident 3 days ago and is on strict bed rest due to severe vertigo. Tom requests to "use the bathroom." You retrieve a urinal and hand it to him. He just stares at you and replies, "I don't have a penis, I have female reproductive organs." How could you have avoided this situation?

DISCUSSION POINTS

- During your last clinical experience, how was cultural competency demonstrated by the nurses?

- What impact does the changing demographic landscape of the U.S. have on your role as a nurse?

- Which health disparities mentioned in this chapter have you seen in your clinicals?

- How does the culture of a hospital effect nurse satisfaction with their job?

- As a nurse manager, how would you address a nurse who was consistently late to work?

- How does assessing the spirituality of patients improve outcomes?

DISCUSSION OF OPENING SCENARIO

1. There is a real concern that when a family member interprets medical information from the patient to the health care team or from the team to the patient, information will get intentionally or unintentionally neglected or miscommunicated. In the opening scenario, the son was only 10 years old and was honoring his culture and mother by not speaking to the nurse

about his mother's *vaginal bleeding*. Additionally, when nurses rely on family to interpret difficult information to the patient, the family is put in the uncomfortable position of being the deliverer of bad news. Consider if the pregnant women lost her unborn baby. Asking the son to deliver that news to his mother may be considered unethical. Moreover, many of the medical terms do not have a direct translation between languages. This causes the "interpreter" to have to describe the information in a way that required an understanding of the medical information; certainly a 10-year-old child does not have this ability.

2. Many technological advances have been made in regard to interpretation and language translation in the health care setting. Sometimes human translators are used in person (i.e., a translation service) or via remote access (i.e., iPads, computers, video, or cell phones). Because phone-based translation services can be confusing to elderly patients, institutions commonly provide access to video remote interpreting services where they can look at a computer screen and see the person with whom they are communicating.

3. As a result of the cultural norm of Chinese to respect their elders, the boy did not communicate necessary information about his mother's vaginal bleeding to the nurse. As a result of the patient not being able to communicate this information in a reliable way to the nurse, her own life and that of her unborn baby were at risk.

EXPLORING THE WEB

- The ANA Web site has a cultural competency self-assessment tool that you can access to reflect on your cultural competency. www.nursingworld.org/practice-policy/innovation/clinical-practice-material/diversity-awareness Accessed March 21, 2019.

- Read the position statement on equity for LGBTQ families and youth from The **Child Welfare League of America (CWLA), Donaldson Adoption Institute (DAI), North American Council on Adoptable Children (NACAC), Voice for Adoption (VFA),** the **National Center for Adoption and Permanency (NCAP),** Foster Club, and RESOLVE: The National Infertility Association. www.cwla.org/wp-content/uploads/2017/05/Child-Welfare-Leaders-Position-Statement-LGBTQ-Equality.pdf accessed April 14, 2019.

- This site contains information about cultural beliefs and medical issues pertinent to the health care of recent immigrants to the United States. Who are the most recent immigrants, and what are their cultural needs? www.ethnomed.org Accessed April 21, 2019.

- Identify the eligibility requirements for following nursing professional organizations (all accessed April 6, 2019):

- Canadian Nurses Association: www.cna-aiic.ca/en

- **National Alaskan Native American Indian Nurses Association (NANAINA):** www.nanainanurses.org

- National Black Nurses Association, Inc.: www.nbna.org

- National Association of Hispanic Nurses: www.nahnnet.org

- Philippine Nurses Association of America, INC.: http://mypnaa.org

- Transcultural Nursing Society: www.tcns.org

- U.S. Census Bureau: www.census.gov

- **Islamic Information Center of American (IICA):** www.icofa.com

- U.S. Citizenship and Immigration Services: www.uscis.gov

- American-Arab Antidiscrimination Committee: www.adc.org

- **American Civil Liberties Union (ACLU):** www.aclu.org

- American Indian Heritage Foundation: www.indians.org

- American Jewish Community: www.ajc.org

- Anti-Defamation League: www.adl.org

- Asian and Pacific Islander Partnership for Health: www.apiahf.org

- National Association for the Advancement of Colored People: www.naacp.org

- International Council of Nurses: www.icn.ch

- Global Health Council: www.globalhealth.org

- World Health Organization: www.who.org

- United States Committee for Refugees and Immigrants: www.refugees.org

INFORMATICS

Go to: www.thinkculturalhealth.hhs.gov/education/nurses Accessed January 18, 2019. Click on, Begin Program, and then click on, Register. Here you will enter your email address and create a password. Select the program, Culturally Competent Nursing Care: A Cornerstone of Caring. Now finish entering the required registration information. You can print a certificate of completion for your instructor after completing the program.

QSEN Exercises:
Go to QSEN.org and do the following:

1. In the search box type the word "culture." Identify the topic(s) or concept(s) that you see the most. Click on one of the topics and read the related materials.

2. How does this article relate to culture, health disparities, generational differences, or spirituality?

LEAN BACK

- What do you see in the clinical setting that represents culturally competent care? What do you see that does not?

- How can you apply what you have learned in this chapter directly to your practice as a nurse?

- How does cultural awareness impact health outcomes of patients?

- What are some cultural influences on Health and health behaviors?

- Assess the importance of client culture/ethnicity when planning, providing, and evaluating care.

- Evaluate and document how client language needs were met the next time you are at clinical.

REFERENCES

Adepoju, O. E., Preston, M. A., & Gonzales, G. (2015). Health care disparities in the post-affordable care act era. *American Journal of Public Health*, *105*(Suppl 5), S665–S667.

Agency for Healthcare Research and Quality. (2015). *Learn about CUSP*. Rockville, MD: Agency for Healthcare Research and Quality. Retrieved from www.ahrq.gov/professionals/education/curriculum-tools/cusptoolkit/modules/learn/index.html

Akerjordet, K., Furunes, T., & Haver, A. (2018). Health-promoting leadership: An integrative review and future research agenda. *Journal of Advanced Nursing*, *74*, 1505–1516. Retrieved from https://doi.org/10.1111/jan.13567

American Association of Critical-Care Nurses (AACN). (2016). *AACN standards for establishing and sustaining healthy work environments: A journey to excellence* (2nd ed.) [Executive Summary]). Aliso Viejo: CA: AACN. Retrieved from www.aacn.org/~/media/aacn-website/nursing-excellence/healthy-work-environment/execsum.pdf?la=en

American Cancer Society. (2018). *Cancer facts & figures 2018*. Atlanta: American Cancer Society. Retrieved from www.cancer.org/content/dam/cancer-org/research/cancer-facts-and-statistics/annual-cancer-facts-and-figures/2018/cancer-facts-and-figures-2018.pdf

American Nurses Association. (2015). *Nursing: Scope and standards of practice* (3rd ed.). Silver Springs, MD: Nursesbooks.org.

American Nursing Association. (2018). *Nursing advocacy for LGBTQ+ populations: position statement*. Retrieved from www.nursingworld.org/~49866e/globalassets/practiceandpolicy/ethics/nursing-advocacy-for-lgbtq-populations.pdf

Arndt, M. (2015). The first men in leadership positions in the American Association of Nurse Anesthetists. *Nursing Forum*, *50*(1), 20–30. doi:10.1111/nuf.12057

Artiga, S., & Ubri, P. (2017). *Living in an immigrant family in America: How fear and toxic stress are affecting daily life, well-being, & health*. Henry J. Kaiser Family Foundation. Retrieved from www.kff.org/disparities-policy/issue-brief/living-in-an-immigrant-family-in-america-how-fear-and-toxic-stress-are-affecting-daily-life-well-being-health

Atashzadeh-Shoorideh, F., Zakaryaee, N. S., & Fani, M. (2018). The barriers and facilitators in providing spiritual care for parents who have children suffering from cancer. *Journal of Family Medicine and Primary Care*, *7*, 1319–1326. Retrieved from www.jfmpc.com/text.asp?2018/7/6/1319/246521

Attum, B. (2019). *Cultural competence in the care of Muslim patients and their families*. Retrieved from https://knowledge.statpearls.com/chapter/0/40656?utm_source=pubmed

Aurilio, L. A. (2017). Creating an inclusive culture for the next generation of nurses. *Nurse Leader*, *15*(5), 315–318.

Barling, J., & Frone, M. R. (2017). If only my leader would just do something! Passive leadership undermines employee well-being through role stressors and psychological resource depletion. *Stress and Health*, *33*(3), 211–222. doi:10.1002/smi.2697

Berkery, E., Tiernan, S., & Morley, M. (2014). The relationship between gender role stereotypes and requisite managerial characteristics: The case of nursing and midwifery professionals. *Journal of Nursing Management*, *22*, 707–719. doi:10.1111/j.1365-2834.2012.01459.x

Bernal, H., & Froman, R. (1993). Influences on the cultural self-efficacy of community health nurses. *Journal of Transcultural Nursing*, *4*(2), 24–31.

Burkhard, M. A., & Nathaniel, A. K. (2014). *Ethics and issues in contemporary nursing* (4th ed.). Stamford, CT: Cengage Learning.

Campinha-Bacote, J. (2003). Many faces: Addressing diversity in health care. *Online Journal of Issues in Nursing*, *8*(1). Retrieved from http://search.ebscohost.com/login.aspx?direct=true&db=ccm&AN=106884953&site=ehost-live

Campinha-Bacote, J. (2009). *Reported reliability and validity of the IAPCC-R*. Retrieved from www.transculturalcare.net/iapcc-r.htm

Carson, V., & Koening, H.. (Eds.). (2008). *Spiritual dimensions of nursing practice* (Revised ed.). West Conshohocken, PA: Templeton Foundation Press.

Center for Disease Control. (2017). *National Diabetes Statistics Report, 2017*. Retrieved from www.diabetes.org/assets/pdfs/basics/cdc-statistics-report-2017.pdf

Center for Disease Control. (2019a). *User guide to the 2016 period linked birth/infant death public use file*. Retrieved from ftp://ftp.cdc.gov/pub/Health_Statistics/NCHS/Dataset_Documentation/DVS/periodlinked/LinkPE16Guide.pdf

Center for Disease Control. (2019b). *Cultural & health literacy*. Retrieved from www.cdc.gov/healthliteracy/culture.html

Center for Disease Control and Prevention. (2019). *Infant mortality*. Retrieved from www.cdc.gov/reproductivehealth/maternalinfanthealth/infantmortality.htm#chart

Chen, S. X., Ng, J. C. K., Buchtel, E. E., Guan, Y., Deng, H., & Bond, M. H. (2017). The added value of world views over self-views: Predicting modest behavior in Eastern and Western cultures. *The British Psychological Society*, *56*, 723–749. doi:10.1111/bjso.12196

Chicca, J. (2018). Connecting with generation Z: Approaches in nursing education. *Teaching and Learning in Nursing*, *12*(3), 180–184. doi:10.1016/j.teln.2018.03.008

Choi, D., Colbert, A. E., & Oh, I. (2015). Understanding organizational commitment: A meta-analytic examination of the roles of the five-factor model of personality and culture. *Journal of Applied Psychology*, *100*(5), 1542–1567. doi:10.1037/apl0000014

Christensen, S. S., Wilson, B. L., & Edelman, L. S. (2018). Can I relate? A review and guide for nurse managers in leading generations. *Journal of Nursing Management, 26,* 689–695. doi:10.1111/jonm.12601

Cox, D., & Jones, R. P. (2017). *America's changing religious identity.* Retrieved from www.prri.org/research/american-religious-landscape-christian-religiously-unaffiliated

Cronenwett, L., Sherwood, G., Barnsteiner, J., Disch, J., Johnson, J., Mitchell, P., Sullivan, D. T. & Warren, J. (2007). Quality and safety education for nurses. *Nursing Outlook, 55*(3), 122–131. doi:10.1016/j.outlook.2007.02.006

Cuevas, A. G., O'Brien, K., & Saha, S. (2017). What is the key to culturally competent care: Reducing bias or cultural tailoring? *Psychology & Health, 32*(4), 493–507.

De Chesnay, M. (2016). Teaching nurses about vulnerable populations. In M. De Chesnay & B. A. Anderson (Eds.), *Caring for the vulnerable: Perspectives in nursing theory, practice, and research* (pp. 429–439). Burlingon, MA: Jones & Bartlett Learning.

De Meester, K., Verspuy, M., Monsieurs, K. G., & VanBogaert, P. (2013). SBAR improves nurse-physician communication and reduces unexpected death: A pre and post intervention study. *Resuscitation, 84*(9), 1192–1196. doi:10.1016/j.resuscitation.2013.03.016

Deng, F. (2015). Comparison of nursing educations among different countries. *Chinese Nursing Research, 2,* 96–98. doi:10.1016/j.cnre.2015.11.001

Ellison, D. (2015). Communication skills. *Nursing Clinicals of North America, 50*(1), 45–57. doi:10.1016/j.cnur.2014.10.004

Ely, D. M., & Hoyert, D. L. (2018). Differences between rural and urban areas in mortality rates for the leading causes of infant death: United States, 2013–2015. *NCHS Data Brief,* no 300. Hyattsville, MD: National Center for Health Statistics.

Fontenot, A. E. (2018). *2020 census program memorandum series.* Washington, DC: U.S. Census Bureau. Retrieved from www2.census.gov/programs-surveys/decennial/2020/program-management/memo-series/2020-memo-2018_02.pdf

Fowler, M. D. M. (2015). *Guide to the code of ethics for nurses with interpretive statements* (2nd ed.). Silver Springs, MD: Nursesbooks.org.

Frey, W. H. (2018). *The US will become 'minority White' in 2045, census projects.* Retrieved from www.brookings.edu/blog/the-avenue/2018/03/14/the-us-will-become-minority-white-in-2045-census-projects

Garneau, A., & Pepin, J. (2015). Cultural competence: A constructivist definition. *Journal of Transcultural Nursing, 26*(1), 9–15. doi:10.1177/1043659614541294

Gates, G. J. (2017). *In U.S., more adults identifying as LGBT.* Retrieved from https://news.gallup.com/poll/201731/lgbt-identification-rises.aspx

Ginger, J. (2012). *Transcultural nursing: Assessment and intervention* (6th ed.). Philadelphia, PA: Elsevier.

Ginger, J., & Davidhizar, R. E. (2008). *Transcultural nursing: Assessment and intervention* (5th ed.). St. Louis, MO: Mosby Year Book.

Giske, T., & Cone, H. (2015). Discerning the healing path—How nurses assist patient spirituality in diverse health care settings. *Journal of Clinical Nursing, 24,* 2926–2935. doi:10.1111/jocn.12907

Gomes, M., Hash, P., Orsolini, L., Watkins, A., & Mazzoccoli, A. (2016). Connecting professional practice and technology at the bedside. *Computers, Informatics, Nursing, 34*(12), 578–586. doi:10.1097/CIN.0000000000000280

Harold, C. M., & Holtz, B. C. (2015). The effects of passive leadership on workplace incivility. *Journal of Organizational Behavior, 36*(1), 16–38. doi:10.1002/job.1926

Healthy People 2020. (2019). *Access to health services.* Washington, DC: U.S. Department of Health and Human Services, Office of Disease Prevention and Health Promotion. Retrieved from www.healthypeople.gov/2020/topics-objectives/topic/Access-to-Health-Services

Henderson, A. (2015). Leadership and communication: What are the imperatives? *Journal of Nursing Management, 23,* 693–694. doi:10.1111/jonm.12336

Herdman, T. H., Kamitsuru, S., & North American Nursing Diagnosis Association. (2018). *Nursing diagnoses: Definitions & classification 2018–2020* (11th ed.). New York: Thieme Publishers.

HRSA. (2017). *Nursing workforce projections by ethnicity and race 2014–2030.* Retrieved from https://bhw.hrsa.gov/sites/default/files/bhw/health-workforce-analysis/research/projections/hrsa-bhw-rn-lpn-fact-sheet-12-17.pdf

Hughes, K. H., & Hood, L. J. (2007). Teaching methods and an outcome tool for measuring cultural sensitivity in undergraduate nursing students. *Journal of Transcultural Nursing, 18*(1), 57–62.

Jeffreys, M. R., & Smodlaka, I. (1996). Steps of the instrument design process. An illustrative approach for nurse educators. *Nurse Educator, 21*(6), 47–52.

Jenkins, M. L., Wikoff, K., Amankwaa, L., & Trent, B. (2009). Nursing the spirit. *Nursing Management, 20*(8), 29–36.

Kates, J., Ranji, U., Beamesderfer, A., Salganicoff, A., & Dawson, L. (2017). *Health and access to care and coverage for lesbian, gay, bisexual, and transgender individuals in the U.S. (issue brief).* Kaiser Family Foundation. Retrieved from http://files.kff.org/attachment/Issue-Brief-Health-and-Access-to-Care-and-Coverage-for-LGBT-Individuals-in-the-US

Ko, A., & Turner, J. (2017). Culturally sensitive care for Asian immigrants: Home healthcare perspectives. *Home Healthcare Now, 35*(9), 507–513. doi:10.1097/NHH.0000000000000608

Kosoko-Lasaki, O., Cook, C. T., O'Brien, R., Kissell, J., Purtilo, R., & Peak, F. (2006). Promoting cultural proficiency in researchers to enhance the recruitment and participation of minority populations in research: Development and refinement of survey instruments. *Evaluation and Program Planning, 29*(3), 227–235.

Kreps, G. L. (2016). Communication and effective interprofessional health care teams. *International Archives of Nursing and Health Care, 2,* 051. Retrieved from https://clinmedjournals.org/articles/ianhc/international-archives-of-nursing-and-health-care-ianhc-2-051.pdf

Lee, B. A., Martin, M. J. R., & Hall, M. (2017). Solamente Mexicanos? Patterns and sources of Hispanic diversity in U.S. metropolitan areas. *Social Science Research, 68,* 117–131.

Lee, S., Liu, M., & Hu, M. (2017). Relationship between future time orientation and item nonresponse on subjective probability questions: A cross-cultural analysis. *Journal of Cross-Cultural Psychology, 48*(5), 698–717. doi:10.1177/0022022117698572

Leininger, M. M. (2006). Cultural care diversity and universality theory and evolution of the ethno nursing method. In M. M. Leininger & M. R. McFarland (Eds.), *Culture care diversity and universality: A worldwide nursing theory* (2nd ed., pp. 1–42). Sudbury, MA: Jones & Bartlett. doi:10.1016/j.ssresearch.2017.08.006

Lockhart, L. (2018). What to do if your workplace is toxic. *Nursing Made Incredibly Easy, 12*(6), 54–55. doi:10.1097/01.NME.0000546257.61537.14

Mannix, J., Wilkes, L., & Daly, J. (2015). Grace under fire: Aesthetic leadership in clinical nursing. *Journal of Clinical Nursing, 24*, 2649–2658. doi:10.1111/jocn.12883

Marin, D. B., Sharma, V., Sosunov, E., Egorova, N., Goldstein, R., & Handzo, G. F. (2015). Relationship between chaplain visits and patient satisfaction. *Journal of Health Care Chaplaincy, 21*(1), 14–24. doi:10.1080/08854726.2014.981417

Marion, L., Douglas, M., Lavin, M., Barr, N., Gazaway, S., et al. (2017). Implementing the new ANA Standard 8: Culturally congruent practice. *The Online Journal of Issues in Nursing, 22*(1). Retrieved from http://ojin.nursingworld.org/MainMenuCategories/ANAMarketplace/ANAPeriodicals/OJIN/TableofContents/Vol-22-2017/No1-Jan-2017/Articles-Previous-Topics/Implementing-the-New-ANA-Standard-8.html

Mead, M. (1935). *Sex and temperament in three primitive societies*. New York: Morrow & Company.

Mendez, A. (2015). Culture and religion in nursing: Providing culturally sensitive care. *British Journal of Nursing, 24*(8), 459. doi:10.12968/bjon.2015.24.8.459

Meyer, O. L., & Zane, N. (2013). The influence of race and ethnicity in clients' experiences of mental health treatment. *Journal of Community Psychology, 41*(7), 884–901.

Miller, K., Briody, C., Casey, D., Kane, J. K., Mitchell, D., et al. (2016). Using the comprehensive unit-based safety program model for sustained reduction in hospital infections. *American Journal of Infection Control, 44*(9), 969–976. doi:10.1016/j.ajic.2016.02.038

Munnich, E., & Wozniak, A. (2017). *What explains the rising share of U.S. men in registered nursing?* [Working paper series] Washington, DC: Washington Center for Equitable Growth. Retrieved from http://equitablegrowth.org/working-papers/rising-sharemen-nursing

Murcia, S. E., & Lopez, L. (2016). The experience of nurses in care for culturally diverse families: A qualitative meta-synthesis. *Revista Latino-Americana de Enfermagem, 24*, e2718. doi:10.1590/1518-8345.1052.2718

Napholz, L. A. (1999). A Comparison of self-reported cultural competency skills among two groups of nursing students: Implications for nursing education. *The Journal of Nursing Education, 38*(2), 81–83.

National Conference of State Legislatures (NCSL). (2016). *Federal and state recognized tribes*. Retrieved from www.ncsl.org/research/state-tribal-institute/list-of-federal-and-state-recognized-tribes.aspx

National Institute of Health. (2015). *NIH funds consortium for childhood oral health disparities research*. Retrieved from www.nih.gov/news/health/sep2015/nidcr-18.htm

National Patient Safety Foundation. (2015). *Free from harm: Accelerating patient safety improvement fifteen years after to err is human*. Boston, MA: National Patient Safety Foundation. Retrieved from www.ihi.org/resources/Pages/Publications/Free-from-Harm-Accelerating-Patient-Safety-Improvement.aspx

National State Boards of Nursing. (2016). Registered nurse results. *Journal of Nursing Regulations, 7*(1), S12–S53. doi:10.1016/S2155-8256(16)31058-4

Nhamo, M. M., & Macleod, C. I. (2018). Lesbian, gay, and bisexual (LGB) people's experiences of nursing health care: An emancipatory nursing practice integrative review. *International Journal of Nursing Practice, 24*(1), 1–10. doi:10.1111/ijn.12606

O'Brien, A., Weaver, C., Settergren, T. T., Hook, M. L., & Ivory, C. (2015). EHR documentation: The hype and the hope for improving nursing satisfaction and quality outcomes. *Nursing Administration Quarterly, 39*(4), 333–339.

Pant, B. (2016). Different cultures see deadlines differently. *Harvard Business Review*. Retrieved from https://hbr.org/2016/05/different-cultures-see-deadlines-differently

Parker, K., Horowitz, J. M., Morin, R., & Lopez, M. H. (2015). *Chapter 1: Race and multiracial Americans in the U.S. census*. Retrieved from www.pewsocialtrends.org/2015/06/11/chapter-1-race-and-multiracial-americans-in-the-u-s-census

Parsian, N., & Dunning, T. (2009). Developing and validating a questionnaire to measure spirituality: A psychometric process. *Global Journal of Health Science, 1*(1), 2–11.

Perng, S., & Watson, R. (2012). Construct validity of the nurse cultural competence scale: A hierarchy of abilities. *Journal of Clinical Nursing, 21*, 1678–1684.

Pew Research Center. (2015). *America's changing religious landscape*. Retrieved from www.pewforum.org/2015/05/12/americas-changing-religious-landscape

Pew Research Center. (2019). *Religious landscape study*. Retrieved from www.pewforum.org/religious-landscape-study

Puchalski, C. M., & Romer, A. L. (2000). Taking a spiritual history allows clinicians to understand patients more fully. *Journal of Palliative Medicine, 3*, 129–137. doi:10.1089/jpm.2000.3.129

Purnell, L. (2008). The Purnell model for cultural competence. In L. Purnell & B. Paulanka (Eds.), *Transcultural health care: A culturally competent approach* (3rd ed.). Philadelphia: F. A. Davis Company.

Purnell, L. D. (2014). *Guide to culturally competent health care* (3rd ed.). Philadelphia, PA: F. A. Davis Company.

QSEN Institute. (2018). *Quality and safety education for nurses*. Retrieved from http://qsen.org

Quinn-Szcesuil, J. (2018). *Recognizing implicit bias in health care settings*. Minority Nurse. Retrieved from https://minoritynurse.com/recognizing-implicit-bias-health-care-settings

Rew, L., Becker, H., Cookston, J., Khosropour, S., & Martinez, S. (2003). Measuring cultural awareness in nursing students. *Journal of Nursing Education, 42*(6), 249–257.

Rickes, P. S. (2016). Generation in flux: How Gen Z will continue to transform higher education space. *Planning for Higher Education Journal, 44*(4), 21–45.

Rosenthal, L. (2013). Enhancing communication between night shift RNs and hospitalists: An opportunity for performance improvement. *The Journal of Nursing Administration, 43*(2), 59–61. doi:10.1097/NNA.0b013e31827f200b

Santos, C. E., Goldstein, A. L., & Tracey, T. J. G. (2017). Development and evaluation of the gender expression attitudes towards transgender clients scale. *The Counseling Psychologist, 45*(3), 353–386. doi:10.1177/0011000017702966

Schim, S. M., Doorenbos, A. Z., Miller, J., & Benkert, R. (2003). Development of a cultural competence assessment instrument. *Journal of Nursing Measurement, 11*(1), 29–40.

Seemiller, C., & Grace, M. (2016). *Generation Z goes to college*. San Francisco, CA: Jossey-Bass.

Semega, J. L., Fontenot, K. R., & Kollar, M. A. (2017). *Income and poverty in the United States: 2016 current population reports*. Washington, DC: US

Census Bureau. Retrieved from www.census.gov/content/dam/Census/library/publications/2017/demo/P60-259.pdf

Shen, Z. (2015). Cultural competence models and cultural competence assessment instruments in nursing a literature review. *Journal of Transcultural Nursing, 26*(3), 308–321.

Shepherd, S. M., Willis-Esqueda, C., Paradies, Y., Sivasubramaniam, D., Sherwood, J., & Brockie, T. (2018). Racial and cultural minority experiences and perceptions of health care provision in a mid-western region. *International Journal for Equity in Health, 17*(1), 33. doi:10.1186/s12939-018-0744-x

Sherman, R. O. (2015). Recruiting and retaining generation Y perioperative nurses. *The Official Voice of Perioperative Nursing Journal, 101*(1), 138–143. doi:10.1016/j.aorn.2014.10.006

Smiley, R. A., Lauer, P., Berg, J. G., Shireman, E., Reneau, K. A., & Alexander, M. (2018). The 2017 national nursing workforce survey. *Journal of Nursing Regulation, 9*(3), S1–S88. doi:10.1016/S2155-8256(18)30131-5

Spector, R. (2009). *Cultural diversity in health and illness.* Upper Saddle River, NJ: Pearson Prentice Hall.

The Joint Commission. (2016). Implicit bias in health care. *Quick Safety (issue 23).* Retrieved from www.jointcommission.org/resources/news-and-multimedia/newsletters/newsletters/quick-safety/quick-safety-issue-23-implicit-bias-in-health-care/

The Joint Commission. (2018). The increasing need for cultural and religious sensitivity. *Dateline @ TJC.* Retrieved from www.jointcommission.org/dateline_tjc/the_increasing_need_for_cultural_and_religious_sensitivity

The National Council of State Boards of Nursing. (2015). *Resource manual on the licensure of internationally educated nurses.* Retrieved from www.ncsbn.org/16_IEN_manual_WEB.pdf

The State of Queensland. Multicultural Health. (2013). *A guide for health professionals.* Retrieved from www.health.qld.gov.au/multicultural/health_workers/cultdiver_guide

Think Cultural Health. (2018). *The National CLAS Standards.* Retrieved from https://minorityhealth.hhs.gov/omh/browse.aspx?lvl=2&lvlid=53

Thornton, R., Glover, C. M., Cené, C. W., Glik, D., Henderson, J. A., & Williams, D. R. (2016). Evaluating strategies for reducing health disparities by addressing the social determinants of health. *Health Affairs, 35*(8), 1416–1423. doi:10.1377/hlthaff.2015.1357

U.S. Census Bureau. (2015). *Census bureau reports at least 350 languages spoken in U.S. homes.* Retrieved from www.census.gov/newsroom/press-releases/2015/cb15–185.html

U.S. Census Bureau. (2017). *American community survey 1-year estimates.* People Reporting Ancestry. Retrieved from https://factfinder.census.gov/faces/tableservices/jsf/pages/productview.xhtml?src=bkmk

U.S. Census Bureau. (2018a). *Popclock.* Retrieved from www.census.gov/popclock

U.S. Census Bureau. (2018b). *Race.* Retrieved from www.census.gov/topics/population/race/about.html

U.S. Census Bureau. (2019a). *2013–2017 American community survey 5-year estimates.* Hispanic or Latino Origin by Specific Origin. Retrieved from https://factfi0nder.census.gov/faces/tableservices/jsf/pages/productview.xhtml?pid=ACS_11_5YR_B03001&prodType=table

U.S. Census Bureau. (2019b). *Quick facts United States.* Retrieved from www.census.gov/quickfacts/fact/table/US/RHI125217

U.S. Department of Health and Human Services. (2017). *Sex, race, and ethnic diversity of U.S. Health Occupations (2011–2015).* Retrieved from https://bhw.hrsa.gov/sites/default/files/bhw/nchwa/diversityushealthoccupations.pdf

U.S. Department of Health and Human Services, Office of Minority Health. (2018). *The National CLAS Standards.* Retrieved from https://minorityhealth.hhs.gov/omh/browse.aspx?lvl=2&lvlid=53

U.S. National Library of Medicine. (2018). *Health services research information central: Health disparities.* Retrieved from www.nlm.nih.gov/hsrinfo/disparities.html#1095Search%20Queries%20Using%20NLM%20Resources:%20Health%20Disparities

Vespa, J., Armstrong, D. M., & Medina, L. (2018). *U.S. Department of Commerce. Demographic turning points for the United States: Population projection for 2020 to 2060.* Retrieved from www.census.gov/content/dam/Census/library/publications/2018/demo/P25_1144.pdf

Vigil, J. M., Coulombe, P., Alcock, J., Stith, S. S., Kruger, E., & Cichowski, S. (2017). How nurse gender influences patient priority assignments in U.S. emergency departments. *Pain, 158*(3), 377–382.

Wang, L. H. (2018). *2020 census will ask white people more about their ethnicities.* Retrieved from www.npr.org/2018/02/01/582338628/-what-kind-of-white-2020-census-to-ask-white-people-about-origins

Xu, J. Q., Murphy, S. L., Kochanek, K. D., Bastian, B., & Arias, E. (2018). Deaths: Final data for 2016. In *National Vital Statistics Reports* (Vol. 67(5)). Hyattsville, MD: National Center for Health Statistics.

Zaidi, D. (2018). Influences of religion and spirituality in medicine. *AMA Journal of Ethics, 20*(7), E609–E612. doi:10.1001/amajethics.2018.609

SUGGESTED READINGS

Almutairi, A. F., Dahinten, V. S., & Rodney, P. (2015). Almutairi's Critical Cultural Competence model for a multicultural healthcare environment. *Nursing Inquiry, 22*(4), 317–325.

Campione, J., & Famolaro, T. (2018). Promising practices for improving hospital patient safety culture. *The Joint Commission Journal on Quality and Patient Safety, 44*(1), 23–32. doi:10.1016/j.jcjq.2017.09.001

Carrion, I. V., Nedjat-Haiem, F., Macip-Billbe, M., & Black, R. (2016). "I told myself to stay positive" perceptions of coping among Latinos with a cancer diagnosis living in the United States. *American Journal of Hospice and Palliative Medicine, 34,* 233e240.

Casey, B. R., Chisholm-Burns, M., Passiment, M., Wagner, R., Riordan, L., & Weiss, K. B. (2019). *The role of the clinical learning environment in preparing new clinicians to engage in quality improvement efforts to eliminate health care disparities.* doi:10.33385/NCICLE.0001 Retrieved from http://ncicle.org

Kaiser Family Foundation. (2018). *Key health implications of separation of families at the border (as of June 27, 2018).* Retrieved from www.kff.org/disparities-policy/fact-sheet/key-health-implications-of-separation-of-families-at-the-border

Lim, A. F., & Borski, B. D. (2016). Supporting LGBT nurses. *Nursing Management,* 47(8), 48–52. doi:10.1097/01.NUMA.0000473515.84420.ad

Loftin, C., Hartin, V., Branson, M., & Reyes, H. (2013). Measures of cultural competence in nurses: An integrative review. *Scientific World Journal,* 1–10. doi:10.1155/2013/289101

Spence Cagle, C., & Wells, J. N. (2017). Culturally sensitive care. *Clinical Journal of Oncology Nursing,* 21(1), E1–E8. doi:10.1188/17.CJON.E1-E8

Stanley, D., Beament, T., Falconer, D., Haigh, M., Saunders, R., et al. (2016). The male of the species: A profile of men in nursing. *Journal of Advanced Nursing,* 72(5), 1155–1168. doi:10.1111/jan.12905

U.S. Department of Health and Human Service. (2019). *Healthy People 2020. Lesbian, gay, bisexual, and transgender health.* Retrieved from www.healthypeople.gov/2020/topics-objectives/topic/lesbian-gay-bisexual-and-transgender-health

25

NCLEX-RN Preparation

Janice Tazbir[1,2,3,4], Patricia Kelly Vana[3,4]

[1] University of Chicago Medicine, Chicago, IL, USA
[2] Anderson Continuing Education, Sacramento, CA, USA
[3] Retired, Purdue University Northwest, College of Nursing, Hammond, IN, USA
[4] Health Education Systems, Inc. (HESI), Houston, TX, USA

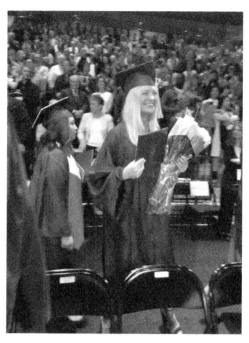

Graduation Day at last!.
Source: Used with permission from Jade Tazbir.

I attribute my success to this—I never gave or took any excuse. Florence Nightingale

Cook, E. (1913). The Life of Florence Nightingale, by Sir Edward Cook. (p 57).
London, UK: Macmillan.

OBJECTIVES

Upon completion of this chapter, the reader should be able to:

1. Review the Present and Next Generation National Council Licensure Examination-RN (NCLEX-RN).

2. Identify that the NCLEX-RN exam is a computer adaptive exam and reflects current nursing practice.

3. Identify rules for passing and failing and the steps of applying for the NCLEX-RN exam.

4. Identify the NCLEX-RN test question formats and samples.

5. Review variables related to NCLEX-RN success.

6. Outline components of organizing a review to prepare for the NCLEX-RN.

7. Identify NCLEX-RN review materials.

8. Identify elements of NCLEX-RN preparation, i.e., content review, ARKO Test Taking Practice, Maslow's ABC-SAFE test taking tips, and anxiety management.

9. Review Nutrition, Sleep, and Wardrobe tips to prepare for NCLEX-RN.

10. Identify medications and diets commonly tested on the NCLEX-RN.

OPENING SCENARIO

Jade graduated from her nursing education program today. Happy and proud to graduate, yet nervous because she knows that she must pass the National Council of State Boards of Nursing Licensure Examination (NCLEX-RN) to practice as a professional nurse. She plans to focus her efforts now on preparing to take the NCLEX-RN Licensure Examination, following a calendar she created using her multiple study guides. She is working on multiple areas of examination preparation. Jade knows continuing to gain

knowledge, using test taking strategies, practicing exam questions, and controlling her anxiety are important ways to be successful on the NCLEX-RN.

1. *How should she prepare for the examination?*

2. *How does she sign up for the examination?*

3. *What's on the examination?*

4. *Where should she focus her preparation for the examination?*

5. *How can she decrease her anxiety?*

Graduates from educational programs in the United States (U.S.) and Canada will take the **National Council of State Boards of Nursing Licensure Examination for Registered Nurses** (NCLEX-RN) examination prepared under the supervision of the National Council of State Boards of Nursing. The NCLEX-RN examination is a source of fear for practically every nursing graduate. The idea that one exam, with anywhere between 75 and 265 questions, will determine your ability to practice nursing is truly daunting. How can nursing graduates best prepare for success on this exam? There is no magic or easy way. This chapter will explore the present and next generation NCLEX-RN examination. It will identify the NCLEX-RN exam as a computer adaptive exam, identify how it is constructed, identify rules for passing and failing the exam, and identify the steps of applying for the NCLEX-RN exam. The chapter will discuss NCLEX-RN test question formats and samples and review variables related to NCLEX-RN success, for example, a Study Calendar, Preparation Courses, and Exit Exams. It will outline components of organizing a review to prepare for the NCLEX-RN and identify NCLEX-RN review courses. The chapter will identify elements of NCLEX-RN preparation, content review, ARKO Test Taking Practice and Maslow's **Airway, Breathing, or Circulation** (ABC)-SAFE test taking tips, and anxiety management. It will review Nutrition, Sleep, and Wardrobe tips to prepare for NCLEX-RN and identify medications and diets commonly tested on NCLEX-RN. In other words, this chapter will help you pass the NCLEX-RN exam.

The NCLEX-RN Examination

The **National Council of State Boards of Nursing** (NCSBN) is the central organization for the independent member state boards of nursing, which includes the boards of nursing of the 50 states, the District of Columbia, Guam, the Virgin Islands, and Canada. The member boards of nursing are divided into

areas, which supervise the selection of test item writers, representing nursing educators and clinicians, whose names are suggested by the individual state boards of nursing. This provides for regional representation in the testing of nursing practice. The NCLEX-RN examination ensures a basic level of safe registered nursing practice to the public that is essential for working as a professional RN. RNs are the single largest health care profession in the United States and in Canada. There are close to 3.1 million RNs holding licenses to practice in the United States (U.S.) and over 400,000 in Canada (Canadian Institute for Health Information, 2018).

Every 3 years, there is a practice analysis sent out to entry level nurses, or nurses with less than 1 year's experience as an RN. The practice analysis surveys where nurses work, what they do, and who they are. The majority of survey respondents (89.0%) recently indicated their gender as female and reported predominantly working in the medical/surgical (27.6%) and critical care (23.3%) settings (NCSBN, 2017). From the survey, the most common activities that nurses perform on a daily basis are ranked in multiple ways. Using these ranked activities, nurse clinicians and educators collaborate and write NCLEX-RN test questions taking the ranked activities and the NCLEX-RN test plan into account. All test items are validated in at least two approved nursing textbooks or references and go through extensive statistical testing prior to use on the NCLEX-RN exam.

The level of passing on NCLEX-RN is based on a mathematical computation called a logit. A **logit** is a unit of measurement used to report relative differences between candidate ability estimates and item difficulties on the NCLEX-RN, (NCSBN, 2019) www.ncsbn.org/1216.htm, accessed April 15, 2019. The harder the NCLEX-RN question is, the higher the logit score. This standard is reviewed and published every 3 years along with the test plan. The passing standard is often referred to as the "passing line." The **passing** standard will remain at the current level of 0.00 logits that was instituted on April 1, 2016 and will remain in effect through March 31, 2022 (Passing Standard (n.d.). Retrieved from www.ncsbn.org/2630.htm). The 2019 NCLEX-RN test plan can be found at www.ncsbn.org/2019_RN_TestPlan-English.pdf, accessed April 15, 2019. Recent passing rates for nurses taking can be viewed at www.ncsbn.org/Table_of_Pass_Rates_2018.pdf, accessed April 15, 2019.

The NCLEX-RN is taken after graduation and prior to practice as an RN. It is wise to schedule the exam date soon after graduation. In 2009, a study by Wooi, Went, and Luand found that the NCLEX-RN pass rate is inversely related to lag time for both RN and **licensed practical nurse** (LPN) candidates. Overall, candidates were *less likely to pass* the NCLEX-RN *the longer they waited* to take the NCLEX-RN. This underscores the importance of exam readiness and taking the exam as soon as possible after graduation. The NCLEX-RN examination is given across North America at professional Pearson VUE testing centers. Steps to apply for the NCLEX-RN are outlined below. **Every candidate should review the National Council of State Boards of Nursing (2020). NCLEX-RN Examination Test Plan for the National Council Licensure Examination for Registered Nurses.** Retrieved January 10, 2019 from www.ncsbn.org/2019_NCLEX-RN_TestPlan.pdf

The NCLEX-RN Examination Test Plan is formulated on four categories of client needs that RNs commonly encounter, that is, Safe and Effective Care Environment, Health Promotion and Maintenance, Psychosocial Integrity, and Physiological Integrity. Integrated processes in the four categories of client needs include the nursing process, caring, communication and documentation, and teaching/learning (NCSBN, 2019). See Table 25.1 to view the percent of test items in each category of client needs and a related example of client need activity that may be tested on NCLEX-RN. Licensure ensures a basic level of safe registered nursing practice to the public and is essential for working as a professional RN. RNs are the single largest health care profession in the United States and in Canada.

NCLEX-RN, Next Generation

Since July, 2017, NCSBN has presented a Special Research Section as part of NCLEX-RN administration. This Special Research Section explored testing based on the **Clinical Judgment Model** (CJM) (Figure 25.1). Nursing clinical judgment research conducted by NCSBN created a CJM. The CJM was designed to explore new ways of testing clinical judgment in the nursing profession as part of the licensure examination. The NCSBN-CJM aligns with the Information-Processing Model (which likens thinking to a computer where the mind takes information, organizes and stores it for retrieval later) and the Intuitive-Humanistic Model (where knowledge is gained from nursing experience that enriches the clinical decision-making process) and can be used to assess the Dual Process Reasoning Theory (where two thinking processes go on at once, the first thinking process is a knee jerk reaction and the second thinking process is an analytical cognitive process

Table 25.1   NCLEX-RN Test Plan

Client Need Integrated Processes throughout Client Needs include: Nursing Process, Caring, Communication and Documentation, and Teaching/Learning	Percent of test items	Example of Client Need activity that may be tested on NCLEX-RN[a]
Safe and Effective Care Environment		
• Management of Care	17–23%	Provide care within the legal scope of practice
• Safety and Infection Control	9–15%	Protect the client from injury (e.g., falls, electrical hazards)
Health Promotion and Maintenance	6–12%	Provide prenatal care and education
Psychosocial Integrity	6–12%	Assess the client for abuse or neglect and intervene, as appropriate
Physiological Integrity		
• Basic Care and Comfort	6–12%	Assess and manage the client with an alteration in elimination
• Pharmacological and Parenteral Therapies	12–18%	Administer blood products and evaluate the client's response
• Reduction of risk potential	9–15%	Insert, maintain, or remove a nasal/oral gastrointestinal tub
• Physiological Adaptation	11–17%	Monitor and care for clients on a ventilator

[a] *Note:* each of the Client Needs above have a list of sample client need activities in the NCLEX-RN Examination Test Plan. These activities can be reviewed as part of NCLEX-RN exam preparation.

Source: Data from National Council Licensure Examination for Registered Nurses. Retrieved January 10, 2019 from https://www.ncsbn.org/2019_NCLEX-RN_RN_Test-Plan.pdf. These activities can be reviewed as part of NCLEX-RN exam preparation.

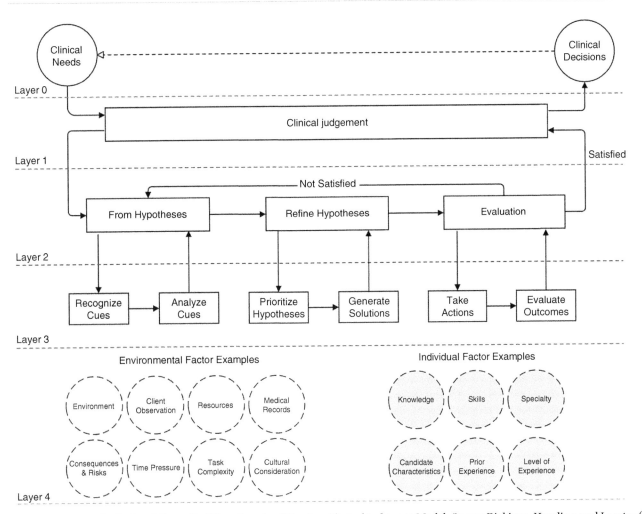

FIGURE 25.1 The National Council of State Boards of Nursing-Clinical Judgment Model. *Source:* Dickison, Haerling, and Lasater (2019).

that "puts the pieces together.") The **clinical judgment model** is defined as "the observed outcome of critical thinking and decision-making" (NCSBN, 2019, accessed May 13, 2019, at, www.ncsbn.org/NGN_Winter19.pdf). The CJM uses nursing knowledge to observe and present situations, identify and prioritize patient care, and generate evidence-based solutions to deliver safe patient care. The CJM hopes to close the gap between what is measured in the exam and what is taught in clinical nursing education.

Nurse educators can use this action model as a guide to developing test questions that assess clinical judgment. The CJM has four layers and uses nursing knowledge to observe and present situations, identify and prioritize patient care, and generate evidence-based solutions to deliver safe patient care. An example of how nurses can use the NCSBN-CJM to construct effective assessments of clinical judgment is shown in Table 25.2, which provides a hypothetical action model for a pediatric setting. Nurse educators can use this action model as a guide to developing test questions that assess clinical judgment. Students may use this model to better understand the kind of thinking required for the new generation NCLEX and the kind of thinking that models real world practice. For example, Layer Three of the NCSBN-CJM identifies the need to use one's cognitive thinking operations to recognize and analyze cues, prioritize hypotheses, generate solutions, take action, and evaluate outcomes. Layer Four of the Model notes Individual and Environmental Factors reviewed in arriving at the expected behaviors/actions of a Clinical Judgment. To summarize, the model takes the student through the cognitive operations (layer 3) of using the nursing process to use factor conditioning (layer 4) or the "what is" to formulate expected behaviors/actions. Students may use this model to better understand the kind of thinking required for the new generation NCLEX and the kind of thinking that models real world practice.

The NCLEX-RN Special Research Section is given to selected candidates, based on the amount of time that the candidate has left in their NCLEX-RN appointment, as it takes approximately 30 minutes to complete the Special Research Section. This Special Research Section is administered following the regular NCLEX-RN exam and does not count as part of the NCLEX-RN score. By participating in the Special Research Section, candidates are making valuable contributions to the future development of NCSBN examinations. Once an NCLEX-RN candidate finishes their exam, an introductory screen indicates the beginning of the Special Research Section.

Table 25.2   Hypothetical Action Model for a Pediatric Case Study

Cognitive operations (NCSBN-CJM Layer 3)	Factor conditioning (NCSBN-CJM Layer 4)	Expected behaviors/actions
Recognize cues	Environmental cues	Recognize signs and symptoms of dehydration
	Location: emergency department	Identify history of diabetes
	Parent present	Recognize abnormal vital signs
	Client observation cues	Hypothesize dehydration
	Present age: 8 to 10 years	Hypothesize diabetes
	Present: signs and symptoms of dehydration (dry mucous membranes, cool extremities, capillary refill 3 to 4 s)	
	Present or imply: lethargy	
	Medical record cues	
	Present or imply: history of diabetes	
	Present or imply: vital signs	
	Time pressure cues	
	Set time pressure to vary with onset and acuity of symptoms	
Analyze cues	Requires knowledge of pediatric development	Describe relationship between blood sugar level and dehydration
	Requires knowledge of dehydration symptoms	Use evidence to determine client issues
	Requires knowledge of diabetes symptoms	
Prioritize hypotheses	Give vital sign monitors as resources	Prioritize dehydration
	Set time pressure to vary with vital signs	Address dehydration
		Avoid glucose
Generate solutions	Requires knowledge of pediatric developmentally appropriate approach	
	Requires knowledge of dehydration treatment and intervention	
	Requires knowledge of diabetes treatment and intervention	
Take actions	Experience: requires experience of administering isotonic fluid	Administer isotonic fluid
Evaluate outcomes	Experience: Requires experience of administering isotonic fluid	Reassess vital signs
		Reassess lethargy
	Client observation cues	
	Show client awake and talking	
	Imply improvement in vital signs based on actions	

Note. NCSBN-CJM = National Council of State Boards of Nursing-Clinical Judgment Model.
Source: Dickison, Haerling, and Lasater (2019).

This Special Research Section will continue to be numbered in accordance with the completed exam, for example, if a candidate's exam ended with question 153, the first question on the Special Research Section will be numbered 154. Despite the consecutive numbering, these new questions have no impact on NCLEX-RN scoring or results. Candidates do not have to start or complete the Special Research Section. They may exit once their actual exam is over. All questions on the NCLEX-RN and the Special Research Section are confidential. NCSBN is researching several question types, including: extended multiple response items; extended drag and drop items; CLOZE items (consist of a passage of text that has various answers embedded within it, including multiple choice, short answers, and numerical answers); enhanced hot-spot items; dynamic exhibit items; and constructed response items (NCSBN, 2019).

NCLEX-RN Computer Adaptive Testing (CAT)

The NCLEX-RN exam is a computer adaptive exam. Candidates receive between 75 and 265 questions in the NCLEX-RN examination during the exam session. Of these questions, 15 questions are being piloted to determine their psychometric value and validity for use in future NCLEX-RN examinations. The 15 pilot questions will not count toward the student's score. The 15 pilot questions are always in the first 75 questions to ensure every candidate completes them. The other questions will determine the student's ability estimate on the NCLEX-RN. Students cannot determine whether they have passed or failed the NCLEX-RN examination from the number of questions they receive during their session. As stated in the 2019 RN Test Plan (2019), "since the practice of nursing requires application of knowledge, skills, and abilities, the majority of items are written at the application or higher levels." With this in mind, candidates need to practice comprehensive questions written at high cognitive levels. Each test question is presented to the student. If the student answers the question correctly, a slightly more difficult item will follow. The level of difficulty will increase with each item until the candidate misses an item. If the student misses an item, a slightly less difficult item will follow, and the level of difficulty will decrease with each item until the student has answered an item correctly. This process continues until the student has achieved a definite passing or definite failing score.

At the NCLEX-RN testing center, candidates are verified by their photo identification (driver's license or passport), fingerprints, and palm vein recognition. Every time a candidate leaves the testing room for a break, the candidate verification process must occur, again, before the student re-enters the testing room each time. Each candidate is oriented to the computer before the examination starts. This computer orientation is included in the 6-hr testing window. Candidates are allowed up to 6 hr to complete the NCLEX-RN, which means that they could take the entire 6 hr to complete as few as 75 test items. However, because candidates do not know how many test items they will be required to answer, they should progress through the exam as though they will have to answer all 265 items. This means they should allow an average of 1 min per question. A 10-min break is mandatory after 2 hr of testing. An optional 10-min break may be taken after another 90 minutes of testing. Because the exam is geared to the candidate's skill level, each candidate will have a unique **Computer Adaptive Test** (CAT). Note there is a NCLEX-RN licensure examination tutorial available at: www.pearsonvue.com/nclex, accessed April 15, 2019.

NCLEX-RN Rules for Passing and Failing

The decision as to whether a candidate passes or fails the NCLEX-RN is guided by three different rules:

Rule 1: The 95% Confidence Interval

The 95% Confidence Interval is the rule most commonly used for NCLEX-RN candidates. The computer will stop administering items when it is 95% certain that the candidate's ability is either clearly above or clearly below the passing standard.

Rule 2: The Maximum-Length Exam

Some candidate's ability levels will be very close to the passing standard. When this is the case, the computer continues to administer items until the maximum number of items is reached. At this point, the computer disregards the 95% confidence interval rule and considers only the final ability estimate. If the final ability estimate is above the passing standard, the candidate passes; if the final ability estimate is at or below the passing standard, the candidate fails.

Scenario 3: Run-Out-Of-Time (R.O.O.T)
If a candidate runs out of time before reaching the maximum number of items and the computer has not determined with 95%

certainty whether the candidate has passed or failed, an alternate rule is imposed. If the candidate has not answered the minimum number of required items, the candidate automatically fails. If at least the minimum number of required items were answered, the computer looks at the last 60 ability estimates (or questions): if the last 60 ability estimates were above the passing standard, the candidate passes. If during the last 60 ability estimates, the candidate drops below the passing standard, even once, the candidate fails. This does not mean that the candidate must answer the last 60 items correctly. Each ability estimate is based on all the previous items the candidate has answered (National Council of State Boards of Nursing (2020). Retrieved from www. ncsbn.org/2630.htm, accessed April 15, 2019).

After completion of the NCLEX-RN exam, candidates may access their "unofficial" results two business days after taking the exam by paying a fee through the Pearson VUE website (National Council of State Boards of Nursing, 2020), accessed May 13, 2019 at www.ncsbn.org/1225.htm. These are unofficial results and do not authorize one to practice as an RN. Only the state nursing regulatory body to which a candidate applied can release the official results. Results will be sent to the candidate within 6 weeks after the exam. Successful candidates are notified that they have passed. Unsuccessful candidates are provided with a diagnostic profile that describes their overall performance on a scale from low to high and their performance on the questions testing their abilities to meet client needs (NCSBN.org, 2019).

NCLEX-RN Application Steps

Steps to apply for the NCLEX-RN are outlined below. Every candidate should review the Candidate NCLEX-RN bulletin at: www.ncsbn.org/2019_Bulletin_Final.pdf, accessed April 15, 2019. Steps in the NCLEX-RN application include:

1. Apply to the Board of Nursing in the state you plan to practice first. Each state has its own application process that is unique to the state. Once the candidate has applied, most states contact the candidate. At this point, fingerprinting and a background check are performed at fingerprinting vendors specific to the state. The **last step** in the state application process is sending the certificate of completion from the school attended. Register for the NCLEX-RN exam with Pearson VUE (www.pearsonvue.com/NCLEX-RN). This can be done before, during, or after state application. Once you pay for the exam, you have 365 days to take the exam.

2. Once the state verifies the candidate's background check and graduation from an accredited school of nursing and the candidate has registered and paid for the NCLEX-RN exam, the candidate will be sent an **Authorization To Test** (ATT) electronically.

3. Once the candidate obtains the ATT, they can schedule the NCLEX-RN exam at any Pearson VUE Center. Since the NCLEX-RN is a national exam, multiple nursing students apply and take the NCLEX-RN every spring and fall. Multiple other professions also use Pearson VUE to administer their exams, so it is wise to be willing to travel

to another Pearson VUE Center to take the NCLEX-RN exam at a date early and convenient to the candidate.

NCLEX-RN Test Question Formats and Samples

There are several formats for NCLEX-RN test questions. Questions may include but are not limited to multiple choice (one answer), multiple response (select one or more answers), fill in the blank calculation, hot spots, exhibit, drop and drag/ordered response, audio, and graphics. All questions may include multimedia, such as charts, graphics, and audio. Examples of all the formats used in the test questions are available in the 2019 National Council of State Boards of Nursing National Council Licensure Examination for Registered Nurses (NCLEX-RN) Test Plan, retrieved January 10, 2019 from www.ncsbn.org/2019_RN_TestPlan-English.htm. More sample questions are available at, ncsbn.org/9010.htm, accessed April 10, 2019. Also, the NCSBN's Learning Extension website offers a Weekly "NCLEX-RN-Style" Question of the week at ww2.learningext.com/qotw.htm, accessed April 10, 2019.

Variables Related to NCLEX-RN Success

Several factors have been identified in research studies as being associated with performance on the NCLEX-RN examination. To date, there is no evidence of what specifically makes an NCLEX-RN candidate successful. Recent studied variables associated with NCLEX-RN performance include students who speak English as a second or additional language or have low end-of-program **Grade Point Average** (GPA) and **Health Education Systems, Inc** (HESI) Exit Exam scores (Kaddoura et al., 2017); students with poor performance on adult medical-surgical, pharmacology, and community health standardized tests (Yeom, 2013); and students who performed poorly on the HESI-A2 (Twidwell & Records, 2017).

Other variables that can help predict NCLEX-RN success include self-efficacy and control of test anxiety. **Self-efficacy** has been defined as an individual's judgment of his or her capabilities to organize and execute courses of action (Resnick, 2018). Self-efficacy has been correlated to academic performance and NCLEX-RN success. Students with higher levels of self-efficacy perform at higher academic levels than other students do and increased self-efficacy has a significant positive effect on passing the NCLEX-RN (Fiske, 2017). Test anxiety has also been studied extensively and has been shown to be related to NCLEX-RN pass rates and academic performance in general. Variables related to NCLEX-RN performance are listed in Table 25.3.

NCLEX-RN Review Materials

NCLEX-RN review materials are available from live courses to integrated online courses and often focus on nursing content, test taking skills, or both. The test questions may be arranged in the NCLEX-RN book by clinical content area, or they may be presented in one or more comprehensive examinations covering all areas of the NCLEX-RN. Many NCLEX-RN review books are presently available at www.amazon.com. Review materials should be formatted in a way that is easy to approach for the candidate. One mistake that nursing students commonly

Table 25.3   Variables Related to NCLEX-RN Performance

Health Education Systems Incorporated (*HESI*) Exit Exam Performance	Assessment Technologies Institute (ATI) Exit Exam Performance
Kaplan Diagnostic and Readiness Test Performance	Grades in Science, Medical-Surgical Nursing, Pharmacology, and Community Health Nursing Courses
Verbal SAT Score	*English Language Proficiency*
ACT Score	High School Rank and Grade Point Average (GPA)
HESI-A2	End of Program Grade Point Average (GPA)
Anxiety	Self-Efficacy

Source: Compiled by J. Tazbir & P. Kelly Vana.

Evidence from the Literature

Source: Fiske, E. (2017). Contemplative Practices, Self-efficacy, and NCLEX-RN Success. *Nurse Educator, 42*(3), 159–161. doi:10.1097/nne.0000000000000327

Discussion: Even though graduates have completed nursing programs, not all graduates are successful on the NCLEX-RN Examination. When contemplative practices such as meditation and guided imagery were added to an NCLEX-RN Preparatory Course, the differences in self-efficacy scores were statistically significant and participants reported that the activities were useful and they would use them again.

Implications for Practice: Contemplative practices such as meditation and guided imagery improves self-efficacy and can help in the NCLEX-RN review process.

Table 25.4 NCLEX-RN Review Courses and Course Resources

NCLEX-RN Review Course	Examples of NCLEX-RN Review Resources
National Council of State Boards of Nursing (NCSBN) Learning Extension	https://ww2.learningext.com/students, accessed April 10, 2019. 1,500+ question test bank Content and tutoring courses online
Health Education Systems, Inc. (HESI)	https://evolve.elsevier.com, accessed April 10, 2019. Live 3-day course and online courses available, Focus is on content and test questions
Assessment Technologies Institute (ATI)	www.atitesting.com, accessed April 10, 2019. 3-day live review course and an on-line course version with 3,000+ questions and sample exams
Kaplan	www.kaptest.com/NCLEX-RN, accessed April 10, 2019. Live and online courses available 3-day live Review course. Focus is on using the Kaplan Decision Tree, extensive on line resources, multiple preparation tests, and an over 2,500 test question bank
Hurst Review Services	www.hurstreview.com, accessed April 10, 2019. 3-day review with on line resources, 500+ test question bank
NRSNG	www.nrsng.com, accessed April 10, 2019. Nursing content review by body system with multiple study sources and practice exams
UWorld	www.uworld.com, accessed April 10, 2019. 2,000+ question bank with in depth explanations available on line

Source: Compiled by J. Tazbir & P. Kelly Vana.

make is to purchase a plethora of resources, and then not use them. Whatever resource is used, be sure to use it to its full potential. NCLEX-RN review courses are a great way to help a candidate organize their NCLEX-RN preparation, improve confidence, and improve test taking skills (Table 25.4). The quality of these programs can vary, and students may want to ask former nursing graduates and faculty for recommendations as well as visit websites for more specifics about each course.

Exit Examinations

Many nursing programs administer an exit examination to students at the completion of their nursing program. These exit exams are created to mimic the NCLEX-RN exam and predict if candidates will pass the exam. Two common exit exams are the **Assessment Technologies Institute** (ATI) Exit Exam and the Health Education Systems, Inc., (HESI) Exit Exam. These high stakes exit exams are used because of their predictiveness related to the NCLEX-RN. When taking these types of exit exams, they must be taken very seriously. When exit examinations are part of a nursing program, finding out how scoring can affect NCLEX-RN readiness is prudent as some nursing programs may delay graduation until a certain score is achieved on the exit exam. As a new graduate, take time to review strengths and weaknesses in these exit exams and ensure that you complete remediation; this will help you prepare for the NCLEX-RN.

Real World Interview

Tips for upcoming testers.... know that no matter how much you study you will see things you do not know and know that the exam is designed that way... you cannot possibly know everything. Do not freak out. Answer the best you can with what you do know. Do not think that you are failing if you get what you might think is a "basic knowledge" question in the middle of the exam. Know that you may not get any math, hot spots, or audio sections.... (Was a little sad since I love math). Know that even the Chancellor's Medal recipient (me) with a 4.0 throughout nursing school who had studied for boards since November felt horrible leaving the exam and I was questioning myself and wondering if I passed and I was looking up information after leaving for peace of mind. Trust in your instincts, they are right. Do not second guess yourself. Trust in the people who are teaching you that they know what they are doing. Work hard and breathe. Passing in 75 is possible... most of my friends passed with between 75 and 83 questions. I guess also remember why you want to be a nurse... this is not easy... actually this is an extremely challenging process and one of the hardest things I have ever done in my life. We only have to do it once, and nothing easy is ever worth anything anyway. Take the leap—you can do it.

MICHELLE ZIRKLE, MDIV., BS,
AND NOW FINALLY..... BSN, RN!!!!!
Schererville, IN

Three Elements of NCLEX-RN Preparation

When students prepare to take the NCLEX-RN, they will use a plan that includes three elements, that is, NCLEX-RN learning needs analysis, ARKO test taking practice, and anxiety management. To begin, complete the NCLEX-RN Learning Needs Analysis (Table 25.5). This will help you identify where you need to focus your preparation.

Next, list all NCLEX-RN areas needing content review. Plan to review one content area daily, focusing on areas of weakness first. Establish an NCLEX-RN 8-week preparation calendar (Table 25.6) that permits you to organize your review and cover completely all the material to be reviewed. Choose the week you want to take NCLEX-RN, within 8 weeks after graduation. Starting with your projected test date, work backwards 8 weeks. List all areas of test content weakness identified on your NCLEX-RN Learning Needs Analysis. Consider taking one of the NCLEX-RN Review Courses (Table 25.4). Reflect on your test taking practices and anxiety level. Plan your time, using the NCLEX-RN Daily Preparation Calendar (Table 25.7) to organize your study. Review and strengthen identified areas of test content weakness. Identify your personal best time to study. Are you a day person? Are you a night person? Study when you are well rested. Arrange to study one or more hours daily. Practice testing, scoring, and reading the rationales of at least 60 test questions daily. Also add time for "life," such as birthdays, work schedules, and life events, to your test preparation calendar. By creating and sticking with your test preparation calendar, achieving your goal is much easier. Students who use these techniques should increase their ability to do well in the NCLEX-RN.

NCLEX-RN Study Schedule

Your study schedule may look like the following:

Day 1: Practice 60 adult health test questions. Score the test, analyze your performance, and review test question rationales.

Table 25.5 NCLEX-RN Learning Needs Analysis

Anxiety level (circle)
1   2   3   4   5   6   7   8   9   10

Weak content areas identified on NCLEX-RN Test Plan in Table 25.1, Exit Exam, or other comprehensive exam:

_____

Nursing courses below B:

_____

Content weaknesses identified through review of activities of integrated processes in NCLEX-RN Test Plan (Table 25.1):

_____

Variable Weaknesses Identified (Table 25.3):

_____

Weak content areas identified in any common patient conditions:

* Adult Health—e.g., Cancer, Myocardial Infarction, Cardiac Arrhythmias, Chronic Obstructive Pulmonary Disease, Diabetes, Pneumonia, COVID-19, Human Immunodeficiency Virus (HIV), Hepatitis, Cholecystectomy, Lobectomy, Nephrectomy, Cardiac Arrest, Thyroidectomy, Shock, Hypertension, CerebroVascular Accident (CVA), Appendectomy, Tuberculosis, and so on.

_____

* Women's Health—e.g., Antepartum Care, Intrapartum Care, Postpartum Care, Newborn Care, Gynecological Disorders, Autoimmune Disorders, Osteoporosis, and so on.

_____

* Mental Health—e.g., Schizophrenia, Bipolar disorders, Anxiety, Personality Disorders, Eating Disorders, Abuse, Suicide, Eating Disorders, Substance Abuse, Dementia, Drug Abuse, Defense Mechanisms, and so on.

_____

* Children's Health—e.g., Leukemia, Cardiovascular Surgery, Fractures, Cancer, Tonsillectomy, Asthma, Poisoning, Wilms' Tumor, Diabetes, Cleft Palate, Growth and Development, Developmental Milestones and Toys, Immunization Schedules, Child Abuse, Unhealthy Eating, and so on.

_____

Weak content areas identified in any of the following:
* Management, Delegation, and Priority Setting
* Therapeutic Communication
* Medications (Table 25.10)
* Diagnostic Tests and Laboratory Values
* Common Food Sources for Various Nutrients and Diets (Table 25.11)
* Isolation Techniques, i.e., Standard, Airborne, Droplet, Contact Isolation

Source: J. Tazbir & P. Kelly Vana.

Table 25.6 NCLEX-RN 8 Week Preparation Calendar

8 Weeks to Test	Plan for 3 elements of successful test preparation
	• NCLEX-RN learning needs analysis (Table 25.5),
	• Test taking practice, and
	• Anxiety management.
	Consider taking one of the NCLEX-RN Review Courses and Course Resources (Table 25.4)
	Review NCLEX-RN Learning Analysis CC List all NCLEX-RN areas needing content review. Plan to review one weak content area daily.
	Set up Review of your NCLEX-RN Daily Preparation Calendar (Table 25.7), Monday through Friday, for next 8 weeks. Identify content for each day
	Practice 60 test questions 5 days weekly in weak content areas. Score the test and review all test question rationales.
	Plan to schedule content review at time when you are freshest, e.g., morning, afternoon, evening
	Answer NCSBN Learning Extension's weekly NCLEX-RN test question at wwwlearningext.com
	Practice Management, Delegation, and Priority Setting NCLEX-RN questions for the Exam.
	Continue this process until you are doing well in all areas of the Exam
	Practice Anxiety Management Strategies, e.g., PERMA, Yoga, Deep Breathing, Regular Exercise, Meditation, Visualization, Yoga, Positive Thinking, Self-Efficacy, Declaring Your Intention, Listening to Classical Music, etc.
	Practice test taking with the Test taking ARKO Strategies and ABC-Safe Tips
	Build time into weekly schedules for Life Enjoyment with Family and Friends
7 Weeks to Test	Plan to review one weak content area daily from your NCLEX-RN Content Learning Needs Analysis (Table 25.5).
	Practice 60 test questions 5 days weekly in weak content areas. Score the test and review all test question rationales. Include some Delegation and Priority Setting Test questions.
	Answer NCSBN Learning Extension's weekly NCLEX-RN test question at wwwlearningext.com
	Practice Anxiety Management Strategies
6 Weeks to Test	Plan to review one weak content area daily from your NCLEX-RN Content Learning Needs Analysis (Table 25.5).
	Practice 60 test questions 5 days weekly in weak content areas. Score the test and review all test question rationales. Include some Delegation and Priority Setting Test questions.
	Answer NCSBN Learning Extension's weekly NCLEX-RN test question at wwwlearningext.com
	Practice Anxiety Management Strategies
5 Weeks to Test	Plan to review one weak content area daily from your NCLEX-RN Content Learning Needs Analysis (Table 25.5).
	Practice 60 test questions 5 days weekly in weak content areas. Score the test and review all test question rationales. Include some Delegation and Priority Setting Test questions.
	Answer NCSBN Learning Extension's weekly NCLEX-RN test question at wwwlearningext.com
	Practice Anxiety Management Strategies
4 Weeks to Test	Plan to review one weak content area daily from your NCLEX-RN Content Learning Needs Analysis (Table 25.5).
	Practice 60 test questions 5 days weekly in weak content areas. Score the test and review all test question rationales. Include some Delegation and Priority Setting Test questions.
	Answer NCSBN Learning Extension's weekly NCLEX-RN test question at wwwlearningext.com
	Practice Anxiety Management Strategies
3 Weeks to Test	Plan to review one weak content area daily from your NCLEX-RN Content Learning Needs Analysis (Table 25.5).
	Practice 60 test questions 5 days weekly in weak content areas. Score the test and review all test question rationales. Include some Delegation and Priority Setting Test questions.
	Answer NCSBN Learning Extension's weekly NCLEX-RN test question at wwwlearningext.com
	Practice Anxiety Management Strategies
2 Weeks to Test	Plan to review one weak content area daily from your NCLEX-RN Content Learning Needs Analysis (Table 25.5).
	Practice 60 test questions 5 days weekly in weak content areas. Score the test and review all test question rationales. Include some Delegation and Priority Setting Test questions.
	Answer NCSBN Learning Extension's weekly NCLEX-RN test question at wwwlearningext.com
	Practice Anxiety Management Strategies
1 Week to Test	Plan to review one weak content area daily from your NCLEX-RN Content Learning Needs Analysis (Table 25.5).
	Practice 60 test questions 5 days weekly in weak content areas. Score the test and review all test question rationales. Include some Delegation and Priority Setting Test questions.
	Answer NCSBN Learning Extension's weekly NCLEX-RN test question at wwwlearningext.com
	Practice Anxiety Management Strategies
Night Before Test	Relax and listen to classical music. Don't do any heavy studying.
	Don't eat or drink any alcohol or stimulants.
	Go to bed early and get a good night's sleep
Day of Test	Have a light, but nutritious breakfast. Listen to classical music on your way to the test site. Be sure to take all allotted breaks during test. Think positive and breathe deep if you start to feel anxious. Expect to have 265 questions to answer.

Source: P. Kelly Vana & J. Tazbir.

Table 25.7   NCLEX-RN Daily Preparation Calendar^a

	M	T	W	T	F	S	S
6 a.m.							
7 a.m.							
8 a.m.	X	X	X	X	X		
9 a.m.							
10 a.m.							
11 a.m.							
12 p.m.							
1 p.m.							
2 p.m.							
3 p.m.							
4 p.m.							
5 p.m.							
6 p.m.							
7 p.m.							
8 p.m.							
9 p.m.							
10 p.m.							
Etc.							

^a Choose the time daily that you are freshest to prepare for NCLEX-RN.
Source: J. Tazbir & P. Kelly Vana.

Review any content weaknesses from your NCLEX-RN Learning Needs Analysis (Table 25.5), for example, Exit Exam, NCSBN NCLEX-RN Test Plan Client Needs, Activities of Integrated Processes, including the nursing process, caring, communication and documentation and teaching/learning (Table 25.1), Delegation and Priority Setting Tips, etc. Practice anxiety management tips, for example, deep breathing, regular exercise, journaling, and positive thinking, as needed. Continue this process until you are doing well in adult health questions.

Day 2: Practice 60 women's health test questions. Repeat the Day 1 schedule until you are doing well in women's health questions.

Day 3: Practice 60 children's health test questions. Repeat the Day 1 schedule until you are doing well in children's health questions.

Day 4: Practice 60 mental health test questions. Repeat the Day 1 schedule until you are doing well in mental health questions.

Day 5: Continue with content review and test question practice in all weak content areas. Practice deep breathing, regular exercise, journaling, and positive thinking. Continue this process until you are doing well in all areas of the exam. Study when you are most alert.

ARKO Test Taking Practice, the Second Element of NCLEX-RN Preparation

ARKO test taking practice is the second element needed for successful NCLEX-RN test completion. A strategy to improve test-taking skills includes practicing many high-quality test questions daily using the ARKO test-taking strategy and then reading the answer rationales on any questions you miss. The ARKO test-taking strategy includes:

- A Is the question stem asking for you to take Action or take no Action?

- R Reword the question.

- K Identify any Key words in the question stem.

- O Option elimination.

Apply the ARKO test-taking strategy to this test question:

  What should the nurse do first for a patient post spinal tap who complains of a headache?

  A. Insert a Foley catheter.

  B. Assess the patient's pupils.

  C. Obtain the patient's blood pressure.

  D. Place the patient flat.

Applying the ARKO test-taking strategy to the question above:

- A   Stem asks for nurse to take Action—i.e., What should the nurse do first?

- R   Reword the question as follows: What is a priority nursing action for a patient with a spinal tap who has a headache?

- K   Keywords are "first," "spinal tap," and "headache."

- O   Option elimination.
  Note the following:

Option A has nothing to do with a headache and will put the patient at risk for **catheter associated urinary tract infection** (CAUTI). Option B does not give us useful information about this patient with a spinal tap and a headache.

Option C is useful to assess blood pressure for signs of hypertension, but is not a priority.

Option D will reduce cerebrospinal fluid leakage by placing the patient flat, which is a common cause of headache after a spinal tap.

The correct answer is D.

Maslow's ABC-Safe Test Tips

As you review test questions, it is helpful to review the five categories of Maslow's Hierarchy of Needs (1943), that is physiological needs, safety needs, love and belonging needs, esteem needs, and self-actualization needs (Figure 25.2). NCLEX-RN predominately includes test questions that apply nursing's ability to meet patient needs related to Maslow's two most basic categories of needs, **ABC-SAFE,** i.e., physiological needs, e.g., **Airway, Breathing, Circulation,** food, water, etc.; and **Safety** needs, e.g., security of health, security of body, etc. When answering test questions, look for answers that meet patient needs in that order, physiological needs of **ABC** first, and then **Safety** needs (**ABC-Safe**). After these two basic categories of patient needs are met, other patient needs can be addressed, such as love and belonging needs, esteem needs, and self-actualization needs.

Application of Maslow's Hierarchy to a test question (Figure 25.2):

The nurse is unable to obtain a pedal pulse with doppler examination of the cold painful leg of a patient who has been casted a few hours ago for a fractured tibia. What is the priority intervention for this patient?

- A.   Administer Dilaudid 1.0 mg IVP, as ordered.

- B.   Obtain blankets to warm the cool extremity.

- C.   Notify the health care provider.

- D.   Split the cast with a cast cutter, per protocol.

Apply Maslow's Hierarchy to the question's options:

- A.   Comfort might be achieved with the pain medication, Dilaudid, but achieving the basic physiological need of arterial blood circulation is a higher priority.

- B.   Warmth might be achieved with blankets, but achieving the basic physiological need of arterial blood circulation is a higher priority.

- C.   Notifying the health care provider needs to be done, but this is not the priority choice.

- D.   Splitting the cast with a cast cutter, per protocol, is the correct answer. The patient identified in the question has no pedal pulse, his leg is cold and painful, and he has a new cast. This may be compartment syndrome caused by a tight cast as evidenced by the loss of pulse in the extremity.

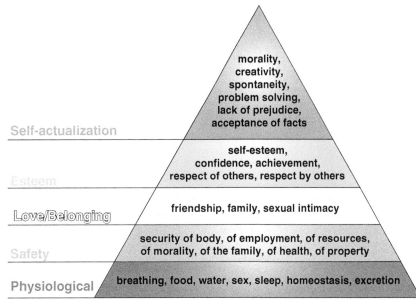

FIGURE 25.2   Maslow's Hierarchy of Need. *Source:* Maslow's Hierarchy of Human Needs (Finkelstein 2006). Public Domain.

The physiological need here is restoration of arterial blood flow before permanent tissue damage occurs. Splitting the cast with a cast cutter, following the cast cutting protocol in place on many orthopedic patient care units, will allow the extremity to re-establish blood flow quickly and is within the nurse's scope of practice. Then the nurse will notify the health care provider. The correct answer is D.

Consider sharing your test preparation plan and study calendars with a nursing friend. Ask them to check in with you to make sure you are sticking with it. By sharing your test preparation plan and study calendars, accountability is added. As you study, be sure to practice lots of test questions. Identify a quiet environment and avoid interruptions. Practice test questions and review content daily at a time that is a good study time for you, for example, early morning, afternoon, late at night, etc. After you have completed your daily test questions, score the test, review the answers, and read the rationales for any weak content areas. Repeat this process until you are doing well in all weak clinical content areas and in all areas of the NCLEX-RN examination test plan. Completing preparation for the NCLEX-RN examination in this way should improve your examination performance. Use methods of memory improvement that work for you. Mnemonic devices, where letters represent the first letters of items, are a useful means of recalling information as you study (Table 25.8).

Anxiety Management, the Third Element of NCLEX-RN Preparation

Anxiety management is an often overlooked, but essential part of NCLEX-RN preparation. Begin with a true assessment of yourself and how you manage anxiety. Does anxiety affect your sleeping, eating, studying, relationships, or performance on exams? If the answer is yes, to any of these questions, anxiety management is a way to alleviate these issues. From a physiological standpoint, small amounts of anxiety heighten awareness and can be a great motivator. However, when anxiety is overwhelming, it can cause many physiological imbalances as well as the inability to concentrate and effectively study. The anxiety management strategies presented here are only a fraction of the available options, for example, deep diaphragmatic breathing, regular exercise, journaling, positive thinking, mental imagery, listening to classical music, etc. Choose an anxiety management strategy that works for you. Consider looking into University and community resources. Most Universities have meditation classes, yoga, stress management workshops, one-on-one counseling, just to name a few resources. Additionally, if anxiety is interfering with your

test taking skills, consider visiting the Disability Center on campus to see if there are options available through the **Americans with Disabilities Act** (ADA) to allow a private testing environment or additional time to test while a student. If you require special accommodations for the NCLEX-RN, testing accommodations can only be authorized by the **State Board of Nursing** (SBON). See your individual SBON to determine the process for requesting special accommodations. Do not schedule your exam until confirmation of your special accommodations and the Authorization to Test (ATT) email lists the accommodations granted. If you have accommodations, you need to schedule your exam over the phone, not through the website (NCSBN NCLEX-RN Candidate Bulletin, 2020).

Maintaining PERMA

While in school, balance is difficult to achieve as studying seems to take all one's free time. If one studies all the time and disassociates themselves from the rest of their human needs, imbalance will occur. Maintaining PERMA (Seligman, 2019) is a way to help maintain balance. To do well in life, we need Positive (P) emotions; more Engagement (E) in our work, friendships, and love; better human Relationships (R); more Meaning (M) and purpose in life; and we want to be moving toward Achievement (A) of our goals. Maintaining PERMA in your life should also help in preparing for NCLEX-RN. An example of using PERMA for preparing for NCLEX-RN is as follows:

Positive Emotions—Each day I will remind myself how far I have come in the nursing program and how lucky I am to be here.

Engagement—I will be engaged in class while in class, engaged in studying when I study and engaged in my family and support system when I am with them.

Relationships—I will make time each day for people important to me, including myself.

Meaning—I will find meaning in each day as I become the person and the nurse I want to be.

Achievement—I will keep my "eye on the prize" of achieving NCLEX-RN success, no matter what it takes.

Avoidance of Negative Thinking

It is important to avoid negative thinking as you prepare for the NCLEX-RN. Hurst & Hurst (2018) suggest these tips to avoid negative thinking:

Table 25.8   A Mnemonic Device

A Mnemonic Device

It is "**OK**" to have your blood tested while on anticoagulants. This is a memory device to assist you in remembering the antidote for Coumadin overdose, that is, the antidote for Oral Coumadin is Vitamin K (Oral K=**OK**). Remembering this can help you recall this information as well as eliminate the antidote for the intravenous anticoagulant, Intravenous Heparin. Heparin's antidote is Protamine Sulfate.

Source: P. Kelly Vana.

1. Thought stopping. When a negative thought comes into your head, recognize it as negative and STOP it. Literally say, "get out of my head."

2. Positive affirmations. Saying is believing. Tell yourself, "I am smart, I trust myself, and I am a great nurse!" every day, multiple times a day.

3. Enforcing boundaries. When negative thoughts keep on coming, enforce a boundary, such as, only for the next 10 minutes will I think about these negative things. Once you do this, negative thoughts seem much less powerful.

4. Writing and destroying. When your thoughts are tied to emotions like fear of failing the NCLEX-RN, write out all your fears on a piece of paper and then symbolically destroy it. Rip it to shreds or safely burn the paper.

5. Just because. Remember, "Just because" I did poorly in an exam doesn't mean I am stupid or I'm not going to be a good nurse. Using your reasoning skills can help you think through a situation logically.

Declaring an Intention

When studying and preparing for the NCLEX-RN, it is useful to declare an intention. An **intention** is a purpose or aim. Intentions can and will change. One day, your intention may be to "find peace"; other days, it may be to, "do whatever it takes to be successful on NCLEX-RN." By declaring an intention, you give purpose to your actions. This will help you stay focused on your goal, passing the NCLEX-RN, and help you avoid negative thinking.

Meditation

People often have multiple things, such as "mind chatter" on their minds. This "mind chatter" that we may incessantly have on our minds was called chitta vritti or monkey mind by Pantanjuli & Gherwal (1979). Just like a monkey hopping from tree to tree, our minds are often chattering away at us. Realizing that we have this constant "mind chatter" and finding ways to slow our thoughts allows us to focus better on the task at hand. When studying, students should attempt to find a quiet environment to minimize noise and distractions. Put the timer on your phone for the amount of time you plan to study and do not pick up the phone again, not to check texts or social media, until the alarm rings. If using a computer, do not have multiple windows open that allow you to "drift" and end up shopping for shoes instead of studying. Commit yourself fully and be present when studying. This also allows "on" and "off" times for studying, and allows you to not think about studying when you are "off."

Meditation is a proven way to decrease stress and anxiety and slow down and clear your mind. When meditating, your thoughts slow down, your breath slows and deepens, and your focus is on the present. Meditation can be helpful even if only done for 1 or 2 minutes a day. Guided meditations are a great way to start meditating. In guided meditation, all you do is find a comfortable spot and listen to the meditation guide. There are many meditation apps available for free or a nominal cost. These include:

- The Mindfulness App
- Headspace App
- Calm App
- Smiling Mind App
- Insight Timer App

All apps are available at www.healthline.com/health/mental-health/top-meditation-iphone-android-apps#the-mindfulness-app, accessed April 10, 2019.

Visualization is a type of meditation with an emphasis on the future. Seeing is believing. By visualizing an event in the future, we cannot only "see" it in our minds eye, but we can shape how it unfolds. By visualizing, we can build in success and confidence in an event that hasn't taken place to try to make our visualization become reality. Try this simple exercise and repeat often:

1. Find a quiet spot where you can sit comfortably, uninterrupted

2. Close your eyes and "see" yourself:
   - Driving to the Pearson VUE center
   - Checking in with a receptionist
   - Sitting down to take the NCLEX-RN exam
   - Taking up to 265 questions
   - Walking out of the center not knowing if you passed or not
   - Dealing with the of uncertainty of waiting till your results are available
   - Waking up and checking the state website and seeing your name, your license number, and your license status as active

3. Remember the great feeling this exercise leaves you with, the satisfaction and joy of achieving the goal of becoming a Registered Nurse

4. When you are tired, stressed, or wondering why you are doing all of this NCLEX-RN preparation, remember how it "feels" to be an RN

Nutrition, Sleep, and Wardrobe

You will function best in the NCLEX-RN if you are well nourished. Plan to eat three well-balanced meals a day for at least 3 days prior to the examination. Be careful when choosing the food that you consume within 24 hr of the examination. Avoid alcohol, stimulants, and foods that will make you thirsty or cause intestinal distress. Minimize the

Evidence from the Literature

Source: Flavin. (2016). 7 Expert Tips to Survive Stress and Get Through Nursing School. Retrieved from www.rasmussen.edu/degrees/nursing/blog/7-expert-tips-to-survive-stress-get-through-nursing-school

Discussion: Tips for surviving nursing school are abundant, most of these tips work for school as well as for studying for NCLEX-RN. Flavin (2016) published 7 Expert Tips to Survive Stress and Get Through Nursing School that include:

1. Practice an after-class-recap, or going through the materials that were just covered in class after class.
2. Find a solid study group.
3. Mix exercise into your study sessions.
4. Begin a study session with a simple meditation.
5. Journal before bed.
6. Figure out what enhances your mood.
7. Eat well and nurture your body.

Implications for Practice: Utilizing these tips can improve your stress levels while in nursing school. These practices help incorporate healthy practices into students' life styles and will ultimately help with studying for the NCLEX-RN Examination and success.

potential of a full bladder midway through the examination by limiting the amount of fluids you drink and by allowing sufficient time at the test site to use the bathroom before entering the room.

Plan to allow enough time in your schedule the week before the examination to provide yourself with the sleep you need to function effectively. Plan your wardrobe ahead of time. Shoes and clothes that fit you comfortably will not distract your thought processes during the examination. Consider dressing in layers that can be easily removed in case the testing room is too cool or too hot. Your clothes for the test day should be ready to wear by the night before the examination. If you wear glasses or contact lenses, take along an extra pair of glasses. If you are taking medications on a regular basis, continue to do so during this period of time.

Some Final Tips and a Medication Study Guide

Table 25.9 has some final tips on organizing for the NCLEX-RN. Table 25.10 is a medication study guide to aid you in your NCLEX-RN preparation. Table 25.11 has common food sources for various nutrients and diets. Use these Tables to prepare for NCLEX-RN. Be sure to organize your study.

In this chapter you have learned about the present and next generation NCLEX-RN exam, everything from how it is constructed to instructions on how to sign up. Multiple study tips and aids have been provided to help you to be successful. Now it is up to you to implement what you have learned and plan for your NCLEX-RN exam success.

Case Study 25.1

Analyze your NCLEX-RN learning needs, based on Table 25.5. Use Table 25.7, the NCLEX-RN Daily Preparation Calendar, to identify your best time to practice NCLEX-RN questions and review content and practice test taking. Complete your study schedule for the next 4–8 weeks. When is the best time to study? Note the NCLEX-RN licensure examination tutorial (Pearson Education, Inc., 2011) and the NCSBN NCLEX-RN weekly Question of the week at The Learning Extension (NCSBN, n.d. Retrieved May 15, 2019 from: https://ww2.learningext.com). Did you get the correct answer to the Question of the week?

Are you planning to take an NCLEX-RN Review course?

Real World Interview

I believe some students deny their anxiety about taking the NCLEX-RN by saying it is not a big deal. If they fail it, they can always retake it. However, it *is* a big deal—you have given years of your life preparing to become a registered nurse, and you want to be successful the first time you take the licensing exam. My advice to you is to use your HESI Exit Exam score sheets to identify your weaknesses. Study carefully all subject content areas for which you received a score of less than 850, particularly if the content area is medical-surgical or management, each of which makes up a large part of the licensing exam.

Susan Morrison, RN, PhD, FAAN
Nurse Consultant
Houston, Texas

Table 25.9   Final NCLEX-RN Tips

Remember Maslow ABC-SAFE as you answer questions. Patients' Physiological Needs are met first—e.g., Patients with Airway, Breathing, or Circulation (ABCs) Problems,

- Patients with Airway Problems
  - Altered Level of Consciousness (LOC)
  - Unconscious
  - Foreign Object in Airway
- Patients with Breathing Problems
  - Asthma
  - Chronic Obstructive Pulmonary Disease (COPD)
- Patients with Circulation Problems
  - Cardiac Arrest
  - Shock
- Patients' Safety Needs are met second—
  - Patients who have Tuberculosis
  - Patients who are Infectious
  - Patients who are threatening Suicide
- Think ABC-SAFE. Physiological needs (ABC's) are met first and foremost, followed by Safety needs. These ABC-SAFE needs must be met before higher needs can be met.
- Love and Belonging needs, Esteem needs, and Self-Actualization needs are addressed later. Don't consider a test question answer that meets the patient's love and belonging needs, esteem needs, or self-actualization needs until the patient's ABC-SAFE needs have been met.
- Remember the Nursing Process when answering test questions: Assess your patient first, then Plan, Implement, and Evaluate.
- Keep all your patients safe—Anticipate problems and maintain an open airway; side rails up; IV access line in place on unstable patient; monitor vital signs, pulse oximeter, cardiac rhythm, urine output, as needed.
- Follow Delegation Guidelines for RNs, LPNs, and Nursing Assistive Personnel (NAP). Observe the Rights of Delegation including, the right task, the right circumstance, the right person, the right direction/communication, and the right supervision (see Chapter 18).
  - The RN assures quality care of all patients, especially complex patients. RNs can delegate care of stable patients with predictable outcomes.
  - The RN uses patient care data such as vital signs, collected either by the nurse or others, to make clinical judgments. The RN continuously monitors and evaluates patient care and gives care involving standard, unchanging procedures to LPNs and NAP.
  - The RN never delegates patient Assessment, Teaching, Evaluation (ATE), or Judgment.
  - LPNs perform medication administration (oral meds and intramuscular and subcutaneous injections), sterile dressings, Foley insertions, and so on.
  - NAPs perform basic care—e.g., vital sign measurement, bathing, transferring, ambulating, communicating with patients, and stocking supplies.
  - In some states, with approval of the state board of nursing and documented competency of education and experience, LPNs can insert IVs, pass nasogastric tubes, and so on.
  - In some states, with approval of the state board of nursing and documented competency of education and experience, NAP can perform venipuncture, do blood glucose tests, insert Foley catheters, and so on.
- When delegating care, don't mix a patient with Human Immunodeficiency Virus (HIV), Tuberculosis, or other infectious disease, with a patient who has decreased immunity, e.g., a patient with diabetes, patient on steroids, a very young patient, a very old patient, etc.
- In answering test questions, remember the following:
  - When choosing patient care priorities, choose the first answer you would do if you were alone and could only do one thing at a time. Don't think that one RN will do one thing and another RN will do another thing.
  - Assume that you have the practitioner's order for any possible choices on the exam.
  - The NCLEX-RN exam is usually looking for the correct *nursing* action. Review exam questions carefully to see if there is a nursing action that can be completed before choosing an answer of, "call the health care provider."
  - Taking action to help the patient first is usually the top priority answer to NCLEX-RN test questions.
  - Assume that you have perfect staffing, plenty of time, and all the necessary equipment for any possible test question choices on the exam. Choose the answer that indicates the best nursing care possible.
  - Assume that you are able to give perfect care "By the book." Don't let your personal clinical experience direct you to choose a test answer that is less than high-quality care.
  - Remember to care for the patient first and then check the equipment.
- Know the most common medical-surgical, maternal-child, and mental health care disorders. For each disorder, know the medications, diet, laboratory and diagnostic tools, procedures, and evidence-based nursing care and treatments commonly used.
- Know common medications (see Table 25.10).
- Know common laboratory norms—e.g., arterial blood gas (ABG), sodium, potassium, blood sugar, hemoglobin A1C, complete blood count, hematocrit, prothrombin time, partial thromboplastin time, international normalized ratio (INR), cardiac enzymes, lactate levels, blood urea nitrogen (BUN), creatinine, digoxin level, dilantin level, lithium level, and the specific gravity of urine.
- Know how to utilize medication protocols such as sliding scale Insulin and heparin protocols.
- Know communication techniques—look for answers that give patients support and allow the patient to keep talking and verbalize concerns and problems. Be a comforting nurse, not a therapist. Avoid advice.
- Know common food sources for various nutrients and diets (Table 25.11).
- Know the common defense mechanisms.

(Continued)

Table 25.9 **(Continued)**

- Know growth and development, such as the developmental tasks for each childhood stage, toys for each childhood stage, and so on.
- Know immunization schedules (Centers for Disease Control and Prevention, 2019, available at www.cdc.gov/vaccines/schedules/index.html, accessed April 15, 2019.

Prepare mentally with the following:
- Anxiety management strategies
- Regular exercise
- Maintaining PERMA
- Avoiding automatic negative thoughts

- Meditation
- Visualize your name with RN next to it on your name tag.
- Remember—you graduated from an accredited nursing program. You can do it!

Source: P. Kelly Vana.

Table 25.10 **Medication Study Guide**

(Add to Medication Study Guide below as you study)
General Tips
1. Drowsiness and changes in Vital Signs (VS) are a side effect of many medications given for their analgesic, antiemetic, antiseizure, tranquilizer, sedative/hypnotic, antihistamine, or anxiolytic effects.
2. If medication has side effect of drowsiness/changes in vital signs,
   - Monitor Airway, Level of Consciousness (LOC), Blood Pressure (BP), Pulse (P), Respirations (R), Pulse Oximetry

   - Consider the need for:
     - Side Rails Up/Fall Precautions
     - Intravenous (IV) Line inserted to safeguard patient
     - Cardiac Monitor
     - Avoid Driving and Alcohol
3. If medication given for Cardiac or Hypertension Problem Monitor for:
   - Blood Pressure (BP) and Pulse (P)
     - Postural Hypotension
4. Many medications cause renal, liver, heart, brain, and/or bone marrow side effects. Monitor related labs.
5. Learn the generic and trade names, action, nursing implications, related labs to monitor, and side effects of all the medications in this table. Be familiar with Chemotherapy guidelines also.

prefix, root, suffix	generic name(Trade name)	Category	Nursing implications
cort- pred- -sone	dexamethasone (Decadron) prednisone (Deltasone) methylprednisolone (Depo-Medrol, Medrol)	Corticosteroid	• Anti-inflammatory effects, (e.g., decreased inflammation in arthritis) • Monitor labs for ↑Sodium, ↑Sugar, ↓Potassium • Monitor for depression or psychiatric disturbances • Wean off (taper) med to avoid Adrenal Shock
-olone	hydrocortisone (Solu-Cortef)		
-onide	budesonide (Uceris, Pulmicort)		
		Antibiotics	• Check allergy • Monitor liver and renal labs • Check culture and sensitivity report • Monitor many antibiotics for C. diff side effect[b]
ceph- cef-	cephalexin (Keflex) ceftriaxone(Rocephin) cefepime (Maxipime)	cephalosporin	• Monitor for Steven Johnson syndrome[a] • Monitor CBCs • Side effect = diarrhea, *C. diff*
-cillin	penicillin amoxicillin (Amoxil)	beta-lactams	• Monitor for any signs of anaphylaxis/hypersen-sitivity reaction • Side effect = diarrhea, *C.diff*

(Continued)

Table 25.10 (Continued)

- floxacin	ciprofloxacin (Cipro) levofloxacin (Levaquin) moxifloxacin (Avelox)	fluoroquinolone	• Monitor CK→ possible side effect of tendon rupture • Monitor QT→ QT prolongation • Monitor glucose levels • Side effect: altered mental status, seizures, diarrhea, C. *diff*
-cycline	tetracycline (Sumycin) doxycycline (Vibramycin)	tetracycline derivatives	• Side effect: Can cause staining of developing teeth and photosensitivity • Monitor for thrombophlebitis and irritation at IV site • Monitor for adequate hydration
-mycin	gentamycin (Garamycin) tobramycin amikacin vancomycin (Vancocin)	Aminoglyco-sides and glycopeptides	• Monitor peak and trough levels • Monitor renal labs and intake and output • Monitor for ototoxicity
sulfa-	sulfamethoxazole (Gantanol) sulfasalazine (Azulfidine)		• Check for sulfa allergy • Monitor potassium • Maintain adequate fluid intake to prevent stone forma-tion • Monitor for Steven Johnson syndrome. • Monitor glucose levels • Monitor for rash, blood dyscrasias, and CNS changes
	Antifungals		
-azole	fluconazole (Diflucan) miconazole (Monistat) voriconazole (Vfend) itraconazole (Sporanox)	antifungals	• Monitor QT→ QT prolongation and ECG changes • Monitor renal/hepatic function • Monitor K+ levels • Monitor for signs of rash or dermatologic changes • Monitor for vision changes
	Antivirals		
-vir;	abacavir (Ziagen) acyclovir (Zovirax) valacyclovir (Valtrex) valganciclovir (Valcyte)	antivirals	• Perform HLA-B*5701 testing prior to initiation of abacavir. If test (+), drug is contraindicated. • Monitor hepatic/renal function. • Hep B/Hep C screen prior to initiation. • Monitor for signs of hypersensitivity reaction • Assess risk factors for heart disease
-tadine	amantadine (Symmetrel) rimantadine (Flumadine)		• Monitor renal function • Do not stop abruptly • Monitor for CNS effects such as depression/hallucination • Monitor BP • Not recommended for prophylaxis or treatment of influ-enza A due to issues of resistance
	Heart Medication		
Dig-	digoxin (Lanoxin)	anti-arrhythmic	• Monitor K level; Monitor digoxin levels • Educate on signs of toxicity (yellow vision, nausea/vomit-ing, altered mental status and halo vision around lights) • Monitor ECG and/or apical pulse • Patient prone to Digoxin toxicity if K is low
-caine	lidocaine (Xylocaine)	Anti-Arrhythmic; Local Anesthetic	• Side effect = skin discoloration (topical), CNS changes • Monitor ECG, BP, and respiratory rate • Monitor for CNS toxicity • Patient in supine position = Decreased hypotensive effects

Table 25.10 **(Continued)**

-one	amiodarone (Cordarone) dronedarone (Multaq)	Anti-Arrhythmic	• Monitor for cardiac and CNS changes • Monitor for pulmonary toxicity • Monitor bradycardia, hypotension. • Monitor thyroid function • Avoid extravasation; vesicant. • Monitor Steven-Johnson syndrome and Toxic Epidermal Necrolysis (TEN).
	Anticoagulants		
-arin	warfarin (Coumadin) heparin	Oral anticoagulant parenteral anticoagulant	• Coumadin is an oral med; takes days to take effect; • monitor INR; antidote is Vitamin K • Monitor for signs of bleeding • Heparin is a parenteral med; • Onset of action is immediate; • monitor PTT; • antidote is Protamine Sulfate • Monitor for signs of bleeding
	BP Meds		• Monitor BP • Normal BP is Less than 120/80 mmHg • Monitor postural hypotension
-dipine	amlodipine (Norvasc) nifedipine (Adalat, Procardia)	Dihydro-pyridine Calcium Channel Blocker	• Side effects = hypotension, peripheral edema, angina, weight
-pril	lisinopril (Zestril) captopril (Capoten) ramipril (Altace)	ACE Inhibitors	• Side effects = dry cough, hypotension • Adverse effect = angioedema • Monitor for hyperkalemia, increased serum creatinine and other metabolic abnormalities
-olol	metoprolol tartrate (Lopressor) metoprolol succinate (Toprol XL) propranolol (Inderal)	Beta Blocker	• Side effects = Bradycardia, fatigue, postural hypotension, depression, and bronchospasm • Monitor BP, HR, and rhythm • Monitor for altered glucose levels • Monitor for fluid status changes.
-pres	clonidine (Catapres) hydralazine (Apresoline)	alpha$_2$ agonist vasodilator	• Side effects = CNS depression, bradycardia (clonidine), tachycardia (hydralazine), hypotension • Monitor standing and supine BP • Do not stop clonidine abruptly • If epidural: monitor for infection and catheter blockage (clonidine) • Transdermal patch must be taken off before an MRI, cardioversion, or defibrillation (clonidine) • monitor for fluid retention
-sartan	telmisartan (Micardis) losartan (Cozaar) valsartan (Diovan)	Angiotensin II Receptor Antagonist (ARB)	• Side effects: hypotension, angioedema • Monitor blood pressure • Monitor for abnormalities in electrolytes and renal function
-zosin	doxazosin (Cardura) prazosin (Minipress)	Alpha$_1$ Blocker	• Side effect = priapism, orthostatic hypotension, angioedema, dizziness • Monitor BP, Intake and Output, and CNS changes
Nitr-	nitroglycerin (Nitrostat) nitroprusside sodium (Nipride)	vasodilators	• Monitor for hypotension, bradycardia • Side effect = headache, dizziness. Flushing • Nitrate free interval recommended • Thiocyanate toxicity: Can occur and may be life-threatening when levels reach 200 mg/L (nitroprusside)

(Continued)

Table 25.10   (Continued)

	Thrombolytic		
-ase	alteplase		Give IV within 4.5 hrs of ischemic CVA symptoms if patient meets inclusion criteria; Can also be used for treatment of MI, PE, DVT[b], or arterial occlusion • Monitor BP closely during administration • Many contraindications exist – must closely review list to ensure proper patient selection • Observe the patient for signs of bleeding while on alteplase • Observe patient for hypersensitivity during infusion
	Bronchodilator		
-phylline	aminophylline theophylline	Phosphodie-sterase inhibitor	• Avoid extravasation; vesicant • monitor temperature • side effects = irritability, dizziness, headache
-terol	albuterol(Proventil)	beta$_2$ agonist	• Check for rapid pulse and Nausea and Vomiting • Monitor Blood Pressure
	Diuretic		• Monitor electrolytes (especially check for low K level) and glucose • Monitor renal function (Creatinine and BUN) • Monitor Intake/Output • Watch for signs of excessive diuresis • High IV doses can cause ototoxicity
-semide	furosemide (Lasix) torsemide (Demadex) bumetanide (Bumex)	Loop Diuretic	• Monitor electrolytes • Monitor uric acid • Monitor renal/hepatic function • ototoxicity seen at drug rates of >4 mg/min for intermittent infusions • Monitor BP and diuresis
-thiazide	chlorothiazide (Diuril) hydrochlorothiazide (Microzide)	Thiazide Diuretic	• Monitor electrolytes/ uric acid • Monitor BP • Monitor renal/hepatic function • possible phototoxicity.
	Analgesics		• Monitor drowsiness
-coxib	celecoxib (Celebrex)	NSAID	• Monitor renal function • Monitor for GI bleed • Sulfa allergy contraindicated • Monitor blood pressure.
-profen	ibuprofen (Advil) ketorolac (Toradol)	NSAID	• Monitor for renal function. • Monitor for GI bleed/active bleed • Check allergies
-ine	morphine codeine	Opioid analgesic	• Addictive; • Side effects = drowsiness, constipation, itching • Monitor respiratory rate/respiratory depression
-triptan	almotriptan (Axert) sumatriptan (Imitrex)	Anti-migraine	• Monitor ↑blood pressure, CNS depression • Side effects = vision loss, dizziness, hypertension
	Other Medications		
-prazole	pantoprazole (Protonix) omeprazole (Prilosec) lansoprazole (Prevacid)	Proton Pump Inhibitor (PPI)	• Side effect = C. diff. • Monitor magnesium and Vitamin B12
-statin	atorvastatin (Lipitor) pravastatin (Pravachol)	Anti-cholesterol	• Monitor leg cramps/muscle pain • Monitor **creatine kinase (CK)** due to possible rhabdomyolysis.

Table 25.10 (Continued)

-dronate	alendronate (Fosamax) ibandronate (Boniva)	Bisphos-phonates	• Bone/joint/muscle pain, GI irritation 30–60 min before food/medications. • Must be taken in upright position, avoid laying down for 30–60 min. • In rare cases osteonecrosis of the jaw has occurred
-setron	Granisetron (Kytril) ondansetron (Zofran)	Antiemetic and Antinauseant	• Monitor drowsiness • Monitor QT → QT prolongation • Side effects = drowsiness, constipation, headache.
	Antidepressants		**Monitor drowsiness**
-triptyline	amitriptyline (Elavil) nortriptyline (Pamelor)	TriCyclic Antidepressant (TCA)	• Side effects = blurred vision, constipation, xerostomia, urinary retention • Monitor mental status, suicide ideation, and orthostatic hypotension
-ipramine	desipramine (Norpramin) trimipramine (Surmontil)	TriCyclic Antidepressant (TCA)	• Side effects = blurred vision, constipation, xerostomia, urinary retention • Monitor mental status, suicide ideation, and orthostatic hypotension
-zodone	nefazodone (Serzone), trazodone (Desyrel)	Antidepressant	• Side effects = blurred vision, constipation, xerostomia, urinary retention • Monitor mental status, suicide ideation
-azine	prochlorperazine (Compazine) chlorpromazine (Thorazine)	Antiemetic and Antipsychotic	• Monitor drowsiness, hypotension, and anticholinergic effects • May increase risk for falls
-eridone	iloperidone (Fanapt) risperidone (Risperdal)	Atypical antipsychotic	• Monitor orthostatic hypotension • Side effect = corrected **QT interval(QTc)** prolongation; • extrapyramidal symptoms
-atadine	desloratadine (Clarinex.) loratadine(Claritin);	Antihistamine, Anti-Allergy	• Monitor drowsiness
-azolam	alprazolam (Xanax); midazolam (Versed)	Tranquilizer; Benzodiazepine	• Monitor drowsiness • Monitor Respiratory rate/depression • Avoid abrupt discontinuation
-azepam	diazepam (Valium); lorazepam (Ativan);	Tranquilizer; Benzodiazepine Sedative	• Side effects = anterograde amnesia, Central Nervous System depression • Monitor blood pressure • Monitor respiratory rate/depression. • Avoid abrupt discontinuation
	Antidiabetic Agents		**Monitor blood glucose**
-gliptin	saxagliptin (Onglyza) sitagliptin (Januvia)	DPP-4 inhibitor	• Side effect = arthralgia • Monitor for hypersensitivity reactions • Monitor for angioedema • Monitor for hypoglycemia • Monitor renal function.
-glitazone	pioglitazone (Actos) rosiglitazone (Avandia)	Thiazolidine-dione	• Monitor for heart failure (rapid weight gain, edema, dyspnea). • Monitor hepatic function.

[a] Stevens-Johnson syndrome/toxic epidermal necrolysis (SJS/TEN) is a severe skin reaction most often triggered by particular medications. Severe damage to the skin and mucous membranes makes SJS/TEN a life-threatening disease, developed with information from, https://ghr.nlm.nih.gov/condition/stevens-johnson-syndrome-toxic-epidermal-necrolysis, accessed August 14, 2019.

[b] Clostridium difficile (C difficile) is responsible for 20–30% of antibiotic-associated diarrhea cases and is the most common cause of infectious diarrhea in the health care setting.

Table 25.10   (Continued)

Antipsychotics	Antidepressants	Mood Stabilizers	Cardiac Drugs
Zyprexa	Celexa	Lithium	Diltiazem;
Seroquel	Cymbalta	Depakote	Epinephrine;
Haldol	Lexapro	Tegretol	Norpace (Disopy-ramide);
Prolixin	Zoloft		Rythmol (Propa-fenone);
Abilify	Paxil		Tambocor (Flecainide);
Risperdal	Prozac		Betapace (Sotalol)
	Remeron		
	Venlafaxine		

Note: Miotic eye drops constrict the pupils, Mydriatic eye drops dilate the pupils *Source:* Developed with information from Lina Piech, Pharm.D., BCPS, Advocate Christ Medical Center, Oak Lawn, Illinois, lina.piech@advocatehealth.com, and Patricia Kelly Vana, RN, M.S.N.

Table 25.11   Common Food Sources for Various Nutrients and Diets

Nutrient:	Common Sources:
Iron	Iron in animal foods (heme iron) is best absorbed when eaten in a meal containing Vitamin C: Liver/liver sausage, beef, chicken, eggs, pork Non-heme iron sources (less efficiently absorbed than heme iron): Dark green leafy vegetables, fortified breakfast cereals, kidney beans and other legumes, whole grain breads/cereals
Potassium	Bananas, cantaloupe, oranges/orange juice, potatoes, honey dew, apricots, grapefruit, prunes/prune juice, raisins, dates
Vitamin C (antioxidant)	Citrus fruits (e.g., oranges, grapefruit), strawberries, sweet peppers, tomatoes, lemons, limes
Vitamin D	Exposure to sunshine! Cod liver oil, fatty fish (e.g., tuna, salmon/canned salmon with bones), most milk, cheese, yogurt (Check label)
Vitamin E (antioxidant)	Nuts, salad dressings, vegetable oils, wheat germ, whole grain breads/cereals/starches
Calcium	Milk, cheese, yogurt, dark leafy green vegetables, fortified cereal, fortified orange juice

Therapeutic Diets:	Foods to Avoid on Diet:
Bland/Soft	Generally, avoid caffeine, chocolate, fatty/fried foods, fresh fruit (except banana), raw vegetables, tomato products/acidic foods, spicy foods, whole grain breads/cereals/pasta Eat smaller, more frequent meals.
Diabetic	Generally, avoid foods/beverages containing regular sugar (e.g., cakes, candy, cookies, ice cream, pies, soda, sweetened juices, jams/jellies, syrup) <u>or</u> reduce portion size to meet individualized carbohydrate allowance. Do not skip meals. Learn how to "Carbohydrate Count." Plan meals in advance for consistent carbohydrate intake at meals and to balance medication interactions to promote acceptable blood sugar.
Gluten Free	Avoid foods containing white flour, wheat flour (e.g., breads, rolls, pastries, desserts, crackers, cereals, noodles/pasta), barley, oats, and/or rye Look for "Gluten Free" on the package label.
Low Fat/Low Cholesterol	Avoid bacon, sausage, fried foods, gravies/sauces made with butter, whole milk/whole-milk cheese/cream Remove visible fat from meat; remove skin from poultry.
Low Sodium	Avoid bacon, sausage, corned beef, ham, hot dogs, deli-style meats, cheese, canned soups, snack foods (e.g., potato chips, pretzels, crackers), canned vegetables, prepared salad dressings, condiments (e.g., ketchup, mustard, soy sauce, steak sauce), packaged rice and noodle mixes, some frozen entrees Do not add salt in cooking or at table.
Low Protein	Restrict intake of beef, chicken, eggs, fish, pork, turkey, dairy products, legumes to what MD has ordered for individualized plan Restriction varies. In general, 1 oz. meat = 7 g protein. Plan meals in advance and monitor correct portion sizes.

Selected Diet Needs:	Food Choices:
High Calorie	Increase intake of food such as, avocados, butter, cheese, cream, ice cream, mayonnaise, oil-based salad dressings, olives, peanut butter, nuts

(Continued)

Table 25.11 (Continued)

High Fiber	Increase intake of foods such as, fresh fruit (eat with peel or skin, when appropriate; e.g., apples, pears, peaches), legumes, nuts, peas, whole kernel corn, raw vegetables, whole grain breads/cereals/starches
High Protein	Increase intake of beef, chicken, eggs, fish, pork, turkey, dairy products, legumes to what MD has ordered for individualized plan In general, 1 oz. meat = 7 g protein.

Source: Developed by Georgia Hammerli, RD, LDN, Registered Dietitian, Clinical Nutrition Manager-Unidine, Arlington Heights, Illinois.

KEY CONCEPTS

- Client needs tested on NCLEX-RN include Safe and Effective Care Environment (Management of Care and Safety and Infection Control); Health Promotion and Maintenance; Psychosocial Integrity; and Physiological Integrity (Basic Care and Comfort, Pharmacological, and Parenteral Therapies, Reduction of Risk Potential, and Physiological Adaptation).

- Integrated Processes throughout the four major categories of Client Needs include the Nursing Process, Caring, Communication and Documentation, and Teaching/Learning.

- Each of the NCLEX-RN Client Needs have a list of sample client need activities in the Test Plan that can be reviewed as part of exam preparation.

- The CJM was designed to explore new ways of testing clinical judgment in the nursing profession as part of NCLEX-RN.

- NCLEX-RN candidates receive between 75 and 265 questions in the NCLEX-RN computer adaptive examination during the exam session.

- The decision as to whether a candidate passes or fails the NCLEX-RN is guided by three different rules, i.e., the 95% Confidence Interval Rule, the Maximum-Length Exam Rule, and the Run-Out-Of-Time (R.O.O.T) Rule.

- NCLEX-RN question formats may include but are not limited to multiple choice (one answer), multiple response (select one or more answers), fill in the blank calculation, hot spots, exhibit, drop and drag/ordered response, audio, and graphics. All questions may include multimedia, such as charts, graphics, and audio.

- Examples of all the formats used in the NCLEX-RN test questions are available in the 2019 National Council Licensure Examination Test Plan for Registered Nurses.

- The NCSBN's Learning Extension website offers a Weekly "NCLEX-RN-Style" Question of the week.

- Several academic and non-academic factors have been identified in research studies as being associated with performance on the NCLEX-RN examination. Review these factors in the chapter's tables and consider them, but know that, to date, there is no evidence of what specifically makes an NCLEX-RN candidate successful.

- NCLEX-RN review materials are available from books, live courses, and integrated online courses. They often focus on nursing content, test taking skills, or both.

- NCLEX-RN review courses are a great way to help a candidate organize their NCLEX-RN preparation.

- Exit exams are created to mimic the NCLEX-RN exam and predict if candidates will pass NCLEX-RN.

- When students prepare to take the NCLEX-RN, they will use a plan that includes three elements, i.e., NCLEX-RN learning needs analysis, test taking practice, and anxiety management.

- Use Table 25.5 to complete your NCLEX-RN Learning Needs Analysis.

- Use Table 25.6 to establish an NCLEX-RN 8-week preparation calendar.

- Practice testing, scoring, and reading the rationales of at least 60 NCLEX-RN test questions daily.

- Use Table 25.7, the NCLEX-RN Daily Preparation Calendar, to organize your daily study.

- Test taking practice is the second element needed for successful NCLEX-RN test completion. This strategy includes practicing many high-quality test questions daily using the ARKO test-taking strategy and then reading the answer rationales on any questions you miss.

- Anxiety Management Is the Third Element of NCLEX-RN Preparation

- Small amounts of anxiety heighten awareness and can be a great motivator. However, when anxiety is overwhelming, it can cause many physiological imbalances as well as the inability to concentrate and effectively study

- To do well in life, we need PERMA, i.e., Positive (P) emotions; more Engagement (E) in our work, friendships, and love; better human Relationships (R); more Meaning (M) and purpose in life; and we want to be moving toward Achievement (A) of our goals.

- Mnemonic devices, where letters represent the first letters of items, are a useful means of recalling information as you study (Table 25.8).

- Avoid Negative Thinking as you prepare for NCLEX-RN. Avoidance of negative thinking includes: Thought stopping, Positive affirmations, Enforcing boundaries, and Writing and destroying.

- Avoid "mind chatter," also referred to as chitta vritti or monkey mind by Pantanjuli & Gherwal (1979). When studying, students should attempt to find a quiet environment to minimize noise and distractions.

- There are many meditation apps available for free or a nominal cost.

- By visualizing an event in the future, we cannot only "see" it, but we can shape how it unfolds.

- By declaring an intention, you stay focused on your goal, passing the NCLEX-RN.

- Pay attention to Nutrition, Sleep, and Wardrobe prior to the NCLEX-RN.

- The anxiety management items presented here are only a fraction of the available options, e.g., deep diaphragmatic breathing, regular exercise, journaling, positive thinking, mental imagery, listening to classical music, etc. Choose a strategy that works for you.

- Review Medications and common food sources for the NCLEX-RN.

KEY TERMS

Visualization	Self-efficacy	logit
Intention	Clinical judgment model	

REVIEW QUESTIONS

1. Which of the following isolation measures would the nurse institute when a patient has tuberculosis? Select all that apply.
   a. Use gloves when there is risk of exposure to blood or body fluids.
   b. Use gloves at all times when caring for patients.
   c. Place patient in a private, negative airflow pressure room.
   d. Use a mask at all times while in the patient's room.
   e. Place a mask on the patient when transporting him or her out of the room.

2. The nurse is caring for a patient with Alzheimer's disease. Which of the following factors are associated with this disease? Select all that apply.
   a. Reversible disease
   b. Amyloid plaques
   c. Acute onset
   d. Personality changes
   e. Impaired memory

3. A 3-year-old girl is admitted with epiglottitis. She is drooling, sitting upright, unable to swallow, and looking panicky. Which of the following equipment is most important for the nurse to place at the patient's bedside?
   a. Suction
   b. Croup tent
   c. Tracheotomy set
   d. Padded bedsides for seizure precautions

4. A nurse has just drawn arterial blood gases on a patient. Which of the following is important for the nurse to do?
   a. Apply pressure to the puncture site for 5 min.
   b. Shake the vial of blood before transporting it to the lab.
   c. Keep the patient on bed rest for 1 hr.
   d. Encourage the patient to cough and deep-breathe.

5. The nurse is administering an intramuscular injection to a 1-year-old patient. Which of the following sites is most appropriate for the nurse to select?
   a. Ventral forearm
   b. Ventral gluteal
   c. Vastus lateralis
   d. Dorsal gluteal

6. A low-sodium, low-fat diet has been prescribed for a patient with hypertension. The nurse knows that the patient understands his diet when he selects which of the following menus?
   a. Steak, baked potato, peas, and hot coffee
   b. Macaroni and cheese casserole, tossed salad with dressing, and hot chocolate
   c. Baked chicken, steamed broccoli and cauliflower, steamed rice, and hot tea
   d. Fried chicken, mashed potatoes, green beans, and milk

7. The nurse is caring for a patient who is having a panic attack. Which symptom will the patient be least likely to exhibit?
   a. Choking
   b. Chest pain
   c. Bradycardia
   d. Shortness of breath

8. The nurse is caring for a patient with angina. Nitroglycerin is prescribed for what purpose?
   a. To assist smooth muscles to relax
   b. To decrease venous return to the heart
   c. To increase preload and afterload
   d. To slow and strengthen the heart rate

9. Which special precautions must the nurse take when assisting a patient with self-monitoring of blood glucose?
   a. Wear gloves when performing the test.
   b. Rinse the lancet between uses.
   c. Recalibrate the glucometer before each use.
   d. Give the patient a machine for his use only.

10. The nurse is caring for a postoperative patient who develops a wound dehiscence. Which of the following will the nurse do when this occurs?
    a. Approximate the wound edges with tape.
    b. Irrigate the wound with sterile saline.
    c. Cover the wound with sterile, moist saline dressings.
    d. Hold the abdominal contents in place with a sterile, gloved hand.

REVIEW QUESTION ANSWERS

1. Answers A, C, D, and E are correct.
   Rationale: Droplet precautions include (A) use gloves when there is risk of exposure to blood or body fluids. (C) Place patient in a private, negative airflow pressure room. (D) Use a mask at all times while in the patient's room and (E) place a mask on the patient when transporting him or her out of the room. Incorrect response is (B) using gloves at all times when caring for a patient is NOT correct nor required for droplet precautions.

2. Answers B, D, and E are correct.
   Rationale: Facts regarding Alzheimer's disease include (B) Amyloid plaques (are present on imaging), (D) personality changes, and (E) impaired memory. It is untrue or false regarding Alzheimer's disease that it is (A) a reversible disease. The onset is slow, not acute (C).

3. Answer: C is correct.
   Rationale: (C) Tracheotomy set is emergency equipment that is necessary to have at the bedside with severe respiratory distress. Incorrect responses include (A) suction is important, but not the most important, (B) a croup tent may be helpful later but this patient is too acute for this intervention, and (D) padded bedsides for seizure precautions will not help at all in this situation.

4. Answer: A is correct.
   Rationale: (A) Apply pressure to the puncture site for 5 min. This will prevent arterial bleeding and hematoma formation. Incorrect responses include (B) shaking the vial of blood before transporting it to the lab. Important, but not the most important is (C), to keep the patient on bed rest for 1 hr. (D) Encouraging the patient to cough and deep-breathe is not a priority nor related to the question's subject.

5. Answer: C is correct.
   Rationale: (C) Vastus lateralis is an appropriate place for an IM injection in a pediatric patient? Incorrect responses include: (A) ventral forearm (not appropriate for an IM injection in any patient), (B) ventral gluteal (not appropriate for a patient of this age patient) and (D) dorsal gluteal (not appropriate for patient of this age).

6. Answer: C is correct.
   Rationale: (C) The patient understands his diet if he chooses baked chicken, steamed broccoli and cauliflower, steamed rice, and hot tea. Incorrect responses include (A) steak, baked potato, peas, and hot coffee (high fat), (B) macaroni and cheese casserole, tossed salad with dressing, and hot chocolate (high fat and high sodium), and (D) fried chicken, mashed potatoes, green beans, and milk (high in fat and sodium).

7. Answer: C is correct.
   Rationale: (C) Bradycardia is the least likely symptom to exhibit in a panic attack. Symptoms of panic attacks include (A) choking, (B) chest pain, nd (D) shortness of breath.

8. Answer: A is correct.
   Rationale: (A) The rationale for giving nitroglycerin is to assist smooth muscles to relax (vasodilation). Incorrect responses include (B) to increase venous return to the heart (will decrease), (C) to increase preload and afterload (will decrease), and (D) to slow and strengthen the heart rate (will increase heart rate)

9. Answer: A is correct.
   Rationale: (A) Wear gloves when performing the test. Incorrect responses, that are false, include (B) Rinse the lancet between uses (single use only), (C) recalibrate the glucometer before each use (not performed with each use, usually once a shift), and (D) give the patient a machine for his use only (this is not necessary nor a special precaution).

10. Answer: C is corect.
    Rationale: (C) Cover the wound with sterile, moist saline dressings. Incorrect responses include (A) Approximate the wound edges with tape. This is unsterile and not an appropriate intervention at this time. (B) Irrigate the wound with sterile saline. This will not protect or contain abdominal contents. (D) Hold the abdominal contents in place with a sterile, gloved hand. This is not appropriate. Even though the hand is sterile, this may cause harm to abdominal contents and does not cover and protect the wound.

REVIEW ACTIVITIES

1. Set up a group to study for the NCLEX with several of your friends. Arrange to meet to discuss how your NCLEX review is going. Have each member of the group buy an NCLEX review book from a different publisher. Practice answering 60 questions for 1 hr daily. Don't mark your answers in the review book. Share your review books with each other to increase your exposure to various authors' test questions.

2. Review the medication guide in Table 25.10. Become comfortable with the root/prefix/suffix for different categories to increase your ability to recognize medications. Add nursing implications to the Table as you study.

EXPLORING THE WEB

- Search for NCLEX review books at www.amazon.com How many different books published in the past 3 years did you see on the topic of NCLEX-RN review?

- Go to www.ncsbn.org. Click on NCLEX Examinations. Explore the site.

- Go to www.learningext.com Note: NCSBN's review for the NCLEX-RN is offered through this NCSBN learning extension. This self-paced, online review features NCLEX-style questions, interactive exercises, topic-specific course exams, and a diagnostic pretest that can help you develop a personal study plan. Visit this site every Monday to see its new NCLEX-RN sample test question.

DISCUSSION POINTS

- Consider the NCLEX-RN Review courses presented in this chapter. Have you heard any tips from your Faculty or classmates about which of them are most helpful?

- How can you set up your schedule to increase the likelihood of your passing NCLEX-RN the first time?

DISCUSSION OF OPENING SCENARIO

Jade graduated from her nursing education program today. Happy and proud to graduate, yet nervous because she knows that she must pass the National Council of State Boards of Nursing Licensure Examination (NCLEX-RN) to practice as a professional nurse. She plans to focus her efforts now on preparing to take the NCLEX-RN Licensure Examination, following a calendar she created. She is working on multiple areas of examination preparation. Jade knows continuing to gain knowledge, using test taking strategies, practicing exam questions, and controlling her anxiety are important ways to be successful in the NCLEX-RN.

1. How should she prepare for the examination?

   Use the information in the chapter and the Tables to prepare (Table 25.2 through Table 25.11)

2. How does she sign up for the examination?
   Jade should sign up for the examination following the steps to apply for the NCLEX-RN outlined below. Every candidate should review the Candidate NCLEX-RN bulletin that can be found at: www.ncsbn.org/2019_Bulletin_Final.pdf, accessed April 15, 2019. Steps in the NCLEX-RN application include:

   a. Apply to the Board of Nursing in the state you plan to practice first. Each state has its own application process that is unique to the state. Once the candidate has applied, most states contact the candidate. At this point, fingerprinting and a background check are performed at fingerprinting vendors specific to the state. The last step in the state application process is sending the certificate of completion from the school attended. Register for the NCLEX-RN exam with Pearson VUE, (www.pearsonvue.com/NCLEX-RN). This can be done, before,

   during or after state application. Once you pay for the exam, you have 365 days to take the test.

   b. Once the state verifies the candidate's background check and graduation from an accredited school of nursing and the candidate has registered and paid for the NCLEX-RN exam, the candidate will be sent an ATT electronically.

   c. Once the candidate obtains the ATT, they can schedule the NCLEX-RN exam at any Pearson VUE Center. Since the NCLEX-RN is a national exam, multiple nursing students apply and take the NCLEX-RN every Spring and Fall. Multiple other professions also use Pearson VUE to deliver their exams, so it is wise to be willing to travel to another Pearson VUE Center to take the NCLEX-RN exam at a date early and convenient to the candidate.

3. What's in the test?
   Jade should review Table 25.1 and the question types in the chapter for this information.

4. Where should she focus her preparation for the examination??
   Jade's focus should include reviewing content, practicing test taking, and managing her anxiety related to NCLEX-RN success. She should consider utilizing a Study Calendar, Preparation Courses, Exit Exam, etc.

5. How can she decrease her anxiety?
   The anxiety management items presented here are only a fraction of available options and include: avoiding negative thinking, instead using visualization, meditation, declaring intentions, and maintaining PERMA. Finding what works for you takes practice and exploration.

EXPLORING THE WEB

- Search for NCLEX-RN review books at www.amazon.com How many different books published in the past 3 years did you see on the topic of NCLEX-RN review?

- Go to www.ncsbn.org, Click on NCLEX-RN Examination. Explore the site.

INFORMATICS

- Go to www.learningext.com. Visit this site every Monday to see its new NCLEX-RN sample test question.

- Go to http://qsen.org, accessed August 20, 2019. Search for NCLEX-RN. Did you find any useful resources to help you prepare for the examination?

LEAN BACK

- How can this chapter's information be directly applied to your NCLEX-RN knowledge and studying?

- Does having a plan and using the tips in the chapter help increase your confidence?

- Are there any barriers to you implementing the plans provided in this chapter for NCLEX-RN success?

REFERENCES

Cook, E. (1913). The Life of Florence Nightingale, by Sir Edward Cook. (p 57). London, UK: Macmillan.

Dickison, P., Haerling, K. A., & Lasater, K. (2019). Integrating the National Council of State Boards of nursing clinical judgment model into nursing educational frameworks. *Journal of Nursing Education*, 58(2), 72–78.

Fiske, E. (2017). Contemplative practices, self-efficacy, and NCLEX-RN success. *Nurse Educator*, 42(3), 159–161. doi:10.1097/nne.0000000000000327

Flavin B. (2016). *7 Expert tips to survive stress and get through nursing school*. Retrieved from www.rasmussen.edu/degrees/nursing/blog/7-expert-tips-to-survive-stress-get-through-nursing-school

Hurst, K., & Hurst, K. (2018, November 16). *How to stop negative thinking with these 5 techniques?* Retrieved from www.thelawofattraction.com/5-techniques-stop-negative-thinking

Kaddoura, M. A., Flint, E. P., Dyke, O. V., Yang, Q., & Chiang, L. (2017). Academic and Demographic Predictors of NCLEX-RN Pass Rates in First- and Second-Degree Accelerated BSN Programs. *Journal of Professional Nursing*, 33(3), 229–240. doi:10.1016/j.profnurs.2016.09.005

Maslow, A. H. (1943). A theory of human motivation. *Psychological Review*, 50(4), 370–396. https://doi.org/10.1037/h0054346

NCSBN. (2019). *Computerized Adaptive Testing (CAT)*. Retrieved November 24, 2020, from from https://www.ncsbn.org/1216.htm

National Council of State Boards of Nursing. (2020). *2020 NCLEX Candidate Bulletin [Brochure]*. Chicago, IL: National Council of State

Boards of Nursing. Retrieved from www.ncsbn.org/NGN_Fall18_Eng_05_FINAL.pdf

NCSBN. (2017). *Research Brief*. Volume 73 | May 2018. Retrieved from http://NCSBN.org

Passing Standard. (n.d.). Retrieved from www.ncsbn.org/2630.htm

Patañjali, & Gherwal, R. S. (1979). *Patañjalis Raja-Yoga*. New Delhi: Asian Publication Services.

Pearson Education, Inc. (2011). *Online tutorial for NCLEX-RN® examinations*. Retrieved from www.pearsonvue.com/NCLEX-RN

Resnick, B. (2018). *Middle range theory for nursing*. New York: Springer Publishing Company, LLC.

Seligman, M. E. (2019). Positive Psychology: A Personal History. *Annual Review of Clinical Psychology*, 15(1, 1), –23. doi:10.1146/annurev

Twidwell, J. E., & Records, K. (2017). An Integrative Review on Standardized Exams as a Predictive Admission Criterion for RN Programs. *International Journal of Nursing Education Scholarship*, 14(1). doi:10.1515/ijnes-2016-0040

U.S. Department of Health and Human Services. (2011). *National heart, lung, and blood institute. Calculate your body mass index*. Retrieved from www.nhlbisupport.com/bmi/bminojs.htm

Yeom, Y. (2013). An investigation of predictors of NCLEX-RN outcomes among nursing content standardized tests. *Nurse Education Today*, 33(12), 1523–1528. doi:10.1016/j.nedt.2013.04.004

SUGGESTED READINGS

American Nurses Association. (2010). *Nursing-sensitive indicators*. Retrieved from www.nursingworld.org/MainMenuCategories/ThePracticeofProfessionalNursing/PatientSafetyQuality/Research-Measurement/The-National-Database/Nursing-Sensitive-Indicators_1.aspx

Assessment Technologies Institute. (2011). *About ATI*. Retrieved from www.atitesting.com/About.aspx

Banks, J., McCullough, E., Ketner, D., & Darby, R. (2018). Tailoring NCLEX-RN indicator assessments for historically black colleges and universities: Literature review. *Journal of Professional Nursing*, 34(5), 331–345. doi:10.1016/j.profnurs.2018.05.007

Caputi, L. J. (2019a). Getting ready for the next generation NCLEX. *Nurse Educator*, 44(3), 117. doi:10.1097/NNE.0000000000000672

Caputi, L. J. (2019b). Reflections on the next generation NCLEX with implications for nursing programs. *Nursing Education Perspectives*, 40(1), 2–3. doi:10.1097/01.NEP.0000000000000439

Centers for Disease Control and Prevention. (2011a). *Adult immunization schedule*. Retrieved from www.cdc.gov/vaccines/recs/schedules/adult-schedule.htm

Centers for Disease Control and Prevention. (2011b). *Physical activity for everyone*. Retrieved from www.cdc.gov/physicalactivity/everyone/guidelines/adults.html

Conklin, P. S., & Cutright, L. H. (2019). A model for sustaining NCLEX-RN success. *Nursing Education Perspectives*, 40(3), 176–178. doi:10.1097/01.NEP.0000000000000326

Czekanski, K., Mingo, S., & Piper, L. (2018). Coaching to NCLEX-RN success: A postgraduation intervention to improve first-time pass rates. *The*

Journal of Nursing Education, 57(9), 561–565. doi:10.3928/01484834-20180815-10

DiBartolo, M. C., & Seldomridge, L. A. (2005). A review of intervention studies to promote NCLEX-RN success. *Nurse Educator*, 30(4), 166–171.

Dreher, H. M., Smith Glasgow, M. E., & Schreiber, J. (2019). The use of "high-stakes testing" in nursing education: Rhetoric or rigor? *Nursing Forum*, 54(4), 447–482. doi:10.1111/nuf.12363

Emory, J. (2019). Exploring NCLEX failures and standardized assessments. *Nurse Educator*, 44(3), 142–146. doi:10.1097/NNE.0000000000000601

Evolve Learning System. (2011). *HESI frequently asked questions*. Retrieved from https://evolve.elsevier.com/staticPages/hesi-faq.html

Foreman, S. (2019). Reliability and validity of NCLEX-RN(c) state pass rate standards. *Nursing Education Perspectives*, 40(1), E3–E8. doi:10.1097/01.NEP.0000000000000412

Gallup. (2010). *Nurses top honesty and ethics list for 11th year*. Retrieved from www.gallup.com/poll/145043/Nurses-Top-Honesty-Ethics-List-11-Year.aspx

Gillespie, M. D., & Nadeau, J. W. (2019). Predicting HESI(R) exit exam success: A retrospective study. *Nursing Education Perspectives*, 40(4), 238–240. doi:10.1097/01.NEP.0000000000000410

Gordon, S., & Nelson, S. (2006). *Moving beyond the virtue script in nursing in the complexities of care*. Ithaca, NY: ILR Press.

Havrilla, E., Zbegner, D., & Victor, J. (2018). Exploring predictors of NCLEX-RN success: One school's search for excellence. *The Journal of Nursing Education*, 57(9), 554–556. doi:10.3928/01484834-20180815-08

HealthyMind.com. (2004). *Cognitive distortions.* Retrieved from www.healthymind.com/s-distortions.html

Kasprovich, T., & VandeVusse, L. (2018). Registered nurses' experiences of passing the NCLEX-RN after more than one attempt. *The Journal of Nursing Education, 57*(10), 590–597. doi:10.3928/01484834-20180921-04

Kesselman-Turkel, J., & Peterson, F. (2007). *Test-taking strategies.* Madison, WI: University of Wisconsin Press.

Kramer, D., Hillman, S. M., & Zavala, M. (2018). Developing a culture of caring and support through a peer mentorship program. *The Journal of Nursing Education, 57*(7), 430–435. doi:10.3928/01484834-20180618-09

McGillis Hall, L., Lalonde, M., Visekruna, S., Chartrand, A., Reali, V., & Feather, J. (2019). A comparative analysis of NCLEX pass rates: Nursing health human resources considerations. *Journal of Nursing Management, 27*(6), 1067–1074. doi:10.1111/jonm.12752

McCloskey, R., & Stewart, C. (2019). Predictors of Success in the NCLEX-RN for Canadian Graduates. *Nursing Leadership* (Toronto Ontario), Dec;32(4), 30–45. doi:10.12927/cjnl.2020.26103

Moosvi, K. & Garbutt, S. (2018). Shifting strategies: Using film to improve therapeutic communication and nursing education. *Nursing Education Perspectives, 41*(2), 134–135. doi:10.1097/01.NEP.0000000000000431

National Council of State Boards of Nursing, Inc. (2019). *NCSBN Learning Extension.* Weekly "NCLEX-RN Style" Question and online NCLEX-RN Review course. Retrieved from https://www.learningext.com/#/public-dashboard

NCSBN. (2019a). Retrieved from www.ncsbn.org/NGN_Winter19.pdf

NCSBN. (2019b). Retrieved from www.ncsbn.org/1216.htm

Needleman, J., Buerhaus, P., Mattke, S., Stewart, M., & Zelevinsky, K. (2002). Nurse-staffing levels and the quality of care in hospitals. *New England Journal of Medicine, 346*(22), 1715–1722.

Nibert, A., Young, A., & Adamson, C. (2002). Predicting NCLEX-RN success with the HESI Exit Exam: Fourth annual validity study. *Computers, Informatics, Nursing, 20*(6), 261–267.

Noone, J., Ingwerson, J., & Kunz, A. (2018). Analysis of licensure testing patterns of RN graduates in Oregon. *The Journal of Nursing Education, 57*(11), 655–661. doi:10.3928/01484834-20181022-05

Nursing Theories. (2020). Retrieved from https://www.currentnursing.com/nursing_theory/introduction.html

Oliver, B. J., Pomerleau, M., Potter, M., Phillips, A., Carpenter, S., et al. (2018). Optimizing NCLEX-RN pass rate performance using an educational microsystems improvement approach. *The Journal of Nursing Education, 57*(5), 265–274. doi:10.3928/01484834-20180420-03

Opsahl, A. G., Auberry, K., Sharer, B., & Shaver, C. (2018). A comprehensive educational approach to improving NCLEX-RN pass rates. *Nursing Forum, 53*(4), 549–554. doi:10.1111/nuf.12285

Petrovic, K., Doyle, E., Lane, A., & Corcoran, L. (2019). The work of preparing Canadian nurses for a licensure exam originating from the USA: A nurse educator's journey into the institutional organization of the NCLEX-RN. *International Journal of Nursing Education Scholarship, 16*(1). doi:10.1515/ijnes-2018-0052

Pike, A. D., Lukewich, J., Wells, J., Kirkland, M. C., Manuel, M., & Watkins, K. (2019). Identifying indicators of National Council Licensure Examination for registered nurses (NCLEX-RN) success in nursing graduates in Newfoundland & Labrador. *International Journal of Nursing Education Scholarship, 16*(1). doi:10.1515/ijnes-2018-0060

Presti, C. R., & Sanko, J. S. (2019). Adaptive quizzing improves end-of-program exit examination scores. *Nurse Educator, 44*(3), 151–153. doi:10.1097/NNE.0000000000000566

Rode, J., & Brown, K. (2019). Emotional intelligence relates to NCLEX and standardized readiness test: A pilot study. *Nurse Educator, 44*(3), 154–158. doi:10.1097/NNE.0000000000000565

Rosenthal, H. G. (2004). *Test anxiety prevention.* London: Routledge Publishers.

Schlairet, M. C., & Rubenstein, C. (2019). Senior NCLEX-RN coaching model: Development and implementation. *Nurse Educator, 44*(5), 250–254. doi:10.1097/NNE.0000000000000644

Seligman, M. E. P. (2011). *Flourish: A new understanding of happiness and well-being - and how to achieve them.* Simon & Schuster.

Shatto, B., Shagavah, A., Krieger, M., Lutz, L., Duncan, C. E., & Wagner, E. K. (2019). Active learning outcomes on NCLEX-RN or standardized predictor examinations: An integrative review. *The Journal of Nursing Education, 58*(1), 42–46. doi:10.3928/01484834-20190103-07

Simpson, K. R. (2005). Failure to rescue: Implications for evaluating quality of care during labor and birth. *Journal of Perinatal and Neonatal Nursing, 19*(1), 24–36.

Snowden, K., Foronda, C., Gonzalez, J., Ortega, J., Salani, D., et al. (2018). Developing minority nursing students: Evaluation of an innovative mentorship and leadership program. *The Journal of Nursing Education, 57*(9), 526–534. doi:10.3928/01484834-20180815-04

Spurlock, D. R. J., Patterson, B. J., & Colby, N. (2019). Gender differences and similarities in accelerated nursing education programs: Evidence of success from the new careers in nursing program. *Nursing Education Perspectives, 40*(6), 343–351. doi:10.1097/01.NEP.0000000000000508

Stein, A. M. (2005). *NCLEX-RN review* (5th ed.). Clifton Park, NY: Delmar Cengage Learning.

The National Council of State Boards of Nursing. (2010a). *NCLEX-RN examination test plan for the national council licensure examination for registered nurses.* Retrieved from www.ncsbn.org/2010_NCLEX-RN_RN_TestPlan.pdf

The National Council of State Boards of Nursing. (2010b). *Alternate item formats frequently asked questions.* Retrieved from www.ncsbn.org/2334.htm

The National Council of State Boards of Nursing. (2011a). *NCLEX-RN administration frequently asked questions.* Retrieved from www.ncsbn.org/2325.htm#Why_do_you_need_palm_vein_reading_if_you_have_fingerprints

Victor, J., Havrilla, E., & Zbegner, D. A. (2019). Game show-themed games for NCLEX-RN preparation. *Nurse Educator, 44*(5), 232–234. doi:10.1097/NNE.0000000000000655

Woo, A., Wendt, A., & Liu, W. (2009). NCLEX-RN pass rates. *JONA's Healthcare Law, Ethics, and Regulation, 11*(1), 23–26. doi:10.1097/nhl.0b013e31819a78ce

Wu, Y., Larrabee, J. H., & Putnam, H. P. (2006). Caring behaviors inventory. *Nursing Research, 55*(1), 18–25.

26 Entry into the Profession: Your First Job

Dianne Hoekstra

College of Nursing, Purdue University Northwest, Hammond, IN, USA

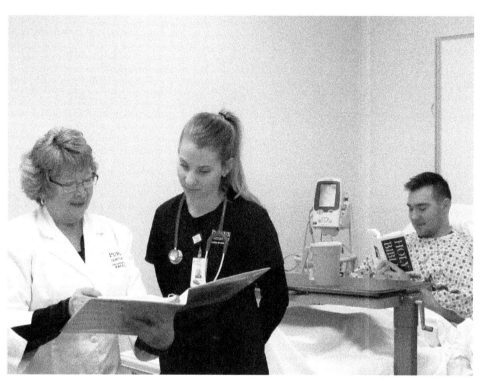

A nurse is precepted as she begins her nursing career-her first job!
Source: K. Walsh, E. Bastic, Allison C. Banasiak

New nurses want to make a difference in patient care, and those in nursing management want to coach them in ways that will enable them to maintain their idealism and vision while they are acquiring the skills and perspectives they need to become effective in the system.

Benner, P. *From* Novice to Expert. *(1984)*

OBJECTIVES

Upon completion of this chapter, the reader should be able to:

1. Examine key elements to consider when choosing a nursing position.
2. Describe typical components of health care orientation.
3. Differentiate between sources of performance feedback.
4. Discuss typical organizational responses to performance.
5. Analyze strategies to enhance the role of the nurse as a manager of a small patient group.
6. Select mechanisms to enhance professional growth.

Kelly Vana's Nursing Leadership and Management, Fourth Edition. Edited by Patricia Kelly Vana and Janice Tazbir
© 2021 John Wiley & Sons Ltd. Published 2021 by John Wiley & Sons Ltd.
Companion Website: www.wiley.com/go/kelly-Nursing-Leadership

OPENING SCENARIO

Congratulations! You have just completed your nursing educational requirements and received notice that you passed your NCLEX exam! You have decided to stay in this geographical area and have received three job offers:

1. *A 12-hr night position in the surgical intensive care unit (ICU) in an urban teaching hospital. This hospital offers a 12-month Transition to Practice (TTP) Program and is a nationally recognized research center for heart disease and cancer.*

2. *An 8-hr rotating shift position on a suburban hospital's medical-surgical floor. This health care organization is in a neighborhood with some shabby homes. This hospital is just starting up a year-long TTP Program for new grads like you. Several of the nursing leaders of this hospital have been featured in the State Board of Nursing publication for innovation and bringing evidence to the bedside.*

3. *A RN position in a local dialysis center. Orientation would involve spending a week rounding with the Nurse Practitioner as well as 2 or 3 months of orientation with the staff nurses. The center is closed on holidays and Sundays. Day shift starts at 5:00 a.m. No TTP program is available.*

4. *Which position would you accept?*

5. *What factors will help you decide which is the best fit for you?*

6. *Consider your career goal, would any of these positions start your career on the path you wish to take?*

Graduation brings the transition from the role of student to that of RN. A nurse's first job is an opportunity to solidify skills learned in school. It is also the time to establish relationships with mentors and to set a foundation for future professional growth. This chapter will discuss important considerations regarding your first job including what to consider when choosing a nursing position, typical components of health care orientation, performance feedback, and how to enhance professional growth.

Choosing a Nursing Position

When choosing your first position as an RN, there are many factors to consider and must be take into account. According to the United States Bureau of Labor Statistics (www.bls.gov/ooh/healthcare/registered-nurses.htm, accessed July, 2019), "employment of RNs is projected to grow 15% from 2016 to 2026, much faster than the average for all occupations. Growth will occur for a number of reasons, including an increased emphasis on preventive care; growing rates of chronic conditions, such as diabetes and obesity; and demand for health care services from the baby-boom population, as they live longer and more active lives." In the current job market, new nurses in some states are in the enviable position of having broad choices for their first job. Nurses in other states are having to relocate to find a position or must alter their expectations of where they will work. Some community health organizations hire newly graduated nurses. And some hospitals will recruit new nurses to specialty areas such as obstetrics and critical care units. More than 80% of RNs obtain their first jobs in hospitals. This changes later in the career of a nurse. Only 60% of U.S. nurses in the workforce are hospital-based. (Clarke, 2016).

Patient Types

One of the most important considerations in selecting a job is choosing your best fit in a patient care environment. New nurses who start their career on a general medical or surgical unit typically manage multiple adult patients with a variety of diagnoses. Consider Julie, a nurse with 8 months of experience, who is working the midnight shift on a busy medical/surgical unit. During her night shift Julie provides care for:

- A gentleman with a recent colectomy related to colon cancer

- A lady with End Stage Renal disease and a non-functioning hemodialysis access

- A lady with an exacerbation of COPD and pneumonia

- A gentleman with poorly controlled diabetes and osteomyelitis in his left foot

- A lady who fell and will have surgery for a fractured hip in the morning

- A gentleman with a low hemoglobin and suspected gastrointestinal bleed

- And a lady with fluid volume overload related to heart failure.

Julie learns diverse technical and assessment skills on this medical/surgical unit. She is developing a working knowledge of many common medications and diagnostic testing during the treatment of a variety of patients.

In contrast, nurses who choose an entry position on a specialty unit focus on patients with specific diseases, body system disorders, or age groups. Specialty units may include pediatrics, critical care, operating rooms, obstetrics, psychiatry, or neonatology units. Nurses working in community home health often have roles similar to those of medical and surgical nurses; seeing a variety of diagnoses among the patients receiving care in their home. New nurses working in the community may have more specialized roles such as those of community health neonatal nurses or outpatient dialysis.

Work Environment

Work environments in health care organizations can vary tremendously. Some new RNs find a smaller hospital easier to navigate and learn co-workers' names. For other nurses, a large, busy, nationally renowned hospital associated with medical and nursing schools is appealing. Large medical centers often offer advantages such as working with residents and many opportunities for learning and personal development. With any option, the nurse becomes part of a team. For example, the nurse whose first job is on an oncology unit in a hospital will learn to be a member of a team and must develop the ability be the leader and manager for their group of assigned patients. A nurse hired to work in home health may work alone for most of the day, seeing patients in their home one at a time. Each area requires mastery of specific skills, organizational skills, and the skill of effective time management.

To find out more about institutions, http://Leapfroggroup. org and Centers for Medicare and Medicaid Services (Hospital Compare) offer information on how well hospitals provide care to their patients; similar to a report card. Hospitals with the American Nurse Credentialing Center (**ANCC**) Magnet Recognition Program® may be attractive to some new RNs. The ANCC has a rigorous application process for Magnet recognition. According to Ostermeyer (2018a,b), these hospitals with Magnet Recognition demonstrate the following benefits:

- High job satisfaction

- Low job turnover rates

- A culture that focuses on improving patient outcomes

- Professional growth by educational opportunities

- Focus on professional autonomy

- Interdisciplinary collaboration

- Leadership opportunities.

Shifts, Salary, and Benefits

Another consideration in weighing possible positions is the available schedule. Many health care organizations now offer a variety of schedules including 8- and 12-hr shifts, full and part time, and part-time weekend only options. Twelve-hour shifts are particularly popular, because a full-time nurse can work as few as three shifts per week helping reduce stress and burnout. For the patient, this means fewer changes in nurs-

ing personnel within a day, but less continuity in nursing personnel from day to day throughout their hospital stay. For the new nurse, a 12-hr shift can be a long work day but it allows increased flexibility in personal time. Some facilities offer rotations between daytime and other shifts. Others award the more popular day shifts by seniority. For the nurse with a family, working 12-hr shifts every weekend allows spending time with children during the week while their spouse cares for the children at the weekends. It is customary in most facilities to work every other weekend.

The Bureau of Labor Statistics identifies the median annual salary for Registered Nurses in 2018 as \$71,730, or \$34.48 per hour. While pay is an obvious element in choosing your first job, the best-paying job offer is not necessarily the wisest choice, even from a financial point of view. Consider the employee benefits and advancement opportunities available for each potential employer. Hospitals in the same geographical area tend to offer competitive salaries at the start of employment. It is important to ask about an employer's salary policy. Does the health care organization you are considering give a raise after you have passed your NCLEX, or would any potential raise be held until your first-year anniversary? Are nurses paid extra for having an advance degree or for any other nursing certifications? How are pay scales structured? Is it based on time of service or merit based? Glass Ceiling (http://jobs.glassceiling.com/jobs/seeker/salary) and other websites can offer a glimpse of salaries to aid in the search.

Differentials

Differentials are a percentage of the hourly salary added to the nurse's hourly pay for working off shifts, such as midnights, evenings, or weekends. Think of a health care organization by considering, what are the differentials for weekend work or working night or evening shifts? Confirm that nurses are paid for orientation shifts and any required educational courses. When comparing offers between two health care organizations, ask how many hours are paid for a typical workweek. Some employers pay for a full 8- or 12-hr shift by allowing for a 30-min overlap at change of shifts. Other organizations do not expect staff nurses to overlap, resulting in a shorter shift. Thus, at some facilities, a typical pay week includes 40 hr, whereas at others, nurses routinely work 37.5 hr per week.

The benefits and salary gap in hospitals compared to nonhospital settings has increased, which is partly related to the larger number of Baccalaureate prepared nurses employed in hospitals (Buerhaus, Skinner, Auerbach, & Staiger, 2017). Consider the retirement benefits for all of your potential employers. Does the employer contribute a percentage into the retirement plan? Are financial counselors and advisors available for your consultation? Starting to save for retirement early will allow you to take full advantage of compounding interest. Your future retired self will thank you for starting to plan for retirement now.

Case Study 26.1

Adam, a newly licensed RN is considering two different positions. One is a full-time 8-hr night shift position on a Pediatric Oncology unit. The second is a rotating 12-hr shift position on an Adult Telemetry unit with a Neurology focus.

Adam decides to spend a shift shadowing a nurse on each of these units. During the two shadowed shifts, Adam observes the usual routine for the nurses working on the unit for a night shift. He asks about the typical nurse-to-patient ratio. He looks for teamwork and collaboration among the nurses and the unlicensed assistive personnel (UAP). Adam watches carefully for signs of incivility such as eye rolling, and for the use of please and thank you. He attempts to identify the resources that he would have at his disposal while providing patient care. Are there Respiratory Therapists available for patients with breathing issues? Are there Residents or in-house physicians, known as Hospitalists, available for consultation and orders? Is a Pharmacist available for questions and for patient medication needs around the clock? While shadowing on the Pediatric Oncology unit, he observes the nurses pulling together and working as a team after two pediatric patients are admitted from the ER and the transfer of one patient to the Pediatric Intensive Care Unit (ICU). He really appreciates the layout of the Pediatric Unit, which allows the nurses to be near the assigned patients, yet not isolated from each other. Adam also had a good experience shadowing on the Adult Neuro Telemetry unit where the nurses are assigned to work with one UAP each shift. The unit is set up so that each RN and UAP pair is stationed in an enclave near their assigned patients. Adam did not notice any obvious signs of incivility, but felt the nurses were isolated from each other. Which position would you select? Why? Why not the other position?

Self-Scheduling

When choosing a position, it is important to find out about the process for changing to a different schedule or department after hiring. Often, nurses accept a position at a health care organization, but perhaps not in the department or specialty of first choice. Some hospitals restrict new nurses from changing positions or shifts for a set period of time, usually a minimum of 6 months.

Consider the following questions to ask about scheduling:

- What are the weekend commitments?

- How many holidays are nurses expected to work each year and how is preference selected?

- Is there additional pay for holidays or weekends?

- Does the unit use a **self-scheduling** system (in which nurses select their own schedule according to unit guidelines), or is time assigned by the manager?

- How much notice is required to request a day off for personal reasons?

- How much vacation is offered?

- What is the process for requesting vacation days?

- Are there benefits for furthering your education (many institutions will pay up to 100% tuition reimbursement)?

- Is there additional pay or benefit to for receiving certification (such as Advanced Cardiac Life Support)?

- Is there a financial support for continuing education?

- How long is orientation?

Shadowing

Fortunate nurses may have to choose between two seemingly perfect job offers. Many organizations allow new graduates to spend time **shadowing** nurses in different roles and departments before making a career decision (Sherman, 2018). Shadowing consists of following an experienced nurse at an institution for a short period of time (it may be a couple hours or up to a shift) to experience the care provided, the patient population of the unit, and the unit culture.

Orientation Considerations

Different health care organizations can have very different approaches to new employee orientation and education. Because orientation is a key component of the transition between being a student nurse and becoming a first-time manager of patients, it is important to establish what the organization offers before accepting the position. Some potential questions to consider appear in Table 26.1 Questions to Consider Regarding Orientation.

Table 26.1 Questions to Consider Regarding Orientation

How long should I expect to be in orientation? What if I need more time?

Is orientation tailored to my learning needs, or is it the same for all newly graduated nurses?

Does orientation occur at the beginning, or is it offered in stages throughout the first year?

What ongoing education will be available to me after the orientation phase?

Will I be paid for time spent in education programs? Will I be paid for required on-line education activities that I complete at home?

Will I be assigned to work with one preceptor or multiple?

In case of short staffing on the unit, will I be pulled from the orientation activities to provide patient care on my unit?

Is there a Nurse Residency or Transition to Practice Program?

Is Simulation part of the Nursing Orientation for the newly graduated RN?

When will I be evaluated and receive feedback? By whom?

Source: D. Hoekstra.

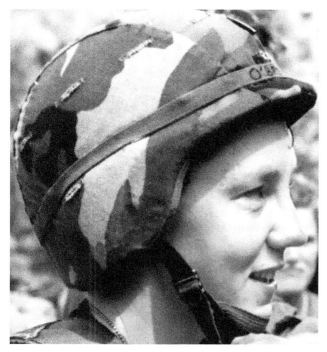

FIGURE 26.1 Photo of 1LT Karen O'Brien, Army Nurse Corp, circa 1987.
Source: Used with permission from K. O'Brien.

New nurses may feel pressure to find just the right setting for their first job, particularly if they have a long-term goal of working in a subspecialty. Instead of focusing on which unit the nurse is working, the true priority in the first job is understanding hospital policy and procedures, refining assessment and technical skills, and learning organizational and time

management in the delivery of nursing care. These skills, coupled with a positive work record regarding attendance, flexibility, and attitude, will ensure the new nurse of many future opportunities.

No matter the place or unit of employment, as a professional nurse you have committed to providing the very best evidence-based care to your patients. They deserve no less. Nurses frequently find that the second or even third choice position is a truly wonderful place to work! Discovering great teamwork and collaboration, a supportive nurse manager, and patients who truly need you and appreciate your care, are more important than the initially desired unit or position. Perhaps your first job does not fit the ideal picture that you imagined; however, you need to make the best of it, to learn and grow personally and professionally.

Components of Health Care Orientation

Orientation fosters a smooth transition from graduate to practicing nurse. At its completion, a new nurse should be able to demonstrate competency in the basic skills needed for safe patient care.

General Orientation

Many health care organizations divide nursing orientation into general sections and unit-specific sections. General orientation includes information and skills measurement, which all nurses new to the health care organization need, regardless of their eventual unit assignment. Two examples of information discussed at general orientation are infection control standards and an introduction to policies regarding medication administration (Table 26.2).

Table 26.2 Sample of the First Week of Orientation for All Nurses on Inpatient Nursing Units

	Orientation for inpatient nurses (to be offered the third week of each month)	
	Topics	**Presenter and location**
Monday	Welcome, mission statement, introduction of administrators, attendance policy, dress code and professionalism, health insurance benefits, retirement benefits, hospital codes	Human resources Administrators Human resources conference Room
Tuesday	Proactive patient care Patient transfers De-escalation and Restraint Alternatives Infection control Glucometer testing PFR mask face fitting	Nurse educators, physical Therapy, infection control nurses Education classroom
Wednesday	Medication administration safety; diabetes standards; wound care and pressure ulcer prevention; role of pharmacy; role of case managers; centers of excellence for stroke, MI, neurology, and chest pain; blood administration; organ donation.	Nurse educators, certified diabetes educators (CDE), wound ostomy continence nurses (WOCN), case managers, pharmacists Education classroom

On the third Thursday and Friday of the month.
Computer training for Nurses. Located in Computer Classrooms.

Fourth Monday of the month (subsequent to above orientation classes)
Simulation and Skills Lab for Nurses. Located in Nursing Education Sim Lab.

Fourth Tuesday of the month (subsequent to above orientation classes)
New Nurse Necessities for new RNs working in Med/Surg and Telemetry. Located in Education Classroom.

Source: D. Hoekstra.

Real World Interview

"I finished my Baccalaureate degree in Nursing in January 1986 from Loyola University of Chicago. The next few weeks flew by as I prepared for and took my NCLEX licensure exam. After that, I packed up what little I had and headed for the AMEDD Officer's Basic Course in San Antonio, TX. About 3 weeks into training, I received notification via mail from the IL State Board of Nursing saying I had passed my exam! This meant I could move on to my first duty station at Fort Carson, in Colorado Springs, CO, where I would begin my career as Second Lieutenant Karen Lynn O'Brien, RN and Army Nurse Corps Officer.

As a new nurse and officer, I had developed some pictures in my mind about how everything would look and feel. How I would look and act; what the hospital would be like. When I arrived at Ft. Carson in search of the building where I would begin my Army In-Processing, I happened to drive past the hospital. The hospital at Fort Carson was a cantonment hospital left over from World War 1. These types of hospitals were a series of two-story buildings connected by ramps and long hallways and had open bay wards with very few private or semi-private rooms. I wondered what I had gotten myself into! This looked nothing like the hospitals in and around Chicago where I had done my clinical practicums. Where were the high rises, the sparkling hallways, the fancy electronic beds?

I was assigned to a male medical surgical unit and the head nurse (nurse manager) was Major Tom Anderson. He was small in stature, his uniform crisp and white, and gold insignia polished. His organization and nursing skills were as polished and crisp as his uniform. He taught me so much about how to manage during a shift, how to be a leader, and how to care compassionately for patients. I learned quickly I did not need fancy equipment, or a new modern building to practice as a nurse. Expert nursing care required excellent nursing skills and the ability to communicate and adapt to different surroundings. I learned to take the opportunities afforded to me and bloom where I was planted. After approximately 6 months in the cantonment hospital, we moved to a brand-new facility called Evans Army Community Hospital.

This facility DID have all of the bells and whistles and was sparkling. I was glad I had my first experience in the old hospital; it wasn't pretty but it helped prepare me for what was to come.

Eighteen months into my time at Ft. Carson, I received orders to move to Ft. Bragg, North Carolina, where I joined the 28th Combat Support Hospital. I had a joint assignment with the fixed hospital facility on post, Womack Army Community Hospital, where I would work day to day, but would also be released for field training exercises. During the field training exercises, we would set up and run a field hospital with emergency rooms, operating rooms, ICUs, and a variety of care wards. I reveled in these opportunities and grew from these experiences. I became a better nurse and stronger leader. I bloomed where I was planted.

I continued my army career in the Reserves with the 801st Combat Support Hospital at Ft. Sheridan, IL, and continued training in the field environment one weekend a month and 2 weeks in the summer for what became the inevitable. In 2003, as a Major in the U.S. Army Reserves, I was called upon to deploy overseas with the 801st. I was able to provide care to men and women of all branches of service in Kuwait and Iraq for almost a year and a half. During my time in Iraq, I worked in an ICU with patients with neurological injuries. I was a Major then, and the young officers were not accustomed to an officer of my rank functioning as a staff nurse on their unit. They were surprised that I wanted to participate in patient care, and not be in charge! During this time, I was reminded that basic nursing care is foundational to holistic care and is never insignificant. Even under difficult circumstances, washing an injured soldier and providing comfort care was moving and gratifying. Again, I may have bloomed where planted, but I think I also helped others to bloom."

Lieutenant Colonel Karen L. O'Brien, USAR, Ret.

LTC O'Brien currently is a PHD, RN, CNE,
Associate Dean and Associate Professor at Purdue University Northwest College of Nursing, photo at start of chapter.

General orientation also typically includes explanations of human resource policies and opportunities to hear from representatives of various departments within the organization. New employees from other departments and specialties may be included in these presentations. Recent concerns about patient safety have expanded orientation to include information about Joint Commission (JC) standards and National Patient Safety Goals.

Frequently, organizations offer portions of general orientation as written materials or computer-based learning. This allows a more flexible orientation schedule. It is particularly beneficial for new employees who are available to attend orientation only outside daytime hours.

Most facilities offer general orientation first, followed by unit-specific classroom orientation. In this case, new nurses may not actually spend a shift on their unit for 2 weeks after starting work. Other nurse educators plan orientation so that nurses go to their home unit very early, reserving some of the general content for later in the orientation schedule. The health care organization works to get information to the new graduates in a meaningful way. These are specific questions you may ask when interviewing.

Most organizations tailor their general orientation to individual learners. Thus, an experienced nurse may opt to challenge particular orientation classes by successfully completing the demonstration, the written test, or demonstrating competency in some other fashion. For example, experienced nurses who previously worked at a health care organization utilizing EPIC electronic health records (**EHRs**) may take a 1-day EPIC computer training class versus a 2-day class. Or consider Ashley who, while in school, worked part time as a nursing assistant on a Medical/Surgical Renal unit. Ashley has now been hired to work as an RN on this same unit. Ashley is already very familiar with the staff, the geographical layout, and the general routine on the unit. Ashley will need to adapt to the care provided by the RN versus the UAP.

Using Simulated Learning for New

Using simulated learning for newly hired RNs is another way to support transition into a new position. Hospitals are realizing the benefits of simulation and investing in interactive high and low fidelity manikins and equipment. For new nurses, simulations can bridge the gap between knowledge already gained in their nursing program and the skills needed to care for multiple, complex patients. Even for nurses with experience, education in a simulation lab can introduce the experienced nurse to protocols and polices with their new employer. Simulations allow a wide range of clinical scenarios to be analyzed in the safety of a lab where patients cannot be harmed (Twibell et al., 2012). Simulation also allows the nurse educator to verify knowledge base, assessment skills, technical skills, critical thinking, and reasoning skills of the novice nurse.

Unit-Specific Orientation

Unit-based orientation, whether it follows the general orientation or is interspersed throughout, focuses on the specific competencies a novice nurse needs to care for the diagnoses and ages of patients typical to the assigned unit. These competencies include technical skills as well as beginning mastery of unit-specific processes. Content covered may include topics such as what paperwork is necessary for new admissions and how to acquire equipment needed for patient care, such as getting an IV pump.

Most organizations have developed unit-specific competency tools that list those skills orientees that need to demonstrate. These lists provide a useful road map with which to plan a learner-specific orientation. Competency tools are often used on an annual basis by all nurses as a mechanism to demonstrate competence with certain clinical skills. Table 26.3 is a portion from a Medical Surgical department's unit-based orientation tool. Additionally, the new RN must achieve the skills and requirements set forth in the job description for the position. Job descriptions are discussed in further detail later in this chapter.

Socialization

Socialization to the new workplace is an important part of orientation. Social support has been shown to be an essential element in positively influencing retention of new nurses. Having someone to talk to and receive emotional and practical support is highly beneficial. Nurse unit managers and preceptors play a key role in introducing the new nurse to co-workers and other members of the inter-professional team, both on and off the unit. This helps the new nurse identify relationships within the unit and between the unit and the larger health care organization. In practice areas where staff are infrequently together, such as a home health agency, socialization can be difficult. Some nurse managers may arrange a luncheon or coffee hour to introduce new staff members to the work group (Gardiner & Sheen, 2016).

Working with Your Preceptor

Ideally, the nurse manager assigns each new orientee to a **preceptor**. The manager understands the need to match the teaching style of the preceptor to the new nurse's learning needs. In some organizations, the learner follows the preceptor's schedule so that orientation to the unit is consistent. Ashley and her preceptor will spend several weeks working the day shift before moving to midnights, Ashley's assigned shift.

The preceptor is the first nurse who intensely invests in the new RN, planning patient assignments on a daily basis, nurturing confidence and competence, and overseeing the development of skills and clinical judgment Allowing autonomous practice with appropriate preceptor presence, preceptors socialize newly graduated nurses into new roles, unit processes, and workplace norms. The preceptor and newly graduated nurse may work together for a variable length of

Evidence From the Literature

Citation: Murphy, L. J., & Janisse, L. (2017). Optimizing transition to practice through orientation: A quality improvement initiative. *Clinical Simulation in Nursing, 13*(11), 583–590.

Discussion: A study at a Canadian hospital utilized skill-based stations, high-fidelity simulations, hands-on case studies, and a head-to-toe patient assessment demonstration as part of the first week of RN orientation. Examples of skills reviewed at the stations included PICC dressing changes, blood sampling, PPE donning and doffing, blood transfusion, wound care management, management of an unwitnessed fall, and documentation of a patient admission process.

Implications for practice: The authors of the article reported a decrease in the time spent in orientation by one full day, saving their facility thousands of dollars in 1 year and allowing the new nurse to move to unit-based learning more quickly.

Table 26.3   Sample of a Medical-Surgical RN Skills Assessment and Orientation Checklist

The skills assessment and orientation checklist consists of procedures, skills, and responsibilities of the RN. The first column is a self-assessment of the new RN's experience related to the skill. The remaining columns are to be dated and completed by the Preceptor and Manager in conjunction with the Orientee. Below is just a portion of a checklist for a new inpatient RN.

Self-Assessment is scored by the Orientee:

1 = can perform skill without supervision

2 = need for observation of or practice with this skill

3 = need for basic instruction on this skill

Self-assessment	Skills statement	Oriented to procedure	Clinical experience provided	Criteria met satisfactorily
	Prepare and administers NG or PEG Bolus tube feedings			
	Prepare and administer NG or PEG Continuous tube feedings			
	Medication administration via NG or PEG tube			
	Medication administration—oral			
	Medication administration—IV push and IVPG			
	Medication administration—Subcutaneous and IM			
	Evaluation and documentation of patient response to medications			
	Provides and documents patient teaching related to initial dose of medication, i.e. purpose and side effects			
	Assessment and documentation of peripheral and PICC IV sites			
	Assessment and documentation of care for Wound Vac			
	Set up of PCA pump for continuous and bolus pain medication			
	Assessment and documentation for a patient receiving PCA pain management			

Source: D. Hoekstra.

time from weeks to months. Research suggests that preceptors not only should be experienced clinicians but should have skilled communication, relational abilities, and a positive attitude toward nursing and the organization. Good preceptors are familiar with the organization's policies and procedures, willing to share knowledge with their orientees, and able to model behaviors for their orientees. New nurses report high anxiety levels in the first weeks of employment. Preceptors who consistently convey caring behaviors can reduce anxiety and facilitate learning for the newly graduated nurse (Twibell et al., 2012).

In some larger organizations, one preceptor is assigned to a group of new nurses. Together, several orientees work with the preceptor to master core competencies before being assigned

Evidence From the Literature

Citation: Gardiner, I., & Sheen, J. (2016). Graduate nurse experiences of support: A review. *Nurse Education Today,* *40*(2016), 7–12.

Discussion: In their review of a newly graduated nurse's support, Gardiner and Sheen (2016) noted that newly graduated nurses experience stress from interactions with other nurses. Most negative interactions stemmed from other nurses being perceived as unavailable or disinterested in helping the newly graduated nurse. Unfortunately, some newly graduated nurses reported experiencing bullying or horizontal violence directly. Horizontal violence is defined as hostile or aggressive behavior toward an individual within the same work group. Such behaviors may be displayed as power games, with one individual being ignored or excluded.

Implications for Practice: Horizontal violence is present in nursing. New nurses should be aware of the signs of horizontal violence and report it when it occurs.

to their home unit. For example, several new graduates hired for medical or surgical floors may all be assigned temporarily to one unit, with one preceptor. In some organizations this is called an Educational Unit. This has the advantage of providing peer support to the new nurses and may be more efficient and less expensive than a traditional one-on-one relationship.

Experienced nurses accrue clinical knowledge over time and lose track of what they have learned, according to Patricia Benner (1984, 2001). Experienced nurse preceptors sometimes forget to explain all of the steps and thoughts going through their brain during patient care. The new Nurse needs to ask questions! "So tell me what you were thinking when. . ..." is a suggested way to phrase a question to your preceptor.

A helpful technique that may be used is role-play with their preceptor. Ask the preceptor, "Before we go into the patient's room, can we talk through what I need to do?" Ask for feedback frequently and immediately after a complex situation. Be direct with your questions to your preceptor; "What can I do differently next time? What should I do differently tomorrow?" All feedback should be private, not at the nurse's station or in front of patients.

The preceptor should behave toward you, the preceptee, with kindness and patience. Trust yourself to listen to your needs and expectations. Caution–if you see your preceptor using unsafe, unethical, or non-caring nursing practices, do not adopt these behaviors into your practice just because "my preceptor did it too." As an RN, you are responsible for your practice alone. If you find it difficult to work with your assigned preceptor, make this known early in the orientation process. By using "I feel" statements, have a private discussion with your preceptor, Nursing Manager, or Unit Educator to discuss and resolve the situation.

Practice Drift

What if a preceptor takes unsafe shortcuts? A **practice drift** is a phenomenon that occurs when a nurse takes a short-cut, circumventing a policy, regulation, or standard of care in order to accomplish an immediate goal. Practice drifts maybe a solution to an inefficiency and can serve to foster patient's safety by identifying a process that needs improvement. Serious practice drifts may threaten patient safety when the standard of care is ignored, and the Nurse Practice Act violated (Chastain, Burhans, Koch, 2018). Practice drifts need to be discussed with the preceptor. "Could you tell me more about the care provided, because when I was in school we learned it differently." After a discussion, if you have continued concerns you may need to be more direct and specific with your question. After you have attempted to discuss your concerns for patient safety with your preceptor on two occasions, it is time to move up the chain of command and discuss this with the unit manager or educator.

Understand that there are limitations in the use of preceptors in the orientation of new nurses. Not all nurses like to teach, nor do they have the patience to precept a new nurse. Some experienced nurses want to "get the job done" and lack

interest in new employees. Sometimes preceptors are busy with their own heavy workload and are unable to support the new nurse (Gardiner & Sheen, 2016). Facilities may utilize an evaluation or questionnaire for the new nurse to complete regarding the preceptor and their experiences. Nurse Managers or Team Leaders will have routinely scheduled meetings with the new nurse and the preceptor, providing a chance to ensure a smooth interpersonal relationship between orientee and preceptor. Speak to your preceptor directly about any concerns you may have using "I feel" statements.

Caring for Patients

When beginning to care for patients during orientation, you will quickly realize that you are a "real" nurse now. Patients expect you to have the answers. This is intimidating at first. When experiencing an emergency for the first time, it can be unnerving to realize that you are the nurse in charge of this patient. Trust that your nursing education, hospital orientation, critical thinking, and clinical reasoning skills has prepared you for this moment. Gain confidence by keeping your knowledge base up to date and by looking and acting professional. With time and experience, caring for patients changes from daunting to rewarding.

By demonstrating a sense of caring and nursing care knowledge, patients will trust and expect you to provide excellent care. Consider beginning the shift by simply sitting down for just a few moments at the patient's eye level to discuss the plan of care for the day, and listen to the patient. Get to know your patient as a human by asking them questions such as what they do for fun or what is the most important thing you can do for them today. Do not converse with your patient while you are looking at the computer screen. Make eye contact. Knowing your patient will allow you to identify any subtle changes in their presentation later. Never be afraid to ask other, more experienced nurses for advice or help if you are unsure of a situation; not asking for help is where you can get into trouble. Always remember a smile and a great attitude can be the most important part of your nursing uniform.

Working With Physicians and Other Health Care Providers

Sometimes, nurses are intimidated by the physicians and practitioners with whom they work. Establish rapport and introduce yourself to the practitioners you work with. Do not be intimidated. Both you and the practitioner are part of the inter-professional health care team to meet the patient's goals. Every member of the team is important to all patient's welfare; one could not function well without the other. Make every effort to round with the physician or practitioner when on the unit. Nurses who make patient rounds with the physician not only improve patient-care outcomes, but also build relationships with physician partners. Nurse-physician relationships are a key component to nurses' job satisfaction and perceived competence (Twibell et al., 2012).

Case Study 26.2

Jenny is a new nurse on the Surgical Orthopedic unit, working late in the evening. Her patient is very concerned that he did not receive his eye drops for glaucoma today. Jenny knows that this surgeon hates to be bothered after regular business hours. How should Jenny state her concerns with the surgeon?

You may have heard nurses apologizing when calling a health care provider with a question. "I am sorry to bother you Dr. Branson." Don't adopt this habit; never apologize for doing your job. As the primary nurse providing direct hands-on patient care, you are the eyes and ears of the health care provider. If a concern or a question arises, contact the health care provider and ensure the patient's care needs are met. Organize information in the Situation-Background-Assessment-Recommendation (SBAR) format. Ensure a recent set of vital signs and all of the pertinent information is readily available via the EHR during a phone call or when texting a Health Care Provider.

Nurses should be assertive, concise, but sincere when calling practitioners. Never fear calling practitioners because they may "yell." Lateral violence is never acceptable. Nurses are patient advocates and it is part of the role of the RN to act as such. If a health care provider prescribes or discusses something unfamiliar, ask questions. Many practitioners will appreciate questions and love to teach. Be honest and up front.

Respect is two ways, give due respect to health care providers, and expect the same from them. If the health care provider is rude or condescending, respond promptly by acknowledging their action and that it is unacceptable saying, "I don't appreciate being spoken to in that way" or "I would appreciate being spoken to in a civil tone of voice, and I promise to do the same with you."

Always seek clarification from the practitioner if an order is unclear. Always repeat the order to clarify if a phone order or if electronically written. Statements such as, "This order does not seem appropriate for this patient" may put the health care providers on the defensive, while clearer statements such as "I am concerned with this order. It makes me uncomfortable. This is a safety issue" are recommended (TeamSTEPPS®, Agency for Healthcare Research and Quality (AHRQ), 2013). This approach usually results in the practitioner either reevaluating an order or changing it. If the health care provider does not change an order that you think is inappropriate, contact the charge nurse or nurse manager and follow the guidelines of the agency. Never administer any medication if the order is unclear; clear the issue before administration. Remember, diplomacy often works wonders, and it is your RN license that may be at risk. TeamSTEPPS, SBAR, the 2 Challenge Rule, and the CUS assertive statements are discussed in greater detail in Chapter 16.

Nurse Residency and Transition to Practice Programs

Nurse Residency programs are intended to help the new RN transition from being a student to clinical practice. Most programs last 6–12 months beyond the initial orientation period. The terms Nurse Residency and **TTP** are both used in the literature. The Institute of Medicine (now called The National Academy of Medicine), the National Council of State Boards of Nursing (NCSBN), and the Commission on Collegiate Nursing Education (CCNE) all advocate for a Nurse Residency or TTP program for the new RN. Look for these key evidence-based elements of Nurse Residency or TTP programs at your potential employer:

- clinical coaching by a preceptor who is matched for compatibility with the new RN. Preceptors and new RNs should work the same shift on the same unit, and meet weekly to discuss feedback and areas of concern.

- evidence-based classroom experiences with case studies and direct links to clinical experiences in the new RN's specialty and unit.

- hands-on learning of skills in a clinical setting or simulations lab.

- time spent in areas outside the new RN's home unit to understand overall health care organization issues as well as policies and procedures.

- participation in a support group of new RNs peers.

- high visibility of nurse leaders.

- professional socialization and opportunities for development (Twibell et al., 2012).

Spector et al., (2015) studied TTP programs within hospitals and non-hospital facilities. New nurses in hospitals with minimal assistance and support during the first year had more errors and more negative safety practices, felt less competent, experienced more stress, reported less job satisfaction, and had twice the turnover when compared to the hospitals with established TTP programs.

Although the incidence is improving, outpatient clinics, hospice facilities, home health organizations, and nursing homes are less likely to offer a Nurse Residency Program to their newly graduated nurses. The cost of a nurse residency program has been cited as the reason for this lack. However, Silvestre, Ulrich, Johnson, Spector, and Blegen (2017) considered the return on investment for a Nurse Residency program. Their cost analysis shows a positive return on investment when using a structured TTP program, with a cost saving of between $735 and $1,458 per newly graduated RN. These authors estimate these savings are conservative compared to those of other researchers; even small organizations that hire only a few new nurses can expect cost savings when implementing and maintaining a TTP program (Silvestre, et al. 2017).

To further enhance the TTP for any newly licensed nurse, the NCSBN (2017) has developed an on-line e-learning program for both the newly RN and for preceptors. Centered around the QSEN competencies, the program for the newly

Table 26.4   NCSBN On-line e-learning Transition to Practice

5 courses for the newly licensed registered nurse
*Each course is $40 and offers 4.0 contact hours of continuing education. The package including all 5 courses is $150. Courses are self-paced and must be completed within 6 months.

Transition to Practice Course 1	Communication and Teamwork v.1.4
Transition to Practice Course 2	Patient and Family Centered Care v. 1.4
Transition to Practice Course 3	Evidence Based Practice v.1.4
Transition to Practice Course 4	Quality Improvement v. 1.4
Transition to Practice Course 5	Informatics v.1.4

1 course for the preceptor
*Transition to Practice: Course for Preceptors v1.4, 2.0 contact hours, $30
*cost at the time of publication, notice to change

Source: NCSBN Learning Extension. (2017). Transition to Practice [Pamphlet]. Chicago, IL: NCSBN.

licensed nurse reviews and discusses important concepts integral to patient safety and critical thinking, helping newly graduated nurses understand how to apply nursing knowledge, learn new skills, and think critically as they transition to confident professionals. See Table 26.4 NCSBN On-line eLearning Transition to Practice Program.

Identifying Your Own Learning Needs

New RNs begin orientation with varied clinical experiences and competencies. Often, beginning nurses are asked to self-rate their level of knowledge or experience with various patient care skills. It is important for new nurses to identify their own learning needs and ask themselves: What skills do I need to develop to do a good job in this position? New RNs may feel overwhelmed and feel they have much to learn. Orientation is the ideal time for the new RN to observe co-workers and establish learning priorities. Ask questions of the preceptor and/or nurse educator. Be alert for opportunities to grow and learn. If you have never had the opportunity to insert an indwelling Foley catheter, volunteer to complete the task for another nurse on the unit. Take advantage of teaching moments to observe and learn new things. The time is now, before you are assigned your own team of patients. Once the orientation phase is complete, it is more difficult to find the time to observe, practice, and learn new things.

In addition, plan to do your own self-study to prepare for your new patients. Remember Case Study 26.1 with Adam? He accepted a position in a Pediatric Oncology unit. Adam decided to review Pediatric physical assessment skills and medication administration and dosing for the pediatric patient before he started providing care on his new unit. During the first week or two, he also created a list of common medications, lab and diagnostic testing, medical diagnoses, and nursing diagnoses for the patients on his unit. He made note cards on these common findings and kept them in his locker for easy

reference. He also identified the resources available to him during his night shifts. He discovered an on-line medication reference and a link to a reference for nursing skills. He realized that a pharmacist was available for questions around the clock. He intentionally introduced himself to the respiratory therapists who work nights on his unit. Adam developed a plan for his learning needs. Discussing his plan with his preceptor and manager allows their input and suggestions.

Learning Styles

Educators have long realized that people learn in different ways, based in part on their previous experiences. At each stage of the learning process, individuals have different learning styles and may need different interventions from their preceptors or leaders. New RNs orienting to the clinical area need a preceptor who gives specific directions. They need details and demonstration of skills. New nurses benefit if the preceptor or educator breaks tasks down into components so that they can readily see the proper order or priority of items. As new nurses become more experienced, they do well with a teaching style that emphasizes collaboration and relates the new material to the learner's frame of reference.

Taking a learning style inventory can help bring awareness to the orientation process. The VARK questionnaire allows exploration of the methods that works best for your learning style. The VARK model identifies four types of learners: visual, auditory, reading/writing, and kinesthetic. Which type of learner are you? See the Exploring the Web section at the end of this chapter.

It can be difficult to match a teaching style to a learning style. Newly graduated nurses may find it helpful to develop learning objectives that can be shared with a preceptor and with a nurse educator or manager. Together they review and update the learning objectives each week. This will help give direction and purpose to the new graduate.

Performance Feedback

"So, how am I doing?" Everyone wants feedback about their performance, particularly when they are in a new position. Feedback is important because it boosts confidence, encourages positive behavior, stops unproductive actions, and acknowledges a job well done. A concrete mechanism to measure your performance is through the objective assessment materials provided by nurse educators. New nurses must successfully pass the written and technical portions of orientation. For example, many hospitals will require the new RN to successfully pass a medication math and administration test as part of their orientation process. If the organization has a competency-based orientation tool, the new nurse must meet its performance criteria.

Preceptor Assessment

During the orientation period, new nurses value friendly and respectful conversations regarding their performance and progress. Most preceptors and managers recognize new employees for their progress, but sometimes the new nurse needs to request feedback. A new nurse can ask for feedback from preceptors and managers regarding progress toward meeting learning objectives. When feedback is absent or lacking, a cycle of self-doubt and isolation can arise, causing anxiety. Even if the feedback of the new RN is not positive, negative feedback is better than no feedback (Gardiner & Sheen, 2016).

New RNs should meet at regular intervals with their preceptor and manager to review progress. This evaluation time is important to make certain that new nurses are being assigned to clinical experiences that match their learning needs. At each of these private sessions, it is important for the new nurse to solicit feedback. Ask, "How do you think I'm doing? Am I at the level you would expect? What should I focus on next?" Answers to questions such as these allow the orientee to measure progress. Many new graduates take negative evaluation personally. It is important that the preceptor and manager identify that it is the skill or behavior that is inappropriate, and not the nurse as a person.

At these private meetings, the preceptor, manager, and new RN should set goals for the next week or month. For example, "By the end of next week, the new RN will have progressed to independent patient physical assessments, completed a patient admission, and increased the workload to a four-patient assignment."

During these sessions, the newly licensed nurse, the preceptor, and the manager can also review progress on the list of skills and tasks required for the new nurse in that unit. See Table 26.5 "Sample of a Medical-urgical RN Skills Assessment and Orientation Checklist."

For the new nurse who is struggling during the orientation phase, it is during feedback that lack of progress is often clearly identified and documented. As a result, more frequent sessions between the manager, preceptor, and the new RN will occur. On occasion, the decision may be made to switch the new RN to another shift or assign the new RN to work with another preceptor. Human Resources specialists will likely be involved in such decisions. One-on-one sessions with the nurse educator for that unit or speciality may be scheduled. Additional weeks of orientation may be added. Despite all efforts by the manager, educators, and human resources specialists, if the new nurse continues to struggle, a health care organization will dismiss a new nurse who is not meeting goals and expectations. Dismissal is done with great reluctance. The health care organization has invested time and effort into the training and coaching of this new nurse and will not make the decision to dismiss a new nurse lightly.

There should be opportunities for the new nurse to evaluate her preceptor throughout the orientation process (Table 26.5). These evaluations would be reviewed by the manager of the unit. The preceptor may be evaluated by the new RN on the following:

An attitude that is positive, helpful, and motivating

Promotion of the new nurse's socialization within the department and the health care organization

Knowledge of policies, procedures, and guidelines

Organization and planning for learning opportunities

Communication skills.

Formal Performance Evaluation

To maintain accreditation, health care organizations are required to administer performance evaluations for each

---

Table 26.5 **Feedback**

Feedback is information provided for the purpose of improving performance and sharing concerns. Feedback should be:	
Timely	**Given soon after the concerning action, skill or behavior has occurred.**
Respectful	Focuses on behaviors, skills, and actions, not personal attributes.
Specific	Relates to a specific action, skill, or behavior that requires correction or improvement.
Directed Toward Improvement	Provides clear direction for future improvement. May include examples or suggestions.
Considerate	Considers the other's feelings and delivers negative information with fairness and respect.

Source: Adapted from Pocket Guide: TeamSTEPPS. Content last reviewed January 2014. Agency for Healthcare Research and Quality, Rockville, MD. https://www.ahrq.gov/teamstepps/instructor/essentials/pocketguide.html.

employee at regular intervals. Individual facilities set their own policies, identifying the process and time frames. For many, annual evaluations are the norm. The new RN may also be evaluated at 6 months. Evaluation forms are usually standardized within the health care organization, but they also allow for individual performance feedback from the nurse manager.

What should nurses expect from their first formal performance evaluation? The individual and the nurse manager meet in private to review progress since either the previous evaluation or date of hiring. The evaluation should be objective, based on the nurse's performance as measured against the job description. Job descriptions consist of similar components, such as:

- Job title, the department and division; i.e. RN-1, Oncology, Division of Nursing

- OSHA categories identify the risk of exposure to blood and body fluids

- To whom the position reports and who oversees work performance

- Age of the population of patients served

- Mission and values of the organization

- Standards of behavior

- Job duties and responsibilities may be categorized into evidence-based interventions, relationships and caring, critical thinking, technical expertise, leadership, and qualifications. Qualifications will include an RN license in the appropriate state and a bachelors or associates degree

- A description of the physical requirements of the position will also be listed, such as walking most of the designated shift, lifting or carrying objects of 35–40 pounds, using a computer keyboard and mouse to enter and retrieve data.

Most performance evaluations use some sort of checklist, reflecting whether the individual being evaluated meets standards, exceeds standards, or falls below the organization's standards. Checklists are derived from the components of a job description. Formal performance evaluation between the manager and staff member serves several purposes. The evaluation is used to ensure competence in the skills required for safe patient care. It is also an opportunity to recognize the nurse's accomplishments in the evaluation period, which can be a real morale boost. This is the ideal time for the manager to enhance future performance by coaching, setting goals, and identifying learning needs. At the end of the performance evaluation, both the manager and the new RN should have a clear understanding of what needs to happen in the next months or year for that nurse to grow and continue to be successful. Feedback is most useful when it identifies actual examples of good and poor performance and gives suggestions for change. Should the new nurse not meet the mutually agreed upon goals, new goals will be established. Corrective action may be a consequence for a nurse who is consistently not meeting goals. Often the human resources representatives will be involved if the employee is not be meeting the goals and standards set in the job description. Even during the orientation phase, the new nurse who is not meeting goals can be dismissed.

During the feedback and performance evaluation process, a new nurse may realize that their position is not what they hoped and anticipated. Signs that a nurse may consider leaving a position include feelings of stress and negativity, differences in beliefs from the organization, imbalance between job and personal life, no longer being challenged to learn and grow, and abuse or harassment (McGill & Loveless, 2018).

There are ways to leave a job with grace and professionalism. First, ensure another job offer has been received, in writing preferably. The unit manager needs to be the first one informed. Do not share plans with anyone else. The manager should never hear the news through the unit's grapevine. Calmly and clearly let the manager know of plans to leave and when the last day will be. Be thankful. This is not the time to vent anger and burn bridges. It is considerate to give notice at least 2 weeks in advance. Or perhaps finish out the current schedule. A written and signed letter of resignation will be submitted after the discussion with the manager. Meet with representatives in Human Resources (**HR**) to discuss any benefits and retirement details. Discuss plans for any retirement funds and the potential to roll that into an account with a new employer or investment specialist. Once the manager and HR have been informed, then co-workers may learn of the news. Do everything possible to make this transition easy for the manager and co-workers. Regarding any special projects or tasks, ask the manager which co-worker should be trained to take over. Ask for an exit interview with the manager. This is still not a time for any anger. If there are criticisms that should be shared to promote patient care and safety, then share the facts and give specific examples. Be honest and yet positive. When leaving, the goal should be to share concerns and hopefully leave the unit a better place. Leave on good terms, as it is possible that some of these same people may be your co-workers again in the future.

Organizational Responses to Performance

Many health care organizations have a merit-based compensation structure that is tied to performance evaluations. Employees' pay raises are matched to their performance. But most health care organizations are looking for other ways—in addition to money—to create job satisfaction. Recognition is an important way in which health care organizations can motivate employee performance.

Employee Recognition Programs

Many health care organizations have developed formal recognition activities. These may take the form of surprising an employee of the month with balloons and a plaque, bringing in

---

Real World Interview (with a Nurse Manager)

I always say that the key to retaining someone is engaging someone. You have to get people involved on the front end, because if you get buy-in early they become more productive and efficient in the long term. We have a very structured orientation process that is based on experience. We have meetings multiple times with the Orientee, Preceptor, our Nurse Educator, Charge Nurse, and from time to time myself (Clinical Nurse Leader in Telemetry) to discuss how things are going, what barriers there might be, and what we can do as a leadership team to make that orientee successful. I always tell the orientee that THEY drive the bus, we are just there to help get them to where they need to go.

After orientation, we have employee recognition programs, open door policies, and every employee is rounded on by leadership at least monthly, if not more, in order to determine what is going well on the unit and what may need some more attention. This has helped shape us into a strong unit/team, because the employees are very well aware that our leadership team is here for THEM, and we will always listen to what they have to say. They also know we expect that in return.

Elaine Bastek

CLINICAL NURSE LEADER IN TELEMETRY
PALOS HEIGHTS, IL

---

a national speaker for a celebration of Nurses Day, or presenting recognition gifts for years of service. One popular recognition involves selecting an employee from each unit to attend a quarterly luncheon with the organization's administrator. At the luncheon, employees are recognized individually for their contributions to patient care, based on the narratives submitted by the nominating individuals.

Corrective Action Programs

Sometimes, formal performance reviews or feedback indicate the need for significant performance improvement. Most health care organizations have a prescribed **corrective action program**, established steps and processes taken by the nurse manager with the support of Human Resources when the performance of the employee is not meeting the standards delineated in the job description and the health care organization's policies. One of the first steps in helping employees improve their performance is identifying whether their poor performance is developmental or related to a failure to follow policies or procedures. For example, a nurse may be having difficulty completing assignments in an appropriate time frame. It is unlikely that the nurse's problem is related to a lack of understanding of the rules. Instead, the manager needs to coach the employee, assisting the nurse with whatever support will help the nurse improve. It may be that the nurse needs remedial work in some particular technical skill or feedback specifically directed to organizing a patient assignment, either of which can affect the nurse's ability to complete the shift on time.

Progressive Discipline

Another category of corrective action is disciplinary corrective action. In this case, an employee receives feedback for failing to follow the organization's policies. Excessive absenteeism is an example. As with the previous example, the goal is to assist the nurse to improve performance. Most organizations have a series of progressive steps for corrective action

in cases in which employee performance does not improve. With **progressive discipline**, the manager and employee's mutual goal is to take steps to correct performance to bring it back to an acceptable level. Actions taken by the manager follow specific steps and processes that gradually worsen in their impact on the employee who is not meeting standards. To continue with the example of excessive absenteeism, a manager will meet with the nurse and provide a verbal warning to an employee whose attendance is minimally acceptable. If the nurse's attendance problem continues, the nurse may receive a written warning from the manager. Without improvement, this could proceed to a suspension, final warning, and eventually termination. Throughout this entire process, the specialists with Human Resources provide policy and coaching for the manager and the employee. Progressive discipline offers a stepwise process with opportunities for continued feedback and clarification of expectations. In any event, the corrective action applied by the manager must be fair. Employees should be forewarned of the consequences of violating an institution's policies so that there are no surprises. The corrective action should be consistent and impartial—each person is treated the same each time the rule is broken.

It is required and expected that all employees practice within the policies and standards established by the health care organization. This is the standard to which all new RNs are held to within the health care organization. Additionally, the nurse practice act for RNs in your state has legal implications for your practice.

The Nurse as a Manager of a Small Patient Group

The nurse responsible for direct care of a small group of patients is functioning as a leader and manager. Time management and keeping organized are some of the challenges faced by the new RN. Being familiar with the expectations for the care of your patients during the shift is critical.

Time Management

Time management is often a challenge for the new RN. New nurses find themselves in a quicksand-like time trap with too many tasks to be accomplished all at the same time. The health care environment is fast-paced with many interruptions. Taking control of the time available during the shift is challenging. Being organized involves both planning your day and collecting all of the needed supplies prior to beginning a task such as a dressing change. Multitasking is assessing the skin while repositioning the patient. Saying "No, I cannot help you right now, but would love to help you in about 45 min when I finish this," is a tactful method for use with your co-workers when they have a non-critical situation. Bundling or clustering activities is flushing the patient's saline lock after an antibiotic and re-checking the blood pressure at the same time. Do not allow any interruptions when completing critical tasks, such as medication administration. Ensure you know exactly how to complete a skill before entering the room. Check the policy or discuss the skill with your preceptor first. Close the door while you are assessing your patient to limit interruptions. Document your assessment while still at the patient's bedside and all of the information is still fresh in your memory. "Only Handle It Once" (OHIO) is a tip from a mentor of mine many years ago that has reduced procrastination and time wasting. Delegate care often and appropriately.

Eventually every nurse will establish a routine for receiving report from the previous nurse. Some nurses have developed a report sheet that helps to keep them organized. It may be small enough to fold up and fit in a pocket. Or the nurse's report sheet may be several pages long and be kept on a clip board. By writing down key information, such as lab results, assessment findings, and the times medications are due, the nurse is able to stay current with the care their patients require. A brief report sheet also allows quick access to the questions that other members of the health care team may have. Not all patient rooms will have bedside computers, so writing down some key points means the RN does not have to rely on memory (Table 26.6).

Relating to Other Disciplines

Given the complexity of health care organizations in the United States, the successful interconnection among departments is a potential source of tremendous strength. The RN who understands the functions of the team, including respiratory therapists, pharmacists, dieticians, social workers, case managers, and vendors for durable medical equipment, will be able to efficiently incorporate the contributions of the team in planning for effective patient care. In many settings, diagnosis-specific care plans or clinical practice guidelines articulate the anticipated relationships among disciplines. For example, a care plan for a patient admitted for a stroke may include a referral to a speech therapist for an aspiration assessment on day one of admission, a consultation with physical therapy for mobility on day two, and an evaluation for home care needs with the social worker

on day three. It is important for nurses to develop strong relationships with representatives of the many other disciplines whose practices interface with the nursing role.

Delegation to Team Members

"To be 'in charge' is certainly not only to carry out the proper measures yourself but to see that everyone else does so too; to see that no one either willfully or ignorantly thwarts or prevents such measures. It is neither to do everything yourself nor to appoint a number of people to do each duty, but to ensure that each does that duty to which he is appointed" (Florence Nightingale, 1859, p. 42).

As a manager of a small patient group, the nurse is responsible for linking each patient to the resources that the patient needs. This often involves delegation and supervision of other members of the health care team, such as Licensed Practice Nurses (LPNs) and UAPs as they provide direct patient care.

In the current health care environment, lengths of stay (LOS) are shorter despite increased patient acuity and complexity. The nurse who is responsible for a group of patients also needs to work with other nurses and licensed and unlicensed personnel to provide safe patient care. This usually involves delegating specific responsibilities to other staff, including some staff who may be either from an older or a younger generation with different beliefs and working styles. Good communication among staff of all generations is critical in assuring safe patient care and good working relationships. The RN who delegates effectively assigns routine tasks to a co-worker, freeing the nurse for more-complex planning or care. As a starting point, a nurse needs to refer to the nurse practice act for the state in which the nurse practices. This document is specific to each state and limits or defines the responsibilities that may be delegated. For example, in some states, LPNs may draw blood but may not start IV lines. Responsibilities that may be delegated can also vary from hospital to hospital. The nurse needs to follow all such policies in decisions about delegation.

The nurse must also consider the skills and knowledge of co-workers in order to delegate well. This allows the nurse to give teammates the opportunity to work within their competencies. The nurse needs to match the co-worker's skills with the delegated task, while remembering which skills cannot be delegated, such as ongoing evaluation and supervision of tasks.

It is easy to fall into the trap of over-delegating or under-delegating, particularly for new nurses. Some new RNs are hesitant to delegate activities to others, because they are afraid their teammates will resent being asked to do a specific task. They worry they will be seen as lazy or lacking ability. Or they may hesitate to delegate out of a belief that they can do the task better or faster themselves.

Other nurses delegate more care than is appropriate or safe. Nurses who over-delegate may do so because they are poor time managers or because they personally lack the skill required. It may be that they failed to first assess their patients or are unfamiliar with their co-workers' competencies.

The Charge Role

Many hospital-based nurses, especially those who work evening or night shifts, rapidly progress from being assigned responsibility for a small group of patients to being assigned to the charge role for the shift. The charge nurse coordinates care for the whole unit and may also continue to care for a small group of assigned patients. This nurse is responsible for assigning the workload of the nursing staff for the shift.

First-time charge nurses often have high expectations for their own performance, and they can easily become stressed in

Table 26.6 Sample Telemetry Report Sheet

Patient Initials:_____ Sex:_____ Age:_____ Room: _____ Admission Date: _____ Code Status: _____
Allergies _____ Isolation: _____ Diet: _____ Activity: _____
            C/C: _____ Diagnosis: _____

Pertinent Medical/Surgical History:	Psychosocial History:
A FIB / Alzheimer's / Asthma / BPH / CA / CABG / CAD / CHF / CKD / COPD / CVA / Dementia / DM / ESRD / GERD / HIV / HLD / HTN / Hyperthyroid / Hypothyroid / Mastectomy / Pacemaker / PCI / PVD / RA / SCD / Seizures / SLE / TB / Valve Replacement	Smoker: Alcohol: Illicit Drugs:
	ADD/AHDH / Anxiety / Bipolar / Chronic Pain / Confusion / Depression / Hallucinations / Restlessness/Agitation / Suicidal ideations / Schizophrenia /
	Lives at Home / Lives at facility / Other:
	Married / Single / Other:

Medications:

0800/2000	0900/2100	1000/2200	1100/2300
1200/0000	1300/0100	1400/0200	1500/0300
1600/0400	1700/0500	1800/0600	1900/0700

IV: #_____ R / L SL Date: _____	IVF: NS / ½ NS / D5 ⅓ / D5 NS / LR / Abx
Site: AC / FA / Hand / Wrist / UA	IV Rate: _____ ml/hr / _____ u/kg/hr
Central: IJ / Midline / PICC / Port / Trialysis	Drips: Heparin / Blood / TPN / Dilt Titration:

Trach: Equipment at bedside? YES / NO	Mode:	Rate:	TV:	PEEP:	PS:	FiO₂:

Tests: ABG / MRI / X-Ray / CT / Echo EF: ____ / Endo / US / Cath / Swallow Study / Urine / C&S

Circle the appropriate assessment documentation to best fit the patient in your care

Table 26.6   **(Continued)**

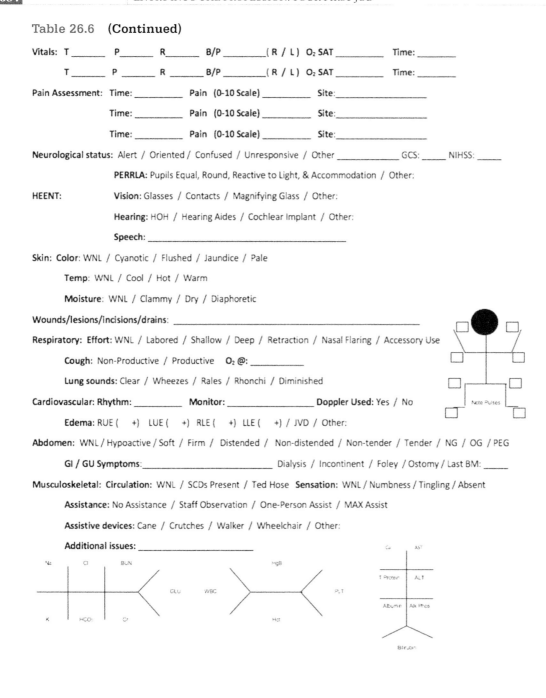

Vitals: T _____   P_____   R_____   B/P _____ (R / L) O₂ SAT _____   Time: _____

T _____   P _____   R _____   B/P _____ (R / L) O₂ SAT _____   Time: _____

Pain Assessment: Time: _____   Pain (0-10 Scale) _____   Site:_____

Time: _____   Pain (0-10 Scale) _____   Site:_____

Time: _____   Pain (0-10 Scale) _____   Site:_____

Neurological status: Alert / Oriented / Confused / Unresponsive / Other _____ GCS: _____ NIHSS: _____

PERRLA: Pupils Equal, Round, Reactive to Light, & Accommodation / Other:

HEENT: **Vision:** Glasses / Contacts / Magnifying Glass / Other:

Hearing: HOH / Hearing Aides / Cochlear Implant / Other:

Speech: _____

Skin: **Color:** WNL / Cyanotic / Flushed / Jaundice / Pale

Temp: WNL / Cool / Hot / Warm

Moisture: WNL / Clammy / Dry / Diaphoretic

Wounds/lesions/incisions/drains: _____

Respiratory: Effort: WNL / Labored / Shallow / Deep / Retraction / Nasal Flaring / Accessory Use

Cough: Non-Productive / Productive   **O₂ @:** _____

Lung sounds: Clear / Wheezes / Rales / Rhonchi / Diminished

Cardiovascular: Rhythm: _____   **Monitor:** _____ **Doppler Used: Yes** / No

Edema: RUE (+) LUE (+) RLE (+) LLE (+) / JVD / Other:

Abdomen: WNL / Hypoactive / Soft / Firm / Distended / Non-distended / Non-tender / Tender / NG / OG / PEG

GI / GU Symptoms:_____   Dialysis / Incontinent / Foley / Ostomy / Last BM: _____

Musculoskeletal: Circulation: WNL / SCDs Present / Ted Hose **Sensation:** WNL / Numbness / Tingling / Absent

Assistance: No Assistance / Staff Observation / One-Person Assist / MAX Assist

Assistive devices: Cane / Crutches / Walker / Wheelchair / Other:

Additional issues: _____

Source: D. Hoekstra.

Articulating Expectations

the new role. It is helpful to recognize that the nursing process—assessing, diagnosing, planning, implementing, and evaluating care—requires organizational and priority-setting skills that directly apply to the charge nurse role. It is a matter of perceiving and delegating patient care needs from the perspective of the unit as a whole. The new charge nurse must let go of the need to be perfect. Instead, the nurse should concentrate on staying organized and focused on what is best for the patients. It is also important to recognize and utilize the available resources for problem solving, such as co-workers or the supervisor.

As a first-time charge nurse, it is important to build relationships with other staff members, as well as co-workers from other disciplines. One way to develop these relationships is by sharing expectations. This may be as simple as sitting down over coffee and agreeing to certain behaviors, such as "We will maintain a patient focus, as evidenced by answering call lights quickly." Some performance expectations may be more generic, applying to relationships more than specific patient

Critical Thinking 26.1

As a new RN, you may be reluctant to delegate care to others. Review the policies established at your health care organization regarding the care that can be delegated to the UAP. What care can be delegated to a sitter? An LPN? How do these policies compare to the State Board of Nursing guidelines and regulations?

Performance feedback is a crucial element of delegation. It is important to openly recognize team members' contributions to safe patient care. In an instance in which the nurse is not satisfied with the outcome of a delegated task, it is equally important to discuss the assignment with the co-worker individually. Perhaps the nurse's directions were unclear, misunderstood, or failed to include an important time frame. Taking the time to provide feedback demonstrates the respect and value a nurse places on his or her teammates' contributions.

Sometimes when one delegates an assignment to a team member, that person may question the parameters of the assignment. If, for example, the nurse in charge of a group of patients delegates a patient's ostomy teaching to another nurse on the team. That nurse may hear that assignment several ways. For example, the nurse may think, "I need to do the ostomy appliance change while the patient's wife is here." Or "I need to assess what

the patient has learned already and report back to the nurse." Or, finally, "I need to develop a teaching plan with the patient and begin to implement it today."

These possibilities demonstrate the importance of delegating clearly and specifically. It is important to remember that even when a task is delegated, the person delegating the task is still responsible to assure that the task is completed correctly. The licensed nurse who delegates a responsibility maintains overall accountability for the patient. However, the other team member bears the responsibility for the delegated activity, skill, or procedure (National Council of State Boards of Nursing (NCSBN), 2016). Communication is key to effective delegation. The person to whom the task is assigned must clearly understand the expectations. In the above scenario, the nurse who is delegating should explicitly tell the second nurse what the expected outcome and time frame are for the delegated task. For example, the delegating nurse might state, "Please construct a teaching plan for this patient's ostomy care today. Be sure to include the patient and his wife to ensure they will be able to perform effective ostomy care at home."

care items, but they still need to be clearly spelled out. For example, "If you disagree with me, you will talk to me about it before you discuss our disagreement with others." These specific expectations help establish a level of trust and prevent the need for mind reading. They open the doorway for clear communication, so that when a problem develops, it is easier to approach the individual involved.

Mechanisms to Enhance Professional Growth

New nurses are more likely to stay in their positions if they are challenged and have opportunities for professional growth. Some health care facilities have a wealth of available educational opportunities. Others, particularly smaller or community-based organizations, may require the nurse to be more creative when looking for education opportunities. The best place to start is with the experts on and around the nursing unit.

Cross-Training

Given today's shortage of nurses, there is increased floating from one's usual unit to another short-staffed unit for one shift. Floating to another unit offers nurses **cross-training** to new areas. Cross-training is another opportunity for individual growth. Although some organizations have strict guidelines to limit the practice of floating and cross-training nurses, other health care facilities expect nurses to routinely float to either

a related unit or an area particularly in need of assistance. It is useful for all staff to recall that a hospital is a business and must have staff available to care for patients at all times.

It is important for nurses in their first job to be articulate about their competencies for a new patient population if they are asked to float. They need to be sure the manager assigning them is aware of their experience level. Nurses should not accept total responsibility for an area or population in which they have not achieved competency. It may be more appropriate to assign an inexperienced nurse to specific tasks to help on the unit rather than asking that nurse to take a typical patient assignment on an unfamiliar unit.

One way to minimize the stress of being asked to float to a different unit is to volunteer ahead of time to cross-train to the new area. This has many advantages. It allows the nurse the opportunity to experience working with different ages or types of patients. Besides learning new skills, it gives a nurse the chance to see how the other half lives. For example, Jessica has worked only on a medical floor. Receiving an admission from the emergency department (**ED**) during her night shift is always a challenge to be worked into Jessica's shift routine. After cross-training to the ED and seeing patients waiting on stretchers in the hall, Jessica has a new appreciation of the need to negotiate for timely acceptance of ED admissions to the floor.

Cross-training has some long-term benefits as well. Since Mario (see Case Study 26.3) is considering a career in a unit for patients with a cardiac condition, Mario volunteers to float to the Cardiac Intermediate Care Unit (**IMCU**). By spending

Case Study 26.3

Mario is working on a Rehab unit at a large community-based hospital. He has an interest in learning more about the care of patients with cardiac conditions. Since the hospital offers a Basic EKG Interpretation course, he asks his manager if he could participate in the course. Since it is not a requirement for his current position, Mario's manager cannot pay him while he attends the classes. She encourages him to attend the classes on his own time and does her best to fit the classes into his work schedule. When Mario speaks with the educator about his interests, the educator recommends some websites and nursing specialty organizations. Mario rounds with the cardiologist while evaluating patients on the unit. Mario also asks for the name of an interventional cardiologist so he can observe the physician perform a cardiac catheterization. When the EKG Tech arrives to the unit, Mario observes the process for obtaining a 12 lead EKG. By expanding his investigation and asking other health care disciplines within his health care organization, Mario is learning about the team approach to a patient with a

cardiac disorder. Can you think of a specific disease that interests you? Identify another Health Care Professional that could serve as a resource for you. Is there a national organization for nurses that specialize in your area of interest? Would you consider volunteering for a patient support group for those who have that disease?

Not all nurses have the motivation or time for a lot of formal professional growth activities. What is important is to stay challenged. Find a particular skill or interest in your position, and expand it. What do you like best of all the skills and care you provide? Is it working with the patient's family? Teaching the new diabetic? Starting an IV? Whatever it is, look for opportunities to become your unit's expert. Professional development increases nurses' knowledge and skill, which increases the quality of care provided to patients. Life-long learning is a requirement for all nurses. Nurses are professionals who have a complex role with great responsibility, requiring long-term continuing development (Benner, 2001/1984).

some time cross-training in this unit, Mario can decide whether he wants to pursue a more permanent job in this more specialized unit.

Cross-training is also beneficial to the nurse seeking a new position. When a nurse is applying for a new job, experience in more than one clinical area enhances a resume and makes the individual a stronger candidate for desired jobs.

Some health care organizations reward nurses who volunteer to cross-train so they can safely float to different areas. At some facilities these rewards may be monetary. Other facilities offer nonmonetary incentives, such as reduced weekend or holiday commitments as rewards for cross-training or floating.

Identifying a Mentor

Developing a mentoring relationship with a more experienced, successful nurse is another helpful strategy for professional growth. A **mentor** coaches a new RN and helps the novice develop skills and career direction. A mentor may introduce the new RN to professional networking opportunities. A good person to assist the new nurse in a workplace ethical dilemma may well be his or her mentor.

How does a new nurse find a mentor? First, the new nurse needs to communicate a willingness to learn and grow. A new RN usually needs to seek out a prospective mentor rather than wait to be approached by one. An ideal mentor is an experienced nurse who is willing to support and counsel other nurses when asked. This may lead to a formal structured relationship or a more informal role-modeling association.

Nurses who have been successful preceptors are often potential mentors because they are committed to helping another nurse learn and grow. Even though the preceptor role is shorter and more defined, the role can easily be expanded to a more informal mentoring relationship. Mentors differ from

preceptors in that mentors invest in newly licensed nurses for years, rather than the weeks or months of guidance provided by a preceptor (Twibell et al., 2012).

The Internet is a newer mentoring resource. Nurses can develop relationships through special-interest chat rooms or by e-mailing experts in other geographical areas. There are forums for questions and answers, often on specific patient populations, disease processes, or operational issues. Want to get some expert advice on a particular patient problem? Spend some time on the Internet.

Developing Professional Goals

After a new nurse has mastered the skills for day-to-day nursing care, what is next? How does a nurse measure professional growth? For many nurses, the answer to these questions is a clinical ladder.

A **clinical ladder** is a program established by a health care organization to encourage nurses to earn promotions and gain recognition and increased pay by meeting specific requirements. Although the criteria may vary, most programs have three or four distinct levels. Some also offer the nurse the opportunity to seek promotion in a specific track, within a clinical, an educational, or a managerial focus. Thus, it is possible for a new nurse to choose a clinical nursing track and move through the organization's promotional levels by meeting those requirements. For example, to be promoted from a new graduate level to a Level II RN, the nurse may be required to complete a specialty course such as Basic EKG interpretation and Advanced Cardiac Life Support (ACLS) and join a unit-based or hospital-based committee. Besides offering opportunity for promotion, these programs offer an objective way to measure a nurse's achievements. Clinical ladders can be time-consuming to complete, yet they provide valuable information.

Does your state require Continuing Education (**CE**) credits? What is the requirement? In some states the requirement is 20 credit hours every 2 years. Some of the education and training offered by your employer may meet some of the state requirements (Table 26.7).

Remember the simple things of being a professional. Dress for success. If not required to wear scrubs, then wear business casual. No yoga pants. No jeans. No sweats. Make sure you are neat with polished and clean shoes. See Table 26.7 Six Ways to Get Promoted at Work. Professionalism needs to extend to your social media posts as well. Think before you post. Remove inappropriate photos with evidence of substance use. Keep your political opinions to yourself. Profanity, sexually explicit, violent, and racially derogatory comments should never be part of your social profile. Your current and future manager may be following you.

Specialty Certifications

Many health care organizations encourage their staff to become certified. Nearly all nursing specialties now offer board certification exams to validate expert knowledge of that particular discipline. Emergency nurses may sit for the Certified Emergency Nurse (**CEN**) exam and the ACLS certification. Nurses who specialize in critical care may take the critical care certifying exam to earn their CCRN. Successfully passing a specialty certification exam is another measure of professional growth and offers the benefit of national recognition of one's credentials. If you want to pursue a specialty in nursing, how much additional education is required? What schools offer that education? How long will it take? Does your employer offer tuition reimbursement for certifications and courses?

Reality Shock and Burnout

In 1974, Kramer described **Reality Shock** and discussed the difficulties that some new graduates have in adjusting to the work environment. Kramer identified the conflict between new graduates' expectations and the reality of their first nursing position. A skilled preceptor or mentor can assist new RNs through this transition by offering opportunities to validate impressions. The support of other new nurses in a similar situation, such as those participating in a Nurse Residency or TTP program, is particularly helpful.

New RNs can experience burnout when they do not feel competent to care for patients safely, especially if experiencing other life stress outside of the workplace as well. Strategies to address burnout and compassion fatigue should be implemented in a timely manner. Debriefing after difficult shifts, team-building events, celebration of meaningful work, and rotating difficult patient assignments, are possible strategies. Peers, managers, or an **Employee Assistance Program**

Table 26.7 Six Ways to Get Promoted at Work

6 Ways to get promoted at work:

1. *Know what your ultimate goal looks like. What can you do right now to start you down the path to your dream nursing job?*

2. *Keep positive while others are trending negative. Avoid the negativity. Avoid the gossip. Remember what you enjoy about your job. Be the one who finds solutions to the problem, not the one who just finds the problems.*

3. *Make the most of your current position. Review the job description for your current nursing position, then strive to exceed that description. You will not stand out by just doing your job.*

4. *Volunteer for different opportunities. Show those in authority that you are willing to take on some extra responsibilities. Make the unit a more pleasant place or make your bosses' job a little easier.*

5. *Show up on time and stay late if necessary.*

6. *When all else fails . . . ask! Speak with your manager or supervisor and let them know you are interested in additional responsibility.*

Note. Adapted from Senior, 2018

Evidence From the Literature

Citation: Melnyk, B. M., Orsolini, L., Tan, A., Arslanian-Engoren, C., Melkus, G. D., et al. (2018). A national study links nurses' perceived physical and mental health to medical errors and perceived worksite wellness. *Journal of Occupational and Environmental Medicine, 60*(2), 126–131.

Discussion: The findings from a study by Melnik et al. lends support for the strong positive association between nurses' health and medical errors. While employers typically understand that healthier engaged nurses translate into higher levels of productivity, less absenteeism, and less expensive health care costs, this study demonstrates that there is much more at stake in terms of patient safety . . . stress leads to depression and reductions in job satisfaction and these outcomes increase risk of patient harm.

Implications for Practice: Nurses need to understand the importance of life balance and stress reduction, not only for personal health, but to be a safer and happier nurse.

Critical Thinking 26.2

Go to the website for QSEN and review the QSEN Competencies and the KSAs (Knowledge Skills and Attitudes) http://qsen.org/competencies/pre-licensure-ksas. Focus on the KSAs for Safety.

How will you. the new RN. provide safe patient care? How can your inter-professional health care team help you to provide safe patient care, for example the physical therapist? The UAP?

Real World Interview

Reflections of a newly graduated nurse—6 months later

1. During your preceptorship, if you feel like you are not learning from your preceptor, SPEAK UP! It is so important to get the most out of your preceptorship because soon you will be on your own. Don't be afraid to talk to your preceptor about your learning needs, and maybe involve upper management in how to address the specific issue, whether it be about learning styles or hands-on nursing skills.

2. Know how long you will be on orientation, and know the steps on how to extend your orientation (if possible) at your facility. If you feel unsafe caring for your patients by yourself, tell your preceptor or your manager. Talk to them about your concerns about being on your own. This could potentially lead to more orientation days if your preceptor/manager does not think you are ready to end your orientation, or they might say the opposite and say you are freaking out for no reason and you'll be fine on the floor by yourself.

3. Do not beat yourself up for not knowing everything. No one knows everything. Instead of thinking about all the things you don't know how to do for your patient, think of all the things you DO know. Having a positive mindset during your workday changes everything, and I can say this is tough for new grads since we feel like we know next to nothing. You will never know everything.

4. Find a floor/unit/co-workers to work on that utilizes teamwork. I work in the Cardiac ICU, and I would not be happy working there if I had no other nurses to support me or my patients in crisis situations. Having co-workers that respond to your calls for help or assistance is essential. You need your co-workers as much as they need you.

5. Don't be afraid of calling or paging the doctor. I know I was terrified of calling the doctor about my patient, with the fear that I would sound stupid or not know what I was talking about. All that changed when I started my job. Working with interns or residents, they are similar to brand new nurses on the floor. They're just getting started with their careers, and their knowledge base is minimal (for

doctors). Interns and residents often depend on the nurses to guide them to a new intervention or tell them what they can and can't do, so do not be afraid to tell your doctor the facts about your patient, and what you would recommend. If they reject your recommendation, it is okay to ask why. Open communication and information sharing between the doctor and nurse makes everyone's work days better.

6. Giving report. Also, not that scary since you spent the last 8–12 hr with your patient. Report seemed like a daunting task in nursing school, but each unit has a way of giving report, so it's important to know what your floor thinks is important. For example, in a cardiac ICU, I need to know the strength of my radial, post tibial, and pedal pulses every 4 hr, along with the patient's heart rhythm, including ectopy. We also check our patient's pupils (PERRLA) every 4 hr. Each floor is different. I've had nurses on stepdown units say they don't want all of the unnecessary information about pupil size during report, and that they just need to know if the patient can get up and walk by themselves. Like I said, each unit is different.

7. Passing medications is not your highest priority. When I started, I always wanted to get my worklist objectives done and get them done on time, because that's what I was taught in nursing school. But your worklist doesn't talk about how your patient just started having chest pain, or how you need a stat EKG done by YOU at the bedside, or how the doctors want labs drawn stat, or how your other patient next door just started having decreased LOC 1 day after his valve replacement. Those medications can wait because your patients are your highest priority.

8. Goggles are a part of your uniform, and you'll never know when you need them. Whether it be blood spurts or your patient who coughs up nastiness. More PPE > less PPE.

9. Reading through notes in your spare time at work really helps to understand what your patient is going through, especially if they're extremely complicated.

Kelley Walsh, BS, RN
Northwestern Memorial Hospital
Chicago, IL

can provide emotional support when new nurses experience moral distress. Many organizations offer Employee Assistance Program through the Human Resources or Employee Benefits departments. Not only will EAP offer support and counseling, many programs also offer referral services for child and elder care. A goal of the EAP is to help with work life balance.

Healthy work cultures encourage new nurses to practice good self-care, such as taking breaks away from the bedside, limiting overtime hours, and achieving life-work balance. Be sure to take care of yourself. Avoid bad work habits such as gossiping, procrastinating then rushing, taking things too personally, being disorganized, putting personal life before work, and isolating yourself. Eat healthy food. Stay hydrated. Ask for help and delegate. Later you can return the favor when a co-worker asks for help, by giving back and lending a helping hand. Exercise and get moving. Schedule some pampering, like a pedicure or massage. Meditate and pray. Air your negative feelings by reflecting in a personal and private journal. Talk with your preceptor. Talk with your former classmates who are probably having similar experiences. New nurses need to anticipate reality shock and burnout. Be prepared. Nurses have a duty to also care for themselves if they hope to provide the best possible care for their patients. Preventing burnout among staff is shown in the current literature as a key strategy in reducing sick time, staffing issues, turnover, as well as improving morale and retaining valuable, skilled personnel in the long run (Twibell et al., 2012; Ostermeyer, 2018a,b; Van Wijlen, 2017).

Unfortunately, mistakes will happen. Every nurse has made mistakes and wishes to push the rewind button and have a do-over. Reach out and consult with the manager, preceptor, and/or mentor for encouragement and support when an error occurs. Confidence and sense of belonging may suffer otherwise. After an error, a new nurse tends to withdraw from relationships, may call in sick, or begin to think about terminating their job. A manager, preceptor, or any nurse peer should reach out to express acceptance and understanding during this difficult time (Twibell et al., 2012).

Reflection

Nursing is a profession with a long-standing tradition of honest and ethical professionals who bring together the science and caring of nursing. This is a high calling. There may be days when you feel like the best nurse, and other days when you do not. Journaling provides a foundation for reflective thinking, can help express emotions, and develop critical thinking skills. Journaling is you providing feedback on yourself. Decide on how, when, and where you want to journal. Some nurses type personal thoughts and insights about the events of the day on a computer immediately after arriving home from work. Others record reflections and emotions in a notebook with a pen just before bed. Questions that may be asked in a journal might include "What went well? What would I do differently next time? What was my 'aha' moment today? Who do I want to be in the future? How will I become that nurse?" A nurse's focus on compassionate patient care can be both rewarding and depleting. Journaling and reflection are valuable resources allowing a nurse to express feelings and promote understanding, self-awareness, self-compassion, and critical-thinking (Dimitroff, 2018).

This chapter has helped you consider many elements when choosing a nursing position. The orientation process and performance feedback were discussed. Strategies to enhance your role as the manager of a patient group were considered and mechanisms to enhance professional growth were discussed. Now is the time to consider what your first step into the professional role of the registered nurse will be. You have worked to get this far and now you will be awarded with the endless opportunities as a registered nurse.

KEY CONCEPTS

- When choosing a first nursing position, it is important to contemplate the different opportunities between specialty and general medical-surgical units.

- In addition to salary and benefits, environment, scheduling, patient type, and orientation options are also important considerations.

- Organizational orientation is both general and unit based. Orientation is a time for developing strong relationships with preceptors and members of other disciplines, as well as for mastering competencies needed for safe patient care.

- Nurse Residency and TTP Programs offered by many health care organizations help the new RN move from the role of a student to that of an RN providing high-quality care. These programs focus on building skills, critical thinking, socialization, debriefing, and peer support.

- Nurses receive performance feedback both informally and as part of periodic evaluations. This input is valuable in developing personal goals.

- Health care organizations have mechanisms to recognize employee contributions. Many of these programs reward success both monetarily and through recognition programs.

- Corrective action programs can be used to coach an employee who is having performance problems and to foster change in an employee who is failing to follow policies.

- Given the increasing complexity of health care today, it is crucial for the first-time nurse to develop strong relationships with team members and representatives of other health care disciplines. The new nurse needs to delegate appropriately and identify specific levels of authority with co-workers. Relationships with co-workers are enhanced when staff members mutually agree to performance expectations.

- Professional growth is important for job satisfaction. Organizational opportunities for growth include clinical ladders and developing mentoring relationships.

- Cross-training is another means to expand experiences and can be helpful in defining future career plans.

- Reality shock and burnout may be experienced when the new RN's expectations do not match reality.

- Nurse Residency programs, mentors, and Employee Assistance Programs are all directed to aid the new RN.

KEY TERMS

Differentials	Practice drift	Cross Training
Self-scheduling	Nurse Residency	Mentor
Shadowing	Transition to Practice	Clinical Ladder
Socialization	Corrective action	Reality shock
Preceptor	Progressive discipline	Employee Assistance Programs

---

REVIEW QUESTIONS

1. Match the terms with the appropriate definition:
   a. Clinical Ladder: 1. RNs select their schedule according to guidelines
   b. Differentials: 2. Percentage added to hourly pay for working off shifts
   c. Self-scheduling: 3. Following nurses in different roles before choosing a job
   d. Shadowing: 4. Program to encourage RNs to earn promotions, recognition, and raises by meeting specific requirements

2. Which of the following should not impact the RN's decision when selecting a new position?
   a. Pay scale and retirement benefits
   b. Small or large hospital setting
   c. Age and medical diagnoses of the patient population
   d. Age of the fellow employees.

3. Which statement by the new RN regarding general orientation requires clarification and correction by the nurse manager?
   a. General orientation includes information all nurses new to a health care organization need.
   b. Portions of the general orientation include employees from non-nursing departments.
   c. The duration of general orientation includes the first year after hire.
   d. General orientation will not include patient care information for a specific diagnostic group of patients.

4. Which of the following is required during the first year of an RN's nursing career? Select all that apply.
   a. Learning to be organized.
   b. Developing a good attendance record.
   c. Refining your assessment skills.
   d. Completing written performance evaluations of the UAP.
   e. Establishing relationship with a preceptor.

5. Preceptors who work with new nursing graduates should have which of the following characteristics? Select all that apply.
   a. Be clinically experienced.
   b. Enjoy teaching.
   c. A commitment to the preceptor role.
   d. The ability to float to specialty units.
   e. A master's degree in nursing education.

6. Sources of performance feedback may include all of the following, except:
   a. Regular meetings with preceptor
   b. Review of goals with the manager
   c. Annual review of competency assessment with review of job description
   d. Weekly meetings with Human Resources (HR) representatives

7. Which of the following is a benefit for the hospital when cross-training nurses to another patient care area?
   a. To keep nurses minimally competent in all patient care specialty areas
   b. To discover interest in employment in another patient care specialty area
   c. To allow the nurse to increase her marketability for future jobs at other facilities
   d. To learn about processes in other patient care areas and the impact those processes have on one's own unit.

8. New RNs should develop rapport with other practitioners such as physicians so that they can accomplish which of the following?
   a. Become effective patient advocates.
   b. Become friends with new colleagues.
   c. Become better patient educators.
   d. Learn more about the role of the RN.

9. Which issue would most likely require corrective action by the nurse manager?
   a. Complaints from patients that the RN has a speech accent that is difficult to understand.
   b. Complaints from a physician that a nurse who is obese is not setting a good example for the patients.
   c. Complaints from second shift RNs that a nurse continuously arrives late for handoff report.
   d. Complaints of unfairness the new RN has about the manager developed work schedule.

10. Nurse residency programs offered by some hospitals have resulted in all of the following benefits, except:
    a. Increased comfort in communicating with the health care team.
    b. Decreased levels of stress with the transition to the RN role.
    c. Better salary and compensation package
    d. Ability to organize and prioritize their care and responsibilities.

REVIEW QUESTION ANSWERS

1. Answers: A = 4, B = 2, C = 1, and D = 3 are correct.
   Rational:

   A. Shadowing: Following nurses in different roles before choosing a job.

   B. Differentials: Percentage added to hourly pay for working off shifts.

   C. Clinical Ladder: Program to encourage RNs to earn promotions, recognition, and raises by meeting specific requirements.

   D. Self-scheduling: RNs select their schedule according to guidelines.

2. Answer: D is correct.
   Rational: Age of the fellow employees should not impact the RN's decision (D). A variety of ages will allow different perspectives. (A) Pay scale, retirement benefits, (B) size of hospital, and (C) patient population should be considerations and should align with future career goals.

3. Answer: C is correct.
   Rational: The duration of general orientation is not a year (C). Nurse residency and TTP programs typically extend a year. General orientation includes information for all new nurses (A), will include employees from non-nursing departments (especially for Human Resources information) (B), and patient specific information will be part of the unit orientation, not general orientation (D).

4. Answers A, B, C, and E are correct.
   Rational: During the first year of a RN's career, evaluating UAP is not required (D). Organizational and assessment skills will be refined and improved (A, C). Developing a good attendance record is required, if not the new RN may receive corrective action and potentially lose the position (B). Establishing a relationship with a preceptor is part of the unit orientation process and will direct the growth of the new RN (E).

5. Answers A, B, and C are correct.
   Rational: A preceptor does not require a Masters degree in nursing education (E) and does not require the ability to float to specialty units (D). The preceptor needs to be willing to share knowledge and teach (B), be experienced in their assigned unit and specialty area (A), and have the clinical experience required to help the new nurse transition (C). Floating to specialty units does not indicate the preceptor is experienced in the new RN's specialty area. Some of the nurses who are best at precepting do not have an advanced degree.

6. Answer: D is correct.
   Rational: Human Resources representatives do not get involved with unit specific performance feedback, and are not involved in feedback with new RNs on a weekly basis (D). The new RN should have regular meetings with the preceptor (A), review goals with the unit manager (B), and an annual competency assessment with review of job description (C) as part of her feedback.

7. Answer: D is correct.
   Rational: When a nurse cross-trains to another patient care area, the nurse learns about processes in other patient care areas and their impact on one's own unit (D). It is not a benefit for the hospital if the nurse who cross-trains remains minimally competent in all areas (A), discovers interest in another unit (B), and seeks to improve her own marketability for future jobs (C).

8. Answer: A is correct.
   Rational: Functioning as an effective patient advocate is the goal for developing rapport with practitioners. (A) Becoming friends (B), better educators (C), and learning more about the RN role (D) will not be accomplished by developing rapport with other practitioners.

9. Answer: C is correct.
   Rational: Corrective action by the nurse manager would be indicated when the second shift RN complains that a nurse is continuously late for handoff report (C). Patient complaints about an accent (A), physician complaints about obesity (B), and complaints of unfairness in the schedule (D) will all be addressed by the nurse manager, but do not require corrective action by the manager.

10. Answer: C is correct.
    Rational: Benefits of Nurse Residency programs have included increased comfort in communication with the health care team (A), decreased stress levels with the transition from student to RN (B), and ability to organize and prioritize care and responsibilities (D). Nurse Residency programs do not result in better salaries and compensation packages for nurses (C).

REVIEW ACTIVITIES

1. You will be graduating from your nursing program in a few months. Identify several possible employment opportunities in your desired location. Prepare examples of questions you will ask as part of choosing a position. What factors are most important to you?

2. You have been working as a new graduate RN for a year and you have done well. Your nurse manager asks you to be the relief charge nurse on your unit for the midnight shift. What type of orientation will you need for this position? How can you work with a mentor to do well in this position?

3. Review a recent nurse salary survey in a nursing journal or website (consider American Nurse Today or Glass Ceiling), (www.jobs. glassceiling.com/jobs/seeker/salary). How do nursing salaries in your area compare?

4. As a new nurse you may be nervous about dealing with physicians, particularly phoning the doctor with patient concerns. While using the SBAR format, role play with your preceptor or a friend from nursing school.

DISCUSSION POINTS

• During your interview with the manager of a unit where you would love to work, you are asked, "Why would you be the best nurse for this job? Where do you see yourself in 5 years?" How would you answer these questions?

• After the interview questions are completed, the manager takes you on a tour of the unit. You look for posters and fliers on the wall that identify or explain quality improvement initiatives. What is the focus of the QI projects on this unit?

• During your last clinical experience, how did you observe the bedside nurse as a leader and manager of a small group of patients. Now put yourself in that role. How would you plan your day? What will be your priority actions at the beginning of your shift?

DISCUSSION OF OPENING SCENARIO

1. *Which position would you accept?*

   After reading this chapter, would you still choose the same position? Is the 12-hr nights on a Surgical ICU in an urban teaching hospital your first choice? Or the 8-hr rotating shifts in a suburban medical/surgical unit suits you. Or maybe the third option, a local dialysis center with no holidays and no Saturdays.

2. *What factors will help you decide which is the best fit for you?*

   The local dialysis center does not offer a Nurse Residency or TTP program, so maybe this is a negative for you. Commuting into the city may not be appealing with your young family. The Med/Surg unit in the local hospital is a great place to learn time management and organization, but will this take you to your dream job?

3. *By considering your career goals, would any of these positions start your career on the path you wish to take?*

   The urban teaching hospital will provide fantastic experience and allow plenty of opportunities for career growth. Maybe this is the type of health care organization that most appeals to you. A local hospital whose nursing leadership is making waves at the state level may also have excellent growth potential.

EXPLORING THE WEB

1. NCSBN On-line e-learning TTP Program. Look at the modules for the new RN and for the Preceptor created by the NCSBN. Some employers will reimburse the new RN for the purchase of these modules. Ask your manager. Retrieved from http://ww2. learningext.com/newnurses.html

2. *ANA http://nursingworld.org—Welcome to the Profession Kit is available to students and new nurses. This kit includes a collection of digital resources to help you through your first year of being nursing. Tips on job hunting, healthy work-life balance, and best practices for patient care can be found in this kit. Download the kit which can be retrieved from www.nursingworld.org/resources/individual/welcome-to-the-profession*

3. The Center for Medicare and Medicaid Services (**CMS**) can provide information on patient care as well. Access CMS Hospital Compare at www.cms.gov/medicare/quality-initiatives-patient-assessment-instruments/hospitalqualityinits/hospitalcompare.html. The Leapfrog group can be found at www.leapfroggroup.org Compare the information provided in these 2 websites for several hospitals in your region. How well do they provide care for patients with heart failure? A knee replacement?

4. Healthy Nurse, Healthy Nation ™ "Leading the way to better health." The Healthy Nurse, Healthy Nation™ Grand Challenge (**HNHN GC**), is a social movement designed to transform the health of the nation by improving the health of the nation's 4 million registered nurses. Retrieved from www. healthynursehealthynation.org/en Log in and complete a risk assessment, then accept the challenge to improve your health.

5. Locate a professional organization in the specialty area that interests you. How does an RN become a member? What are some of the benefits of membership? Is there a specialty certification exam associated with this professional organization? Suggestions for professional organizations include:

   AORN (Association of perioperative Registered Nurses)
   ENA (Emergency Nurses Association)
   ONS (Oncology Nursing Society)
   SPN (Society of Pediatric Nurses)

INFORMATICS

• Visual, Aural, Read/Write, and Kinesthetic (VARK®) (n.d.) (Fleming & Mills, 1992) provides information about learning preferences. What strategies should you be using when you are taking information in? What strategies are best when you are trying to share information with others? By completing the VARK questionnaire you will receive a free report with this information and more. Portions of the website require a fee. However, good insight regarding your learning style is free. Retrieved from http://vark-learn.com/the-vark-questionnaire Consider how your

learning style may impact the teaching for a patient preparing for discharge. How could you modify your discharge teaching to meet the variety of learning styles that your patients may have?

LEAN BACK

- During your experience as a nursing student in clinical practice, have you observed practice drift? How did you feel about the situation? Would you react differently today?

- Think about a stressful time in your life. How did you handle it? Did you talk with your family? Friends?

- Think ahead to your first nursing job. There will likely be some stress involved as you adjust. Plan how you will cope with this stressful time of adjusting. Will you stick to your exercise routine? Talk with friends and family?

- Remember that all employers have employee assistance programs

(EAP) where professionals can help you work through any struggles. These services may be free.

- One of the 6 QSEN competencies is evidence-based practice. How have you used the best available evidence to provide care during your student clinical experiences.

- How will you provide care to your future patients utilizing the best available care? Do you plan to subscribe to a couple of nursing journals? Will you join a professional nursing organization? Will you volunteer to be part of the committee that researches and creates the health care organization's nursing policies?

REFERENCES

Agency for Healthcare Research and Quality. (2013). *TeamSTEPPS®2.0 pocket guide*. Retrieved from www.ahrq.gov/sites/default/files/wysiwyg/professionals/education/curriculum-tools/teamstepps/instructor/essentials/pocketguide.pdf

Benner, P. E. (1984). From novice to expert: *Excellence and power in clinical nursing practice*. Menlo Park, CA: Addison-Wesley.

Buerhaus, P. I., Skinner, L. E., Auerbach, D. I., & Staiger, D. O. (2017). State of the registered nurse workforce as a new era of health reform emerges. *Nursing Economic$*, *35*(5), 229–237.

Chastain, K., Burhans, L., & Koch, G. (2018). The consequences of requirement vs. professional "practice drift.". *Indiana State Board of Nursing Focus*, *56*, 24–29.

Clarke, S. P. (2016). RN workforce update: Current and long-range forecast. *Nursing Management*, *47*(11), 20–25.

Dimitroff, L. J. (2018). Journaling: A valuable tool for registered nurses. *American Nurse Today*, *13*(11), 27–28.

Fleming, N. D., & Mills, C. (1992). Not another inventory, rather a catalyst for reflection. *To Improve the Academy*, *11*(1), 137–155. doi:10.1002/j.2334-4822.1992.tb00213.x www.vark-learn.com

Gardiner, I., & Sheen, J. (2016). Graduate nurse experiences of support: A review. *Nurse Education Today*, *40*(2016), 7–12. Retrieved from http://GlassCeiling.com http://jobs.glassceiling.com/jobs/results/keyword/registered+nurse?radius=25

Kramer (1974). *Reality shock: Why nurses leave nursing*. St. Louis, MO: Mosby.

McGill, M., & Loveless, B. (2018). Knowing when and how to leave your job. *American Nurse Today*, *13*(4), 60–62.

Melnyk, B. M., Orsolini, L., Tan, A., Arslanian-Engoren, C., Melkus, G. D., et al. (2018). A national study links nurses' perceived physical and mental health to medical errors and perceived worksite wellness. *Journal of Occupational and Environmental Medicine*, *60*(2), 126–131.

Murphy, L. J., & Janisse, L. (2017). Optimizing transition to practice through orientation: A quality improvement initiative. *Clinical Simulation in Nursing*, *13*(11), 583–590.

National Council of State Boards of Nursing (NCSBN). (2016). National Guidelines for nursing delegation. *Journal of Nursing Regulation*, *7*(1), 5–12.

National Council of State Boards of Nursing (NCSBN). Learning Extension. (2017). *Transition to Practice* [Pamphlet]. Chicago, IL: NCSBN.

Nightingale, F. (1969/1859). *Notes on nursing: What it is and what it is not*. New York: Dover Publications, Inc.

Ostermeyer, K. (2018a). Tips for combatting nurse burnout. .Retrieved from http://nursing.advanceweb.com/tips-for-combatting-nurse-burnout

Ostermeyer, K. (2018b). *Magnet designation: The honor remains as a nursing gold standard*. Retrieved from http://Advanceweb.com https://www.elitecme.com/wp-content/uploads/ebook/2018/December/MAG_121018/index.html?page=8

Senior, R. (2018). *Top ways to get promoted at work*. Retrieved from www.elitecme.com/resource-center/career-center/top-ways-to-get-promoted-at-work

Sherman, R. O. (2018). The leader coach. *American Nurse Today*, *13*(5), 6–9.

Silvestre, J., Ulrich, B. T., Johnson, T., Spector, N., & Blegen, M. A. (2017). A multisite study on a new graduate registered nurse transition to practice program: Return on investment. *Nursing Economics*, *35*(3), 110–118.

Spector, N., Blegen, M. A., Silvestre, J., Barnsteiner, J., Lynn, M. R., et al. (2015). Transition to practice in hospital settings. *Journal of Nursing Regulation*, *5*(4), 24–38.

Twibell, R., St. Pierre, J., Johnson, D., Barton, D., Davis, C., et al. (2012). Tripping over the welcome mat: Why new nurses don't stay and what the evidence says we can do about it. *American Nurse Today*, *7*(6). Retrieved from www.myamericannurse.com/tripping-over-the-welcome-mat-why-new-nurses-dont-stay-and-what-the-evidence-says-we-can-do-about-it/

United States Bureau of Labor Statistics. (2019). *Occupational outlook handbook*. Bureau of Labor Statistics. Retrieved from www.bls.gov/ooh/healthcare/registered-nurses.htm

Van Wiljen, J. (2017). Healing the healer: A caring science approach to moral distress in new graduate nurses. *International Journal for Human Caring*, *21*(1), 15–19.

Visual, Aural, Read/Write, and Kinesthetic (VARK®). (n.d.). Retrieved from http://vark-learn.com/the-vark-questionnaire

SUGGESTED READING

American Association of Colleges of Nursing (AACN). (2002). *Hallmarks of the Professional Nursing Practice Environment*. Washington, DC: American Association of Colleges of Nursing. Retrieved from www.aacnnursing.org/Portals/42/Student/what-every-nursing-student-should-know-when-seeking-employment.pdf?ver=2017-07-28-083316-627

Gardiner, I., & Sheen, J. (2016). Graduate nurse experiences of support: A review. *Nurse Education Today*, *40*(2016), 7–12.

Tanner, C. A. (2006). Thinking like a nurse: A research-based model of clinical judgment in nursing. *Journal of Nursing Education*, *45*(6), 204–211.

Career Planning and Professional Development

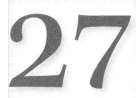

Angela Schooley
Purdue University Northwest, College of Nursing, Hammond, IN, USA

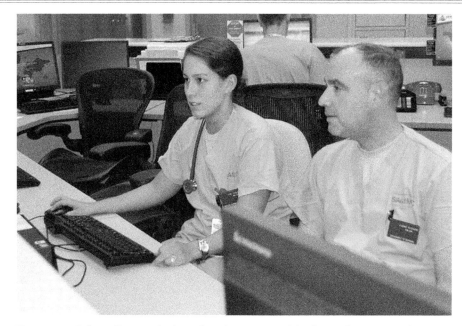

Nurses search for online continuing education opportunities for profession growth.
Source: Corey Toye/U.S. Army.

A career is like a living, breathing, organism that changes and grows over time. It needs continuous nourishment through new experiences, education, risk taking, and challenges.

(*Donna Wilk Cardillo,* 2018, p. 1)

OBJECTIVES

Upon completion of this chapter, the reader should be able to:

1. Identify the importance of career planning as part of professional development.

2. Clarify personal and career values to guide your career.

3. Describe the relationship between career planning, career satisfaction, and safe patient care.

4. Evaluate the various methods available for professional development.

5. Create a career path with 1-, 3-, and 5-year milestones.

6. Initiate and conduct a successful nursing position search.

7. Prepare a professional cover letter and resume.

8. Describe preparation and activities contributing to a productive interview.

9. Define the appropriate steps to follow up after a professional interview.

Kelly Vana's Nursing Leadership and Management, Fourth Edition. Edited by Patricia Kelly Vana and Janice Tazbir
© 2021 John Wiley & Sons Ltd. Published 2021 by John Wiley & Sons Ltd.
Companion Website: www.wiley.com/go/kelly-Nursing-Leadership

OPENING SCENARIO

During nursing orientation, the new nurse is shadowing in the Emergency Room (ER). A patient is rushed in with the paramedics performing chest compressions. The new nurse stands back as a respiratory therapist inserts an endotracheal tube and provides positive pressure ventilations. The new nurse observes and listens as the team coordinates compressions, ventilations, and use of the automated external defibrillator. Another nurse rushes over with the code cart and begins pulling up medications to administer. A resident guides the resuscitation efforts, while yet another nurse documents the activities. The new nurse hears the team inform one another, guide and correct each other, and provide verbal communication of the

interventions by using call-outs. Finally, the patient is stabilized and transferred to the intensive care unit. As the new nurse and the team debrief, the new nurse marvels at the skills, communication, and teamwork observed. The new nurse wonders how the nurses know what to do, how do they learn to work as a team, and how do they cope with the demands of a nursing career?

1. *What steps should a new nurse take to find a position that provides support and opportunities for professional development?*

2. *What factors allow a new nurse to function within the health care team?*

3. *How does a nurse develop the skills needed to be a nurse leader?*

Introduction

This chapter discusses professional development and the critical process of career planning. Career planning clarifies personal values, responsibilities, and career values to guide the nurse in seeking positions and educational opportunities. The vital link between purposeful career planning, satisfaction in the nursing role, and safe nursing practice is explored. Key concepts are covered throughout the chapter such as nursing identity, engagement within the health care system, residency programs, mentoring, committee service, professional organization membership, and obtaining further education. The chapter guides new nurses through creating a career path with 1-, 3-, and 5-year milestones. Tips for initiating and conducting a successful nursing position search, preparing a professional cover letter and resume, and interviewing are also provided throughout the chapter.

The Importance of Career Planning

Career planning allows for reflection on personal and career values to form a path to guide a career in nursing. Developing a **career path** is a process of self-reflection and goal setting, which helps align interests, ethical beliefs, and personal needs to a nursing career. Taking time to create a career path allows the nurse to maximize energies to achieve a fulfilling nursing career. A career path will increase personal satisfaction in a nurse's professional career and prevent personal distress due to competing demands in life (Mills, Woods, Harrison, Chamberlain-Salaun, & Spencer, 2017; Yarbrough, Martin, Alfred, & McNeill, 2017). Purposeful career planning will also improve the nurse's safety at the bedside by reducing role strain, and promoting focus and engagement (Price, Hall, Murphy, & Pierce, 2018). Health care systems seek nurses

possessing the ability to make good clinical decisions and the capability to hone their professional knowledge to become a valuable team member (American Nurses Association (ANA) Career Center Staff, 2014). Throughout this chapter, three scenarios portraying nurses entering the profession at different stages of their lives, and different career goals, are introduced. With each exercise, concepts of career planning, professional development, and successful transition from graduation to a nursing career will be integrated (Table 27.1). While reviewing Table 27.1, ask yourself these questions:

- Do any of the situations presented sound familiar?

- How do you make the choice between different nursing positions?

- What factors do you consider when choosing between positions?

Career Planning Process

Taking the time to create a career path is a vital step at the start of a nursing career. A career path is a visual diagram of 1-, 3-, and 5-year milestones that one hopes to achieve at these time intervals in their career (see Figure 27.1). A career path includes specific and measurable professional development goals to meet each milestone. Employers desire nurses with developed career goals, as this demonstrates the nurse's ambition and intention for growth (ANA Career Center Staff, 2014). Following a career path allows the nurse to seek professional nursing positions, and professional development activities, with the milestones as a guide. A career path allows the nurse purposeful control of their professional life by including career opportunities which complement and balance their personal life.

Table 27.1 Case Study

Scenario	Case study	Values/responsibilities	Career path milestones
Isabella	Isabella is 23 and is a first-generation college student. Her immediate family is supportive of her aspirations to become a nurse. Isabella has worked for 8 years as a nursing assistant on a maternity unit. Isabella is completing her associate degree in nursing (ASN) and is aware that many of the local hospitals require a bachelor's degree in nursing (BSN) within 5 years of hire. After graduation, and obtaining her RN license, she hopes to go back to school in 2–3 years to obtain her bachelor's degree. She is considering a full-time night nursing position offer in the unit she is currently working in.	Provides care for her siblings and mother who suffers from a chronic illness Lives with her parents and siblings, helps with the finances of the household Active in her Catholic Religion Describes herself as a night owl Works well within the team and appreciates their support Enjoys creating a working relationship with her patients	Beginning nursing career possibly on a maternity unit BSN in 3–5 years
Lauren	Lauren, age 32, entered a bachelor nursing program following a 11-year career as a cosmetologist. She completed her cosmetology license during high school, as a teen mom. Lauren is thrilled to have achieved her childhood goal of being a nurse. Lauren needs to create a career path that will allow her to support her family and manage childrearing responsibilities. Lauren has concerns about balancing her career and family life.	Mother to a 12-year-old, recently remarried and planning for more children Husband is police officer, working various shifts, weekends, and holidays Early riser, works best in the morning Treasures the ability to support patient's quality of life. Appreciates working with a team Has very high expectations of herself and her peers	Beginning nursing career Interested in working on a Memory Care Unit
Robert	Robert, age 28, finished his bachelor's degree in nursing. He achieved good grades in the nursing program and has worked on a medical surgical/telemetry unit for 3 years on the night shift. Due to his expertise, many of his peers have encouraged him to consider seeking an advanced practice degree in nursing. He has also been encouraged by his manager to pursue his medical-surgical nursing certification. The idea of further schooling has led Robert to review his career path.	Enjoys mentoring and working in a team Describes himself as lifelong learner and often seeks out more information Prefers to sleep in and stay up late.	Has worked as an RN for 3 years and is would like to seek his medical-surgical nursing certification in the next year and pursue an advanced practice degree as an Acute Care Nurse Practitioner within the next 5 years.

Source: A. Schooley.

Personal Values and Responsibilities

The first step of creating a career path is to perform a self-assessment of personal values, and personal responsibilities. While considering personal values, include personal and family-life obligations. A nursing position that is a poor fit for the nurse's lifestyle will cause role strain between personal and professional life. A balance between work and personal life provides nurses with increased satisfaction with their career (Anselmo-Witzel, Orshan, Heitner, & Bachanc, 2017). Important considerations while seeking a new position or change in career path, are the desire to obtain further professional growth and/or the want to work in another specialty area, the

available job market, the need for shift work, weekends, holidays, retirement planning, salary, and commuting. Personal considerations include marriage, children, family, and social commitments and the possibility of going back to further education. Providing safe nursing care requires the nurse to be physically and emotionally present; the ability to balance home life and nursing is vital to success (Price et al., 2018).

Career Values

After identifying the personal values and family obligations, the nurse needs to identify career values. A key place to start

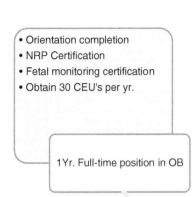

- Orientation completion
- NRP Certification
- Fetal monitoring certification
- Obtain 30 CEU's per yr.

1Yr. Full-time position in OB

3 yr.: Begin BSN degree while remaining in full-time position

- Complete 30 CEU's per yr.
- Apply and enroll in BSN program.
- Maintain NRP and fetal monitoring certification

- Attend classes and complete BSN requirments
- participate in certification review course
- apply and take certification examination

5 yr: Complete BSN education, and pursue Certification for Maternal/Newborn Nursing.

FIGURE 27.1   Career path.
Source: A. Schooley.

Critical Thinking 27.1

Consider the values that may be significant for our new nurses, Isabella, Lauren, and Robert, from Table 27.1.
1. What personal values may be significant for each?
2. What family responsibilities should be considered?

3. Do you envision that Isabella, Lauren, or Robert's values may change over time?
4. What situations may cause a conflict in values between each of the new nurses and their employers?

---

with career planning is to perform a value clarification assessment. Newer nurses entering the work force seek health care systems that provide alignment between personal values and health care system values (Anselmo-Witzel et al., 2017). Nursing is an honorable profession, requiring a deep commitment and nurses have strong views of the type of nurse they want to be. Nurses want to be in a position of providing holistic care to their clients and they need to be supported by administration to have a sense that they are providing good care (Price et al., 2018). Seeking a position in a health care system that shares the same values regarding nursing care will improve a nurse's ability be the nurse envisioned. Consider the questions posed in Table 27.2 to identify personal and career values.

Nursing Identity

Clarifying personal values and career values allows the new nurse to develop their **nursing identity** and choose a position that supports them as a valuable team member. Nursing identity is the ability to see yourself as a competent professional, capable of performing in the nursing role. Working within a health care setting that aligns professional and personal values facilitates the nurse's engagement and feelings of value within the nursing career. Quality and Safety in Nursing Education (QSEN) identifies the need for nurses to have the knowledge, skills, and attitude (KSA) to understand how their own strengths and weaknesses influence the functioning of the health care team (Quality and Safety Education for Nursing (QSEN), 2019).

A strong nursing identity provides the nurse with confidence in assessment, diagnosis, and deciding the appropriate nursing interventions needed using clinical reasoning. New nurses often feel inadequate in their knowledge and skills when starting their career and need to draw on their personal values and strengths to build their confidence and **resilience**. Resilience is the ability to work effectively in high-pressure situations, while remaining positive and persistent (Hart, Brannan, & De Chesnay, 2014). Stress, anxiety, incivility, and lack of confidence in the nursing role are common experiences as nurses face new practice experiences (Awaisi et al., 2015). Resilience and nursing identity are necessary for retention and growth in nursing (Mills et al., 2017). A positive identification with the nursing role increases over time and experience has an impact on the nurse's professional abilities and productivity (Mills et al., 2017).

Engagement

Nurses who feel they are valued team members and are part of their health care system will remain in the nursing profession.

Table 27.2 Values Assessment Questions

Personal values questions	Professional values questions	Personal obligations
What activities have meaning to me in my personal life?	What type of health care setting do I prefer?	Do I have family obligations that require specific days, times of availability?
What makes me feel comfortable in my life?	Do I need to feel that I make a difference in my work?	How long of a commute am I willing to consider?
What makes me feel uncomfortable in my life?	Do I need to feel valued and appreciated by my co-workers?	Do I prefer rising early to embrace the day, or am I more productive at night?
What are some of my strengths?	Do I enjoy working alone, or do I work better with a team?	Do I have personal/religious restrictions regarding holiday or weekend work?
What are some of my weaknesses?	Do I have personal ethical concerns with aspects of nursing that I would like to avoid?	
	Do I enjoy being challenged to learn new skills, and knowledge?	
	Do I deal well with high stress and multiple demands?	

Source: A. Schooley.

Real World Interview

During my orientation, my preceptor told me I was too slow. I was taking a lot of time at the beginning to double and triple check medications and/or assessment findings. I think this is because I am so scared and didn't want to let my patient down. As a new nurse, I found myself doubting my abilities in the beginning because I didn't have a professor by my side to make sure I am practicing safely. It's hard to trust yourself without needing verification, but I think that will fade with time and experience.

ANDREW FRECKE, REGISTERED NURSE
South Bend, Indiana, United States

Evidence from the Literature: Self-efficacy

Citation: Fida, R., Laschinder, H. K., & Leiter, M. P. (2018). The protective role of self-efficacy against workplace incivility and burnout in nursing: A time-lagged study. Health Care Management Review, 43(1), 21-29. doi:10.1097/HMR.00000000000126

Self-efficacy is the belief a person has in their ability to manage difficult situations.

Discussion: Nurses face incivility, burnout, and mental distress related to the demands of their job. Incivility, burnout, and mental distress often result in nurse turnover which is costly to the health care industry and the nursing profession. Higher levels of self-efficacy protect a nurse from mental distress related to the emotional demands of the nursing profession, and incivility experienced.

Implications for Practice: Nurses with self-efficacy were better able to cope with incivility, high work demands, and to avoid burnout. Mentoring new nurses to develop communication skills to manage incivility and modeling coping mechanisms to deal with workplace stressors may prevent turnover and loss of new nurses.

Creating cohesive teams, respectful relationships, and providing professional development opportunities helps nurses feel engaged (Mills et al., 2017). Strong teams include an environment where members experience **psychological safety** (Institute for Healthcare Improvement (IHI), 2017, p. 9). The Institute of Health Improvement (IHI) describes psychological safety as "creating an environment where people feel comfortable and have opportunities to raise concerns or ask questions" (IHI, 2017, p. 9). The concept of psychological safety is vital for new nurses as they bridge the span from nursing education to nursing practice. Engagement also encompasses the employee's feeling of belonging, and interest in the health care system in which they work. Creation of personal connections and opportunities for career training in the health care environment increases a sense of engagement by nurses (Hsing et al., 2018). Interestingly, male nurses may leave the nursing profession earlier in their career if their feeling of engagement is low (Yu, Lou, Eng, Yang, & Lee, 2018). A health care system culture that supports knowledge development and role exploration will retain nurses. Engagement may further be facilitated by inclusion in nurse residency programs, mentoring, and serving on committees.

Nurse Residency Programs

Many health care systems offer residency programs for graduate nurses. Residency programs are intended to bridge the gap between nursing education into the professional role of the nurse by socializing the graduate nurse (Walsh, 2018). The intent behind nurse residency programs is to strengthen the new nurse's commitment to practice by providing skills in clinical judgment and socialization into the nursing role (Institute of Medicine, 2010). Residency programs provide an evidence-based curriculum incorporating, leadership, patient outcomes, and professional development for new nurses (American Association of Colleges of Nursing (AACN), 2019). Residencies usually last a year and vary with different models used: didactic, simulation, and progressive learning with guidance

with a preceptor (Walsh, 2018). Residency programs enhance nurse satisfaction within their nursing career, and also increase retention in the health care system (Walsh, 2018). Common activities that occur in nurse residency programs include:

- Creating an evidence-based project for the unit employed
- Pairing nurses and doctors to follow each other for part of a shift to sensitize each to their roles in the inter-professional team
- Discussing difficult patient situations and finding better approaches
- Working shifts with expert nurses in different units to see how they organize and deliver care
- Simulation exercises to improve clinical judgment and review the nurses' skills
- Discussing and clarifying procedures and policies within the institution

More information can be found about residency programs and programs available by state through the American Association of Colleges of Nursing at: www.aacnnursing.org/Nurse-Residency-Program

Mentoring

Mentoring is a way to improve socialization and belonging of novice nurses into new roles.

Many new nurses report feelings of inadequacy and need more time to feel comfortable in their role and in the health care system. A mentor can support new nurses transitioning into a valuable team member. Many health care systems have a mentoring process in place for new nurses. A mentor is usually an experienced nurse who is formally assigned to provide socialization and practice guidance for the new nurse. During all stages of the nursing career there is a need for autonomy, ongoing learning, and need for support from mentors (Price & Reichert, 2017). Nurses often have many mentors, formally and informally, throughout their careers.

Evidence from the Literature: New Graduate Orientation

Citation: Pasila, K. Elo, S., & Kaarainen, M. (2017). Newly graduated nurses' orientation experiences: A systematic review of qualitative studies. *International Journal of Nursing Studies, 71*, 17-27.

A systematic review of nursing orientation provides qualitative evidence to understand the experiences new graduates face during their introduction to the profession.

Discussion: Nursing is facing a shortage of nurses, which is related to retiring nurses and nurses leaving the profession. Orientation themes include: orientation experiences in general, socialization into the unit culture, cycling experiences to various units, the relationship with the preceptor, stress experienced related to

the nursing role, progress in confidence and abilities within the nursing role, the need for individualization of the orientation process, and creation of an ongoing formal mentorship process.

Implications for Practice: The orientation process and preceptor have a vital role in preparing new nurses for nursing, and remaining in the nursing profession. Poor orientation processes, and ineffective preceptors were directly related to new nurses leaving the health care system, or the profession. Stress related to reality shock and bullying were common experiences during the orientation process. Many new nurses wanted to maintain a formal mentorship relationship with their mentor after the orientation process.

Committees

Committee membership develops engagement by participating in shared governance at the unit level, or system wide level. New nurses benefit from joining policy development committees, quality improvement efforts, and shared governance within their health care system. Valuable relationships may come from work with the committee. Serving on committees provides professional development for the new nurse, as it provides a view of the broader aspects of the nursing role and increases their nursing identity as leaders within the profession. Berwick suggests that all nurses should constantly be striving for quality improvement to increase patient safety and nurses' awareness of potential safety concerns (Frankel et al., 2017). Being on a committee helps the nurse understand the process of how change occurs in the health care system and improves career satisfaction. Being part of the solution is an active and positive way to help change any challenges the nurse may face and increases the sense of engagement.

Providing Safe Patient Care

Nurses' satisfaction in their career is enmeshed with their ability to provide safe and effective patient care (Price et al., 2018). Nurses experience satisfaction from being able to focus on compassionate care, and the positive effects of caring for others (Sacco & Copel, 2017). Nurse staffing, which allows for effective teamwork and manageable patient assignments, improves the nurse's feelings of value and desire to improve the patient care experience. Nurses working in a health care system which supports the nurse's professional abilities demonstrate higher levels of productivity (Mills et al., 2017).

Creating a work life balance for nurses is essential to nurse satisfaction and patient safety. Nurses' ability to have some control over their working hours allows them to be physically and emotionally present during their working hours (Price et al., 2018). A tired nurse, struggling with home life obligations and work expectations, will quickly experience role strain and disengage at the bedside. When nurses are not fully present in their practice area, patients have lower satisfaction, increased errors are made, and productivity decreases (Perlo et al., 2017). Supporting professional development to increase the nurse's confidence in their nursing abilities prevents

Table 27.3 Smart Career Planning Milestones

SMART	Example
Specific	Employment as an RN in a Maternity Unit
Measurable	Function independently in a full-time nightshift staff RN position
Achievable	Employment at hospital that allows recently graduated RNs to work in maternity
Realistic	Presence of other new graduates that were able to achieve goal
Timely	Achieve goal within 1 year

Source: A. Schooley.

negative patient outcomes, and improves patient safety (Dyrbye, Johnson, Johnson, Satele, & Shanafelt, 2018).

Milestone Development

The second step of career planning is identifying the milestones you would like to reach in your career; consider 1-, 3-, and 5-year goals. Milestones should be *smart*: Specific, Measurable, Achievable, Realistic, and Timely (SMART) (see Table 27.3). Drawing the milestones out can assist the nurse with a visual diagram to plan educational activities to develop the skills needed to meet the milestone (see Figure 27.1).

Seeking Employment as a Nurse

There are several ways a new nurse can pursue employment. Networking through family, friends, nursing faculty, fellow nursing students, and acquaintances is one path to discover possible positions. Prospective nurses may use online recruiting sites, the health care facility web page, and their college career office to search for a position. A number of websites specific to nursing positions allow searches by specialty and location and include:

- www.health careerweb.com: *National website, register as a user to create a profile.*

- www.healthcareersinteraction.com: *Recruitment tool, allows the applicant to meet directly with employers and recruiters,*

Critical Thinking 27.2

Note the analysis of the components of SMART in Isabella's milestones listed here.

- *Year One*: Work as a nurse full-time night shift on the maternity unit of a community hospital for 1 year.

- *Year Three*: Work as a nurse for 3 years full-time, while studying part-time for a Bachelor's degree in an online nursing program.

- *Year Five*: Within 5 years, complete BSN degree and pursue certification in maternal/newborn nursing.

Now, develop 1-, 3-, and 5-year SMART milestones for Robert and Lauren. Take time now to create your own 1, 3, and 5 year milestones. Did this process help you clarify strategic career milestones?

some employers offer onsite interviews and on-the-spot job offers, local and regional employers from all Canadian Provinces and the United States.

* www.aone.org: (This site requires membership to use) *Students may purchase a membership.*

* www.jobs.ana.org: *The American Nurses Association Career Center. Allows searching by position and location.*

* www.nurse.com: *A website that allows searching by position and location. Ability to create an account for position notifications and to upload a resume.*

New graduate nurses should consider looking for health care systems offering internships, or residencies before applying for a nursing position. When exploring nurse residency programs, the graduate should consider what the program consists of, who serves as preceptors for the program and their backgrounds, and what the salary is during the internship or residency. New nurses should be aware that internship or residency programs vary with regards to salary, with length of time, and for full-time or part-time requirements. Searching for positions in hospitals with Magnet status is another way to narrow the search. The American Nurses Credentialing Center (ANCC) established the Magnet Services Recognition Program, which has certified many hospitals in the United States and is expanding internationally. A list of all Magnet hospitals is available through the American Nurses Association site at www.nursingworld.org/organizational-programs/magnet/find-a-magnet-facility.

Many hospitals offer RN positions to nurse graduates who are currently employed as nurse externs, or certified nurse assistants (as in Isabella's case). A benefit to working within the health care system during nursing school is that many systems provide new employment opportunities to employees first before opening positions to candidates outside the health care system. Clinical rotations also provide an opportunity to explore the health care system's culture and the fit between the nurse's personal and professional values. The new graduate should consider applying to a unit or health care system that provides a wonderful learning opportunity during nursing clinical experiences When seeking employment, the nurse graduate should consider their preferences for a large city teaching hospital, a smaller community hospital, or possibly a private religion-based health care system.

Researching Potential Employers

Prior to applying for a position, the nurse applicant should access information about the specific health care systems which are of interest. A review of the mission and philosophy of the health care system will allow the applicant to become familiar with the employer's values. Refining the resume to align to the health care systems' values and needs will increase the potential for success in the interview process. Knowledge of the specific health care system is an important step when

pursing employment. The nurse applicant should be aware if the hospital is Magnet status, has religious affiliation, or is a teaching hospital. These types or classifications of hospitals guide the health care system to seek specific skills and qualifications in their employees.

Researching the Position Description

In addition to being familiar with the health care system, the nursing graduate should review the specific descriptions of any posted nursing positions. A careful study of the posted position allows the nurse graduate to streamline their cover letter, resume, and interview to meet the needs of the health care system. Accessing the advertised position description electronically gives applicants the ability to use key words to emphasize their skills and expertise, to display that they are a good fit within the system's requirements on their cover letter and resume. The nursing position description alerts the new nurse to the variety of skills required, expectations regarding floating to different departments, or cross training requirements. The nurse applicant should carefully reflect on their skills and potential for skill mastery in the positions for which they apply.

Many new graduates may hesitate to apply for a position that requires specialized skills or certifications. Reading the description carefully, and looking for the words required versus preferred may provide guidance. The wording "required" indicates only candidates with the specific qualifications will be considered. Focusing on the requirements is important when applying, because some hospitals expect an RN license to apply for an RN position, so new graduates with resumes without a license may not even be considered. The wording preferred may allow for training once hired. Generally, applying for non-advertised positions may not lead to a successful search. Health care systems may keep desirable resumes on file for future reference, if the applicant has the skills required. New nurses should apply for positions of interest, as many units will provide educational opportunities to new nurses, if the applicant appears to have the majority of the skills needed. Nurse applicants should not be discouraged if offered a position that differs from the one they initially applied for. This is common and allows the applicant to "get their foot in the door." Once hired in an institution, nurses can transfer, usually after a year, to the unit initially wanted. Entry-level positions allow the new nurse to gain experiences, allowing options to move into acute care settings, or more specialized settings later.

Recruitment Fairs

Nurse recruitment fairs can be a timesaver for nurse applicants. These types of fairs allow the applicant to meet and learn about many different employers in one location. Many colleges offer professional recruitment fairs during the school year. Health care systems also hold recruitment fairs which are often a beneficial experience for nurse candidates. Recruitment fairs expose the applicant to many opportunities in various health care agencies in a timely manner and with limited effort. Prior to attendance, the applicant should prepare a resume and a brief **elevator speech** to introduce themselves to recruiters. An elevator speech is a quick 30–60 s speech outlining the applicant's qualifications and highlights specific skills that makes an applicant memorable, and employable. For example, Lauren would describe her experience in creating a mobility checklist to prevent falls in elderly patient during her capstone course, while discussing her wish to work in an extended care facility. Prior to attending the recruitment fair, a brief review of participating health care systems is also important, to familiarize the applicant with the positions available, and the values of the employers present at the fair. The applicant should have a hard copy of their resume and have many copies to share with recruiters. A cover letter is not needed when attending a recruitment fair (Cardillo, 2018). The applicant should also keep a notebook to write down the names of the recruiter they talked to, the health care system, position discussed, and contact information for follow up. Requesting business cards is also a helpful strategy when attending a recruitment fair. The nurse applicant should follow up within a week after applying for employment or meeting with a recruiter at a job fair (Hess, 2017). When writing a follow-up letter, or email, the applicant should develop a script reviewing the position they are interested in, their qualifications for the position, and a request for an interview.

Professional Considerations

The applicant should consider the professionalism of their email handle and voicemail messages during the application process. For example, an email handle of IzzyBDancing queen@gmail.com, appears unprofessional, and Isabella should consider a professional handle of IsabellaRN@gmail.com (Gibson, 2019). Applicants do not want a nurse recruiter to receive an outgoing message of, "Hey, this is IzzyB, you know what to do!" Changing the outgoing message to create a good first impression is needed, for example, "This is Isabella, sorry, I cannot take your call, please leave a message." The applicant should also consider the professionalism of their social media presence. Most recruiters will search social media for the applicant. The applicant must remove inappropriate photos, questionable activities, and posts containing vulgar language (Augustine, 2019a). Do keep in mind that posts and pictures on social media never are fully deleted. Recruiters may disqualify an applicant due to questionable social media posts that do not align with the values of the health care system. Nursing students must be mindful of their social media presence and the need to represent the profession in a trustworthy and ethical manner.

Landing the Interview

When contacted for an interview, the applicant should display knowledge about the health care system. A professional, interested candidate is able to link their professional experience, and skills, to the system's nursing position needs, as well as the mission and values. If the nurse applicant has applied for multiple positions, an application spreadsheet may be useful (Figure 27.2).

Preparation of a Cover Letter and Resume

Nurse graduates have a valuable resource in their college's career center. During their education, they should work closely with the career center to develop a resume and cover letter. Many college career centers offer resume writing tips, as well a free editing. Graduates from colleges retain access to the career center through their alumni association. The career center provides templates, and guidance in writing resumes, cover letters,

---

Critical Thinking 27.3

1. Practice writing a short elevator speech for yourself to use a recruitment fairs, and remember to identify the position you are interested in, your individual skills, and an activity/talent/recognition that sets you apart from other graduate nurses.
2. Write a short script to use when following up with a recruiter.

Agency	Contact Information Name, Phone number, email	Resume/Cover letter/Position applied for	Follow-up: date and with whom?	Interview: Date and with whom, location	Thank-you
New Hospital	Andrea Newhouse 214-788-5695 anewhouse@ newhospital.org	Submitted online 02/19 RN Med Surg	Andrea 02/26	Kelly Smith, 03/01, Nursing office on 3rd floor medical surgical unit.	03/03 sent to Kelly Smith

FIGURE 27.2 Applications spreadsheet.
Source: A. Schooley.

Robert Wills
3564 Hammond Place, Lawrence, IN 49685
Cell: (764) 875-9821
February 19, 20XX

Andrea Newhouse, Nurse Recruiter
New Hospital
2300 Hospital Way
Fredericksburg, IN 56732

Dear Andrea Newhouse:

I am seeking a position as a registered nurse. I will be graduating on May 15, 20XX, from the University of XXXX, with a Baccalaureate of Science Degree in Nursing. I will take my NCLEX-RN on June 11, 20XX.

I have been a certified nurse assistant for 3 years on an oncology/medical surgical floor. This employment has provided me with the skills to communicate effectively with patients, work with the health care team by alerting the staff to abnormal vital signs, assisting patients with activities of daily living, and improving patient satisfaction as documented by my unit's positive Hospital Consumer Assessment of Healthcare Providers and Systems (HCAHPS) scores. I feel that these skills, combined with my newly acquired nursing skills, would be an asset to your medical surgical unit.

I would appreciate the opportunity to discuss employment possibilities with you. I will call you next week to schedule an appointment. In the meantime, I can be contacted via phone at Home: (764) 335-3765, or Cell: (764) 875-9821. Or via email: Rwills@nurseschool.edu

Thank you for your time and consideration of my resume.

Sincerely,

Robert Wills
Robert Wills

FIGURE 27.3   Cover letter.
Source: A. Schooley.

Critical Thinking 27.4

1. Identify how each of three nursing students from Table 27.1 should begin their search for a nursing position?
2. How will their career milestones and values guide their search for a nursing position?
3. How should they begin writing their resume's and cover letter?

---

and interview etiquette, as well as recruitment fair opportunities. Career centers often have job opportunities posted as well.

Cover Letter

A well-written cover letter and resume provide the nurse applicant with an opportunity to market themselves and display their professional communication abilities. The cover letter is a brief opportunity to convince the nurse recruiter to consider the applicant as a viable candidate. The cover letter is one page, uses active language, contains three paragraphs, and provides highlights of the candidate's qualifications without repeating information that is found on the resume. Paragraphs are not indented, and the cover letter should contain the applicant's signature in black ink. See Figure 27.3 for an example.

Resume

The nurse manager or human resources personnel will form an opinion of the applicant's skills, and potential as an employee based on the quality of the cover letter and resume. The resume and cover letter should provide a brief and specific outline of the nurses' credentials and skills that qualify for the position. The resume includes a professional summary, professional experience, education, licensure, and certifications (Gibson, 2019). The objective is replaced by the professional summary and should use the key words from the position description, to demonstrate the applicant's qualifications for the position. Professional experiences should include work history organized from most current to oldest, and list specific tasks and responsibilities of previous positions (Gibson, 2019). This section provides the applicant with a perfect opportunity to display their unique talents, or expertise, and to also highlight the skills that align to the advertised position. Use of either first or third person is acceptable when listing skills, for example; Managed an interdisciplinary team. Action verbs are powerful and should be used to describe prior employment (see Web Exercise 6). Careful editing of the resume and cover letter for accuracy, formatting, and grammar is vital. Recommendations of best practice are: keep top and bottom margins 1 in., and keep text left aligned indentations, dates, and places consistent, use only approved abbreviations, for example, IL for Illinois, and check dates for accuracy (American Nurses Association (ANA) Enterprise, 2019; Turner, 2019). Proof reading to avoid typographical, spelling, or grammar errors, is vital to showcase the applicant's written communication skills (Gibson, 2019).

Electronic Submissions

The majority of health care systems request electronic submission of resumes and applications only. Nurse applicants must be aware that many electronic submission systems use Applicant Tracking Systems (ATSs), which search for specific key words and require specific formatting. The applicant should begin submitting the application by having the cover letter and resume tailored to reflect the health care system and advertised position. The resume and cover letter should be created as a Microsoft Word document in preparation for electronic submissions. The applicant should use key words such as "registered nurse" or terms used in the advertised position in their resumes. Using specific key words listed in the position advertisement assists the ATS tracking to match the applicant's resume with the position (Kohler, 2020). ATS systems may discard the applicant's resume due to non-use of keywords (Bell, 2018). Specific suggestions include:

- Use Sans serif font, e.g., Calibri, do not use serif fonts such as Times New Roman or Cambria.

- Font size should be 10–12 (name and information may be larger).

- Use round bullet points only, avoid arrows or symbols, these may be translated into nonsense by the ATS.

- Remove headers and footers for electronic submission.

- Do not use acronyms but do use as many keywords as possible in the resume.

- Use standard resume headings, but avoid boldface, underlining, or italics when submitting electronically. *Use of italics, boldface, and underlining is useful for readability when distributing a hard copy.*

- Avoid a two-column format. Use left alignment of the text, with side margins set at 0.63 in.

- Use a chronological resume format.

Suggestions from: Bell (2018), Gibson (2019), and Kohler (2020).

Other electronic submission systems may require submission into fillable sections, so familiarity with the requested information is vital to submission. Have licensure information, certification information, employment history, and education information on hand when submitting applications electronically. The applicant must follow the directions of the electronic submission site, for example, No cover letter or submit as a word document. Failure to follow the directions may result in dismissal of the applicant's resume.

Writing a Resume

There are three types of resumes, chronological, functional, and a combination of both (ANA Enterprise, 2019; Gibson, 2019). The chronological style lists positions in chronological order, beginning with the most current. This style provides a concise employment history and works well for applicants with a fair amount of work history. Chronological style may be problematic if the applicant has gaps in their work history. This style of resume is an efficient method of highlighting progression from an entry level position to a position with greater responsibilities. See Figure 27.4 for a chronological resume. A functional style of resume gives the applicant the opportunity to illustrate experience in categories of skills within multiple careers and reduces the focus on specific job (Cardillo, 2018). The functional resume emphasizes skills and abilities rather than a sequence of nursing position experiences. While there are benefits to the functional style, ATS systems do not read this style well, and may reject them (Gibson, 2019).

Using a combination of both styles may be used by nurses who are changing their career focus, or who have a gap in employment (Gibson, 2019). The combined resume also lists educational status, professional licensure, certifications, personal attributes, societal contributions, and related work experience. See Figure 27.5 for an example of a combination of chronological and functional resume. Nurse graduates may also want to list clinical rotations with specific locations to highlight the diversity of their clinical experiences.

Employment History

Professional skills listed in the resume should emphasize the professional nursing skills embraced by the health care system and emphasized in the nursing position description. The resume should not include dissatisfaction with previous employers, or positions, informal language or slang, or irrelevant information (Gibson, 2019). Non-nursing positions do not need to be listed, but some State Boards of Nursing require full disclosure

---

Critical Thinking 27.5 Cover Letters and Resumes

You are helping some of the new nurses in Table 27.1, to prepare their cover letters and resumes.
1. What nursing position application method is illustrated in Robert's cover letter?
2. What skills would you list in Isabella's cover letter?

Robert Wills
3564 Hammond Place
Lawrence, IN 49685
Cell: (764) 875-9821
February 19, 20XX

Summary

Newly licensed graduate RN with a variety of clinical and work experience. Professional communication skills, work well with a team, possess strong interpersonal skills. Seeking an entry-level staff nurse position on a medical-surgical patient care unit.

Education

Bachelor of Nursing, University of Indiana, Hamilton, IN

Licensure/Certifications

- Registered Nurse, Indiana, NCLEX scheduled June 14, 2019

- BCLS CPR, American Heart Association, obtained June 2014, expires June 2020.

- Naloxone administration training Red Cross, June 2017

- Institute of Health Improvement Basic Certification, November, 2019

Clinical Rotations

- Senior Practicum, Intensive Care Unit at Calgary Mayo Care Center

- Maternal Child Nursing at Nightingale Health Center

- Medical Surgical Nursing, Medical Surgical Unit: University Health Systems, a level 3 trauma center.

- Community Health Riverdale: Community Health Center

Employment History

2012 to 2017: Shift Leader: Burger Chain Restaurant

- Supervise team members

- Provide excellent customer service

- Maintain safety of food handling

Societal/Professional Contributions

2016–present

- Tutored first-year nursing students in pathophysiology

- President of the Nursing Club

FIGURE 27.4   Chronological resume.
Source: Adapted from Courtesy of Nurse.Org.

of previous employment, so the applicant should be mindful of their State's requirements. While the applicant may not list previous employers on their resume, they should be prepared to list them on the application.

Summary Section

Traditional advice for preparing a resume suggest starting with an objective. Many experts recommend avoiding the objective in favor of a three to five-line statement summarizing the applicant's skills, career experiences, and competencies (ANA Enterprise, 2019).

Education Section

Educational degrees, including the year of graduation and academic institution, should be itemized in the resume. The year of graduation may not be reported on the resume to avoid age discrimination. However, specific date of the graduation will be required for the application (Gibson, 2019).

Resume—Licensure and Certification Section

The resume should include professional licensure with the State issuing the license, the license number, and expiration date. Certification should also be listed with the dates obtained

Lauren Callihan
2426 New Prairie Drive
Apple Blossom, NJ 08080
(609) 444–2212 (home)
Laur24@gmail.net

Summary

Graduate nurse seeking an entry-level position in a Memory Care Unit. Able to provide safe, effective, and professional nursing care for residents to enhance their autonomy and quality of life. Skilled at executing individualized plans of care to promote physical, social, and psychological well-being of the memory care residents.

Education

Bachelor of Science in Nursing, May 2019
University of Pennsylvania, Philadelphia, PA
*90-hour Practicum on the Memory Care Unit at Prairie Grove Community Living Center.

- Developed individualized plans of care for 10 newly admitted residents.

- Revised individualized plans of care for 5 residents due to changes in their psychological and physical conditions.
*Capstone Project: Assisted in developing a mobility checklist to prevent falls in elderly patients.

Professional Experience

- Professional Cosmetologist

  - Provided grooming to elderly clientele at a community living center.

  - Able to handle clients who are unhappy, or scared during haircuts.

  - Skilled at listening and meeting client's needs to improve their self esteem.

- Communication skills

  - Excellent written and verbal communication skills

  - Empathic listener

- Teamwork and Collaboration:

  - Possess strong commitment to teamwork to meet client needs

  - Able to contribute my expertise and follow leadership directives to meet deadlines.

  - Thrive in a team environment and work well with others

  - Enjoy working as a team member as well as independently

Volunteer/Community Service

Boy Scout Leader, Apple Blossom, NJ, 2012–Present

- Coordinate Boy Scout Troop # 445.

- Supervise Boy Scout monthly meetings.

- Perform basic leader duties, including direct supervision of boy scouts ages 9 to 14.

Certification

  - Certified as a Basic Life Support Provider, American Heart Association, 2014–present

  - Computer Informatics certificate, June 2019

Professional Organizations

  - Nursing Student Association, University of Pennsylvania Chapter

  - National Student Nurses Association

  - Sigma Theta Tau Member, Inducted April 23, 2018

FIGURE 27.5 Combined resume.
Source: A. Schooley.

Robert Wills
3564 Hammond Place
Lawrence, IN 49685
Cell: (764) 875-9821
February 19, 20XX
Andrea Newhouse, Nurse Recruiter
New Hospital
2300 Hospital Way
Fredericksburg, IN 56732
Dear Ms Newhouse,
Thank you for the time you spent with me as I interviewed for a position as a registered nurse at New Hospital. I enjoyed meeting the medical-surgical department nurse manager and several of the staff nurses yesterday and was especially impressed with the sense of professionalism among the staff. I believe I would be a good fit for the position in your medical-surgical department. I worked there for a year during my nursing education program and benefited from working with the dedicated nurses,and staff.

I have requested that my transcripts be sent directly to your office. I will have three of my instructors complete the reference forms you gave me. I look forward to hearing from you soon about my second interview and will contact you in two weeks as directed.
Sincerely,
Robert Wills
Robert Wills

FIGURE 27.6   Interview follow-up letter.
Source: Compiled with information from Polifko-Harris (2003).

(such as cardiopulmonary resuscitation (CPR)), the accrediting body, and the expiration date (Gibson, 2019).

Professional Experience Section

Nurse graduates may lack nursing experience, so listing clinical experience may help them display skills experienced. Prospective employers will gain knowledge of clinical exposure during the nursing education program, if the applicant lists clinical experiences with the location (Figure 27.4). Listing every nursing course is not recommended for nursing graduates, as this does not vary significantly between nurse graduates (ANA Enterprise, 2019). The applicant should expand on specialized experiences that are unique to the applicant, for example. Participated in a quality improvement effort with New Hospital focusing on reducing falls in the maternity unit.

The applicant should include additional education experiences such as leadership of a nursing club, serving as a student instructor, or efforts in research with faculty members.

Health care employers are looking for nurses with the ability to be leaders, flexibility, potential and desire for growth, professional communication and behavior, as well as special skills such as bilingual, equipment use certifications, or computer programming skills (ANA Career Center Staff, 2014). The applicant should provide a list of attributes to demonstrate to the potential employer that they are desirable hire. Some examples may include the following:

- Pay attention to detail

- Autonomous, self-directed

- Eager to learn new skills

- Team player, thrives in a team environment

- Demonstrate resilience in resolving conflict

- Demonstrate effective communication skills within the health care team.

- Provide therapeutic communication

- Accept constructive feedback

- Demonstrate reliability in attendance and punctuality

- Perform therapeutic nursing interventions.

Marketable skills in nursing are good communication, teamwork, flexibility, clinical reasoning, problem solving, positivity, and professionalism (ANA Career Center Staff, 2014). The applicant should write their resume to magnify their talents and emphasize what makes them unique form other nursing graduates.

Obtaining References

Contact referencee for permission prior to submitting applications or resumes. Seeking permission, allows the applicant to verify correct contact information, verify the referencee's willingness to provide a positive reference, and alerts them to expect a call, or email. When contacting referencee, the applicant should let them know the health care system, and nursing position they are seeking. Notifying referencees also will prevent undue hardship for the person providing a reference, by allowing them time to review their time with the applicant and prepare answers to potential questions. Nurses should build their network of references and contacts throughout nursing school, and their career by maintain their professional contacts.

Past employment guides who to list as employer references. Past health care employers, such as Isabella and Robert (Table 27.1), should be listed. Nurse graduates should include any character references, including at least one nursing professor. For graduates who have not had many work-life experiences, references from volunteer service and high school contributions are helpful.

Preparation for the Interview

After securing the interview, verify all details, type of interview: face to face, telephone, or video conference, panel interview, as well as time and place. If the interview is to occur at the health care system location, clarify exact room location, where the applicant should report. To prepare for the interview, learn more about the agency and the possible questions they may ask and explore university resources in the career center (Purdue Northwest, 2018–2019). Obtain a copy of the nursing position description before the interview if possible. The applicant should familiarize themselves with the health care agency and the nursing position description. Projecting knowledge about the health care system and the position demonstrates serious interest and will enhance the professional image of the applicant. Researching the system and position also gives the applicant an opportunity to prepare appropriate interview questions. For example, if the nursing position description requires the nurse to demonstrate the use of an intravenous pump, the applicant can clarify what type of intravenous pump is used in the unit. Prior to the interview, the applicant should prepare a folder containing a description of the health care system and its services, extra copies of the resume, questions to ask of the interviewer, blank paper for notes, and any documents such as nursing license, references, or school transcripts, if requested. During the interview the applicant should:

- Arrive on time, not early and not late.

- Smile, make eye contact, and shake hands.

- Be prepared to complete an application or additional paperwork.

- Maintain good eye contact and greet the interviewer formally.

- Wait to sit until the interviewer sits, unless directed to do so.

- Avoid chewing gum, fidgeting, or tapping.

During the interview the ability of the applicant to meet the nursing position requirements will be assessed as part of the interview process. The nurse manager or representatives of the human resources department will verify licensure, assess competency, review employment references, and complete background and criminal checks, as appropriate. The applicant's ability to meet any health requirements or any other nursing position requirements of a nursing position will also be assessed. During the interview process, the interviewer will be assessing the applicant's fit within with the agency's culture and the particular unit's culture.

Desirable traits of nurses are teamwork, resilience, time-management skills, strong communication skills, self-motivation, and strong ethical core values (Gibson, 2018; National Councils of State Boards of Nursing (NCSBN), 2018). These traits will be assessed during the interview by asking questions regarding communication skills, dependability, nursing skills, delegation skills, autonomy, and professional judgment. Some health care systems may use a panel to interview the applicant for the position, to assess such things as ability to work on a team, stay calm, keep focused on questions, establish rapport with the group, etc. For entry-level position interviews, it is customary to have only the nursing manager, or the nurse manager and a nurse recruiter or human resources person present during the interview. In some situations, other staff nurses are included in interviews for new unit staff. Toward the end of the interview, the nursing representatives and the human resources representatives will offer the applicant a competitive hourly rate within approved budget guidelines. At this time, they will assure the completion of any required organizational and governmental paperwork.

Question Preparation

Once the applicant has obtained a time and date for their first interview, they should prepare for their interview. Practice interview skills with a peer, parent, or by using a video. Many colleges offer interview preparation through their Career Center. The Career Center may have a space for mock interviews for students to practice (Purdue University Northwest Career Center, 2018). Types of interviews can vary from one-to-one interviews, panel interviews, telephone interviews, and follow-up interviews, all with varying types of questions involving hypothetical case scenarios. Graduate nurses are applying for an entry-level position, and therefore the questions will be directed at the novice nursing care knowledge. For example, if the applicant is applying for a nursing position on a general medical unit, they should be ready to give the nursing interventions for a patient experiencing chest pain or hypoglycemia. Common questions asked during an interview include recalling a difficult nursing situation and how the applicant would behave. For example, you may be asked,

---

Critical Thinking 27.6

1. Prepare a cover letter for Lauren from Table 27.1.
2. How can Lauren capture the attention of an ATS system, which focuses on particular keywords to be selected for an interview?
3. How should Lauren develop her cover letter and resume so that she is interviewed for a nursing position on an adult memory care unit?

Real World Interview

What advice about the interview process would you give? I asked my friends who had interviewed. They said they asked about a time you went above and beyond in your job, and please describe. I was asked about my strengths and weaknesses. I was also given a scenario of customer service: a patient gave a low score from a previous visit, how would you handle this, and provide service. I said I would acknowledge that the patient was unhappy with their care before, ask how I can make this visit better, and assure them that I want them to be satisfied with my care as their nurse. Prior to the interview, I would practice my answers a little bit, but never rehearse, as you want it to feel natural and genuine. You should also avoid rambling.

ANDREW FRECKE, REGISTERED NURSE
South, Bend, Indiana, United States

"If you are faced with an irritable patient who has been waiting for a long time for pain medication, what would you do?" To respond the applicant should use the STAR acronym and include each component. Describe Specifically (S) what happened; the Task (T), problem, or issue; the Action (A) taken; and the Result (R) of the action. The interviewer is exploring the problem-solving skills and potential for self-correction when faced with difficult situations (Table 27.4). When answering questions, avoid rambling, keep the answers concise and to the point. During an interview it is acceptable to take a few minutes to form an answer, take notes, or to ask the interviewer to repeat the question. The applicant should be positive and engaged during the interview, but should avoid monopolizing the conversation, or giving overly long answers to the questions. In other words, let the interviewer direct and lead the interview.

Questions about work behaviors during the interview are designed to provide the employer with information about how the applicant has handled both negative and positive experiences in the past. Employers are seeking employees who can reflect on their past performance and learn from it. Health care systems are seeking nurses who are eager to learn new skills, are punctual and dependable, and display a sense of discipline and resilience, even in the face of difficult situations (NCSBN, 2018; Registered Nursing.org, 2019). During the introductory phase of the interview, the employer outlines the nursing position and the conditions of employment. The applicant should clarify questions regarding the position at this time.

Working Phase

The working phase of the interview begins with the employer asking the applicant questions regarding the cover letter and resume. Many of the questions during the interview will refer to the nursing position description. The applicant should familiarize themselves with the legal and illegal questions that may be asked. Illegal questions include asking about citizenship, age, religion, gender, cultural heritage, marital status, membership in social organizations, family characteristics, height and weight, or medical history (Government of Canada, 2018; U.S. Equal Employment Opportunity Commission, n.d.). Rather than refusing to answer an illegal question, which may be seen as being uncooperative or confrontational, respond to the intention of the question (Jackson, 2017). For example, should the interviewer ask if you are a citizen, respond by indicating that you are legally eligible to work as a nurse. Responding in this manner will answer the intent of the question without compromising the legal or ethical issues of the nursing position requirements (Jackson, 2017). Legally acceptable questions include reason for applying, your career goals, any problems with the position that the applicant may have, and the applicant's strengths and weaknesses.

When answering questions, the applicant should highlight specific personal and professional accomplishments. The applicant must not appear overly confident, and lacking knowledge of their own limitations (Registered Nursing. org, 2019). Over confidence can raise doubts concerning

---

Table 27.4 STAR Interviews

STAR	Example
Specifics	A patient was overdue for his pain medication. He became angry and accused me of ignoring his pain.
Task	I was busy with other high-priority patients. I was having trouble getting to the pain medication passed.
Action	I called my charge nurse and asked for help. The charge nurse was able to administer the pain medication, talk with him, and help him to relax. I stopped in to tell the patient I was sorry for the delay.
Result	I asked the charge nurse to review my actions with this patient. I also resolved to examine the way I prioritize my patients at the beginning of a shift to determine the best way to meet patient care needs. I resolved to assess pain medication schedules of my patient's so I could plan care for other time-consuming nursing procedures so they would not conflict with pain medication administration.

Source: A. Schooley.

truthfulness and the trainability of the applicant. Interviewers want a newly hired nurse who will fit into the current team and will have the good judgment to ask for help when needed. Applicants who appear overly confident regarding their nursing knowledge and expertise, may lose the nursing position opportunity. All information listed in the resume and application is subject to verification by the employer. The applicant should respond in a calm, problem-solving fashion to all questions. See Table 27.5 for interview questions commonly asked. Questions may be asked about prior employments, or other experiences listed on the resume. When discussing prior employment, or educational experiences, avoid any negative discussion regarding an employer/faculty/or work environment. Keep the entire interview process as positive as possible. The interview process is not a time to discuss any personal problems. Employers are looking for nurses who are dependable and reliable, and they will choose an applicant who has no life drama, over an applicant who lost their last nursing position due to call offs.

Dressing for the Interview

Dress appropriately for the position by wearing professionally acceptable, comfortable, and neatly pressed clothing. For women, this may be a solid-color conservative suit with a modest, coordinated blouse; medium-heeled or flat polished shoes; limited jewelry; and a neat, professional hairstyle. Skirt length should be long enough so you can sit down comfortably. Hosiery should be worn with skirts, even if the weather is warm. Avoid flip flops, or casual sandals. Light, natural makeup is preferable, if makeup is worn. Do not use perfumes or scented lotions, and have neat, short, manicured nails. Avoid visible tattoos, facial jewelry, nose rings, extra earrings, or wild hair or clothing colors or styles.

For men, a suit is preferred with jacket and button-down collared shirt, and pants and jacket should match, if they are not a suit. Avoid bright colors or patterns, keep it simple. Match the socks to dress shoes. Avoid exposing tattoos, piercings, or gages. Hair should be natural hair color and neatly styled and trimmed, and facial hair also should be neatly trimmed. Cologne should be avoided. Nails should be clean and trimmed. A general rule for interview attire is to keep it simple, keep colors plain and muted, and body parts covered.

Food, drinks, gum chewing, and cell phones or any device use during the interview is not acceptable. Do accept water if offered, as nervousness may lead to a dry parched throat. The applicant should turn off their cell phone prior to entering the interview. If the applicant is concerned about bad breath, use a breath mint before entering the interview.

Table 27.5 **Interview Questions**

Question	Potential Response
Tell me about yourself.	Have a short description, with two to three traits that are solid (for example, "I am a positive person and look for new learning experiences.").
Why do you want to work here?	This is where the research pays off, describe several attributes of the work environment, the staff, or the patients (for example, "I enjoyed my rotation on the memory unit, the staff worked as a team, and I am looking for that type of support in my first position." Commenting on organizational strengths also demonstrates that you are serious about your intent and that you understand about the health care system.
What do you want to be doing in 5 years?	Identify a long-term goal and your plans to achieve it with progressive responsibilities and achievements. The Interviewer wants to know that their investment in orienting you will be worthwhile. This question also allows them to see your growth potential.
What are your qualifications?	Discuss experiences that you have had that qualify you for the new position.
What are your strengths?	This is a favorite question. Look at the nursing position description. What qualities do you have that are required? Are you able to work under stress, are you organized, are you eager to learn new skills, do you enjoy new challenges? You may be asked to provide an example of that strength in a work-related scenario.
What would your references say?	You may want to ask your references this question. Would they say you are easily distracted or focused? A team player or solo player? A problem solver or one who ignores problems?
Are you interested in more schooling?	Most who have just graduated may want to say no, but an employer wants someone who is interested in lifelong learning, especially in the nursing profession. This question is really looking at your growth potential.
What has been your biggest success?	Think of a success ahead of time that may fit with the health care system. It does not have to be in nursing. This question should reflect one of your areas of strength.
What has been your greatest failure?	Again, think ahead, but this time make sure you can state what you learned from the negative experience. After all, to fail is to learn, so state what you would do differently next time and why.
Why do you want to leave your current nursing position?	For an RN, you can say that you are seeking new responsibilities, experiences, and challenges. Give an example of a new experience you are looking for.

Source: Compiled with information from Polifko-Harris (2003).

Termination Phase of the Interview

Applicant activity during the interview termination phase is important. The interviewer will close the interview by asking the applicant if they have any questions. Applicants should ask questions at this point. Lack of questions may indicate a lack of serious intent, or interest in the nursing position. The questions posed by the applicant also provide one last opportunity to leave a positive last impression (Maldonado, 2019). Some suggestion questions are outlined in Table 27.6. The applicant should limit their questions to four or five key questions.

Interviewing can be very tiring, but the applicant should take time during the end to review their notes, clarify any questions, and ask what the next step is, for example, when they may hear regarding the position. This question allows the applicant to demonstrate their interest in the position, provides an expected time period, and suggests that the applicant is open to an offer.

Following Up the Interview

Within 24 hr, follow up the interview with a simple thank-you note, or email (Figure 27.5). Writing a thank-you note may feel old-fashioned but is still seen as a professional strength. The note should be short but personalized to each interviewer the applicant met.

After each interview, reflect upon the event, try to be as objective as possible to identify what went well and what did not go well. Debriefing with a friend or colleague may be helpful, but avoid ruminating negatively over the interview. Even a bad interview provides an opportunity for growth and learning. After reflecting, create a strategy for improvement. Employers and applicants are bound to confidentiality. The applicant may seek more information about their weaknesses, and ways to improve, if they are not the successful applicant. The applicant demonstrates their interest in addressing their weaknesses and learning from the interview by asking for this information. For example, the applicant may not be considered for an intensive care nursing position because employers require 2–3 years of medical surgical nursing experience. If the interviewer does not follow up in the time indicated at the interview, the applicant should follow up with a phone call. This demonstrates the applicants continued interest in the position and willingness to learn about weaknesses for future interviews. A script to follow when following up should include, "I am really interested in your position and here is why. . ."

Upon offer of a nursing position, request a follow-up meeting to clarify any questions that need further explanations, such as salary and benefits. Researching salary levels for registered nurses at the United States Bureau of Labor Statistics provides a realistic salary range for the geographical location (www.bls.gov). Applicants must be realistic about their salary expectations relative to experience level and geographical area (Carlson, n.d.). Shift differential is normally offered for night or weekend shifts.

The applicant may also ask additional questions at this time regarding the following:

- What shift will I be scheduled to work?
- Will I be required to rotate shifts?
- How are special requests for time off honored?
- What holidays and weekends am I scheduled to work?
- How is low census handled, how is high census/short staffing handled?
- Is floating to other units expected, or required?

Table 27.6   Sample Questions for the Applicant to Ask During an Interview

- What would be my goal in my first 3 months in the nursing position?
- How will my performance be evaluated, and by whom?
- What is the potential for growth and or advancement in my position? For example, a clinical ladder program, or ongoing certification expectation?
- What challenges do you think I may face in this role, and what qualities do you think I need to overcome them?
- What type of orientation or internship will I receive? What is the expected length?
- What professional development may be needed in the next 2 years to enhance my ability to be a safe, effective nurse on the unit?
- Is this a magnet hospital? What role do I have in quality improvement efforts and improving nurse-sensitive outcomes?

Source: Compiled with informtion from Maldonado (2019).

Critical Thinking 27.7

For many nurse applicants, the interview is the most stressful part of seeking a nursing position. Assume you are seeking employment. Practice answering the questions in Table 27.5. Have a friend interview you using the questions, or even just practice answering them out loud on your own in front of a mirror or video yourself and watch.

1. What questions would represent your level of knowledge and skill?
2. What characteristics would you emphasize when you respond to the questions?

Table 27.7   Nursing Career Theories

Theory	Author, year	Key aspects	Application to beginning nurses
Novice to expert	Benner (1984)	Maturation of nursing competence during a nurse's career Movement from stages are based on experience not time in the profession	Stage 1: Novice Stage 2: Beginner Stage 3: Competency Stage 4: Proficiency Stage 5: Expert
Career development theory	Super (1980)	Career stages are related to the meaning of each stage. Each stage is influenced by the role position, attitude, and responsibility during work in the clinical area.	Exploration < 2 years Establishment 2–5 years Maintenance 5–15 years (marriage, financial issues) Disengagement >15 years Consider quality of life and retirement.

Source: A Schooley.

Upon offer of a nursing position, nurse applicants should carefully consider their personal values and career values, as well as personal responsibilities when considering the position. If commuting is required, consider the additional costs involved with car maintenance, insurance, and gas, when evaluating the offered salary. It is important to know the average salary paid for similar positions with other agencies when negotiating a salary (Carlson, n.d.), and to clearly communicate salary expectations. If the nursing position offer is unacceptable, clearly state the reason. The employer then can counter offer. The applicant always wants to leave the negotiation process on a professional and positive note. In addition, the applicant should thank the interviewer for their time and the opportunity to discuss their career goals and plans. After landing the first nursing position, career planning must continue. The nurse should reconsider the 1-year milestone, and what professional development is needed over the next year (see Figure 27.1). A mentor may help the new graduate develop milestones and identify the education or training needed to attain the milestone.

Career Development Theories

While thinking of possible milestones, consider some theories around career development. Super (1957) introduced the career model to demonstrate the changing of attitudes and personal growth during the five career development stages, refining it in 1980. According to Super's theory, the first years of the nursing career development will include exploration of work experiences, building skills, and exploring different nursing roles. Consideration of practice setting changes should be included in the career path. Nurses in the early career stages require additional training time built into their work schedule due to the increased training needed (Price & Reichert, 2017).

Patricia Benner's work also supports the professional development needed for the new nurse to grow into their professional identity as they proceed from novice to expert (Benner, 1984).

Both Benner and Super indicate that expertise grows with experience, creating a fluidity of the stages discussed in both

theories. Men in nursing have different career needs at different stages than women in nursing and may seek leadership positions earlier (Yu et al., 2018). The establishment phase begins after the 2nd year in the profession (Hsing et al., 2018). In the establishment stage nurses hone their skills, and work at a high level of professionalism due to professional knowledge (Super, 1980). Retention of nurses in the establishment phase is important for the health care system due to the need for nurses, and the cost of investment.

Awareness of the changing needs of nurses within the profession during their career will help the new nurse consider how their career path may be updated and changed as they progress in their profession. During the maintenance stage, nurses may face challenges related to family obligations competing with professional goals (Super, 1980) Nurses in the mid-career phase, between 5 and 10 years, are important to the profession, providing expertise, and mentorship of new nurses (Yarbrough et al., 2017). Mid-career nurses want support and opportunities for professional growth but may struggle with leaving a unit that is highly dependent on their expertise (Price & Reichert, 2017). Nurses during the maintenance stage express a desire for additional education, to build their expertise but also express the need for additional training time to be included into their work schedule (Price & Reichert, 2017). Nurses in their mid-career still express a need for mentoring to meet their career goals and want opportunities to progress to leadership (Yu et al., 2018).

As nurses are exploring roles and expanding their professional growth, we often see some of the same needs expressed by both novice and experienced nurses. Experienced nurses in the later part of their career path seeking **horizontal or lateral moves** may find themselves needing to develop new skills and knowledge. A horizontal move is an upward movement, such as an administrative position, or an advanced practice position. A horizontal move often requires formal higher education, or informal leadership workshops. A move from a night shift staff nurse position to a night shift charge nurse position is one example of a horizontal move.

A lateral move indicates a move within the same role, such as staff nurse, but to a new practice area, requiring new skills or certifications, or such as Advanced Cardiac Life Support (ACLS), or fetal monitoring. Nurses who are dissatisfied with their current position may benefit from a lateral move into another specialty area. Health care systems often support **internal career changes** of nurses to retain their expertise within the system. An internal career change is a lateral or horizontal move within the same health care system in which the nurse is currently employed. Internal career changes are a beneficial opportunity for nurses who are seeking experiences in another specialty area, or to improve their satisfaction in their work environment (Read & Laschinger, 2017). For the nurse, internal career changes allow them to retain seniority and benefits such as insurance and retirement. Internal career moves also benefit the health care system by retaining the nurse's expertise and their investment in the nurse's professional development.

Professional Development

The third step of creating the career path is listing the professional development needed to achieve each milestone. Professional development may require informal education such as continuing education credits (CEU's), or workshops, or formal education resulting in a higher degree, or **specialty certifications**. Specialty certifications provide evidence of practice knowledge, skills, and clinical expertise within a specialty area of nursing care (American Nurses Credentialing Center (ANCC), 2019).

Certifications

Nurses have the ability to achieve multiple types of certifications. Certifications may be in a clinical practice role or in American Heart Association Certifications (AHAC) required for practice. Specialty certifications are nationally recognized certificates obtained through the ANCC or the National Certification Corporation (NCC). Certification in nurse practice roles generally require 2–5 years of experience in the role, and a specified number of clinical practice hours. Specialty certifications are obtained by passing an exam taken at a testing center and require re-certification every 5 years. Practice role certifications are often a good 3-year milestone. Some health care systems offer training sessions for the practice role exams and reimbursement of the cost of the exam. Nurses with specialty certification can add the letters for the certification after their RN title, such as RN (registered nurse), CCRN (Critical care registered nurse) for those RN's that have taken and passed the adult critical care registered nurse exam (Table 27.8).

Table 27.8   Nursing Practice Certifications for Clinical Specialties

Certification agencies	Specialty certifications by professional nursing organizations
American Nurses Credentialing Center (ANCC) www.nursingworld.org/certification	*Clinical nurse specialist* • Adult Gerontology • Ambulatory Care • Cardiac Vascular • Gerontological • Informatics • Medical Surgical • Pediatric • Psychiatric Mental Health • Nurse Executive • Nurse Case Management • Nursing Professional Development • Pain Management *Inte-rprofessional* • National Health Care disaster Also lists for Nurse Practitioners
National Certification Corporation (NCC) www.nccwebsite.org	*Core certifications* • Inpatient Obstetric Nursing • Low Risk Neonatal Nursing • Maternal Newborn Nursing • Neonatal Intensive Care Nursing *Subspecialties* • Electronic Fetal Monitoring • Neonatal Pediatric Transport *Nurse Practitioner certification* • Neonatal Nurse Practitioner • Women's Health Care Nurse Practitioner

Source: Compiled by A Schooley.

Practice in many health care areas requires AHAC beyond Basic Life Support (BLS), which is required for nursing schools. Medical surgical, intensive care, and surgical units often require obtaining Adult Cardiovascular Life Support (ACLS). Movement into the specialty areas of pediatrics or maternity units often requires Pediatric Advance Life Support (PALS), or Neonatal Resuscitation Provider (NRP) certifications. AHAC certifications generally require an online or classroom-based course, passing exams, and simulated demonstration of skills with certified instructors. AHAC classes are normally offered by the health care facility and require re-certification every 2 years to maintain. AHAC certification is an appropriate professional development to include on the career pathway for the first-year nurse. If a nurse is interested in moving into a specialty area, additional AHAC certification training provides the skills needed.

Formal Education

Continuing education is also vital to career planning. Associate Degree Nurses may seek a bachelor's degree to move into a management position or to obtain an advanced practice degree. Advanced practice nursing degrees require formal education at Masters or Doctorate degree levels. Nurses should consider the options of attending a local university to obtain their degree or an online program with more flexibility. Nurses need their health care systems to invest in their education and training, with paid time and release (Price & Reichert, 2017). Commitment to education is vital to retention of nurses within the health care system and the profession (Price & Reichert, 2017).

Informal Education

Informal education often includes obtaining continuing education (CEU) credits by participation in nursing conferences, online learning modules to obtain CEU's, or face-to-face workshops. Many nursing licensing bodies require regular submission of ongoing continuing education units (CEUs) to maintain licensure (Nurse.com, 2019). A CEU credit is equal to 10 hr of participation in an educational course or professional conference (Nurse.Org). Some states require a specific number of CEUs to maintain licensure as a nurse. In addition to the number of CEU's, the State Board of Nursing (SBN) may also mandate a number of nursing education hours focused on specific areas of care. A visit to the States Board of Nursing will guide the professional development activities needed to maintain licensure. On the other hand, continuing education credits (CE) may be offered by health care institutions, nursing programs, or by professional organizations. Nurses must be aware of CE or CEU requirements by the state.

Professional Portfolio

Nurses should begin documenting professional development by tracking continuing education hours immediately at the start of their career. Best practices include keeping a record of orientation material, and writing a list with the name of the in-service, the presenter, the date, and the location, as well as a brief summary of the learning. A portfolio is an excellent tool to show evidence of a nurse's skill, and ongoing professional development (Burns, 2018). Keep documents chronologically in order, and update on a regular basis. Store CEUs or CEs with the course description and handouts. Electronic or hard copy records are acceptable, but keep them accessible as needed for licensure renewal. Service on committees, service awards, and professional memberships should be included in the portfolio. Only verifiable activities should be included in the portfolio.

Professional Nursing Organizations

Membership in professional nursing organizations (PNOs) provides many benefits to nurses. PNOs, such as the American Nurses Association, provide career opportunities, networking, community, and educational opportunities. Educational resources include certification resources for movement into a specialty area, continuing education material, and discounts of professional resources to their members. Scholarship opportunities exist as well as professional practice conferences.

Aside from the valuable educational resources that membership brings, activity in the organization establishes relationships and opportunities for mentoring. Minority nurses may further benefit from professional ethnic nursing organizations, such as the National Black Nurses Association (NBNA). Minority nurses often experience a stronger sense of mentorship, belonging, and support for further education through professional minority organizations (Matza, Garon, & Que-Lahoo, 2018). Nursing identity is supported by becoming part of this larger community, which further enhances the nurse's professional career. A career path provides a visual diagram of your professional milestones, as well as formal and informal educational steps needed to reach each milestone. Creating professional milestones for 1-, 3-, and 5-years, guides the nurse in their career. Following the career path ensures control over a career by including personal and professional values. A nurse's ability to articulate a career path increases professional satisfaction and insulates the nurse from role strain and frustration with the nursing profession caused by a poor employment/employee fit. Awareness of professional needs ensures the nurse is providing safe patient care by aligning personal needs/obligations to the chosen employment position. Careful consideration during career planning enhances the nurse's identity and increases resilience during their professional career.

In summary, in this chapter you have learned the importance of career planning and professional development. You have clarified personal and career values with a 1, 3-, and 5-year career path and have the tools to create a successful job search and interview. The next steps are up to you as you plan your future in nursing where the potentials are endless.

KEY CONCEPTS

- Career planning begins with identifying professional milestones.

- Alignment of personal values and career values provides a guide to career planning.

- Applying for a nursing position begins with the preparation of a professional resume and cover letter.

- Searching for a nursing position includes examining the health care system and determining the nursing competencies needed.

- Successful application, interviewing strategies, and follow up take practice, time, and effort.

- Mindful career planning increases nurse's satisfaction with their career and improves their ability to practice safely.

- Development and revision of career goals at 1-, 3-, and 5-years improves professional growth and allow for changes of the goals related to life events, or professional opportunities.

KEY TERMS

Career Path
Horizontal career change
Internal career changes

Lateral career change
Nursing identity
Psychological safety

Resilience
Specialty certifications

REVIEW QUESTIONS

1. You are being considered for an entry-level nursing position in an intensive care unit. During the interview, the nursing manager describes the following case scenario: During your shift, one of the patients on the unit goes into atrial fibrillation, and you also have another patient returning from cardiac bypass surgery. How should you handle the situation to provide a safe practice environment?
   a. Ask the charge nurse to assist with the patient with atrial fibrillation while you admit the surgical patient.
   b. Inform the nursing supervisor of the patient's condition and the patient assignment, and request assistance.
   c. Prepare a detailed documentation report to give to the nursing manager in the morning.
   d. Call a rapid response to deal with the surgical patient and get them settled.

2. During an interview for a position in the maternity unit, an applicant was asked how they would handle the following situation: The unit is very busy, and a patient arrives alone. Some of the nurses refer to her as a "Nervous Nelly" and tell you to put her in the triage room until you have time to care for her. What would be your initial response?
   a. After noting the smell of marijuana on her clothes, you realize she may be high, and place her in a triage room.
   b. You place her in the triage room and give her some crackers and water.
   c. You assess her reason for coming in, place a transducer to monitor contractions and fetal heartrate, and take the appropriate nursing action.
   d. You ask a nurse why they called her a "Nervous Nelly," because she appears calm to you.

3. You are being considered for an entry-level nursing position in a medical surgical unit. During the interview, the nursing manager describes the following case scenario: During your shift, you hear a rumor that a famous actor is being admitted in the emergency room. One of your peers goes to the electronic medical record to verify this rumor. What is your responsibility?
   a. Advise your peer this is a violation of HIPAA (Health Insurance Portability and Accountability Act) and they could be fired.
   b. Walk away and state you are uninterested in this actor.
   c. Glance over your peer's shoulder while they pull up the chart.
   d. Say nothing to your peer but report the violation to your supervisor.

4. During a job interview, the nurse recruiter presents the following hypothetical question: You are working the evening shift and are given an assignment with a patient on a ventilator that you are unfamiliar with using. The team on the floor includes nurses, respiratory therapists, and certified nursing assistants. What action should you take?
   a. Request a change in assignments until you are in-serviced on the ventilator by another nurse.
   b. Refuse the assignment, because you are putting your nursing license at risk by using unfamiliar equipment.
   c. Ask the respiratory therapist to explain the ventilator to you and demonstrate any procedures that may be different from the ventilator you are familiar with using.
   d. Inform the nursing manager that you are not capable of caring for the patient due to the ventilator.

5. The employer is posing clinical judgment scenarios to the applicant. During your orientation, the charge nurse states the unit is too busy for you to be paired with your preceptor and you will be taking your own assignment. How should you advocate for yourself?
   a. Inform the charge nurse that you are not comfortable taking an assignment and you feel it is a safety concern.
   b. Check the policy of the hospital with respect to the orientation process.

c. Contact the nursing manager to report the violation of the orientation agreement.

d. Check the policy of the orientation process regarding short staffing on the unit.

6. During orientation to the workplace, the staff educator states that nurses are not allowed to refuse an assignment that violates their personal beliefs. You are concerned because this contradicts what you learned in school. What would be the best approach to address your understanding of your rights as a nurse?

a. Research your states' nurse's rights.

b. Ask your preceptor on the unit regarding the policy.

c. Confront the staff educator regarding the policy.

d. Contact a former nursing faculty member.

7. During your interview, you are asked to consider the following scenario: A patient in a rehabilitation unit states they would pay you to bring them food from a fast food restaurant. What would you do?

a. Inform the patient that the hospital policy does not permit food from outside the facility.

b. Suggest that the family sneak the food in the next time they visit.

c. Explore approaches with the dietary department that could meet the patient's need.

d. Offer to pick up the food and bring it in the next time you work.

8. You are assisting a health care provider (HCP) who is performing a sterile procedure. The HCP contaminates the sterile field but appears to not notice the violation. What would be the most appropriate action?

a. Ignore the accidental contamination and allow the HCP to perform the procedure.

b. Notify the HCP, and obtain a different sterile tray so they can proceed with the procedure.

c. Speak to the HCP about the break in sterility after the procedure is complete, and you are away from the patient.

d. Complete an adverse event form regarding the break in sterility and inform the HCP of the reporting the adverse event.

9. During your nursing employment interview, the nurse recruiter asks if you can provide references. Your best response would be which of the following?

a. Contact a high school teacher and a nursing professor to provide references.

b. Give the recruiter the names of possible referenees, such as neighbors and family friends.

c. Provide the names of referenees who have consented to provide a reference, who are able to provide a character or professional reference.

d. Provide the name of your former employer at a fast food chain.

10. You are seeking your first nursing position upon your graduation. You are trying to be pro-active and build a professional image for your social media presence and recruiters. Which of the following actions should you do to present a positive professional image for recruiters? Select all that apply.

a. Ask former employers for a reference

b. Remove photos of partying from social media

c. Create a professional email address

d. Verify voice mail message is professional

e. Remove political views or offensive posts from personal social media.

f. Print your resume on colored paper

REVIEW QUESTION ANSWERS

1. Answer: A is correct.
Rationale: The nurse must quickly provide care for two critical patients (A). The nurse must realize this assignment requires additional help and recognize her own limitation. The charge nurse may notify the nursing supervisor of the changes in acuity (B) after stabilizing the atrial fibrillation patient and allowing the new nurse to complete the admission of the post-op bypass patient. (C) Notification in the morning does not correct the high acuity and lack of staff that is currently a problem. (D) Calling a rapid response for the stabilized post-surgical patient is not appropriate.

2. Answer: C is correct.
Rationale: (C) Assessing the reason for seeking care, monitoring contractions, and fetal heart rate are vital triage activities in the maternity unit. (A) The nurse must provide care to all patients regardless of drug use. (B) Placing her in the triage room, and providing food does not address the reason the patient is seeking care. (D) Seeking more information from the other nurses will prevent you from being non-judgmental and non-biased. You should always treat each patient contact ethically to address the patient's needs.

3. Answer: A is correct.
Rationale: (A) Nurses have to the obligation to protect patient information. Reminding your peer of the policy regarding HIPAA violation allows them to correct their actions and prevent the violation from occurring. (B) Not participating in the HIPAA violation is commendable, but does not prevent the violation, nor relieve you of the responsibility to protect patient data. (C) Glancing over your peer's shoulder violates HIPAA and puts you in violation of the policy as well. (D) The HIPAA violation is reportable and should be reported to the supervisor, but by not addressing the action in a way that can prevent the violation allows the violation to occur.

4. Answer: C is correct.
Rationale: (A) Nurses provide care to ventilated patients within a team, the respiratory therapist has the responsibility to manage the ventilator. (B) Refusing a nursing assignment has legal aspects and should be used only for conditions where patient safety is a concern. (C) Seeking the support and expertise of the Respiratory Therapist to learn about the new ventilator provides an opportunity to develop important nursing skills. (D) Refusing the assignment is an option, but may leave the unit short of nurses. As explained in (B), this action should rarely be used.

5. Answer: A is correct.
    Rationale: (A) Sharing your concern and framing it as a patient safety concern notifies the charge nurse that you do not feel capable of being on your own and allows the charge nurse to consider other options to cover the assignments. (B) Checking the policy does not notify the charge nurse of your discomfort with the change in the orientation policy. (C) Contacting the unit director also does not address the concern occurring. (D) Checking the policy regarding orientation and short staffing will not cause a change in the assignments. As a nurse you must use strong communication skills to advocate for the safety of the patient.

6. Answer: B is correct.
    Rationale: (A) Knowing the State Board of Nursing policy is important to understand the scope of the nursing role and legal obligations within the role. But each health care facility may have their own interpretation/policy regarding the refusal of assignments, which you should be aware of. (B) Asking your preceptor about the facility policy avoids confrontation, and provides an opportunity to familiarize yourself with the conditions regarding assignment refusal in your facility and within the particular unit (C) Confronting the unit director may be interpreted as incivility and may not lead to further information about the policy. (D) While a nursing faculty member may know what the practice act outlines, each facility has their own policy that may vary based on certain conditions. Seeking further clarification from your preceptor is a non-confrontational way to obtain further information.

7. Answer: C is correct.
    Rationale: (A) Providing patient centered care which recognizes the patient's autonomy is an aspect in this scenario. While the policy may prohibit outside food, perhaps the patient is really seeking more control over their care as discussed in option (C). (B) Suggesting that food be snuck in, may harm the patient due to medication interactions. (C) Exploring the patient's wishes with the dietary department may allow for the patient's wishes to be met without ignoring any dietary restrictions. (D) Taking money, or providing special favors that are outside the nurse's scope of practice is an ethical and legal issue that should be avoided.

8. Answer B: is correct.
    Rationale: (A) Nurses have to the obligation to protect patient safety, ignoring the the violation of the pre-procedure checklist and time-out puts the patient at risk. (B) Notifying the HCP in a constructive manner brings to their attention that there was a break in sterility, and allows for immediate correction. (C) Informing the HCP after the procedure does not allow for immediate correction and prevent possible infection risk for the patient. (D) While reporting the adverse event afterward may seem correct, this does not prevent the danger to the patient that can be averted by the nurse.

9. Answer: C is correct.
    Rationale: (A) Providing the name of your high school teacher will not provide the employer with your skills in the nursing role. (B) Nursing positions generally request references beyond character references which would be given by neighbors or family friends. (C) A nursing professor who has evaluated your clinical performance would be appropriate to provide a reference regarding your skills in the nursing role. (D) Nursing positions generally request references who can speak to professional abilities, a former employer may be a good reference, but in this case the employer is requesting information regarding the nursing skills.

10. Answers B, C, D, and E are correct.
    Rationale: (A) is incorrect. Securing references will not improve your social media image but may be needed for filling out applications. (B) Recruiters will look at your social media; you do not want them to believe you have an alcohol issue. Removing these pictures will improve your professional image. (C) A professional email address will improve their first impression of you as a nurse. (D) Verification if a professional outgoing voicemail insures that the recruiter will have a positive first impression. (E) Recruiters will look at your social media; you do not want them to believe you have political views, or unprofessional behaviors that may not represent their organization. (F) is Incorrect. Your resume should be printed on white paper only.

REVIEW ACTIVITIES

Activity 1

When considering Lauren's journey into her nursing career, what may help her feel more confident in her ability as a nurse?

Activity 2

Consider Robert planning for a horizontal move through an advanced practice degree. How can his employer support his move and retain him as a member of the health care team?

Activity 3

Consider Robert, Lauren, and Isabella, choose an immediate or intermediate milestone for each, and identify the requirements to meet that milestone.

Activity 4

While considering Robert, Lauren, and Isabella's future, how does this help you in your personal career planning?

DISCUSSION POINTS

1. Consider the career values that may be significant for nurses, at different stages of their life and careers.

2. What personal values may be significant for each of our new nurses?

3. Consider how personal and professional values may change over time?

4. What workplace situations may cause a conflict in values between each of the new nurses and their employers?

DISCUSSION OF OPENING SCENARIO

1. What steps should a new nurse take to find a position that provides support and opportunities for professional growth? Begin with your personal values and career values. Purposeful career planning prevents role strain between home and work life. Achieving an effective balance allows the nurse to come to work well rested, and present for the patient, and provide safe, error-free care. Career planning allows the nurse to seek further education/professional development to improve their skills and knowledge. Find a position that fits you, will allow you to develop your nursing identity, and become fully engaged in your practice unit. Support through orientation, mentorship, inclusion on committees, and support for ongoing education also help you grow as a nurse.

2. What factors allow a new nurse to function within the health care team? Career planning and clarifying your personal goals helps you find a position that works for you. Some nurses thrive on busy, non-stop, high acuity areas of nursing. Other nurses prefer a steadier paced unit that allows for development of relationships with their patients. Some areas of nursing require high levels of teamwork and communication with careful coordination of care. Other areas of nursing are very autonomous and require less communication within the team but do require self-initiative.

3. How does a nurse develop the skills needed to be a nurse leader? Developing personal milestones will allow for purposeful professional development efforts such as continuing education, or more formal education to achieve the milestones set. Keeping the milestones as a goal point provides a direction for seeking engagement activities, committee participation, seeking mentorship, and participation in professional organizations. Defining specific milestones increases your control over your career and increases satisfaction by aligning your energy and efforts to achieve milestones that are important to your personal career. Seeking mentors to guide you, and continual pursuit of your milestones by engaging in your healthcare community will allow you to develop as a nurse leader. You can also develop as a nurse leader by serving on committees, joining professional organizations, and growing as nurse by seeking further informal and/or formal education.

EXPLORING THE WEB

Exploring the Web Activity 1

Explore the website https://nurse.org/resources/nursing-resume. This resource includes templates and advice on resume writing. Midway down the page there is a section listed as action verbs that may be used to in the resume. Accessed March 2, 2019.

Exploring the Web Activity 2

Explore the U.S. Equal Employment Opportunity Commission. www.eeoc.gov/laws/practices/index.cfm This resource includes examples of questions and inquiries that are illegal to ask during the hiring process. Accessed March 2, 2019.

Exploring the Web Activity 3

The National Student Nurses Association (NSNA) publishes the Imprint Career Planning Guide every January. This online only publication has many resources regarding specialty certifications, furthering your education, and career planning. Look at one of your 3-year milestones and explore one of the resources at: www.nsna.org/career-planning-guides.html Click on, Career Center, and then click on, Nursing Specialties. Scroll through the list to find the minimal education needed, experience needed, and certification requirements to achieve the goal. Accessed January 16, 2019.

Exploring the Web Activity 4

Explore the ANCC website and determine the test content outline for the medical-surgical nursing certification that Robert would like to pursue. www.nursingworld.org/certification Scroll down to the middle of the page, click on "See all ANCC Certifications" scroll two-thirds down the page and click on Medical-Surgical Nursing Certification (RN-BC). Under Apply for Certification click on Eligibility and read through the requirements for eligibility. Is Robert eligible to sit for the certification? Accessed January 20, 2019.

Exploring the Web Activity 5

Explore the website Nurse.com. Nurse.com is a for-profit website offering online continuing education opportunities for nurses. This online site has a webpage titled Nursing CE Requirements by State. This webpage provides a direct link to each SBN and the continuing education requirements. www.nurse.com/state-nurse-ce-requirements Accessed January 21, 2019.

INFORMATICS

Go to, http://qsen.org Accessed December18, 2018. Click on, Education, and then click on, Competencies. Then click on, QSEN Competencies. Then click on, Teamwork and Collaboration. Scroll down and review the definition and KSAs for Teamwork and Collaboration.

1. How do your professional values affect your ability to participate in the healthcare team?

2. Identify the connection between engagement as a team member and patient safety.

LEAN BACK

- What do you see in practice regarding career development that is different from what you read in the text? Why?

- How can this information directly apply to your nursing career?

- After reading this information, what action are you going to take today?

- Will this information matter to you as a future nurse leader?

- How can you apply this information directly to improve your practice as a nurse?

REFERENCES

American Association of Colleges of Nursing (AACN). (2019). *Vizient/AACN nurse residency program*. Retrieved from www.aacnnursing.org/Nurse-Residency-Program

American Nurses Association (ANA) Career Center Staff. (2014). *What recruiters look for*. Retrieved from www.nursingworld.org/resources/individual/recruiters-look-for

American Nurses Association (ANA) Enterprise. (2019). *2019 ANA digital recruitment guide*.

American Nurses Credentialing Center (ANCC). (2019). *Home page*. Retrieved from www.nursingworld.org/ancc

ANA Career Center Staff. (2014). *Recruiters look for*. Retrieved from www.nursingworld.org/resources/individual/recruiters-look-for/

Anselmo-Witzel, S., Orshan, S. A., Heitner, K. L., & Bachanc, J. (2017). Are generation Y nurses satisfied on the job? Understanding their lived experiences. *The Journal of Nursing Administration, 47*(4), 232–237.

Awaisi, H. A., Cooke, H., & Pryjmachuk, S. (2015). The experiences of newly graduated nurses during their first year of practice in the Sultanate of Oman–A case study. *International Journal of Nursing Studies, 52*(11), 1723–1734. doi:10.1016/j.ijnurstu.2015.06.009

Bell, T. (2018). *The secrets to beating an applicant tracking system (ATS)*. IDG Communications. Retrieved from www.cio.com/article/2398753/careers-staffing/careers-staffing-5-insider-secrets-for-beating-applicant-tracking-systems.html

Benner, P. (1984). *From novice to expert: Excellence and power in clinical nursing practice*. Menlo Park, CA: Addison-Wesley.

Burns, M. K. (2018). Creating a nursing portfolio. *Ohio Nurses Review, 93*(3), 16–17.

Cardillo, D. W. (2018). *The ultimate career guide for nurses: Practical advice for thriving at every stage of your career* (2nd ed.). Silver Springs, MD: American Nurses Association.

Carlson, K. (n.d.). *6 tips to salary negotiations*. American Nurse Today. Retrieved from www.americannursetoday.com/tips-salary-negotiations

Dyrbye, L. N., Johnson, P. O., Johnson, L. M., Satele, D. V., & Shanafelt, T. D. (2018). Efficacy of the well-being index to identify distress and well-being in U.S. nurses. *Nursing Research, 67*(6), 447–455. 10.197/NNR.0000000000000313

Frankel, A., Haraden, C., Federico, F., & Lenoci-Edwards, J. (2017). *A framework for safe, reliable, and effective care. White Paper*. Cambridge, MA: Institute for Healthcare Improvement and Safe & Reliable Healthcare. Retrieved from www.ihi.org/resources/Pages/IHIWhitePapers/Framework-Safe-Reliable-Effective-Care.aspx

Gibson, A. (2018). *31 Sample nursing interview questions with answer guide*. Retrieved from https://nurse.org/articles/nurse-behavioral-interview-questions-answers

Gibson, A. (2019a). *Career guide series: The ultimate guide to nursing resumes*. Retrieved from https://nurse.org/resources/nursing-resume

Gibson, A. (2019b). *Nursing resumes: The ultimate guide*. Retrieved from https://nurse.org/resources/nursing-resume/

Government of Canada. (2018). *Canadian Human Rights Commission*. Retrieved from www.canada.ca/en/human-rights-commission.html

Hart, P. L., Brannan, J. D., & De Chesnay, M. (2014). Resilience in nurses: An integrative review. *Journal of Nursing Management, 22*(6), 720–734.

Hess, R. (2017). *Nurse interview tips for millennials, Gen Xers and everyone else—Part 1: Be a Jen, not a Nancy, during nursing interview*. Retrieved from www.nurse.com/blog/2017/05/19/nurse-interview-tips-for-millennials-gen-xers-and-everyone-else-part-1

Institute for Healthcare Improvement (IHI). (2017). *A framework for safe reliable and effective care*. Retrieved from www.ihi.org/resources/Pages/IHIWhitePapers/Framework-Safe-Reliable-Effective-Care.aspx

Institute of Medicine. (2010). *The future of nursing: Leading change, advancing health*. Washington, DC: National Academies Press.

Jackson, A. E. (2017). *Glassdoor: Career advice, interviews. 8 Inappropriate interview questions and how to tackle them like a pro*. Retrieved from www.glassdoor.com/blog/inappropriate-interview-questions

Kohler, C. (2020). *How to write a resume to 'beat the bots': Don't let your resume fall into the ATS black hole*. Retrieved from https://jobs.ana.org/career-resources/articles/?article=40

Maldonado, C. (2019). *Do you have any questions for us? 4 great responses and the best question you can ask at your interview*. Retrieved from https://jobs.ana.org/career-resources/articles/?article=5&category=2&subcategory=3

Matza, M. R., Garon, M. B., & Que-Lahoo, J. (2018). Developing minority nurse leaders: The anchor and the rope. *Nursing Forum, 53*, 348–357. doi:10.1111/nuf.12261

Mills, J., Woods, C., Harrison, H., Chamberlain-Salaun, J., & Spencer, B. (2017). Retention of early career registered nurses: The influence of self-concept, practice environment and resilience in the first five years post-graduation. *Journal of Research in Nursing, 22*(5), 372–385. doi:10.1177/1744987117709515

National Councils of State Boards of Nursing (NCSBN). (2018). *NCSBN welcomes you to the nursing profession*. Chicago, IL: National Council of State Boards of Nursing, Inc. www.ncsbn.org/12096.htm

Nurse.com. (2019). *Nursing CE requirements by state*. Retrieved from www.nurse.com/state-nurse-ce-requirements

Perlo, J., Balik, B., Swensen, S., Kabcenell, A., Landsman, J., & Feeley, D. (2017). *IHI framework for improving joy in work. IHI white paper*. Cambridge, MA: Institute for Healthcare Improvement.

Price, S., & Reichert, C. (2017). The importance of continuing professional development to career satisfaction and patient care: Meeting the needs of novice to mid-to late-career nurses throughout their career span. *Administrative Sciences, 7*(17), 1–13. doi:10.33390/admsci7020017

Price, S. I., Hall, L. M., Murphy, G. T., & Pierce, B. (2018). Evolving career choices narratives of new graduate nurses. *Nurse Education in Practice, 28*, 86–91.

Purdue University Northwest Career Center. (2018). *Career resource guide 2081-2019.* Retrieved from www.pnw.edu/career-center/wp-content/uploads/sites/9/PurdueNW_CRG_18-19.pdf

Quality and Safety Education for Nursing (QSEN). (2019). *QSEN competencies.* Retrieved from http://qsen.org/competencies/pre-licensure-ksas/#teamwork_collaboration

Read, E., & Laschinger, H. (2017). Transition experiences, intrapersonal resources, and job retention of new graduate nurses from accelerated and traditional nursing programs: A cross-sectional comparative study. *Nurse Education Today, 59*, 53–58.

Registered Nursing.org. (2019). *RN interview tips and advice.* Retrieved from www.registerednursing.org/guide/interview

Sacco, T. L., & Copel, L. C. (2017). Compassion satisfaction: A concept analysis in nursing. *Nursing Forum, 53*, 76–83. doi:10.1111/nuf.12213

Super, D. E. (1957). *The psychology of careers: An introduction to vocational development.* New York, NY: Harper.

Super, D. E. (1980). A life-span, life-space approach to career development. *Journal of Vocational Behavior, 16*(3), 282–298.

Turner, J. (2019). A nurse's guide to understanding digital recruitment trends. *Minority Nurse, 0*–16.

U.S. Equal Employment Opportunity Commission. (n.d.). *Prohibited employment policies/practices: Pre-employment inquiries and . . .* Retrieved from www.eeoc.gov/laws/practices/index.cfm

Walsh, A. L. (2018). Nurse residency programs and the benefits for new nurses. *Pediatric Nursing, 44*(6), 275–279.

Yarbrough, S., Martin, P., Alfred, D., & McNeill, C. (2017). Professional values, job satisfaction, career development, and intent to stay. *Nursing Ethics, 24*(6), 675–685. doi:10.1177/0969733015623098

Yu, H.-Y., Lou, J.-H., Eng, C.-J., Yang, C.-I., & Lee, L.-H. (2018). Organizational citizenship behaviour of men in nursing professions: Career stage perspectives. *Collegian, 25*(1), 19–26. doi:10.1016/j.colegn.2017.02.003

SUGGESTED READING

American Heart Association Certifications (AHAC). (2018). *Healthcare professional.* Retrieved from https://cpr.heart.org/AHAECC/CPRAndECC/Training/HealthcareProfessional/UCM_473185_Healthcare-Professional.jsp

Augustine, A. (2019a). *The importance of saying "thank you" after an interview.* American Nurses Association Career Center. Retrieved from https://jobs.ana.org/career-resources/articles/?article=38&category=2&subcategory=10

Augustine, A. (2019b). *Why you should google yourself to monitor your online brand.* American Nurses Association Career Center. Retrieved from https://jobs.ana.org/career-resources/articles/?article=34&category=4&subcategory=7

Fida, R., Laschinder, H. K., & Leiter, M. P. (2018). The protective role of self-efficacy against workplace incivility and burnout in nursing: A time-lagged study. *Health Care Management Review, 43*(1), 21–29. doi:10.1097/HMR.0000000000000126

Hicks, T. P., Sullivan, M., Sexton, J. B., & Adair, K. C. (2019). Transforming culture through resiliency and teamwork: Support positive relationships and value each team member. *American Nurse Today, 14*(2), 41–43.

Pasila, K., Elo, S., & Kaariainen, M. (2017). Newly graduated nurses' orientation experience: A systematic review of qualitative studies. *International Journal of Nursing Studies, 71*, 17–27.

United States Bureau of Labor. (2017). *Occupational employment statistics: occupational employment and wages.* Retrieved from www.bls.gov/oes/2017/may/oes291141.htm#st

Wilkinson, J. (2016). Factors that influence new graduates' preferences for specialty areas. *Nursing Praxis in New Zealand, 32*(1), 8–19.

28 Balancing a Healthy Personal and Professional Life

Cheryl Moredich
Purdue University Northwest, College of Nursing, Hammond, IN, USA

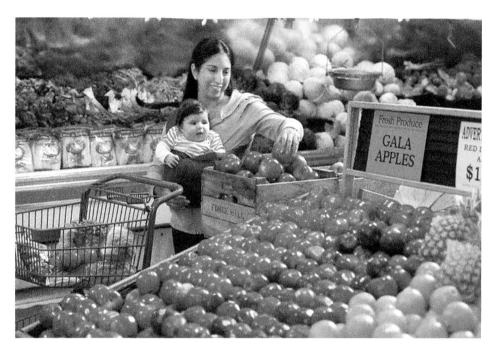

Balancing a healthy personal and professional life requires thought and planning.
Source: Lisa M. Gaetke/National Institute of Health (NIH)

A healthy nurse is someone who actively focuses on creating and maintaining a balance and synergy of physical, intellectual, emotional, social, spiritual, personal and professional wellbeing.

(American Nurses Association (2017)). Healthy Nurse, Healthy Nation.

OBJECTIVES

Upon completion of this chapter, the reader should be able to:

1. Generate a personal definition of health.

2. Formulate a plan for maintaining optimal physical health.

3. Strategize ways to incorporate activities that promote emotional and spiritual health.

4. Recognize ways to create a healthy work-life balance

Kelly Vana's Nursing Leadership and Management, Fourth Edition. Edited by Patricia Kelly Vana and Janice Tazbir
© 2021 John Wiley & Sons Ltd. Published 2020 by John Wiley & Sons Ltd.
Companion Website: www.wiley.com/go/kelly-Nursing-Leadership

OPENING SCENARIO

Sahara gets up early to work the day shift. On her drive to work, she grabs a cup of coffee and a doughnut to sustain her through the morning. It is one of those busy days. The phone is ringing, patients are not stable, family members are demanding, practitioners are slow to answer a page, and the laboratory delivers misinformation. It is now noon, and Sahara skips lunch. In instead, she runs down to the vending machines for a Coke and peanut butter crackers. The evening shift nurse is running late, so Sahara stays until 5 o'clock, even though she is

already late for a community meeting she must attend. She races through a fast-food restaurant for a hamburger, fries, and a milkshake. When she finally arrives home late in the evening, she rewards herself with cookies and a bowl of ice cream and falls into bed. She has given so much throughout the day. There has been little time for exercise, good nutrition, or self.

1. How can Sahara improve her health habits?

2. What will be the effects of this lifestyle over time?

3. How can anyone find balance in life?

Nursing is a caring profession. Throughout a shift, nurses use the nursing process to identify, plan, and implement patient care, always keeping in mind ways to promote health. While nurses are accustomed to caring for individuals entrusted into their care, research indicates that nurses may not be as good at attending to their own health. How can the caregiver be motivated to live a healthier lifestyle? In this chapter, we will explore the concepts of a personal definition of health and formulate a plan for maintaining optimal physical health. Realizing health is not just physical, ways to promote emotional, spiritual, and work-life balance health will be discussed.

Definition of Health

The World Health Organization (2006) describes **health** as a "state of complete physical, social, and mental well-being, and not merely the absence of disease or infirmity". Similarly, nurses view health holistically, considering the influence of the mind, body, and spirit on well-being. Health is in a constant state of flux and is influenced by genetics, lifestyle choices, stress, and environmental factors. All must be in balance to reach the highest level of wellness.

Health promotion is a process of enabling persons to make informed choices about their health. *Healthy People 2020* is an initiative by the U.S. department of Health and Human Services that creates a framework for health promotion and disease prevention priorities. The overarching goals are: (a) attainment of longer lives free of preventable disease, (b) elimination of health disparities, (c) creation of social environments that promote health, and (d) promotion of healthy behaviors across all life stages. The *Healthy People 2020* objectives assist health care providers to choose topics for health education. Nurses provide health education to individuals and groups with the intention of reducing risk and encouraging developmentally appropriate health screening.

Concern over the health habits of registered nurses has emerged. Atkins, Campoli, Havens, Abraham, and Gillum (2018) found that nurses self-report that workplace restraints play a role in poor food choices, physical inactivity, inadequate sleep, and high levels of stress. Also concerning is the high prevalence of obesity among nurses that increases risk of chronic health issues (Kyle et al., 2017). **Workplace barriers** to positive health habits have been reported by nurses, and include nutritionally poor food choices, mandated long hours and off shifts, inadequate sleep, and musculoskeletal injuries. The American Nurses Association (ANA) recognizes that the health of the nation depends on maintaining a healthy workforce. The *Healthy Nurse Healthy Nation Grand Challenge* was initiated by the ANA as a means to nurture healthy lifestyle habits among nurses and eliminate workplace barriers (ANA, 2017a).

It has been suggested that in order to be effective at promoting the health of others, nurses must exemplify a healthy lifestyle. Is there a professional obligation for nurses to role model the same health advice they provide patients? Fie, Norman, and While (2013) revealed that patients were more likely to accept health advice offered by a nurse with a normal

---

Critical Thinking 28.1

Maintaining good health is important to a nurse's overall and ability to cope with job demands. Only when you feel good are you able to deliver optimal patient care.

1. What is your personal definition of health?
2. What motivates or inhibits you from engaging in healthy behaviors?

3. Do you feel an ethical obligation to serve as role models for patients?
4. Go to the web *Healthy Nurse Healthy Nation* page. Would your employer be willing to sponsor the Healthy Nurse Healthy Nation Grand Challenge?

weight. However, a recent systematic review found there is little evidence to support a causal relationship exists between nurses' health behaviors and the patient response (Kelly, Wills, & Sykes, 2017).

Areas of Health

Health is a complex and a dynamic state. The human mind-body-spirit adjusts to external and internal stimuli while attempting to maintain balance. When experiencing stressors, the body responds. As an example, nurses who work a prolonged shift experience not only physical fatigue but a slowed reaction time (Thomas et al., 2016). Being tired lends itself to a change in mood and a potential for social isolation. To maintain a state of optimal health, nurses must attend to their physical, emotional, and spiritual health.

Physical Health

A personal inventory of one's body mass index (BMI), dietary practices, pattern of physical activity, and participation of health screening is an important step toward improving **physical health. Physical health is** a state of physical well-being, the absence of physical disease. Health habits that contribute to maintaining a normal BMI, flexibility, and strong muscles can become routine over time. Nurses can access reliable, evidence-based nutrition, and physical fitness resources online. As such, publications from the U.S. Department of Health and Human Services, U.S. Department of Agriculture, and the United States Preventative Task Force provide a wealth of health information. Nurses can use the information gleaned from these web sources to improve their physical health.

Calculation of Body Mass Index

Body mass index (BMI) can be used to characterize a weight as normal or one that places an individual at risk. Likewise, BMI is a convenient way to estimate body fat and can help determine appropriate caloric intake. A BMI between 18.5 and 24.9 is considered normal. Both dietary intake and level of physical activity contribute to BMI. An online BMI calculator is easily accessible (Obesity Expert Panel 2013) (Table 28.1).

Dietary Intake

Maintaining proper nutrition, one aspect of physical health, helps the body perform at an optimal level. Two resources that guide healthy food choices include the *2015–2020 Dietary Guidelines for Americans* and a web resource called Choosemyplate.gov (Figure 28.1). These resources can be used by the nurse to counsel patients and serve as a good refresher of the food portions and patterns that help individuals achieve a normal BMI. Remember that every food and beverage choice matters. Choose nutrient rich foods in order to stay within recommended caloric intake. Consider filling half of each plate of food with fruits and vegetables. Make sure that at least half the grains consumed are whole grains. Switch to low fat or skim milk and yogurt choices. In all food choices, consider using less sodium, saturated fat, and added sugars (Dietary Guidelines Advisory Committee, 2015). Avoid highly processed foods and choose fresh instead. Take the Dietary Intake Self-Assessment (Table 28.2) to evaluate your choices.

Benefits of Exercise

Being physically active is beneficial to health. Performing even brief moments of moderate or vigorous physical activity improves insulin sensitivity, blood pressure, sleep, cognition, and has been associated with a reduction in anxiety (U.S. Department of Health and Human Services, 2018). The *Physical Activity Guidelines for Americans* clearly outlines the amount of time adults are encouraged to carve out for aerobic and muscle building activities (Figure 28.2). Simply adding 150–300 min of moderate-intensity aerobic exercise each week is recommended. Finally, include muscle-strengthening exercises twice weekly that work all major muscle groups.

In order to make exercise fun, find an activity that you are passionate about and truly enjoy. Finding friends to participate in your activity will help you keep the commitment. Once you find an exercise that suits you, try engaging in that activity a little more each time. Start slowly, and gradually build the intensity

Table 28.1 **Clarification of Body Mass Index**

Classification of body mass index	
Term	**BMI**
Underweight	Less than 18.5
Normal	18.5–24.9
Overweight	25.0–29.9
Obesity Class I	30.0–34.9
Obesity Class II	35.0–39.9
Obesity Class III	Greater than 40.0

Source: Adapted from National Heart, Lungs and Blood Institute, BMI calculator.

Critical Thinking 28.2

Proper nutrition is one aspect in maintaining good health. How can the nurse take control of dietary choices at home and at work?

1. Can you determine one portion of the following foods: peanut butter, pasta, chicken, cheese, milk? What strategy can you use to control your food portions?

2. How can journaling your dietary intake help in your healthy eating journey?

3. Does the institution that you are employed by provide healthy cafeteria choices? If not, as a nurse leader, how could you influence a change?

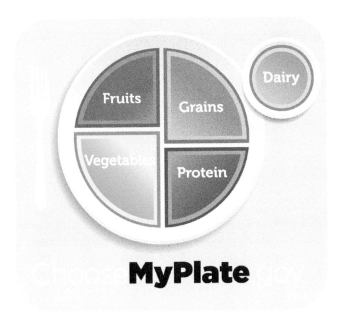

FIGURE 28.1 My plate.
Source: USDA's Center for Nutrition Policy and Promotion at www. health.gov.

Table 28.2 Dietary Intake Self-Assessment

Dietary intake self-assessment	Yes	No
1. I consume 2–3 servings of vegetables each day.	____	____
2. I choose beverages that are low calorie.	____	____
3. I consume 2 fruit servings each day.	____	____
4. Each meal, I make half of each plate fruits and vegetables.	____	____
5. My daily sodium consumption is less than 2,300 mg.	____	____
6. I am easily able to judge a serving size of grains.	____	____
7. I bring unprocessed foods for snacks at work.	____	____
8. I choose lean meats, legumes and nuts for my protein intake.	____	____
9. I know how many calories are in my favorite foods.	____	____
10. I prepare foods using unsaturated fats.	____	____

Source: C. Moredich.

and duration. Remember, even small amounts of physical activity have a health benefit. Physical activity needs to be increased gradually over time, even if you consider yourself physically fit.

When starting an exercise program, safety should always be considered. If you have been mostly sedentary, have chronic health conditions, or have physical limitations, getting a physical exam and approval from your primary care provider is a smart way to start an exercise program (Table 28.3).

Sleep

It is not uncommon for nurses to sleep less than 8 hr per night. Nurses who work nights may find it especially difficult to sleep for an uninterrupted block of time. Many nurses find it a challenge to leave thoughts of patients and the day's activities at work, contributing to insomnia.

There are occupational hazards of nurses being **sleep deprived or suffering from insufficient sleep or sleepiness**. Johnson, Jung, Brown, Weaver, and Richards (2014) found that a direct correlation between a decrease in hours slept and an increase in patient care errors reported by nurses. The drive home after work for a nurse can be equally dangerous. In fact, drivers who report between 4 and 5 hr of sleep per night are at 4.3 times the risk of a motor vehicle crash than those who slept 7 hr or more (Taft, 2016). Nurses who work rotating shifts are at the greatest risk of fatigue compared to those committed to one shift. Nurses who rotate to evenings or nights are almost twice as likely to nod off while driving home (Frank, 2005).

There is no magic formula to guarantee a good night's sleep, but the following suggestions may improve the quality of your sleep life:

- Make sleep a priority. Make a conscious decision to obtain adequate sleep every night.

- Do not use caffeine as a stimulant to stay awake or alcohol as a tool to fall asleep.

- Try drinking warm milk or decaffeinated tea at bedtime. Establish a routine before bed that is repeated nightly.

- Reserve your bed only for sleeping. Using electronics, such as a phone or computer, in bed can interfere with sleep patterns.

- If thoughts of work prevent you from falling asleep, write your worries on a piece of paper. Leave your thoughts on paper, and plan to deal with worries the next day while awake.

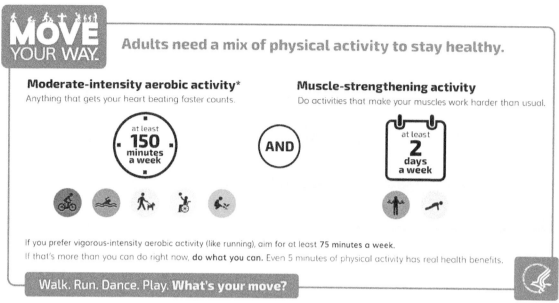

FIGURE 28.2   Physical activity needs of adults.
Source: ODPHP: Physical Activity Guidelines for Americans at www.health.gov.

Table 28.3   Physical Activity Self-Assessment

Physical activity self-assessment	Yes	No
1. I include 30 min of exercise in my daily routine.	____	____
2. I have one exercise I enjoy.	____	____
3. I consider myself to be a physically active person.	____	____
4. I perform muscle strengthening exercise twice each week.	____	____
5. I often take the stairs instead of the elevator.	____	____
6. I track the number of steps I take.	____	____
7. I find ways to exercise on bad weather days.	____	____
8. I feel better when I exercise.	____	____
9. I include stretching in my exercise routine.	____	____
10. I get 150–300 min of moderate-intensity exercise weekly.	____	____

Source: C. Moredich.

Adequate sleep, good nutrition, and proper exercise all go hand in hand. When you are tired, you may eat more to compensate for the lack of sleep. Overeating can lead to unnecessary weight gain. And the weight gain and fatigue can lead to a lack of exercise. Proper balance among the three is critical.

Emotional Health

Our emotions express how we are feeling about an event. Emotions can be intense, and each emotion evokes a strong response. Our challenge as human beings are to acknowledge the emotion and then respond appropriately. It is important to have balance between our thought processes and the emotion we are feeling; otherwise, disharmony occurs. Emotions are what make us human. Truly, emotions are one of our greatest gifts and add spice to our lives (Dossey, Keegan, & Guzzetta, 2005).

Emotional Intelligence

Emotional intelligence is the ability to recognize your own feelings and the feelings of those around you and manage your emotions in a positive manner. Emotional intelligence requires a mix of practice and skill. Emotional intelligence includes these five basic emotional and social competencies:

- *Self-awareness:* Knowing what you are feeling in the moment and using this assessment to guide your decision making.

- *Self-regulation:* Handling your emotions so that they facilitate rather than interfere with the task at hand.

- *Motivation:* Using your deepest preferences to move and guide you toward your goals, to help you take initiative and strive to improve, and to persevere in the face of setbacks.

- *Empathy:* Sensing what people are feeling, being able to take their perspective, and cultivating rapport and attunement with a broad diversity of people.

- *Social skills:* Handling emotions well in relationships and accurately reading social situations and networks, interacting smoothly; using appropriate skills to persuade and lead, negotiate, and settle disputes for cooperation and teamwork (Goleman, 1998).

Engaging in Activities

Just as it is important to find a type of exercise you are passionate about, it is also important to find activities outside nursing that bring you pleasure. Some activities, like meditation, may be purposefully sought out to reduce stress. However, joy from engaging in any activity may bring a sense of stress relief. The list is endless—antique shopping, reading, painting, sewing, photography, and so on. It's never too late to develop a new hobby. New hobbies often spur a new network of persons who share your passion.

Impact of Social Relationships

The positive effects of social support on health outcomes have been documented in the literature (Breedlove, 2005). If these interactions are frequent, that only adds to good health. In other words, the more you see your friends, the healthier you become. The variety of those relationships may also keep you healthy. The greater the diversity of the relationships—such as professional, family, neighborhood, or church relationships— the more likely you are to remain healthy. Engaging in new professional or social activities allows new relationships to form. These relationships give meaning to our lives.

Compassion Fatigue

Being compassionate when caring for others is an attribute most nurses are proud of. However, constant exposure to human suffering can cause the nurse to experience **compassion fatigue**. Compassion fatigue is the inability to feel compassion to those who are suffering from constant exposure to human suffering. Left, unchecked, compassion fatigue can negatively affect the emotional and physical health of nurse, and lead to decreased productivity, job dissatisfaction, and turnover (Salmond, Salmond, Ames, Kamienski, & Holly, 2018). Symptoms include anxiety, irritability, distancing self from patients, developing insomnia and depression (Mattioli, Walters, and Cannon, 2018). Nurses must learn ways to decompress to overcome the stress of human suffering and nurture the mind-body-spirit. Taking time to implement a routine that refreshes and promotes healthy habits will protect the nurse from the loss of energy associated with compassion fatigue. Nurse leaders need to consider the impact compassion fatigue has on the staff. Recommendations for creating a supportive work environment include:

1. Team building and a culture of support

2. Establishing informal debriefing strategies

Table 8.4 Suggested Activities to Relieve Stress

Tell yourself "good job"	Practice breathing	Meditate
Think peaceful thoughts	Read	Take a walk
Forgive your mistakes	Hire a life coach	Join a club
Do a good deed	Attend a support group	Listen to music or sing a song
Laugh	Get a massage	Take a hot bath
Focus on the positive	Say a prayer	Call a friend

Source: C. Moredich.

Real World Interview

I have learned a lot in the 9 months that I have practiced nursing. I used to say yes to overtime each time when asked. I thought I needed the experience and that I owed it to the staff. I have since learned to say no. I have also learned that I need to take care of myself. I used to come home and eat a lot and fall into bed. I gained weight and felt awful. Now I either go for a walk or to the health club after work. I volunteer at my church youth organization part-time whenever I can. I have also developed my own routine in delivering patient care. I am better organized and leave on time. I have gained more confidence in my clinical decisions. For example, I had a patient who I thought should not be extubated from the ventilator. I tried to voice my opinion to the resident on call but was overridden by the attending physician. The charge nurse was also supportive of keeping the patient intubated. As it

turned out, the patient was extubated for a half hour and then reintubated. I felt bad for the unnecessary procedure for the patient, but it did boost my confidence. I know now that in the future I will be even more assertive with physicians concerning the welfare of my patients.

When I am scared in a clinical situation, I try not to let fear paralyze me. I try to think everything through logically. I have found that the better I understand what I am doing, the better nurse I have become. I'm always trying to learn new things. I've been to about five seminars this year, and I subscribe to three nursing journals. I want to learn as much as I can.

Nayiri M. Birazian, RN
New Staff Nurse
Maywood, Illinois

3. Flexibility in assignments to protect a nurse's emotional well-being

4. Encouraging ongoing self-assessment of work-life balance

5. Help staff make personal plans for managing stress (Salmond et al., 2018).

Most health care institutions provide Employee Assistance Programs (EAP) designed to provide counseling to employees who feel they need emotional health support. Many things can be done to relieve the emotional stress of life. See Table 28.4 for a few suggestions.

Spiritual Health

Spirituality, another component of health, can be viewed as the essence of being. It is that which gives meaning and direction in life. Spirituality can be described as a relationship with a higher being, other individuals, or the environment (Dossey, Keegan, & Guzzetta, 2005). Having a strong sense of spirituality may help nurses cope with stressors, resolve problems, and adapt (Ramezanzade et al., 2017). Nurses can gain insight into their own spirituality by taking a self-assessment (Table 28.5).

Professional Health

Healthy nurses are resilient individuals who adapt well in a constantly changing work environment. Resilience is the ability to recover from any situation and move on. You are professionally healthy when you are satisfied with your career choice and have continual opportunities for growth. A professionally healthy individual is goal directed and seeks every opportunity to obtain knowledge and new learning experiences. You can

Table 28.5 Spiritual Health Assessment

Spiritual health assessment	Yes	No
1. I believe in a higher power.	____	____
2. I spend time each day mindfully meditating or praying.	____	____
3. I am open to learning about others' spiritual beliefs.	____	____
4. I am able to help patients talk about their spirituality.	____	____
5. I have found ways to pray with patients when invited to do so.	____	____

Source: C. Moredich.

assess your professional health by using Table 28.6. This tool is designed to assess trends only.

Plan for Your Lifelong Learning

Your first job as a registered nurse will provide you with an opportunity to be mentored by experienced nurses. These nurse mentors will provide guidance as you learn new policies, meet the health care team members, and support you when problems arise. Over time, you will become that nurse mentor. As you embark on your new career, join a professional organization, attend educational opportunities, and learn about nursing governance committees.

Once you start to feel comfortable in your new role, you may want to return to school for an advanced degree. The U.S. Department of Labor Statistics estimates a 31% projected growth in the need for advanced practice nurses between 2016 and 2026 (Bureau of Labor Statistics, U.S. Department of Labor, 2020). Many employers are willing to pay for a portion

---

Critical Thinking 28.3

There is evidence suggesting that people can improve their happiness by practicing positive psychology (Seligman & Csikszentmihalyi, 2000). A *Gratitude Journal* will help you document an expression of appreciation of those events in your life that make you joyful. Take a few minutes each evening to sit and think about the day's activities. Ask yourself, what are the three things that made me happiest today? Write them down in your *Gratitude Journal*. The busier you become, the more important it is to take time to reflect and relax. Be good to you!

Case Study 28.1

You have been working for a home health agency for about 1 year now. One of your best friends at work, another nurse, asks your advice about how to maintain a healthier lifestyle. She states that she is 10 pounds overweight and does not really exercise much. She says she feels like all she does is work and come home and go to sleep. She says she does not have fun in life anymore and that college life was great compared to all the stress at work.

What advice would you give your friend about how to stay healthy? What would your first priority be in offering suggestions? What other major areas of consideration would you explore with your friend?

Table 28.6 Professional Health Assessment

Professional health behavior	Yes	No
1. I have short- and long-term career goals.	____	____
2. I stay current about changes in health care.	____	____
3. I participate in nursing governance opportunities.	____	____
4. I subscribe to a professional nursing journal.	____	____
5. I belong to at least one professional organization.	____	____
6. I use appropriate personal protective equipment.	____	____
7. I use good body mechanics when transferring patients.	____	____
8. I participate in my employer's retirement plan	____	____

Source: C. Moredich.

of an advanced education. Even if tuition reimbursement is not available, think about how an advanced degree may allow you reach your professional goals.

Plan for a Long Healthy Career

An important aspect of professional health is avoidance of occupational hazards. The U.S. Department of Labor Statistics (2018) reports that in 2016, there was an incidence rate of 104.2 cases per 10,000 of registered nurse work injury and illness cases, significantly greater than the rate for all occupations (91.7 cases per 10,000 workers). Nurses experience musculoskeletal injuries from patient lifting and transferring, exposure to infectious agents, and violence in the workplace. It is important that you follow standard precautions and learn proper lifting techniques.

Plan for Your Financial Future

There is no better time than now to invest in your future. Now is the time to begin saving for such things as a home, your children's education, and even retirement, no matter what your age.

Note that a nurse who is making $50,000 annually will make $1,800,000 in a 30-year working career. If this nurse invests $200 per month at 12% interest for the 30 years, the nurse will have more than $1,000,000 in a retirement account at age 65. Savings for retirement are three pronged: (a) Social Security funds, (b) retirement funds, and (c) additional personal savings.

Social Security

Social Security is automatically taken out of every paycheck by your employer. The benefits from Social Security will not cover all retirement expenses, especially with today's projected life span and inflation. You will need other retirement money. You should annually check the accuracy of your Social Security account by reviewing the information available online from the Social Security Administration.

Retirement Funds

The most common retirement funds are the 401K or 403b plans. The primary difference between the two is that the 403b is a plan offered by a nonprofit organization and the 401K is offered by a for-profit organization. For purposes of this discussion, the term 403b will be used.

Both the employee and employer contribute money to a 403b. This is a great way to save, because many health care institutions will match the funds that you contribute. After your money is put into the fund, it is tax sheltered, meaning that you do not pay any taxes on the amount contributed until it is withdrawn. For example, if you earn $58,000 per year and contribute $5,800 to the 403b, you will be taxed on only $52,200 of income. If the money is withdrawn before you reach the age of 59 1/2, you will pay a 10% federal penalty. This is an incentive to keep the money in the account until retirement; the plan should be considered a long-term investment.

Personal Savings

After investing in retirement funds, you also have a few more options for investment. You can open a money market account. This is similar to a bank checking account, although it often requires a larger minimum amount of money to open the account. The interest rate is higher than that of a passbook savings account or a traditional bank checking account, and you have check-writing privileges. This is a place for money that you may need to access quickly

You also have the option to invest in stock mutual funds, bond mutual funds, individual stocks, or individual bonds outside your retirement account. The key to successful investment is to diversify, meaning to spread your money around in many different types of investment options, including stocks, bonds, mutual funds, and so on. There are many ways to learn more about investments. Try taking a course on personal finance or hire a financial planner.

In this chapter you have reflected on your health in many aspects. Just as our patients are unique and have different needs, so do we as nurses. You have identified a personal definition of health and have been introduced in many ways to optimize your physical, spiritual, emotional, and financial health. The onus is now on you to improve your health and maintain balance into the future.

KEY CONCEPTS

- Nurses can provide self-care by maintaining a healthy lifestyle.

- Health is not just the absence of disease, but a balance among the mind-body-spirit.

- Maintaining good health is important to a nurse's overall and ability to cope with job demands.

- Physical health includes good nutrition, proper exercise, and adequate sleep.

- Emotional health is mastered when we acknowledge our emotions and respond appropriately.

- Maintaining many different types of relationships helps keep you healthy.

- Spiritual well-being provides direction and meaning in life.

- Healthy nurses are resilient individuals who adapt well in a constantly changing work environment.

- Learning to save money toward retirement provides nurses a sense of financial health.

KEY TERMS

Health	Resilience	Emotional intelligence
Physical health	Compassion fatigue	Sleep deprived

REVIEW QUESTIONS

1. You are trying to maintain a healthy diet. Which of the following would you include in your daily consumption? Select all that apply.
   a. Peanut butter
   b. Four glasses of fruit juice
   c. Green leafy vegetables
   d. White bread
   e. Nuts
   f. Whole milk

2. You have just calculated your BMI to be 28. How much exercise would be appropriate for you?
   a. 30 min 3 days a week
   b. 30 min every day
   c. 60 min 3 days a week
   d. 60 min daily

3. You work in the operating room and notice that your hands have become very itchy and have small papules. What would be the most appropriate first action to take?
   a. Wear only non-latex gloves in the future
   b. Ignore the situation
   c. Make a conscious effort to apply hand cream after washing your hands
   d. Apply a corticosteroid cream

4. The CNS for your unit has just passed you in the cafeteria. You are generally on very good terms with her. She does not acknowledge your presence. The most probable explanation for this is which of the following?
   a. You must have done something wrong with one of your patients yesterday.
   b. She has something else on her mind and didn't see you.
   c. She doesn't want to acknowledge you in front of other nursing leaders because you are only a staff nurse.
   d. She doesn't want to acknowledge you because you are one of the worst nurses on your unit.

5. Lack of attention to spiritual health can lead to which of the following? Select all that apply.
   a. Lack of sleep
   b. Job dissatisfaction
   c. Burnout
   d. Increased sense of well-being
   e. Suboptimal patient care
   f. Shorter life span

6. Social support is essential to health because it does which of the following?
   a. Facilitates weight loss
   b. Provides an opportunity to relate to others
   c. Improves intellect
   d. Improves creative thinking

7. Research has shown that sleep deprivation can lead to a significant increase in which of the following?
   a. Salary
   b. Job satisfaction
   c. Spirituality
   d. Patient care errors

8. Retirement financial planning includes all but which of the following?
   a. Social Security
   b. Playing the lottery
   c. Retirement funds
   d. Personal savings

9. Examples of activities promoting emotional health include all but which of the following?
   a. Drinking coffee
   b. Reading books
   c. Engaging in a hobby
   d. Becoming a member of an organization

10. Establishing professional goals is an example of which of the following?
    a. Aggression
    b. Physical health
    c. Healthy People 2020 indicators
    d. Professional health

REVIEW QUESTION ANSWERS

1. Answers A, C, and E are correct.
   Rational: Peanut butter, green leafy vegetables, and nuts are healthy to include in your diet. (B) Four glasses of fruit juice have a great deal of sugar and calories, (D) white bread has little nutritional value, and (F) whole milk has a high fat content.

2. Answer: A is correct.
   Rational: 30 min 3 days a week. A BMI of 28 is normal so (B, C, D) are greater than needed.

3. Answer: A is correct.
   Rational: Wear only non-latex gloves in the future because this may be a sign of a latex allergy. (B) Ignoring the situation will not help. (C) Making a conscious effort to apply hand cream after washing your hands will not help a latex allergy, and (D) applying a corticosteroid cream may not be necessary if latex is not worn.

4. Answer: B is correct.
   Rational: She would almost certainly have acknowledged you if she had seen you (B). The other responses (A, C, D) are all unlikely explanations for her not acknowledging your presence.

5. Answers A, B, C, E, and F are all correct.
   Rational: Spiritual distress will decrease your sense of well-being (D). Ignoring your spiritual health can lead to (A) inability to sleep, (B) job dissatisfaction, (C) burnout, (E) suboptimal patient care, and (F) even shorten your life span.

6. Answer: B is correct.
   Rational: The correct response is B. Social support provides you with the opportunity to relate to others (B). Social support does not help with weight loss (A), or have any effect on your intellect or creative thinking (C, D).

7. Answer: D is correct.
   Rational: Patient care errors are more likely to occur if you have been deprivied of sleep (D). Sleep deprivation cannot improve (A) salary, (B) job satisfaction, or (C) spiritual well-being.

8. Answer: B is correct.
   Rational: Playing the lottery is purely a game of chance (B). A, C, and D are all financial tools that will provide an income in retirement.

9. Answer: A is correct.
   Rational: Drinking coffee will not improve your emotional well-being (A). Examples of activities promoting emotional health include (B) reading, (C) taking up a new hobby, and (D) joining an organization.

10. Answer: D is correct.
    Rational: Professional health will aid you to reach your professional goals (D). (A) Aggression, (B) physical health, and (C) *Healthy People* 2020 indicators are not examples of professional health.

REVIEW ACTIVITIES

1. Try doing a short relaxation exercise. Take a deep breath in and let it out. Take slow, deep breaths that originate from the diaphragm. Tighten the muscles in your right arm for 30 s and release. Your arm should feel totally limp and relaxed. Do the same with your left arm. Tighten the muscles in your right leg for 30 s and release. Repeat with the left leg. Pull in your stomach muscles for 30 s and release. Tighten the muscles in your buttocks and release. Continue to breathe in and out deeply. You can practice this brief exercise anytime or anywhere. If you are having a particularly hectic day, take a minute to do a relaxation exercise. You can vary the exercise by flexing any group of muscles you want.

2. Your best friend is getting married next month, and you are the maid of honor. You have been invited to a shower to be held out of town in honor of your friend this next weekend. You have already purchased a nonrefundable airline ticket to attend the shower. You work in a very small Intensive Care Unit (ICU). You have been working 10- and 12-hr shifts and are near exhaustion. Your head nurse calls you 2 days before you are to leave for the shower and asks you to work the weekend. One of the staff has been involved in a serious car accident, and there is no one else to work. What would you do? If you work this weekend, you would disappoint your best friend and lose the money for your ticket. You are already exhausted, and you do not know how effective you would be at work. You know you need the break.

   If you do not work, you would be letting the rest of the staff down. They have been there for you, and now it is your turn to help them. You find it very hard to say no. You are a young nurse and you feel you should "pay your dues." How could you relax when you know that you are needed elsewhere?

   You are interviewing for your first job. You are attending the human resource session of orientation. Which investment benefits would you be most concerned about and why?

DISCUSSION POINTS

- As you develop your plan for being healthy, what barriers might get in the way of reaching your physical fitness or dietary plan? How might you remove those barriers?

- What new social activity would you like to begin that will feed your mind-body-spirit?

- Do you have a good work-life balance? If not, what change will you make to improve your healthy down time to make you more resilient?

- Starting to think about saving for retirement now will help you be financially secure in the future. Make an appointment with your Human Resources representative to make sure you are taking advantage of savings plans that are available to you.

DISCUSSION OF OPENING SCENARIO

1. How can Sahara improve her health habits?

   A personal commitment to making healthy choices is important to balancing your mind-body-spirit. In this opening scenario, Sahara make unhealthy food choices. Hurriedly, she chose foods that were convenient instead of nutrient dense meals. By thinking ahead, Sahara could plan her meals. Instead of hurrying, she could open a delicious lunch she packed the night before. By adding some fresh fruit for a late afternoon snack, she would not feel so hungry on the drive home. Sahara also needs to take care of her emotional needs. Could she stop in the middle of her busy day to leave the unit and take a walk as she listens to her music? Or, could she simply sit and practice some deep breathing? As a final thought, instead of food, how else could Sahara reward herself after a long day? Could she put in a yoga video and stretch her body?

2. What will be the effects of this lifestyle over time?

   This type of lifestyle will put Sahara at risk for many problems: obesity, arthritis, hypertension, depression, burn-out to name a few. What seems like a not so bad lifestyle will compound over time and cause devastating effects to Saraha.

3. How can anyone find balance in life?

   We have seen that balance is not easy and it takes consistent effort. To do anything well we must educate ourselves and be aware of our habits. We need to know when we feel imbalance in any aspect of our lives; we must actively work on the issue, otherwise it will cause further imbalance.

EXPLORING THE WEB

1. Go to the web site for the Healthy Nurse, Healthy Nation, www.nursingworld.org/practice-policy/work-environment/health-safety/healthy-nurse-healthy-nation Read about the Healthy Nurse, Healthy Nation Grand Challenge. Take the steps to complete the survey and join the Challenge.

2. Go to the web site for Healthy People 2020 www.healthypeople.gov Read about the work in progress for Healthy People 2030 and consider getting involved.

3. Go to the website for Calculating your BMI www.nhlbi.nih.gov/health/educational/lose_wt/BMI/bmicalc.htm and assess your current BMI.

4. Go to the web site www.choosemyplate.gov and find the amount of food in one portion of your favorite foods.

5. Go to the web site for Physical Activity Guidelines for Americans www.hhs.gov/fitness/be-active/physical-activity-guidelines-for-americans/index.html and discover Handouts to share with your patients.

6. Go to the web site for 2015–2020 Dietary Guidelines for Americans health.gov/dietaryguidelines/2015/guidelines and review the key elements of healthy eating patterns.

7. Go to the web page National Sleep Foundation /www.sleepfoundation.org/sleep-topics/sleep-disease and read the article on shift work disorders.

INFORMATICS

Quality and Safety Education for Nurses (QSEN) competencies necessitate effective communication within nursing and inter-professional teams that foster open communication, mutual respect, and shared decision-making (Cronenwett et al., 2007). Incivility exists when workplace communication includes excessive criticism, intimidation, public humiliation, and isolating. Acts of lateral violence need to be recognized and addressed to foster a culture of respect (Germann & Moore, 2017). Go to the ANA web site and review the information on violence, incivility and bullying: www.nursingworld.org/practice-policy/work-environment/violence-incivility-bullying

- Read the position statement (consider posting at work)
- Understand the 4 types of violence
- Consider taking the pledge
- LEAN BACK
- How can you apply the information learned in this chapter to reach a healthier you?
- What workplace barriers to positive health habits can you remove?
- How can you inspire others to be better caregivers to self?

REFERENCES

American Nurses Association. (2017a). *Healthy Nurse, Healthy Nation.* Retrieved from www.healthynursehealthynation.org/en/about/about-the-hnhn-gc

American Nurses Association. (2017b). *Resources to support Nurses to take control of their health.* Retrieved from www.nursingworld.org/practice-policy/hnhn/2017-year-of-the-healthy-nurse

Atkins, H., Campoli, M., Havens, T., Abraham, S., & Gillum, D. (2018). Self-care habits of nurses and the perception of their body image. *The Health Care Manager, 37*(3), 211–219.

Breedlove, G. (2005). Perceptions of social support from pregnant and parenting teens using community-based doulas. *The Journal of Perinatal Education, 14*(3), 15–22.

Bureau of Labor Statistics, U.S. Department of Labor. (2020). *Occupational Outlook Handbook, Registered Nurses*. Retrieved from www.bls.gov/ooh/healthcare/registered-nurses.htm

Cronenwett, L., Sherwood, G., Barnsteiner, J., Disch, J., Johnson, J., . . . Warren, J. (2007). Quality and safety education for nurses. *Nursing Outlook*, 55(3), 122–131. doi:10.1016/j.outlook.2007.02.006

Dietary Guidelines Advisory Committee. (2015). *Dietary Guidelines for Americans 2015–2020 ... - health.gov*. Retrieved from https://health.gov/dietaryguidelines/2015/guidelines/

Dossey, B. M., Keegan, L., & Guzzetta, C. E. (2005). *Holistic nursing: A handbook for practice*. Sudbury, MA: Jones & Bartlett Publishers.

Fie, S., Norman, I., & While, A. (2013). The relationship between physicians' and nurses' personal physical activity habits and their health promotion practice: A systematic review. *Health Education Journal*, 72, 102–119.

Frank, M. B. (2005). Practicing under the influence of fatigue (PUIF): A wake-up call for patients and providers. *Advances in Neonatal Care* National Association of Neonatal Nurses,, 5(2), 55–61.

Germann, S. and Moore, S. (2017). *Lateral violence, a nursing epidemic? Reflections of Nursing Leadership*. Retrieved from www.reflectionsonnursingleadership.org/features/more-features/Vol43_1_lateral-violence-a-nursing-epidemic

Goleman, D. (1998). *Working with emotional intelligence*. New York: Bantam Doubleday Dell Publishing Group.

Johnson, A., Jung, L., Brown, K., Weaver, M., & Richards, K. (2014). Sleep deprivation and error in nurses that work the night shift. *The Journal of Nursing Administration*, 44(1), 17–22. doi:10.1097/NNA.0000000000000016

Kelly, M., Wills, J., & Sykes, S. (2017). Do nurses' personal health behaviors impact on their health promotion practice? A systematic review. *International Journal of Nursing Studies*, 76, 62–77.

Kyle, R., Wills, J., Mahoney, C., Hoyle, L., Kelly, M., & Atherton, M. (2017). Obesity prevalence among healthcare professionals in England: A cross sectional study using the Health Survey for England. *BMJ Open*, 7, e018498. doi:10.1136/bmjopen-2017-018498

Mattioli, D., Walters, L., & Cannon, E. (2018). Focusing on the caregiver: Compassion fatigue awareness and understanding. *Medsurg Nursing*, 27(5), 323–328.

Obesity Expert Panel. (2013, November). *Managing Overweight and Obesity in Adults: Systematic Evidence Review from the Obesity Expert Panel Published [Review of National Heart, Lung and Blood Institute]*. pp. 1-501. Retrieved from www.nhlbi.nih.gov/sites/default/files/media/docs/obesity-evidence-review.pdf

Ramezanzade, T. E., Orooji, A., Bikverdi, M., & Alizade, T. B. (2017). Investigation of clinical competence and its relationship with professional ethics and spiritual health in nurses. *Health, Spirituality and Medical Ethics*, 4(1), 2–9.

Salmond, E., Salmond, S., Ames, M., Kamienski, M., & Holly, C. (2018). Experiences of co passion fatigue in direct care nurses: A qualitative systematic review. *Joanna Briggs Database System Rev Implement Rep 2018*, 16, 1–72.

Seligman, M., & Csikszentmihalyi, M. (2000). Positive psychology: An introduction. *American Psychologist*, 55(1), 5–14.

Taft, B. (2016). *Acute sleep deprivation and risk of motor vehicle crash involvement*. Washington, DC: AAA Foundation for Traffic Safety.

Thompson, B., Stock, M., Banuelas, V., & Akalonu, C. (2016). The Impact of a Rigorous Multiple Work Shift Schedule and Day Versus Night Shift Work on Reaction Time and Balance Performance in Female Nurses: A Repeated Measures Study. *JOEM*, 58(7), 737–743.

U.S. Department of Health and Human Services. (2018). *Physical activity guidelines for Americans* (2nd ed.). Washington, DC: U.S. Department of Health and Human Services.

U.S. Department of Labor Statistics. (2018). Occupational injuries and illnesses among registered nurses. Retrieved from www.bls.gov/opub/mlr/2018/article/occupational-injuries-and-illnesses-among-registered-nurses.htm

World Health Organization. (2006). *Definition of Health*. Retrieved from https://8fit.com/lifestyle/the-world-health-organization-definition-of-health

SUGGESTED READINGS

Frankl, V. (1984). *Man's search for meaning*. New York: Simon & Schuster, Inc.

Hunt, L. (2005). Sit-down comedy. Meet Ivy Push, nursing's funny girl. *American Journal of Nursing*, 105(7), 110–111.

Lyndon, A. (2016). *Burnout Among Health Professionals and Its Effect of Patient Safety. Agency for Healthcare Research and Quality Patient Safety Network*. Retrieved from https://psnet.ahrq.gov/perspectives/perspective/190/burnoutamong-health-professionals-and-its-effect-on-patientsafety

Moreo, J. (2007). *You are more than enough*. New York: Stephens Press, LLC.

Phiri, L., Draper, C., Lambert, E., & Kolbe-Alexander, T. (2014). Nurses' lifestyle behaviors, health priorities and barriers to living a healthy lifestyle: A qualitative descriptive study. *BMC Nursing*, 13(380)), 2–11. Retrieved from: www.biomedcentral.com/1472-6955/13/38

Ruiz, D. M. (1997). *The four agreements: A practical guide to personal freedom, a Toltec wisdom book*. San Rafael, CA: Amber Allen Publishing.

Thompson, B., Stock, M., Banuelas, V., & Akalonu, C. (2016). The impact of a rigorous multiple work shift schedule and day versus night shift work on reaction time and balance performance in female nurses: A repeated measures study. *Journal of Occupational and Environmental Medicine*, 58(7), 737–743.

U.S. Bureau of Labor Statistics. (n.d.). *Occupational Outlook Handbook*. Retrieved from www.bls.gov/ooh/healthcare/nurse-anesthetists-nurse-midwives-and-nurse-practitioners.htm

U.S. Department of Health and Human Services and U.S. Department of Agriculture. 2015–2020 Dietary Guidelines for Americans, 8th Edition. Available at http://health.gov/dietaryguidelines/2015/guidelines

Wagner, L. (2017). *The four seasons of grieving: A nurse's healing journey with nature*. Indianapolis: Sigma Theta Tau.

Nursing Career Opportunities

Jade Tazbir[1], Janice Tazbir[1,2,3,4]
[1] University of Chicago Medicine, Chicago, IL, USA
[2] Anderson Continuing Education, Sacramento, CA, USA
[3] Health Education Systems, Inc. (HESI), Houston, TX, USA
[4] Retired, Purdue University Northwest, College of Nursing, Hammond, IN, USA

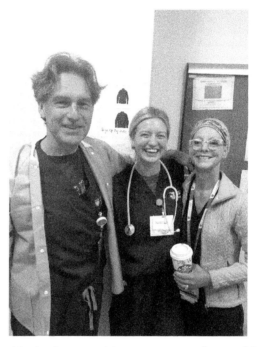

Nurses have a multitude of opportunities at every age and stage of their career.
Source: Used with permission from Johnny Tazbir, Jade Tazbir and Janice Tazbir.

So never lose an opportunity of urging a practical beginning, however small, for it is wonderful how often in such matters the mustard-seed germinates and roots itself.

—— Florence Nightingale in Cook, E. (1913). The Life of Florence Nightingale, by Sir Edward Cook. (p. 57). London, UK: Macmillan.

OBJECTIVES

Upon completion of this chapter, the reader should be able to:

1. Understand the current job market for nurses.

2. Describe different career paths for entry level nurses.

3. Identify nursing career resources and how to use them.

4. List nursing career options including education, certification, job outlook, and salaries for select nursing careers.

5. Apply information to obtain employment as a Registered Nurse.

Kelly Vana's Nursing Leadership and Management, Fourth Edition. Edited by Patricia Kelly Vana and Janice Tazbir
© 2021 John Wiley & Sons Ltd. Published 2021 by John Wiley & Sons Ltd.
Companion Website: www.wiley.com/go/kelly-Nursing-Leadership

OPENING SCENARIO

Jaclyn recently graduated nursing school and passed her NCLEX exam. She has her diploma, licensure, and a resume in hand, yet feels confused about the next steps. She knows that she wants to begin her search for a nursing career, but does not know where to begin.

1. Where should she look for a career?

2. What kind of nursing career does would fit her best?

3. How can she best evaluate options so that she has the right career?

4. What is the current market for nursing and nursing opportunities?

Confusion is a common feeling among graduate nurses as they enter the job search. A new graduate will often wonder where to begin their job search. In a career like nursing, there are seemingly endless opportunities and it can be stressful to choose a first job that will help you meet your goals (Figure 29.1). In this chapter, you will learn about the current job market, different career paths and options, career resources for nursing, and how to take advantage of them.

Understanding the Current Job Market

There are approximately 3 million licensed nurses in the United States and 61% of nurses work in a hospital setting, 18% work in ambulatory healthcare services, 7% in nursing and residential care facilities, and the remaining 8% work in either government positions or educational services (U.S. Bureau of Labor Statistics, 2020). Employment of registered nurses is expected to grow by a mammoth 15% from 2016 to 2026, which makes it one of the fastest growing professions (U.S. Bureau of Labor Statistics, 2020). Statistical data from the American Association of Colleges of Nursing (AACN) and the National League for Nursing (NLN) (NLN, 2020 reveal the latest data on nursing as a profession:

- Nursing is the United States' largest healthcare profession, with more than 3.1 million registered nurses (RNs) nationwide.

- Registered nurses comprise one of the largest segments of the U.S. workforce as a whole and are among the highest-paid large occupations.

- Nurses comprise the largest single component of hospital staff, are the primary providers of hospital patient care, and deliver most of the nation's long-term care.

- Most health care services involve some form of care by nurses. From 1980 to 2004, the percentage of employed RNs working in hospitals decreased from 66 to 56.2% as health care moved to sites beyond the hospital and nurses increased their numbers in a wide range of other settings.

- There are over four times as many RNs in the United States as physicians.

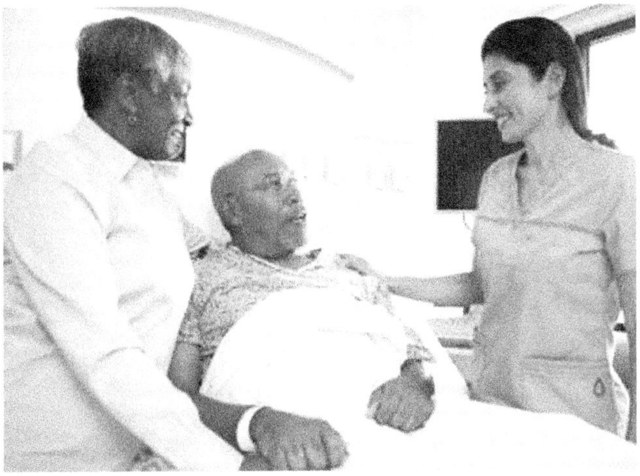

Aging Workforce and Population

Also, according to an NCSBN National Nursing Workforce Survey in 2015, the average age of an RN was 48.8. Fifty-five percent of the RN workforce is age 50 or older, and more than 1 million registered nurses are predicted to reach retirement age within the next 10–15 years, that is approximately one-third of the current workforce. Reasons for expected growth in nursing include an aging patient population, more nurses facing retirement, and a nursing faculty shortage, which translates that more nurses will be needed in the coming years and the patients we care for will be aging.

Changing Opportunities

Throughout its history, nursing has always responded to changes in society's health care needs. From the days of Florence Nightingale and her service in the mid-1800s, to Lillian Wald and public health nursing in the early 1900s, to Martha

FIGURE 29.1 Most nurses choose to work in acute care hospitals but choices for nurses are virtually endless.
Source: U.S. Bureau of Labor Statistics

Rogers in the 1930s and 1940s, suggesting that nurses prepare themselves to handle the health issues that arise from space travel, nursing has met society's changing health care needs by expanding the roles of nurses. For decades, nurses in acute care settings have been taking on advanced and expanded roles on evening, night, and weekend shifts.

Many of the changes in nursing have evolved naturally and logically. Positions such as a staff nurse, nurse manager, director of nursing, and case manager, and organizations such as visiting nurse associations and public health organizations, are a direct reflection of these evolutions. Nursing has established itself in hospitals, ambulatory clinics, practitioners' offices, and community and school settings. An issue confronting nursing, however, has been identifying what the appropriate entry-level educational degree should be and what a nurse really is, because of the many levels of educational preparation. These include a 2-year associate degree, a 3-year diploma, and a 4-year baccalaureate degree. Many 4-year baccalaureate schools of nursing have changed the traditional 4-year pathway to a degree and are admitting students who already have a non-nursing baccalaureate degree or an associate degree. In deciding which education option to pursue, students should consider their future, that is, where they want to be in 5–10 years. If advanced practice is a desired goal, then a baccalaureate education is the required first step toward that goal.

Additionally, our practice environment is changing as hospitals face financial pressure to discharge patients quickly in order to save money and free up hospital beds. This translates to increases in long-term care facilities, outpatient care centers, and home health areas with an increased demand for registered nurses. Despite the high demand for registered nurses, nursing remains a competitive job market. As the older generations of nurses begin to retire, the market will continue to open for young nurses. In order to stand out in this competitive field, it is wise to gain experience while in nursing school or while looking for a job. Experience can be gained by volunteering at hospitals, working as an RN fellow or patient care tech, or getting a CNA license. Caution must be taken not to over stretch responsibilities and to keep school as the main focus.

Demand

While there are many jobs nationally, demand varies by geography. Some states and metropolitan areas have a higher demand for nurses than others (Figure 29.2). States with the highest employment level for registered nurses are large states with a high population, including- California, Texas, New York, Florida, and Pennsylvania (U.S. Bureau of Labor Statistics, 2020). States yielding the highest concentration of jobs

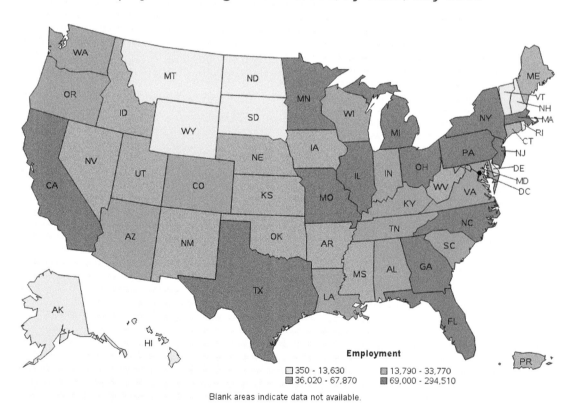

Blank areas indicate data not available.

FIGURE 29.2   Employment of Registered Nurses by State.
Source: Bureau of Labor Statistics, U.S. Bureau of Labor Statistics, U.S. Department of Labor, *Occupational Outlook Handbook*, Registered Nurses, Retrieved August 6, 2019 at www.bls.gov/ooh/healthcare/registered-nurses.html.

are South Dakota, West Virginia, Delaware, Missouri, and Mississippi. A nurse may consider visiting this information in considering relocating to a different part of the country.

Wages

Nursing wages vary vastly by location as well. The U.S. Bureau of Labor Statistics (2020) reports 2017 data for states with the highest average income for nurses as California - $98,400, Hawaii - $88,230, Massachusetts - $85,770, Alaska - $85,740, and Oregon - $82,940. The U.S. Bureau of Labor Statistics occupational outlook handbook employment and Wages for Registered Nurses page is a helpful resource for new graduates and senior nursing students, because you can identify the state you live in as well as identify the demand for nurses in that state, including the average wages.

Choosing a Career Option

The average nurse will work many years and hold many positions. Knowing that your first job won't be your last, thinking about your career as a timeline is just a beginning. As all nursing career paths hold their own benefits and unique experience to be gained, the question to begin asking yourself is which path seems best for you and your dream nursing career. Reflecting on what aspects of nursing school you enjoyed the most and which clinical experiences you enjoyed the most are excellent first steps toward finding a career that suits you. Then, think about your personal morals and ethics when it comes to health care. Would you prefer to work at a Catholic hospital? How would you feel if you worked at a Catholic hospital and a woman was denied an abortion? Or conversely, how would you feel if you worked at a different hospital and they agreed to give a woman an abortion? It is important to ask yourself these questions so you can work for a hospital whose values align with your own. Then, start considering what kind of environment you would like to work in— hospital, non-hospital, military, and once you begin to narrow down your interests, the job search will become much less confusing. Knowing yourself and your personality traits can also help you figure out where you might fit best. For example, when comparing ICU nurses to community health nurses, they found significant differences in the two groups. While ICU nurses were more comfortable with uncertainty, were highly sensitive to patterns, and scored very high on facets of flexibility, community health nurses were more introspective, had a strong need to understand the details, were more political in nature, and very plan-oriented (Nursing specialty personality test (n.d) Retrieved August 6, 2019 from www.healthecareers. com/article/career/nursing-specialty-personality-test).

Choosing a Career Path

Career path refers to the growth of the employee in an organization. A career path basically means the various positions an employee moves on one by one as he grows in an organization. The employee may move vertically most of the time but also move laterally or cross functionally to move to a different type of job role.

A career path is used interchangeably with a "career ladder." Most successful companies chalk out a career path/career ladder for the employees in order to provide them with a realistic picture of their position in the coming years in order to retain them. Having a clear idea about future positions and job responsibilities, the employee and the company can work to identify areas where relevant training is required for the individual's growth.

Critical Thinking 29.1

What percentage of nurses work in a hospital setting? Do you see yourself as that majority or someone that is seeking a less traditional setting?

- Name 3 states that have the highest wages for nurses. Note that the states with the highest wages also have a very high cost of living. Consider the cost of living before getting lured by high salaries.

- How do the salaries (and cost of living) compare in your area? Is it worth considering relocating?

Critical Thinking 29.2

While trying to figure out what job is best for you, consider these important questions:

1. What aspects of nursing interest me the most?
2. What clinical experiences did I enjoy the most and why?
3. What are my ethics and morals regarding health care?
4. Do I want to work in a hospital setting or outside of a hospital setting?
5. Do I want to work in a nursing home or long-term care facility?
6. Do I want to be a travel nurse?
7. Do I want to work for an insurance or government agency?
8. Do I want to be a Military nurse?

Case Study 29.1

- Consider your answers to the questions in Critical Thinking 29.2.
- Where did your strengths lie in your clinical rotations?
- What experiences did you enjoy, and which did you dislike?

- Decide whether you want to work in a hospital setting and, if so, what kind of hospital, or if you would prefer to work in a non-hospital environment.
- Speak with a professional mentor about each opportunity.
- Write down the pro's and con's of each potential position to help you figure which fits you best.

A great way to learn more about nursing jobs and opportunities is to form relationships with your clinical preceptors, the nurse managers on the floors for clinicals, and professors. These people can offer unparalleled advice, may be willing to write recommendation letters, offer shadowing opportunities, and possibly secure job opportunities in a hospital or setting where clinical rotations took place. Ask nurses during clinicals how they like working on that floor and how they got their job, tips for interviews and applications, and for any other advice they can offer a new nurse. Consider making a linkedin profile and adding managers and nurses you know from clinicals, professors, and alumni from your school. Networking can be a great way for a new nurse to open doors to many opportunities.

Applying and Interviewing

Once licensed and applying to jobs online, circle back to the hospitals you have clinical experience through nursing school and email past preceptors and managers to see if there are any job openings. It is easier to get an interview if someone currently working at the hospital can offer a personal recommendation. Also, contact the hospital's Human Resources or Talent Acquisition department and network with the staff. They have the ability to offer advice, schedule interviews internally, and speed up the job-hunting process substantially.

To prepare for the interview process, gather clinical stories and experiences, and practice talking about them in a professional way. New graduate nurses are often asked questions during interviews such as:

1. What made you want to become a nurse?

2. What makes you interested in this floor/unit?

3. Recall a time where you dealt with a difficult patient or co-worker and how did you handle it?

4. What has been the most complicated patient you have had so far and how did you deal with it?

5. How do you deal with stress and working in a fast-paced environment?

As you can probably gather, most of the questions will be dealing with clinical experiences and how you handled them, how you deal with difficult people and stressful environments, and why you want to be doing this job in the first place. Nurses are expected to be quick problem solvers, adept in stressful situations, and competent, pleasant people to be around and work with. If you can relay your experiences and knowledge to the interviewer in a professional and friendly manner, this allows the interviewer to gain much about your clinical reasoning, judgment, and interpersonal skills. Always keep track of the interviewer's name and title and a way to reach them for follow up. Remember to email or mail a professional "thank-you." Kindness and courtesy go a long way, and this will help you stand out in a crowd. Bring a copy of your resume printed on resume paper and a binder with questions to ask your interviewer, as well as notes on clinical experiences to draw on if you get nervous or tongue-tied. Dress modestly and professionally, and wear comfortable shoes, because you will most likely get to walk around the unit with the manager and meet other employees. When speaking with other employees during a staff interview, be professional but allow your personality to shine through. Ask questions about the culture of the floor, their job satisfaction, and how they oriented when they started working on the unit. Remember to smile, be yourself, and allow them to see the results of your schooling and experience. Don't let anxiety get in the way of a great interview—completing nursing school and passing the NCLEX exam lets employers know

Evidence From the Literature

Citation: Fowler, J. (2019). From staff nurse to nurse consultant Continuing professional development part 11: Using reflection. *British Journal of Nursing (Mark Allen Publishing)*, *28*(6), 394. https://doi.org/10.12968/bjon.2019.28.6.394

Discussion: Is this excellent continuing professional development series, Fowler reminds us that reflection is something

that we ask of our patients often, but we need to use reflection with ourselves.

Implications for Practice: Reflecting on practice can help a nurse see where they have been and where they want to go. If this important step is left out, nurses often stay where they are, eventually leading to burn out.

Real World Interview

"When I started nursing, I was an associate degree nurse and had no idea what a career path was. After a couple of years, I wanted to go back for my BSN. Once I went back for my BSN, I realized the many opportunities I could have and began a career path. I decided to go to graduate school because I wanted to teach nursing. Once I became a professor I decided I wanted to be in management so I went back to school for my DNP. I have had a few roles in nursing education management. By continuing to grow and stretch, I have accomplished more than I could have dreamed of as that beginning RN."

Cheryl Moredich RN, DNP
Program Coordinator for RN-BSN at PNW
Hammond, IN

Case Study 29.2

Recall clinical learning experiences you have had so far in your career as a nursing student. If you do not do so already, begin to keep a clinical journal where you reflect on the day and what you have learned. Refer to these experiences and comprise a list of your five most challenging, unique, and informative exposures. Add to the list as you see fit and keep it in a safe place to refer to for interviews.

that you have worked hard to get to the position you are in, and although you are new and have much to learn, you have the latest and most accurate knowledge of nursing and patient care through your studies.

Career Resources

Nursing students and new grads are often familiar with nursing opportunities within a hospital setting. Clinical rotations familiarize nursing students with different units and specialties, including Pediatrics, Intensive Care, Geriatrics, Emergency Medicine, and Cardiac nursing. However, there are many non-hospital nursing jobs that many students are not as aware of. Many non-hospital nursing jobs require some clinical experience, but that is not always the case. It is important to understand different clinical roles a nurse may have, because nurses are not only needed in the hospital setting, but outside of the hospital as well.

Online Resources

Searching for nursing opportunities can be overwhelming, but there are many online resources, including:

www.nursingworld.org/resources/individual

https://jobs.ana.org

www.bls.gov/oes/current/oes291141.htm

www.nursingworld.org/membership/member-benefits/professional-development-resources

Certification www.nursingworld.org/continuing-education/ce-subcategories/certification-review

Obtaining Employment

The next step is applying what you have learned in this chapter to obtain a professional nursing position. Use the checklist in Table 29.1 to prepare for employment.

If you need an advanced degree to reach your career goals, a wise option would be to work at a hospital that offers tuition reimbursement for graduate school. This way, while you are working, earning money and gaining experience, you can also work toward your Master's or Doctorate degree in nursing. In Table 29.2, find a comprised list of a few hospitals in each state that offer tuition reimbursement or educational assistance to their nursing staff. Consider applying to some of these hospitals and consider whether you will live at home or around your hometown after school or move to another city or state while reviewing these hospitals. Keep in mind that some hospitals offer complete tuition reimbursement, while other offer partial reimbursement or only offer to eligible employees. For more information, contact the hospitals that peak your interest and ask about their education reimbursement program. Remember that this list is not definitive and that it is subject to change. If you are wondering about a hospital that is not on this list, call and ask if they offer educational assistance or tuition reimbursement to employees.

Certification

Professional **certification** in nursing is a measure of distinctive nursing practice. The rise in consumerism in the face of a compelling nursing shortage and the profession's movement to elevate nursing as a career option have given prominence to the value of certification in nursing (Shirey, 2005). Certification in nursing represents an example of professional credentialing and is a voluntary process undertaken by practicing

Table 29.1 Job Search Checklist

- Update your resume and cover letter. Make sure your resume has the necessary keywords that hiring managers are looking for in your field.

- Figure out if you need a resume objective—in some cases it actually makes your resume look outdated.

- As you apply for various jobs, you might want to tailor your resume or even create a Curriculum Vitae to align with the job description—it could make or break your chances of getting an interview.

- Make sure your LinkedIn profile looks as good as your resume and you have plenty of endorsements from colleagues. Do some clean up and remove anything on this list.

- Start searching for jobs and do your research on the top companies for women, paid parental leave (if you think you may need it in the future), and employers who offer flexibility (if that's important to you).

- Get in touch with headhunters and recruiters.

- Network, even if you hate to network. Or, you can attend conferences instead of networking events.

- Do lots of interview prep, and make sure you're prepared to answer the most common interview questions, especially tough ones like "Tell me about yourself" and "Where do you see yourself in 5 years?" If your first round is a call, follow these phone interview tips.

- Don't forget to prepare questions to ASK your interviewer—not doing so could make you look unengaged or uninterested in the role.

- As tedious as it is, you must send a thank you after every interview and make sure you follow up the right way.

- Ask at least three colleagues to be references in case you are asked for them, and be sure that they know a call may be coming. You should be confident that they will share a glowing review of your work with the hiring manager!

- Figure out your salary request and prepare to negotiate. This is the time to make sure you get paid what you're worth! If you're not sure what a fair salary is, do your research on salaries by company and position.

Source: Adapted from: Fairygodboss. (2017, July 27). Don't Begin Job Searching Without Reading This Checklist. Retrieved March 9, 2020, from https://fairygodboss.com/career-topics/job-search-checklist.

Table 29.2 Select Hospitals with Educational Assistance/Tuition Reimbursement

Alabama: Brookwood Baptist Health, Encompass Health, East Alabama Medical Center, Jackson Hospital, Russell Medical Center, Red Bay Hospital

Alaska: Alaska Native Medical Center, Kodiak Hospital Auxiliary, Alaska Medical Employee Association

Arizona: Northern Arizona Healthcare, Mount Graham Regional Medical Center, Yavapai Regional Medical Center, Honor Health Hospital System, Kingman Medical Center, Yuma Regional Medical Center

Arkansas: University Hospital of Arkansas, White River Health System

California: Citrus Valley Health Partners, City of Hope, Emanuel Medical Center, Presbyterian Intercommunity Hospital, Twin Cities Community Hospital, Glendale Memorial Hospital and Health Center, University of California Davis Health System

Colorado: Children's Hospital Colorado, Craig Hospital, HealthONE Hospitals, Centura Health, UCHealth University of Colorado Hospital

Connecticut: Saint Mary's Hospital, Backus Hospital, Yale New Haven Hospital

Delaware: Beebe Healthcare, Christiana Care Health System, Bayhealth Hospitals

District of Columbia: Howard University Hospital, MedStar Georgetown University Hospital

Florida: Nicklaus Children's Hospital, North Florida Regional Medical Center, Tallahassee Memorial HealthCare, Florida Hospital

Georgia: Piedmont Healthcare, Archbold Medical Group

Idaho: St. Luke's Boise Medical Center

Illinois: OSF Healthcare System, Franciscan Health, Rush University Medical Center, Sinai Health System, University of Chicago Hospital

Indiana: Marion General Hospital

Iowa: Mercy Health Network, Sioux Center Health, University of Iowa Hospitals and Clinics

Kansas: Coffeyville Regional Medical Center

Kentucky: Baptist Health Hospital, University of Kentucky Hospital and UK Children's Hospital

Louisiana: East Jefferson General Hospital, Ochsner Hospital Network

Maine: Maine Medical Center

Maryland: Johns Hopkins Bayview Medical Center, Calvert Health Medical Center, Carroll Hospital, University of Maryland St. Joseph Medical Center, Adventist HealthCare, Greater Baltimore Medical Center

Massachusetts: Boston Medical Center, Brigham and Women's Hospital, Massachusetts General Hospital

Table 29.2   (Continued)

Michigan: Dickinson County Healthcare System, Munson Medical Center, Sparrow Health System, Spectrum Health Pennock

Minnesota: Health East Care System, Mayo Clinic Health System Mankato, Park Nicollet Health Services

Mississippi: Baptist Health Systems

Missouri: Saint Louis University Hospital, Saint Francis Medical Center

Montana: Billings Clinic, Providence St. Patrick Hospital, Wheatland Memorial Healthcare

Nebraska: CHI Health, Nebraska Medicine

Nevada: Valley Health System

New Hampshire: Dartmouth-Hitchcock Medical Center, Wentworth-Douglass Hospital

New Jersey: Atlantic Health System, Jefferson Health

New Mexico: Christus St. Vincent Health System, University of New Mexico Health System

New York: Health Quest, Northwell Health, New York Presbyterian Hudson Valley Hospital

North Carolina: Duke University Health System, Caromont Health, Wayne UNC Healthcare

North Dakota: CHI St. Alexius Health, Cavalier County Memorial Hospital and Clinics

Ohio: Cleveland Clinic, University Hospitals Cleveland Medical Center

Oklahoma: INTEGRIS Health Oklahoma, St. John Medical Center

Oregon: OSHU Hospital, Providence Portland Medical Center, Providence St. Vincent Medical Center, Salem Hospital

Pennsylvania: Penn State Hershey Medical Center, Fox Chase Cancer Center, Penn Medicine

Rhode Island: Rhode Island Hospital and Hasbro Children's Hospital, Roger Williams Medical Center

South Carolina: MUSC Health-University Medical Center, Spartanburg Regional Healthcare System

South Dakota: Avera Hospitals and Health Centers

Tennessee: HCA Healthcare

Texas: Menninger Clinic, Texas Health Resources, Valley Baptist Health System

Utah: University of Utah Health Care, Intermountain Medical Center

Vermont: University of Vermont Medical Center, Central Vermont Medical Center

Virginia: Novant Health UVA Health System Culpeper Medical Center, University of Virginia Medical Center

Washington: PeaceHealth Southwest Medical Center, Seattle Children's Hospital

West Virginia: Charleston Area Medical Center, West Virginia University Medicine

Wisconsin: Aurora St. Luke's Medical Center, Aspirus Wausau Hospital

Wyoming: Cheyenne Regional Medical Center

Source: Adapted from Student Debt Relief, Student Loans, Hospitals that Pay For Nursing School, www.studentdebtrelief.us

---

Critical Thinking 29.3

What is a hospital in your state that offers a tuition reimbursement program? How much does tuition reimbursement affect your decision in a position?

1. What other benefits mean the most to you now? In 5 years? In 10?

---

nurses. It is a marker of the knowledge and experience of a professional RN and is more than just a symbolic title, whether at the BSN or advanced degree level. It is also a means of validating a nurse's knowledge in a specific practice area (Watts, 2010). The American Board of Nursing Specialists (ABNS) defines the certification process as formal recognition of the specialized knowledge, skills, and experience demonstrated by the achievement of standards identified by a nursing specialty to promote optimal health outcomes (Stromberg et al., 2005).

Certification attests to the education, skills, and training of a registered nurse, and this recognition is achieved through testing for standard knowledge by examination (Hittle, 2010).

Certification should not be confused with credentialing and/or privileging, which is the process by which a physician, advanced practice nurse, or other health care provider obtains authorization from a health care organization to practice in a particular health care setting. The credentialing and/or privileging process involves an objective evaluation of a subject's current licensure, training or experience, competence, and ability to provide particular health care services.

Information about specialty nursing certification is available (American Nurses Credentialing Center, 2017) (Table 29.3).

Nursing Careers Options

Nursing has a plethora of career options, many of which you may not even be aware of. It is important to keep current on what types of careers there are in nursing. as it is ever changing. Below is information to discover more about different nursing career options. Important information such as description, salary, and certifications are outlined in Table 29.4, and the following paragraphs describe less common nursing careers in more detail. Remember, this list only offers a glimpse into the world of nursing careers-—there are many more career paths. The purpose of this section is to introduce different ideas and nursing practices that you may not be as familiar with as a student. Keep in mind the discussion questions you answered earlier in this chapter while reading the following table and paragraphs.

Travel Nursing

Travel nursing is another unique career path for nurses, and many new graduates find themselves drawn to the idea of a nursing career that allows them the freedom to travel the country and branch out into different nursing specialties. Travel nurses also enjoy the benefits of a larger than average salary and housing compensation. While travel nursing offers many benefits, a nurse considering this career needs to understand that your agency may require you to stay longer than expected if a patient assignment runs over, you may have to sacrifice sick time and vacation pay, and being on call might be a part of the contractual agreement. Also, frequently switching hospitals and settings may make it difficult to form solid working relationships and establish friendships outside of work. You are expected to quickly adapt to the culture and procedures of every hospital you work at. Like any job, travel nursing has pros and cons. Finding a travel agency to work for can be overwhelming but can make a world of a difference when it comes to job satisfaction. Some things to consider when looking at travel nursing companies are:

Volume and Variety of Nursing Jobs

A travel nursing agency with many contracts gives you a better chance of finding a placement that fits your wants and needs. Ask about how many contracts are usually available and what states they tend to be in. The average length of a contract is 13 weeks but can range anywhere from 1 to 6 months or more. Finding out what kind of contracts are available and what kind

Table 29.3   Certifications Available from American Nurses Credentialing Center

Nurse Practitioners (NP)	Specialties
<ul><li>Acute Care NP</li><li>Adult NP</li><li>Adult Psychiatric & Mental Health NP</li><li>Diabetes Management—Advanced</li><li>Family NP</li><li>Family Psych & Mental Health NP</li><li>Gerontological NP</li><li>Pediatric NP</li><li>School NP</li></ul>*Clinical Nurse Specialists*<ul><li>Adult Health CNS</li><li>Adult Psychiatric & Mental Health CNS</li><li>Child Adolescent Psych & Mental Health CNS</li><li>CNS Core Exam</li><li>Diabetes Management—Advanced</li><li>Gerontological CNS</li><li>Home Health CNS</li><li>Pediatric CNS</li><li>Public/Community Health CNS</li></ul>*Other Advanced-Level*<ul><li>Diabetes Management—Advanced</li><li>Forensic Nursing—Advanced</li><li>Nurse Executive—Advanced</li><li>Public Health Nursing—Advanced</li></ul>	<ul><li>Ambulatory Care Nursing</li><li>Cardiac Rehabilitation Nursing</li><li>Cardiac Vascular Nursing</li><li>Case Management Nursing</li><li>College Health Nursing</li><li>Community Health Nursing</li><li>General Nursing Practice</li><li>Gerontological Nursing</li><li>High-Risk Perinatal Nursing</li><li>Home Health Nursing</li><li>Informatics Nursing</li><li>Medical-Surgical Nursing</li><li>Nurse Executive</li><li>Nursing Professional Development</li><li>Pain Management</li><li>Pediatric Nursing</li><li>Perinatal Nursing</li><li>Psychiatric & Mental Health Nursing</li><li>School Nursing</li></ul>

Source: Based on from American Nurses Credentialing Center (2011). ANCC Nurse Certification.

Table 29.4 **Select Job Titles and Information**

Job Title	Description	Certification/education	More information	Salary	Job Outlook
Nurse Navigator	Nurses who advocate for and coordinate care for patients battling serious illness, such as cancer	NCLEX, Oncology Nurse Navigator- Certified Generalist (ONN-CG), Oncology Patient Navigator- Certified Generalist (OPN-CG), or Oncology Nurse Navigator- Certified Generalist Thoracic [ONN-CG(T)]	After receiving NCLEX Certification, the Academy of Oncology Nurse and Patient Navigators offers 3 different certifications, which you can choose from if you wish.	$84,700	15%
Public Health Nurse	Defined as the practice of promoting and protecting the health of populations using knowledge from nursing, social, and public health sciences (American Public Health Association, Public Health Nursing Section, 1996).	NCLEX, no further certification required but nurses can acquire their Certified in Public Health (CPH) certification		$56,000	15%
Dermatology Nurse	nursing specialty where you have the opportunity to work in a hospital, dermatology clinic, or plastic surgeon's office providing care for patients with skin conditions such as skin cancer, acne, burns, psoriasis, or just providing aesthetic treatments such as lasers or chemical peels.	NCLEX, Dermatology Nurse Certification Examination given by the Dermatology Nurses' Association.	The job outlook for dermatology nurses may grow to be even higher than 15%, due to advancements in cosmetic dermatology	$52,035	15%
Cardiac Cath Lab Nurse	Cardiac Cath Lab Nurses assist doctors with cardiac catheterization procedures.	NCLEX certification, preference given to Critical Care Registered Nurses, or CCRNs.		$71,297	15%
Emergency Room Nurse	ER nurses work as part of a medical care team providing the first line of care for people with traumatic injuries, pain, or need other urgent medical attention.	NCLEX certified, depending on the state or hospital, there may be other requirements such as certification as a Critical Care Registered Nurse (CCRN)		$64,690	15%
Fertility Nurse	Fertility Nurses care for patients and couples in areas concerning fertility and conception	NCLEX certification, the National Certification Corporation offers certifications in areas such as obstetrics, gynecology, and neonatal care, and the Nurses' Professional Group (NPG) offers training in reproductive endocrinology and infertility (REI) through a nursing certification course	Fertility Nurses can work anywhere from a hospital to an egg donation center.	$65,382	15%
ICU Nurse	ICU nurses provide care to unstable patients with life threatening injuries or illnesses.	NCLEX certification, possibly Critical Care Registered Nurse certified (CCRN)		$72,531	15%
Labor and Delivery Nurse	L&D nurses assist female patients before, during and after childbirth as well as care for any complications that arise during the birth.	NCLEX certification	No additional certifications are required to become a Labor and Delivery nurse, but the National Certification Corporation (NCC) offers field specific certifications for L&D nurses.	$67,490	15%

Table 29.4   (Continued)

Burn Nurse	Burn nurses care for patients with varying burn levels and body percentages cover. Burn nurses plan, evaluate, and document for these clients as well as providing wound care.	NCLEX, some units may require Advanced Burn Life Support (ABLS) or Advanced Cardiovascular Life Support (ACLS)	Many employers prefer to hire Burn Care nurses who have ICU experience.	15%

Note. Compiled with information from: U.S. Bureau of Labor Statistics. (2020, March 31). Glassdoor (2020, June 10).

you are seeking is an important thing to consider when contemplating travel nursing.

Exclusivity of Contracts

Some travel nursing agencies have contracts with state-of-the-art hospitals and medical centers, which allows new nurses to gain experience at prestigious hospitals.

Company Longevity and Expertise

It is usually better to find a travel nursing agency that has longevity because that means they have connections, expertise, and an outstanding staff of recruiters and managers.

How Knowledgeable and Friendly are the Recruiters?

A recruiter is an important ally for travel nurses. It is important to have a recruiter you trust and can build a relationship with, because they are your key advocate while working as a travel nurse.

Are they Certified by The Joint Commission?

The Joint Commission is the gold standard of health care staffing and having their Gold Seal of Approval means that the travel nursing agency has proven their ability to staff and provide health care services with outstanding competency. Some agencies with the Joint Commission Gold Seal of Approval include American Traveler, Medical Solutions, TaleMed, and Millenia Medical (The Joint Commission, 2018).

Benefits

Ask agencies you are interested in what their average pay rates are, although pay differs according to contracts. Ask the agency what compensation is taxable and what is non-taxable, and what their benefits include. Inquire as to what the orientation process is like at each new hospital you work at. It is crucial to know their policy on professional liability insurance, continuing education courses, housing and travel stipends, and remember to ask when the insurance coverage starts and whether they will pay for and assist you to be licensed in each state or if their contracts offer a certain amount of guaranteed hours in that state.

Bonuses

Remember to ask agencies if they offer sign-on bonuses, seasonal bonuses, completion bonuses, or overtime pay.

Support Provided on the Job

While working in unfamiliar states and hospitals, it is important to understand what kind of support will be provided to you while working and living in another state. Ask if they will be available in case of an issue or emergency while on the job and if they have licensing and housing support that will help prepare you to thrive during your assignment. If an agency answers "no" to questions like these, consider an agency who can provide this type of support.

Client Satisfaction

Last, but certainly not least, how satisfied are the clients with this agency? Are the nurses satisfied with their contracts and the way they are managed? Look into the agency's reviews and testimonials on sites such as Glassdoor to determine the satisfaction level of their staff (AMN Healthcare Inc., 2018).

After visiting a couple of travel nursing agencies websites and speaking with recruiters, you should have a better idea of whether or not travel nursing would be a satisfying job choice for you. Travel Nurses have an average salary of $78,120 (Glassdoor, 2018), but it varies based on the company you work for and the locations you take on assignments at. As a new nurse, exploring options is vital to finding a job that fits you and your needs.

Aesthetic Nursing

Another option in the ever-evolving world of nursing is the career path of an aesthetic nurse. An aesthetic nurse is an RN with training in different cosmetic procedures, including Botox injections, collagen replacement therapy, chemical peels, and microdermabrasion. Nursing has always taken a holistic approach to healing, and aesthetic nursing offers care for patients who may be typically healthy or may have genetic abnormalities or disfigurements due to accidents, and those for whom we can enhance their aesthetic sense of self. The medical aesthetics industry is currently a $16 billion-dollar industry and many patients are seeking advanced medical treatments to improve the way they look and feel (National Laser Institute, 2018). Nursing skills such as assessment and intervention are used to properly address the patient's concerns and leave them with results that allow them to feel better about themselves as a whole. Aesthetic nursing combines the art and science of a nursing career and can be achieved by acquiring a certification, or Certified Aesthetic Nurse Specialist (CANS). The requirements to take the exam are that the applicant must be a registered nurse; work in collaboration with a Board Certified physician in: plastic/aesthetic surgery, surgery, ophthalmology, dermatology, or facial plastic surgery; have a minimum of 2 years' experience working with the above physician, 1,000 practice hours working in the past 2 years; and have the supervising physician endorse your application. The exam is taken through the Plastic Surgical Nursing Certification Board and covers Aesthetic injectables, Laser, Light, and Energy-based therapies, and Clinical Skin Care. It also covers nursing activities including monitoring patient status, both physical and psychosocial before, during, and after treatment, as well as planning and administering procedures and patient teaching (Plastic Surgery Nursing Certification Board, 2015). Many nurses who work in aesthetics do procedures on their own as well as assist surgeons in the OR as a circulating and recovery nurse. Aesthetic nurses often begin their careers by working as a Cosmetic or Plastic Surgery nurse and developing a working relationship with a surgeon they trust and who will mentor them. Once they feel comfortable in their foundational knowledge, classes and training are available through nurse trainers working for companies like Allergan, Galderma, and the National Laser Institute. After their 1,000 hr and 3 years of practice, you become eligible to sit for the CANS exam and receive your license to safely practice as an Aesthetic nurse. Recertification is required every 3 years and continuing education is mandatory due to the ever growing and changing field. Aesthetic nurses require advanced knowledge of facial anatomy, nerves, and blood vessels. It requires an artistic eye and is a fabulous option for nurses who want to combine their artistic and aesthetic eye with their knowledge of science and patient care, and even offers an opportunity to partner with a doctor or surgeon and start a business. There are also opportunities down this career path to become a clinical trainer for a company like Galderma or Allergan—the companies who make the majority of injectable products. The average salary for aesthetic nurses is $65,000 (Payscale, 2020).

Military Nursing

Military nursing is another viable option for nurses and is a possible career path for nurses wanting to go the extra step to serve their country. Military nurses work for either the Army Nurse Corps, the Army National Guard, the Navy Nurse Corps, or the Air Force. Offering medical care to soldiers and their families is an extremely fulfilling job, and there are many other benefits. The military nursing career outlook is expected to rise to between 19% and 26% in the next decade, so there will be a litany of jobs to choose from (Nursejournal, 2018). You will most likely be working at a military base, military hospital, V.A. hospital or clinic, or a military clinic and you could be somewhere in the United States, or in a foreign country. Hazard pay is also usually provided when assigned to work in combat zones. The average salary for military nurses is $73,347 (http://Registerednursing.org, 2018). Duties of military nurses

outside of treating soldiers and their families includes setting up military triage in war zones, providing vaccines to people in developing countries, and assisting in humanitarian efforts that the U.S. military is engaged in (http://Registerednursing.org, 2018). It is a career path for strong, dedicated individuals who would not hesitate to work in war zones, potentially dangerous circumstances, and being deployed during natural disasters or times of war and hardship. Military nurses receive amazing benefits including, sign-on bonuses and raises, housing stipends, vacation time, retirement benefits, and have the opportunity to rise in rank as military personnel. Military nursing is also a great opportunity if you have student loans to repay, as many branches of the military offer up to $120,000 in loan forgiveness (CreditDonkey, 2018). If military nursing seems like something you'd be interested, there are steps to take after you complete your nursing program and pass the NCLEX. You have the opportunity to either work and gain some experience first or enlist as a military nurse as a new graduate. The choice is entirely up to you, and military nursing is seen by many as a great way for new nurses to both gain experience and pay off loans. Once you make the decision to enlist, contact a local recruiter for whichever branch you are interested in working for, make sure you are eligible to enlist, and then fill out an application packet. The process is not quick, as it usually takes about a year for your application to be approved from the time you fill it out. Once you are accepted, it is mandatory that military nurses complete a course to become a commissioned officer. This course is 5–10 weeks long and teaches you the skills necessary for a career as a military nurse, including leadership, military skills, and physical training. The longer you work and the more experience you gain, you can rise up in Military Ranking and earn more money and benefits (http://Nurse.org, 2018).

Developmental Disability Nursing

Developmental Disability nurses work with patients who have developmental disabilities such as Autism Spectrum Disorder, Down Syndrome, Cerebral Palsy, and many other developmental disorders. They typically work with patients from the time they are newborns to adults, working to improve their quality of life along the way, creating a bond with the patient and family while acting as an advocate for them (http://registerednurse.org). To become a Developmental Disability nurse, you must graduate from nursing school, pass NCLEX, and then work for 2 or more years with patients who have developmental disabilities. You can accomplish this by checking local hospital systems to see if they have programs for developmentally disabled patients or adult day services and if they have any openings, volunteer or working. Even volunteering can be a wonderful opportunity to meet the staff, patients, and apply for a job once they see you are a good fit. Once you have 2 years of experience, you can become certified through the Developmental Disabilities Nurses Association (DDNA). This certification is not required for most jobs, but it shows that you took the extra step to prove your competency and expertise with this unique population. Many Developmental Disability nurses work in direct patient-care—usually in clinics, group homes, or directly in family's homes. They work closely with all other providers for their patients, as well as social workers, support staff, and language and physical therapists to help patients achieve the best quality of life possible. The salary range is between $42,000 and $86,000 per year, and the reason it varies is the experience of the nurse and their geographical location (http://registerednurse.org). Most DD nurses also receive a gas stipend, due to the home care aspect that usually accompanies the job.

Flight Nursing

Flight nurses, or transport nurses, are RNs who provide treatment to patients while they're being airlifted to a hospital during a medical emergency. They are part of a medical care team on the flight, including medics and physicians. The goal is to keep the patient stable until they arrive at the hospital and can receive further care. Flight nurses work in both military environments and civilian environments. Flight nurses require 5 or more years of experience in an ICU, ER, or Trauma setting. so they can hone their skills and perfect their critical care knowledge. They must be strong and fearless leaders, have an ability to work in a small, confined space and under immense pressure, and be open to working abnormal hours including overtime and on-call rotation. There is a certification for flight nurses, Certified Flight Registered Nurse. Many certifications require 2 years of experience, but the CFRN does not, so you can sit for the exam whenever you see fit. Flight nurses are also expected to have their Advanced Cardiac Life Support (ACLS), Pediatric Advanced Life Support (PALS), Transport Professional Advanced Trauma Course (TPATC), and Certified Emergency Nurse (CEN) or Critical Care Nurse (CCRN).

The military is always looking for flight nurses and large hospitals need an outstanding transport team to bring patients to them safely. The average salary of a flight nurse is around $68,000. Transport nursing is great for nurses who like the critical care/emergency care and are looking for a dynamic and unique environment to work in (http://registerednurse. org, 2018).

Legal Nurse Consultants

Legal Nurse Consultants are highly experienced and educated nurses, usually with a Masters or Doctoral degree, who after many years of gaining clinical experience, are considered experts in their field and are hired to work for insurance companies, hospitals, law offices, and government agencies to go to court and assist attorneys in the litigation process for malpractice claims or other insurance claims with their medical expertise. Legal Nurse Consultants can also be self- employed and start their own company. Understanding standards of care, the nursing process, and disease processes is vital to the role

and a basic understanding of the legal system is required. There is a certification available for Legal Nurse Consultants, called the LNCC (Legal Nurse Consultant Certification). You can study for it online via the Center for Legal Studies under Legal Nurse Consultant Training Course. A nurse is eligible to take the exam after 5 years of nursing experience, proof of 2,000 hr practicing legal consulting in the last 5 years, and a current RN license. Renewal is required every 5 years. When working on a claim, Legal Nurse Consultant roles include but are certainly not limited to reviewing charting, medical records, collaborating with the legal team of the facility being claimed against, and doing utilization reviews. Legal Nurse Consultants are able to set their own hours and hourly pay in many cases, are able to work from home often, and have the opportunity to branch out into a new field and learn how to apply their nursing expertise in a different way. The payscale is wide, and ranges from around $58,000 per year all the way up to over $200,000 (Payscale, 2020) (http://Registerednursing.org, 2018).

Nurse Managers

Nursing managers are nurses, usually with a BSN degree, who oversee and lead the nursing staff of a specific unit of a hospital. Their role requires organization, critical thinking, and understanding of competent and effective care of both patients and their staff, so that their staff functions well and provides better patient care. They understand the nursing and business aspects of the unit and manage schedules, budgets, call offs, hiring, and unit projects. Most of the time, 5 years of nursing experience is required to become a nursing manager and they are often hired straight from the floor or unit they work on, once they express interest and the previous manager either leaves or needs an assistant. There are two options for certifications, the CENP (Certified in Executive Nursing Practice) and the (CNML) Certified Nurse Manager and Leader. The CENP is geared toward nurses working in or seeking an executive position, such as Nursing Administration, and the CNML is geared toward nurses looking to stay in a managerial role. Nursing managers work on the unit they oversee, and usually have an office on the unit that they work in as well as circulating the floor, talking with patients and nurses. The average salary for nursing managers is $79,725 a year (http:// Registerednursing.org).

Transcultural Nurses

Transcultural Nursing is nursing with a specific focus on world cultures and comparative cultural care, with an aim to provide culturally congruent nursing care and eliminate disparities. Transcultural nurses understand and recognize cultural differences in their health care beliefs, customs, and values and the way these beliefs affect their understanding and treatment of disease, sickness, and death. They aim to be culturally competent and inclusive in their care and, as a result, treat patients who are migrants, refugees, or immigrants. Transcultural nurses can work in foreign countries or in diverse cities with many immigrants. They work to integrate their nursing philosophies into the standard of nursing care at hospitals and clinics they work at. Transcultural nurses can have any nursing degree, but in order to obtain additional certification from the Transcultural Nursing Society will have to receive a Master's or Doctorate degree first. Transcultural nursing is projected to grow in the coming years because: (a) nursing as a profession is growing rapidly, and (b) with the global refugee crisis and increased number of immigrants coming into the US, nursing is working toward the ability to provide culturally competent and effective care to these new populations in the U.S. (http://registerednursing.org).

Certified Registered Nurse Anesthetists

Certified Registered Nurse Anesthetists (CRNA), are highly intelligent and skilled nurses who prepare anesthesia and deliver it to patients before surgical procedures, as well as monitor the patients during anesthesia and closely watching their recovery afterwards. They work alongside surgeons, anesthesiologists, dentists, and other health care professionals and assist in their practice. To become a CRNA, enroll in and complete a program for Nurse Anesthetists—which can take between 2 and 4 years—and afterwards, take your NBCRNA exam: National Boards of Certification and Recertification of Nurse Anesthetists. CRNAs comprise some of the highest paid nurses—their average salary is $157,000 per year but can reach up to $242,000 per year. The BLS has projected the job outlook for CRNAs to be 31% by 2024, which is an outstanding growth. Many hospitals are looking to use CRNAs in place of anesthesiologists due to cost and availability, so seeking a job as a Certified Registered Nurse Anesthetist may be difficult, but it is a path to career stability, high salary, and satisfying work (http://nurse.org, 2018).

Wound, Ostomy, Continence Nurse Specialist

The field of enterostomal therapy was initiated in 1958 at the Cleveland Clinic, with the first enterostomal therapists (ETs) being non-nurses. The first nursing training program was started in 1961, and in 1972 new standards for the schools of enterostomal therapy were established. The year 1976 marked a significant change when the governing body of the International Association of Enterostomal Therapists determined that only RNs would be admitted to enterostomal therapy educational programs. After this, the scope of practice was expanded beyond just caring for ostomies to include skin care, management of draining wounds and fistulas, pressure sores, and incontinence. At this point, the entry requirements into an enterostomal therapy nursing education program (ETNEP) changed to a Bachelor's degree with a major in nursing.

Nurses with this training and education practice both in hospitals and community-based settings such as visiting nurse associations, public health, nursing homes, and long-term care facilities. Over the past 20 years, these specialists have truly become the clinical experts in managing patients with ostomies, alterations in skin integrity, and wounds.

Public Health Nursing

Public health nurses integrate community involvement and knowledge about the entire population with personal, clinical understandings of the health and illness experiences of individuals and families within the population (Core Competencies for Basic Midwifery Practice, 2012). According to the American Public Health Association, "the primary focus of public health nursing is improving the health of the community as a whole rather than just that of an individual or family" (American Public Health Association, 2013).

The work of a public health nurse is essentially primary prevention, such as preventing disease, injury, disability, and premature death. Public health nurses work collaboratively as a team with other public health professionals, such as health educators, epidemiologists, physicians, advanced practice nurses, nutritionists, etc.

To become a public health nurse usually requires a Bachelor's degree in nursing from an accredited 4-year college. Some communities will employ public health nurses with an Associate Degree in Nursing. Public health nurses are found in a variety of settings, including schools and the workplace, the latter called occupational health nurses. Public health nurses also often work for government agencies, non-profit groups, and community health centers.

Certified Nurse-Midwife (CNM)

Midwifery has existed from the beginning of humankind, and throughout history has played a vital and integral role in a community's growth. In the 1920s, Mary Breckenridge (a British midwife), along with other British midwives, worked with the Frontier Nursing Services in Kentucky to provide services for the rural population. The first American midwifery program was established in 1932, with the curriculum adapted and modified from the British model. In 1955, the American College of Nurse-Midwives (ACNM) was formed, with its main goals focused on setting standards for practice and education.

Currently, there are numerous midwifery educational programs. Since 1980, CNMs have been allowed to practice in a variety of settings, including hospitals, homes, and birthing centers, providing care for women throughout the childbearing cycle as well as postpartum. Nurse-midwives and collaborating practitioners agree upon the protocols and procedures. Health education, including the teaching of self-care skills and preparation for childbirth and child rearing, comprises a large part of clinical activities in addition to the actual delivering of babies. The American College of Nurse-Midwives asserts that the CNM can provide "services to women and their babies in the areas of prenatal care, labor and delivery management, postpartum care, normal newborn care, well-women gynecology, and family planning (Core Compenencies for Basic Midwifery Practice, 2012).

Clinical Nurse Specialist (CNS)

By the turn of the twentieth century, the greatest percentage of APNs were the CNSs, whose origins can be traced back to 1938. Reiter first coined the term *nurse clinician* in 1943 to designate a nurse with advanced clinical competence and recommended that such clinicians get their preparation in graduate nursing education programs. Educators first developed the clinical nurse specialist (CNS) role because of their concern for improving nursing care. They believed that nursing care improvement was dependent upon increasing expertise at the bedside, giving both direct and indirect care, and incorporating role modeling and consultation. The CNS role has evolved to include many specialties. The first CNS Master's program in psychiatry was started by Peplau in 1955 at Rutgers University.

Nurse Entrepreneur

Nurse entrepreneurs use their nursing experience in a creative way to market and promote their ideas, knowledge, or certain products. This can include anything from nursing education and review courses to badge reels and hoodies. Becoming a nurse entrepreneur allows you to share with others from your own knowledge and experience, as well as have independence and autonomy.

The first step to becoming a nurse entrepreneur is completing your nursing degree and passing the NCLEX. Then, practicing as an RN in order to learn about the health care industry, nursing as a profession, and the opportunities within it. Aside from basic nursing knowledge, nurse entrepreneurs benefit from having an understanding of business and leadership skills. Some nurses accomplish this by obtaining a dual Master's degree in Nursing and Business Administration, and some obtain informal training or a Business degree. However, there are no specific requirements, aside from a degree and active license, to become a nurse entrepreneur.

The NNBA, or the National Nurses in Business Association is a resource for nurses in business and provides mentoring, insight to trends in health care, and continuing education. Business opportunities within nursing include, but are not limited to, diabetes education, CPR/BLS certification, home care, podcasts/public speaking, and products such as badge reels and stethoscope holders. Creativity is key when becoming a nurse entrepreneur. With the rise in popularity of social media and blogs, many nurses find their business through the internet. No matter where you decide to go as a nurse entrepreneur, you can be sure to find a path. Nursing is a diverse field with many opportunities. A few current examples of nurse entrepreneurs include:

NurseTim   https://nursetim.com

Nurse Blake   www.nurseblake.com

Nurse Jamie   https://nursejamie.com

Seattle Sutton   www.seattlesutton.com

Direction for the Future

In examining the evolution of nursing and the direction in which it is heading, the ANA believes that more effective utilization of RNs to provide primary health care services is part of the solution to the cost and accessibility problems in health care today.

The twenty-first century holds a great deal of promise, but there are many questions to be answered regarding the cost, accessibility, and quality of the health care system in the United States. Nursing has a wonderful opportunity to be a leader in a changing health care delivery system. Few other professions provide as many options. There is a world of emerging opportunities as you prepare to enter the workforce. Many of the jobs you will hold in the future do not even exist at this time. Take your time, research the possibilities, organize your plan, and live your dream. As Sophia Palmer said in 1897 at the first convention of the American Society of Superintendents of Training Schools for Nursing, "Organization is the power of the day. Without it, nothing great is accomplished" (Feldman, 2000).

Evidence from the Literature

Citation: Colichi, R. M. B., Lima, S. G. S. E., Bonini, A. B. B., & Lima, S. A. M. (2019). Entrepreneurship and Nursing: Integrative review. *Revista brasileira de enfermagem, 72*(suppl 1), 321–330. https://doi.org/10.1590/0034-7167-2018-0498

Discussion: An integrative literature review in the following databases: Cumulative Index to Nursing and Allied Health Literature (CINAHL), EMBASE, SCOPUS, Web of Science, PubMed, Medline, Latin American and Caribbean Literature in Health Sciences (LILACS), Nursing Database (BDENF), Index Psychology and National *Information Center of Medical* Sciences of Cuba (CUMED), was used to identify the knowledge produced on business entrepreneurship in nursing. It was found that there is a need to prepare nurses with adequate skills to increase the capacity to integrate into the labor market and to improve their own well-being and that of society.

Implications for Practice: Nurses aren't adequately prepared in school with the knowledge of business entrepreneurship in nursing. Nursing education and nurses in general need to increase their knowledge of business entrepreneurship to better prepare themselves for entrepreneurial opportunities in the future.

In this chapter you have been given information on the current job market and different career paths for entry level nurses. Career resources and information on obtaining employment has been shared. Select nursing career opportunities have been shared to give you a glimpse of what nursing has to offer. Hopefully, this chapter has opened your eyes to the myriad of choices nursing has to offer.

KEY CONCEPTS

- Confusion is a common feeling among graduate nurses as they enter the job search.

- There are approximately 3 million licensed nurses in the United States.

- Employment of registered nurses is expected to grow to a mammoth 15% from 2016 to 2026. Registered nurses comprise one of the largest segments of the U.S. workforce as a whole and are among the highest-paid large occupations.

- Nurses comprise the largest single component of hospital staff, are the primary providers of hospital patient care, and deliver most of the nation's long-term care.

- From 1980 to 2004, the percentage of employed RNs working in hospitals decreased from 66 to 56.2% as health care moved to sites beyond the hospital and nurses increased their numbers in a wide range of other settings.

- There are over four times as many RNs in the United States as there are physicians.

- Fifty-five percent of the RN workforce is age 50 or older, and more than 1 million registered nurses are predicted to reach retirement age within the next 10–15 years, that is approximately one-third of the current workforce.

- While there are many jobs nationally, demand varies by geography.

- Networking can be a great way as a new nurse to open doors to many opportunities.

- Nursing possesses myriad emerging practice opportunities.

- Certification is a process readily available to any RN.

- Entrepreneurship and other nontraditional positions such as travel nursing have proven very successful for nurses.

- Nursing practice has become increasingly specialized.

- To prepare for the interview process, gather clinical stories and experiences and practice talking about them in a professional way.

- Nurses are expected to be quick problem solvers, adept in stressful situations, and competent, pleasant people to be around and work with.

- Searching for nursing opportunities can be overwhelming, but there are many online resources.

- Use the checklist found in Table 29.1 to prepare for employment.

- Professional certification in nursing is a measure of distinctive nursing practice.

- Nursing has a plethora of career options, many of which you may not even be aware of.

- Travel nursing is another unique career path for nurses.

- The twenty-first century holds a great deal of promise, but there are many questions to be answered regarding the cost, accessibility, and quality of the health care system in the United States.

- Numerous types of APNs are now practicing in both the hospital and community settings.

- For any RN, a plan to develop professional opportunities is essential.

KEY TERMS

Clinical ladder   Certification

REVIEW QUESTIONS

1. Traveling nurses should do which of the following?
   a. Carry a notarized copy of their home state license.
   b. Become a Basic Life Support (BLS) instructor.
   c. Obtain state licenses for each state in which they will be practicing.
   d. Work for only one travel company.

2. The hospital-based case manager's primary focus is which of the following?
   a. Providing care and services that focus on outcome.
   b. Making sure all the patient's expenses are taken care of.
   c. Guiding medical and nursing protocols.
   d. Ensuring that each patient has a primary nurse.

3. To be a successful nurse entrepreneur, it is imperative that the individual nurse do which of the following?
   a. Obtain a sizable loan from a bank to help with start-up costs.
   b. Attain credit card approval.
   c. Understand how the stock market functions.
   d. Develop a solid business plan.

4. Which of the following is the best method of determining the effectiveness of an APN's practice?
   a. Patient satisfaction guide
   b. Fewer hospital admissions
   c. Improved patient outcomes
   d. Number of research studies

5. APNs provide both nursing and health care services. APNs can best fulfill this mission by doing which of the following?
   a. Performing and then publishing research
   b. Responding to patients' health care needs
   c. Maintaining as many certifications as possible
   d. Managing patients in both the hospital and outpatient settings

6. The CNS/NP role is multidimensional and provides a unique opportunity to practice in a variety of settings. Select all that apply to the CNS/NP role.
   a. The CNS/NP role is mostly primary care based.
   b. The CNS/NP role often has an unclear overlap in responsibilities.
   c. Both roles are vested in utilizing research to advance care.
   d. The CNS role is more geared toward systems management and enhancement.
   e. The CNS/NP role requires ACLS.

7. What are some factors that may influence the development of clinical competence? Select all that apply.
   a. Management preparation
   b. Experience, motivation, and theoretical knowledge
   c. Working within the intensive care setting
   d. Opportunities, environment
   e. Personal characteristics
   f. Motivation and initiative

8. Which of the following is true about certification?
   a. Mandatory in most states
   b. Achieved through an examination that attests to the education and training of a registered nurse
   c. Usually covered when you apply for your state license
   d. One of the first processes you will complete after passing the NCLEX

9. Which of the following is correct concerning a public health nurse?
   a. You would interface with pharmaceutical representatives and companies routinely.
   b. You would work primarily with injured patients in a home environment.
   c. You would be required to work with ventilatory dependent patients.
   d. The work is essentially primary prevention, i.e., preventing disease, injury, disability, and premature death.

10. It is important that nursing not only encourages and welcomes new graduates in the field, but also implements strategies to retain nurses already employed. From research, it is known that the major predictor of intent to leave a nursing job is job dissatisfaction. A significant strategy that will enhance job satisfaction and the desire to continue in nursing is which of the following?
    a. Encourage certification at the earliest opportunity.
    b. Maintain a 40-hr work week.
    c. Work at several institutions within the first several years of employment.
    d. Practice in a setting that creates and maintains a positive work environment

REVIEW QUESTION ANSWERS

1. Answer: A is correct.
   Rationale: (A) Traveling nurses should carry a notarized copy of their home state license. This will quickly verify their RN status in case of any computer glitches that may arise. It is not necessary for a traveling nurse to (B) become a Basic Life Support (BLS) instructor, (C) obtain state licenses for each state in which they will be practicing, or (D) to work for only one travel company.

2. Answer: A is correct.
   Rationale: (A) Providing care and services that focus on outcome is the primary function of a case manager. (B) Making sure all the patient's expenses are taken care of, (C) guiding medical and nursing protocols, and (D) ensuring that each patient has a primary nurse, are all inappropriate.

3. Answer: D is correct.
   Rationale: (D) To become a nurse entrepreneur, it is imperative to develop a solid business plan. (A) To obtain a large loan, (B) attain credit card approval, or (C) understand the stock market, are not essential to becoming a nurse entrepreneur.

4. Answer: C is correct.
   Rationale: (C) Improved patient outcomes are the best way to determine APN effectiveness. (A) patient satisfaction is essential, but doesn't determine effectivenss. (B). Fewer hospitalizations may or may not show effectiveness, and (D) number of research studies doesn't show effectiveness.

5. Answer: B is correct.
   Rationale: (B) Responding the patients' health care needs is the primary function of an APN. (A) Research and publications are helpful but not essential to these roles, (C) more certifications doesn't always mean you are responding to patients' needs, and (D) it doesn't matter the setting, patients are the priority.

6. Answers A, B, C, and D are correct.
   Rationale: It is true that (A) the CNS/NP role is mostly primary care based, (B) the CNS/NP role often has an unclear overlap in responsibilities, (C) both roles are vested in utilizing research to advance care, and (D) the CNS role is more geared toward systems management and enhancement. It is untrue that (E) the CNS/NP role requires ACLS.

7. Answers A, B, C, D, E, and F are correct.
   Rationale: All may influence clinical competence (A) Management preparation, (B) experience, motivation, and theoretical knowledge, (C) working within the intensive care setting, (D) opportunities, environment, (E) personal characteristics, and (F) motivation and initiative, are all correct.

8. Answer: B is correct.

   Rationale: (B) Certification is achieved through an examination that attests to the education and training of a registered nurse. It is not (A) mandatory in most states, (C) covered when you apply for your state license, or (D) one of the first processes you will complete after passing NCLEX.

9. Answer: D is correct

   Rationale: Public health nursing deals essentially with (D) primary prevention, i.e., preventing disease, injury, disability, and premature death. Incorrect responses include (A) you would interface with pharmaceutical representatives and companies routinely is incorrect because you work on primary prevention. (B) Your primary work would not include injured patients in a home setting, nor (D) would you be required to work with ventilators.

10. Answer: D is correct

    Rationale: (D) Practice in a setting that creates and maintains a positive work environment will enhance job satisfaction. (A) Encourage certification at the earliest opportunity, (B) maintain a 40-hr work week, (C) work at several institutions within the first several years of employment, may not enhance job satisfaction.

REVIEW ACTIVITIES

1. What are three different types of nursing careers and what are the certifications needed to obtain that career?

2. What is the average job outlook for RN careers? What about the specialty that interests you most?

3. Review Table 29.4 and choose 3 nursing careers that interest you. Do further research for these chosen careers and check openings for them in your area. What is the average salary? What are the required credentials? Do they align with the information in the table?

4. Review nursing issues/programs, information, services, and certification at ANA's website (www.nursingworld.org). What did you see there?

DISCUSSION POINTS

• What is the current job market for nurses in your area?

• What career path appeals to you and why for entry?

• What nursing career resources have you used and which do you need to learn more and how to use them?

• After reviewing the list nursing career options including education, certification, job outlook, and salaries for select nursing careers in Table 29.4, which interest you the most and why?

• How can you apply the information in the chapter to obtain employment as a Registered Nurse?

• Review Table 29.1 Job Search Checklist, are you prepared? What else can be added to this list?

• What kind of Certification is a process readily available to any RN?

DISCUSSION OF OPENING SCENARIO

1. *Where should she look for a career?*

   There are many places for her to look. She can network with colleagues, clinical instructors, and managers at clinical rotation sites. There are many online sources and she needs to start with a good resume and Linkedin profile.

2. *What kind of nursing career would fit her best?*

   What kind of nursing career fits a nurse is very individual, based on the nurses needs and interests. This chapter explores many career choices to consider.

3. *How can she best evaluate options so that she has the right career?*

   She can make pro and con lists for positions considered and look at how the positions fit in her career path.

4. *What is the current market for nursing and nursing opportunities?*

   The current market for nursing and nursing opportunities is excellent. Realize that different areas of the country have higher or lower than average nursing opportunities. If moving is an option for you, you will always have access to excellent nursing opportunities.

EXPLORING THE WEB

Understanding online resources is crucial in any career, especially nursing. There are many sites to help students and nurses gain awareness about different types of nursing careers, interview success, certifications, and where nurses are most in demand. Below, you will find a list of nursing websites which you may find helpful as you search for a job. Visit each site and review the resources available regarding nursing opportunities.

• National League for Nursing: www.nln.org

• American Nurses Association (ANA): www.nursingworld.org

• ANA certification listing: www.nursingworld.org

• Discover Nursing: www.discovernursing.com

• Center for Nursing: www.nursingcenter.com

- National Council of State Boards of Nursing: www.ncsbn.org

- General nursing interest site: www.allnurses.com

- Information on a wide variety of health careers. www.explore-healthcareers.org

- American Association of Nurse Anesthetists: www.aana.com

- Flight nursing: www.flightweb.com

- Traveling nurses: www.healthcareers-online.com

- American Academy of Nurse Practitioners: www.aanp.org

- Nurse Practitioner Central: www.npcentral.net

- https://allnurses.com

- www.nursingworld.org

INFORMATICS

Visit www.nursingcenter.com and click on the "career resources" tab. Next, click on "advice for new nurses." Choose a category—they include preparing for and taking the NCLEX, job search, orientation, keys to success, teamwork, and professionalism. After choosing a category that interests you, select one of the free articles, read it, and write a brief summary of what you have learned from the article. Under the "career resources" tab, you can also choose "job search" and enter in your data to find open RN positions near you. Take time to explore this website and remember to utilize it as a resource when preparing for the NCLEX and searching for a job!

LEAN BACK

- Did this chapter give insight and ideas into nursing careers you had not considered?

- Has this helped you clarify your values and what is most important to you as you consider career choices?

- Are you considering working toward a position in a couple of years? What can you do today to help make that a reality?

REFERENCES

American Nurses Credentialing Center. (2017). *Certification general testing and renewal handbook [Brochure]*. Silver Springs, MD: American Nurses Credentialing Center. Retrieved from www.nursingworld.org/~4aae16/globalassets/certification/certification-policies/ancc-generaltestingrenewalrequirements4-1-2017_final.pdf

American Public Health Association, Public Health Nursing Section. (2013). *Brochure*. Washington, DC: American Public Health Association. Retrieved from www.apha.org/-/media/files/pdf/membergroups/phn/nursingdefinition.ashx?la=en&hash=331DBEC4B79E0C0B8C644BF2BEA571249F8717A0

Cook, E. (1913). *The Life of Florence Nightingale*, by Sir Edward Cook. (p. 57). London, UK: Macmillan.

Glassdoor. (2020, May 30). *Salary: Travel Nurse*. Retrieved from www.glassdoor.com/Salaries/travel-nurse-salary-SRCH_KO0,12.htm

Hagstrom, M. (2020). *10 Things to Look for in a Top Travel Nurse Agency*. Retrieved from www.travelnursing.com/news/career-development/top-10-things-to-look-for-in-a-travel-nurse-agency/

Louie, K. (2019, July 01). Guide to Certified Registered Nurse Anesthesia. Retrieved from www.onlinefnpprograms.com/aprn-career-guide/certified-registered-nurse-anesthetist/

National Laser Institute. (2019, April 25). *Medical Aesthetics Trends in 2019*. Retrieved from https://nationallaserinstitute.com/blog/cosmetic-laser-training/medical-aesthetics-trends-2019/

Credit Donkey. (2019, October 01). *Loan Forgiveness for Nurses*. Retrieved from www.creditdonkey.com/loan-forgiveness-nurses.html

Plastic Surgical Nursing Certification Board. (2015). *Certified Plastic Surgical Nurse Examination [Brochure]*. Beverly, MA: Plastic Surgical Nursing Certification Board. Retrieved from https://psncb.org/multimedia/files/CPSN/Test-Specifications.pdf

U.S. Bureau of Labor Statistics. (2020, March 31). *29-1141 Registered Nurses*. Retrieved from www.bls.gov/oes/current/oes291141.htm

Writers, R. S. (2019d, August 19). *Military Nurse Careers & Salary Outlook, 2019*. http://NurseJournal.org. Retrieved from https://nursejournal.org/military-nursing/military-nurse-careers-salary-outlook

SUGGESTED READINGS

Bellack, J. P., & Dickow, M. (2019). Why nurse leaders derail: Preventing and rebounding from leadership failure. *Nursing Administration Quarterly, 43*(2), 113–122. doi:10.1097/NAQ.0000000000000345

Bowles, J. R., Batcheller, J., Adams, J. M., Zimmermann, D., & Pappas, S. (2019). Nursing's leadership role in advancing professional practice/work environments as part of the quadruple aim. *Nursing Administration Quarterly, 43*(2), 157–163. doi:10.1097/NAQ.0000000000000342

Cardillo, D. (2019). Passionate about nursing professional development. *Journal for Nurses in Professional Development, 35*(1), 50–51. doi:10.1097/NND.0000000000000511

Chai, X., Cheng, C., Mei, J., & Fan, X. (2019). Student nurses' career motivation toward gerontological nursing: A longitudinal study. *Nurse Education Today, 76*, 165–171. doi:10.1016/j.nedt.2019.01.028

Chicca, J., & Bindon, S. (2019). New-to-setting nurse transitions: A concept analysis. *Journal for Nurses in Professional Development, 35*(2), 66–75. doi:10.1097/NND.0000000000000530

Choi, J., & Park, M. (2019). Effects of nursing organisational culture on face-to-face bullying and cyberbullying in the workplace. *Journal of Clinical Nursing, 28*(13–14), 2577–2588. doi:10.1111/jocn.14843

Colichi, R. M. B., Lima, S. G. S. E., Bonini, A. B. B., & Lima, S. A. M. (2019).

Entrepreneurship and nursing: Integrative review. *Revista Brasileira de Enfermagem, 72*(suppl. 1), 321–330. doi:10.1590/0034-7167-2018-0498

Dols, J. D., Chargualaf, K. A., & Martinez, K. S. (2019). Cultural and generational considerations in RN retention. *The Journal of Nursing Administration, 49*(4), 201–207. doi:10.1097/NNA.0000000000000738

Dunbar, G., Kawar, L. N., & Scruth, E. A. (2019). The transition from expert to novice and Back to expert: Ensuring competent and safe practice. *Clinical Nurse Specialist CNS, 33*(3), 106–109. doi:10.1097/NUR.0000000000000442

Fowler, J. (2019). From staff nurse to nurse consultant continuing professional development part 11: Using reflection. *British Journal of Nursing (Mark Allen Publishing), 28*(6), 394. doi:10.12968/bjon.2019.28.6.394

Gorman, V. L.-A. (2019). Future emergency nursing workforce: What the evidence is telling us. *Journal of Emergency Nursing: JEN: Official Publication of the Emergency Department Nurses Association, 45*(2), 132–136. doi:10.1016/j.jen.2018.09.009

Ispir, O., Elibol, E., & Sonmez, B. (2019). The relationship of personality traits and entrepreneurship tendencies with career adaptability of nursing students. *Nurse Education Today, 79*, 41–47. doi:10.1016/j.nedt.2019.05.017

Joo, K. R. (2019). Ten lessons learned on the road to earning a doctor of nursing practice degree. *Worldviews on Evidence-Based Nursing, 16*(3), 247–248. doi:10.1111/wvn.12366

Major, R., & Tetley, J. (2019). Effects of dyslexia on registered nurses in practice. *Nurse Education in Practice, 35*, 7–13. doi:10.1016/j.nepr.2018.12.012

Maughan, E. D. (2019). Breaking the glass cage: The power of data, courage, and voice. *NASN School Nurse (Print), 34*(2), 95–99. doi:10.1177/1942602X18815444

McNally, S., Azzopardi, T., Hatcher, D., O'Reilly, R., & Keedle, H. (2019). Student perceptions, experiences and support within their current bachelor of nursing. *Nurse Education Today, 76*, 56–61. doi:10.1016/j.nedt.2019.01.032

Mohamed, L. K. (2019). First-career and second-career nurses' experiences of stress, presenteeism and burn-out during transition to practice. *Evidence-Based Nursing, 22*(3), 85. doi:10.1136/ebnurs-2019-103069

Noone, J., & Young, H. M. (2019). Creating a Community of Writers: Participant perception of the impact of a writing retreat on scholarly productivity. *Journal of Professional Nursing: Official Journal of the American Association of Colleges of Nursing, 35*(1), 65–69. doi:10.1016/j.profnurs.2018.07.006

Pham, T. T. L., Teng, C.-I., Friesner, D., Li, K., Wu, W.-E., et al. (2019). The impact of mentor-mentee rapport on nurses' professional turnover intention: Perspectives of social capital theory and social cognitive career theory. *Journal of Clinical Nursing, 28*(13–14), 2669–2680. doi:10.1111/jocn.14858

Quail, M. T. (2019). Considering toxicology: Specialists in poison information. *Nursing, 49*(3), 45–47. doi:10.1097/01.NURSE.0000553275.18719.44

Wilson, C. (2019). Own your practice. *Journal for Nurses in Professional Development, 35*(2), 115–116. doi:10.1097/NND.0000000000000516

Wyllie, A., Levett-Jones, T., DiGiacomo, M., & Davidson, P. (2019). Exploring the experiences of early career academic nurses as they shape their career journey: A qualitative study. *Nurse Education Today, 76*, 68–72. doi:10.1016/j.nedt.2019.01.021

Zangerle, C. (2019). Risk, resilience, and creating balance: An interview with Gail Latimer. *The Journal of Nursing Administration, 49*(7–8), 345–346. doi:10.1097/NNA.0000000000000763

APPENDIX 1

Janice Tazbir[1,2,3,4]

[1] University of Chicago Medicine, Chicago, IL, USA
[2] Anderson Continuing Education, Sacramento, CA, USA
[3] Retired, Purdue University Northwest, College of Nursing, Hammond, IN, USA
[4] Health Education Systems, Inc. (HESI) Houston, Texas

These photos illustrate some of the equipment, posters, and ways nurses identify goals and demonstrate leadership while delivering and monitoring patient care to assure patient-centered, evidence-based, high-quality, safe patient care. The posters are displayed in the Surgical Intensive Care Unit (**SICU**) nurse's conference room and/or on the Patient Care Unit at the University of Chicago Medicine. Having visual reminders is an effective and valuable way to involve all members of the inter-professional team in setting goals, assuming leadership, taking initiatives, and reminding them of the continual need for excellence in nursing. Nurses and other members of the inter-professional team lead patient care delivery. Photos are gratefully used with permission from Peggy Zemansky, Manager of SICU at UCM.

1. Managing for Daily Improvement

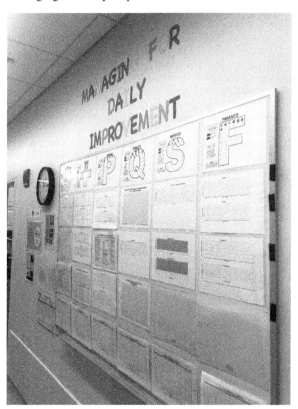

Kelly Vana's Nursing Leadership and Management, Fourth Edition. Edited by Patricia Kelly Vana and Janice Tazbir
© 2021 John Wiley & Sons Ltd. Published 2021 by John Wiley & Sons Ltd.
Companion Website: www.wiley.com/go/kelly-Nursing-Leadership

The Poster Board used to highlight Managing for Daily Improvement. The Poster Board identifies information about the following five quality measures:

- Safety (Are there any patient falls or staff injuries?),

- People (Is staffing adequate?),

- Quality (How are we doing with our quality measures like the number of Catheter Associated Urinary Tract Infections (CAUTI)?),

- Service (Are staff participating in councils and committees, are there any needs?)

- Finance (Does any equipment need to be fixed or purchased? Has there been an unusual amount of overtime needed lately?).

The Poster Board is in the staff room and is used daily in Unit Huddles to review information about Safety, People, Quality, Service, and Finance. The information is used to identify both strengths and weaknesses, and plan for improvement. This builds a patient care environment that is continually improving.

2. Magnet Mission Poster

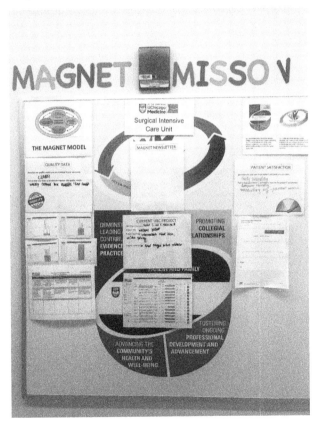

This is a photo of the Magnet Mission Poster, which is hung in the SICU nurse's area at the University of Chicago Medicine Hospital. Included on the poster is information about items such as elements of the Magnet Model, Patient Satisfaction, the Nursing Professional Practice Model, Quality Data, Evidence-Based Practice, and other projects. This info is reviewed by all the unit's nurses and other inter-professional staff, both informally and in meetings, etc., in order to deliver patient-centered, evidence-based, high-quality, safe patient care.

3. Stop Light Report and the MESS Board

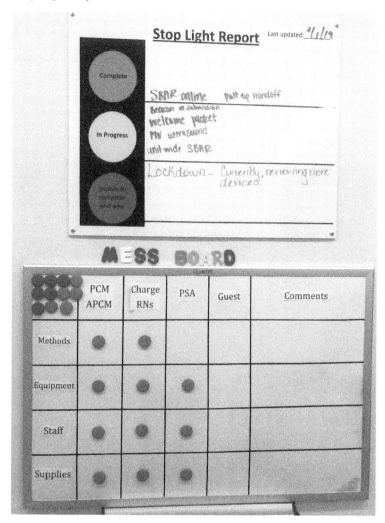

This photo identifies the Stop Light Report and the MESS Board in the SICU Nurse's conference room.

The Stop Light Report identifies nursing unit projects that are complete, in progress, or unable to be completed and why. An example is "SBAR-online." For example, the nurse giving the unit's end of shift report identifies for each patient, as needed, any information regarding the patient's current Situation, Background, Assessment, and any Recommendations for follow up. This information is documented and updated each shift electronically to ensure ongoing nursing assessment of patient needs, adjustment of the plan of care to meet the patient's emerging needs, continuity of care, and clear communication between the inter-professional team and between nursing shifts. All patients have an SBAR online that nurses use for inter-professional communication and shift report. It is updated each shift.

The "**MESS**" Board identifies **Methods, Equipment, Staff, and Supplies** and addresses the Patient Care Manager/Assistant Patient Care Manager, Charge RNs, or Patient Support Associates (**PSAs**) and Guests to the unit. The green dots identify "Go" (things are running smoothly). Red dots identify that there are issues that have been identified as a problem.

4. Shift Huddle Guidelines and the Huddle Process

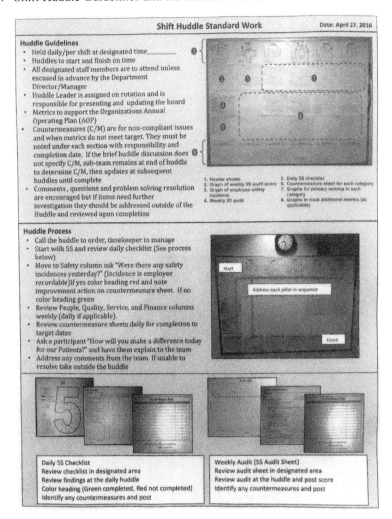

This poster identifies Shift Huddle Guidelines and the Huddle Process. Huddles are used to review daily the above Managing for Daily Improvement Poster Goals related to the Safety, People, Quality, Service, and Finance Pillars, in order to assure patient-centered, evidence-based, high-quality, safe patient care. Huddles are performed each shift at a designated time.

5. University of Chicago Medicine Hospital (**UCMC**) Annual Operating Plan

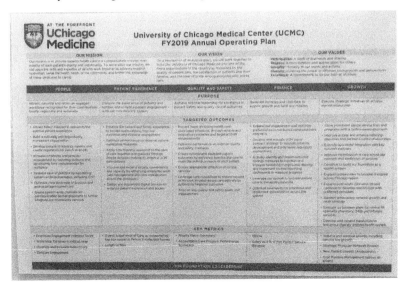

The University of Chicago Medicine Hospital (UCMC) Annual Operating Plan is posted as part of the Magnet Mission Poster and displayed in the Surgical Intensive Care Unit nurse's conference room at UCMC. Included on the poster is information about the UCMC Mission, Vision and Values, as well as the Purpose, Targeted Outcomes, and Key Metrics related to People, Patient Experience, Quality and Safety, Finance, and Growth. This information is reviewed by all the unit's nurses and other inter-professional staff, both informally and in huddles, etc., in order to deliver patient-centered, evidence-based, high-quality, safe patient care.

6. Standard Pathway for Prevention of Catheter-Associated Urinary Tract Infections (**CAUTI**)

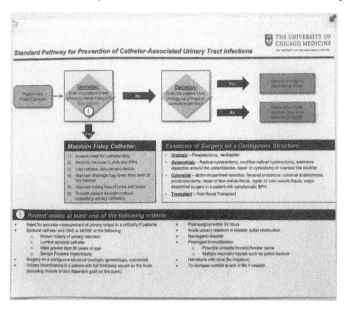

This is the Standard Pathway for Prevention of Catheter-Associated Urinary Tract Infections (CAUTI), which includes nursing decision criteria for insertion of a catheter, as well as criteria for ongoing maintenance and prevention of CAUTI.

7. Clean Hands Reminder

I'll bee watching you......

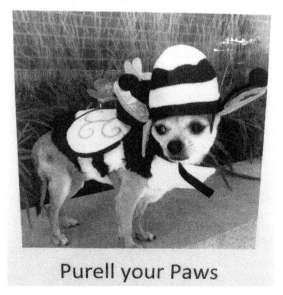

Purell your Paws

This is a cute picture of a small dog, Zoey, owned by Peggy Zemansky, the unit manager, reminding all members of the interprofessional team to use Purell hand sanitizer pre- and post-patient care.

8. Advanced Airway Cart

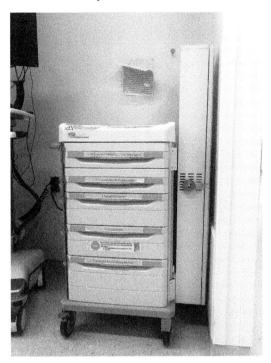

This is an Advanced Airway Cart which is available on the Unit in case of difficult airway placement. The Advanced Airway cart has labeled drawers, like a crash cart, but with equipment that may be used in critical airway situations. The cart contents are verified each shift. The Advanced Airway Cart is checked each shift to endure its readiness in case of an emergency.

9. Zero Tolerance Policy

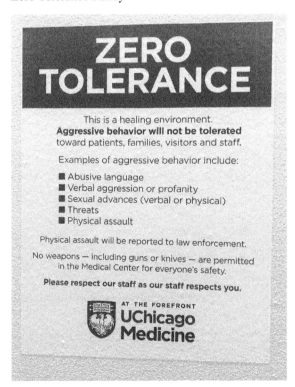

The Zero Tolerance Policy is used to remind all patients, family, visitors, and staff that there is Zero Tolerance for aggressive behavior and actions by anyone.

10. Surgical Intensive Care Unit Center Quality Measures Performance

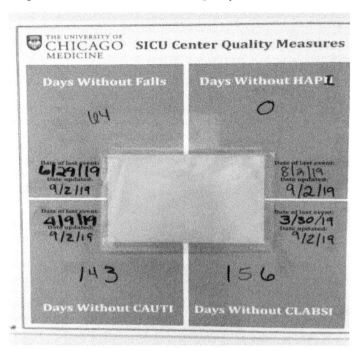

This is a photo of a poster identifying the Surgical Intensive Care Unit's Center Quality Measures Performance on Days without Falls, Days without Hospital Acquired Pressure Injury (**HAPI**), Days without Catheter-Induced Urinary Tract Infections (**CAUTI**), and Days without Central Line-Associated Blood Stream Infections (**CLABSI**). Keeping these indicators present on the unit reminds everyone on the health care team about quality and safety vigilance.

11. University of Chicago Medicine Hospital's Nursing Councils

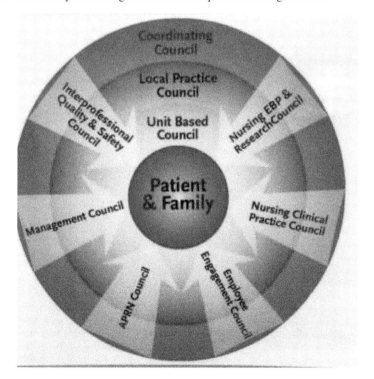

This poster identifies the University of Chicago Medicine Hospital's Nursing Councils which assist in meeting the Hospital's commitment to the Patient and Family or patient-centered care.

12. Staff Education about Prevention of Patient Heel Pressure Injuries

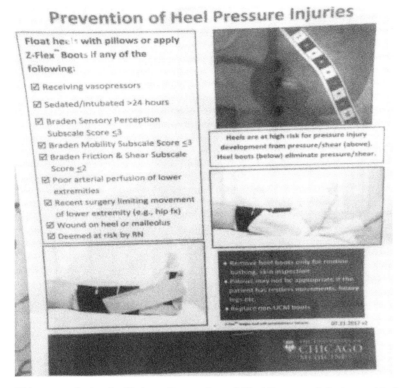

This poster is for Staff about Prevention of Heel Pressure Injuries and helps visually to remind staff how to prevent patient heel pressure injuries.

13. Patient and Family Centered Care Model.

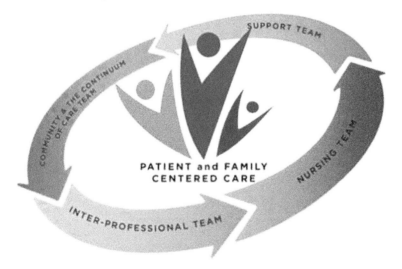

The University of Chicago Medicine Nursing Department's Commitment Model demonstrates the provision of Patient and Family Centered Care by the support team, nursing team, inter-professional team, the community, and the continuum of care team.

14. Hand Hygiene Reminder for Families and Friends

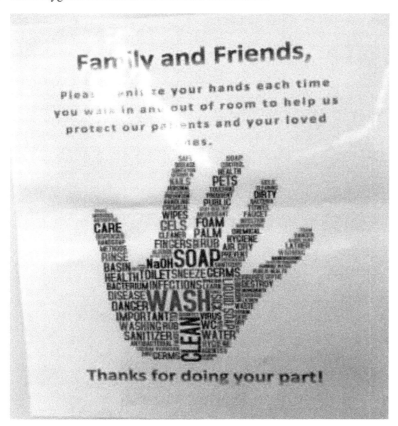

This photo of the Hand Hygiene Reminder for Families and Friends Poster illustrates the need for good hand hygiene. This reminds Family and Friends to sanitize their hands each time they walk in and out of patient's room and reminds visitors that they play a part in protecting family and friends in the hospital's fight against infections.

15. Patient Fall Protocol

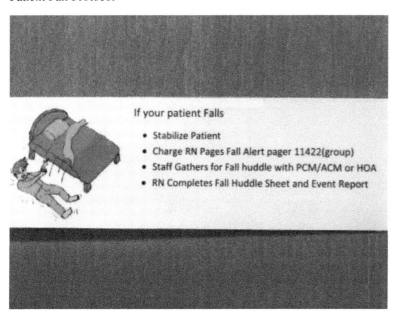

This is a photo of the Patient Fall Protocol, demonstrating that patient falls are monitored closely. After stabilizing a patient who has fallen, the charge nurse must be made aware and pages a Fall Alert. A staff huddle is then performed with the nurse manager, and the RN must complete a Fall Huddle sheet and an Event Report.

16. Patient Transfers

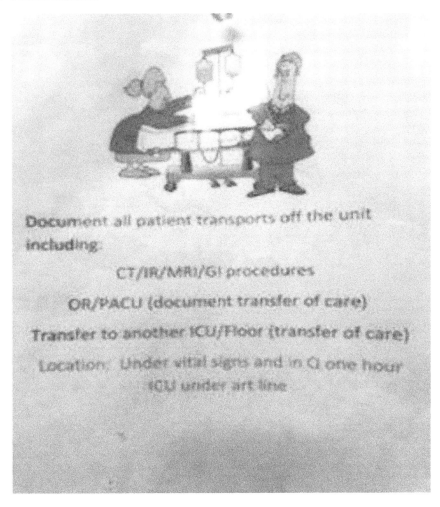

This photo about Patient Transfers is a staff reminder to document all patient transfers off the unit. These transports may include CT, computerized tomography, IR, interventional radiation, MRI, magnetic resonance imaging, OR, operating room, PACU, post-anesthesia care unit, and ICU, intensive care unit.

17. ExtraCorporeal Membrane Oxygenation (**ECMO**)

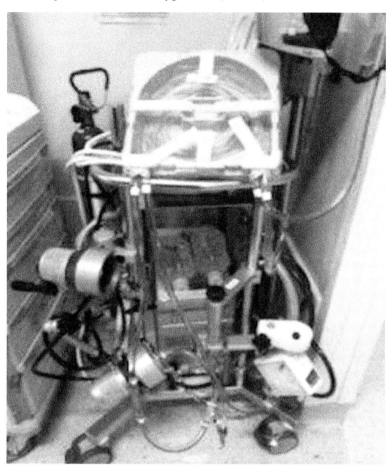

This is a photo of an ExtraCorporeal Membrane Oxygenation (ECMO) machine used to support critically ill patients. It provides prolonged cardiac and respiratory support to persons whose heart and lungs are unable to provide an adequate amount of gas exchange or perfusion to sustain life.

18. Suction Set-Up

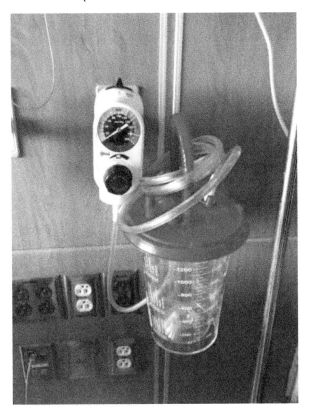

This is a photo of a Suction Set Up, which is emergency equipment available at the patient's bedside.

19. Patient Information Board

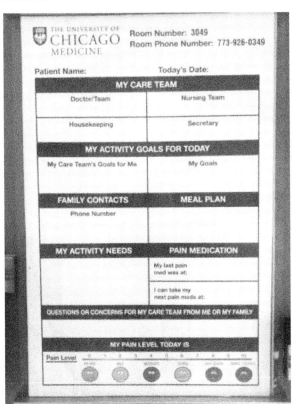

This is a photo of a Patient Information Board that is present in every patient room to help communicate with the patient and family. It is updated each shift.

20. Computer with Bar Code Scanner

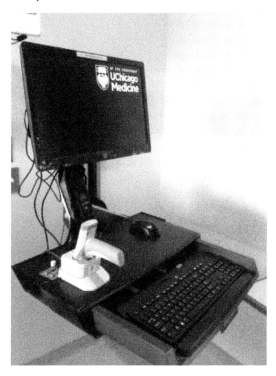

This is a Computer with Bar Code Scanner, which is available in acute hospitals in the United States and many developed countries. They are used in many hospitals for bedside documentation, patient wristband scanning for medication administration, etc.

21. Admission Supplies

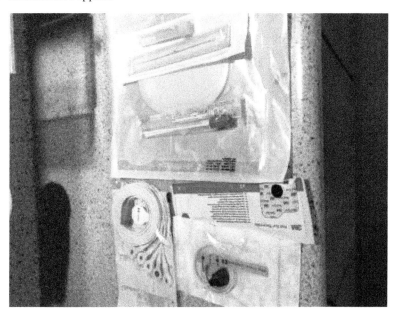

This photo of Admission Supplies shows supplies gathered in anticipation of a patient's admission: swabs for C-Diff and MRSA, EKG patches and leads, pulse oximetry, and a protective coccyx dressing.

22. Electronic Sling

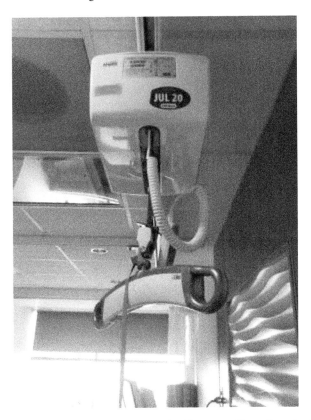

This is a photo of an Electronic Sling, a ceiling sling device that allows the nurse to safely move patients from bed to chair. Always check the weight load on this equipment prior to use.

23. Code Cart/Crash Cart

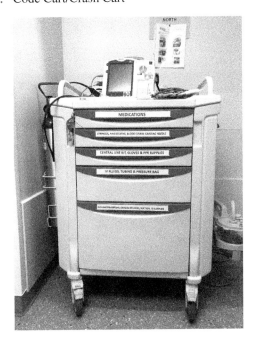

Code cart or crash carts are kept on every unit in case of a medical emergency. A defibrillator is placed on top of the cart and always plugged in while not in use. The drawers are labeled for quick access to items and include: medications, central line kit, gloves & PPE supplies. IV fluids, tubing and pressure bag. There is a suction set up on the cart as well as an oxygen tank. Equipment on and in the code cart/crash cart are verified each shift. Nurses should familiarize themselves with the cart and its contents.

Preparation to Assume New Position as Bedside Staff Nurse Leader and Manager of Various Types of Patients

Carolyn Ruud

Northwestern Delnor Hospital, Geneva, IL, USA
Chamberlain College of Nursing, Addison, IL, USA
Aurora University, Aurora, IL, USA

Review patient care for most common types of patients cared for on your unit, for example:

Medical Unit Patient Examples
Chronic Obstructive Pulmonary Disease; Pneumonia; Oncology; Diabetes; Fractures; Infection, e.g., Urinary Tract Infection, etc.;
Complex medication regimes, e.g., Intravenous Immunoglobulin (**IVIG**);
Unable to care for self; Needs Nursing Home Placement

Surgical Unit Patient Examples
Renal disease with dialysis; Abdominal surgery; Gynecological surgery;
Trauma with chest tubes, etc.; Organ failure, e.g., liver, kidney, etc.

Cardiac Telemetry Unit Patient Examples
Myocardial Infarction; Congestive Heart Failure; Pneumonia; Angiogram; Angioplasty with simple intervention; Carotid Endarterectomy;
Substance Abuse with withdrawal

Neurology Unit Patient Examples
Spinal surgery; Stable Craniotomy; Cerebral Vascular Accident (**CVA**);
Altered mental status, i.e., rule out CVA

Critical Care/Trauma Unit Patient Examples
Pneumonia; Infection; Ventilator, Shock, Complex CVA, Craniotomy;
Unstable Bilevel Positive Airway Pressure (**BiPAP**), at risk for intubation;
Requires hemodynamic monitoring; Unstable trauma

Stepdown Unit Patient Examples
Needs hemodynamic monitoring (At risk for deterioration);
Has stable Bilevel Positive Airway Pressure (BiPAP);
Needs The Clinical Institute Withdrawal Assessment for Alcohol (**CIWA**) Protocol or The Clinical Opiate Withdrawal Scale (**COWS**) Protocol;
Is post complex angioplasty intervention; has Myocardial Infarction without vasoactive agents

Nursing Protocol for All Above Patients

Review evidence-based clinical practice guidelines for patients you will care for on your unit. A good way to keep up with clinical practice guidelines is to belong to your nursing practice association. They provide regular updates and practice guidelines and also provide current and archive journals. Review the clinical practice guidelines in this Appendix to learn more about evidence-based practice for nurses.

Review the most common medications used for these patients on your unit, for example: Albuterol, Apixaban, Atorvastatin, Budesonide-Formoterol, Cetirizine, Carvedilol, Cephalexin, Coumadin, Diazepam, Digoxin, Diphenhydramine, Dopamine, Dobutamine, Enoxaparin, Famotidine, Ferrous sulfate, Glycopyrrolate, Heparin, Hydralazine, Hydrocodone-Acetaminophen, Hydromorphone, Insulin, Ipratropium, Ketorolac, Labetalol, Furosemide, Levothyroxine, Levophed, Epinephrine, Metoclopramide HCl, Montelukast, Morphine, Nitroglycerine, Amlodipine, Ondansetron, Pantoprazole, Penicillin, Potassium, Clopidogrel, Pravastatin, Lisinopril, Compazine, Metoprolol, Simvastatin, Tissue Plasminogen Activator (TPA).

Consider what health care structures and processes are needed to achieve good patient care outcomes:

- Structures (supplies, unit structures, and equipment, etc.)

- Electronic documentation for point of care documentation—if nurse uses computer on wheels, the computer needs to be functional with a plan for real time computer back up and repair

- Unit-based Council where the voice of all staff (Nurses and Unlicensed Assistive Personnel (UAP) can proactively discuss, formulate, and develop best practices for the unit)

- Multiple, well-located supply areas for staff to avoid "hunting" for supplies

- Processes (staffing guidelines, patient care routines, clinical practice guidelines, etc.)

- Use an evidence-based rounding process, e.g., hourly rounding decreases falls, improves patient outcomes, and increases patient satisfaction

- Outcomes—Monitor patient satisfaction and patient outcomes. Assume leadership rounding to improve patient care outcomes.

Work on becoming an expert nurse and certified in your area of practice, for example, ACLS, CCRN, CEN, CPN, OCN, ONC, RN-BC, etc. See list of certifications at, https://nurse.org/articles/nursing-certifications-credentials-list/, accessed July 5, 2019.

Develop a professional style of inter-professional teamwork and communication, dress, speech, etc.

Develop good rapport and communication with other staff on your unit. Some units develop a "Buddy for the Day" System. A Buddy for the Day is your go-to person for help with patient care during the shift, for coverage for breaks and lunch, and for consistency with patients. Charge nurses and other staff have many competing priorities and when you need to have help, they may not be able to help. A Buddy for the Day System allows the RN and UAP to have uninterrupted breaks and lunch and allows patients to regularly see a "Buddy," who is a familiar face from their team when their assigned RN and/or UAP is not available. Working on units that do not use the Buddy for the Day System for breaks and lunch means that nurses and UAP may not be able to go on uninterrupted breaks. The Literature supports that best practice is to have an uninterrupted break.

Preparation to Assume New Position as Bedside Staff Nurse Leader and Manager of Patients on Labor and Delivery Unit

Beth L. A. Richard
Northwestern Delnor Hospital, Geneva, IL, USA
Waubonsee Community College, School of Nursing, Aurora, IL, USA

A. Identify the 5 most common types of patients cared for on this unit.

Patients:

- with Spontaneous Labor

- with Induced Labor

- scheduled for Cesarean Section

- with Post-Partum Hemorrhage needing the Massive Transfusion Protocol

- who are Antepartum (Preterm Labor, Preeclampsia [mild, moderate, and severe]), Type 1 & Type 2 Diabetes and Cholestasis)

- who are Outpatients (with decreased fetal movements, trauma to abdomen, pregnancy induced hypertension, Urinary Tract Infections, and preterm labor)

B. Review patient care clinical Practice Guidelines for these types of patients, e.g.,
The Association of Women's Health, Obstetric and Neonatal Nurses (**AWHONN**) Position Statement on Fetal Monitoring (2015).
AWHONN. *Guidelines for Professional Registered Nurse Staffing for Perinatal Units, 2019.*
Guidelines for Oxytocin Administration after Birth: AWHONN Practice Brief Number 2, 2014.
California Maternal Quality Care Collaborative (**CMQCC**) Toolkits, e.g.,

- Pre-Eclampsia Toolkit, 2014

- OB Hemorrhage Toolkit, 2015

Carlson, N. Current Resources for Evidence-Based Practice, July/August 2016.

C. Review common medications used for patients on your unit

- Pitocin

- Cytotec

- Magnesium Sulfate

- Ropivacaine/Fentanyl

- Labetalol/Hydralazine

- Insulin

- Astramorph

- Pepcid

- Betamethasone

- Penicillin

D. The Charge Nurse is tasked with utilizing the team to make decisions for the safest care and best patient outcomes by assigning more expert nurses vs. novice nurses to a high acuity patient or maybe an expert and novice nurse both assigned so the novice nurse is able to gain experience and knowledge from the expert nurse.

E. Inter-Professional Teamwork is the backbone of patient care. Without this teamwork, we do not give excellent patient care to our patients. The team bonds better when all members are working in tandem.

F. All communication is done professionally. RNs utilize the Situation, Background, Assessment, and Recommendation (SBAR) format when reporting information to a Physician or another member of the inter-professional team. New novice nurses on the unit can get help and guidance from competent to expert nurses on the unit in using this important communication skill.

G. The Health Insurance Portability and Accountability Act (HIPAA) Guidelines are followed by all members of the inter-professional team to protect patient privacy and confidentiality. All team members are encouraged to stay off their personal phones, social media, and Facebook while in a patient care area

H. Your dress code varies with your nursing role. Professional nursing scrubs are worn by nurses working at the bedside who all wear royal blue scrubs, which differentiates the nurses from other hospital health care workers; professional business attire is worn by those nurses working in management, quality, and other non-patient care areas.

I. This hospital has achieved Magnet Recognition, which identifies hospitals whose nursing leaders have aligned their nursing strategic goals to improve the organization's patient outcomes and provide a roadmap to high-quality, safe, patient-centered care and nursing excellence on all patient care units, including the Labor and Delivery Unit.

J. Expert nurses drive themselves forward to achieve nursing certifications and give excellent care to their patients. Consider what type of nurse are you going to be? Will you be an Obstetric (OB) nurse, Pediatric nurse, or Medical-Surgical nurse, etc.? Your answer will guide your choice of certifications based on your practice. Labor and Delivery nurses are certified in Basic Life Support (BLS), Advanced Cardiac Life Support (ACLS), and in the Neonatal Resuscitation Program (NRP). These nursing certifications are required to work on the Labor and Delivery unit. Mother/Baby Couplet Care nurses are certified in BLS and NRP. BLS and NRP certifications are required for nurses to work on the Mother/Baby Couplet Care unit. External Fetal Monitoring, Low Risk Maternal Newborn, and Inpatient OB are examples of certifications that both a Labor and Delivery nurse and a Mother/Baby Couplet Care nurse may have when working at the bedside to improve patient outcomes. The OB unit also has International Board-Certified Lactation Consultants on staff who can be supported by Mother/Baby Couplet Care nurses who obtain a breastfeeding counselor certification.

WEB RESOURCES

California Maternal Quality Care Collaborative (CMQCC) Toolkits. (2014). Preeclampsia Toolkit , available at www.cmqcc.org/resources-tool-kits/toolkits/preeclampsia-toolkit, accessed September 4, 2019.

California Maternal Quality Care Collaborative (CMQCC) Toolkits. OB Hemorrhage Toolkit (2015), available at www.cmqcc.org/resources-tool-kits/toolkits/ob-hemorrhage-toolkit, accessed September 4, 2019.

Carlson, N. (July/August, 2016). Current Resources for Evidence-Based Practice. Journal of Obstetric, Gynecologic, & Neonatal Nursing (JOGNN), 45(4), e9–e14. doi: https://doi.org/10.1016/j.jogn.2016.06.002, retrieved from www.jognn.org/article/S0884-2175(16)30206-4/pdf, accessed September 4, 2019.

Merrill, L. (February–March, 2013). Nursing for Women's Health, 17(1), 42–51. Magnesium Sulfate During Anticipated Preterm Birth for Infant Neuroprotection. doi: https://doi.org/10.1111/1751-486X.12005

The Association of Women's Health, Obstetric and Neonatal Nurses (AWHONN) position statement on fetal monitoring. (June 2015). Journal of Obstetric, Gynecologic, & Neonatal Nursing (JOGNN), 44, 683-686. doi: 10.1111/1552-6909.12743. available at www.jognn.org/article/S0884-2175(15)35318-1/pdf, accessed September 4, 2019.

The Association of Women's Health, Obstetric and Neonatal Nurses (AWHONN). Guidelines for Oxytocin Administration after Birth: AWHONN Practice Brief Number 2. 2014. JOGNN, 44, 161–163; 2015. doi: 10.1111/1552-6909.12528 C 2014 s

AWHONN. Guidelines for Professional Registered Nurse Staffing for Perinatal Units (2019). Available at www.awhonn.org/store/ViewProduct.aspx?id=5152716, retrieved September 11, 2019.

Daily RN Shift Timeline for Nursing Care of Patients on Labor and Delivery (L&D) Unit

Beth L. A. Richard
Northwestern Delnor Hospital, Geneva, IL, USA
Waubonsee Community College, School of Nursing, Aurora, IL, USA

RN accountable to lead patient achievement of safe, high-quality, patient-centered care outcomes

0700	Huddle with Oncoming shift of RNs; support staff including Unit Clerks, Patient Care Technicians (**PCT**), Obstetrical Surgical Technicians (**OBT**); and the Charge Nurse. Unit Clerks work closely with the Charge RN over the course of the day, by answering phone calls and keeping the Charge RN appraised of any new outpatients coming over from provider offices for evaluation. The PCTs are the helping hands of the Mother/Baby Couplet nurses, who delegate patient care within the PCT scope of practice to assist in care of the Mother/Baby Couplet, i.e., completing the newborn baby's bath or helping mom up to the bathroom. The OBT has multiple roles and functions as a Patient Care Technicians (PCT) in L&D, assisting with patients going to the bathroom or needing position changes; the OBT also assist in the Operating Room for both scheduled and emergency Cesarean Sections patients. They are responsible for keeping standard supply levels in L&D and the operating rooms.
0710–0730	Shift Handoff Report, previous shift RN, and oncoming shift RN
0715–1900	Rounding, Assessment, and Documentation of Mother and Fetus well-being, coping, and pain every 15, 30, or 60 min, throughout shift, depending on stage of labor and how Mother and Fetus are coping. Assessment and documentation to include: monitoring of patient's labor with assessment of patient, IV, labor progression, and vital signs based on needs of patient and stage of labor. Temperature is checked every 4 hours until amniotic sac is ruptured, then temperature is monitored hourly, along with vaginal bleeding assessment and fetal monitoring.

Turn patient every 30 min throughout entire labor process unless fetus is not tolerating a position; in that case, turn patient immediately.

Diet of Clear liquids or NPO, depending on stage of labor, Document Intake and Output

Patient is included in the plan of care by discussing patient desires for her birth experience and pain management. Patients are encouraged to be active participants in their own care. Nurse does a visual sweep of the room for safety equipment each time the nurse enters the room, e.g., emergency equipment and suction for Mom and baby. Check that all patient's personal belongings are within reach, for example call light, water, TV remote, cell phone, glasses, tissues, etc.

For patients who are new admissions, the RN completes a physical assessment, history: current pregnancy, past pregnancies, surgical history, past medical history, and social history. The RN starts the patient's IV; draws their blood for lab work; and obtain consents signed for the epidural, consents for medications for the newborn, and consents for an obstetrical delivery, as ordered.

The RN communicates with the Charge RN if assistance is needed with admitting a new patient and/or if any unusual findings are assessed, for example an abnormal Blood Pressure of above 160 systolic or 110 diastolic. This finding would prompt the Charge RN to assess the need for a new staffing assignment(s) based on the patient's higher acuity and the RN's need for help with any special procedures, monitoring, preparation of medications, or STAT Cesarean Section.

For patients who need Induction Of Labor (**IOL**), the RN will assess and record mother and fetal vital signs and status. The RN starts IV Pitocin for IOL and offers patients support for their pain and labor (position changes, walking on unit while on wireless fetal monitoring system, etc.), based on patient need.

When a patient requests an epidural, the RN may collaborate with more than one physician at once, such as the OB and the Anesthesiologist. The OB will give the order that the patient may have the epidural and the nurse will manage the mother and fetus related to the OB standing protocol for monitoring uterine contractions and fetal heart rate. The nurse is integral to the monitoring process to help keep mother and fetus safe during the epidural and continuation of the labor process.

0715–1900	For patients who request epidural placement, the RN will prepare the patient with a loading dose of a crystalloid solution per anesthesia standing protocol and position the patient for epidural placement. The RN will obtain a signed patient epidural consent and have it ready for the Anesthesiologist to sign. During the epidural process, the medications that Anesthesia uses will sometimes decrease the mother's BP to a dangerously low BP, e.g., 80 systolic or 50 diastolic. A loading dose of crystalloid solution is one way to proactively prevent a dramatic drop in BP. The Anesthesiologist generally remains at the bedside or in the nurses station until the mother and fetus are stable. The patient's BP is checked every 2 min for 20 min' post placement of the epidural. The Anesthesiologist has standing protocols for medications like ephedrine, if needed to increase the BP.

If the patient experiences a dramatic drop in BP, the lowered mean arterial pressure decreases placenta perfusion and impacts the O_2/CO_2 gas exchange. This can lower the fetal heart rate to less than 110 beats per minute. If the fetal heart rate remains 110 beats per minute or lower for longer than 10 min, the fetus is bradycardic. The Charge RN is an expert and leader on the unit to assist the primary RN with tasks or communication that would be difficult for her to complete while the primary RN is at the bedside caring for the patient. The Charge RN can contact the OB and give an SBAR report to the OB while interventions are being completed per the OB standing protocol. Examples of these interventions would be to turn the Pitocin off if there is a category II fetal heart rate strip that is requiring intervention, giving a crystalloid bolus, or changing the patient's position. |
| 0730 | Document vital signs for mother, fetal heart rate, and frequency and timing of uterine contractions. |
| 0735–0800 | |
| | Establish baseline of patient care for the day
Update OB and Neonatal Nurse Practitioner (NNP) on progress of labor and any need for the presence of the NNP for delivery. Develop the plan of care as an inter-professional team. Is the newborn going to be less than 35 weeks gestation at delivery, indicating a need for the NNP? Has there been fetal heart rate decelerations? Will the physician be placing forceps or a vacuum on the fetal head to help facilitate a vaginal delivery?
Assess the patient's needs and show her different methods of pain management and labor support. If the patient is 6 cm dilated and in active labor, the nurse may delegate to the OBT to set up the delivery cart to assist the OB in delivery of the newborn. |
| 0945–1045 | |
| | Ongoing Patient Assessment and labor support
Complete patient assessments and daily care documentation |
| 1045–1200 | Ongoing Patient Assessment and labor support. Rounding Huddle with OB, NNP, and Charge Nurse, keeping all of them abreast of patient labor progression and patient needs.
• Is the patient ready for an epidural or for a pain medication?
• Evaluate maternal and fetal heart rate for Pitocin or Cytotec effectiveness
• Is the tocodynamometer, which monitors contractions externally, giving a clear clinical picture re frequency and length of contractions? If the clinical picture is unclear, does the nurse need to ask for an Intra-Uterine Pressure Catheter (IUPC) to monitor the safe administration of Pitocin and Cytotec and keep the fetus safe? Safety becomes an issue related to the mothers' uterus possibly rupturing and the fetal O_2/CO_2 gas exchange becoming compromised when there are not enough rest periods between contractions and tachysystole of 6 or greater contractions within a 10-minute window ensues. Tachysystole does not support a safe environment for the mother's uterus or the fetus. Pitocin is a high-risk medication, administered with extreme care and accuracy while the patient's uterine contractions are being monitored.
• The physician is notified of tachysytole and the nurse would SBAR the assessment of the uterus and request use of the tachysytole protocol, as appropriate, if the OB was not present at the bedside. The nurse may request the OB to come to the bedside for an assessment of the patient.
• Report any new patient findings immediately such as spontaneous rupture of membranes and what the amniotic fluid looks like, for example, is it clear fluid, meconium fluid, or bloody fluid? How much fluid is present? Small, moderate, large, or copious amounts? Report fetal heart rate status and any nursing interventions while reviewing the fetal heart rate strip. |
| 1830–1900 | Final Hourly Rounding, Documentation, Check Orders, Intake and Output, and wrap up of delivery. If the patient is not delivered, then a thorough SBAR bedside report will be given to the oncoming nurse along with introduction to their new patient for the shift. |
| 1900 | Handoff and completion of shift (documentation, new orders, etc.) |

In addition to the above, depending on type of patient:

• On Post Delivery Mother/Baby Couplet unit, assessments to include: mother's fundal assessment, vitals, bleeding, patient teaching about postpartum care, e.g., peri care, appropriate amount of bleeding once discharged home, care of newborn, e.g., feedings, circumcision care, bottle feeding or breastfeeding, etc.

The Labor and Delivery RN is responsible for patient achievement of safe, high-quality, patient-centered care outcomes. The nurse makes critical decisions to keep the mother and baby safe while working within the nursing scope of practice and protocols and establishing rapport with each OB that babies mothers on the unit. The OB actively engages the L&D nurse as their eyes and ears while the OB is away from the bedside. It is the responsibility of the Labor and Delivery nurse to be proactive with patient care and keep the OB updated with all crucial information related to the progress of the patient in Labor.

DAILY RN SHIFT TIMELINE (EXAMPLE) FOR NURSING CARE OF PATIENTS ON MEDICAL, SURGICAL, INTENSIVE/CRITICAL CARE AND STEPDOWN UNITS, LABOR AND DELIVERY, MOTHER/BABY, PEDIATRIC, AND PSYCHIATRIC UNITS

Carolyn Ruud
Northwestern Delnor Hospital, Geneva, IL, USA
Chamberlain College of Nursing, Addison, IL, USA
Aurora University, Aurora, IL, USA

RN accountable to lead patient achievement of safe, high-quality, patient-centered care outcomes

0700	Huddle with Oncoming shift of RNs. Unlicensed Assistive Personnel (**UAP**) have their own huddle at 0600, an hour before day shift so they are answering lights, etc., during 0700 huddle. The night nurses are answering lights during the 0600 UAP huddle.
0705–0730	Shift Handoff Report at the bedside between night shift RN, the oncoming day shift RN, and the patient. The White Board in the patient's room is updated with patient's name, Doctor's name, and significant family contact information. Patient's care goals for the day are reviewed with patient and placed on the White Board.
0730–0800	Assess patients and give report to UAP. Delegate patient care expectations and identify reporting times and parameters. Identify Regular and PRN Times for UAP to Report Patient Problems, Vitals, Blood Sugars, etc., to RN. UAP also checks their worklist on electronic documentation system.
0800–1100	Vital Signs, Medications, Documentation UAP check and record vitals and blood glucose and report abnormal findings to RN. RN verifies breakfast ordered and trays are delivered to all patients' bedsides. RN gives medications. Insulin is given when the Diabetic patient's breakfast tray arrives, based on blood glucose. UAP and/or RN assist patient to eat, as needed. Begin hourly patient rounds and use the 5 Ps (Pain, Position, Potty, Pump, Possessions) as a reminder when rounding. UAP and RN alternate hourly rounds and decide who rounds on even hours and who rounds on the odd hours. Also, housekeeping staff, dietary hostesses, and any other staff are encouraged to check the 5 Ps when entering patient rooms. This provides more eyes on the patient for safety. Document patient assessments. Check morning labs, orders, and plan of care. RN assesses need to talk to MD regarding new orders for safe, high-quality patient-centered care. Has anything been missed? What are the barriers to patient discharge? What is needed to assure the plan of care is moving forward? RN uses the hospital chain of command, if needed, to assure patient's need for high-quality, safe, patient-centered care is met. RN rounds with primary physicians, consultants, and/or Nurse Practitioners as they arrive on unit. All arrive at different times. RN is available for rounds to provide consistency in the plan of care, support the patient needs for clarification, and assure good patient outcomes. (Charge nurse is the back up for rounds, but it is preferred that the primary care nurse rounds). Discharge rounds with Social Services, nurse case manager, charge nurse, and, on some units, the physician, nurse practitioner, and dietary, to discuss barriers to patient discharge (timing of rounds depends on unit). Check, does patient have any discharge planning needs? Is follow up needed? Discharge rounds allow an average time of 2–3 minutes for each patient and discuss the reason the patient was hospitalized, any barriers to discharge, and any need for consultants. The RN assesses that the unit structures (e.g., staffing, supplies, Code Blue Cart, etc.) and work processes (team work, staffing, evidence-based standards, informatics, clear communication, etc.) are in place to achieve high-quality, safe, patient-centered outcomes. RN and UAP regularly check if the patient has any needs and RN takes action to assure that safe, high-quality, patient-centered care structures and processes are in place to achieve high-quality patient outcomes. For example, on each unit, the Code Blue Cart is checked by the charge RN when coming on shift, for example, is the Code Blue Cart handy? Is it completely stocked, as needed?

RN does ongoing assessment and checks the following, in addition to the 5 Ps:
- Is patient NPO for lab, tests, surgery, etc. If so, assure Dietary is aware of this. The dietary hostesses deliver food to rooms and need to know which patients are Diabetics, who is NPO, who is a 1 : 1 feed patient, to assure patient safety, etc.
- Is patient oriented and safe? ABCs Okay? Need Side Rails? Help with Bathing? Oral Hygiene? Linen Change? Eating? Dressing Change? Comfort? Oxygen? Ambulation? If patient on Bedrest, plan discussed with UAP to turn patient at least every 2 hr and offload patient's bony prominences. Does patient need a specialty bed to prevent skin breakdown? Check if patient needs foam boots to prevent heel ulcers.
- Does patient need help to prevent Hazards of Immobility, maintain good skin care, turn, cough, and deep breathe Q2H?
- Does patient need help to ambulate 4–5 times daily and/or be put in chair for all meals, unless contraindicated? Are Sequential Compression Devices in place?

0900–1000	Break as time allows (bathroom, drink)
0900–1100	AM patient care by UAP (RN assists, as needed, with complicated patients (baths, ambulation, treatments).
1100–1200	Continue patient care, procedures, patient rounds, assessment, and documentation.
1200–1400	Check Vital Signs
	30 min lunch-use assigned Buddy RN to monitor and coordinate patient care in RN absence
	UAP check Blood Sugars
	Pass Medications, Check New Orders, Check new lab and test results
1300–1900	Patient Admissions, Discharges, and Transfers to unit (may occur anytime during shift). Patient medications, treatments, documentation. Check for new orders. Assure fluid balance. Intake and Output are recorded and assessed.
1500–1600	Vital signs review and patient care, as needed. If this is an 8-hr shift, RN or UAP handoff to oncoming RN and/or UAP, using the same best practice processes listed earlier. If this is a 12-hr shift, continue the day.
1630–1700	Pass Medications, assure patient receives dinner and feed patient, if needed.
1700–1750	UAP report to RN on delegated patient care activities, Intake and Output, Vitals, etc.
	UAP Handoff at patient bedside. Update White Board. Complete the shift (documentation, new orders, intake and output, etc.)
1800–1850	Final Hourly Rounding, Documentation, Check new Orders, Complete shift, etc.) Reflect on your shift and ask yourself, what can I do to improve my patient care and prepare for tomorrow?
1800–1900	UAP Huddle
	RN Huddle
1900–1930	Handoff to oncoming nurse

5 Ps refers to hourly assessment of Patient Pain, Position (Need to change position every 2 hr), Potty (Need for bathroom assistance), Pump (Check IV site and IV fluid rate), Possessions (Check access to call light, cell phone, glasses, tissues, dentures, hearing aids, TV remote, etc.)

Note that, in addition to above, add to daily schedule on any of below units:
- On Medical Patient unit, assessments to include: vital signs, level of consciousness, airway, breathing and circulation, turn, cough, and deep breathe Q2H, intake and output, and intravenous (IV) and skin assessments. Follow up on abnormal labs and act based on orders or guidelines or protocols.
- On Surgical Patient unit, assessments to include: vital signs, level of consciousness, airway, breathing and circulation, check dressing status, turn, cough, and deep breathe Q2H, ambulation 3–5 or more times daily, fluid balance, intravenous (IV) assessments, and intake and output.
- Intensive/critical care units/stepdown (higher acuity units): assessments include vital signs more frequently or the same as on other units, depending on patient stability; intravenous (IV) and skin assessments, patient response to ventilator, continuous infusions of IV medications and cardiac, neurological, and pulmonary monitoring as well as skin and tissue perfusion monitoring and intake and output.
- On Labor and Delivery Patient unit, assessments to include: monitor patient's labor with assessment of Fetal heart rate, IV, labor progression, vaginal assessment, vaginal bleeding, blood pressure, etc.
- On Mother/Baby Patient unit, assessments to include: Mother/Baby assessment, vaginal assessment, vaginal bleeding, patient teaching about vaginal care and breast feeding, as well as care of newborn.
- On Pediatric Patient unit, assessments to include: child safety, toys, necessity of child's education during hospitalization.
- On Psychiatric Patient unit, assessments to include: assure patient safety, share information on counseling times, activity times on unit, etc.

Clinical Practice Guidelines

Carolyn Ruud
Northwestern Medicine Delnor Hospital, Geneva, IL, USA
Chamberlain College of Nursing, Addison, IL, USA
Aurora University, Aurora, IL, USA

Joanna Briggs Institute EBP Database, available at www.libraries.rutgers.edu/indexes/jbi, retrieved September 14, 2019.

U.S. Department of Veteran's Affairs, Clinical Practice Guidelines, available at www.healthquality.va.gov/, accessed September 14, 2019. There are Guidelines and Algorithms for Chronic Disease in Primary Care, Mental Health, Pain, Rehabilitation, Women's Health, and Military-Related Diseases.

Association of Rehabilitation Nurses Clinical Practice Guidelines, Multiple Sclerosis, available at https://rehabnurse.org/advance-your-practice/clinical-practice-guidelines, accessed September 15, 2019.

Cochrane Collaboration, available at www.cochrane.org/, retrieved September 14, 2019.

Joanna Briggs Institute EBP Database, available at www.libraries.rutgers.edu/indexes/jbi, retrieved September 14, 2019.

Registered Nurses' Association of Ontario, RNAO Best Practice Guidelines, available at http://careersinnursing.ca/new-nursing-and-students/becoming-registered-nurse/standards-and-best-practices, accessed September 15, 2019.

American Medical Association, Guideline Central, available at www.guidelinecentral.com/summaries/specialties/nursing/, accessed September 15, 2019.

Duke University Medical Center, Clinical Practice Guidelines, available at https://guides.mclibrary.duke.edu/nursing/guidelines, accessed September 15, 2019.

American Association of Neuroscience Nurses *Clinical Practice Guidelines,* available at http://aann.org/publications/clinical-practice-guidelines, accessed September 15, 2019.

Agency for Healthcare Research & Quality (AHRQ) research tools, available at www.ahrq.gov/, accessed September 23, 2019.

Appraisal of Guidelines for Research & Evaluation (AGREE) II, available at www.agreetrust.org/, accessed September 23, 2019.

American Nurses Association Research Toolkit, available at www.nursingworld.org/practice-policy/workforce/improving-your-practice/research-toolkit/, accessed September 23, 2019.

Health Sciences & Human Services Library, University of Maryland, available at https://guides.hshsl.umaryland.edu/c.php?g=94009&p=609190, accessed September 23, 2019.

Health links at the University of Washington, available at https://depts.washington.edu/hprc/evidence-based-programs/workplace-wellness-2/healthlinks/, accessed September 23, 2019, offers a guide to finding, learning and constructing questions in the pursuit of EBP.

Institute for Healthcare Improvement (IHI), available at www.ihi.org/, accessed September 23, 2019, is a primary resource for tools and methods to identify, design, and implement best practices. As the leading innovator in health care improvement, IHI is an invaluable resource for health and health care practices.

McMaster University, available at https://secretariat.mcmaster.ca/university-policies-procedures-guidelines/, accessed September 23, 2019, holds a library of resources aligned with the principles of EBP.

National Guideline Clearinghouse, available at www.ahrq.gov/gam/index.html, is coordinated by the AHRQ and provides structured, standardized summaries of clinical practice guidelines related to a wide range of clinical issues from regional, national, and international organizations. In many cases, links to the full documents are provided.

Oncology Nursing Society Evidence Based Resource Area, available at www.ons.org/explore-resources?display=source&source=1506&ref=RO, website contains a wealth of resources related to evidence based nursing practice, including an overview, tutorials, and a toolkit. Many resources are applicable in a wide range of settings, in addition to oncology settings.

Oxford Centre for Evidence-based Medicine, available at www.cebm.net/2009/06/oxford-centre-evidence-based-medicine-levels-evidence-march-2009/, provides in-depth strategies, resources, and references about appraising and using evidence in health care. Although intended primarily for physicians, the information is applicable to all health care providers with an interest in EBP.

PubMed's, available at www.ncbi.nlm.nih.gov/pubmed/, article database includes over 22 million citations from journal articles and online books related to biomedicine and health. A detailed tutorial about use of the database for conducting searches is provided. When available, links to full text articles are provided.

Registered Nurses Association of Ontario, available at https://rnao.ca/bpg, provides information and resources on development and utilization of nursing best practice guidelines. Although intended for members, the information is accessible to health care providers with an interest in best practices literature.

University of Texas Health Science Center School of Nursing Ace Star website, https://nursing.uthscsa.edu/onrs/starmodel/star-model.asp, for the Academic Center for Evidence-Based Practice (ACE) serves as a resource to bridge research to practice, to advance nursing roles, nursing knowledge and practice through education and resources.

The Turning Research Into Practice (*TRIP*) *database*, available at www.ncbi.nlm.nih.gov/pmc/articles/PMC1852635/, is a search engine that serves to help the user "find evidence fast" by entering keywords to search journal and database articles.

Emergency Nurses Association, www.ena.org/

Glossary of Terms

A Culture of Safety is one where everyone feels responsible for safety, pursues it on a daily basis, and is comfortable reporting unsafe conditions and behaviors.

A High Reliability Organization is an organization that achieves a culture of safety in dangerous environments, such as aviation, nuclear energy, and health care.

Academic practice partnerships are partnerships that allow academic institutions and health care organizations to create strategic relationships based on the advancement of their mutual interests related to practice, education, and research. These strategic relationships can be informal or formally defined and are important for increasing the pool of baccalaureate prepared nursing applicants, fostering the pursuit of Magnet designation, building a robust nursing workforce, and developing excellent clinical leaders.

Accountability is defined as to be answerable to oneself and others for one's own choices, decisions, and actions as measured against a standard. Nursing accountability includes the preparedness and obligation to explain or justify to relevant others (including the regulatory authority) the relevant judgments, intentions, decisions, actions, and omissions, as well as the consequences of those judgments, intentions, decisions, actions, and omissions. Being accountable as a nurse means being answerable for what one has done or said, or not done and standing behind that decision or action.

Action Plans are part of Root Cause Analyses and Strategic Planning. They are established based on priorities. Action plans include timelines, financial resources, and individuals responsible for the implementation.

Activity Log is a time management tool that can assist the nurse in determining how time is used. The activity log should be used for several days. The nurse should record every activity, from the beginning of the shift until the end, as well as periodically noting their feelings while doing the activities—alert, energetic, tired, bored, and so on.

Advanced Directive is a document that outlines the patient's wishes for what care should be provided if the patient cannot provide consent due to dementia, terminal illness, or lack of capacity.

Adverse Events also called serious safety events, occur during health care delivery when an error affects the patient, resulting in prolonged hospitalization or disability.

Advocacy is the process of exercising one's voice to communicate issues of concern and the need for action. This process promotes both self-interest and the interest of others, whether in the work setting, throughout the organization, or in the larger society.

Affective Domain is the learning domain involving feelings, emotions, beliefs, values, and willingness to engage (or participate). Learning in the affective domain cannot be directly observed but is demonstrated through attitudes and behaviors.

Affinity Diagram is a diagram that places similar items together so that the team can see where their individual ideas from brainstorming are alike.

Aggregate Reviews are when a series of similar adverse events or near misses are examined by an interprofessional team to determine if a pattern of breakdowns exists in the health care system that has caused such adverse events.

Alert Fatigue describes how busy workers (in the case of health care, clinicians) become desensitized to safety alerts, and as a result ignore or fail to respond appropriately to such warnings; also applies to alarms and notifications.

An Assignment is the "routine care, activities, procedures that are within the authorized scope of practice of the RN or LPN/LVN or part of the routine functions" of the UAP (NAP); "the distribution of work that each staff member is responsible for during a given work period."

Kelly Vana's Nursing Leadership and Management, Fourth Edition. Edited by Patricia Kelly Vana and Janice Tazbir
© 2021 John Wiley & Sons Ltd. Published 2021 by John Wiley & Sons Ltd.
Companion Website: www.wiley.com/go/kelly-Nursing-Leadership

An Incident Report is a document used by health care organizations for staff reporting of any adverse event such as a fall, medication error, or close call.

Ancillary Services Team completes specific tasks for the patient for a limited period of time, such as a Radiology Tech who completes a chest X-ray.

Assault is threatening to touch another person in an offensive manner without that person's permission.

Assistive Personnel (AP) is a term used to describe the personnel trained to "function in a supportive role, regardless of title, to whom nursing responsibility may be delegated. This includes but is not limited to certified nursing assistants or nursing aides (CNAs or NAs), patient care technicians, CMAs (certified medication aides), and home health aides (formerly referred to as 'unlicensed' assistive personnel (UAP))"

Authentic Leadership is one of the standards in American Association of Critical-Care Nurses (AACNs) Healthy Work Environment standards that requires core competencies of self-knowledge, strategic vision, risk taking and creativity, and interpersonal communication effectiveness and inspiration.

Authority Gradient refers to one's position within a group or profession.

Authority is the right to act or to command the action of others. Authority occurs when a person who has been given the right to delegate, based on the State Nurse Practice Act, also has the official power from an agency to delegate.

Autocratic leadership behavior is where the leader makes decisions using his/her power to command and control others; it is characterized by centralized decision making.

Autonomy is respect for an individual's right to self-determination and respect for individual liberty.

Balanced Scorecard is a framework to implement and manage strategy. It links a vision to strategic objectives, measures, targets, and initiatives. It balances financial measures with performance measures and objectives related to all other parts of the organization. This tool is used by hospital leadership to identify, track, and manage their strategy for achieving desired quality outcomes.

Battery is touching another person without that person's consent.

Benchmarking is the public reporting of data that helps patients make more informed choices about where to obtain their health care based on their individual needs and preferences.

Beneficence is the duty to do good to others and to maintain a balance between benefits and harms

Bias are factors outside of a research study which could affect the results.

Bibliographical Databases are a collection of bibliographical records which include descriptive information such as article title, abstract, journal information, but it does not include the full text of the article or item.

Bibliographical Records are records created with the purpose of being easily retrieved on command by keywords or subject headings. Each bibliographical record has information describing that article broken down into different sections which are called fields. These fields include article title, journal title, abstract, subjects, author names, etc.

Bioethics are health care ethics.

Blunt End The blunt end of a triangle refers to the many factors and decisions made before an actual error occurs. These factors and decisions may greatly influence the type and frequency of errors.

Boolean Operators are specific words that connect two terms with the goal of narrowing or broadening literature search results in electronic databases.

Brainstorming is a way to gather a lot of ideas very quickly.

Break-Even Point is when income and expenses are equal.

Brief provides a list of responsibilities of effective team leaders as well as checklists for sharing the plan. Prior to a start, the team meets to share the plan, assign roles, establish expectations, and anticipate outcomes and issues.

Budget is a plan that provides formal quantitative expression for acquiring and distributing funds over the ensuing time period (generally 1 year).

Call-Out Communication is a communication technique used in TeamSTEPPS® to communicate important information. It informs all team members simultaneously during an emergency and helps team members anticipate the next steps.

Call-Out is a communication technique informing all team members of the patient status simultaneously and allows the team to anticipate the next steps.

Career Path is a visual diagram developed by a process of self-reflection and goal setting, which helps align interests, ethical beliefs, and personal needs to a nursing career. A career path basically means the various positions an employee moves to one by one as the employee grows in an organization. The employee may move vertically most of the time but may also move laterally or cross-functionally to move to a different type of job role.

Certification is a formal recognition of the specialized knowledge, skills, and experience and is demonstrated by the achievement of standards identified by a nursing specialty to promote optimal health outcomes.

Check-Back is a closed loop communication technique which ensures that the message the sender intended was received by the intended recipient. The recipient acknowledges the communication by repeating back the information.

Clinical Indicators are clinical outcome data measured over time to assess the quality and safety of health care at a system level.

Clinical Information System (CIS) is an information system designed specifically for use in the hospital environment. It draws information from multiple systems into an electronic patient record.

Clinical Judgment (or Professional Clinical Judgment) is the "outcome of critical thinking or clinical reasoning, i.e., the conclusion, decision, or opinion you make after thinking about the issues."

Clinical Judgment Model is the observed outcome of critical thinking and decision making.

Clinical Ladder is a program established by a health care organization to encourage nurses to earn promotions, recognition, and increased pay by meeting specific requirements. Most programs have three or four distinct levels. Promotion in a specific track, such as a clinical, an educational, or a managerial track is possible in some organizations.

Clinical Librarians are those who specialize in supporting education needs of all members of the interprofessional health care team as well as patients in the health care environment.

Clinical Value Compass is a visual tool for evaluating the balance or imbalance between patient clinical and functional status, cost, and patient satisfaction outcomes.

Closed Loop Communication is a communication technique used in TeamSTEPPS to ensure that the message received is the same as what was intended by the sender. The sender initiates communication with a receiver by providing a request, information, or clinician order. The receiver acknowledges the communication with a repeat-back. The sender then confirms the accuracy of the acknowledgement by saying "that's correct."

Coercive Power is power that comes from the ability to punish others for their behavior.

Cognitive Domain is the learning domain involving the development of intellectual/mental skills including, remembering, understanding, and the acquisition of knowledge. The cognitive domain results cannot be directly observed but may be seen through behaviors.

Coinsurance Amounts is the fixed percentage of money a patient must pay for a health care services bill after the deductible is satisfied.

Collaboration is a process of sharing, involving both professionals within nursing (intra-professional) and other members of the health care team (inter-professional).

Collaborative Team Member is a team member who uses behaviors that ensure the partnership with the inter-professional team is one of trust and mutual respect.

Collective Bargaining Agent is an agent that works on behalf of employees to formalize collective bargaining through unionization.

Collective Bargaining is the practice of employees bargaining as a group with management for wages, benefits, and working conditions.

Commitment to Resilience is when leaders in the health care organization think about what could go wrong in a complex system and attempt to create backup systems to catch errors before any harm comes to the patient.

Communication is an interactive process that occurs when a person (the sender) sends a verbal or nonverbal message to another person (the receiver) and receives feedback.

Comorbidities are diseases or conditions that coexist with a primary disease but also stand on their own as specific diseases.

Compassion Fatigue is the inability to feel compassion for those who are suffering from constant exposure to human suffering.

Competence is the "ability to accomplish specific skills safely and effectively under various circumstances" and true competency is confirmed as nurses who "consistently display appropriate behaviors and sound judgments at the point of care."

Competency is a complex integration of knowledge including professional judgment, skills, values, and attitudes.

Complex Adaptive System is a system that is complex, nonlinear, interactive, and self-organizing with the capacity for self-renewal. This system can learn and adapt as a network of interacting, interdependent agents who cooperate in common goals and create new patterns of operating.

Complexity Leadership is a form of leadership described as transformational, collaborative, self-reflective, and relationship based. Complexity leaders see people in organizations as self-organizing and self-renewing and envision work occurring through relationships.

Computer Literacy is defined as the knowledge and understanding of computers, combined with the ability to use them effectively.

Confidentiality refers to the act of limiting disclosure of private matters. After a patient has disclosed private information to a health care provider, the provider has a responsibility to maintain the confidentiality of that information.

Conflict is two or more parties experiencing a breakdown in communication and/or human relations.

Connection Power is power that comes from personal and professional connections with others.

Consideration is the dimension of consideration that involves activities that focus on the employee and emphasizes relating and getting along with people. Leader behavior focuses on the well-being of others. The leader is involved in creating a relationship that fosters communication and trust as a basis for respecting other people and their potential contributions

Constitution is a written set of basic laws that specifies the powers of the various segments of a country's government and how those segments relate to each other.

Content Analysis is the analysis of specific information, facts, evidence, or content in any given context or medium.

Context Analysis is a review of both the situation in which the educational need arises and the instructional environment in which the education will occur. It is essentially a review of the circumstances that created the need for the education.

Contingency Teams are formed for emergencies, such as the code blue team or the rapid response team.

Contingency Theory is another approach to leadership. Contingency theory acknowledges that factors in the environment influence outcomes as much as leadership style and that leader effectiveness is contingent upon or depends upon something other than the leader's behavior. The premise is that different leader behavior patterns will be effective in different situations.

Continuing Education is the systematic attempt to facilitate change in professional practice and ensure ongoing professional competence and increase employability and promote optimal patient outcomes.

Controlled Vocabularies are standardized systems of words and concepts which provide a consistent framework for retrieving information. The reason it is called controlled is because there is a system of rules which define how terms and concepts are organized.

Coordinating Team involves those who are responsible for the day-to-day management and direction of care provided by the core team and the unit manager.

Copayment is money paid for health care services by an insurance policy holder each time they receive a health care service.

Copayments are fixed health care fees paid by the patient to the health care provider at the time of service. This amount is paid in addition to the money the health care provider will receive from the insurance company; a payment made by a patient (especially for health services) in addition to that made by an insurer.

Core Team includes those who are providing direct and continuous patient care and it is located on the unit where the patient is assigned. In a hospital setting, the staff nurse and the unlicensed assistive personnel are part of the core team.

Corrective Actions are established steps and processes taken by the nurse manager with the support of Human Resources when the performance of the employee is not meeting the standards delineated in the Job Description and facility policies.

Cost Shifting is where health care providers raise prices for the privately insured to offset the lower health care payments from both Medicare and Medicaid, as well as from the often nonpayment of health care premiums from the uninsured.

Critical Appraisal is the act of evaluating evidence for its quality and relevance to a specific topic.

Cross Training is floating from one's usual unit to another short-staffed unit for one shift.

Crucial Conversations are discussions when the stakes are high, opinions vary, and emotions run strong.

Culture of Safety is a commitment made by health care organizations to provide a safe patient environment by involving senior leadership, caregivers, patients, and families to work together toward continual improvement. In this type of organizational culture, safety is the highest priority.

Culture is the sum of all the characteristics, values, thinking, and behaviors of people in organizations, including more specific workplace characteristics within the larger organization.

Daily Safety Huddle is a short, stand-up meeting that is typically used once at the start of each workday in a clinical setting. The huddle gives teams a way to actively manage quality and safety, including a review of important work. Huddles enable teams to look back to review performance and to look ahead to flag concerns proactively.

Database Alerts is an online tool where a database will notify the user when a research citation has been released.

Debrief is where the team exchanges information about what went well, reinforcing these positive behaviors, and making plans for improvement.

Deductible is money paid for health care services yearly by an insurance policy holder before an insurance company will pay for any expenses.

Deductibles are predetermined out-of-pocket fees paid by a patient for health care services before reimbursement through health insurance begins to be paid.

Defamation is the tort that occurs when a person intentionally communicates or publishes false information, including written (libel) or verbal (slander) remarks that may cause damage to a person's reputation.

Deference to Expertise is the practice of seeking advice from the person with the most experience or expertise in a specific situation, regardless of their position in the organizational hierarchy.

Delegates or Delegatees are terms used interchangeably for the personnel who have been delegated to do some work by another health care professional. A delegate, as described by the National Council of State Board of Nursing (NCSBN), is "one who is delegated a nursing responsibility . . . and is competent to perform it, and verbally accepts the responsibility" and the term could refer to an "RN, LPN/LVN, or UAP."

Delegation is the transfer of responsibility for the performance of a task from one individual to another while retaining accountability for the outcome. NCSBN definition is, "To allow a delegatee (e.g., NAP) to perform a specific nursing activity, skill, or procedure that is beyond the delegatee's general traditional role and not routinely performed."

Democratic Leadership Behavior is a form of leadership that is participatory, with authority delegated to others. To be influential, the democratic leader uses expert power and the power base afforded by having close, personal relationships.

Desired Optimal Outcomes are the best possible objectives to be achieved given the resources at hand.

Differentials are a percentage of the hourly salary added to the nurse's hourly pay for working off-shifts, such as midnights and weekends.

Digital Health shows promise in reducing the cost of health care due in part to remote processes and the ability to treat a higher number of patients and includes mobile apps, e-Health, telemedicine, Electronic Health Records, and consumer data.

Direct Cost is a cost directly related to patient care within a manager's unit, such as the cost of nurses' wages and the cost of patient care supplies.

Disease Management is a system of coordinated health care interventions and communications for populations with conditions in which patient self-care is significant. Each state may have a different (similar) definition.

Economics are based on the analysis of the distribution, production, and consumption of goods and services.

Education Evaluation evaluates the content, context, and learner retention of the education event itself.

E-Health is the intersection of medical informatics, public health, and business, referring to health services and information delivered or enhanced through the internet and related electronic technologies.

E-Learning is an umbrella term for various terms and concepts related to electronic learning such as digital, online, web-based, and mobile learning.

Electronic Databases are collections of information which can be searched and retrieved by a computer or mobile device such as a phone/tablet. Types of information in electronic databases include research studies, clinical trials, clinical practice guidelines, and more.

Electronic Health Record system (EHR) is a digital version of a patient's chart.

Emotional Intelligence (EI) refers to the ability to harness and focus the strengths of human emotions. For leaders, EI enhances the skill to lead effectively by encouraging, inspiring, and empowering others. Key components of EI are: (a) self-awareness, (b) self-regulation, (c) social skills (recognition of other's emotion), (d) empathy, and (e) motivation.

Emotional Intelligence is a component of leadership and refers to the capacity to accurately perceive and express emotion, to use feelings to inform and guide thinking, to understand the meanings of emotions, and to manage emotions for personal and social growth. It also includes the ability to recognize your own feelings and the feelings of those around you and manage your emotions in a positive manner.

Employee Assistance Programs are offered by the Human Resources and Employee Benefits Departments within organizations to help employees by providing counseling and aiding with work–life balance.

Employee-Centered Leadership are leadership behaviors that focus on the human needs of employees, developing work groups, and setting high-performance goals.

Enterprise is an organization of any size, established as a business venture.

Ergonomics is the scientific study of the relationship between work being performed, the physical environment where the work is performed, and the tools used to help perform the work.

Error is defined as a deviation from generally acceptable performance standards. Most medical errors do not result from individual recklessness. Instead, many medical errors are caused by faulty health care systems, processes, and conditions that lead people to make mistakes or fail to prevent them.

Ethical Dilemma occurs when there is a conflict between two or more ethical principles and there appears to be no "correct" decision.

Ethics is a branch of philosophy dealing with what is morally right or wrong from a range of perspectives.

Expert Power is power derived from the knowledge and skills that nurses develop over time.

Failure Modes and Effect Analysis (FMEA) is a rigorous process in which a team of clinicians identify and eliminate known and potential failures, errors, or problems before they occur. Failures are prioritized according to the seriousness of the consequences, how frequently they occur, and how easily they can be detected.

Fair and Just Culture is a Just Culture that recognizes that competent professionals make mistakes; recognizes that many errors represent predictable interactions between human operators and the systems in which they work; recognizes that individual practitioners should not be held accountable for system failings over which they have no control; acknowledges that even competent professionals will develop unhealthy norms (shortcuts, "routine rule violations"); and has no tolerance for reckless behavior. A Fair and Just Culture helps staff speak up when things go wrong and facilitates a learning organization.

False Imprisonment is the act of physically preventing or leading a patient to incorrectly believe the patient is prevented from leaving a place.

Fidelity refers to loyalty within the nurse–patient relationship.

Filters are online tools used in electronic databases to restrict information retrieved to specific characteristics such as publication date, article type, language, etc.

Financial Performance refers to the accomplishments of an organization expressed in terms of overall profits and losses during a time.

Fixed Cost is a cost that exists irrespective of the number of patients for whom care is provided.

Flowchart is a visual representation of a work process.

FOCUS Methodology is a standardized approach to problem-solving and Quality Improvement that helps the health care team look at an entire process which has many dimensions.

Formal Leadership is being in a position of leadership and authority in an organization.

Fraud is deception designed to result in personal or financial gain, such as submitting a bill for services that were never provided to the patient.

Full Text Databases are electronic databases where the records are all full text.

Good Samaritan Laws are laws that have been enacted to protect the health care professional from legal liability for actions rendered in an emergency when the professional is giving service without being paid.

Grapevine is an informal avenue in which rumors circulate. It ignores the formal chain of command.

Gross Domestic Product (GDP) is an economic measure of a country's national income and output within a year and reflects the market value of goods and services produced within the country.

Groupthink is when the desire for harmony and consensus within the group or team overrides the member's efforts to appraise the situation.

Hawthorne Effect is the phenomena of being observed or studied which results in changes in behavior.

Health Care Consumers are patients that "purchase" health care services.

Health Care Reforms are major changes in health care policy or the development of a new health care policy or program.

Health Disparities are the inequalities of access to health care across populations.

Health Literacy is the degree to which individuals have the capacity to obtain, process, and understand basic health information and services needed to make appropriate health decisions.

Health The World Health Organization describes **health** as a "state of complete physical, social, and mental well-being, and not merely the absence of disease or infirmity."

Healthcare Failure Mode and Effect Analysis (HFMEA) is a step-by-step method that examines activities having a high possibility for a negative outcome, identifies possible ways the system can fail in those activities, and recommends actions to improve patient and staff safety when doing those activities.

Healthcare Transparency is truth in reporting the ability to discover information about health care costs, medical errors, or practice preferences, preferably before receiving the service.

Henry Street Settlement House was founded in New York as a site for poor and immigrant children and families to receive social services and health care.

Hierarchy refers to the perceived level of power across groups.

High Reliability Organizations (HRO) are organizations that are able to correct errors and adapt to unexpected events through identifying and discussing potential sources of system failure, questioning assumptions, learning from errors and near misses, and deferring to others' expertise when needed. They operate in complex, high-hazard situations for extended periods without serious accidents or catastrophic failures. HROs relentlessly prioritize safety over other performance pressures.

Holistic Care is a foundational feature of nursing in which healing involves a mind-body-spirit-emotion-environment approach.

Horizontal Career Change is an upward career movement, such as an administrative position, or an advanced practice position.

Horizontal Violence are behaviors exhibited by a single nurse or group of nurses, such as hostility, or aggressive or harmful actions toward another nurse or group of nurses.

Huddles are planned and sometime impromptu (such as in a case where there is a patient fall) short meetings are encouraged throughout the patient care delivery process to monitor and modify the plan as needed.

Human Factors is a science that examines the relationship between human beings and the systems with which they interact with the goal of minimizing errors.

Image of Nurses are characterizations about nurses that reflects and influences nurses' professional identity.

Indirect Cost is a cost not explicitly related to care within a manager's unit but it is a cost necessary to support care.

Informal Leader is leadership outside the scope of a formal leadership role or as a member of a group rather than as the head or leader of the group.

Information Literacy is defined as the understanding of the architecture of information; the ability to navigate among a variety of print and electronic tools to effectively access, search, and critically evaluate appropriate resources; and the ability to synthesize accumulated information into an existing body of knowledge and practice.

Information Power is power based on information that someone can provide to the group.

Informed Consent is the process of communication, or conversation between a doctor or nurse and a patient that apprises the patient of the nature, risks, and alternatives of a health care procedure or treatment. The final step of this process is the patient's signature on the consent form.

Initiating Structure is behavior that emphasizes the work to be done, a focus on the task, and production. Leaders who focus on initiating structure are concerned with how work is organized and on the achievement of goals.

Intention is a purpose or aim.

Internal Career Change is a lateral or horizontal move within the same health care system in which the nurse is currently employed.

Interpersonal Communication involves communication between individuals, person-to-person, or in small groups.

Inter-Professional refers to other members of the health care team whose discipline is different from one's own.

Intrapersonal communication can be thought of as self-talk. As the name suggests, it is what individuals do within themselves, and it can present as doubts or affirmations.

Invasion of Privacy is the public revelation of private information about another in an objectionable manner; even if the information is true and nondefamatory.

Job-Centered Leaders are leaders that focus more on schedules, costs, and efficiency rather than focusing on the human needs of employees.

Just Culture focuses on identifying system flaws that may have led to an error rather than focusing on the failure of a single individual.

Justice is the principle of fairness that is served when an individual is given that which he or she is due, owed, deserves, or can legitimately claim.

Keyword Literature Searching is the type of searching that occurs when individuals use specific words or phrases to do a literature search on a literature search topic. There are no defined rules or structure to keyword literature searching.

Knowledge Workers are those who bring specialized, expert knowledge to an organization. They are valued for what they know.

Knowledge-Based Performance refers to problem solving in new and unfamiliar situations. In this dangerous situation, clinicians may try to figure out how to perform based on what they already know, using trial and error, or even guessing at the solution.

Laissez-Faire Leadership is leadership that is passive and permissive, and the leader defers decision making to others.

Latent Errors are hidden problems within health care systems that contribute to adverse events.

Lateral Career Change is a move within the same role, such as staff nurse, but to a new practice area, requiring new skills or certifications.

Leadership is commonly defined as a process of influence in which the leader influences others toward goal achievement.

Learner Analysis is the process of identifying not only who the learner is, but their unique characteristics and needs, and the ways their characteristics and needs can influence the education process.

Learning Domain refers to the specific knowledge, abilities, and values that result from the learning. There are three domains of thinking and performance used to describe learning and the intended outcome of that learning: affective, cognitive, and psychomotor.

Learning Objectives are statements that define the expected outcomes or goals of the learning process written in measurable terms.

Learning Organization is a learning organization where people continuously learn and enhance their capabilities to improve and create.

Legitimate Power is power derived from the position of authority that a nurse holds in a group.

Lesson Plan is a formally developed document that provides a blueprint for an education session. A lesson plan typically has five components: Objectives, Outline, Time frame, Teaching strategies, and Evaluation.

Licensed Independent Practitioner (LIP) is a person that may independently practice and prescribe under their license in a given state.

Living Will is a written advance directive voluntarily signed by the patient that specifies the type of care the patient desires if and when the patient is in a terminal state and cannot sign a consent form or convey this information verbally.

Logit is a unit of measurement used to report relative differences between candidate ability estimates and item difficulties on the National Council of State Boards of Nursing Licensure EXamination for Registered Nurses (NCLEX-RN).

LPNs/LVNs Licensed Practical Nurse/Licensed Vocational Nurses (LPN/LVNs) are licensed nurses that perform routine uncomplicated nursing care in a dependent role under the delegation (or "direction" depending on the state) and supervision of RNs or other licensed care providers such as nurse practitioners, physicians, dentists, or others. Their roles vary depending on practice site and state.

Maintenance Hygiene Factors must be maintained to avoid job dissatisfaction, according to Herzberg. These factors include such items as salary, working conditions, status, quality of supervision, and relationships with others.

Malpractice is a form of negligence where a professional's wrongful conduct in the discharge of his or her professional duties, or failure to meet standards of care for the profession, results in harm to another individual entrusted to the professional's care.

Management Process includes planning, organizing, coordinating, and controlling which are the classic functions that compose the management process.

Margin is the amount by which revenue from sales or services exceeds costs in a business.

Marketing Plan outlines actions that will be taken to achieve an organization's missions and goals. As part of a strategic plan, a marketing plan communicates all the plans across the organization and ensures that all stakeholders have the needed information.

Mentor is a relationship with a more experienced, successful nurse who coaches the novice RN in developing skills and career direction; introduces the new RN to professional networking opportunities; and assists with ethical dilemmas, stress, and burnout.

Mobile Applications are software applications designed for gathering information through the use of a mobile device such as a smartphone or a tablet.

Morality refers to the distinction between right and wrong or good and bad behavior.

Motivation Factors are factors associated with motivation. Herzberg proposed two types of motivation factors: hygiene maintenance factors and motivation factors. Motivation factors included achievement, recognition, responsibility achievement, recognition, responsibility, and advancement, and they contribute to job satisfaction.

Motivation is a source of influence for personal choices made to satisfy needs.

Multi-Voting is a way to achieve team consensus about which problem from an affinity diagram should be improved first.

Near Miss Safety Event is a near miss safety event occurring when a safety event doesn't reach the patient because it is caught by chance or because the process was engineered with a detection barrier.

Needs Assessments are processes conducted to identify strategic priorities, determine desired results, and guide decisions based on gaps in knowledge skills and practices.

Negligence is the failure to provide the care or behave in a way that a reasonable person would ordinarily perform in a similar situation.

Nonmaleficence is the principle of doing no harm.

Nurse Residency and Transition to Practice are terms used interchangeably in the literature to refer to a program for new RNs that extends for 6–12 months after the orientation phase is completed. Focus is on additional skill building, critical thinking, socialization, debriefing, and peer support as the new RN moves from the role of a nursing student to a RN.

Nurse Training Schools were based in hospitals where students typically worked full time while hearing lectures in their off-duty hours.

Nursing History is the story of nursing care given from antiquity to the present day.

Nursing Identity is the ability to see oneself as a competent professional, capable of performing in a nursing role.

Nursing Informatics (NI) is a nursing specialty that integrates nursing science with multiple information and analytical sciences to identify, define, manage, and communicate data, information, knowledge, and wisdom in nursing practice. NI supports nurses, consumers, patients, the inter-professional health care team, and other stakeholders in their decision making in all roles and settings to achieve desired outcomes.

Nursing Technicians could, as conceived by Montag, perform the technical rather than the professional components of nursing.

Onboarding is a series of events that includes orientation but is much more in-depth to encompass the process of learning the employee's role and how that role contributes to the overall organization.

Organizational Culture includes an organization's expectations, experiences, philosophy, and values. It is based on shared attitudes, beliefs, customs, and written and unwritten rules.

Organizational Power is power based on an organizational hierarchy, one's position in that hierarchy, and one's understanding of the organization's structures and functions.

Orientation is the process in which employees are familiarized with the organization, staff roles, the inter-professional work team, and the conditions of employment.

Outcome Component of Health refers to the results of good care delivery achieved by using quality structures and quality processes and includes the achievement of outcomes such as patient satisfaction, good health and functional ability, and the absence of health care acquired infections and morbidity.

Outcome Measurements indicate an individual's clinical state, such as the severity of illness, course of illness, and identifies the effect of interventions on the individual's clinical state.

Outcomes are the end results of all the structures and work processes, as well as the relationships among them.

Pareto Principle is the principle stating that 20% of focused effort results in 80% of outcome results, or conversely, that 80% of unfocused effort results in 20% of outcome results. Pareto's Principle, named after Vilfredo Pareto, was invoked by the total quality management (TQM) movement and is now reemerging as a strategy for balancing life and work through prioritization of effort.

Paternalism is the practice of a person in authority making decisions for a subordinate in the subordinate's supposed best interest.

Patient Experience encompasses all the interactions that patients have with the health care system.

Patient Handoff is the transfer and acceptance of patient care responsibility.

Patient Satisfaction is a quality measure that is measured using surveys that are distributed to patients after they are discharged from the hospital. These surveys ask patients to rate how satisfied they were with various aspects of the care they received, including responsiveness of their nursing staff, how well their pain was managed, cleanliness of the environment, and other topics.

Patient-Centered Care (PCC) is care that occurs when members of the health care team view their patients through this holistic and humanistic lens, respect the patient's input as being equally important to their own, and allow patients to guide how their care is delivered.

Patient-Centered Education is a set of planned learning activities in which nurses work with patients and their families or caregivers to share information that will alter patient health behaviors, with the goal of improving their health status and/or slowing the deterioration of their health.

Person Approach to Safety is the perspective that each health care staff member is responsible for keeping patients safe and in order to do that, no one can make mistakes while doing their jobs.

Personal Accounts are online tools in electronic databases or websites that provide a customized space for the user to store things such as saved searches, set up database alerts, and more.

Personal Power is power based on characteristics within the individual.

Philosophy is the rational investigation of the truths and principles of knowledge, reality, and human conduct.

Physical Health is a state of physical well-being; the absence of physical disease.

PICOT (Patient/Population, Intervention, Comparison, Outcome, and Time) is a model used to assemble clinical questions within the Evidence-Based Practice (EBP) process.

Plan Do Study Act Cycle (PDSA) is a test of change on a small scale that develops a plan to test a change (Plan), carries out the test (Do), observes and learns from the consequences (Study), and determines what modifications should be made to the test (Act).

Politics are the processes of forming alliances, exercising power, and protecting and advancing particular ideas or goals.

Position Power is the degree of formal authority and influence associated with the leader. High position power is favorable for the leader, and low position power is unfavorable.

Power of Attorney is a legal document executed by an individual (principal) granting another person (agent) the right to perform certain activities in the principal's name.

Power is the ability to acquire and use influence to achieve one's goals.

Practice Drift is a phenomenon that occurs when a nurse takes short-cuts, circumventing policy, regulation, or a standard of care in order to accomplish an immediate goal.

Preceptor is the first staff nurse who intensely invests in the new RN. Preceptors should be matched with new RNs with similar learning styles. The preceptor and new RN will work the same schedule to enhance learning and socialization.

Precursor Safety Event occurs when a health care error reaches the patient and results in no harm or minimal detectable harm.

Preferred Provider Organization (PPO) are contracts with the hospitals and health care practitioner providers (both practitioners and hospitals) and payers (self-insured employers, insurance companies, or managed care organizations) to provide health care services to a defined population for predetermined fixed fees.

Preoccupation With Failure is when leaders want to study errors and undesirable outcomes to improve care.

Primary Care provides integrated, accessible health care services by clinicians who are accountable for addressing a large majority of personal health care needs, developing a sustained partnership with patients, and practicing in the context of family and community.

Privacy refers to the right of individuals to keep information about themselves from being disclosed to anyone.

Process Component of Health includes the quality activities, procedures, tasks, and processes performed within the health care structures, such as hospital admissions, surgical operations, and nursing and medical care delivery following standards and guidelines to achieve quality outcomes.

Process is a series of steps and decisions that interact to produce a result.

Professional Identity reflects the profession's history as well as the profession's status.

Professional Power is conferred on members of a profession by others with whom they work and by the larger society to which they belong.

Progressive Disciplines are actions taken by the manager following specific steps and processes that gradually worsen in their impact on an employee who is not meeting standards.

Psychological Safety is creating an environment where people feel comfortable and have opportunities to raise concerns or ask questions.

Psychomotor Domain is the learning domain that involves utilizing motor skills and performing a behavior or skills that are directly observable. This type of learning can also be thought of as learning by doing.

Public Communication is communication that happens when individuals and groups engage in dialogue in the public sphere in order to deliver a message to a specific audience.

Quality and Safety Education for Nurses (QSEN) The Quality and Safety Education for Nurses (QSEN) Institute is a collaborative of health care professionals focused on education, practice, and scholarship to improve the quality and safety of health care systems. Their goal is to prepare future nurses at the baccalaureate and graduate levels with the knowledge, skills, and attitudes necessary to continuously improve the quality and safety of the health care systems within which they work. QSEN has identified six core competencies for new graduates: patient-centered care, teamwork and collaboration, evidence-based practice, quality improvement, safety, and informatics.

Quality Improvement (QI) is the use of data to monitor the outcomes of care structures, processes, and improvement methods to design and test changes to continuously improve the quality and safety of health care systems.

Quality is the standard of something as measured against other things of a similar kind, or the degree of excellence of something. In health care, quality care is the extent to which health care services provided to individuals and patient populations improve desired health outcomes. In order to achieve this, health care should be Safe, Timely, Effective, Equitable, and Patient-centered (STEEP).

Rapid Response Team (RRT) is a team of expert health care clinicians who provide additional care for patients on acute care units who are experiencing unexpected acute changes in their conditions.

Reading Literacy is defined as being able to perform simple everyday reading.

Reality Shock is difficulty that new RNs have in adjusting to the work environment and includes the new nurse's conflict between expectations and reality.

Referent Power is power derived from how much others respect and like an individual, group, or organization with which one is associated.

Relative Value Unit (RVU) is a measure of value used by The Centers for Medicare and Medicaid Services (CMS) to calculate reimbursement fees for three types of provider resources, i.e., provider work RVUs, practice expense RVUs, and professional liability insurance RVUs.

Reliability is the quality of performing consistently and well.

Reluctance to Simplify is a disinclination to apply a one-size-fits-all solution to a problem.

Resilience is the ability to recover from any situation and move on. It is the ability to work effectively in high-pressure situations, while remaining positive and persistent.

Respect for Others is to consider others to be of high regard.

Reward Power is power that comes from the ability to give others something they value in response to their behavior.

Risk Management Programs are programs in health care organizations that are designed to identify and correct systemic problems that contribute to errors in patient care or to employee injury. The emphasis in risk management is on quality improvement and protection of the institution from financial liability.

Root Cause Analysis (RCA) is an error analysis tool used in health care to investigate the underlying main cause of serious adverse events or near misses. An RCA uses a systems approach to identify both active and latent errors.

Rule-Based Performance is the rule-based performance mode characterized by the performance of prepackaged actions taken because of the recognition of a familiar situation. In health care, the clinician applies a learned rule to an appropriate situation.

Safety is a process that minimizes the risk of harm to patients and providers through both system effectiveness and individual performance. It is the condition of being protected from or unlikely to cause danger, risk, or injury. In health care, safety is the prevention of errors and adverse effects.

SBAR is a helpful tool for handoffs. Situation reflects what is going on with the patient. Background is the clinical background or context. Assessment refers to my assessment of the problem, what I think the problem is. Recommendation and Request includes recommending and requesting what I think should be done to correct the problem. These four areas are used to organize a health care report.

Security refers to the means to controlling access and protecting information from accidental or intentional disclosure to unauthorized persons and from alteration, destruction, or loss.

Self-Awareness is the ability to look at yourself critically and identify your strengths and your weaknesses.

Self-Efficacy is an individual's judgment of his or her capabilities to organize and execute courses of action.

Self-Scheduling is a system wherein nurses select their own schedule according to guidelines established by the unit, as opposed to a work schedule created by the unit manager or designee.

Sensitivity to Operations is when leadership is aware of the day-to-day operations of the health care organization.

Sentinel Events are a subcategory of adverse events. A sentinel event is a patient safety event that is not primarily related to the natural course of the patient's illness or underlying condition, reaches the patient, and results in death, permanent harm, or severe temporary harm.

Serious Safety Event also called adverse events, occur when an error reaches the patient and results in moderate to severe harm or even death.

Shadowing is allowing a potential nurse employee to spend time following a staff nurse in a desired role or department. Allows the potential employee to experience the care provided to that unit's patient population and the unit's culture.

Shared Decision Making is working with patients and giving patients greater autonomy to make decisions that affect their own health.

Sharp End is the sharp end of a triangle and the point of care where nurses and other clinicians interact with patients. Errors are often noticed at the sharp end and they occur at the point of interface between humans and a complex system.

Simplification of the work process is the reduction of a work process to its essential steps, making it easier to understand and complete. It is the act of reducing a work process to its basic components.

Simulation is part of an immersive learning strategy often used to demonstrate high risk, low volume situations and allows the provider to maintain essential skills needed to adapt and respond to a specific scenario. During scenario-based simulation training, the learner can acquire such important skills as interpersonal communication, teamwork, leadership, decision-making, the ability to prioritize tasks under pressure, and stress management.

Situation Monitoring involves continuous scanning and evaluation of what is going on around you. Four components of situation monitoring involve the status of the patient, the team members, the environment, and the progress toward meeting the established goal.

Situational Leadership is a theory that addresses follower characteristics to identify an effective leader behavior.

Skill-Based Performance refers to the mode of functioning humans use for routine, familiar tasks that can be done without thinking about them.

Sleep Deprived refers to suffering from insufficient sleep or sleepiness.

SMART Goal Formats are goals that are Specific, Measureable Achievable, Realistic, and Time-bound.

Socialization is social support shown to the new RN by her preceptor and manager. Introduces the new RN to employees and the culture of the unit. May include social events outside of the work environment.

Soft Skills are skills that include negotiation, collaboration, problem-solving, and so forth.

Specialty Certifications are evidence of practice knowledge, skills, and clinical expertise within a specialty area of nursing care.

Stakeholders are providers, employers, customers, patients, and payers who may have an interest in, and seek to influence, the decisions and actions of an organization.

Standardization are work processes using a single set of terms, definitions, practices, and/or clinical tools, such as bundles, checklists, or protocols.

Statute is a written law passed by a legislative body and signed into law by the chief executive of that government, usually after a period of deliberation that includes testimony from witnesses at committee hearings and debate among the legislative members.

Strategic Planning is a continuous, systematic process of making decisions today with the greatest possible knowledge of their effects on the future. The final product of the strategic planning process is the creation of a strategic plan.

Structure Component of Health includes resources or structures needed to deliver quality health care, for example, human and physical resources, such as nurses and nursing and medical practitioners, hospital buildings, medical records, and pharmaceuticals.

Structure refers to the physical and organizational characteristics of a hospital such as its buildings, human resources, financing, and equipment.

Subject Headings are concepts or terms within a controlled vocabulary which can be used for locating information and often answer some of the challenges posed with keyword literature searching.

Substitutes for Leadership are variables that may influence followers to the same extent as the leader's behavior and may eliminate the needs for leader behavior. Examples include structured routine tasks and intrinsic satisfaction in the work itself.

Supervision is "the active process of directing, guiding, and influencing the outcome of an individual's performance of a task." This type of supervision refers to clinical supervision and not managerial supervision (hiring, firing, as in a managerial role). Supervision of licensed or unlicensed nursing personnel means the provision of guidance and evaluation for the accomplishment of a nursing task or activity with the initial direction of the task or activity; periodic inspection of the actual act of accomplishing the task or activity; and the authority to require corrective action.

Support Services Team creates a comfortable, safe, and clean health care environment for all patients and staff.

Swiss Cheese Model depicts the potential errors inherent in every step of a process. The holes in the Swiss Cheese represent opportunities for a process to fail, and each slice is a defensive layer to prevent an error in the process. More layers of cheese and smaller holes allow more errors to be stopped or caught. When the holes in the Swiss Cheese line up, an error occurs.

Synergism is a component of the orientation and onboarding process where the organization facilitates integration into a work group and the overall organizational culture to provide a sense of fit and belonging. This synergism is achieved often through the use of a preceptor and team-based learning.

System Approach to Safety is a system of patient care that takes into account human error and strives to keep the harm potentially caused by an error from reaching patients.

Task Structure is a term used to define work. High task structure involves routine, predictable work tasks, whereas low task structure indicates work that is creative, artistic, not routine, and less predictable.

Taxonomy is a system that provides the order of principles to create groupings or classification.

Teach Back is a method of teaching which confirms learner knowledge, where the learner "teaches back" the new information in their own words and/or can demonstrate the correct way to perform a task. This method allows the teacher to evaluate the learner's comprehension of the education.

Team in health care is two or more people with a full set of complementary skills who interact dynamically, interdependently, and adaptively toward a common and valued goal, have specific roles or functions, and have a time-limited membership. That common and valued goal is the best possible outcome for the patient. Team members: (a) operate with a high degree of interdependence, (b) share authority and responsibility for self-management, (c) are accountable for the collective performance, and (d) work toward a common goal and shared reward(s).

Team Huddle is a brief, in-person, scheduled meeting with relevant team members to anticipate and prepare to meet patient needs so the work day runs more smoothly.

TeamSTEPPS provides team strategies and tools to enhance performance and patient safety. It is an evidence-based framework developed by the Agency for Healthcare Research and Quality (AHRQ).

Teamwork is defined as two or more people who interact interdependently with a common purpose, working toward measurable goals.

Telehealth is the delivery of health-related services and information for health promotion, disease prevention, diagnosis, consultation, education, and therapy, via telecommunications technologies and computers to patients and providers at another location.

Theory X is a theory of human behavior that views employees in an organization as needing security, direction, and minimal responsibility.

Theory Y is a theory of human behavior that views employees in an organization as needing to contribute creatively, motivated by ties to the group, the organization, and the work itself.

Theory Z is an approach to motivating people in an organization by investing in the people and considering both home and work issues when providing career development.

Therapeutic Patient-Centered Education is education managed by health care providers trained in the education of patients, and designed to enable a patient (or a group of patients and families) to manage the treatment of their condition, support daily self-management, and prevent avoidable complications, while maintaining or improving quality of life.

Time Management is a set of related common-sense skills that helps you use your time in the most effective and productive way possible.

To Assign is to allocate "routine care, activities, and procedures that are within the authorized scope of practice of the RN or LPN (LVN) or part of the routine functions" of the NAP.

Tort is a civil wrong resulting in injury to another person.

Transactional Leader is the leader who is more focused on day-to-day operations and the traditional functions of a managerial role.

Transformational Leadership is a theory that defines leadership as the process in which leaders and followers raise one another to higher levels of motivation and morality.

Transparency is functioning in a way that makes it is easy for others to see what actions are performed. Transparency implies openness, communication, and accountability and allows health care organizations to evaluate their performance more completely, learn from errors, and take action more quickly.

Truncation is a literature search technique where a character is used to replace the end of the word. Using this technique retrieves all words with the common root. For example, nurs* will retrieve articles about nurse, nurses, nursing, etc.

UAP (Unlicensed Assistive Personnel), NAP (Nursing Assistive Personnel) Or AP (Assistive Personnel) the UAP job class is "an umbrella term to describe . . . paraprofessionals who assist individuals with physical disabilities, mental impairments, and other health care needs with their activities of daily living and provide care—including basic nursing procedures—all under the supervision of the registered nurse, licensed practical nurse (in some states), and other health care professionals." The National Council of State Boards of Nursing (NCSBN) uses the terms, NAP or UAP, to delineate employees that aid the licensed nurse with nursing activities. The American Nurses Association's (ANA) and the NCSBN Joint Statement on Delegation, Decision Tree for Delegation to Nursing Assistive Personnel uses the term NAP. The NCSBN states that the term UAP can be used to identify this helpful group which includes certified nursing assistants, patient care technicians of various types (such as psychiatric, rehabilitation), home health aides, certified medication aides, home health aides, and certified medical assistants. These broad inclusive terms designate supportive unlicensed health care personnel who assist nurses and who may or may not hold various training certifications.

Union is a formal and legal group that acts as a collective bargaining agent to formally present worker desires to management.

Value is the regard that something held to deserve due to its importance, worth, or usefulness.

Value-Based Payment is payment for services based on achieving specific quality and cost outcomes.

Values Clarification is the process of analyzing one's own values to better understand what is truly important.

Variable Cost is a cost that varies with volume and it will increase or decrease depending on the number of patients.

Veracity refers to truth and loyalty within the nurse–patient relationship.

Virtual Reality (VR) is a type of simulation using a three-dimensional computer environment that offers a variety of simulations to practice essential aspects of a clinical situation.

Visiting Nurses are nurses who go to the homes of the poor to provide nursing care and coordinate support.

Visualization is a type of meditation with an emphasis on the future.

Wildcards is a literature search technique used when only one character needs to be replaced in a literature search. For example, Nurse+ will retrieve articles about nurse in the singular or plural form.

Work Around is the use of short cuts to streamline care without realizing the potential impact on safety.

Workplace Advocacy is a type of nursing collective action besides collective bargaining, by which nurses' voices can be heard and it is a less structured process than that which is formalized by a union contract.